Home Health Considerations

 MEDICATIONS

 DRUG CLASSIFICATIONS, xxvii

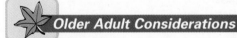 **Older Adult Considerations**

 Patient Teaching

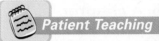 **Therapeutic Dialogues**

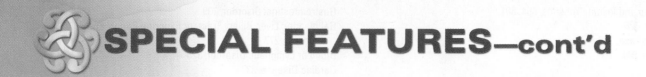

SPECIAL FEATURES—cont'd

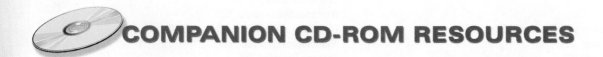

COMPANION CD-ROM RESOURCES

NCLEX®-STYLE REVIEW QUESTIONS for each chapter

DORLAND'S AUDIO PRONUNCIATIONS

HELPFUL PHRASES FOR COMMUNICATING IN SPANISH

ANATOMY & PHYSIOLOGY BODY SPECTRUM

FLUIDS & ELECTROLYTES MODULE

ANIMATIONS
Classification of Joints: Hinge Joint
Classification of Joints: Gliding Joint (Hand)
Cardiac Cycle During Systole and Diastole
Auscultation of Heart Valves
Pulse Variations
Blood Flow: Circulatory System
Pulmonary Circulation
Patterns of Respiration
Percussion Tones throughout the Chest
Anatomic Location of Sinuses
The Menstrual Cycle
Lymphatic Drainage of Breast
Reflex Arc
Sensory Pathways and Clinical Evaluation of the Central Nervous System
Motor Pathways and Clinical Evaluation of the Central Nervous System

VIDEO CLIPS
Inspection: Gait (Older Adult Female)
Inspection: General Muscular Strength (Adult Male)
Auscultation: Abdomen, Bowel Sounds (Adult Male)
Percussion: Abdomen (Adult Male)
Percussion: Liver (Adult Male)
Auscultation: Cardiac, with Diaphragm and Bell (Adult Female)
Inspection and Palpation: Pulses, Lower Extremities (Adult Female)
Inspection and Palpation: Breathing and Respiratory Excursion, Anterior Chest (Adult Male)
Palpation: Tactile Fremitus, Posterior Chest (Adult Female)
Inspection and Palpation: Standing Position (Younger Adult Male)
Inspection: External Genitalia (Younger Adult Female)
Evaluation: Central Vision and Visual Acuity (Adult Male)
Inspection: Ear Canal (Adult Male)
Inspection: Fine Motor Coordination, Upper Extremities (Older Adult Male)
Inspection: Fine Motor Coordination, Lower Extremities (Older Adult Female)

AUDIO CLIPS
S1 at Various Locations
S2 at Various Locations
The Third Heart Sound (S3)
The Fourth Heart Sound (S4)
Murmurs: High, Medium, and Low
Murmurs: Blowing, Harsh or Rough, and Rumble
Systolic Murmur
Diastolic Murmur
Pericardial Friction Rub
Vesicular Breath Sounds
Bronchial Breath Sounds
High-Pitched Crackles
Low-Pitched Crackles
High-Pitched Wheeze
Low-Pitched Wheeze

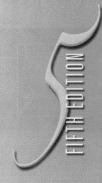

ADULT HEALTH NURSING

Barbara Lauritsen Christensen, RN, MS

Nurse Educator
Mid-Plains Community College
North Platte, Nebraska

Elaine Oden Kockrow, RN, MS

Formerly, Nurse Educator
Mid-Plains Community College
North Platte, Nebraska

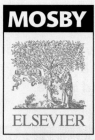

MOSBY

ELSEVIER

evolve

To access your Student Resources, visit the web address below:

http://evolve.elsevier.com/Christensen/adult

Evolve® Student Resources for *Christensen: Adult Health Nursing,* 5th ed. offer the following features:

- **NCLEX®-style Review Questions**
  Test your knowledge with interactive activities.

- **Body Spectrum Electronic Anatomy Coloring Book**
  Provides 80 anatomy illustrations that can be colored online or printed out for coloring and study offline. Choose from a varied color palette and learn anatomy in this fun, interactive format. Test your knowledge by completing quizzes after each part is colored.

- **Helpful Phrases for Communicating in Spanish**
  A useful tool for English-as-a-Second-Language situations.

- **WebLinks**
  An exciting resource that lets you link to hundreds of websites carefully chosen to supplement the content of the textbook. The WebLinks are regularly updated, with new ones added as they develop.

- **Additional Resources**
  To bring the content alive with animations, assessment videos, a glossary of audio pronunciations, and more!

The CD-ROM included with every copy of
Adult Health Nursing, 5th ed.
**offers learning tools for study and review, useful
language references, a self-study Fluids & Electrolytes
module, multimedia resources, and more!**

http://evolve.elsevier.com/Christensen/adult/

To my beloved children and grandchildren,
Jennifer Holly, David Joseph,
Alexander Edison, Emma Elizabeth, Ava,
Jessica Heather, Eigo, Gus,
Mirabella, and Jason Heath,
whose presence in my life brings fulfillment, pride,
wonderment, and contentment.

To my siblings:
Shirlee, Ann, Lowell Chris, and Garnet.
I could not have had a more loving, generous,
and helpful circle of loved ones. Our parents
continue to positively influence us all.

BARBARA LAURITSEN CHRISTENSEN

To Annetta Oden, in thankful appreciation
for your loving devotion to my father,
Charles Oden.

To my siblings:
Dean and Helga, Barbara,
Phyllis and William,
Sharon and Wayne,
whose love and devotion have been a lifetime
source of strength and inspiration.

ELAINE ODEN KOCKROW

MOSBY
ELSEVIER

11830 Westline Industrial Drive
St. Louis, Missouri 63146

ISBN-13: 978-0-323-03936-9
ISBN-10: 0-323-03936-7

NCLEX®, NCLEX-RN®, AND NCLEX-PN® are federally registered trademarks and service marks of
the National Council of State Boards of Nursing, Inc.

Executive Publisher: Barbara Nelson Cullen
Managing Editor: Robin Levin Richman
Associate Developmental Editor: Catherine Ott
Publishing Services Manager: Jeffrey Patterson
Senior Project Manager: Mary Stueck
Designer: Teresa McBryan

Printed in Canada

Last digit is the print number: 9 8 7 6 5 4 3

Contributors & Reviewers

CONTRIBUTORS

CRAIG E. NIELSEN, MS, NP, BC, ACRN
Senior Instructor of Medicine
University of Colorado at Denver,
    Health Sciences Center
Denver, Colorado

LINDA Y. NORTH, MSN, EdS, PhD
Dean of Health Sciences
Southern Union State Community
    College at Opelika
Opelika, Alabama

ALITA K. SELLERS, PhD, RN
Chairperson, Health Sciences
    Division
West Virginia University at
    Parkersburg
Parkersburg, West Virginia

MARTHA E. SPRAY, MS, BSN, RN
Formerly, Practical Nursing Instructor
Mid-East Ohio Vocational School
    District
Zanesville, Ohio

REVIEWERS

RUTH ANN ECKENSTEIN, RN, BS, MEd
Oklahoma Department of Career and
    Technology Education
Stillwater, Oklahoma

SHELIA L. ESCH, RN
Louisiana Technical College—Florida
    Parishes Campus
Greensburg, Louisiana

ELIZABETH HAMEL, RN, BSN
Garden City Community College
Garden City, Kansas

CHARLA K. HOLLIN, RN, BSN
Rich Mountain Community College
Mena, Arkansas

SHEENA R. NEWMAN, MSN, RN
Louisiana Technical College—Florida
    Parishes Campus
Greensburg, Louisiana

MARY RUSSO, RN, MSN
Lincoln Land Community College
Jacksonville, Illinois

JOLON VAUGHN, RN, BSN
Sikeston Public School Practical
    Nursing Program
Sikeston, Missouri

We want to thank the following former contributors to previous editions of this book: **M. Christine Neff** (Chapter 1), **Patricia Helmer Oles** and **Karen H. Richardson** (Chapter 13), and **Elizabeth Schenk** (Chapter 14).

Adult Health Nursing, fifth edition, was developed to educate the practical/vocational nursing student in medical-surgical nursing with an overview of anatomy and physiology. This **full-color** companion text to *Foundations of Nursing* continues to fill the needs of educators and students. It is a text that is accessible, accurate, up-to-date, clearly written, user-friendly, and portable.

Everything in this new fifth edition was revised to incorporate the most accurate, current, and clinically relevant information available. *Adult Health Nursing* and *Foundations of Nursing*, whether used together or separately, are the perfect texts to meet all the educational needs of LPN/LVNs in all health care settings.

Keeping the strengths of the first four editions, we have added new features to stay current with the many changes in the practice of nursing. The role of the LPN/LVN as health care provider continues to expand along with the needs of society and the technological advances in the health care system. With this revision, *Adult Health Nursing* will continue to be an excellent educational tool for providing the knowledge base necessary for the expanded role of LPN/LVNs.

Finally, it is our belief that nursing will always be both an art and a science. This philosophy is reflected throughout the text.

ORGANIZATION AND STANDARD FEATURES

The organization of the fifth edition continues to follow the strengths of the previous edition, based on positive comments from educators and students.

Table of Contents

As in the previous editions, the text begins with an introductory chapter on anatomy and physiology to give students the basis for comprehension of the disorders content to follow. This is followed by Chapter 2: "Care of the Surgical Patient," and continued with all of the body systems disorders chapters. The chapters in systems disorders are arranged in an orderly flow. New and additional content has been added to ensure that students have access to the most current information.

- Chapter 6: "Care of the Patient with a Gall Bladder, Liver, Biliary Tract, or Exocrine Pancreatic Disorder" has been updated to reflect **revised hepatitis classifications**.
- Chapter 8: "Care of the Patient with a Cardiovascular or a Peripheral Vascular Disorder" includes

new information on **serum tests for chronic heart failure** (BNP).
- **Sacroneural stimulators for urinary incontinence** are discussed in Chapter 10: "Care of the Patient with a Urinary Disorder."
- Chapter 11: "Care of the Patient with an Endocrine Disorder" **discusses new diabetes medications, both oral hypoglycemics and insulins**.
- The latest research findings and concerns about **Hormone Replacement Therapy (HRT)** and its issues are addressed in Chapter 12: "Care of the Patient with a Reproductive Disorder."
- **New treatment modalities** are presented in Chapter 16: "Care of the Patient with **HIV/AIDS**."

Nursing Process

The **nursing process** as applied to specific disorders is integrated throughout. The special nursing process summary section appears at the end of each chapter, enabling the reader to see more clearly its application to the chapter content as a whole.

We have emphasized the role of the LPN/LVN in the nursing process as follows:
- The LPN/LVN will participate in planning care for the patient based on the patient's needs.
- The LPN/LVN will review the patient's plan of care and recommend revisions as needed.
- The LPN/LVN will follow defined prioritization for patient care.
- The LPN/LVN will use clinical pathways/care maps/care plans to guide and review patient care.

Chapter Openers

Each chapter begins with the following:
- **Objectives:** These learning objectives are divided into Anatomy and Physiology and Medical-Surgical categories as appropriate. Many of the learning objectives have been revised for greater inclusion of chapter content.
- **Key Terms:** Selected terms are accompanied by a phonetic pronunciation and a page number where the content may be found. Students are also directed to the free CD-ROM for audio pronunciation clips of selected terms. Key terms are in color the first time they appear in the narrative and are briefly defined in the text, with complete definitions in the Glossary. Terms that were assigned simple phonetic pronunciations were selected because they are either (1) difficult med-

ical, nursing, or scientific terms or (2) other words that may be difficult for students to pronounce. The goal is to help the student reader with limited proficiency in English to develop a greater command of the pronunciation of scientific and nonscientific English terminology. It is hoped that a more general competency in the understanding and use of medical and scientific language may result.

- **Overview of Anatomy and Physiology:** Precedes the medical-surgical content, allowing the reader to correlate easily normal anatomy and physiology with common disease conditions.

Chapter Organization

Disorders chapters typically are organized in the following format for more effective learning:

- Etiology/Pathophysiology
- Clinical Manifestations
- Assessment (with subjective and objective data)
- Diagnostic Tests
- Medical Management
- Nursing Diagnoses and Nursing Interventions (including relevant medications)
- Patient Teaching
- Prognosis

Throughout the chapters, an ⊙ icon in the margin directs the student to the free CD-ROM for additional resources, such as animations and video clips, to reinforce the content.

End-of-Chapter Features

Each chapter ends with the following:

- **Key Points:** These are correlated with the objectives and serve as a useful chapter review.
- **Chapter Challenge:** NCLEX®-style study questions are a handy self-study tool. New alternate format questions such as fill-in-the-blank and multiple-response have been added to the multiple-choice questions, reflecting the most current question formats of the NCLEX-PN®. Answers to the Chapter Challenge are located in the back of the textbook. The student is also directed to the free CD-ROM for additional NCLEX®-style review questions in an interactive format with rationales for both correct and incorrect answers.
- **Evolve Resources,** such as regularly updated WebLinks reflecting chapter content, are indicated with an *evolve* icon.

References and Suggested Readings

These are grouped by chapter and listed at the end of the book for easy access. **Additional Resources** such as websites and agencies are included where applicable.

SPECIAL FEATURES

The following special features are designed to foster effective learning and comprehension through substance and form, with the added benefit of a creative and appealing design:

- **Skills** are presented in a logical step-by-step format with accompanying full-color illustrations. Clearly defined Nursing Actions followed by Rationales in bold type show the student how and why skills are performed. Emphasis is placed on accurate, effective documentation of data.
- **Nursing Care Plans,** developed around specific case studies, include nursing diagnoses with an emphasis on patient goals and outcomes and questions to promote **critical thinking.** This valuable tool serves as a guideline for the student in the clinical setting. The critical thinking aspect will empower the student to develop clinical decision-making skills. Answers to the critical thinking questions are located in the Instructor's Resource Manual section of the Instructor's Electronic Resource CD.
- **Safety Considerations,** *new to this edition,* emphasize the importance of maintaining safety in patient and resident care to protect patients, family, health care providers, and the public from accidents and the spread of disease.
- **Health Promotion Considerations,** *new to this edition,* emphasize a healthy lifestyle, preventive behaviors, and screening tests to assist in the prevention of accidents and disease.
- **Clinical Pathways** throughout the text reflect collaborative care.
- **Nursing Diagnoses** are screened and set apart in the text. This step of the nursing process presents nursing diagnoses and appropriate nursing interventions in a clear, easy-to-understand format to aid the nurse educator and student in participating in the development of a nursing care plan. The most current NANDA-approved nursing diagnoses are used.
- **Complementary & Alternative Therapies** boxes in nearly every chapter give a breakdown of specific nontraditional therapies, along with precau-

tions and possible side effects. A complete discussion of complementary and alternative therapies is given in Chapter 17 of *Foundations of Nursing*.

- **Cultural and Ethnic Considerations** teach students about specific cultural preferences and how to address the needs of a culturally diverse patient and resident population when planning nursing care.
- **Therapeutic Dialogue** boxes focus on communication strategies through real-life examples of nurse-patient dialogue.
- **Patient Teaching,** appearing frequently in the text, helps develop awareness of the vital role of patient/family teaching in health care today.
- **Older Adult Considerations** bring a gerontologic perspective to nursing care, focusing on the nursing interventions unique to the older adult patient or resident.
- **Home Health Considerations** discuss the issues facing patients and caregivers in the home setting.
- **Medications Tables** developed for specific disorders provide quick access to action, dosage, side effects, and nursing considerations for commonly used medications.

Two new appendices have been added to the fifth edition. The **Joint Commission on Accreditation of Health Care Organizations (JCAHO) Lists of Dangerous Abbreviations, Acronyms, and Symbols** promotes safety in clinical practice in such areas as avoiding dosage errors. **Laboratory Reference Values** provide quick, time-saving access to important information.

TEACHING AND LEARNING PACKAGE

Instructor's Electronic Resource CD

We recognize that educators today have limited time in which to prepare classroom and clinical activities. Therefore, we provide an expanded **Instructor's Electronic Resource CD** that covers both *Adult Health Nursing* and *Foundations of Nursing,* fifth editions, and include the following:

- **Computerized Test Bank** with over 1300 NCLEX®-style *Foundations of Nursing* and *Adult Health Nursing* questions. Questions are both multiple-choice and in alternate formats, such as fill-in-the-blank and multiple-response. Each question consists of the following: (1) stem, (2) possible answers, (3) topic, (4) nursing process step, (5) objective, (6) cognitive level, (7) NCLEX® category of patient needs, (8) correct answer, (9) rationale for correct answer, and (10) text page reference.
- **PowerPoint Presentation** of approximately 1000 *Adult Health Nursing* text and graphic slides.
- **Instructor's Resource Manual,** with Objectives, Key Terms, Classroom Activities, Clinical Activities, Chapter Outlines, Key Points, and Additional Resources. Answers to the textbook Nursing Care Plan critical thinking questions and the

Adult Health Nursing Study Guide Answer Key are also provided in the IRM.

- **Open-Book Quizzes,** completely rewritten for every chapter of the fifth edition of *Adult Health Nursing,* with textbook page numbers where content may be found for each question.
- **Electronic Image Collection** with over 400 images from *Adult Health Nursing* and 50 images from supplemental sources.
- **WebLinks** supplement the content of the text.

Lesson Plan Manual

An exciting new instructor's resource, Elsevier's **TEACH (Total Education and Curriculum Help)** Lesson Plan Manual is keyed chapter by chapter to the textbook and provides instructors with customizable lesson plans and lecture outlines based on learning objectives. This Lesson Plan Manual provides the ultimate tool for busy new LPN/LVN instructors, or instructors who want to revitalize their classroom presentations.

Companion CD

New to this edition of *Adult Health Nursing* is a free CD-ROM bound into the text, providing students with an unparalleled selection of study tools and multimedia resources. Interactive NCLEX®-style review questions for each chapter reinforce content and help students identify areas of weakness, with rationales provided for both correct and incorrect answers. The interactive Anatomy & Physiology Body Spectrum coloring book, Fluids & Electrolytes Module, animations, video clips, and audio clips increase comprehension of difficult concepts and terminology. A selection of Helpful Phrases for Communicating in Spanish assists ESL students in studying and all nursing students in communicating with Spanish-speaking patients and their families.

Study Guide

Designed to promote learning, understanding, and application of the content in the textbook, the *Study Guide for Adult Health Nursing,* **fifth edition,** is **completely revised,** with a **new author, Kim Cooper, MSN.** Each chapter ties specific activities to specific objectives rather than simply listing objectives and activities separately. Illustrations from the text are incorporated into some of the exercises. Types of activities include the following, among others:

- *New* **multiple-choice and multiple-response questions** for every chapter
- *New* **critical thinking questions** with clinical scenarios
- Labeling
- Terminology
- Compare and contrast
- Short-answer

Page numbers where content may be found are located next to the appropriate activity as a study aid. The complete answer key is located in the Instructor's

Resource Manual section of the Instructor's Electronic Resource CD. The Study Guide also includes a complete set of Performance Checklists for all of the Skills in the text.

Virtual Clinical Excursions

This interactive workbook CD-ROM package guides the student through a multifloor virtual hospital in a hands-on clinical learning experience. Students can assess and analyze information, diagnose, set priorities, and implement and evaluate care. NCLEX®-style review questions provide immediate testing of clinical knowledge.

Evolve Resources

Both instructors and students will find many useful internet-based tools and resources on *Adult Health Nurs-*

ing's companion Evolve website. For instructors, the Evolve Learning System allows you to reinforce and expand on the concepts you deliver in class. You can use Evolve to:

- Publish your class syllabus, outline, and lecture notes
- Set-up "virtual office hours" and Email communication
- Share important dates and information through the online class *Calendar*
- Encourage student participation through *Chat Rooms* and *Discussion Boards*

For students, interactive quizzes and multimedia resources reinforce classroom teaching and provide an opportunity to strengthen their understanding of information in each chapter. All student resources are also available to instructors.

Acknowledgments

This edition has been completed through diligent research and response to reviewers, educators, and student nurses. We are grateful for the success of the past four editions and look forward to continuing to contribute to the education of student nurses.

For the completion of a textbook, one must have the cooperation of gifted and creative individuals. We wish to recognize those persons who have assisted with this text.

We would like to acknowledge the talented editorial and production staff at Elsevier: Robin Levin Richman, Managing Editor, Nursing, for her positive attitude, astute observations, and meticulous attention to detail; Catherine Ott, Associate Developmental Editor, Nursing, for her steadfastness of purpose, professionalism, and sincere interest; Giselle DeGrandis, Editorial Assistant, Nursing, for her prompt attention to all requests, and Mary Stueck, Senior Project Manager, Book Production, for her organizational skills, prompt attention to our requests, and conscientious effort.

We are particularly grateful for the diligent effort and conscientious attention to detail provided by our contributors and reviewers throughout the completion of this edition.

We wish to acknowledge Debbie Beebout, our typist, for her patience and attention to detail.

Our thanks to the pharmacists at Great Plains Regional Medical Center: James L. Manning, RP; John G. Guzallis, RP; Paula Stobbs, RP; Cindy Way, RP; and Andrew Sokolowski, RP, for their generous professional assistance in pharmacology consultation. We would also like to thank the administrators at Great Plains Regional Medical Center for their generous use of various GPRMC forms.

We wish to thank Dr. Jennifer H. Christensen for her expertise and helpfulness in providing counsel and current data.

We are very appreciative of the many nurse educators and student nurses who have used our first four editions to achieve their goal of excellence in the field of nursing.

We wish to thank our families for their love, kindness, and interest that provided us with strength and encouragement to complete this laborious task.

Last, we wish to express to each other our gratitude for the gift of friendship that is sterling and has provided us with courage, strength, enthusiasm, energy, and purpose.

BARBARA LAURITSEN CHRISTENSEN

ELAINE ODEN KOCKROW

LPN Threads

Adult Health Nursing, fifth edition, shares some features and design elements with other LPN titles on the Elsevier list. The purpose of these LPN Threads is to make it easier for students and instructors to use the variety of books required by the relatively brief and demanding LPN curriculum.

The shared features in *Adult Health Nursing*, fifth edition, include the following:

- A **reading level evaluation** performed on every manuscript chapter during the book's development to increase the consistency among chapters and to make the reading easy to understand
- Cover and internal **design similarities**; the colorful, student-friendly design encourages reading and learning of this core content
- Numbered lists of **Objectives** that begin each chapter
- **Key Terms** with phonetic pronunciations and page number references at the beginning of each chapter; the key terms are in color the first time they appear in the chapter
- **Critical Thinking Questions** at the end of every Nursing Care Plan.
- Bulleted lists of **Key Points** at the end of each chapter
- A **Bibliography** list at the end of the text
- A **Glossary** at the end of the text

And for Instructors . . .

- A **Computerized Test Bank** with the following categories of information: Topic, Step of the Nursing Process, Objective, Cognitive Level, NCLEX® Category of Client Need, Correct Answer, Rationale, and Text Page Reference
- A **PowerPoint slide presentation** on the *Instructor's Electronic Resource* CD-ROM
- **Open-Book Quizzes** on the *Instructor's Electronic Resource* CD-ROM
- **Study Guide answer key** in the Instructor's Manual on the *Instructor's Electronic Resource* CD-ROM; the Study Guide itself contains text page number references where students can find the answers
- **Tips for teaching English as a Second Language (ESL) students** in the Instructor's Manual

In addition to content and design threads, these LPN textbooks benefit from the advice and input of the Elsevier LPN Advisory Board.

LPN Advisory Board

To the Student

Designed with the student in mind, *Adult Health Nursing*, fifth edition, will help you learn medical-surgical nursing with its visually appealing and easy-to-use format. Here are some of the numerous special features that will help you understand and apply the material.

FREE CD-ROM

The free CD-ROM packaged in your copy of *Adult Health Nursing*, fifth edition, contains the following sections: NCLEX®-style review and study questions, an audio pronunciation guide of selected Key Terms, Helpful Phrases for Communicating in Spanish, interactive Anatomy & Physiology Body Spectrum coloring book, Fluids & Electrolytes Module, animations, video clips, and audio clips. Using these resources as you study can help you master the material in this book.

Chapters open with **Anatomy and Physiology** and **Medical-Surgical Objectives**, **Key Terms** with Pronunciations, and **Overview of Anatomy and Physiology**

Eye-catching **full-color art** and **design** throughout.

***NEW* Health Promotion Considerations** focus on wellness and disease prevention.

***NEW* Safety Considerations** highlight guidelines and precautions for LPN/LVNs caring for vulnerable populations (older adults, children).

Therapeutic Dialogue illustrates communication strategies through real-life nurse-patient dialogue.

Nursing Diagnoses and Nursing Interventions are highlighted in the narrative.

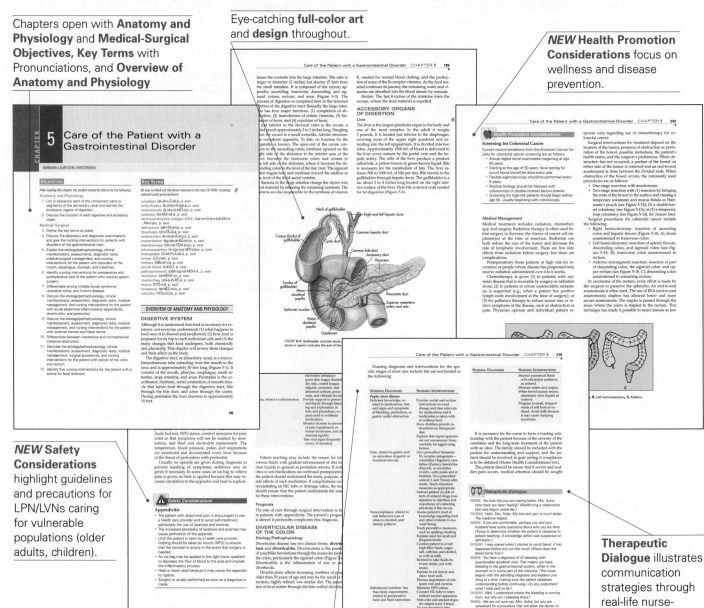

Complementary & Alternative Therapies describe specific therapies, precautions, and possible side effects.

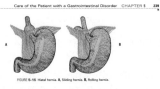

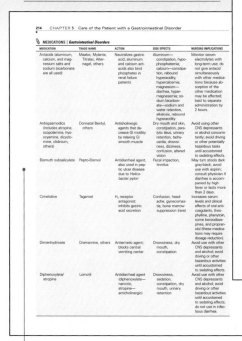

Older Adult Considerations discuss how aging affects specific disorders.

Cultural and Ethnic Considerations discuss how to address the health needs of a culturally diverse patient population when planning care.

Medications tables make it easy to locate action, dosage, precautions, and nursing considerations for commonly used drugs.

Nursing Care Plans with **Critical Thinking Questions** are developed around specific case studies.

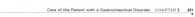

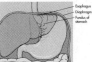

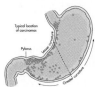

Home Health Considerations present issues facing patients and caregivers in the home care setting.

Chapters end with a summary of **Key Points** and **Chapter Challenge** NCLEX®-style study questions for student practice.

Contents

APPENDIXES

Drug Classifications

ACE inhibitors Prevent the synthesis of angiotensin II, a potent vasoconstrictor; used to treat hypertension and heart failure

acetylcholinesterase inhibitors Promote the accumulation of acetylcholine, resulting in prolonged cholinergic effects

adrenergic Produce effects similar to the neurotransmitter norepinephrine; see Chapter 13

adrenergic blocking agents Inhibit the adrenergic system, preventing stimulation of the adrenergic receptors

aldosterone receptor antagonists Block stimulation of mineralocorticoid receptors by aldosterone, thus reducing high blood pressure by preventing sodium reabsorption

aminoglycosides Gentamicin, tobramycin, and related antibiotics; particularly effective against gram-negative microorganisms; noted for potentially dangerous toxicity

analgesics Narcotic and nonnarcotic; relieve pain without producing loss of consciousness or reflex activity

androgens These steroid hormones produce masculinizing effects

angiotensin II receptor antagonists Also known as ARBs (angiotensin receptor blockers); act by binding to angiotensin II receptor sites, preventing angiotensin II (a very potent vasoconstrictor) from binding to receptor sites in vascular smooth muscle, brain, heart, kidneys, and adrenal gland, thus blocking the blood pressure–elevating and sodium-retaining effects of angiotensin II

anesthetics For example, local anesthesia, general anesthesia; cause a loss of sensation with or without a loss of consciousness

antacids Reduce the acidity of the gastric contents

antianginals Used to prevent or treat attacks of angina pectoris

antianxiety Used to treat anxiety symptoms or disorders; also known as minor tranquilizers or anxiolytics, although the term *tranquilizer* is avoided today to prevent the misperception that the patient is being tranquilized

antiarrhythmics Used to correct cardiac arrhythmias (any heart rate or rhythm other than normal sinus rhythm)

antibiotics Used to treat infections caused by pathogenic microbes; the term is often used interchangeably with antimicrobial agents

anticholinergic Block the action of acetylcholine in the parasympathetic nervous system; also known as cholinergic blocking agents, antispasmodics, and parasympatholytic agents

anticoagulants Do NOT dissolve existing blood clots, but do prevent enlargement or extension of blood clots

anticonvulsants Suppress abnormal neuronal activity in the CNS, preventing seizures

antidepressants Relieve depression

antidiabetics Also known as hypoglycemics; include insulin (used to treat type 1 diabetes mellitus) and oral hypoglycemic agents (used in the treatment of type 2 diabetes mellitus)

antidiarrheals Relieve or control the symptoms of acute or chronic diarrhea

antiemetics Used to prevent or treat nausea and vomiting

antifungals Used to treat fungal infections

antiglaucoma Used to reduce intraocular pressure

antigout Used in the treatment of active gout attacks or to prevent future attacks

antihistamines Used to treat allergy symptoms; may also be used to treat motion sickness, insomnia, and other nonallergic reactions

antihypertensives Used to treat elevated blood pressure (hypertension)

antilipemics Used to reduce serum cholesterol and/or triglycerides

antimicrobials Chemicals that eliminate living microorganisms pathogenic to the patient; also called antibiotics or antiinfectives

antineoplastics Also called chemotherapy agents; used alone or in combination with other treatment modalities such as radiation, surgery, or biologic response modifiers for the treatment of cancer

antiparkinson's Used in the treatment of Parkinson syndrome and other dyskinesias

antiplatelets Prevent platelet clumping (aggregation), thereby preventing an essential step in formation of a blood clot

antipsychotics Used in the treatment of severe mental illnesses; also known as major tranquilizers or neuroleptics, although the term *tranquilizer* is avoided today to prevent the misperception that the patient is being tranquilized

antipyretics Used to reduce fevers associated with a variety of conditions

antispasmodics Actually anticholinergic agents

antithyroid Used to treat the symptoms of hyperthyroidism; also known as thyroid hormone antagonists

antituberculins Used to prevent or treat an infection caused by *Mycobacterium tuberculosis*

antitussive Used to suppress a cough by acting on the cough center of the brain

antiulcer agents These drugs, such as histamine-2 antagonists, decrease the volume and increase the pH of gastric secretions

antivirals Used to treat infections caused by pathogenic viruses

bronchodilators Stimulate receptors within the tracheobronchial tree to relax and dilate the airway passages, allowing a greater volume of air to be exchanged and improving oxygenation

beta blockers Inhibit the activity of sympathetic transmitters, norepinephrine, and epinephrine; used to treat angina, arrhythmias, hypertension, and glaucoma

calcium channel blockers Also called calcium ion antagonists, slow channel blockers or calcium ion influx inhibitors; inhibit the movement of calcium ions across the cell membrane; used to decrease arrhythmias, slow rate of contraction of the heart, and cause dilation of blood vessels

carbapenems Antibiotics (imipenem, ertapenem, meropenem) that have a broad spectrum of activity against gram-positive and gram-negative bacteria; they act by inhibiting cell wall synthesis

carbonic anhydrase inhibitors Interfere with the production of aqueous humor, thereby reducing intraocular pressure associated with glaucoma

cell-stimulating agents Improve immune function by stimulating the activity of various immune cells

cholinergic Also known as parasympathomimetics; produce effects similar to those of acetylcholine

cholinesterase inhibitors These enzymes destroy acetylcholine, the cholinergic neurotransmitter

coating agent This drug, sucralfate, forms a complex that adheres to the crater of an ulcer, protecting it from aggravation by gastric secretions

colony-stimulating factors Stimulate progenitor cells in bone marrow to increase numbers of leukocytes, thereby improving immune function

From Clayton, B.D. and Stock, Y.N. (2004). Basic Pharmacology for Nurses, 13th edition. St. Louis: Mosby.

corticosteroids These hormones are secreted by the adrenal cortex of the adrenal gland

cycloplegics Anticholinergic agents that paralyze accommodation of the iris of the eye

cytotoxics Agents that cause direct cell death; often used for cancer chemotherapy

decongestants Reduce swelling in the nasal passages caused by a common cold or allergic rhinitis

digestants Combination products containing digestive enzymes used to treat various digestive disorders and to supplement deficiencies of natural digestive enzymes

digitalis glycosides A class of drugs, also known as cardiac glycosides, that increase the force of contraction and slow the heart rate, thereby improving cardiac output

diuretics Act to increase the flow of urine

emetics Used to induce vomiting

estrogens Steroids that cause feminizing effects

expectorants Liquefy mucus by stimulating the natural lubricant fluids from the bronchial glands

fluoroquinolones Ciprofloxacin and related agents; widely used broad-spectrum antibiotics

gastric stimulants Used to increase stomach contractions, relax the pyloric valve, and increase peristalsis in the gastrointestinal tract; result in a decrease in gastric transit time and more rapid emptying of the intestinal tract

glucocorticoids Also known as adrenocorticosteroids; are used to regulate carbohydrate, fat, and protein metabolism

gonadal hormones Hormones produced by the testes in the male and ovaries in the female

herbals Plant products usually sold as food supplements; may have pharmacologic effects that are not evaluated or regulated by the FDA

histamine (H2) antagonists Decrease the volume and increase the pH of gastric secretions both during the day and the night

HMG-CoA reductase enzyme inhibitors Also known as the statins; antilipemic agents that inhibit hydroxymethyl-glutaryl coenzyme A (HMG-CoA) reductase enzyme, the enzyme that stimulates the conversion of HMG-CoA to mevalonic acid, a precursor in the biosynthesis of cholesterol, thus reducing the potential for atherosclerosis

hyperuricemics Used to decrease the production or increase the excretion of uric acid

hypnotics Used to produce sleep

insulins Hormone required for glucose transport to the cells

lactation suppressants Used to prevent physiologic lactation

laxatives Act by a variety of mechanisms to treat constipation

low molecular weight heparins Derivatives of heparin; anticoagulants for the prophylactic treatment of pulmonary thromboembolism and deep vein thrombosis

macrolides Erythromycin, azithromycin, and related antibiotics

MAO inhibitors Agents that block monoamine oxidase, thereby preventing the degradation and prolonging the action of norepinephrine and serotonin

mineralocorticoids Steroids that cause the kidneys to retain sodium and water

miotics Cause constriction of the iris

mucolytics Reduce the thickness and stickiness of pulmonary secretions by acting directly on the mucous plugs to dissolve them

muscle relaxants Relieve muscle spasms

mydriatics Cause dilation of the iris

neuromuscular blockers Skeletal muscle relaxants used to produce muscle relaxation during anesthesia; reduce the use and side effects of general anesthetics; used to ease endotracheal intubation and prevent laryngospasm

nitrates Metabolize to nitric oxide, a potent vasodilator used to treat angina

nonsteroidal antiinflammatory drugs (NSAIDs) These "aspirin-like" drugs are chemically unrelated to the salicylates but are prostaglandin inhibitors

opioids Centrally acting analgesic agents related to morphine

oral contraceptives Used for birth control; administered orally

oral hypoglycemics Used in type 2 diabetes mellitus to improve glucose metabolism and lower blood glucose levels

progestins Steroids regulating endometrial and myometrial function; used alone or in combination with estrogen for oral contraception

protease inhibitors Saquinavir, ritonavir, indinavir, and related drugs; block the maturation of human immunodeficiency virus; used to treat HIV infections

salicylates Effective as analgesics, antipyretics, and antiinflammatory agents

sedatives Given to an individual to produce relaxation and rest; do not necessarily produce sleep

selective serotonin reuptake inhibitors (SSRIs) Antidepressants that act by specifically blocking the reuptake of serotonin, thus prolonging its action

serotonin antagonists Used to block serotonin; prevent emesis induced by chemotherapy, radiation therapy, and surgery

statins (HMG-CoA reductase inhibitors) Block the synthesis of cholesterol

stool softeners or fecal softeners Draw water into the stool, thereby softening it

sympatholytics Interfere with the storage and release of norepinephrine

sympathomimetics Mimic the action of dopamine, norepinephrine, and epinephrine

thrombolytics A specific group of drugs (alteplase, anistreplase, streptokinase, urokinase) given to dissolve existing blood clots

thyroid hormone antagonists Used to counteract or block the action of excessive formation of thyroid hormones

thyroid hormones Used when thyroid hormones are not being produced or are not produced in sufficient quantities to meet the body's physiologic needs

tricyclic antidepressants Inhibit the reuptake of norepinephrine and serotonin (include doxepin, amitriptyline, and imipramine)

uricosuric agents Act on the tubules of the kidneys to enhance the excretion of uric acid

urinary analgesics Produce a local anesthetic effect on the mucosa of the ureters and bladder to relieve burning, pain, urgency, and frequency associated with urinary tract infections (UTIs)

urinary antimicrobials Substances excreted and concentrated in the urine in sufficient amounts to have an antiseptic effect on the urine and the urinary tract

uterine relaxants Used primarily to prevent preterm labor and delivery

uterine stimulants Increase the frequency or strength of uterine contractions

vaccines Suspensions of either live, attenuated, or killed bacteria or viruses administered to induce immunity against infection of specific bacteria or viruses

vasodilators Relax the arteriolar smooth muscle, causing a dilation of the blood vessels.

CHAPTER 1

Introduction to Anatomy and Physiology

M. CHRISTINE NEFF and BARBARA LAURITSEN CHRISTENSEN

Objectives

After reading this chapter, the student should be able to do the following:

1. Define the key terms as listed.
2. Use each word of a given list of anatomical terms in a sentence.
3. Define the difference between anatomy and physiology.
4. Identify and define three major components of the cell.
5. Discuss the stages of mitosis and explain the importance of cellular reproduction.
6. Differentiate among tissues, organs, and systems.
7. Describe the four types of body tissues.
8. Discuss the two types of epithelial membranes.
9. List the 11 major organ systems of the body and briefly describe the major functions of each.
10. Differentiate between active and passive transport processes that act to move substances through cell membranes and give two examples of each.
11. List and discuss in order of increasing complexity the levels of organization of the body.
12. Define the term *anatomical position*.
13. List and define the principal directional terms and sections (planes) used in describing the body and the relationship of body parts to one another.
14. List the nine abdominopelvic regions and the abdominopelvic quadrants.

Key Terms

 Be sure to check out the bonus material on the free CD-ROM, including selected audio pronunciations.

active transport (p. 9)
anatomy (p. 1)
cell (p. 5)
cytoplasm (CĪ-tō-plăzm, p. 5)
diffusion (dĭ-FŪ-zhŭn, p. 10)
dorsal (p. 1)
filtration (p. 10)
homeostasis (hō-mē-ō-STĀ-sĭs, p. 5)
membrane (p. 13)
mitosis (mī-TŌ-sĭs, p. 8)
nucleus (p. 6)
organ (p. 4)
osmosis (ŏz-MŌ-sĭs, p. 10)
passive transport (p. 10)
phagocytosis (făg-ō-sī-TŌ-sĭs, p. 9)

physiology (fĭz-ē-ŌL-ø-jē, p. 1)
pinocytosis (pĭ-nō-sī-TŌ-sĭs, p. 9)
system (p. 4)
tissue (p. 4)
ventral (p. 1)

To care for an individual with a disease process, the nurse must understand the normal functioning of the human body. To accomplish this task, the nurse must study basic human anatomy and physiology. **Anatomy** is the study, classification, and description of structures and organs of the body. **Physiology** explains the processes and functions of the various structures and how they interrelate with one another. The normal, healthy human body can be compared with a finely tuned machine, with each part performing a special function to accomplish a given goal. As with the machine, when the human body malfunctions, the repairer must understand how it functions internally. The inability to make the necessary repairs to return the body to homeostasis may result in illness, disease, or death.

ANATOMICAL TERMINOLOGY

To study the human body, certain terms must be mastered to specifically locate a structure. To understand the following terms, the student should consider the body in a normal anatomical position, that is, standing erect with the face and palms facing forward (Figure 1-1):

Anterior (or **ventral**): To face forward; the front of the body. The chest is located anterior to the spine (Figure 1-2).

Posterior (or **dorsal**): Toward the back. The kidneys are posterior to the peritoneum.

Cranial: Toward the head. The brain is located in the cranial portion of the body.

Caudal: Toward the "tail"; the distal portion of the spine. A caudal anesthetic may be given to a patient.

Superior: Toward the head or above. The neck is superior to the shoulders.

Inferior: Lower, toward the feet, or below another. The foot is inferior to the ankle.

Medial: Toward the midline. The sternum (breastbone) is located in the medial portion of the chest.

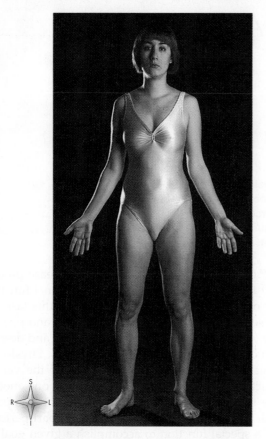

FIGURE **1-1** Anatomical position. The body is in an erect or standing posture with the arms at the sides and palms forward. The head and feet also point forward. The right and left sides of the body are mirror images of each other.

Lateral: Toward the side. The outer area of the leg, the area located on the side, is called lateral.

Proximal: Nearest the origin of the structure; nearest the trunk. The elbow is proximal to the forearm.

Distal: Farthest from the origin of the structure; farthest from the trunk. The fingers are distal to the hand.

Superficial: Nearer the surface. The skin of the arm is superficial to the muscles below it.

Deep: Farther away from the body surface. The bone of the upper arm is deep to the muscles that surround and cover it.

BODY PLANES

To facilitate the study of individual organs or the body as a whole, it is helpful to divide it into three imaginary planes: the sagittal, the coronal, and the transverse (see Figure 1-2).

1. The **sagittal** plane runs lengthwise from the front to the back. A sagittal cut gives a right and left portion of the body. A midsagittal cut gives two equal halves.
2. The **coronal** (frontal) plane divides the body into a ventral (front) section and a dorsal (back) section.

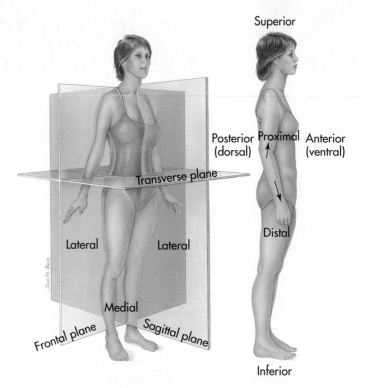

FIGURE **1-2** Directions and planes of the body.

3. The **transverse** plane cuts the body horizontally to the sagittal and the frontal planes, dividing the body into caudal and cranial portions.

BODY CAVITIES

The body, contrary to its external appearance, is not a solid structure. It is made up of open spaces or cavities that in turn contain compact, well-ordered arrangements of internal organs. It contains two major cavities that are, in turn, subdivided and contain compact, well-ordered arrangements of internal organs. The two major cavities are called the ventral and dorsal body cavities (Figure 1-3 and Table 1-1)

Ventral Cavity

The ventral cavity consists of the **thoracic** or chest **cavity** and the **abdominopelvic cavity** (see Figure 1-3).

The diaphragm (a muscle directly beneath the lungs) separates the ventral cavity into the thoracic (chest) and abdominal cavities. The thoracic cavity, a space that you think of as your chest cavity, contains the heart and lungs. Its midportion is a subdivision of the thoracic cavity, called the mediastinum, which contains the trachea, heart, and blood vessels; its other subdivisions are called the right and left pleural cavities, which contain the lungs.

The abdominal cavity contains the stomach, liver, gallbladder, spleen, pancreas, small intestine, and parts of the large intestine. A subdivision called the **pelvic cavity** contains the lower portion of the large

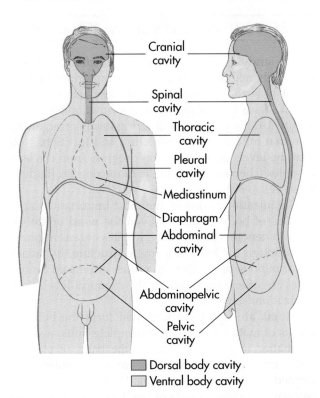

FIGURE **1-3** Location and subdivisions of the dorsal and ventral body cavities as viewed from the front (anterior) and from the side (lateral).

Table 1-1	*Body Cavities*
BODY CAVITY	**ORGAN(S)**
VENTRAL BODY CAVITY	
Thoracic Cavity	
Mediastinum	Trachea, heart, blood vessels
Pleural cavities	Lungs
Abdominopelvic Cavity	
Abdominal cavity	Liver, gallbladder, stomach, spleen, pancreas, small intestine, parts of large intestine
Pelvic cavity	Lower (sigmoid) colon, rectum, urinary bladder, reproductive organs
DORSAL BODY CAVITY	
Cranial cavity	Brain
Spinal cavity	Spinal cord

intestine (lower sigmoid colon, rectum), urinary bladder, and internal structures of the reproductive system.

The abdominal and pelvic cavities are not separated by any structures and therefore may be referred to as the abdominopelvic cavity (see Table 1-1).

Dorsal Cavity

The dorsal cavity is composed of the cranial and spinal cavities. The cranial cavity houses the brain, whereas the spinal cavity contains the spinal cord. The dorsal cavity is smaller than the ventral cavity.

ABDOMINAL REGIONS

For convenience in locating abdominal organs, anatomists divide the abdomen into nine imaginary regions. The following is a list of the nine regions (Figure 1-4) identified from right to left and from top to bottom:

1. Right hypochondriac region
2. Epigastric region
3. Left hypochondriac region
4. Right lumbar region
5. Umbilical region
6. Left lumbar region
7. Right iliac (inguinal) region
8. Hypogastric region
9. Left iliac (inguinal) region

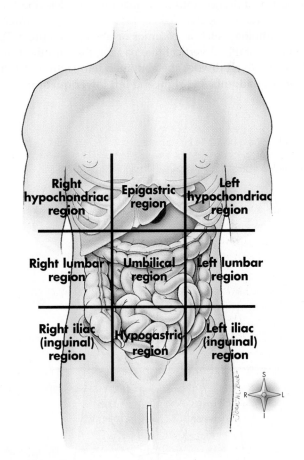

FIGURE **1-4** The nine regions of the abdominopelvic cavity. The most superficial organs are shown. Can you identify the deeper structures in each region?

The most superficial organs located in each of the nine abdominal regions are shown in Figure 1-4. In the right hypochondriac region the right lobe of the liver and the gallbladder are visible. In the epigastric area, parts of the right and left lobes of the liver and a large portion of the stomach can be seen. Viewed superficially, only a small portion of the stomach and large intestine is visible in the left hypochondriac area. Note that the right lumbar region includes parts of the large and small intestine (see Figure 1-4). The superficial organs seen in the umbilical region include a portion of the transverse colon and loops of the small intestine. Additional loops of the small intestine and a part of the colon can be seen in the left lumbar region. The right iliac region contains the cecum and parts of the small intestine. Only loops of the small intestine, the urinary bladder, and the appendix are seen in the hypogastric region. The left iliac region shows portions of the colon and the small intestine.

ABDOMINOPELVIC QUADRANTS

Physicians and other health professionals frequently divide the abdomen into four quadrants to describe the site of abdominopelvic pain or locate some type of internal pathology such as a tumor or abscess (Figure 1-5). A horizontal and vertical line passing through the umbilicus (navel) divides the abdomen into **right** and **left upper quadrants** and **right** and **left lower quadrants.**

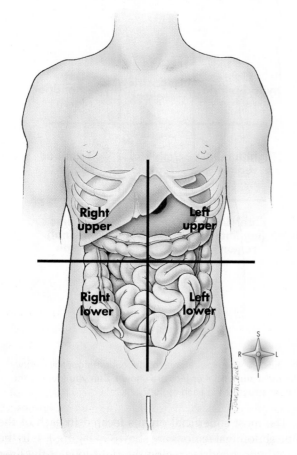

FIGURE **1-5** Horizontal and vertical line passing through the umbilicus (navel) divides the abdomen into right and left upper quadrants and right and left lower quadrants.

STRUCTURAL LEVELS OF ORGANIZATION

Before studying the structure and function of the human body and its many parts, it is important to think about how those parts are organized and how they might logically fit together into a functioning whole. Figure 1-6 illustrates the differing levels of organization that influence body structure and function. Note that the levels of organization progress from the least complex (chemical level) to the most complex (body as a whole).

Organization is one of the most important characteristics of body structure. Even the word *organism,* used to denote a living thing, implies organization.

Although the body is a single structure, it is made up of billions of smaller structures. Atoms and molecules are often referred to as the chemical level of organization (see Figure 1-6).

Atoms are small particles that form the building blocks of matter, the smallest complete units of which all matter is made. When, on the basis of electron structure, two or more atoms unite, a **molecule** is formed. A molecule can be made of like atoms—the oxygen molecule is made of two identical atoms—but more often it is made of two or more different atoms. For example, a molecule of water (H_2O) contains one atom of oxygen (O) and two atoms of hydrogen (H) (see Figure 1-6).

The existence of life depends on the proper levels and proportions of many chemical substances in the cytoplasm of cells. The structural levels of organization in the body are cells, tissues, organs, and systems.

Cells are considered to be the smallest living units of structure and function in our body. Although long recognized as the simplest units of living matter, cells are far from simple. They are extremely complex.

Tissues are somewhat more complex than cells. By definition a tissue is an organization of many similar cells that act together to perform a common function. Cells are held together and surrounded by varying amounts and varieties of gluelike, nonliving intercellular substances.

Organs are more complex than tissues. An organ is a group of several different kinds of tissues arranged so that they can together perform a special function. For instance, the lungs shown in Figure 1-6 are an example of organization at the organ level.

Systems are the most complex units that make up the body. A system is an organization of varying numbers and kinds of organs arranged so that they can together perform complex functions for the body. The organs of the respiratory system shown in Figure 1-6 permit air to enter the body and travel to the lungs, where the eventual exchange of oxygen and carbon dioxide occurs. Organs of the respiratory system include the nose, the windpipe or trachea, and the complex series of bronchial tubes that permit passage of air into the lungs.

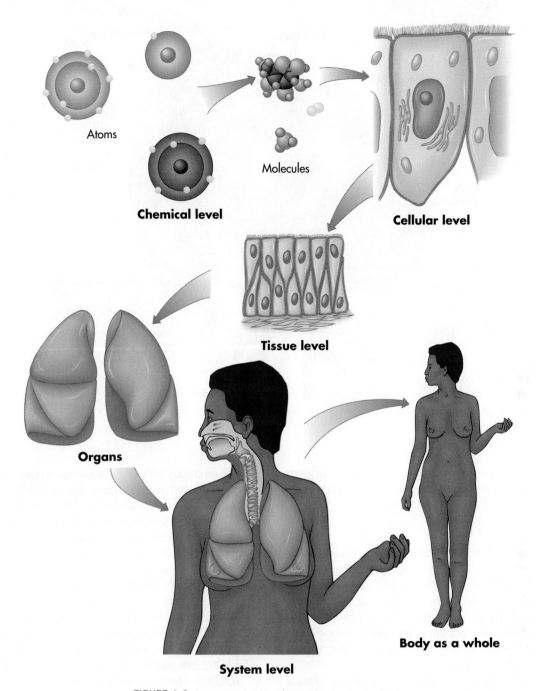

FIGURE **1-6** Structural levels of organization in the body.

CELLS

Nearly 300 years ago Robert Hooke discovered the first cell while examining plant fragments under the microscope. The structures reminded him of tiny, individual miniature prison cells, hence the name cell (the fundamental unit of all living tissue) (Figure 1-7). All cells are microscopic but differ widely in size and shape. Regardless of size or shape, they exhibit five unique characteristics of life—growth, metabolism, responsiveness, reproduction, and homeostasis (a relative constancy in the internal environment of the body, naturally maintained by adaptive responses that pro-

mote healthy survival). Many living things are so simple that they consist of just one cell. The human body, however, is so complex that it consists not of a few thousand or millions or even billions of cells, but trillions of these tiny powerhouses of life.

Cells contain cytoplasm, or "living matter," a substance that exists only in cells. Cytoplasm is composed largely of a gel-like substance that contains water, food, minerals, enzymes, and other specialized materials. The term *cyto-* is a combining form from the Greek and denotes a relationship to a cell. Each cell in the body is surrounded by a thin membrane, the plasma

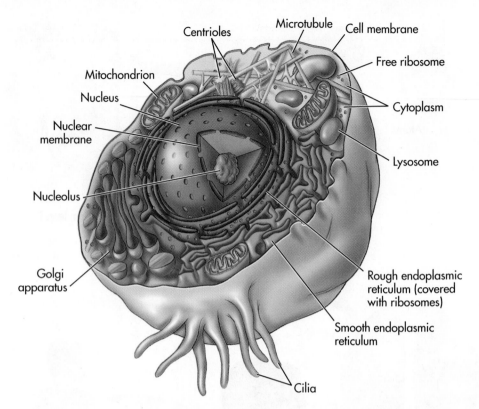

FIGURE **1-7** A typical cell.

membrane. This membrane separates the cell contents from the dilute saltwater solution called **tissue fluid** that bathes every cell in the body.

Structural Parts of Cells

The three main parts of a cell are the plasma membrane, the cytoplasm, and the nucleus (see Figure 1-7).

Plasma membrane. As the name suggests, the plasma membrane is the membrane that encloses the cytoplasm and forms the outer boundary of the cell. It is an incredibly delicate structure—only about 7 nm (nanometers), or 3/10,000,000 inch, thick! Yet it has a precise, orderly structure.

Despite its seeming fragility, the plasma membrane is strong enough to keep the cell whole and intact. It also performs other life-preserving functions for the cell. It serves as a well-guarded gateway between the fluid inside the cell and the fluid around it. The plasma membrane is **selectively permeable.** This means the membrane permits certain substances to enter and leave at will while not allowing other substances to cross. This membrane separates the cell contents from the dilute saltwater solution called interstitial fluid, or simply tissue fluid, which bathes every cell in the body. The plasma membrane also identifies a cell as coming from one particular individual. Its surface proteins serve as positive identification tags because they occur only in the cells of that individual. A practical application of this fact is made in **tissue typing,** a procedure performed

before an organ from one individual is transplanted into another. Carbohydrate chains attached to the surface of cells often play a role in the identification of cell types.

Cytoplasm. Cytoplasm is the internal living material of cells. Cytoplasm (protoplasm) is a sticky, fluidlike substance that lies between the plasma membrane and the nucleus of the cell. Situated within the cytoplasm are numerous organelles (tiny functioning structures). These organelles were not discovered until the development of the powerful electron microscope.

Cytoplasm is composed of 70% water with traces of proteins, lipids, carbohydrates, minerals, and salts. (Table 1-2 lists major cell structures and their functions.)

Nucleus. The nucleus is the largest organelle within the cell. It is responsible for cell reproduction and control of the other organelles. The nucleus is surrounded by a membrane called the nuclear membrane. It contains nucleoplasm, a refined form of cytoplasm. The nucleus contains two specialized structures, the nucleolus and chromatin granules. The nucleolus is critical in the formation of protein. The chromatin granules are composed of protein and deoxyribonucleic acid (DNA). DNA contains the genetic code, or blueprint, of the body.

Endoplasmic reticulum. Throughout the cytoplasm lies a system of membranes, or canals, called the endoplasmic reticulum (ER). ER functions as a miniature circulating system for the cell by carrying substances from one part of the cell to another. There are two types of ER: (1) smooth, found in cells

Table 1-2 | *Some Major Cell Structures and Their Functions*

CELL STRUCTURE	FUNCTION(S)
Plasma membrane	Serves as the boundary of the cell; protein and carbohydrate molecules on outer surface of plasma membrane perform various functions (e.g., they serve as markers that identify cells of each individual or as receptor molecules for certain hormones)
Endoplasmic reticulum (ER)	Ribosomes attach to rough ER to synthesize proteins; smooth ER synthesizes lipids and certain carbohydrates
Ribosomes	Synthesize proteins; they are a cell's "protein factories"
Mitochondria	Synthesize adenosine triphosphate (ATP); they are a cell's "powerhouses"
Lysosomes	Serve as cell's "digestive system"
Golgi apparatus	Synthesizes carbohydrate, combines it with protein, and packages the product as globules of glycoprotein
Centrioles	Function in cell reproduction
Cilia	Short, hairlike extensions on the free surfaces of some cells capable of movement
Flagella	Single projections of cell surfaces; much larger than cilia; an example in humans is the "tail" of a sperm cell
Nucleus	Dictates protein synthesis, thereby playing an essential role in other cell activities, namely, active transport, metabolism, growth, and heredity
Nucleoli	Play an essential role in the formation of ribosomes

that deal with fatty substances; and (2) rough, found in cells that manufacture proteins.

Ribosomes. Ribosomes are tiny structures floating free in the cytoplasm or attached to the rough ER. They are called **protein factories** because they are responsible for the production of enzymes and other proteins.

Mitochondria. The mitochondria are the power-houses of the cells. They are bean-shaped with a fold-like interior membrane. They take food and convert it to a complex energy form, adenosine triphosphate (ATP), for use by the cell. ATP is described as the "energy currency" of the cells because it supplies the energy for all activities.

Lysosomes. Lysosomes are small saclike structures containing enzymes that digest food compounds and microbes that have invaded the cell.

Golgi apparatus. The Golgi apparatus is usually located near the nucleus. It is the "packaging plant" of the cell. It packages certain carbohydrate and protein compounds into globules. Then it moves outward toward and through the cell membrane, where it breaks open and releases its contents.

Centrioles. The centrioles are paired, rod-shaped organelles. During cell division (mitosis) they aid in the formation of the spindle, a structure necessary for cell reproduction.

Protein Synthesis

Protein is a vital component of every cell in the body. To produce protein, nucleic acids exist in the cytoplasm and the nucleus of the cell.

Two important nucleic acids are (1) deoxyribonucleic acid (DNA) (Figure 1-8), which is located in the

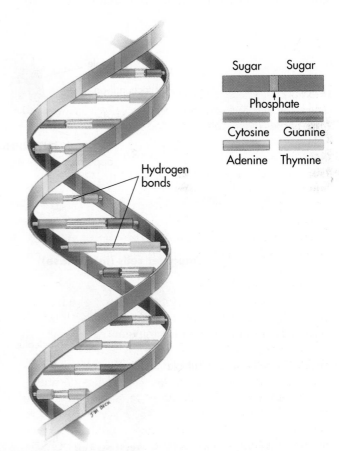

FIGURE **1-8** DNA molecule. Note that each side of the DNA molecule consists of alternating sugar and phosphate groups. Each sugar group is united to the sugar group opposite it by a pair of nitrogenous bases (adenine-thymine or cytosine-guanine). The sequence of these pairs constitutes a genetic code that determines the structure and function of a cell.

nucleus; and (2) ribonucleic acid (RNA), which is located in the cytoplasm. The DNA encodes the message for protein synthesis and sends it to the RNA, which transports it to the ribosomes, where the protein is produced. Hence DNA is called the **chemical blueprint** and RNA is called the **chemical messenger.**

Cell Division

All cells in the body, except sex cells, reproduce by mitosis (type of somatic [pertaining to nonreproductive cells] cell division in which each daughter cell contains the same number of chromosomes as the parent cell). Each daughter chromosome contains the complete genetic information of the original chromosome and forms during the interphase by the duplication of the DNA molecule (Figure 1-9). The original cell divides to form two daughter cells that retain the characteristics of the original cell.

The chromosomes (spindle-shaped rods) in the nucleus of the cell carry the genes that are responsible for the organism's traits. The traits carry such hereditary factors as hair and eye color. These chromosomes are composed of DNA. Before the cell divides, the DNA

must replicate itself so that each new daughter cell contains the original DNA. At the completion of cell division, the daughter cells contain both the nucleus and cytoplasm of the original cell. Each body cell in humans contains 46 chromosomes. These chromosomes exist in pairs. One member of each pair was received from the father of the offspring at the time of fertilization, and one was received from the mother. These paired chromosomes, except for the pair that determines sex, are alike in size and appearance and carry genes for the same traits.

During mitosis the cell goes through four phases: prophase, metaphase, anaphase, and telophase.

Prophase. In the nucleus the chromosomes form two strands called **chromatids.** In the cytoplasm the centrioles form a network of spindle fibers.

Metaphase. The nucleus membrane and nucleolus disappear, and the chromosomes are aligned across the center of the cell. The centrioles are at the opposite ends of the cell, and spindle fibers are attached to each chromatid.

Anaphase. The chromosomes are pulled to the opposite ends of the cell and cell division begins.

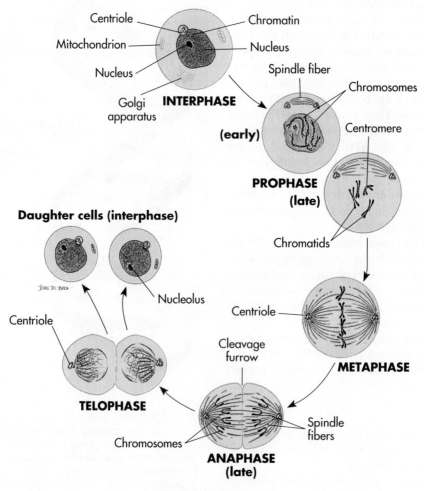

FIGURE **1-9** Mitosis.

Telophase. At this final phase of cell division, the two nuclei appear and the chromosomes disperse. At the end of this phase, two new daughter cells appear.

Movement of Materials across Cell Membranes

For a cell to survive, it must receive food and oxygen and secrete its waste products. To accomplish this task, a number of processes allow for mass movement of substances into and out of the cells. These transport processes are classified under two general headings: **passive transport** and **active transport.**

The difference between the two categories is based on whether energy is required to effect the movement of something through the cell membrane. Active transport (the movement of materials across the membrane of a cell by means of chemical activity that allows the cell to admit larger molecules than would otherwise be able to enter) processes require the expenditure of energy by the cell. Passive transport processes do not require energy expenditure. The energy required for active transport processes is obtained from an important chemical substance called ATP. ATP is produced in the cell from nutrients and is capable of releasing energy that in turn enables the cell to do work. The breakdown of ATP and use of the energy that is released are required for active transport processes to occur.

Active transport is an extremely important process. It allows cells to move certain ions or other water-soluble particles to specific areas.

Active transport processes. As stated, active transport is the movement of material across the membrane of a cell by means of a chemical activity that allows the cell to admit larger molecules that would otherwise be unable to enter. Certain enzymes play a role in active transport, providing a chemical "pump" that helps move substances through the cell membrane. For example, insulin binds with glucose and transports the glucose into the cell. Other active transport processes (Table 1-3) include the following:

* Phagocytosis (Greek for "cell-eating"): The process that permits a cell to engulf or to surround any foreign material and to digest it. This function is often performed by the white blood cells in the human body.
* Pinocytosis: The process by which extracellular fluid is taken into the cell. The cell membrane develops a saclike indentation filled with extracellular fluid, then closes around it and digests it.
* Sodium-potassium pump: One type of active transport pump that operates in the plasma membrane of all human cells. It is essential for healthy cell survival. As its name suggests, the **sodium-potassium pump** actively transports sodium ions (Na^+) and potassium ions (K^+)—but in opposite directions. It transports sodium ions *out of* cells and potassium ions *into* cells. By so doing, the sodium-potassium pump maintains a lower

Table 1-3 | *Active Transport Processes*

PROCESS	DESCRIPTION		EXAMPLES
PHAGOCYTOSIS	Movement of cells or other large particles into cell by trapping it in a section of plasma membrane that pinches off to form an intracellular vesicle; type of endocytosis		Trapping of bacterial cells by phagocytic white blood cells
PINOCYTOSIS	Movement of fluid and dissolved molecules into a cell by trapping them in a section of plasma membrane that pinches off to form an intracellular vesicle; type of endocytosis		Trapping of large protein molecules by some body cell
CALCIUM PUMP	Movement of solute particles from an area of low concentration to an area of high concentration (up the concentration gradient) by means of a carrier molecule	ATP	In muscle cells, pumping of nearly all calcium ions to special compartments or out of the cell

Modified from Thibodeau, G.A. & Patton, K.T. (2003). *Anatomy and physiology.* (5th ed.). St Louis: Mosby.

| Table 1-4 | *Passive Transport Processes* |

PROCESS	DESCRIPTION		EXAMPLES
SIMPLE DIFFUSION	Movement of particles through phospholipid bilayer or through channels from an area of high concentration to an area of low concentration—that is, down the concentration gradient		Movement of carbon dioxide out of all cells; movement of sodium ions into nerve cells as they conduct an impulse
DIALYSIS	Diffusion of small solute particles, but not larger solute particles, through a selectively permeable membrane; results in separation of large and small solutes		During procedure called peritoneal dialysis, small solutes diffuse from blood vessels but blood proteins do not (thus removing only small solutes from the blood)
OSMOSIS	Diffusion of water through a selectively permeable membrane in the presence of at least one impermeable solute		Diffusion of water molecules into and out of cells to correct imbalances in water concentration

Modified from Thibodeau, G.A. & Patton, K.T. (2003). *Anatomy and physiology.* (5th ed.). St Louis: Mosby.

sodium concentration in intracellular fluid than in the surrounding extracellular fluid. At the same time, this pump maintains a higher potassium concentration in the intracellular fluid than in the surrounding extracellular fluid.

- Calcium pump: For example, active calcium carriers, or **calcium pumps,** in the membranes of muscle cells allow the cell to force nearly all of the intracellular calcium ions (Ca^{++}) into special compartments or out of the cell entirely. This is important because a muscle cell cannot operate properly unless the intracellular Ca^{++} concentration is kept low during rest.

In passive transport (the movement of small molecules across the membrane of a cell by diffusion) processes, no cellular energy is required to move substances from a high concentration to a lower concentration; in active transport processes, cellular energy is required to move substances from a low concentration to a high concentration.

Passive transport processes. The primary passive transport processes (Table 1-4) include the following:

- Diffusion: A process in which solid particles in a fluid move from an area of higher concentration to an area of lower concentration, which results in an even distribution of the particles in the fluid (Figure 1-10).
- Osmosis: The passage of water across a selectively permeable membrane, with the water

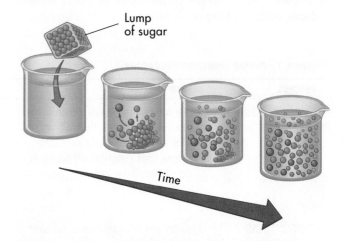

FIGURE **1-10** Diffusion. The molecules of a lump of sugar are very densely packed when they enter the water. As sugar molecules collide frequently in the area of high concentration, they gradually spread away from each other toward the area of lower concentration. Eventually the sugar molecules are evenly distributed.

molecules going from the less concentrated solution to the more concentrated solution (Figure 1-11).

- Filtration: The movement of water and particles through a membrane by a force from either pressure or gravity. This membrane contains spaces through which liquid passes but that are too

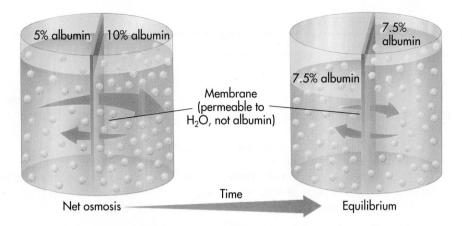

FIGURE **1-11** Osmosis. Osmosis is the diffusion of water through a selectively permeable membrane. The membrane shown in this diagram is permeable to water but not to albumin. Because there are relatively more water molecules in 5% albumin than in 10% albumin, more water molecules osmose from the more dilute into the more concentrated solution (as indicated by the *large arrow* in the diagram on the left) than osmose in the opposite direction. The overall direction of osmosis, in other words, is toward the more concentrated solution. Movement across the membrane continues until the concentrations of the solutions equalize.

small to permit solid particles to pass. Movement is from areas of greater to areas of lesser pressure.

TISSUES

Tissues are groups of similar cells that work together to perform a specific function. The body is composed of the following four main types of tissues, which make up the body's many organs:

- Epithelial tissue
- Connective tissue
- Muscle tissue
- Nervous tissue

Consult Table 1-5 for a summary of tissue locations and functions.

Epithelial Tissue

Epithelial cells are packed closely together and contain no blood vessels. Epithelial tissue covers the outside of the body and some of the internal structures. There are four types or forms of epithelial tissue: (1) simple squamous, (2) stratified squamous, (3) simple columnar, and (4) stratified transitional. Table 1-5 gives the locations and functions of each of these types.

Epithelial tissue serves several important functions in the body. Some of the more important are listed in the following:

- **Protection:** Covering the body and many of its organs, it serves as a protective barrier against invasion.
- **Absorption:** Certain specialized epithelial cells can absorb material in the body (e.g., the lin-

ing of the small intestine can absorb digested nutrients).

- **Secretion:** Mucus is secreted in areas such as the respiratory and digestive tracts.

Connective Tissue

As the name suggests, connective tissue "connects," or joins, tissues or structures of the body. Connective tissue is the most abundant and widely distributed tissue in the body. It also supports and protects body structures and exists in varying forms. It can be thin and delicate or tough and cordlike; it also exists in liquid form (blood). Mast cells, plasma cells, and white blood cells are found in connective tissue. Red blood cells are not usually found in connective tissue unless blood vessels have been injured. Unlike the closely packed epithelial tissue, the connective tissue cells are spaced among varying amounts of intercellular fluid, which is composed of protein complexes and tissue fluid.

Some of the most important forms of connective tissue are **areolar** connective tissue, **adipose** (fat) tissue, **fibrous** connective tissue, **bone, cartilage, blood,** and **hematopoietic** tissue. Consult Table 1-5 for the locations and functions of these tissues.

Muscle Tissue

Muscle tissue is composed of cells that contract in response to a message from the brain or spinal cord. There are three types of muscle cells: (1) **skeletal** (striated, voluntary), (2) **cardiac** (striated, involuntary), and (3) **visceral** (smooth, involuntary) (Figure 1-12).

Table 1-5 | *Tissues*

TISSUE	LOCATION	FUNCTION
EPITHELIAL		
Simple squamous	Alveoli of lungs	Absorption by diffusion of respiratory gases between alveolar air and blood
	Lining of blood and lymphatic vessels	Absorption by diffusion, filtration, and osmosis
Stratified squamous	Surface of lining of mouth and esophagus	Protection
	Surface of skin (epidermis)	Protection
Simple columnar	Surface layer of lining of stomach, intestines, and parts of respiratory tract	Protection; secretion; absorption
Stratified transitional	Urinary bladder	Protection
CONNECTIVE*		
Areolar	Between other tissues and organs	Connection
Adipose (fat)	Under skin	Protection
	Padding at various points	Insulation; support; reserve food
Dense fibrous	Tendons; ligaments	Flexible but strong connection
Bone	Skeleton	Support; protection
Cartilage	Part of nasal septum; covering articular surfaces of bones; larynx; rings in trachea and bronchi	Firm but flexible support
	Disks between vertebrae	
	External ear	
Blood	Blood vessels	Transportation
MUSCLE		
Skeletal (striated voluntary); see Figure 1-12, *A*	Muscles that attach to bones	Movement of bones
	Eyeball muscles	Eye movements
	Upper third of esophagus	First part of swallowing
Cardiac (striated involuntary); see Figure 1-12, *B*	Wall of heart	Contraction of heart
Visceral (nonstriated involuntary or smooth); see Figure 1-12, *C*	In walls of tubular viscera of digestive, respiratory, and genitourinary tracts	Movement of substances along respective tracts
	In walls of blood vessels and large lymphatic vessels	Changing of diameter of blood vessels
	In ducts of glands	Movement of substances along ducts
	Intrinsic eye muscles (iris and ciliary body)	Changing of diameter of pupils and shape of lens
	Arrector of muscles of hairs	Erection of hairs (gooseflesh)
NERVOUS	Brain; spinal cord; nerves	Irritability; conduction

*Connective tissues are the most widely distributed of all tissues.

Skeletal muscle cells are striated (have a striped appearance) and attach to bones to produce voluntary movement. Skeletal muscle is also known as **voluntary muscle** because willed or voluntary control of skeletal muscle contractions is possible.

Cardiac muscle cells are striated with fibers that branch to form many networks, or webs. These networks are found only in the walls of the heart, and the regular but involuntary contractions of cardiac muscle produce the heartbeat. They generally do not function at will (involuntary). They typically contract independently of the will.

Smooth (visceral) muscle cells are nonstriated and have a smooth appearance. These cells appear in the viscera, or internal organs, such as the walls of the blood vessels, stomach, intestines, and uterus. Contractions of smooth (visceral) muscle propel food and fluid through the digestive tract and help regulate the

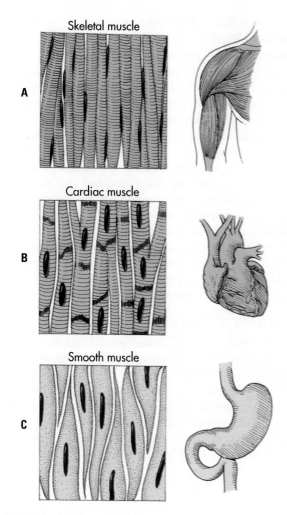

FIGURE **1-12** Types of muscles. **A,** Skeletal muscle. **B,** Cardiac muscle. **C,** Smooth muscle.

diameter of blood vessels. Contraction of smooth muscle in the tubes of the respiratory system, such as the bronchioles in the lungs, can impair breathing and result in asthma attacks and labored respiration. Generally, they are involuntary because they are not under conscious or willful control, but some control can be exerted through the use of biofeedback techniques (see Figure 1-12).

Nervous Tissue

The function of nervous tissue is to provide rapid communication between body structure and control of body functions. Nervous tissue is composed of two types of cells: neurons and glial cells. The neurons are the nerve cells and are responsible for the transmission of impulses or messages. They are the functional or conducting units of the system. The glial cells are connecting and supporting cells; they support and nourish the neurons.

Neurons have three parts: (1) dendrites, which carry impulses toward the cell body; (2) cell body; and (3) axons, which carry impulses away from the cell body (see Figure 14-1).

MEMBRANES

Membranes are thin sheets of tissue that serve many functions in the body. They cover body surfaces, line and lubricate hollow organs, and protect and anchor organs and bones. The two major types of membranes are the epithelial and the connective tissue membranes.

Epithelial Membranes

Epithelial membranes are usually composed of a thin layer of epithelial cells with an underlying layer of connective tissue for strength. Epithelial membranes may be divided into two subgroups: mucous membranes and serous membranes.

Mucous membranes. Mucous membranes secrete **mucus** (a thick, slippery material), which keeps the membranes moist and soft and protects against bacterial invasion. They line the body surfaces that open to the outside environment. Examples include the nose, mouth, and urinary, respiratory, gastrointestinal, and reproductive tracts. The epithelial component of the mucous membrane varies, depending on its location and function. In the esophagus, for example, a tough, abrasion-resistant, stratified squamous epithelium is found. A thin layer of simple columnar epithelium covers the walls of the lower segments of the digestive tract.

Mucous membranes get their name from the fact that they produce a film of mucus that coats and protects the underlying cells. Besides protection, mucus also serves other purposes. For example, it acts as a lubricant for food as it moves along the digestive tract. In the respiratory tract it serves as a sticky trap for contaminants.

Serous membranes. Serous membranes secrete a thin, watery fluid that prevents friction when organs rub against one another. They line the body surfaces that do not open to the outside environment. Examples include the lungs (pleura), intestines (peritoneum), and heart (pericardium). Like all epithelial membranes, a serous membrane is composed of two distinct layers of tissue. One of the layers, the epithelial sheet, is a thin layer of simple squamous epithelium. The other layer, the connective tissue layer, forms a very thin sheet that holds and supports the epithelial cells.

The serous membrane that lines body cavities and covers the surfaces of organs in those cavities is in reality a single, continuous sheet covering two different surfaces. The **parietal** membrane is the portion that lines the wall of the cavity like wallpaper; the **visceral** membrane covers the surface of the viscera (organs within the cavity).

Table 1-6   *Major Systems and Functions of the Body*

SYSTEM	FUNCTION
Integumentary (skin)	Covers the body and is the body's first line of defense
Musculoskeletal	Provides the body's framework and allows for movement
Cardiovascular (Circulatory)	Is the major transportation system for nutrition, water, oxygen, and wastes
Lymphatic	Helps to protect and maintain the internal fluid environment of the body by producing, filtering, and conveying lymph and producing various blood cells
Digestive	Processes food and water and removes waste products
Respiratory	Delivers oxygen and removes carbon dioxide
Urinary	Removes excess water and waste products
Nervous	Contains the body's control center and is responsible for the coordination of all of the body's activities
Endocrine	Protects the individual by detecting changes in the environment Releases hormones that regulate the body's activities
Reproductive	Enables the procreation of life

Connective Tissue Membranes (Synovial Membranes)

Connective tissue membranes are smooth and slick and secrete synovial fluid (a thick, lubricating fluid). These membranes line the joint spaces between bones and prevent friction between the ends of the bones, thus allowing free movement of the joints.

Unlike serous and mucous membranes, connective tissue membranes do not contain epithelial components. The synovial membranes lining the spaces between bones and joints that move are classified as connective tissue membranes. These membranes are smooth and slick and secrete a thick, colorless lubricating fluid called **synovial fluid.** The membrane itself, with its specialized fluid, helps reduce friction between the opposing surfaces of bones in movable joints. Synovial membranes also line the small, cushionlike sacs called **bursae** that are found between some moving body parts.

ORGANS/SYSTEMS

When several kinds of tissues are united to form a more complex function than any tissue alone, they are called organs. Examples are the heart, stomach, and kidneys. These organs functioning together for the same general purpose make up organ systems, which maintain the whole body. Systems perform a more complex function than any one organ can perform alone (Tables 1-6, 1-7; Figure 1-13).

Table 1-7   *Organ Systems and Their Functions*

STRUCTURE	FUNCTION
INTEGUMENTARY SYSTEM	
Skin	Protection
Hair	Regulation of body temperature
Nails	Synthesis of chemicals
Sense receptors	Sense organ
Sweat glands	
Oil glands	
SKELETAL SYSTEM	
Bones	Support
Joints	Movement (with joints and muscles)
	Storage of minerals
	Blood cell formation

Table 1-7 *Organ Systems and Their Functions—cont'd*

STRUCTURE	FUNCTION
MUSCULAR SYSTEM	
Voluntary or striated muscles	Movement
Involuntary or smooth muscles	Maintenance of body posture
	Production of heat
NERVOUS SYSTEM	
Brain	Communication
Spinal cord	Integration
Nerves	Control
Sense organs	Recognition of sensory stimuli
	System functions by production of nerve impulses caused by stimuli of various types
	Control is fast acting and of short duration
ENDOCRINE SYSTEM	
Pituitary gland	Secretion of special substances (hormones) directly into the blood
Pineal gland	Same as nervous system—communication, integration, control
Hypothalamus	Control is slow and of long duration
Thyroid gland	Examples of hormone regulation: growth, metabolism, reproduction, and fluid and electrolyte balance
Parathyroid glands	
Thymus gland	
Adrenal glands	
Pancreas	
Ovaries (female)	
Testes (male)	
CARDIOVASCULAR (CIRCULATORY) SYSTEM	
Heart	Transportation
Blood vessels	Regulation of body temperature
	Immunity (body defense)
LYMPHATIC SYSTEM	
Lymph nodes	Transportation
Lymphatic vessels	Immunity (body defense)
Thymus	
Spleen	
RESPIRATORY SYSTEM	
Nose	Exchange of waste gas (carbon dioxide) for oxygen in the lungs
Pharynx	Area of gas exchange in the lungs called alveoli
Larynx	Filtration of irritants from inspired air
Trachea	Regulation of acid-base balance
Bronchi	
Lungs	

Continued

Table 1-7 | *Organ Systems and Their Functions—cont'd*

STRUCTURE	FUNCTION
DIGESTIVE SYSTEM	
Primary Organs	
Mouth	Mechanical and chemical breakdown (digestion) of food
Pharynx	Absorption of nutrients
Esophagus	Undigested waste product that is eliminated is called **feces**
Stomach	Appendix is a structural but not a functional part of digestive system
Small intestine (duodenum, jejunum, ileum)	Inflammation of appendix is called **appendicitis**
Large intestine (ascending, transverse, descending, sigmoid)	
Rectum	
Anal canal	
Accessory Organs	
Teeth	
Salivary glands	
Tongue	
Liver	
Gallbladder	
Pancreas	
Appendix	
URINARY SYSTEM	
Kidneys	Clearing or cleaning blood of waste products; waste product excreted from body is called urine
Ureters	Electrolyte balance
Urinary bladder	Water balance
Urethra	Acid-base balance
	Urethra has urinary and reproductive functions (in male)
REPRODUCTIVE SYSTEM	
Male	
Gonads (testes)	Survival of species
Genital ducts (epididymis, vas deferens, ejaculatory duct, urethra)	Production of sex cells (male are sperm; female are ova)
	Transfer and fertilization of sex cells
Accessory glands (prostate, seminal vesicles, Cowper's glands)	Development and birth of offspring
	Nourishment of offspring
Supporting structures (penis and scrotum)	Production of sex hormones
Female	
Gonads (ovaries)	
Accessory organs (uterus, fallopian tubes, oviducts, vagina)	
External genitalia (vulva)	
Mons pubis	
Labia majora	
Labia minora	
Clitoris	
Accessory glands	
Skene's glands	
Bartholin's glands	
Mammary glands (breasts)	

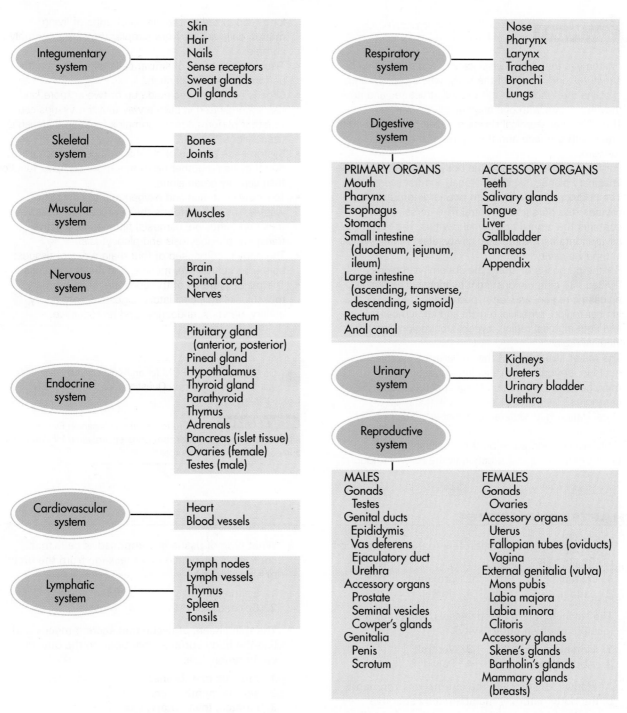

FIGURE **1-13** Body systems and their organs.

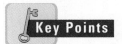
Key Points

- Anatomy is the study, classification, and description of structures and organs of the body, whereas physiology explains the function of the various structures and how they interrelate with one another.
- The normal anatomical position of the body is standing erect with the face and the palms of the hands forward.
- For the purposes of study, the body is divided into three imaginary planes: sagittal, coronal, and transverse.
- The body can be divided into two large groups of cavities: the dorsal and ventral. The dorsal cavity contains the cranial and spinal cavities. The ventral cavity contains the thoracic cavity, abdominal cavity, and pelvic cavity.
- For the purposes of study, the abdominal region is divided into nine regions: right hypochondriac region, epigastric region, and left hypochondriac region; right lumbar region, umbilical region, and left lumbar region; and right inguinal region, hypogastric region, and left inguinal region.
- The major structures of the cell are the cytoplasm, nucleus, endoplasmic reticulum, ribosomes, mitochondria, lysosomes, Golgi apparatus, and centrioles.
- Organization is an outstanding characteristic of body structure.
- Cells are considered to be the smallest "living" units of structure and function in the body. Although

long recognized as the simplest units of living matter, cells are far from simple; they are extremely complex.
- Tissues are groups of similar cells that work together to perform a specific function.
- Organs are structures made up of two or more kinds of tissues organized in such a way that the tissues can together perform a more complex function than can any tissue alone.
- Systems are a group of organs arranged in such a way that they can together perform a more complex function than can any organ alone.
- To receive nutrition and oxygen and to rid itself of wastes, the cell performs these processes: passive transport (diffusion, osmosis, filtration) and active transport (phagocytosis and pinocytosis).
- The body is composed of four main types of tissues: epithelial, connective, muscle, and nervous tissues.
- The major systems of the body are integumentary, musculoskeletal, circulatory, digestive, respiratory, urinary, nervous, endocrine, and reproductive.

🔘 Go to your free CD-ROM for an Audio Glossary, animations, video clips, and Review Questions for the NCLEX-PN® Examination.

evolve   Be sure to visit the companion Evolve site at http://evolve.elsevier.com/Christensen/adult/ for WebLinks and additional online resources.

CHAPTER CHALLENGE

1. The anatomical term that refers to the distal portion of the spine is:
   1. medial.
   2. caudal.
   3. proximal.
   4. dorsal.

2. The trachea, heart, blood vessels, and lungs are located in which body cavity?
   1. Dorsal
   2. Abdominopelvic
   3. Ventral
   4. Pelvic

3. A relative constancy in the internal environment of the body naturally maintained by adaptive responses that promote healthy survival is called:
   1. homeostasis.
   2. mitosis.
   3. lysosomes.
   4. protein synthesis.

4. A process in which solid particles in a fluid move from an area of greater concentration to an area of lesser concentration, resulting in an even distribution of the particles in the fluid, is called:
   1. phagocytosis.
   2. pinocytosis.
   3. osmosis.
   4. diffusion.

5. The movement of materials across the membrane of a cell by means of chemical activity requiring the expenditure of energy by the cell is called:
   1. passive passport.
   2. active transport.
   3. telophase.
   4. transcription.

6. What type of tissue is composed of cells that contract in response to a message from the brain or spinal cord?
   1. Epithelial
   2. Connective
   3. Membrane
   4. Muscle

7. The thin sheets of tissue that secrete mucus and line the body surfaces that open to the outside environment are:
   1. mucous membranes.
   2. serous membranes.
   3. striated, involuntary.
   4. visceral, involuntary.

8. An active transport process that permits a cell to engulf or surround foreign material and digest it is called:
   1. mitosis.
   2. pinocytosis.
   3. phagocytosis.
   4. filtration.

9. A type of cell division of somatic cells in which each daughter cell contains the same number of chromosomes as the parent cell is called:
   1. flagella.
   2. mitosis.
   3. ER synthesis.
   4. mitochondria.

10. A group of several different kinds of tissues arranged so that they can together perform a special function is called:
    1. cells.
    2. organ.
    3. tissue.
    4. system.

11. Groups of similar cells that work together to perform a specific function are called:
    1. cells.
    2. organ.
    3. tissue.
    4. system.

12. The hypogastric region of the abdominopelvic cavity is:
    1. inferior to the umbilical region.
    2. lateral to the left iliac region.
    3. medial to the right iliac region.
    4. both 1 and 3.

13. The two major cavities of the body are the:
    1. thoracic and abdominal.
    2. abdominal and pelvic.
    3. dorsal and ventral.
    4. anterior and posterior.

14. The structure that divides the thoracic cavity from the abdominal cavity is the:
    1. mediastinum.
    2. diaphragm.
    3. lungs.
    4. stomach.

Match the directional terms in Column B with its *opposite* term in Column A.

COLUMN A

15. _____ Superior

16. _____ Distal

17. _____ Anterior

18. _____ Lateral

19. _____ Deep

COLUMN B

a. posterior
b. superficial
c. medial
d. proximal
e. inferior

Match the function in Column B with the correct system in Column A.

COLUMN A

20. _____ Integumentary

21. _____ Skeletal

22. _____ Muscular

23. _____ Nervous

24. _____ Endocrine nutrients

25. _____ Cardiovascular

26. _____ Lymphatic

27. _____ Respiratory

28. _____ Digestive

29. _____ Urinary

30. _____ Reproductive

COLUMN B

a. Provides movement, body posture, and heat
b. Uses hormones to regulate body functions
c. Transports fatty nutrients from the digestive system to the blood
d. Physical and chemical change in nutrients and absorption of nutrients.
e. Cleans the blood of metabolic wastes and regulates electrolyte balance
f. Protection of underlying structures, sensory reception, and regulation of body temperature
g. The transport of substances from one part of the body to another
h. Ensures the survival of the species rather than the individual
i. Uses electrochemical signals to integrate and control body functions
j. Exchanges oxygen and carbon dioxide and regulates acid-base balance
k. Provides a rigid framework for the body and stores minerals

CHAPTER 2

Care of the Surgical Patient

ELAINE ODEN KOCKROW and BARBARA LAURITSEN CHRISTENSEN

Objectives

After reading this chapter, the student should be able to do the following:

1. Define the key terms as listed.
2. Identify the purposes of surgery.
3. Distinguish among elective, urgent, and emergency surgery.
4. Discuss the factors that influence an individual's ability to tolerate surgery.
5. Explain the procedure for turning, deep breathing, coughing, and leg exercises for postoperative patients.
6. Explain the importance of informed consent for surgery.
7. Discuss considerations for the older adult surgical patient.
8. Describe the role of the circulating nurse and the scrub nurse during surgery.
9. Discuss the preoperative checklist.
10. Discuss the initial nursing assessment and management immediately after transfer from the postanesthesia care unit.
11. Differentiate among general, regional, and local anesthesia.
12. Explain conscious sedation.
13. Identify the rationale for nursing interventions designed to prevent postoperative complications.
14. Discuss the nursing process as it pertains to the surgical patient.
15. Identify the information needed for the postoperative patient in preparation for discharge.

Key Terms

 Be sure to check out the bonus material on the free CD-ROM, including selected audio pronunciations.

ablation (ăb-LĀ-shŭn, p. 21)
anesthesia (ăn-ĕs-THĒ-zē-ă, p. 42)
atelectasis (ă-tĕ-LĔK-tă-sĭs, p. 54)
cachexia (kă-KĔK-sē-ă, p. 52)
catabolism (kă-TĂB-ō-lĭsm, p. 58)
conscious sedation (sĕ-DĀ-shŭn, p. 45)
dehiscence (dē-HĬS-ĕns, p. 52)
drainage (p. 50)
embolus (ĔM-bō-lŭs, p. 36)
evisceration (ĕ-vĭs-ĕr-Ā-shŭn, p. 52)
extubate (ĕks-TOO-bāt, p. 50)
exudate (ĔKS-ū-dāt, p. 50)

incentive spirometry (ĭn-SĔN-tĭv spĭ-RŌM-ĕ-trē, p. 31)
incisions (ĭn-SĬZH-ŭn, p. 39)
infarct (ĬN-făhrkt, p. 36)
informed consent (p. 28)
intraoperative (ĭn-tră-ŎP-ĕr-ă-tĭv, p. 21)
palliative (PĂL-ē-ă-tĭv, p. 21)
paralytic ileus (păr-ă-LĬT-ĭk ĬL-ē-ŭs, p. 57)
perioperative (pĕr-ē-ŎP-ĕr-ă-tĭv, p. 21)
postoperative (pōst-ŎP-ĕr-ă-tĭv, p. 21)
preoperative (prē-ŎP-ĕr-ă-tĭv, p. 21)
prosthesis (prŏs-THĒ-sĭs, p. 48)
singultus (SĬNG-gŭl-tŭs, p. 58)
surgery (p. 20)
surgical asepsis (ā-SĔP-sĭs, p. 49)
thrombus (THRŎM-bŭs, p. 36)

Surgery is defined as that branch of medicine concerned with diseases and trauma requiring operative procedures. Surgery became a medical specialty in the mid-nineteenth century. Surgery gave physicians the means to treat conditions that were difficult or impossible to manage only with medicine. However, early surgeons had little knowledge of the principles of asepsis, and anesthesia techniques were primitive and unsafe. Indeed, a surgeon's success was based on speed. However, the discovery of anesthesia in the 1840s made it possible for surgeons to operate on a patient who was free of pain. Nurses working in the first operating rooms cleaned the rooms and equipment, performed technical tasks such as obtaining supplies, and occasionally accompanied the patient to the surgical ward to deliver nursing care.

With the advent of antiseptic and later aseptic practices, surgery became a treatment of choice for many conditions. The development of safer anesthetic gases allowed surgeons to conduct longer operative procedures. All surgery was conducted in hospital settings.

Although modern-day suites have moved surgery from the Dark Ages, patients often view the surgical process as mysterious and frightening.

Surgery is classified as elective, urgent, or emergency. Elective surgery is not necessary to preserve life and may be performed when the patient chooses. Urgent surgery is required to keep additional health problems from occurring. Emergency surgery is performed immediately to save the individual's life or preserve the function of a body part. Although a surgical procedure may also be labeled as either major or minor surgery, all surgeries have an element of risk.

Surgery is performed for various purposes, which include diagnostic studies, ablation (an amputation or excision of any part of the body or removal of a growth or harmful substance), palliative (therapy designed to relieve or reduce intensity of uncomfortable symptoms without cure), reconstructive, transplant, and constructive (Table 2-1). See Table 2-2 for frequently used surgical terminology.

Traditionally, surgical procedures were performed in a hospital setting. With the discovery of new technologies and today's emphasis on decreasing health care costs, the surgical suite may now be in a variety of settings. Although each facility may use different terms for its surgery setting and process, there are common variations (Box 2-1).

PERIOPERATIVE NURSING

Perioperative nursing refers to the role of the nurse during the preoperative (before surgery), intraoperative (during surgery), and postoperative (following surgery) phases of a patient's surgical experience. The concept of perioperative nursing stresses the importance of providing continuity of care for the surgical patient using the nursing process. In many hospitals, perioperative nurses assess a patient's health status preoperatively, identify specific patient needs, teach and counsel, attend to the patient's needs in the operating room, and then follow the patient's recovery. However, in other institutions, different nurses care for the surgical patient during each phase of the surgical experience. Certain aspects of perioperative nursing care may be delegated to appropriate personnel (Box 2-2). The

Table 2-1 *Classification for Surgical Procedures*

TYPE	DESCRIPTION/EXAMPLES
ADMISSION STATUS	
Ambulatory (outpatient)	Patient enters setting, has surgical procedure, and is discharged on the same day (e.g., breast biopsy, cataract extraction, hemorrhoidectomy, scar revision)
Same-day admit	Patient enters hospital and undergoes surgery on the same day and remains for convalescence (e.g., carotid endarterectomy, cholecystectomy, mastectomy, vaginal hysterectomy)
Inpatient	Patient is admitted to hospital, undergoes surgery, and remains in hospital for convalescence (e.g., amputation, heart transplant, laryngectomy, resection of aortic aneurysm)
SERIOUSNESS	
Major	Involves extensive reconstruction or alteration in body parts; poses great risks to well-being (e.g., coronary artery bypass, colon resection, gastric resection)
Minor	Involves minimal alteration in body parts; often designed to correct deformities; involves minimal risks compared with those of major procedures (e.g., cataract extraction, skin graft, tooth extraction)
URGENCY	
Elective	Performed on basis of patient's choice (e.g., bunionectomy, plastic surgery)
Urgent	Necessary for patient's health (e.g., excision of cancerous tumor, removal of gallbladder for stones, vascular repair for obstructed artery [e.g., coronary artery bypass])
Emergency	Must be done immediately to save life or preserve function of body part (e.g., removal of perforated appendix, repair of traumatic amputation, control of internal hemorrhaging)
PURPOSE	
Diagnostic	Surgical exploration that allows physician to confirm diagnosis; may involve removal of tissue for further diagnostic testing (e.g., exploratory laparotomy [incision into peritoneal cavity to inspect abdominal organs] breast mass biopsy)
Ablation	Excision or removal of diseased body part (e.g., amputation, removal of appendix, cholecystectomy)
Palliative	Relieves or reduces intensity of disease symptoms; will not produce cure (e.g., colostomy, debridement of necrotic tissue)
Reconstructive	Restores function or appearance to traumatized or malfunctioning tissue (e.g., internal fixation of fractures, scar revision, breast reconstruction)
Transplant	Replaces malfunctioning organs (e.g., cornea, heart, joints, kidney)
Constructive	Restores function lost or reduced as result of congenital anomalies (e.g., repair of cleft palate, closure of atrial-septal defect in heart)

■

Box 2-1 **Common Variations of Surgical Settings**

- **Inpatient:** Patient hospitalized for surgery
- **One-day (same-day surgery):** Patient is admitted the day surgery is scheduled and dismissed the same day
- **Outpatient:** Patient, not hospitalized, who is being treated; individual is admitted either to a short-stay unit or directly to the surgical suite.
- **Short-stay surgical center ("surgicenter"):** Independently owned agency; surgery performed when overnight hospitalization is not required (also called ambulatory surgical center or one-day surgery center)
- **Short-stay unit:** Department or floor where a patient's stay does not exceed 24 hours (sometimes referred to as outpatient)

Table 2-2 **Surgical Terminology**

TERM	INTERPRETATION WITH EXAMPLE
Anastomosis	Surgical joining of two ducts or blood vessels to allow flow from one to another; to bypass an area (e.g., *Billroth I*, joins together stomach and duodenum)
-ectomy	Surgical removal of (e.g., *cholecystectomy*, removal of the gallbladder)
Lysis	Destruction or dissolution of (e.g., *lysis of adhesions*, removal of adhesions)
-orrhaphy	Surgical repair of (e.g., *herniorrhaphy*, repair of a hernia)
-oscopy	Direct visualization by a scope (e.g., *cystoscopy*, direct visualization of the urinary tract by means of a cystoscope)
-ostomy	Opening is made to allow the passage of drainage (e.g., *ileostomy*, formation of an opening of the ileum onto the surface of the abdomen for passage of feces)
-otomy	Opening into (e.g., *thoracotomy*, surgical opening into the thoracic cavity)
-pexy	Fixation of (e.g., *cecopexy*, fixation or suspension of the cecum to correct its excessive mobility)
-plasty	Plastic surgery (e.g., *mammoplasty*, reshaping of the breasts to reduce, lift, reconstruct)

Box 2-2 **Delegation Considerations in Perioperative Nursing**

- The skills of assessment that are part of preparing the patient for surgery require the critical thinking and knowledge application unique to a nurse. For these skills delegation is inappropriate. Assistive personnel (AP) may obtain vital signs and weight and height measurements. Instruct AP on proper precautions for these delegated procedures as needed.
- The skills of preoperative teaching require the critical thinking and knowledge application unique to a nurse. For this skill, delegation is inappropriate. AP can reinforce and assist patients in performing postoperative exercises.
  - Review with AP any precautions unique for a particular patient (e.g., turning method).
  - Be sure staff know when to inform the nurse if the patient is unable to perform the exercises correctly.
- Coordinating the patient's preparation for surgery requires the critical thinking and knowledge application unique to a nurse. However, AP may administer an enema or douche, obtain vital signs, apply antiembolic stockings, and assist patient in removing clothing, jewelry, and prostheses.
  - Instruct AP in proper precautions when preparing a patient for surgery.
  - Instruct AP in proper observations and precautions if the patient has an IV catheter in place.
- The skills of sterile gowning and gloving can be delegated to a surgical technologist or the nurse who has acquired the proper skills.
- The skill of initiating and managing postoperative care of the patient requires the critical thinking and knowledge application unique to a nurse. AP may obtain vital signs, apply nasal cannula or oxygen mask, and provide basic comfort and hygiene measures.

nurse's major responsibility is safe, consistent, and effective nursing interventions during each phase of surgery.

INFLUENCING FACTORS

Regardless of the surgical procedure scheduled, the process is a stressful experience for the patient. Observing a patient's mannerisms and listening to questions help identify the patient's feelings and concerns. Fear of the unknown can best be addressed by providing information and support; the nurse should assist patients to express their concerns so that support and reassurance can be offered.

Numerous factors affect the individual's ability to tolerate surgery.

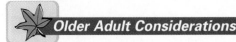

Older Adult Considerations

Undergoing Surgery

- Older adults undergoing surgery have higher morbidity and mortality rates than younger people.
- Surgery places a greater stress on older than on younger persons. The physiologic status of the older individual and coexisting conditions need to be carefully evaluated before surgery. Medical management is often preferred unless a condition is life threatening.
- Older patients tend to recover more slowly from surgery. Recovery can be affected by the level of mental functioning, individual coping ability, and the availability of support systems.
- Risks of aspiration, atelectasis, pneumonia, thrombus formation, infection, and altered tissue perfusion are increased in the older adult.
- Disorientation or toxic reactions can occur in the older adult after the administration of anesthetics, sedatives, or analgesics. These reactions are often present for days after administration of the medication.
- Preoperative and postoperative teaching may require extra time. Teaching should be given at the older person's level of understanding. Directions should be repeated and reinforced frequently.

Box 2-3 | ABCDE Mnemonic Device to Ascertain Serious Illness or Trauma in the Preoperative Patient

A Allergy to medications, chemicals, and other environmental products such as latex. All allergies are reported to anesthesia and surgical personnel before the beginning of surgery. If allergies exist, an allergy band must be placed on the patient's arm immediately.
B Bleeding tendencies or the use of medications that deter clotting, such as aspirin or products containing aspirin, heparin, or warfarin sodium. Herbal medications may also increase bleeding times or mask potential blood-related problems.
C Cortisone or steroid use.
D Diabetes mellitus, a condition that not only requires strict control of blood glucose levels but is also known to delay wound healing.
E Emboli; previous embolic events (such as lower leg blood clots) may recur because of prolonged immobility.
Patients whose immune systems are suppressed are at a much higher risk for development of postoperative infection and have a diminished capacity to fight that infection.

Age

The young and the old do not tolerate major surgical treatment as well as other age groups. Their altered metabolic needs may not respond to physiologic changes quickly. Of specific concern in these age groups is the body's response to temperature changes, cardiovascular shifts, respiratory needs, and renal function. To assist patients to return to their maximal level of health, nursing assessments and appropriate interventions should be ongoing (Older Adult Considerations box).

Physical Condition

Healthy patients have smoother and faster recovery periods than patients who have coexisting health problems. The nurse assesses each body system to identify actual and potential problems. Once problems are identified, the nurse selects measures to decrease potential postsurgical complications (Box 2-3).

Nutritional Factors

The body uses carbohydrates, proteins, and fats to supply energy-producing glucose to its cells. Whereas carbohydrates and fats are the primary energy producers, protein is essential to build and repair body tissue. During stressful conditions the body's need for energy and repair increases. Nutritional needs vary with a patient's age and physical requirements; patients who maintain a sound, nutritional diet tend to recover more quickly.

A completed diet history identifies the patient's usual eating habits and nutritional patterns. Because dietary practices are influenced by a patient's ethnic, cultural, religious, and socioeconomic background, the history highlights food preferences and dislikes. With this information, foods high in energy-producing nutrients can be offered. Because surgery may decrease a patient's appetite and alter metabolic functions, the nurse observes the patient for signs of malnutrition. If malnutrition is promptly identified, tube feedings, intravenous (IV) therapy, or parenteral hyperalimentation can be initiated (see Chapter 21, *Foundations of Nursing*).

PSYCHOSOCIAL NEEDS

As patients and families plan for surgery, they frequently express concern about possible outcomes. Although improved health is the ultimate goal, fears may not be easily identified or understood (Box 2-4).

SOCIOECONOMIC AND CULTURAL NEEDS

Because the United States is a nation of diverse individuals, patients are from different social, economic, religious, ethnic, and cultural origins. Even geographic location affects the way an individual responds. Therefore it is important to allow patients and families to express themselves openly.

Patients from different cultures (see Chapter 7, *Foundations of Nursing*) may react to the preoperative experience in different ways. Nursing from a multicultural perspective assists nurses to have a frame of reference in approaching patients with respect and to

Box 2-4 | *Common Fears Associated with Surgery*

- **Fear of loss of control** is associated primarily with anesthesia. The patient becomes almost totally dependent on the health care team during the surgical experience—even for most basic needs such as breathing and life support—while under the influence of anesthesia.
- **Fear of the unknown** may result from uncertainty about the surgical outcome or may stem from a lack of knowledge regarding the surgical experience.
- **Fear of anesthesia** may include fears of unpleasant induction of or emergence from anesthesia. The patient may fear waking up during the operation and feeling pain while under the effects of anesthetic. This fear is often related to loss of control and fear of the unknown.
- **Fear of pain or inadequate postoperative analgesia.** Reassure the patient and significant others that the pain will be controlled.
- **Fear of death** constitutes a legitimate fear. Even with the great strides in surgery and anesthesia, no anesthetic or operation is perfectly safe for all patients.
- **Fear of separation from the usual support group.** The patient is separated from spouse, family, or significant others, as well as other support groups, and is cared for by strangers during much of this highly stressful period.
- **Fear of disruption of life patterns.** Surgery and recovery interfere in varying degrees with activities of daily living and social activities, as well as with work and professional activities.
- **Fear of change in body image and mutilation.** Surgery disrupts body integrity and threatens body image.
- **Fear of detection of cancer** is a concern that produces a high anxiety level.

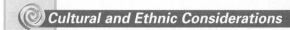

Cultural and Ethnic Considerations

The Surgical Patient

- Use of the patient's language helps to place an anxious patient at ease. The nurse should use an interpreter when possible, learn some key phrases in foreign languages, and use references such as medical dictionaries, which usually have key phrases listed in an appendix.
- Because eye contact may be avoided and considered disrespectful by some Southeast Asians and American Indians, the nurse may decide to limit it.
- Chinese-Americans may not ask for pain medication and may need teaching to help explain how comfort and relief from pain promote healing and a quicker recovery.
- American Indians are often stoic when ill. Complaints of pain to the nurse may be in general terms such as, "I am uncomfortable." Undertreatment of pain is common. May have a basic lack of trust.
- Among Arab-Americans, verbal consent often has more meaning than written consent because it is based on trust. Must explain fully the need for written consent. Very expressive regarding pain; pain may cause intense fear. Prepare the patient for painful procedures and develop a plan of care to prevent pain from occurring.
- African-Americans may be open to expression of pain but may avoid medication because of fear of addiction. If terminal diagnosis, news is best expressed through a family care conference or by speaking with the patient's religious representative.
- If the patient is Vietnamese-American, having an interpreter, often a hired one, is very important, depending on the sensitivity of the subject under discussion, because of modesty. A female family member is expected to be at bedside to provide care and comfort. Men are the decision makers and support for the family; therefore, speaking with the male head of the family may be necessary.

individually tailor care that promotes recovery (Cultural and Ethnic Considerations box).

MEDICATIONS
Review of the patient's current medication regimen is essential. Polypharmacy (concurrent use of multiple medications) occurs in all age groups but is more common with older adults. Studies have shown that patients age 65 and older use an average of two to six prescribed medications and one to three over-the-counter (OTC) medications on a regular basis. The use of multiple medications predisposes patients to adverse drug reactions and interactions with other medications in the perioperative setting.

A number of pharmacologic categories are used routinely during the patient's surgical experience. These include anesthesia agents, antimicrobials, anticoagulants, hemostatic agents, oxytocics, steroids, diagnostic imaging dyes, diuretics, central nervous system agents, and emergency protocol medications. It has been reported that a seriously ill patient may receive as many as 20 medications in a perioperative setting at one time. Large numbers of medications increase the chance of interactions.

It is also common for patients to use herbal remedies as alternative or complementary medicines. Ask patients about their use of herbal remedies, either as dietary supplements or as medicines. Unless specifically asked, some patients may not consider their natural remedies as medicines. Even though herbs are natural products, they act like medications and may interact or potentiate other medications or interfere with surgical procedures (Table 2-3).

Some medications may be canceled when a patient goes to surgery. However, it is important to know the purposes and actions of drugs because specific

Table 2-3 *Preoperative Considerations for Commonly Ingested Herbs*

HERB	COMMON USES	PREOPERATIVE CONSIDERATIONS
Feverfew	Migraine prevention	Has anticoagulation factors Preoperative assessment should include clotting studies Discontinue before surgery
Ginger	Motion sickness Cough Menstrual cramps Intestinal gas	Risk of prolonged clotting times Preoperative assessment should include clotting studies Discontinue before surgery
St. John's wort	Antidepressant Antiviral properties Antiinflammatory action	Should not be used with other psychoactive drugs, mono-amine oxidase inhibitors, or serotonin reuptake inhibitors Discontinue before surgery because of possible drug interactions
Valerian root	Sedative or tranquilizer effect Sleep aid	Should not be used with sedatives or anxiolytics May increase effects of central nervous system depressants

medications may be given to patients with diseases such as diabetes. The anesthesiologist, in collaboration with the patient's physician and surgeon, will determine whether these medications should be taken the day of surgery and whether they should be taken postoperatively.

Remember to assess for allergies to drugs that may be given during any phase of the surgical experience. Ask patients to tell you what exactly happened when they took a drug reported as an allergen. It is also important to enquire about nondrug allergies, including allergies to foods, chemicals, pollen, antiseptics used to prepare the skin for surgery, and latex rubber products. The patient with a history of allergic responsiveness has a greater potential for demonstrating hypersensitivity reactions to anesthesia agents. Many facilities require that the patient receive an allergy identification band to be worn before going to surgery. Flag the front of the patient's chart to alert all health care providers to the patient's allergy status.

EDUCATION AND EXPERIENCE

As individuals age, life experiences influence problem-solving abilities and coping methods. Tailoring information to a patient's educational level permits fear to be replaced with accurate knowledge. The nurse can encourage patients to repeat or summarize what has been presented. This process validates not only what the patient heard, but also how the information was interpreted.

There is evidence that a relationship exists between preoperative fear and postoperative behavior. The preoperative anxiety level has been shown to influence the amount of anesthesia required, the amount of postoperative pain medication needed, and the speed of recovery from surgery.

The nurse must determine each patient's perceptions, emotions, behavior, and support systems that

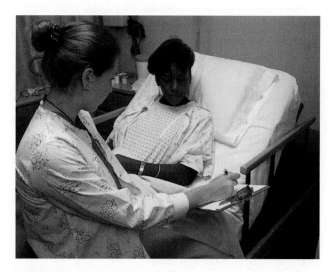

FIGURE **2-1** Often, knowledge deficits occur when the patient is undergoing her first surgical experience.

may help or interfere with the ability to progress through the surgical period. The unhurried and understanding nurse who actively listens to the patient, the family, and significant others invites confidence and helps to promote reduction of anxiety levels (Figure 2-1).

While the patient attempts to understand the approaching surgery, family members and support people are also trying to cope. Families may have additional burdens: financial obligations, living changes, and added personal responsibilities. The patient often expresses a feeling of helplessness. In addition to nursing and medical personnel, support can be provided to patients and their families by ministerial staff, social workers, or patient advocates during this stressful time (Patient Teaching: Preoperative Care box).

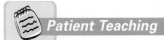

Patient Teaching

Preoperative Care

Examples of helpful information for preoperative patients and families:

- Preoperative tests, reason, preparation
- Preoperative routines, sequence of events
- Special equipment needed
- Transfer to operating room (time, checking procedures)
- Recovery room
  Place where patient will awaken
  Frequent monitoring of vital signs
  Return to room when vital signs are stable
- Probable postoperative therapies
  Need for increased mobility as soon as possible
  Need to keep respiratory passages clear
- Anticipated treatments (e.g., IV, dressing changes, incentive spirometry)
- Pain medication routines (timing sequence, "as needed" [prn] status), other modalities of management such as patient-controlled analgesia (PCA) and epidural analgesia

PREOPERATIVE PHASE

A thorough health assessment is needed before surgery. Acute or chronic diseases hinder the body's ability to repair itself or adjust to surgical treatment. Disorders of the systems identified in Table 2-4 present high-risk conditions for surgery. Each system is further affected by the patient's age, health condition, nutritional status, and mental state.

Assessment questions to ascertain the patient's use of chemicals, alcohol, and abusive substances assist the health team to select medications tolerated by the body. Postoperative care is also adjusted to compensate, when possible, for potential complications. If the patient has been a smoker, alveoli may be impaired and the patient's lung capacity reduced. Mucus and anesthesia by-products may be trapped in the lung, causing atelectasis and pneumonia. Breathing exercises and treatments for the smoker postoperatively aid in lung expansion and decrease the risk of respiratory complications.

Additional preoperative questions identify the patient's allergies, past surgeries, and infection and disease history. When questioning the patient about medication practices, the nurse asks the patient to name prescription drugs currently taken, as well as over-the-counter drugs and home remedies used. The nurse also records the patient's vital signs, height, and weight before surgery to have a baseline for postoperative comparison.

PREOPERATIVE TEACHING

Patient teaching before surgery helps decrease the stress that patients feel. Because fear of the unknown is a primary stressor of preoperative patients, providing information decreases the stress associated with not knowing. Preoperative information helps (1) lessen anxiety, (2) reduce the amount of anesthesia needed, (3) decrease postsurgical pain, and (4) reduce corticosteroid production. By decreasing postsurgical complications through preoperative teaching, wound healing occurs more rapidly.

In providing preoperative teaching, the nurse should include the patient and family and remember that basic terminology and information are easier to understand than complex explanations. The nurse should frequently stop to verify the patient's understanding of information shared, ask questions, and encourage responses. Questions that can be answered "yes" or "no" should be avoided. "Do you have any questions?" is not as clarifying as, "What questions do you have?" If printed materials or videotapes are routinely used in preoperative teaching sessions, it is important to document what the patient read, heard, or saw. Older adults may have difficulty reading small print or hearing taped messages. If the patient does not understand English, an interpreter may be needed to explain information presented. The nurse should also emphasize that a nurse will be with the patient throughout the entire surgical experience.

If the surgical procedure to be performed has potential long-term effects, support groups may be contacted to offer support preoperatively. Cancer organizations, amputation support group, and enterostomal therapist associations are examples of large national organizations that offer peer support for surgical and nonsurgical patients.

Ideally, preoperative teaching is provided 1 or 2 days before surgery, when anxiety is not as high. In some instances the patient may not be admitted to the hospital until early in the morning on the day of surgery. Although preoperative preparation varies, most institutions have an established teaching program. Preoperative teaching is begun by clarifying the sequence of preoperative and postoperative events. Generally, the nurse should instruct the patient about the surgical procedure, informed consent, the method of skin preparation, and gastrointestinal cleanser to be used. In general, the nurse clarifies what the physician has explained. The nurse reviews the time of the surgery and information about the recovery area. Although most patients return to their previously assigned units after surgery, a few may be transferred to an intensive care area, specialty unit, or outpatient area. If a transfer will occur, it is helpful to take the patient and family on a tour of the new unit. The nurse reinforces that vital signs, dressings, and tubes are assessed every 15 to 30 minutes until the patient is

Table 2-4 *Surgical Effects on Body Systems*

DISEASE/DISORDER	SURGICAL EFFECTS
CARDIOVASCULAR (Chapter 8)	
Recent myocardial infarction, dysrhythmias, and heart failure Hypertension	Hypotension and cardiac dysrhythmias are the most common cardiovascular complications of the surgical patient, and early recognition and management of these complications before they become serious enough to diminish cardiac output depend on frequent assessment of the patient's vital signs.
ENDOCRINE (Chapter 11)	
Liver disease	Liver disease alters metabolism and elimination of drugs administered during surgery and impairs wound healing because of alterations in protein metabolism.
Diabetes mellitus	Diabetes increases susceptibility to infection and may impair wound healing from altered glucose metabolism and associated circulatory impairment. Fluctuating blood levels may cause central nervous system malfunction during anesthesia.
GASTROINTESTINAL (Chapter 5)	
Hiatal hernia Ulcers	Preoperative and postoperative medication may be necessary to control gastric acidity.
Esophageal varices	Risk of hemorrhage may increase due to risk of initiating hemorrhage with intubation.
IMMUNE (Chapter 15)	
AIDS Allergies Immune deficiency	Disease slows the body's ability to fight infection. Immunologic disorders increase risk of infection and delay wound healing after surgery.
NEUROLOGICAL (Chapter 14)	
Seizures	Patients need a check of the therapeutic levels of their medications.
Myasthenia gravis	Exclusion of the use of muscle relaxants may be warranted due to decreased ability to reverse their effects.
Cerebral vascular accident	Impaired verbal communication, defective perception of the body, paralysis, and visual disturbances place patient at high risk for injury.
RESPIRATORY (Chapter 9)	
Tumors	Lung motility is decreased and gas exchange slowed.
Chronic obstructive pulmonary disease Emphysema Asthma	Anesthetic agents reduce respiratory function, increasing risk for severe hypoventilation.
URINARY (Chapter 10)	
Renal failure Tumors	Impaired kidney function decreases excretion of anesthesia and alters acid-base balance.

awake and stable. A checklist frequently is used to provide a systematic preoperative teaching plan.

PREOPERATIVE PREPARATION

Preparation for surgery depends on the patient's age, physical and nutritional status, type of surgery, and the preference of the surgeon. When the surgery is performed in a short-stay or ambulatory setting, the workup normally occurs a few days in advance. If the patient is admitted to the hospital, testing may be conducted to assess for potential problems. If the presenting problem has been diagnosed, preparation frequently includes both in-

hospital testing and evaluation of test results previously completed in the physician's office.

Laboratory Tests and Diagnostic Imaging

Testing before surgery depends on the institution's policies, physician's directives, and condition of the patient. The nurse follows standing orders to complete this overall process. Laboratory tests commonly reviewed before surgery include a urinalysis; complete blood count; and blood chemistry profile to assess endocrine, hepatic, renal, and cardiovascular functions. Serum electrolytes are evaluated if extensive surgery is planned or the patient has extenuating problems. One of the essential electrolytes examined is potassium; if potassium is not available in adequate amounts, dysrhythmias can occur during anesthesia and the patient's postoperative recovery may be slowed by general muscle weakness. A chest roentgenogram evaluation and electrocardiogram are used to identify disease processes or previous respiratory or cardiac damage. Additional tests are conducted to assess the organ being evaluated. Blood chemistry profile (LDH, gamma GT, alkaline phosphatase, total bilirubin) and urine bilirubin levels verify the hepatic functioning ability.

Informed Consent

The Patient's Bill of Rights affirms that patients must give informed consent (permission obtained from the patient to perform a specific test or procedure) before the beginning of any procedure. In signing the consent form, the patient is competent and agrees to have the procedure that is stated on the form. Information is to be clear, the risks explained, expected benefits identified, and consequences or alternatives for the presenting problem stated. Witnesses are required to meet the legal requirements of the state. A witness is only verifying that this is the person who signed the consent and that it was a voluntary consent. The witness (often a nurse) is not verifying that the patient understands the procedure. Ideally, the surgeon discusses the surgical procedure with the patient in advance. In some institutions the surgical consent is completed in the physician's office or in the admissions department before the patient is admitted to the unit. Informal consent should not be obtained if the patient is disoriented, unconscious, mentally incompetent, or, in some agencies, under the influence of sedatives. Know agency policy (see Figure 2-1 in *Foundations of Nursing*).

If the patient does not see or hear well, the nurse should allow additional time to explain the surgery. For individuals who do not understand English or persons who are deaf, an interpreter may be necessary. The patient should never be coerced into signing a consent that is not understood or that contains information that differs from what was originally explained. If necessary, the nurse should contact the physician and indicate that the patient does not understand the procedure.

In an emergency the patient may not be able to give consent for surgery. Every effort is made to locate family members to assume this responsibility. Occasionally telephone permission may be obtained. In cases in which verbal consent is received, the hospital will have standard guidelines. If the patient's life is in danger and family members cannot be located, the surgeon may legally perform surgery. In cases in which family members object to surgery that the physician believes is essential, a court order may be obtained for

the procedure. This practice is used very carefully, for example, when a child's life is in danger. Know agency policy.

Gastrointestinal Preparation

At midnight before surgery, the patient is usually placed on nothing by mouth status (NPO); this keeps the gastrointestinal (GI) tract empty when the patient is anesthetized, thereby decreasing the chance of vomiting or aspiration of emesis after surgery. An NPO sign is posted over the patient's bed, and all fluids are removed from the room. The nurse should reinforce with both the patient and family the importance of not ingesting foods or fluids. If the patient fails to comply with the NPO order, the physician is notified.

Patients can have oral care while NPO. The nurse should caution the patient not to swallow fluids used during oral care. A wet cloth on the lips helps relieve dryness. If patients need to be hydrated or if special IV medications are needed, parenteral fluids or medication may be ordered. Depending on the nature of the surgery, many patients postoperatively resume foods and fluids the day of their surgeries.

Because anesthesia relaxes the bowel, a bowel cleanser may be ordered to evacuate fecal material and lessen postoperative GI problems (nausea and vomiting). Frequently used bowel cleansers are the cleansing enema or a general laxative. A GI lavage solution, GoLYTELY (an isosmotic solution), rapidly evacuates the bowel. GoLYTELY is contraindicated, however, in patients with GI obstruction, gastric retention, bowel perforation, toxic colitis, or megacolon. If a bowel preparation is used, the nurse charts the type of preparation used, the patient's tolerance to the procedure, and results. Before bowel surgery, medication (neomycin, sulfonamides, erythromycin) may be given over a period of days to detoxify and sterilize the GI tract. This lessens the chance of fecal contamination during surgery.

Skin Preparation

Preoperatively the patient may have removal of hair at the surgical site and then shower, unless contraindicated, using an antiseptic soap such as Hibiclens. Assess for allergies. There is debate about the best method to remove hair. A lower rate of infection occurs with either no shave or a hair clip than with any other method. Use of a depilatory (a substance or procedure that removes hair) agent has also proved to have a low wound infection rate. If shaving is used, it should be performed close to the actual time of the surgical procedure.

Some surgical departments prepare the patient either in a surgical holding room or in the operating room itself. This is done because the increased time for growth of bacteria has been found to raise the potential for infection. Each agency or facility should have policies and protocols regarding the timing, method, and people responsible for the preoperative skin preparation of surgical patients.

Hospital policies differ regarding the description of skin areas to be prepped. Review agency policy to determine the area to be shaved (Figure 2-2). The surgeon may give specific orders concerning the area to be prepared.

Before the skin preparation the nurse must carefully assess the surgical site for skin impairment (e.g., infection, irritation, bruises, or lesions). Anything unusual should be recorded and reported to the surgeon.

Surgical shaving of the operative site must be completed with utmost care. The nurse must maintain skin integrity. The goal is to remove the hair without causing injury to the skin (Skill 2-1).

In the operating room the nurse scrubs the skin thoroughly with a detergent solution and then ap-plies an antiseptic solution to kill more adherent and deeper-residing bacteria. The surgeon may place a special transparent sterile drape directly over the skin before making an incision.

Special concerns for patients undergoing a surgical skin preparation are as follows:

- Small children may be easily frightened by this procedure, and it may need to be done in the operating room.
- Older adults will need a detailed explanation to relieve their anxiety.
- Older adults have less subcutaneous tissue, less skin elasticity, and more delicate skin tissue. Extreme care needs to be taken when shaving the older adult.
- Older adults are usually more susceptible to infections.

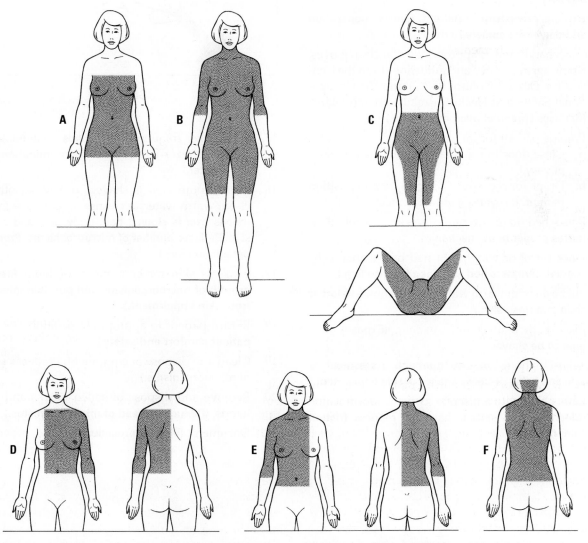

FIGURE **2-2** Skin preparation for surgery on various body areas. The shaded area indicates the area that should be shaved. **A,** Abdominal surgery. **B,** Open heart surgery. **C,** Perineal surgery. **D,** Chest or thoracic surgery. **E,** Breast surgery. **F,** Cervical spine surgery.

Skill 2-1 — Performing a Surgical Skin Preparation

■ Nursing Action (Rationale)

1. Refer to medical record, care plan, or Kardex for special interventions. **(Provides basis for care.)**

2. Obtain equipment. **(Organizes procedure.)**
   a. Appropriate light
   b. OR prep kit
      - Basin
      - Razor
      - Sponge with soap
      - Waterproof pad
      - Cotton-tipped applicators
   c. Clean gloves

3. Introduce self. **(Decreases patient's anxiety.)**

4. Identify patient. **(Identifies correct patient for procedure.)**

5. Explain procedure to patient. **(Seeks cooperation and decreases anxiety.)**

6. Wash hands and, if appropriate, don clean gloves. Know agency policy and guidelines from the Centers for Disease Control (CDC) and the Occupational Safety and Health Administration (OSHA). **(Reduces spread of microorganisms.)**

7. Prepare patient for intervention:
   a. Close door to room or pull curtain. **(Provides privacy.)**
   b. Drape for procedure if necessary and position patient. **(Provides good body mechanics.)**

8. Raise bed to comfortable working level. **(Promotes proper body mechanics.)**

9. Place towel or waterproof pad under area to be shaved. **(Protects bed and linen from soiling.)**

10. Fill basin with warm water. **(Allows nurse to lather soap and rinse skin.)**

11. Place bath blanket over patient. **(Exposes only area to be shaved.)**

12. Adjust lighting. **(Allows thorough assessment of skin and helps decrease chance of skin impairment.)**

13. Lather skin with antiseptic soap and warm water. **(Cleanses skin, softens hair, and reduces friction from razor.)**

14. Hold razor at a 30- to 45-degree angle to skin. **(Minimizes chances of cutting or nicking skin.)**
    a. Shave small areas while holding skin taut.
    b. Use short, smooth strokes. **(Prevents pulling skin.)**
    c. Shave hair in same direction it grows (see illustration). **(Removes hair close to skin surface.)**

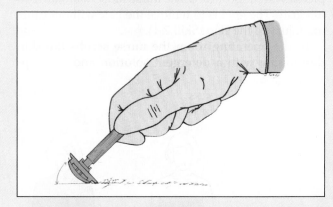

Step **14**

15. Rinse razor frequently. **(Removes accumulation of hair from razor and prevents contamination from dirty water.)**

16. When entire area is shaved, use washcloth and clean, warm water to cleanse area. Dry skin. **(Removes excess shaved hair, body oils, and soil on skin. Reduces number of microorganisms. Promotes patient comfort.)**

17. Reassess skin for cuts, nicks, or hair. **(Prevents growth of microorganisms and possible infections from skin impairment.)**

18. Return patient to appropriate position. **(Provides patient comfort and safety.)**

19. Clean and dispose of equipment. **(Reduces spread of microorganisms.)**

20. Remove and dispose of soiled gloves and wash hands. **(Reduces spread of microorganisms.)**

21. Document. **(Verifies procedure.)**

Latex Allergy Considerations

Focused assessment of risk factors will help you identify patients who need the nursing diagnosis of risk for latex allergy response. In assessing the patient's experience, identify those at risk for a systemic reaction; for example, patients may relate stories of complicated anesthesia events, hives from blowing up a balloon, or severe swelling of the labia with a urinary catheterization.

With the advent of universal precautions (now called standards precautions) in the late 1980s, the use of latex gloves dramatically increased, and latex allergies became much more common. Basically, every health care worker wears gloves. Most gloves are powdered to facilitate donning. The powder absorbs protein allergens from latex gloves and deposits them on skin and into surgical wounds; it also aerosolizes the protein allergens. Aerosolized latex allergens are carried in ventilation systems, causing need for further prevention measures.

Latex allergy is classified into three categories: irritant reaction and types IV and I allergic reactions. The irritant reaction, which is most commonly seen, is actually a nonallergic reaction. The type IV allergic reaction to latex is a cell-mediated response to the chemical irritants found in latex products. The true latex allergy is the type I allergic reaction, and it occurs shortly after exposure to the proteins in latex rubber. The type I reaction is an IgE-mediated systemic reaction that occurs when latex proteins are touched, inhaled, or ingested.

Factors influencing the diagnosis of risk for latex allergy response are the person's susceptibility and the route, duration, and frequency of latex exposure. Risk factors for latex allergy response include the following:

- History of anaphylactic reaction of unknown etiology during a medical or surgical procedure
- Multiple surgical procedures (especially from infancy)
- Food allergies (specifically kiwi, bananas, avocados, chestnuts)
- A job with daily exposure to latex (medical, nursing, food handlers, tire manufacturers)
- History of reactions to latex (balloons, condoms, gloves)
- Allergy to poinsettia plants
- History of allergies and asthma

To provide a latex-safe environment for susceptible patients, all surgical patients should be screened for the risk for latex allergy response before admission. Identification of patients at risk is the initial step in providing prevention.

When a patient with a suspected or known latex allergy is scheduled for surgery, all potential risk areas (latex use) are avoided and the patient is admitted directly to the OR as the first case of the day if possible. Many facilities have converted isolation rooms into latex-safe environments for care of the perioperative patient with latex allergy. Ensure that everyone on the health care team is aware that a patient is, or may be, latex allergic. Place a medical alert band or allergy

Box 2-5   *Responding to a Patient's Risk for Latex Allergy*

LATEX-ALERT PATIENT (HIGH RISK FOR ALLERGIC RESPONSE)
- No required premedications
- No special pharmaceutical protocols required
- Use nonlatex gloves
- Use latex-safe supplies
- Keep a latex-safe supply cart available in patient's area

LATEX-ALLERGY PATIENT (SUSPECTED OR KNOWN ALLERGIC RESPONSE)
- Administer prophylactic treatment with steroids and antihistamines preoperatively
- Prepare a latex-safe environment, include latex-safe supply cart and crash cart
- Apply cloth barrier to patient's arm under a blood pressure cuff
- Use medications from glass ampules
- Do not puncture rubber stoppers with needles
- Wear synthetic gloves
- Use latex-free syringes
- Use latex-safe (polyvinyl chloride) IV tubing
- Do not use latex preparation on IV bags

band around the patient's wrist and clearly flag the chart about the latex reaction status. Remove all natural rubber latex products from a known or suspected latex-allergic patient's care area. Use latex-free pharmaceutical measures to prepare the patient's medication. Have a crash cart standing by stocked with latex-free equipment, supplies, and drugs for treating anaphylaxis. As ordered, give prophylactic treatment with glucocorticoid steroids and antihistamines to latex-allergic patients preoperatively. Box 2-5 lists interventions for the perioperative care of patients with *risk for latex allergy response.*

Respiratory Preparation

If a general anesthetic is administered, ventilating the lungs is vital postoperatively to prevent atelectasis and pneumonia. Because the lungs do not expand fully during surgery, mucus and gases remain in the lungs until expelled. Pulmonary exercises can assist in expanding the lungs and removing these by-products. Preoperative introduction to the use of the incentive spirometer is of great value to the patient.

Spirometry, referred to as incentive spirometry, is a procedure in which a device (spirometer) is used at the bedside at regular intervals to encourage the patient to breathe deeply (Skill 2-2). Inspired measurement can be seen and used to encourage the patient to attain the established goal.

The respiratory therapist will calculate the patient's maximum inspiratory capacity based on height, age, and sex, taking into consideration the type of surgery performed. At rest the usual tidal capacity is 500 mL of

Skill 2-2 | Incentive Spirometry/Positive Expiratory Pressure Therapy and "Huff" Coughing

■ Nursing Action (Rationale)

1. Refer to physician's orders, care plan, or Kardex. **(Health care facilities frequently require a medical order for incentive spirometry.)**

2. Assess patient's respiratory status and lung sounds. Indications for spirometry are (a) asymmetric chest wall movement, (b) increased respiratory rate, (c) increased production of sputum, and (d) diminished lung expansion postoperatively. **(Alerts health care personnel to those patients at risk for respiratory complications during illness or after surgery.)**

3. Explain procedure, and instruct patient in the correct use of the spirometer. Frequently this is accomplished by the respiratory therapist. However, it may be the nurse's responsibility to follow up and promote proper technique. **(Understanding will improve compliance with use.)**

4. Obtain supplies and equipment. **(Organizes procedure.)**
   a. Incentive spirometer/positive expiratory therapy (PEP) device
   b. Emesis basin
   c. Tissues
   d. Bedside trash bag
   e. Clean gloves (if soiling is likely)

5. Wash hands and don gloves (if soiling is likely). Know agency policy and guidelines from the CDC and OSHA. **(Reduces spread of microorganisms.)**

6. Place prescribed incentive spirometer at the bedside. **(Prepares equipment for procedure.)**

7. Place patient in semi-Fowler's or full Fowler's position. **(Promotes optimal lung expansion.)**

8. Place tissues, emesis basin, and bedside trash bag within easy reach. **(Enables sanitary disposal of respiratory secretions that may be expectorated during procedure.)**

9. Incentive spirometry
   a. Instruct patient to completely cover mouthpiece with lips (use a nose clip if patient is unable to breathe through the mouthpiece) and to (a) inhale slowly until maximum inspiration is reached, (b) hold breath 2 or 3 seconds, and (c) slowly exhale (see illustration). **(Promotes maximum inspiration.)**
   b. Instruct patient to relax and breathe normally for a short time. **(Prevents patient from hyperventilating and provides a resting period to prevent fatigue.)**

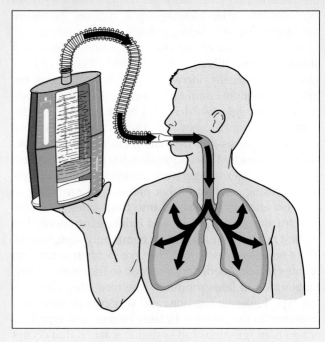

Step **9a**

   c. Instruct and encourage the patient to gradually increase depth of inspiration. **(Promotes maximum lung expansion.)**
   d. Offer oral hygiene after spirometry is completed. **(Patients often find this very refreshing.)**
   e. Store spirometer in an appropriate place, such as the bedside table, until next scheduled time. **(Provides a convenient place for repeated use.)**

10. Positive expiratory pressure therapy and "huff" coughing
   a. Wash hands. **(Reduces transmission of microorganisms.)**
   b. Set PEP device for setting ordered. **(The higher the setting, the more effort will be required by the patient.)**
   c. Instruct the patient to assume semi-Fowler's or high Fowler's position, and place noseclip on patient's nose (see illustration). **(Promotes optimum lung expansion and expectoration of mucus.)**
   d. Have patient place lips around mouthpiece. Patient should take a full breath and then exhale two or three times longer than inhalation. Pattern should be repeated for 10 to 20 breaths. **(Ensures that all breathing is done through mouth and that the device is used properly.)**

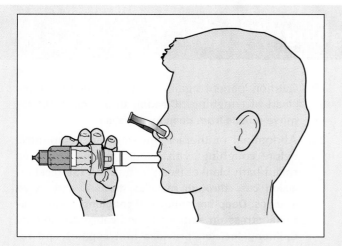

Step **10c**

e. Remove device from mouth, and have patient take a slow, deep breath and hold for 3 seconds. **(Promotes lung expansion before coughing.)**

f. Instruct patient to exhale in quick, short, forced "huffs." **("Huff" coughing, or forced ex-**

piratory technique, promotes bronchial hygiene by increasing expectoration of secretions.)

11. Position patient as desired or as ordered. **(Helps maintain patient comfort and promote maximum chest expansion.)**

12. Place call light within easy reach. **(Maintains patient safety.)**

13. Remove and dispose of soiled gloves and wash hands. **(Reduces spread of microorganisms.)**

14. Assess respiratory status and evaluate patient's response to spirometry. **(Provides a basis for repeated use.)**

15. Document in nurse's notes: patient's respiratory status before and after incentive spirometry, type of spirometry, and any adverse effects from the procedure. **(Verifies patient care. Some agencies require such documentation for third-party reimbursements.)**

16. Do patient teaching (Patient Teaching: Incentive Spirometry).

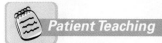
Patient Teaching

Incentive Spirometry

- After incentive spirometer exercises, patients should practice cough control techniques.
- Teach patient to examine sputum for consistency, amount, and color changes.
- Have patient return demonstration of correct procedure for use before discharge.
- Administer breathing treatments before patient's meals to prevent nausea and vomiting.

inspired air. In a tall, healthy young male, a tidal capacity of 4300 mL is not uncommon.

To encourage patient use, place the spirometer in the bed or close by on the bedside stand. The usual rate of use is 8 to 10 breaths hourly during waking hours.

There are four primary purposes for the use of the incentive spirometer:

- To prevent or treat atelectasis
- To improve lung expansion
- To improve oxygenation
- To prevent postoperative pneumonia

Incentive spirometry encourages patients to breathe in their normal inspiratory capacities. Because of postoperative pain, a postoperative inspiratory capacity of one half to three fourths of the preoperative volume is acceptable.

There are two general types of incentive spirometers:

1. **Flow-oriented inspiratory spirometer.** This type of incentive spirometer is inexpensive and mea-

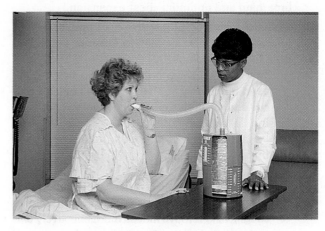

FIGURE **2-3** Volume-oriented spirometer.

sures inspiration but not volume. It contains one or more clear plastic cylinder chambers that contain freely movable, colored, lightweight plastic balls. The patient is instructed to place the mouthpiece in the mouth and inhale slowly and deeply, which raises the balls in the cylinders. The patient is encouraged to keep the colored balls floating as long as possible. The cylinders are marked to measure the degree of elevation so that the degree of elevation and the length of time the patient can maintain elevation can be recorded.

2. **Volume-oriented spirometer.** This form of incentive spirometer maintains a known volume of inspiration. The patient is encouraged to breathe with normal inspired capacity (Figure 2-3).

Skill 2-3 | Teaching Controlled Coughing

■ Nursing Action (Rationale)

1. Refer to medical record, care plan, or Kardex for special interventions. **(Provides basis for care.)**

2. Obtain equipment. **(Organizes procedure.)**
   a. Pillow or bath blanket
   b. Gloves
   c. Emesis basin
   d. Facial tissues
   e. Chair/bed

3. Introduce self. **(Decreases patient anxiety.)**

4. Identify patient. **(Ensures correct patient for procedure.)**

5. Explain procedure. **(Seeks cooperation.)**

6. Wash hands and don clean gloves according to agency policy and guidelines from the CDC and OSHA. **(Reduces spread of microorganisms.)**

7. Assist patient to upright position. Place pillow between bed or chair and patient. **(Facilitates deep breathing and optimum chest expansion.)**

8. Demonstrate coughing exercise for patient (see illustration). **(Allows patient to observe nurse and time to ask questions.)**
   a. Take several deep breaths. **(Deep breaths expand lungs fully so that air moves behind mucus and facilitates effect of coughing.)**
   b. Inhale through nose.
   c. Exhale through mouth with pursed lips.
   d. Inhale deeply again and hold breath for count of three.
   e. Cough two or three consecutive coughs without inhaling between coughs. **(Consecutive coughs help remove mucus more effectively and completely than one forceful cough.)**

9. Caution patient against just clearing throat instead of coughing. **(Clearing throat does not remove mucus from deep in airways.)**

10. Abdominal or thoracic incision can be splinted before coughing with hands, pillow, towel, or rolled bath blanket (see illustration). **(Surgical incision cuts through muscles, tissues, and nerve endings. Deep breathing and coughing place additional stress on suture line and cause discomfort. Splinting incision provides firm support and reduces incisional pulling.)**

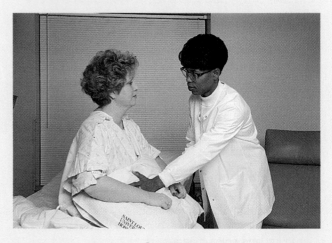

Step **10**

11. Encourage patient to practice coughing while splinting incisional area once or twice an hour during waking hours. Assist patient as indicated. **(Helps effectively expectorate mucus with minimal discomfort.)**

12. Remind patient to use tissues and emesis basin for any mucus expectorated. **(Reduces spread of microorganisms.)**

13. Teach patient to examine sputum for consistency, amount, and color change. **(Any change in sputum consistency, amount, and color could indicate respiratory complications such as pneumonia.)**

14. Provide wash cloth and warm water for washing hands and face, provide for oral hygiene, and return patient to comfortable position. **(Provides for patient comfort.)**

15. Remove and dispose of soiled gloves and wash hands. **(Reduces spread of microorganisms.)**

16. Document exercises performed and patient's ability to perform them independently. **(Verifies care given and patient teaching.)** (Patient Teaching: Controlled Coughing Technique).

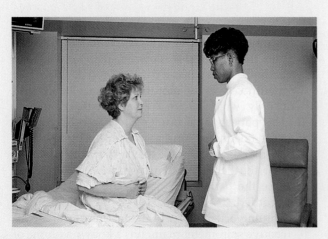

Step **8**

Before surgery the nurse should assist the patient to practice coughing (Skill 2-3), turning, and deep breathing (Skill 2-4). Because coughing increases intracranial pressure, it is usually contraindicated in cranial and spinal-related surgeries. Coughing is also contraindicated for patients having cataract surgery (Box 2-6). Some physicians believe coughing may actually cause alveolar collapse and order only incentive spirometry. Patients are frequently ambulated within a few hours of surgery to return cardiovascular and respiratory functions to normal more quickly.

Cardiovascular Considerations

Accompanying the need to turn, cough, and deep breathe is the need to practice leg exercises (see Skill 2-4). Because blood stasis occurs when the patient is lying flat, leg exercises should be encouraged to assist venous blood flow. With the venous

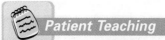
Patient Teaching

Controlled Coughing Technique

- For the patient entering the hospital for same-day surgery, teaching controlled coughing may need to be done in the physician's office, in the preoperative area, or postoperatively before the patient is discharged.
- The home health nurse may need to reinforce the importance of coughing one or two times an hour during waking hours for the patient at home.
- Young children or older adults may not fully understand the importance of controlled coughing, and continual reinforcement of teaching and assistance may be needed.
- Family members of a young child should be taught the procedure to assist the child. This will also help family members meet their needs by assisting in the care of the child.

Skill 2-4 | Teaching Postoperative Breathing Techniques, Turning, and Leg Exercises

■ Nursing Action (Rationale)

1. Refer to medical record, care plan, or Kardex for special interventions. **(Provides basis for care.)**

2. Obtain equipment. **(Helps organize procedure.)**
   a. Support pillow, towel, or folded bath blanket
   b. Gloves
   c. Emesis basin
   d. Facial tissues

3. Introduce self. **(Decreases patient anxiety.)**

4. Identify patient. **(Verifies correct patient for procedure.)**

5. Explain procedure to patient. **(Seeks cooperation and decreases anxiety.)**

6. Wash hands and don clean gloves. Know agency policy and guidelines from the CDC and OSHA. **(Reduces spread of microorganisms.)**

7. Prepare patient for intervention.
   a. Close door to room or pull curtain. **(Provides privacy.)**
   b. Drape for procedure if necessary.

8. Raise bed to comfortable working level. **(Promotes proper body mechanics.)**

9. Premedicate with pain medication, if indicated. **(Helps elicit patient compliance.)**

Postoperative Breathing Techniques

10. Place pillow between patient and bed or chair. **(Allows for fuller chest expansion. [Bed or chair itself is too firm to provide expansion.])**

11. Sit or stand facing patient. **(Allows patient to observe nurse.)**

12. Demonstrate taking slow, deep breaths. Avoid using shoulder and chest while inhaling. Inhale through nose. **(Prevents panting and hyperventilation. Moistens, filters, and warms inhaled air.)**

13. Hold breath for count of three and slowly exhale through pursed lips. **(Allows for gradual expulsion of air.)**

14. Repeat exercise 3 to 5 times. Have patient practice exercise. **(Allows patient to observe appropriate technique. Allows nurse to assess patient's technique and correct errors.)**

15. Instruct patient to take 10 slow, deep breaths every 2 hours until ambulatory. **(Helps prevent postoperative complications.)**

16. If there is an abdominal or chest incision, instruct patient to splint incisional area using pillow or bath blanket, if desired, during breathing exercises. **(Provides support and additional security for patient.)**

Leg Exercises

17. Lifting one leg at a time and supporting joints, gently flex and extend leg 5 to 10 times (see illustration). **(Stimulates circulation and helps prevent formation of thrombi.)**

18. Repeat exercise with opposite extremity. Lifting leg while supporting joints, gently flex leg 5 to 10 times. **(Stimulates circulation and helps prevent thrombi formation.)**

Continued

Skill 2-4 Teaching Postoperative Breathing Techniques, Turning, and Leg Exercises—cont'd

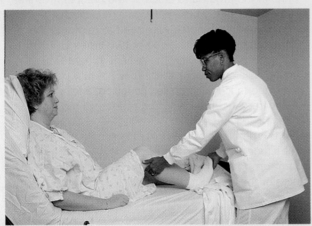

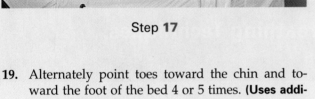

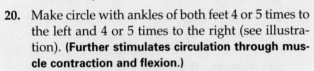

Step **17**

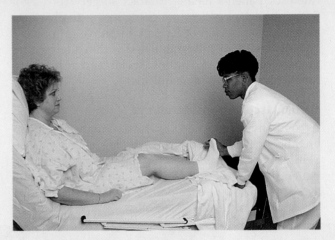

Step **20**

19. Alternately point toes toward the chin and toward the foot of the bed 4 or 5 times. **(Uses additional muscle flexion and contraction to stimulate circulation.)**

20. Make circle with ankles of both feet 4 or 5 times to the left and 4 or 5 times to the right (see illustration). **(Further stimulates circulation through muscle contraction and flexion.)**

21. Assess pulse, respiration, and blood pressure. **(Aids in determining complications from exercise.)**

Turning Exercises

22. Instruct patient to assume supine position to right side of bed. Side rails on both sides of bed should be in up position. **(Positioning begins on right side of bed so that turning to left side will not cause pa-**

tient to roll toward bed's edge. Side rails in the raised position promote patient safety.)

23. Instruct patient to place left hand over incisional area to splint it. **(Supports and minimizes pulling on suture line during turning.)**

24. Instruct patient to keep left leg straight and flex right knee up and over left leg. **(Straight leg stabilizes patient's position. Flexed right leg shifts weight for easier turning.)**

25. Instruct patient to turn every 2 hours while awake. **(Reduces risk of vascular and pulmonary complications.)**

26. Remove and dispose of soiled gloves and wash hands. **(Reduces spread of microorganisms.)**

27. Document. **(Records patient education and verifies procedure.)**

blood slowing, a thrombus (an accumulation of platelets, fibrin, clotting factors, and cellular elements of the blood attached to the anterior wall of a vessel, sometimes occluding the lumen of the vessel) may form. If a thrombus is dislodged, it can travel as an embolus to the lungs, heart, or brain, where the vessel can be occluded. Without an adequate blood supply, an infarct (localized area of necrosis) can occur. Antiembolism stockings (thromboembolic disease stockings [TEDS]), Jobst pump, or sequential compression devices (SCDs) with intermittent external pneumonic compression system may be ordered to provide support and to prevent venous thrombus in the lower extremities (Skill 2-5; Figures 2-4 and 2-5).

The following points should be considered when applying antiembolic stockings:
- Postoperative patients with abdominal or thoracic incisions will not be able to bend and pull on own stockings.
- Stockings may be difficult to fit and maintain in the obese patient and the very thin patient.
- Stockings may be difficult to apply for the elderly patient; the nurse or family members will assist the patient.

Vital Signs

Vital signs mirror the body's response to anesthesia and surgery. The nurse instructs the patient before surgery that it is normal for blood pressure, tempera-

Box 2-6 *Surgeries for Which Coughing Is Contraindicated or Modified*

1. **Intracranial.** Coughing increases intracranial pressure (ICP), leading to cerebral spinal fluid leak.
2. **Eye.** Coughing increases ICP, which then increases intraocular pressure, causing pressure on suture line.
3. **Ear.** Mouth must be kept open if coughing occurs to prevent pressure backup through eustachian tube to middle ear, causing pressure on suture line.
4. **Nose.** Mouth must be kept open if coughing occurs to prevent dislodgement of clot with subsequent bleeding.
5. **Throat.** Vigorous coughing may dislodge a clot with subsequent bleeding.
6. **Spinal.** Coughing increases spinal canal pressure.

ture, pulse, and respiration to be monitored until stable. The schedule for monitoring vital signs depends on the protocol of the hospital and the stability of the patient. Preoperative vital signs serve as the baseline for deciding when stability has returned or problems arise. Postoperative vital signs are discussed later in this chapter.

Genitourinary Considerations

After general anesthesia, the urinary bladder's tone is decreased. Therefore the nurse should know the patient's normal bladder habits and identify when the bladder is full and distended. The nurse informs the patient preoperatively that the lower part of the abdomen will be palpated at intervals to check for bladder fullness (Figure 2-6). Once patients are awake and tolerating fluids, the nurse should encourage an adequate intake. Occasionally a urinary catheter is in-

---

Skill 2-5 Applying Thromboemolic Deterrent Stockings (TEDS)/ Sequential Compression Devices (SCDs)

■ Nursing Action (Rationale)

1. Refer to medical record, care plan, or Kardex for special interventions. **(Provides basis for care.)**

2. Obtain equipment. **(Organizes procedure.)**
   a. TEDS or SCDs
   b. Clean gloves (when appropriate)
   c. Tape measure

3. Introduce self. **(Decreases patient's anxiety.)**

4. Identify patient. **(Identifies correct patient for procedure.)**

5. Explain procedure. **(Seeks cooperation and decreases anxiety.)**

6. Wash hands and, if appropriate, don clean gloves. Know agency policy and guidelines from the CDC and OSHA. **(Reduces spread of microorganisms.)**

7. Prepare patient.
   a. Close door to room, pull curtain, and drape for procedure, if necessary. **(Provides privacy.)**

8. Raise bed to comfortable working level. **(Promotes proper body mechanics.)**

9. Examine legs and assess risk for conditions. **(Helps nurse determine presence of pigmentation around ankles, pitting edema, or peripheral cyanosis, which may indicate inadequate circulation.)**

10. Assess patient for calf pain or positive Homans' sign. **(May indicate presence of thrombophlebitis.)**

11. Measure legs for stockings according to agency policy and order stockings. **(Promotes the correct size to accomplish purpose of stockings.)**

Thromboembolic Deterrent Stockings

12. Assist patient to supine position to apply stockings before patient rises. **(Prevents veins from becoming distended or edema from occurring.)**

13. Turn stockings inside out as far as heel. Place thumbs inside foot part, and slip stocking on until heel is correctly aligned (Figure 2-4, *A* and *B*). **(Positions stocking for appropriate application.)**

14. Gather fabric and ease it over ankle and up the leg (Figure 2-4, *C*). **(Prevents bunching of stocking, which can cause local pooling of blood.)**

15. Pull leg portion of stocking over foot and up as far as it will go, making certain that gusset lies over femoral artery. Adjust stocking to fit evenly and smoothly with no wrinkles (Figure 2-4, *D*). **(Allows appropriate fit and application, which are vital for maintaining even pressure. Prevents irritation and impediments to circulation.)**

16. Repeat Steps 12 to 15 for opposite extremity. **(Ensures appropriate application.)**

Sequential Compression Devices (see Figure 2-5)

17. Place sleeve under patient's leg, with fuller portion at top of thigh. **(Ensures that fuller portion is placed under larger part of leg.)**

Continued

18. Apply sleeve with opening at front of knee and closed portion behind knee. **(Ensures appropriate placement and desired effect.)**

19. When in place, make sure there are no wrinkles or creases in stockings. Fold Velcro strips over to secure stockings. **(Allows proper functioning of stockings and prevents irritation.)**

20. Attach tubing to SCD after both sleeves are applied. Align arrows for correct connection and appropriate effect. Plug in unit. **(Allows air to inflate stockings in sequential order.)**

21. Assess patient periodically. **(Determines presence of edema or cyanosis.)**

22. Assess stocking at regular intervals. **(Ensures that top has not rolled down or loosened and that no wrinkles are present.)**

23. Remove and dispose of soiled gloves and wash hands. **(Reduces spread of microorganisms.)**

24. Document. **(Verifies patient care.)**

25. Do patient teaching (Patient Teaching: Use of TEDS/SCDs).

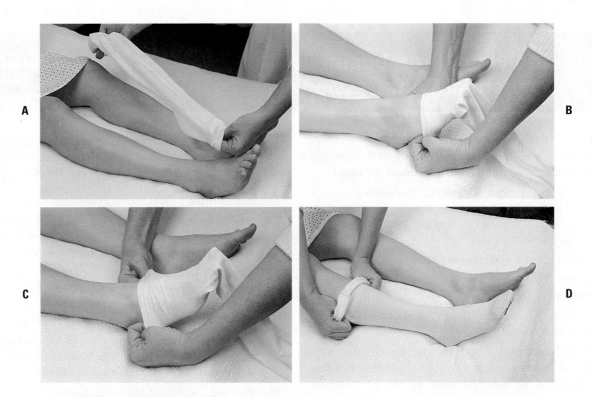

FIGURE **2-4** Applying antiembolism stockings. **A,** Turn the elastic stocking inside out by placing one hand into the sock, holding the toes of the sock with the other hand, and pulling. **B,** Place the patient's toes into the foot of the elastic stocking, making sure that the sock is smooth. **C,** Slide remaining portion of the sock over the patient's foot, making sure that the toes are covered. Sock will now be right-side out. **D,** Slide the sock up over the patient's calf until the sock is completely extended. Be sure that the sock is smooth and that no ridges are present.

serted to monitor urinary output. This procedure is normally reserved for patients undergoing urinary surgery or those who may have difficulty voiding. If a catheter is inserted, it is usually removed 1 to 2 days postoperatively to reduce the chance of bladder infection. Once it is removed, the nurse should encourage the patient to drink 8 ounces of fluids per hour while awake unless contraindicated. The nurse also monitors intake and output values until voiding returns to the patient's normal pattern. Urinary retention and urinary tract infections are common postoperative complications.

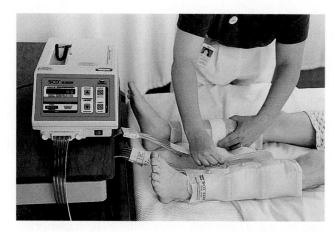

FIGURE **2-5** Application of sequential compression stockings.

Surgical Wounds

With today's technologies, incisions (cuts produced surgically by a sharp instrument to create an opening into an organ or space in the body) are closed in a variety of ways: suture, staples, Steri-Strips, or transparent strips. If the nurse knows the type of closure, its appearance can be explained to the patient. Some surgeries require the removal of exudate. For these patients a drain may be in place. The nurse can explain the purpose of the drain and the need for close monitoring. Although not all incisions require dressings, the nurse will assess the wound's appearance. Wound and drainage systems are described in more detail in Chapters 13 and 18 of *Foundations of Nursing*.

Pain

Patients fear pain more than any other postsurgical complication. The nurse must impress upon the patient that pain relief is an important part of care. Various methods are used to reduce discomfort. If the patient is considering nontraditional analgesia (imagery, biofeedback, relaxation techniques), the nurse should review these techniques and allow practice time. The

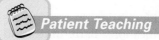 *Patient Teaching*

Use of TEDS/SCDs

- Teach patient to correctly apply antiembolism stockings.
- Teach patient appropriate care of the stockings. (Wash in warm water and mild soap, do not wring dry and lay over flat surface to dry.)
- Instruct patient not to massage legs because of the risk of dislodging a thrombus.
- Teach patient the signs of possible complications. (If too restrictive, edema and pain could result.)

majority of patients elect to obtain comfort through traditional analgesia. Postoperative pain is what the patient says it is, so it is important to reassure patients that addiction to analgesics very rarely occurs in the time frame needed for comfort. For the patient who is apprehensive about intermittent injections, patient-controlled analgesia (PCA) and opioids into the epidural space (patient controlled epidural or PCE) are safe and effective methods of postoperative pain management. When the patient is allowed oral intake, oral analgesics coupled with nontraditional methods are often effective (see Chapter 16, *Foundations of Nursing*).

Tubes

Depending on the surgery, patient teaching includes information about nasogastric tubes, wound evacuation units, and IV and oxygen therapy. Allowing patients to view these items and understand their purposes lessens the fear associated with each. (See Chapters 13 and 20, *Foundations of Nursing*, for more detailed discussion of the tubes and drains used in the postoperative patient.)

Preoperative Medication

Preoperative medication reduces the patient's anxiety, decreases the amount of anesthetic needed, and reduces respiratory tract secretions. The nurse should

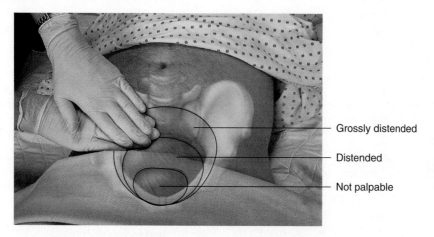

Grossly distended

Distended

Not palpable

FIGURE **2-6** Assess the bladder by palpating the lower abdomen for distention.

provide the patient with information on what to expect from preoperative medications. Barbiturates and tranquilizers (phenobarbital and diazepam [Valium]) are sometimes given for sedation to reduce the amount of the anesthetic required. Opioid analgesics (meperidine and morphine) may be administered by intermittent injection or PCA if the patient has pain before surgery; this also reduces the amount of anesthetic required. An introduction to PCA preoperatively is advantageous because the patient is better able to comprehend the concept and operation of this equipment. Anticholinergics such as atropine reduce spasms of smooth muscles and decrease gastric, bronchial, and salivary secretions (Table 2-5; also see Box 2-3). The patient frequently becomes drowsy, no-

tices a dry mouth, and may experience vertigo after the preoperative medication is given. The nurse should ask the patient to void before receiving a preoperative medication.

If preoperative medication is given on the nursing unit, the patient must remain in bed. The nurse institutes safety measures such as putting the bed in low position and raising side rails and monitors the patient every 15 to 30 minutes until the patient leaves for surgery. In many institutions the preoperative medication is given by the anesthesiologist or anesthetist in the preoperative holding area. These patients should be reassured and provided a quiet environment on the nursing unit while they are waiting to be transported to the surgical suite.

Table 2-5 *Perioperative Medications and Their Purposes*

GENERIC NAME	TRADE NAME	DOSE AND ROUTE	ACTION	NURSING IMPLICATIONS
BENZODIAZEPINES				
Midazolam	Versed	3-5 mg IM	Decreases anxiety and produces sedation	Monitor for respiratory depression, hypotension, drowsiness, and lack of coordination
Diazepam	Valium	5-20 mg po		
Lorazepam	Ativan	1-4 mg IM or IV	Induces amnesia May induce substantial amnesia	
OPIOID ANALGESICS				
Morphine	Morphine	5-15 mg IM, IV	Decreases anxiety	Monitor for respiratory depression, nausea, vomiting, orthostatic hypotension, and pruritus
Meperidine	Demerol	50-150 mg IM, IV	Provides analgesia Allows decreased anesthetics	
Fentanyl citrate	Sublimaze	50 mcg/mL IM or slow IV		
H₂ RECEPTOR ANTAGONISTS				
Cimetidine	Tagamet	300 mg IV, IM, po	Reduces gastric acid volume and concentration	Monitor for confusion and dizziness in older adults
Famotidine	Pepcid	20 mg IV		
Ranitidine	Zantac	50 mg IV, IM, po		
ANTIEMETICS				
Metoclopramide	Reglan	10 mg IV	Enhances gastric emptying	Monitor for sedation and extrapyramidal reaction (involuntary movement, muscle tone changes, and abnormal posture) Instruct patient to report any difficulty breathing
Droperidol	Inapsine	2.5-10 mg IM	Tranquilizer	
Ondansetron HCl (5-HT₃ receptor antagonist)	Zofran	4 mg IV	Prevents postoperative nausea and vomiting	
ANTICHOLINERGICS				
Atropine sulfate	Atropine sulfate	0.4-0.6 mg IM, IV	Reduces oral and respiratory secretions to decrease risk of aspiration	Monitor for confusion, restlessness, and tachycardia
Glycopyrrolate	Robinul	0.1-0.3 mg IM, IV	Decreases vomiting and laryngospasm	Prepare patient to expect dry mouth

Table 2-5 *Perioperative Medications and Their Purposes—cont'd*

GENERIC NAME	TRADE NAME	DOSE AND ROUTE	ACTION	NURSING IMPLICATIONS
ANTIBIOTICS				
Cefazolin sodium	Ancef	500 mg/50 mL vial	Bactericidal Wound infection Minimize risk of wound infection	If large doses are given, therapy is prolonged, or patient is at high risk, monitor for signs and symptoms of superinfection, including abdominal pain, moderate to severe diarrhea, severe anal or genital pruritus, and severe mouth soreness
Cefotaxime sodium	Claforan	1 g 30-90 min IM or IV preoperative	Bactericidal	
Ceftriaxone	Rocephin	1 g 0.5-2 hr IM or IV preoperative	Bactericidal as perioperative prophylaxis	Determine patient's history of allergies If dosing continues, space drug evenly around the clock Advise patient to complete therapy
ADRENOCORTICAL STEROID				
Methylprednisolone	Depo-Medrol Solu-Medrol	Adults: 40-25 mg IV q 4-6 hr	Decreases inflammation	Determine if patient has hypersensitivity to drug Determine if patient has diabetes mellitus and anticipate an increase in antidiabetic drug regimen because of raised blood glucose level
NONSTEROIDAL ANTIINFLAMMATORY DRUGS (NSAIDs)				
Ketorolac	Toradol	50 mg/mL IM; 30 mg/mL IV push over at least 15 sec	Reduces intensity of pain Reduces inflammation	Assess the duration, location, onset, and type of pain the patient is having Evaluate patient for therapeutic response
ANTICOAGULANTS				
Enoxaparin sodium	Lovenox	30 mg/0.3 mL to 150 mg/ mL in pre-filled syringes	Produces anticoagulation Prevents new clot formation or secondary embolic complications	Do not give IM but give subcutaneously Tell the patient not to take aspirin or similar OTC drugs
Heparin sodium	Heparin	10 units/mL to 15,000 units/ 500 mL Heparin sodium flush syringes: 10 units/ml < 100 units/ mL; vials		Cross-check heparin dose with another nurse before administering Use constant rate IV infusion pump Monitor the patient's PTT diligently Assess the patient's gums for erythema

Continued

Table 2-5 *Perioperative Medications and Their Purposes—cont'd*

GENERIC NAME	TRADE NAME	DOSE AND ROUTE	ACTION	NURSING IMPLICATIONS
ANTICOAGULANTS—cont'd				
Heparin sodium—cont'd		10 units/ mL to 100 units/mL		and gingival bleeding; skin for bruises or petechiae and urine for hematuria
Warfarin sodium	Coumadin	5 mg vials IM; 1-10 mg oral tablets		Observe patient for evidence of hemorrhage such as abdominal or back pain, a decrease in BP, an increase in pulse rate, and severe headache
				Urge patient to not ingest alcohol or make drastic dietary changes
				If administration continues, urge patient to notify the physician if he experiences black stools; bleeding; brown, dark or red urine; coffee-ground vomitus; or red-speckled mucus from a cough

Surgery cancels all medications ordered before surgery except for conditions of long-standing duration, such as phenytoin (Dilantin) for seizure control (Table 2-6). The surgeon will reorder medication necessary following surgery.

Anesthesia

Anesthesia means the absence of feelings (pain) (*an*, meaning "without," and *esthesia*, meaning "awareness of feeling"). Anesthesia may be divided into three categories: general, regional, and local.

Types of anesthesia

General anesthesia. Modern anesthetic agents are much easier to reverse and allow the patient to recover with fewer untoward effects. **General anesthesia** results in an immobile, quiet patient who does not recall the surgical procedure. The patient's amnesia acts as a protective measure from the unpleasant events of the procedure. Surgery using general anesthesia involves major procedures requiring extensive tissue manipulation.

An anesthesiologist gives general anesthetics by IV and inhalation routes through the four stages of anesthesia. **Stage I** begins with the patient awake and as the administration of anesthetic agents begins. The stage is completed when the patient loses consciousness. **Stage II** begins with the loss of consciousness and ends with the onset of regular breathing and loss of eyelid reflexes. This is referred to as the excitement of delirium phase because it is often accompanied by involuntary motor activity. The patient must not receive any auditory or physical stimulation during this period, because it can stimulate a release of catecholamines, which can result in an undesirable increase in heart rate and blood pressure. **Stage III** begins with the onset of regular breathing and ends with the cessation of respirations. This stage is known as the operative or surgical phase. **Stage IV** begins with the cessation of respirations and must be avoided, or it will necessitate the initiation of cardiopulmonary resuscitation and may lead to death. These stages were defined with the use of ether and are sometimes difficult to ascertain with newer anesthetic agents.

A more useful designation of stages includes the three phases of **induction, maintenance,** and **emergence. Induction phase** includes the administration of agents and endotracheal intubation. The **maintenance phase** includes positioning the patient, preparation of the skin for incision, and the surgical procedure itself. Appropriate levels of anesthesia are maintained dur-

Table 2-6 *Medications with Special Implications for the Surgical Patient*

DRUG CLASS	EFFECTS DURING SURGERY
Antibiotics	Antibiotics potentiate action of anesthetic agents. If taken within 2 weeks before surgery, aminoglycosides (gentamicin, tobramycin, neomycin) may cause mild respiratory depression from depressed neuromuscular transmission.
Antidysrhythmics	Antidysrhythmics can reduce cardiac contractility and impair cardiac conduction during anesthesia.
Anticoagulants	Anticoagulants alter normal clotting factors and thus increase risk of hemorrhaging. They should be discontinued at least 48 hours before surgery. Aspirin is a commonly used medication that can alter clotting mechanisms.
Anticonvulsants	Long-term use of certain anticonvulsants (e.g., phenytoin [Dilantin], phenobarbital) can alter metabolism of anesthetic agents.
Antihypertensives	Antihypertensives interact with anesthetic agents to cause bradycardia, hypotension, and impaired circulation. They inhibit synthesis and storage of norepinephrine in sympathetic nerve endings.
Corticosteroids	With prolonged use, corticosteroids cause adrenal atrophy, which reduces the body's ability to withstand stress Before and during surgery, dosage may be temporarily increased.
Insulin	Diabetic patient's need for insulin after surgery is reduced because patient's nutritional intake is decreased. Stress response and intravenous (IV) administration of glucose solutions can increase dosage requirements after surgery.
Diuretics	Diuretics potentiate electrolyte imbalances (particularly potassium) after surgery.
Nonsteroidal anti-inflammatory drugs (NSAIDs)	NSAIDs inhibit platelet aggregation and may prolong bleeding, increasing susceptibility to postoperative bleeding.
Herbal therapies (ginger, ginkgo, ginseng)	These herbal therapies have the ability to affect platelet activity and increase susceptibility to postoperative bleeding. Ginseng may increase hypoglycemia with insulin therapy. (See Chapter 17 of *Foundations of Nursing*, Complementary and Alternative Therapies.)

Adapted from Potter, P.A. & Perry, A.G. (2003). *Basic nursing essentials for practice.* (5th ed.). St Louis: Mosby.

ing this phase. During the **emergence phase,** anesthetics are decreased and the patient begins to awaken. Because of the short half-life to today's medications, emergence is often in the operating room.

To induce anesthesia, an IV agent is often given, although an inhalation agent may be used. Unconsciousness is achieved in 10 to 20 seconds after the dose. Barbiturates provide sedation, amnesia, and hypnosis but must be used in combination with other agents to achieve pain relief and muscle relaxation. To prevent possible aspiration and other respiratory complications, the anesthesiologist puts an endotracheal tube into the patient's airway. Endotracheal intubation is usually performed following administration of short-acting or, occasionally, long-acting muscle relaxants (Figure 2-7).

An anesthesia provider or operating room nurse may assist with cricoid pressure (a technique to reduce the risk of the aspiration of stomach contents during induction of general anesthesia: the esophagus is compressed to prevent passive regurgitation; this technique cannot, however, stop active vomiting) and endotracheal cuff inflation during intubation. For patients at risk for aspiration, cricoid pressure can prevent silent regurgitation and aspiration of gastric contents during induction and intubation. The maneuver is begun while the patient is awake. Patient reassurance is important to provide support during this period of mild discomfort. Once initiated, pressure must be held constant until the cuff has been inflated or aspiration can happen rapidly.

When induction is completed, anesthesia may be maintained through a combination of inhalation and IV medications. The patient also receives a continuous supply of oxygen and adjunct medications such as opioid analgesics (analgesia) and muscle relaxants. A combination of smaller amounts of several medications allows a significant reduction in the dose that would be required to produce anesthesia with a single medication.

The duration of anesthesia depends on the length of surgery. Surgical risks influence the duration of surgery. The greatest risks from general anesthesia are the side effects of anesthetic agents, including cardiovascular depression or irritability, respiratory depression, and liver and kidney damage.

The emergence from anesthesia occurs when the procedure is completed and reversal agents are given. The oropharynx is suctioned to decrease the risk of aspiration and laryngeal spasm following extubation. Extubation is often accomplished before transfer to the PAC (postanesthesia care) unit.

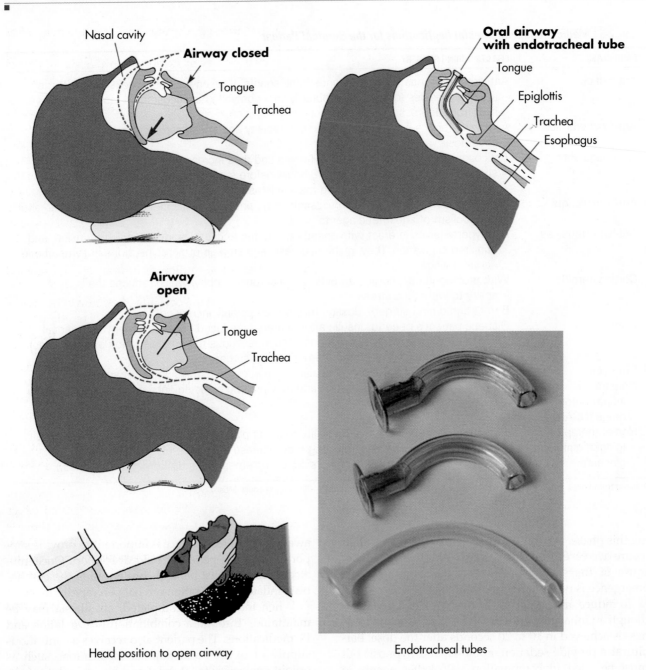

FIGURE **2-7** Possible airways used during surgery.

Regional anesthesia. Induction of **regional anesthesia** results in loss of sensation in an area of the body. The method of induction influences the portion of sensory pathways that is anesthetized. There is no loss of consciousness with regional anesthesia, but the patient is usually sedated. The anesthesiologist gives regional anesthetics by infiltration and local application. Figure 2-8 demonstrates common locations for the introduction of medication to achieve the regional block.

Infiltration of anesthetic agents may involve one of the following induction methods:

- **Nerve block:** Local anesthetic is injected into a nerve (e.g., brachial plexus in the arms), blocking the nerve supply to the operative site.

- **Spinal anesthesia:** The anesthesiologist performs a lumbar puncture and introduces local anesthetic into the cerebrospinal fluid in the spinal subarachnoid space. Anesthesia can extend from the tip of the xiphoid process down to the feet. Positioning of the patient influences movement of the anesthetic agent up or down the spinal cord. This is often used for lower abdominal, pelvic, and lower extremity procedures; urologic procedures; or surgical obstetrics.

- **Epidural anesthesia:** This is a safer procedure than spinal anesthesia because the anesthetic agent is injected into the epidural space outside the dura mater and the depth of anesthesia is not

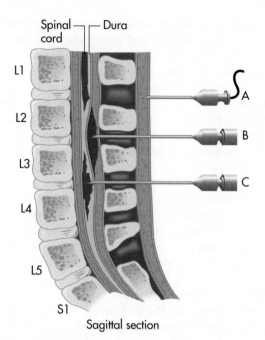

FIGURE **2-8** Spinal column—side view with spinal and epidural anesthesia needle placement. *A*, Epidural catheter. *B*, Single injection epidural. *C*, Spinal anesthesia. (Interspaces most commonly used are L4-5, L3-4, and L2-3.)

as great as that with spinal anesthesia. Because epidural anesthesia provides an effective loss of sensation in the vaginal and perineal areas, it is often used for obstetric procedures. The epidural catheter may be left in so that the patient may receive medication via continuous epidural infusion following surgery.

- **Intravenous regional anesthesia (Bier block):** Local anesthetic is injected via an IV line into an extremity below the level of a tourniquet after blood has been withdrawn. The drug is allowed to infiltrate only tissues in the intended surgical area. The extremity is pain free while the tourniquet is in place. Advantages include a short onset and short recovery time. However, the tourniquet may only be inflated for 2 hours or tissue damage will occur.

There are risks involved with infiltrative anesthetics, particularly in the case of spinal anesthesia, because the level of anesthesia may rise, which means that the anesthetic agent moves upward in the spinal cord and breathing may be affected. This migration of anesthetic depends on the drug type, amount, and patient position. The patient may experience a sudden decrease in blood pressure, which results from extensive vasodilation caused by the anesthetic block to sympathetic vasomotor nerves and pain and motor nerve fibers. If the level of anesthesia rises, respiratory paralysis may develop, requiring resuscitation by the anesthesiologist. Elevation of the upper body prevents respiratory paralysis. The patient requires

careful monitoring during and immediately after surgery.

The patient under regional anesthesia is awake throughout the surgery unless the physician orders a tranquilizer that promotes sleep and/or amnesia. Because the patient is responsive and capable of breathing voluntarily, it is unnecessary for the anesthesiologist to use an endotracheal tube. Operating room personnel often gain a false sense of security because of the patient's relative alertness. Nurses must remember that burns and other trauma can occur on the anesthetized part of the body without the patient being aware of the injury. It is therefore necessary to frequently observe the position of extremities and the condition of the skin. It is also important that operating room staff use caution regarding topics discussed in surgery.

Local anesthesia. Local anesthesia involves loss of sensation at the desired site (e.g., growth on the skin or the cornea of the eye). The anesthetic agent (e.g., lidocaine) inhibits nerve conduction until the drug diffuses into the circulation. It may be injected or applied topically. The patient experiences a loss in pain sensation and touch, and in motor and autonomic activities (e.g., bladder emptying). Local anesthesia is commonly used for minor procedures performed in ambulatory surgery. Physicians may infiltrate the operative area with local anesthetics to promote postoperative pain relief.

Conscious sedation. Conscious sedation (administration of central nervous system depressant drugs and/or analgesia to relieve anxiety and/or provide amnesia during surgical, diagnostic, or interventional procedures) is routinely used for procedures that do not require complete anesthesia but rather a depressed level of consciousness. A patient under conscious sedation must independently retain a patent airway and airway reflexes and be able to respond appropriately to physical and verbal stimuli.

Advantages of conscious sedation include adequate sedation and reduction of fear and anxiety with minimal risk, amnesia, relief of pain and noxious stimuli, mood alteration, elevation of pain threshold, enhanced patient cooperation, stable vital signs, and rapid recovery. A variety of diagnostic and therapeutic procedures are appropriate for conscious sedation (burn dressing changes, cosmetic surgery, pulmonary biopsy and bronchoscopy, and many others).

Nurses assisting with the administration of conscious sedation must demonstrate competency in the care of these patients. Knowledge of anatomy, physiology, cardiac dysrhythmias, procedural complications, and pharmacologic principles related to the administration of individual conscious agents is essential. Nurses must also be able to assess, diagnose, and intervene in the event of untoward reactions and demonstrate skill in airway management and oxygen delivery. Resuscitation equipment must be readily available if conscious sedation is being used.

Positioning the patient for surgery. During general anesthesia the nursing personnel and surgeon often wait to position the patient until the stage of complete relaxation is achieved. The choice of position is usually determined by the surgical approach (Figure 2-9). Ideally the patient's position provides good access to the operative site and sustains adequate circulatory and respiratory function. It should not impair neuromuscular structures. The patient's comfort and safety must be considered. The team must take into account age, weight, height, nutritional status, physical limitations, and preexisting conditions and document them for staff who care for the patient postoperatively.

It is sometimes difficult for nurses in postoperative divisions to appreciate the discomfort a patient may feel after surgery (e.g., discomfort of the left arm or side of a patient whose right kidney was removed). Normal range of joint motion is maintained in an alert person by pain and pressure receptors. If a joint is extended too far, pain stimuli provide a warning that muscle joint strain is too great. In a patient who is anesthetized,

normal defense mechanisms cannot guard against joint damage, muscle stretch, and strain. The muscles are so relaxed that it is relatively easy to place the patient in a position the individual normally could not assume while awake. The patient often remains in a given position for several hours. Although it may be necessary to place a patient in an unusual position, the nurse should attempt to maintain correct alignment and protect the patient from pressure, abrasion, and other injuries (corneal abrasion). Attachments to the operating room table allow protection and padding of extremities and bony prominences. Positioning should not impede normal movement of the diaphragm or interfere with circulation to body parts. If restraints are necessary, the nurse pads the area to be restrained to prevent skin trauma (see *Foundations of Nursing,* Chapter 14).

Preoperative Checklist

The nurse completes the preoperative checklist before the patient leaves the nursing unit (Figure 2-10). When the nurse signs the preoperative checklist, that nurse assumes responsibility for all areas of care included on the list. If the preoperative medication is to be given on

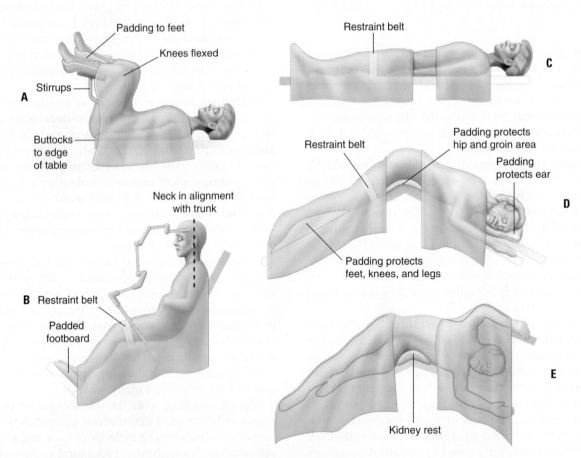

FIGURE **2-9** Common perioperative positions and the padding provided to relieve pressure in each position. **A,** Lithotomy position, used for vaginal and perineal procedures. **B,** Sitting position, used for neurological procedures. **C,** Supine position (the most common position). Potential pressure points are the occiput, scapula, olecranon, thoracic vertebrae, sacrum, coccyx, and calcaneus. **D,** Jackknife position, used for gluteal and anorectal surgeries. **E,** Lateral kidney position, used for procedures requiring a retroperitoneal approach.

PRE-OP ASSESSMENT FORM

(Please check carefully and initial)

Extra
Copies on back
of post-op
Assessment
Sheet

Date *November 10, 2004*

1. DNR Status _____ ✓ *SW*
2. Medical Admission Permit Signed _____ ✓ *SW*
3. Surgical Permit Signed & Witnessed _____ ✓ *SW*
4. Surgical Site Identified/Marked _____ ✓ *SW*   *Left Lower Quadrant*
5. Blood Transfusion Permit _____ ✓ *SW*
6. Sterilization Permit Signed & Witnessed _____ *not applicable*
7. IV Started - Fluids _____ *ns* _____ Site _____ *L.T.A* Patent _____ ✓ *SW*
8. Bone Bank Protocol _____ *Ø* _____ Recipient _____ *Ø* _____ Donor _____ *Ø*
9. Allergies, list: _____ *penicillin*
10. Identification Band _____ ✓ *SW* _____ Blood Bracelet _____ ✓ *SW*
11. Pre-Op Prep Done _____ *to be done in Intraoperative* _____ Checked By RN _____
12. Pre-Op Bath *Hibiclens Shower* _____ Hospital Gown _____ ✓ *SW* _____ Bath Blanket _____ ✓ *SW*
13. Remove: Dentures _____ *Ø* _____ Glasses/Contacts _____ ✓ *SW* _____ Jewelry/Nail Polish/Hair Pins/Make-up _____ ✓ *SW*
14. TED stockings when ordered _____ ✓ *SW* Side Rails Up _____ ✓ *SW* _____ Patient Labels _____ ✓ *SW*
15. Pre-Op Vital Signs Time: *1000* T *98⁶* P *80* R *20* BP *120/80* Pain Intensity 0-10 *Ø SW*
16. Pre-Op Medications _____ *to be administered in Interopative*
17. Insert Foley Catheter _____ ✓ *SW*
18. Physical Disability, such as Amputations, Glass Eye, etc. _____ *Ø*
19. Systemic Diseases _____ *NIDDM   SW*
20. History and Physical _____ ✓ *SW*

See Guidelines for pre-op testing policy number 600 - P 118. Testing completed per policy.

21. Lab Reports: _____ *CBC, Hg, Hct*

EKG _____ *on chart   SW* _____ Chest X-Ray _____ *on chart   SW*

NURSING STAFF IDENTIFICATION
SW   Susan Welker

Great Plains Regional
Medical Center
601 West Leota Street - P.O. Box 1167
North Platte, Nebraska 69103-1167

22. Infectious Process Present _____ Yes _____ ✗ No
    Type of Infection _____
23. Additional Comments _____ *pre & post op nursing interventions explained*
24. Chart Signed Off _____ ✓ *SW*

LABEL

FIGURE **2-10** Preoperative assessment form.

the nursing unit, the nurse completes the preoperative checklist before administering the medication.

Any prosthesis (an artificial replacement for a missing part of the body), contact lenses, dentures, jewelry, and other valuables are removed and either given to family members or placed in a secure area. Some hospitals allow dentures to be left in and worn to surgery and removed at a later time. The removal of dentures preoperatively is according to agency policy. If rings are worn, they should be secured with tape and the disposition of personal items charted. The patient should void before the preoperative medication is administered, or 1 hour before surgery is scheduled. Although the majority of patients become drowsy after administration of a preoperative medication, a few will either become hyperactive or demonstrate no side effects. The patient should be reminded to remain in bed, and the side rails should be raised. The call light should be placed within reach and its location identified for the patient.

Transport to the Operating Room

Personnel in the operating room notify the nursing unit when it is time for surgery. The transporter checks the patient's identification bracelet against the patient's medical record to be sure the correct person is going to surgery. When a patient is to be transported by a gurney, the nurses and transporter assist the patient in safely transferring from bed to gurney. The ambulatory surgery patient may walk to the operating room, allowing more control over the event. The trip to surgery should be as smooth as possible so that the sedated patient does not experience nausea or dizziness.

The family is provided an opportunity to visit before the patient is transported to the operating room. The nurse then directs the family to the appropriate waiting area. If family members plan on leaving the facility during the procedure, ensure that there is a way to contact them and supply them with phone numbers of the nurse's station and patient's room.

Preparing for the Postoperative Patient

If the patient has been hospitalized before surgery and will be returning to the same nursing unit, the nurse prepares the bed and room for the patient's return. Furniture should be arranged so that the gurney can easily be brought to the bedside. The bed should be in the high position. Bed rails should be down on the receiving side and up on the other side. A postoperative bedside unit should include the following:

- Sphygmomanometer, stethoscope, and thermometer
- Emesis basin
- Clean gown
- Washcloth, towel, and facial tissues
- IV pole and pump
- Suction equipment
- Oxygen equipment
- Extra pillows for positioning
- Bed pads to protect bed linen from drainage
- PCA pump

The nurse will be better prepared for postoperative care if the room is readied before the patient returns.

INTRAOPERATIVE PHASE

Intraoperative (within the surgical suite) care centers on the care and protection of the patient. When the patient enters the operating room (Figure 2-11), the nurse identifies the patient both verbally and by the identification band and medical records. Nursing interventions should include warm, personal contact with the patient to humanize the often cold, aseptic, and highly technical environment of the operating room. During surgery and particularly anesthesia, patients are unable to protect themselves from many sources of possible harm. Essential elements for monitoring and promoting patient safety are a keen awareness of the potential for harm, recognition of body areas most susceptible to injury, strict adherence to principles of positioning and asepsis, and monitoring sites for impairment or early signs of injury. Small or potentially dangerous objects such as needles and syringes should not be left near the patient. Side rails and safety straps should be used, even for the fully conscious patient; safety reminder devices may occasionally be necessary to protect the delirious, semicomatose, or disoriented patient from injury.

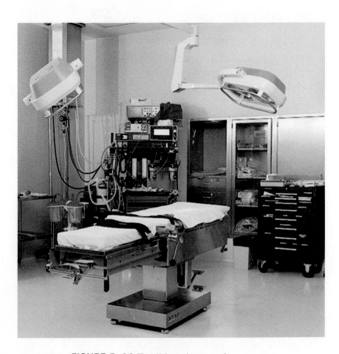

FIGURE **2-11** Traditional operating room.

HOLDING AREA

In many hospitals the patient enters a surgical care unit called a **preanesthesia care unit** (sometimes called a holding area) outside the operating room, where the nurse completes the preoperative preparations. Nurses in this unit are usually part of the operating room staff and wear surgical scrub suits.

The nurses or anesthesiologist will insert an IV catheter into the patient's vein to establish a route for fluid replacement and IV medications. A large-bore IV catheter is used for optimal infusion of all fluids and possible blood products. Preoperative medications are administered.

If hair around the surgical site needs to be removed, this is done in a private area near the operating room immediately before surgery. The nurse should consult the physician's order sheet and the agency policy and procedure manual (see Skill 2-1, Figure 2-2).

Because the temperature in the operating room is usually cool, the patient should be offered an extra blanket for warmth and relaxation. The patient's stay in the holding area is brief.

THE ROLE OF THE NURSE

In the intraoperative phase the nurse assumes one of two roles during the surgical procedure: scrub nurse or circulating nurse (Box 2-7).

Everyone (nurses, physicians, anesthetists) in the operating room must be alert to contamination of sterile items and must aid in maintaining aseptic conditions. Surgical asepsis (protection against infection before, during, or after surgery by the use of sterile technique) is provided to prevent microbial contamination of the operative site. Maintaining a sterile environment in the surgical suite is crucial if the wound is to remain free of contamination. The goal of surgical asepsis is to prevent or minimize postoperative wound infections. The patient is at risk for introduction of infecting organisms through catheters, drains, or the surgical wound. Standards and guidelines for surgical scrubs and skin preparation should be strictly followed. The success and ease with which the operation is accomplished greatly depend on group dynamics as professionals work to achieve common goals (Figure 2-12).

Box 2-7 | *Responsibilities of the Circulating Nurse and of the Scrub Nurse*

RESPONSIBILITIES OF THE CIRCULATING NURSE

- Prepares operating room with necessary equipment and supplies and ensures that equipment is functional.
- Arranges sterile and unsterile supplies; opens sterile supplies for scrub nurse.
- Sends for patient at proper time.
- Visits with patient preoperatively; explains role, verifies operative permit, identifies patient, and answers any questions.
- Performs patient assessment.
- Confirms patient assessment.
- Checks medical record for completeness.
- Assists in safe transfer of patient to operating room table.
- Positions patient on operating room table in accordance with type of procedure and surgeon's preference.
- Places conductive pad on patient if electrocautery is to be used.
- Counts sponges, needles, and instruments with scrub nurse before surgery.
- Assists scrub nurse and surgeons by tying gowns. May prepare patient's skin.
- Assists scrub nurse in arranging tables to create sterile field.
- Maintains continuous astute observations during surgery to anticipate needs of patient, scrub nurse, surgeons, and anesthesiologist.
- Provides supplies to scrub nurse as needed.
- Observes sterile field closely for any breaks in aseptic technique and reports accordingly.

- Cares for surgical specimens according to institutional policy.
- Documents operative record and nurse's notes.
- Counts sponges, needles, and instruments when closure of wound begins.
- Transfers patient to gurney for transport to recovery area.
- Accompanies patient to the recovery room and provides a report.

RESPONSIBILITIES OF THE SCRUB NURSE

- Performs surgical hand scrub.
- Dons sterile gown and gloves aseptically.
- Arranges sterile supplies and instruments in manner prescribed for procedure.
- Checks instruments for proper functioning.
- Counts sponges, needles, and instruments with circulating nurse.
- Gowns and gloves surgeons as they enter operating room.
- Assists with surgical draping of patient.
- Maintains neat and orderly sterile field.
- Corrects breaks in aseptic technique.
- Observes progress of surgical procedure.
- Hands surgeon instruments, sponges, and necessary supplies during procedure.
- Identifies and handles surgical specimens correctly.
- Maintains count of sponges, needles, and instruments so none will be misplaced or lost in wound.

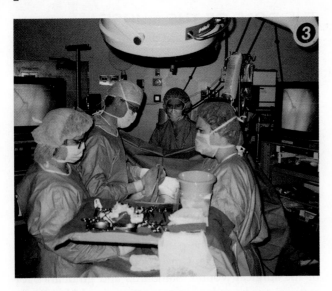

FIGURE **2-12** Safe, effective intraoperative care requires a team effort.

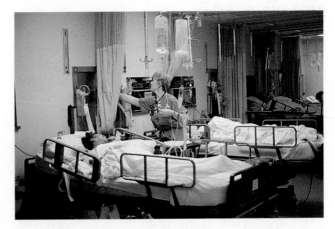

FIGURE **2-13** Nurse in postanesthesia care unit.

During the postoperative phase the operating room (OR) nurse assists in transferring the patient to the postanesthesia care unit (PACU) (Figure 2-13). Information about the patient's status, including a review of IV fluids, medications, and blood products administered; the surgical dressing; the nature of any complication in the OR; and unusual risks for hemorrhage or cardiac irregularities are reviewed with the recovery room staff. The OR nurse is an important resource in planning the patient's postoperative care.

POSTOPERATIVE PHASE

IMMEDIATE POSTOPERATIVE PHASE

Once surgery is completed, the patient is transported to the recovery room (or PACU) or the intensive care area. Evaluation of the patient follows the ABCs of immediate postoperative observation: airway, breathing, consciousness, and circulation. Table 2-7 lists interventions associated with the ABCs. Vital signs are assessed every 15 minutes during the recovery period, and respiratory and GI functions are monitored. The wound is evaluated for any drainage (the removal of fluids from a body cavity, wound, or other source of discharge by one or more methods) and/or exudate (substances that have slowly seeped from cells or blood vessels through small pores or breaks in cell membranes (e.g., perspiration, pus, and serum). When the patient has a patent airway and stable vital signs, is conscious, and responds to stimuli, the anesthesiologist or surgeon approves the transfer of the patient to the nursing unit. As the patient regains consciousness, relief of pain is often the first need expressed. Frequently, medication is given in the recovery area. Doc-

umentation from the surgical suite and recovery room is reviewed by staff on the nursing unit to assess how well the patient tolerated the surgical process. Body temperature is carefully monitored. Hypothermia, a core temperature of less than 98.6° F (37° C), occurs in 60% to 80% of all postoperative patients. Contributing factors include body exposure in a cold operating room, the effects of cold solutions, and a consequence of some anesthetics. Warm blankets are usually applied to the body, especially around the feet; adding warmth around the head is helpful. A newer method is convective warming therapy, in which a disposable cover inflated with warm air from a heating unit is placed over the patient; warm air passes out through the underside, providing constantly moving warm air.

The patient in the PACU is monitored for temperature and vital signs every 15 minutes until vital signs are stable, or more often if they are unstable. The frequency of monitoring and length of time over which monitoring must be done are dictated by facility PACU policy. Patients are monitored until they are discharged from the PACU. This is usually at least 1 hour. Patients must have a minimum temperature of greater than 96.8° F (36° C) before they are discharged from the PACU. The heat loss that occurs in the operating room can continue in the PACU if the patient is not warmed sufficiently. Warming requires the maintenance of temperature without overwarming and causing excessive vasodilation, which can cause fluid shifts and a decrease in blood pressure. The PACU nurse must also realize that malignant hyperthermia can occur in the PACU and the patient should be repeatedly assessed for manifestations of this condition. Malignant hyperthermia is a genetic disorder characterized by uncontrolled skeletal muscle contractions leading to potentially fatal hyperthermia. It occurs in predisposed patients when they receive a combination of certain anesthetic agents. Unless the triggering event is stopped and the body is cooled, death is the result.

Table 2-7 | *Interventions Associated with the ABCs of Immediate Recovery*

ASSESSMENT MODE	INTERVENTION
A—Airway	Maintain patency: keep head tilted up and back; may position on side with the face down and neck slightly extended.
	Note presence or absence of gag/swallowing reflex; stay at bedside until gag reflex returns.
	Suction until awake and alert.
	Provide oxygen if necessary.
B—Breathing	Evaluate depth, rate, sounds, rhythm, and chest movement.
	Assess color of mucous membranes.
	Place hand above patient's nose to detect respirations if shallow.
	Initiate coughing and deep breathing exercises as soon as patient is able to respond.
	Chart time oxygen is discontinued.
	Monitor oxygen saturation levels (Sao_2) by pulse oximetry checks.
C—Consciousness	Able to extubate (the process of removing endotracheal tube from airway).
	Patient responds to commands.
	Patient verbalizes responses.
	Patient reacts to stimuli.
C—Circulation	Monitor T, P, R, and BP every 10 to 15 minutes; take axillary, tympanic, or rectal temperature if warranted.
	Assess rate, rhythm, quality of pulse.
	Evaluate color and warmth of skin and nailbeds.
	Check peripheral pulses as indicated.
	Assess incision/dressing (monitor wound drainage output).
	Monitor IVs: solution, rate, site.
	Cardiac monitors are usually in place when the patient has had general anesthesia.
S—System review	Assess neurological functions, muscle strength, and response.
	Monitor drains, tubes; color and amount of output.
	Check for pressure, type, and condition of dressings.
	Evaluate pain response; may need to give analgesic and monitor patient response.
	Observe for allergic reactions.
	Assess urinary output if Foley catheter is in place.

LATER POSTOPERATIVE PHASE
Immediate Assessments

When the patient returns to the nursing unit, a thorough postsurgical assessment follows. Vital signs, the IV and incisional sites, any tubes, and postoperative orders are reviewed. A review of each body system identifies when body functions return and provides a guideline for further assessments. Unless otherwise indicated, the nurse monitors vital signs and makes general assessments using the "times four" factor—every 15 minutes times 4; every 30 minutes times 4; every hour times 4; then every 4 hours, or until assessments are within expected ranges. The times-four gauge is the maximal time that should elapse between assessments. Table 2-8 details body temperature responses, to surgery. A postoperative flow sheet (Figure 2-14) is frequently used to document the patient's progress.

Significant observations are critical for the patient after surgery. Although the patient may respond, the level of functioning is impaired. Side rails should be kept in the up position and the call light within reach. Until the patient is fully conscious, a pillow should not be placed under the head. The nurse should either position the patient on the side, depending on the type of surgery, or raise the head of the bed to a 45-degree angle. By positioning the head higher than the chest, the chance of the patient's aspirating vomitus lessens. Because nausea and vomiting are normal in the first 12 to 24 hours, an emesis basin should remain at the bedside. If the patient vomits, the amount should be measured and carefully described in the documentation. Any red or coffee-ground emesis should be reported immediately. Frequently the patient remains on NPO status for the first few hours after surgery. Fluids are introduced gradually. The usual fluid regimen ordered by the physician includes ice chips followed by clear or full liquids.

Postoperative complications can occur suddenly; therefore any change should be noted. Because the patient is often cold, additional blankets should be provided for comfort; however, sweating should not be induced. Vital signs, coupled with the patient's behavior, are first-line observations. A pulse that increases and becomes thready—coupled with a declining blood pressure, cool and clammy skin, reduced urine output, and restlessness—may signal hypovolemic shock. Hypo-

Table 2-8 *Temperature Assessment and Intervention*

CAUSE	ASSESSMENT AND INTERVENTION
HYPOTHERMIA **Within First 12 Hours**	
Response to surgery, anesthesia, and body exposure	Monitor temperature readings. Assess for warmth. Provide warm blankets. Do not expose for long periods. Assess orientation.
HYPERTHERMIA **24 to 48 Hours**	
Dehydration Decreased lung activity Inflammatory response to surgery	Monitor temperature readings. Monitor IV rate. Encourage fluids. Assess I&O. Have patient turn, cough, and breathe deeply. Provide incentive spirometer. Assess lung sounds. Observe incision.
After Day 2	
Infection: respiratory, wound, urinary, or circulatory	Monitor temperature readings. Assess lung sounds and expectoration of sputum. Evaluate incision and drainage. Monitor I&O. Encourage fluids of 6 to 8 oz/hr unless contraindicated. Note urine color, odor, amount, and consistency, and patient's complaints of burning on micturition. Perform leg exercises q2h and ambulate q4h.

volemic shock in the postoperative period is frequently caused by internal hemorrhage—a life-threatening emergency (Box 2-8).

A drop in blood pressure slightly below a patient's preoperative baseline reading is common after surgery. However, a significant drop in blood pressure, accompanied by an increased heart rate, may indicate hemorrhage, circulatory failure, or fluid shifts. Do not diagnose impending hypovolemic shock on the basis of one low blood pressure reading. If you are concerned about a dropping blood pressure, measure pressure every 5 minutes for 15 minutes to determine the variability. Decreased blood pressure can also mean that the anesthetic is wearing off or that the patient is experiencing severe pain.

In addition to hypotension, manifestations of shock include tachycardia; restlessness and apprehension; and cold, moist, pale, or cyanotic skin. When a patient appears to be going into shock, the nurse intervenes as follows: (1) administering oxygen or increasing its rate of delivery, (2) raising the patient's legs above the level of the heart, (3) increasing the rate of IV fluids (unless contraindicated because of fluid excretion problems), (4) notifying the anesthesia provider and the surgeon, (5) providing medications as ordered, and (6) continuing to assess the patient and response to interventions.

Incision

The incisional dressing is monitored, because bleeding or excessive drainage may also signal postoperative hemorrhage. Normally dressings are not changed but are reinforced during the first 24 hours. To accurately measure the amount of drainage, the nurse circles the drainage markings on the dressing and writes the time and date. A surgical incision may separate; this action of dehiscence (the separation of a surgical incision or rupture of a wound closure) may occur within 3 days to over 2 weeks postoperatively. Wound separation that occurs in the first 3 days is usually related to technical factors, such as the sutures. Separation from 3 to 14 days postoperatively is usually associated with postoperative complications such as distention, vomiting, excessive coughing, dehydration, or infection. Wound separation after 2 weeks is usually associated with metabolic factors, such as cachexia (ill health, malnutrition, and wasting as a result of chronic disease), hypoproteinemia, increased age, malignancy, radiation therapy, and obesity. If internal organs protrude through the incision, wound evisceration (protrusion of an internal organ through a wound or surgical incision, especially in the abdominal wall) has occurred. Both wound dehiscence and evisceration require prompt attention (Figure 2-15). If the patient feels a sudden "give," sutures may have broken. The nurse should contact the physician immediately. Cover the wound with a sterile towel moistened with sterile physiological saline (warm). Tension on the abdomen may be decreased by having the patient flex knees slightly and by placing the patient in Fowler's position. Reassure patient and advise that surgery will be required. Prepare the patient for surgery. Sterile technique procedures—including the dressing change and care of the surgical incision with phases of wound healing—are discussed in Chapters 12 and 13 of *Foundations of Nursing*.

Ventilation

Immediate postoperative hypoventilation can result from drugs (anesthetics, narcotics, tranquilizers, sedatives), incisional pain, obesity, chronic lung disease, or

POST-OP ASSESSMENT FORM

SURGEON: *DR. J. Bernard*		REPORT FROM: *S Welker RN*		ALLERGIES: *NKA*	
Date: *1-27-05*	Anesthesia Note: *General*		PROCEDURE: *Reverse Colostomy-Sigmoid Colostomy*		
ARRIVAL ON FLOOR *1440*	BLOCK LEVEL: _____			CBI CREDIT ——— *resection (seg mem)*	

PRE-OP MEDS	INTRA OP MEDS	POST OP MEDS	CBI INTAKE ———	IV FLUIDS & CREDITS
Versed 2mg	*Fentanyl 250 mcg*	*Versed 1 mg*	OUTPUT *Foley 650 cc*	*NS - 125 cc*
pepcid 20mg	*Hagyl 750 mg*	*Morphine 1 mg*		*700 cc*
	Zofran 4 g	*2 10 min/6 mg/*	DRAINS *Jackson Pratt Ø*	EBL ———
			PACKS *NA*	IV INTAKE *3300 cc*

Time	BP-P-R	TEMP	PAIN INTENSITY 0-10	SAO2	NURSING OBSERVATIONS
1440	$^{144}/_{83}$ 84-12	96^6	Ø	95%	*1440 Returned from pacunit to Room 356 B per gurney- awake-*
1500	$^{166}/_{82}$ 86-16	96^8	5	94%	*alert-oriented x 4. Color pink-skin warm and dry. IV infusing*
1515	$^{152}/_{82}$ 86-16			96%	*in Left Wrist @ 125 mL/hr. Site without edema or erythema.—*
1530	$^{145}/_{78}$ 84-18	96^9	4	96%	*Pedal pulses 4+ bilaterally. Capillary refill <2 seconds.—*
1545	$^{140}/_{79}$ 86-16	96^3	4	96%	*Lung sounds clear. O2 4L per nasal Cannula. Incentive —*
1600	$^{139}/_{73}$ 86-18	96^4	4	97%	*spirometer to 1500 mL. Abd. dressings dry & intact ō SM —*
1630	$^{144}/_{80}$ 87-18	96^8	4	95%	*am't of serosanguineous exudate. Area marked. Bowel sounds —*
1730	$^{149}/_{78}$ 87-18	97^2	4	90%	*absent. Jackson Pratt draining serosanguineous exudate. Foley—*
1830	$^{129}/_{71}$ 86	97^5	4	99%	*Catheter draining light, yellow urine. TED hose on bilaterally-*
					flowtrons in place. ————————
					1600 active ROM to Lower extremities. ————————
					1730 Walked 100 fut c̄ assistance. C/o dizzyness & nausea —
					returned to bed. ————————
					1800 IV NS changed to D5 ½ NS @ 125 mL/hr. Site s̄ —
					erythema or edema. Luann Richardson SPN ————
					1900 Above assessment remains unchanged. ————
					Luann Richardson SPN. ————————

NURSING STAFF SIGNATURE AND INITIALS	
LR Luann Richardson SPN	

Great Plains Regional
Medical Center
601 West Leota Street - P.O. Box 1167
North Platte, Nebraska 69103-1167

N-12 (Rev. 7/03)   topel   LABEL

FIGURE **2-14** Postoperative assessment form.

Box 2-8 | *Possible Causes of Postoperative Shock*

- Moving patient from operating table to gurney
- Jarring patient (gurney) during transport
- Reactions to drugs and anesthesia
- Loss of blood and other body fluids
- Cardiac dysrhythmias
- Cardiac failure
- Inadequate ventilation
- Pain

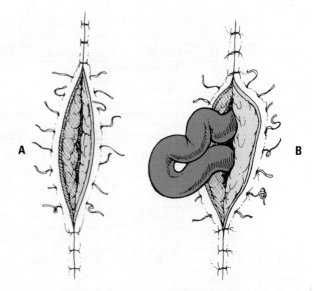

FIGURE **2-15 A,** Wound dehiscence. **B,** Evisceration.

pressure on the diaphragm. Inadequate ventilation leads to hypoxemia. Arterial oxygenation saturation (SaO_2) can be monitored either by arterial blood gas measurements or by pulse oximetry.

Because lung ventilation is vital, the nurse assists the patient to turn, cough, and breathe deeply every 1 to 2 hours until the chest is clear. Having practiced this combination preoperatively, the patient is usually able to adequately remove trapped mucus and surgical gases. To ease the pressure on the incision, the nurse helps the patient support the surgical site with a pillow, rolled bath blanket, or the heel of the hand. Analgesics, as prescribed, are given to control pain before coughing and deep breathing exercises. Early mobility and frequent position changes facilitate secretion clearance and improve the distribution of ventilation and perfusion in the lungs. Respiratory infections are frequently caused by shallow breathing and poor coughing. The nurse should listen for wheezing or crowing sounds from patients who have undergone head or neck surgery; this response occurs when edema places pressure over the trachea, resulting in respiratory insufficiency.

If the patient feels chest pain or has a fever, productive cough, or dyspnea, **atelectasis** (an abnormal condition characterized by the collapse of lung tissue) or pneumonia may be developing. Sudden chest pain combined with dyspnea, tachycardia, cyanosis, diaphoresis, and hypotension are signs of a pulmonary embolism. The head of the bed should be raised to decrease dyspnea, and signs and symptoms must immediately be reported. Frequently oxygen therapy is instituted to assist with respirations.

Whenever air exchange is reduced, postoperative recovery slows. Medication, suctioning, and oxygen therapy may be needed to assist the patient with respiratory distress. Mechanical devices, such as incentive spirometers, are used to stimulate deep breathing (see Skill 2-2). Frequently the incentive spirometer is used when the patient can deep breathe independently; the instrument visually measures the amount of air inhaled. Volume-oriented spirometers assist patients in deep breathing. Patients are encouraged to take 10 deep breaths every hour while awake.

If respiratory complications develop, the physician may order respiratory therapy to provide intermittent positive pressure breathing (IPPB) treatments to deliver a mixture of air and oxygen; medication can be added to enhance respirations. Chest percussion and postural drainage—a form of chest physiotherapy that combines positioning and percussion movements to lung areas to help dislodge and move secretions—are also utilized. Patients are not left unattended during postural drainage treatments, since they may experience respiratory distress.

Pain

Although internal organs do not have many nerve endings, a skin incision does produce painful responses. Because pain is normal postoperatively, the nurse should offer patients prescribed analgesics. The nurse should ask the patient every 3 to 4 hours if something is needed for pain because some patients will not ask for an analgesic. Acute pain begins to subside within 24 to 48 hours. Pain medication is subsequently adjusted to meet the patient's need. In the early stages of recovery, comfort interventions help ease pain. Anxiety may affect pain perception. After the acute phase ends, comfort measures may be the only interventions required (Box 2-9).

A patient's level of pain can be difficult to evaluate. Request patient to rate the pain on a scale of 0 to 10. There are standard pain indexes (restlessness, moaning, grimacing, diaphoresis), but some patients may not outwardly exhibit signs. Objective pain factors are detectable signs that the body is responding to "pain": vital sign changes (BP lowers in the immediate postoperative period and elevates in response to pain after about 12 hours, and pulse increases), restlessness, diaphoresis, pallor. The patient's description of dis-

---

Box 2-9 *Postoperative Comfort Measures for Pain*

DECREASE EXTERNAL STIMULI
- Darken room; close drapes.
- Keep TV/radio off or low.
- Monitor hall traffic/noise.
- Assess staff interruptions.
- Check room for noise—dripping water, buzzing lights, constant intercom messages.

REDUCE INTERRUPTIONS
- Plan care to allow rest.
- Post "Do Not Disturb" sign.
- Unplug telephone.
- Restrict visitors.
- Pull curtains around bed.

ELIMINATE ODORS
- Discuss offending odors and assess elimination.
- Remove from room all dressings that are soiled with exudate.
- Post "No Smoking" sign.
- Alert housekeeping—omit room-cleaning products.
- Install air-circulating unit.
- Alert dietary department to reduce foods with odors.

NURSING INTERVENTIONS
- Question normal relaxation patterns/practices.
- Have patient practice deep breathing and relaxation techniques.
- Plan rest periods.
- Provide back rub.
- Provide conversation and ask about concerns/fears.
- Encourage diversional activities.
- Reposition and support with pillows, bed rolls.
- Check tube placement.
- Offer warm fluids if indicated.
- Reduce room clutter.
- Provide restful environment.

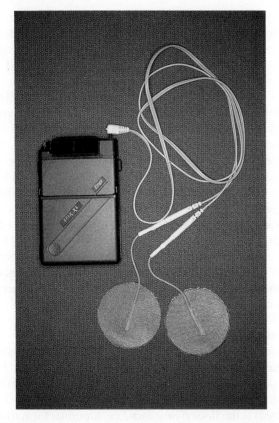

FIGURE **2-16** Transcutaneous electric nerve stimulation (TENS).

comfort represents subjective pain factors. The way the pain is affecting the patient emotionally is termed **suffering.** Pain behaviors are influenced by the patient's culture and past experiences. Behaviors include moaning, grimacing, and favoring a body area.

The effectiveness of analgesic measures differs with each person; if relief is not obtained, changing the medication or administration schedule may provide effective pain control. Each patient interprets pain differently and has a personal pain tolerance level; therefore, if a patient expresses pain, it is real for that person. Remember that only the patient bearing the pain is an expert about that pain. McCaffery states, "Pain is whatever the experiencing person says it is, existing whenever he says it does." Patients experiencing chronic pain may

have more difficulty obtaining relief than individuals with acute episodes (McCaffery, 2003).

The success of pain management depends on the nature of the surgery, emotional state of the patient, and postoperative complications. Commonly used analgesic measures are nurse-administered narcotics, patient-controlled IV medication administration (see Chapter 16, *Foundations of Nursing*), and pain control via a transcutaneous electric nerve stimulation (TENS) unit (Figure 2-16). The patient-controlled anesthesia (PCA) system is a pump that has a predetermined amount of analgesic contained within the unit; the system is programmed to allow only a given amount of medication to be dispensed. The patient can self-administer an analgesic by pressing a control button. The PCA system should be monitored closely every 3 to 4 hours. Attached to the skin, the TENS unit applies electric impulses to the nerve endings and blocks transmission of pain signals to the brain.

Urinary Function

Anesthesia retards urinary function. The bladder area is assessed every 2 hours for distention. It routinely takes 6 to 8 hours for voiding to occur after surgery. If patients do not void within 8 hours, catheterization may be necessary. Catheterization should be used as a last measure. The nurse may have the patient listen to running water; place the hands in warm water; or walk to the bathroom, if able, to facilitate voiding. Helping male patients stand often encourages voiding. To accurately evaluate the hydration level of the patient, the intake and output (I&O) are measured as long as it is deemed necessary (this will depend on the type of surgery). Usually I&O are measured while a Foley catheter is in place, while the patient is receiving IV therapy, and immediately after a Foley catheter has been removed. Urine measurement continues until the patient is voiding without difficulty. Fluid deficit may result from inadequate replacement of body fluids lost during surgery or from continued fluid losses. Fluid excess may occur from large volumes of fluids replaced by IV fluids when kidney function is inadequate (evidenced by oliguria). A urine output of 30 mL per hour is considered an acceptable level postoperatively. Unless the patient has had urinary tract surgery, urine should be clear and yellow and have an ammonia odor.

Venous Stasis

Performing leg exercises every 2 hours and using antiembolic stockings aid the circulatory system, because venous stasis (a disorder in which the normal flow of fluid through a vessel of the body is slowed or halted) is the underlying cause of thrombus formation. Assessment of the feet and legs includes palpating for pedal pulse and noting the skin's color and temperature. If edema, aching or cramping, sensitivity, or pain occurs in the calf (Homans' sign) or leg, a thrombus should be suspected. The patient should remain in bed until the physician can do an evaluation. The nurse should teach the patient not to cross legs when in bed and encourage sitting up as another means of preventing venous stasis.

Another device that helps prevent deep vein thrombosis is the intermittent external pneumatic compression system. Surgical patients are at the greatest life-threatening risk of developing deep vein thrombosis and pulmonary embolism. Not only does surgery injure blood vessels, but anesthesia and inactivity also cause venous stasis.

Surgery, however, is not the only risk factor. Others include pregnancy, myocardial infarction (MI), heart failure, stroke (brain attack), cancer, sepsis, and immobility. The most effective method of decreasing the occurrence of deep vein thrombosis is with low-dose subcutaneous heparin therapy. Heparin is an anticoagulant but is contraindicated in trauma and general surgery patients. Antiembolism elastic stockings and ambulation have also been found useful in preventing deep vein thrombosis.

The external intermittent pneumatic compression system (SCD) (see Skill 2-5) is being used on patients who are at risk of developing deep vein thrombosis and pulmonary embolism. This device includes an air pressure pump and cuffs, one for each calf or foot.

Continuous inflation and deflation of the cuffs decreases pooling of venous blood in the legs and improves venous return to the heart. The pressure cuffs will automatically inflate to 40 mm Hg or the prescribed setting and deflate in cycles, with inflation lasting about 12 seconds and deflation lasting about 48 seconds. This intermittent external pneumatic compression system is contraindicated for any patient with acute thrombophlebitis or deep vein thrombosis.

When ambulating the patient, the nurse should disconnect the pump tubing, although sometimes the cuffs are kept in place on the calves. The device should not be disconnected for more than 30 minutes. If the patient has diagnostic examinations that require leaving the nursing unit for longer than 30 minutes, the compression pump, the cuffs or sleeves, and the instructions on operation should travel with the patient.

The treatment should continue for 72 hours postoperatively or until the patient is ambulating well. The cuffs should be removed once a day to assess for impairment of skin integrity and to provide skin care. Document the use of intermittent external pneumatic compression system and any reaction such as numbness or tingling (see Figure 2-5).

Activity

Early ambulation has been a significant factor in hastening postoperative recovery and preventing postoperative complications. Numerous benefits are derived from the exercise of getting in and out of bed and walking during the early postoperative period. Ambulation is usually contraindicated when there is a severe infection or thrombophlebitis (Box 2-10).

Assessment. Before assisting the patient to ambulate for the first few times after major surgery, an assessment is made of the patient's level of alertness to follow directions, cardiovascular status, and motor status:

1. Level of alertness: ask patient simple questions or to follow simple commands.
2. Cardiovascular status.
   a. Assess pulse and respiratory rate and depth while patient is supine, then after sitting.
   b. Observe skin color for pallor while patient is sitting.
   c. Note complaints of vertigo when patient is sitting.
3. Motor status.
   a. Assess muscle strength of patient's legs.
   b. Assess sitting ability.
      (1) Assist patient to sitting position on side of bed.
      (2) Ask patient to maintain an erect position while being gently pushed sideways.

It is also important to know of any preoperative limitations to ambulation. The patient with arthritis or arteriosclerosis may take longer to move and to adjust

Box **2-10** | *Effects of Early Postoperative Ambulation*

- Increased rate and depth of breathing
  Prevention of atelectasis and hypostatic pneumonia
  Increased mental alertness from increased oxygenation to brain
- Increased circulation
  Nutrients required for healing are more available to wound
  Prevention of thrombophlebitis
- Increased micturition (urinary elimination)
  Increased kidney function
  Prevention of urinary retention
- Increased metabolism
  Prevention of loss of muscle tone
  Restoration of nitrogen balance
- Increased peristalsis
  Promotion of expulsion of flatus
  Prevention of abdominal distention and gas pain
  Prevention of constipation
  Prevention of paralytic ileus

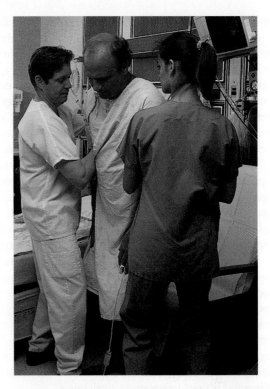

FIGURE **2-17** Progression in levels of postoperative activity promotes tissue perfusion.

to standing and walking. The patient who used a walker preoperatively will need assistance for a longer time before using the walker again. Family members are important in assisting patients with any physical limitation and in providing emotional support during postoperative recovery.

Nursing interventions. Nursing interventions follow:
1. Encourage muscle-strengthening exercises before ambulation:
   a. Have patient bend knees, lower knees, press back of knees hard against bed.
   b. Have patient alternately contract and relax calf and thigh muscles 10 times using the following cycle: contract, relax, rest.
2. Have patient sit on side of bed (legs dangling) to become accustomed to upright position before ambulating the first time. Be sure pulse has stabilized (returned to baseline) before ambulation is attempted.
3. Clamp NG tube while patient ambulates, then reconnect.
4. Keep urinary tube connected to drainage bag; carry bag or pin bag to inside of robe. Keep drainage receptacle below level of bladder to prevent reflux of urine.
5. Attach IV bag to a movable pole.
6. Use two people to assist in ambulating an unsteady patient receiving IV fluids (Figure 2-17).
7. Encourage patient to walk farther at each ambulation.

The word *ambulate* means to move from place to place, to walk. Sitting in a chair is not ambulation. After ambulating, the patient may sit in a chair, but should be advised to stand and walk at intervals and to elevate the legs while sitting to prevent venous pooling in the extremities. Sitting in a chair for long periods is to be avoided.

GASTROINTESTINAL STATUS

Abdominal distention frequently occurs after surgery. Because anesthesia and surgical manipulation slow peristalsis, it may take 3 to 4 days for bowel activity to return. Listening for bowel sounds in the lower abdomen can help gauge the return of function. Normal peristalsis is gauged by hearing 5 to 30 gurgles per minute. When listening for bowel sounds, the nurse should listen for 1 minute. If peristalsis decreases or stops, a **paralytic ileus** (a decrease in or absence of intestinal peristalsis that may occur after abdominal surgery, peritoneal trauma, and severe metabolic disease and other conditions) may have developed. If inactivity continues, an NG or nasointestinal tube to suction is usually ordered to help remove the gas formed in the stomach and small intestine. When listening for bowel sounds in patients who have an NG or nasointestinal tube, the nurse should turn off the suction machine but should *never* leave the room without turning the machine on.

Abdominal distention can be verified by measuring the patient's abdominal girth. Accurate measurement is ensured by marking on the skin the placement for the tape measure, which is at the level of the umbilicus. The nurse should assess and chart the expelling of flatus, bowel sounds, and abdominal girth. Occasionally analgesics (meperidine) and other medications may slow peristalsis; charting the patient's GI habits aids in identifying etiological factors.

Encouraging activity (turning every 2 hours, early ambulation) assists GI activity. A rectal tube may be inserted, or the physician may order an "up and down" flush (Harris flush) to relieve pain from intestinal gas. A Harris flush is a mild colonic irrigation using 100 to 200 mL of enema solution. After instillation, the enema container is lowered and the solution siphoned back into the container. This process may be repeated. For the patient who has difficulty with flatus, limiting iced beverages and encouraging warm liquids may help resolve the discomfort. The patient may have fluids and food withheld until flatus is expelled. As the patient returns to previous eating habits, bowel function slowly resumes its preoperative state. Constipation is also a frequent problem after surgery. The same aids for abdominal distention assist in alleviating constipation. If feces are not passed within 2 to 3 days after the patient has resumed solid foods, a suppository or tap water enema may be ordered. Ambulation is encouraged to promote peristalsis.

Singultus (hiccup) is an involuntary contraction of the diaphragm followed by rapid closure of the glottis. Singultus results from irritation of the phrenic nerve. The condition is seen most often in men. Sedatives may be necessary in extreme cases. Because abdominal distention may be the cause, the nurse assesses the patient's abdomen for proper GI function. Although abdominal distention usually occurs from gas in the intestinal tract, the cause may be internal bleeding. The nurse should evaluate the patient for signs of shock: vital signs, skin condition, and level of consciousness.

FLUIDS AND ELECTROLYTES

Fluid is lost during surgery through blood loss and increased insensible fluid loss through the lungs and skin. For at least the first 24 to 48 hours after surgery, fluids are retained by the body as part of the stress response to trauma and the effect of anesthesia.

Sodium and potassium depletion can occur in the postoperative patient from the loss of blood or body fluids during surgery or the loss of GI secretion by vomiting and through NG tubes. Potassium is also lost during catabolism (tissue breakdown), especially after severe trauma or crush injuries. Loss of gastric secretions can result in chloride loss, producing metabolic alkalosis. Electrolytes are often added to IV solution in the form of potassium chloride (KCl). Potassium may irritate the vein when administered by an IV route. Advise patient that a stinging sensation may occur.

Fluid tolerance and electrolyte values are closely monitored during the postoperative period. When the patient returns from the recovery room, therapy will be in progress. Until the patient is past the nausea and vomiting period and can tolerate oral fluids, parenteral therapy should be maintained. The IV line is observed for patency and ordered fluid rate, and the IV site is monitored for erythema, edema, heat, and pain. Because IV therapy may become infiltrated because of movement or inadvertent dislodgment of the needle when the patient ambulates, the site should be assessed every 1 to 2 hours or when the patient complains of discomfort. The assessment for rate of infusion is extremely important for older patients, who may experience fluid overload and pulmonary edema very quickly.

Muscles and nerves require ongoing nourishment to function adequately, and parenteral fluids contain the necessary glucose and electrolytes. Depending on the type of surgery and nutritional needs of the patient, IV therapy lasts from a few hours to a few days. As long as parenteral fluids are received, the nurse should record the patient's I&O. If there is concern about the patient's overall nutritional state, the patient should be weighed daily.

As oral fluids are introduced, patients should be encouraged to drink small amounts frequently (6 to 8 oz/hr). The nurse reviews the diet history to note fluids normally enjoyed. Unless otherwise ordered, patients usually begin by ingesting clear liquids (7-Up, water, tea, broth, gelatin) and progress as the GI system returns to normal functioning. If the patient has difficulty drinking the amount of fluid recommended, fluids can be offered more frequently and without a straw. (A straw, although convenient, reduces the amount of fluids ingested.) Unless there are other problems (e.g., decreased renal excretion because of renal failure, age), patients should be encouraged to drink 2000 to 2400 mL in 24 hours. Because iced and carbonated beverages cause GI disturbances in some individuals, these fluids should be avoided until active peristalsis is noted. If nausea and vomiting persist, an antiemetic such as promethazine (Phenergan), benzquinamide (Emete-Con), or prochlorperazine (Compazine) is usually ordered to be administered intramuscularly (IM), intravenously, or rectally.

NURSING PROCESS *for the Surgical Patient*

The role of the licensed practical nurse/licensed vocational nurse (LPN/LVN) in the nursing process as stated is that the LPN/LVN will:
- Participate in planning care for patients based on patient needs.
- Review patient's plan of care and recommend revisions as needed.
- Review and follow defined prioritization for patient care.
- Use clinical pathways/care maps/care plans to guide and review patient care.

Assessment

General assessment of the preoperative patient includes obtaining a nursing history. This consists of any prior surgery, allergies, current medications, use of other drugs or alcohol, and smoking status. The nurse also assesses the patient's physical condition, at-risk data, emotional status of the patient and family members, and preoperative diagnostic data. It is important for the patient and family to understand the surgical procedure and the expected outcomes. In the intraoperative stage the nurse completes any procedures such as the skin preparation or catheterization. During surgery and recovery, the nurse continually assesses the patient's condition. The nurse also provides postoperative care to prevent and detect complications and return the patient to wellness.

Nursing Diagnosis

Nursing diagnoses establish direction for care that will be provided during one or all surgical phases. Nursing diagnoses may focus on preoperative, intraoperative, and postoperative risks. Preventive care is essential for effective management of the surgical patient.

See Boxes 2-11 and 2-12 for nursing diagnoses for the preoperative and the postoperative patient.

Box 2-11 *Preoperative Nursing Diagnoses*

Airway clearance, ineffective, related to:
- Diminished cough
- Increased pulmonary congestion

Anxiety, related to:
- Knowledge deficit of impending surgery
- Threat of loss of body part

Coping, compromised family, related to:
- Temporary role change of patient
- Impending severity of surgery

Fear, related to:
- Impending surgery
- Anticipation of postoperative pain

Knowledge, deficient regarding implications of surgery, related to:
- Lack of experience with surgery
- Information misinterpretation

Nutrition, imbalanced: less than body requirements, related to:
- Preoperative malnourishment

Nutrition, imbalanced: more than body requirements, related to:
- Excess intake of food

Powerlessness, related to:
- Emergency nature of surgery

Skin integrity, risk for impaired, related to:
- Preoperative radiation
- Immobilization during surgery

Sleep pattern, disturbed, related to:
- Fear of surgery
- Preoperative hospital routines

Expected Outcomes/Planning

The plan of care begins before surgery and follows through the postoperative period to provide the best nursing interventions possible. It is important for the nurse to include the patient in health care planning. A patient informed about the surgical experience is less likely to be fearful and is better able to prepare for expected outcomes.

Goals and expected outcomes for the surgical patient may include the following:

Goal: Patient achieves physical comfort.

Outcome: Patient verbalizes relief of pain.

Box 2-12 *Postoperative Nursing Diagnoses*

Airway clearance, ineffective, related to:
- Diminished cough
- Retained secretions
- Prolonged sedation

Body temperature, risk for imbalanced, related to:
- Lowered metabolism

Breathing pattern, ineffective, related to:
- Incisional pain
- Analgesia effects on ventilation

Communication, impaired verbal, related to:
- Endotracheal tube placement
- Airway tube placement

Coping, ineffective, related to:
- Constraints imposed by surgery
- Postoperative therapies

Fluid volume, risk for deficient, related to:
- Wound drainage
- Inadequate fluid intake

Grieving, anticipatory, related to:
- Patient's critical condition

Infection, risk for, related to:
- Surgical wound incision
- Presence of Foley catheter and wound drainage tubes

Mobility, impaired physical, related to:
- Pain
- Postoperative activity restrictions
- Casts or dressings
- Surgical incision
- NG tube placement

Oral mucous membrane, impaired, related to:
- Irritation of NG or endotracheal tube
- NPO status

Self-care deficit, bathing/hygiene, dressing/grooming, feeding, toileting, related to:
- Postoperative activity restrictions
- Pain

Skin integrity, risk for impaired, related to:
- Wound exudate
- Impaired mobility
- Decrease in nutritional intake

Implementation

Nursing interventions before surgery physically and psychologically prepare the patient for the surgical procedure. The nurse acts as an advocate for the patient during and after surgery to ensure that the patient's dignity and rights are protected at all times (Nursing Care Plan: Postoperative Patient box).

Evaluation

The effectiveness of the plan of care is evaluated by the nurse. The plan is revised as needed. An example of a goal and an evaluative measure is the following:

Goal: Patient achieves physical comfort.

Evaluative measure: Observe patient for nonverbal signs of discomfort, such as guarding the painful area and grimacing.

DISCHARGE: PROVIDING GENERAL INFORMATION

Preparation for the patient's discharge is an ongoing process throughout the surgical experience that begins during the preoperative period. The informed patient is therefore prepared as events unfold and gradually assumes greater responsibility for self-care during the

---

NURSING CARE PLAN
The Postoperative Patient

Mr. S. is a 40-year-old obese patient weighing 280 pounds, who was admitted with bowel obstruction and a scheduled right hemicolectomy. Mr. S. has hypertension and a history of poor wound healing.

NURSING DIAGNOSIS *Ineffective airway clearance, related to incisional pain*

Patient Goals/Expected Outcomes	Nursing Interventions	Evaluation/Rationale
Patient will cough deeply in 24 hours. Patient's lung sounds will clear after coughing.	Medicate with analgesia to control pain.	Providing pain relief will enable patient to cough and deep breathe without discomfort.
	Raise head of bed to full Fowler's position during exercises.	In Fowler's position the diaphragm falls, which permits lung expansion.
	Splint incision with rolled bath blanket.	Splinting incision provides abdominal support while coughing.
	Have patient turn, cough, and deep breathe every hour while awake.	Turning, coughing, and deep breathing will aid in mobilizing secretions.
	Use incentive spirometer hourly.	Adequate lung expansion can prevent atelectasis.
	Take vital signs q4h and note evidence of dyspnea or restlessness.	
	Monitor IV fluids.	
	Offer sips of fluid every hour if permissible.	Increased fluid intake helps prevent thickening of mucus.

NURSING DIAGNOSIS *Ineffective breathing pattern, related to poor body mechanics*

Patient Goals/Expected Outcomes	Nursing Interventions	Evaluation/Rationale
Patient will effectively use incentive spirometer. Patient's respirations will be even and unlabored.	Encourage deep breathing q 1-2 hr while awake.	Adequate lung expansion can prevent atelectasis.
	Reposition q2h; support joints and incision.	Turning helps promote lung expansion.
	Continue oxygen at 2 L per cannula; cleanse nares q4h; post "No Smoking" sign.	Additional oxygen ensures adequate tissue oxygenation. "No Smoking" signs promote safety.
	Encourage use of incentive spirometer.	Adequate lung expansion can prevent atelectasis.
	Record respirations q4h, noting depth, rate, and quality.	Regular assessments will detect early signs and symptoms of respiratory complications.
	Assess skin and nailbed; report slow blanching color and condition q4h.	A change in color of skin and nailbeds signal poor oxygenation.
	Darken room; decrease stimuli, monitor pain, and offer analgesic prn.	Comfort measures promote rest and relaxation and decrease pain level.

NURSING CARE PLAN

The Postoperative Patient—cont'd

Mr. S. is a 40-year-old obese patient weighing 280 pounds, who was admitted with bowel obstruction and a scheduled right hemicolectomy. Mr. S. has hypertension and a history of poor wound healing.

NURSING DIAGNOSIS *Risk for infection, related to open surgical incision and draining wound*

Patient Goals/Expected Outcomes	Nursing Interventions	Evaluation/Rationale
Patient's wound will not be erythematous or produce purulent exudate. Patient's vital signs will remain within normal range.	Use good handwashing technique.	Handwashing will help prevent transmission of microorganisms.
	Monitor wound q4h, noting amount and color of drainage; assess skin for warmth, color, and sensation.	Regular assessments will reveal early signs and symptoms of wound infection.
	Mark drainage on dressing q4h; reinforce prn.	Containing wound drainage within dressing provides comfort to the patient and enables the nurse to correctly determine the type of drainage.
	Use surgical asepsis when changing dressing.	Surgical asepsis prevents the transmission of microorganisms.
	Monitor vital signs q4h.	Regular assessments of vital signs reveal early signs and symptoms of wound infection
	Monitor white blood cell (WBC) level as ordered.	Elevation of the WBCs indicates an infectious process and its severity.

? CRITICAL THINKING QUESTIONS

1. On the second postoperative day, Mr. S. is taking shallow breaths and is experiencing difficulty in complying with coughing and deep breathing. His temperature is 101.8° F, and he has adventitious breath sounds bilaterally in the bases. List several nursing interventions to assist Mr. S.
2. Mr. S. is in his third postoperative day, and the nurse notes an erythematous incision with moderate amounts of purulent exudate from the Penrose drain site. List the correct nursing interventions.
3. What signs and symptoms would the nurse note when assessing Mr. S. for dehydration secondary to elevated temperature and decreased fluid intake?

---

postoperative period. As the day of discharge approaches, the nurse should be certain that the patient has vital information (Box 2-13).

If the physician has not provided information about particular diet or activity prescriptions or restrictions, the nurse should either obtain this information or encourage the patient to do so. Attention to complete discharge instruction may prevent needless distress for the patient. Written instructions are important for reinforcing verbal information. The nurse should specifically document in the record the discharge instructions provided to the patient and family (Figure 2-18). Information related to patient's mental status (ability to understand importance of teaching for patient and family members should be documented). For the patient, the postoperative phase of care continues and extends into the recuperative period. Assessment and evaluation of the patient after discharge may be accomplished by a follow-up call or by a visit from a home health nurse.

| Box 2-13 | **Vital Information for the Discharged Patient**

- Care of wound site and any dressings
- Action and possible side effects of any medications; when and how to take them
- Activities allowed and prohibited; when various physical activities can be resumed safely (e.g., driving a car, returning to work, sexual intercourse, leisure activities)
- Dietary restrictions or modifications
- Symptoms to be reported (e.g., development of incisional tenderness or increased drainage, discomfort in other parts of the body)
- Where and when to return for follow-up care
- Answers to any individual questions or concerns

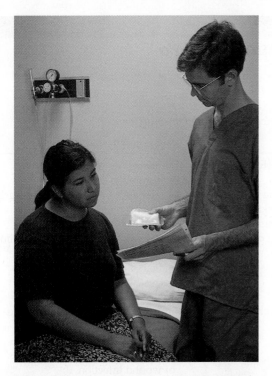

FIGURE **2-18** Reviewing discharge planning instructions.

AMBULATORY SURGERY DISCHARGE

The patient leaving an ambulatory surgery setting must be able to provide a degree of self-care and must be mobile and alert. Postoperative pain and nausea and vomiting must be controlled. Overall, the patient must be stable and near the level of preoperative functioning before discharge from the unit. On discharge, both specific and general instructions are given to the patient and family—verbally and reinforced with written directions. The patient may not drive and must be accompanied by a responsible adult at the time of discharge. A follow-up evaluation of the patient's status is made by telephone, and any specific questions and concerns are addressed.

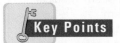
Key Points

- The time before, during, and after surgery is called the perioperative period. It is divided into preoperative, intraoperative, and postoperative phases.
- Perioperative nursing interventions are given to the surgical patient before, during, and after surgery.
- In addition to the nature of nursing interventions provided, previous illness and past surgeries influence the ability to tolerate surgery.

- Older adult patients are at surgical risk from their declining physiologic status.
- All medications taken before surgery are automatically discontinued after surgery unless a physician reorders the medications, except for conditions of long-standing duration such as phenytoin (Dilantin) for seizure control.
- Family members are important in assisting patients with physical limitations and in providing emotional support during the postoperative recovery.
- Preoperative assessment of vital signs and physical findings provides an important baseline with which to compare perioperative and postoperative assessment data.
- A patient's feelings about surgery can have a significant effect on relationships with nursing staff and the patient's ability to participate in care.
- Nursing diagnoses of the surgical patient may pose implications for nursing care during one or all phases of surgery.
- Informed consent should not be obtained if a patient is confused, unconscious, mentally incompetent, or under the influence of sedatives. Know agency policy.
- Structured preoperative teaching positively influences postoperative recovery.
- A routine preoperative checklist is a guide for final preparation of the patient before surgery.
- The responsibility of nurses within the operating room focuses on protecting the patient from potential harm.
- Assessment of the postoperative patient centers on the body systems most likely to be affected by anesthesia, immobilization, and surgical trauma.
- Because a surgical patient's condition may change rapidly during immediate postoperative recovery, the nurse monitors the patient's status at least every 15 minutes.
- The PAC unit nurse reports to the nurse on the postoperative unit information pertaining to the patient's current physical status and risk for postoperative complications.
- From the time of admission, the nurse plans for the surgical patient's discharge.
- Discharge planning identifies home care measures to promote recovery that involve both patient and family.
- Evaluation of all perioperative care is at times difficult, because the patient may be discharged from the nurse's care before the outcome is ready for evaluation.

Go to your free CD-ROM for an Audio Glossary, animations, video clips, and Review Questions for the NCLEX-PN® Examination.

evolve Be sure to visit the companion Evolve site at http://evolve.elsevier.com/Christensen/adult/ for WebLinks and additional online resources.

CHAPTER CHALLENGE

1. Mr. F. has cancer of the larynx and is scheduled for a laryngectomy. This is an example of which type of surgery?

   1. Minor
   2. Elective
   3. Emergency
   4. Major

2. Ms. S. is being discharged, and the nurse is teaching her how to do daily dressing changes at home. The most important point to include in the teaching plan is:

   1. discussion of surgical asepsis.
   2. discussion of hand hygiene.
   3. instruction in sterilization.
   4. demonstration of gloving.

3. To assist Mr. B. in the prevention of postoperative pulmonary complications, preoperatively the nurse should:

   1. ask his physician to prescribe IPPB treatment.
   2. teach him to do leg exercises.
   3. teach him to use an incentive spirometer.
   4. tell him that if he does not cough, he may need to be suctioned.

4. Mr. T. has undergone surgery for lysis of adhesions. He is transferred from the PAC unit to his own room on the surgical floor. In the immediate postoperative period, when he is received on the surgical floor, the nurse should obtain blood pressure, pulse, and respiration every:

   1. 15 minutes.
   2. 5 minutes.
   3. 20 minutes.
   4. 30 minutes.

5. The nurse is assessing the bowel sounds of her patient, Mr. J., who had a suprapubic prostatectomy 2 days ago. To correctly assess that he does not have bowel sounds present, the nurse would need to auscultate each quadrant for:

   1. 1 minute.
   2. 3 minutes.
   3. 10 minutes.
   4. 15 minutes.

6. Ms. C. is recovering from a right lobectomy. The nurse is going to assist in splinting her incision so she can cough and breathe deeply. The most therapeutic administration of an analgesic for Ms. C. would be:

   1. after the procedure so she can rest.
   2. 15 minutes before the procedure.
   3. 1 hour before the procedure.
   4. 30 minutes before the procedure.

7. A patient reports having an allergy to penicillin. Which of the following questions would elicit the most useful information for the nurse?

   1. When did the reaction occur?
   2. What infection did you have that required penicillin?
   3. What type of allergic reaction did you have?
   4. Did you notify your physician of the allergy?

8. Which patient is at greatest risk for surgical and anesthetic complications?

   1. A 3-year-old boy scheduled for a hernia repair
   2. An 80-year-old scheduled for an exploratory laparotomy
   3. An 18-year-old scheduled for an emergency appendectomy
   4. A 42-year-old scheduled for a breast biopsy

9. Mr. J., an alert 75-year-old, is to undergo elective surgery. The operative permit must be signed in the presence of a witness by:

   1. Mr. J.
   2. Mr. and Mrs. J.
   3. either Mr. or Mrs. J.
   4. Mr. J. and the surgeon.

10. A nursing intervention to assist the patient in coping with fear of pain would be to:

    1. describe the degree of pain expected.
    2. explain the availability of pain medication.
    3. inform the patient of the frequency of pain medication.
    4. divert the patient when talking about pain.

11. The patient tells the nurse that "blowing into this tube thing [incentive spirometer] is a ridiculous waste of time." The nurse explains that the specific purpose of the therapy is to:

    1. directly remove excess secretions from the lungs.
    2. increase pulmonary circulation.
    3. promote lung expansion.
    4. stimulate the cough reflex.

12. When preparing the patient for surgery, the nurse should:

    1. provide the patient with sips of water for a dry mouth.
    2. remove the patient's makeup and nail polish.
    3. remove the patient's gown before transport to the operating room.
    4. leave all of the patient's jewelry intact.

13. A patient who is being prepped for surgery asks the nurse to explain the purpose of the medications (Demerol and Vistaril) he has been given. The nurse should inform the patient that these particular medications:

    1. reduce preoperative fear.
    2. promote gastric emptying.
    3. reduce body secretions.
    4. facilitate the induction of the anesthesia.

14. A patient who receives general or regional anesthesia in an ambulatory surgery center:

    1. will remain in the unit longer than a hospitalized patient.
    2. is allowed to ambulate as soon as being admitted to the recovery area.
    3. must be near the level of preoperative functioning before dismissal.
    4. is immediately given liberal amounts of fluid to promote the excretion of the anesthesia.

Continued

15. Following abdominal surgery, the patient is suspected of having internal bleeding. Which of the following findings is most indicative of this complication?

    1. Increased blood pressure
    2. Incisional pain
    3. Abdominal distention
    4. Increased urinary output

16. An obese patient is at risk for poor wound healing postoperatively because:

    1. ventilatory capacity is reduced.
    2. fatty tissue has a poor blood supply.
    3. risk for dehiscence is increased.
    4. resuming normal physical activity is delayed.

17. The nurse should ask each patient preoperatively for the name and dosage of all prescription and over-the-counter medications, including herbal remedies, taken before surgery because they:

    1. may cause allergies to develop.
    2. are automatically ordered postoperatively.
    3. may create greater risk for complications or interact with anesthetic agents.
    4. should be taken the morning of surgery with sips of water.

18. A patient who smokes two packs of cigarettes per day is most at risk postoperatively for:

    1. infection.
    2. pneumonia.
    3. hypotension.
    4. cardiac dysrhythmias.

19. Family members should be included when the nurse teaches the patient preoperative exercises so that they can:

    1. supervise the patient at home.
    2. coach the patient postoperatively.
    3. practice with the patient while waiting to be taken to the operating room.
    4. relieve the nurse by getting the patient to exercise every 2 hours.

20. When the patient is deep breathing and coughing it is important to have the patient sitting because this position:

    1. facilitates expansion of the thorax.
    2. is more comfortable.
    3. increases the patient's view of the room and is more relaxing.
    4. helps the patient to splint with a pillow.

3 Care of the Patient with an Integumentary Disorder

LINDA Y. NORTH

Objectives

After reading this chapter, the student should be able to do the following:

Anatomy and Physiology

1. Define the key terms as listed.
2. Discuss the primary functions of the integumentary system.
3. Describe the differences between the epidermis and dermis.
4. Discuss the functions of the three major glands located in the skin.

Medical-Surgical

5. Define the key terms as listed.
6. Discuss the general assessment of the skin.
7. Identify general nursing interventions for the patient with a skin disorder.
8. Discuss how to use the nursing process in caring for patients with skin disorders.
9. Discuss the viral disorders of the skin.
10. Discuss the bacterial, fungal, and inflammatory disorders of the skin.
11. Identify the parasitic disorders of the skin.
12. Describe the common tumors of the skin.
13. Identify the disorders associated with the appendages of the skin.
14. State the pathophysiology involved in a burn injury.
15. Discuss the stages of burn care with appropriate nursing interventions.
16. Identify the methods used to classify the extent of a burn injury.

Key Terms

Be sure to check out the bonus material on the free CD-ROM, including selected audio pronunciations.

alopecia (ăl-ō-PĒ-shē-ă, p. 102)
autograft (AW-tō-grăft, p. 110)
contracture (kŏn-TRĂK-chŭr, p. 107)
Curling's ulcer (KŬR-lingz ŬL-sĕr, p. 107)
debridement (dă-BRĒD-mŏń, p. 109)
eschar (ĔS-kăr, p. 109)
excoriation (ĕks-kŏr-ē-Ā-shŭn, p. 79)
exudate (ĔKS-ū-dāt, p. 76)
heterograft (xenograft) (HĔT-ĕr-ō-grăft; ZĒ-nō-grăft, p. 110)

homograft (allograft) (HŌ-mō-grăft; ĂL-ō-grăft, p. 110)
keloids (KĒ-loidz, p. 99)
macules (MĂK-ūlz, p. 83)
nevi (NĒ-vī, p. 99)
papules (PĂP-ūlz, p. 87)
pediculosis (pĕ-dīk-ū-LŌ-sĭs, p. 97)
pruritus (proo-RĪ-tŭs, p. 68)
pustulant vesicles (PŬS-tū-lănt VĔS-ĭ-kŭlz, p. 83)
rule of nines (p. 105)
suppuration (sūp-ū-RĀ-shŭn, p. 85)
urticaria (ŭr-tĭ-KĀ-rē-ă, p. 89)
verruca (vĕ-ROO-ka, p. 99)
vesicle (VĔS-ĭ-k'l, p. 75)
wheals (wēlz, p. 89)

The skin, or **integument,** a major organ, is the outer covering of the body, and together with its appendages—hair, nails, and special glands—makes up the integumentary system. Skin is essential to life. Society has long held healthy skin in high esteem, probably because it is so easily viewed by others. People spend many hours grooming their hair, cleansing their skin, and manicuring their nails. A closer look reveals that the integument is really the body's protector—its first line of defense against infection and injury. The skin is pliable yet tough; it resists abrasions, and, as it wears, it is constantly renewed from layers directly beneath it. It also insulates and cushions deeper organs. It prevents loss of body fluids and regulates body temperature. The skin also is the body's sensory contact with the environment because it is sensitive to heat, cold, touch, pressure, and pain.

OVERVIEW OF ANATOMY AND PHYSIOLOGY

FUNCTIONS OF THE SKIN

Although the skin covers the outside of the body, its main function is homeostasis and protection of the internal organs. Each day it is subjected to temperature and humidity changes, trauma, ecchymosis, abrasions, contact with pathogens, and wear and tear. In an attempt to protect and maintain the body, the skin carries out the functions listed in Box 3-1.

Box 3-1 *Functions of the Skin*

PROTECTION FROM THE ENVIRONMENT
- Pathogenic organisms, foreign substances, natural barrier against infection
- Temperature regulation
- Prevention of dehydration
- Excretion of waste products
- Vitamin D synthesis

Protection

Within the skin are sensory receptors that receive information about the environment. Messages about heat, cold, pressure, and touch are received and relayed to the central nervous system for interpretation. Healthy skin protects the body from absorbing many chemicals and foreign substances. Additionally, as long as it remains intact, skin provides protection from many microorganisms in the environment. Internal organs are cushioned and protected by a subcutaneous layer of adipose (fat) tissue. The skin aids in elimination of waste products, prevents dehydration, and serves as a reservoir for food and water.

Temperature Regulation

Skin assists the body in maintaining a constant temperature under varying internal and external conditions. It accomplishes this by allowing blood vessels near the surface to constrict when the environment is cold to preserve heat and allowing them to dilate when it is hot to release excess body heat. Sweat glands release moisture, which results in cooling as the moisture evaporates. A layer of adipose tissue works as an insulator by retaining heat.

Vitamin D Synthesis

Cholesterol compounds located in the skin are converted to vitamin D when exposed to the ultraviolet rays of the sun. This vitamin is necessary for healthy bone development. Prolonged exposure to the sun's rays, which is ultraviolet radiation, should be avoided because of the increased possibility of developing skin cancer.

STRUCTURE OF THE SKIN

Skin consists of two layers: the outer **epidermis** and inner dermis, or corium. Beneath these layers of skin lies the subcutaneous layer, or superficial fascia (Figure 3-1).

Epidermis

The **epidermis** (the superficial fascia [avascular layers of the skin] made up of an outer, dead, cornified portion and a deep, living cellular portion) is composed of stratified squamous (from the Latin *squama,* meaning "scale") epithelium. It is divided into layers, or strata.

The cells of the epidermis are tightly packed and have no distinct blood supply. The inner layer is called the **stratum germinativum;** it is the only layer of the epidermis able to undergo cell division and reproduce itself. It receives its blood supply and nutrition from the underlying dermis through a process called **diffusion.** This provides a constant new supply of cells for the upper layers and enables the skin to repair itself from injury. As these cells are pushed to the surface, they undergo a series of changes. The internal structures of the cells are destroyed and the cells die. When they reach the outermost layer, called the **stratum corneum,** they are flat and the cell structure is filled with a protein called **keratin** (horn), sometimes called the horny layer. The keratin makes the cells dry, tough, and somewhat waterproof. Another layer in the epidermis contains highly specialized cells called **melanocytes;** these cells give rise to the pigment called **melanin** (a black or dark brown pigment occurring naturally in the hair, skin, iris, and choroid of the eye), which is responsible for the skin's color. The greater the concentration of melanin, the darker the skin. Sometimes irregular patches of concentrations of melanin occur, producing "freckles." The amount of melanin a person has is inherited from the parents. Although skin color is inherited, exposure to the sun and other extraneous factors can influence skin color.

Dermis

The **dermis,** or **corium,** is often called the true skin. It is well supplied with blood vessels and nerves and also contains glands and hair follicles. It varies in thickness throughout the body but tends to be thickest in the palms and soles. The dermis is composed of connective tissue with cells scattered among collagen and elastic fibers. The collagen gives strength to the dermis, whereas the elastic connective fibers give it flexibility. The cells throughout this layer are bathed in tissue fluid called interstitial fluid. With the normal aging process, the dermis loses some of its elastic connective fibers, and the subcutaneous tissue directly beneath it loses some of its adipose tissue; wrinkling of the skin results. Located in the upper portion of the dermis are small fingerlike projections called **papillae** that project into the lower epidermal layer. Without the dermal papillae, the epidermal layer would be unable to survive.

Subcutaneous Layer

The subcutaneous layer, sometimes called the **superficial fascia,** is the layer of tissue directly beneath the dermis that connects the skin to the muscle surface. This layer is composed of adipose tissue and loose connective tissue. It serves the following several important functions: (1) stores water and fat, (2) insulates the body, (3) protects the organs lying beneath it, and (4) provides a pathway for nerves and blood vessels. The distribution of subcutaneous tissue throughout

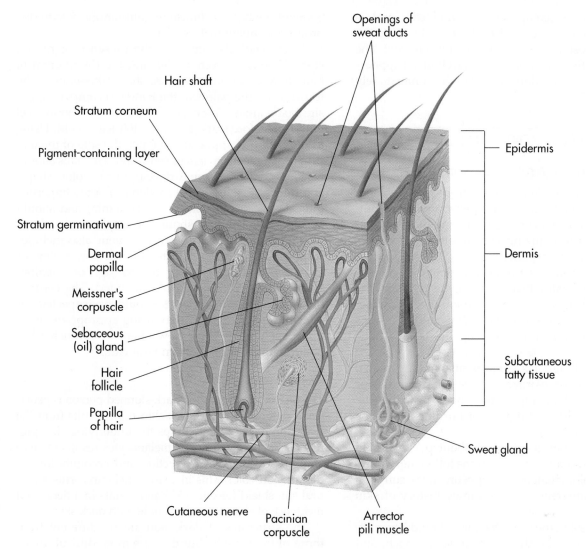

FIGURE **3-1** Structures of the skin.

the body provides shape and contour. A woman's body usually contains more subcutaneous tissue than a man's; thus her body is softer and more rounded.

APPENDAGES OF THE SKIN
Sudoriferous Glands

The **sudoriferous** (sweat) **glands** are coiled tubelike structures located in the dermis and subcutaneous layers. The tubes open into pores on the skin surface. There are approximately 3 million sweat glands located throughout the integumentary system. These glands excrete sweat, which cools the body's surface. Sweat is composed of water, salts, urea, uric acid, ammonia, sugar, lactic acid, and ascorbic acid.

Ceruminous Glands

Ceruminous glands are modified sudoriferous glands. They secrete a waxlike substance called **cerumen** and are located in the external ear canal. It is thought that cerumen protects the canal from foreign body invasion.

Sebaceous Glands

The **sebaceous** (oil) **glands** secrete their substance, **sebum** (an oily secretion), through the hair follicles distributed on the body. Their function is to lubricate the skin and hair that covers the body. Sebum also inhibits bacteria growth.

Hair and Nails

Hair is composed of modified dead epidermal tissue, mainly keratin. It is distributed all over the body in varying amounts. The root of the hair is enclosed in a follicle deep in the dermis. The shaft of the hair protrudes from the skin. Surrounding the hair follicle is a band of muscle tissue called **arrector pili** (see Figure 3-1). A sensation of cold or fear causes these muscles to contract, making the hair stand upright and dimpling the skin surrounding it. The effect is called piloerection, or "gooseflesh."

Nails are also composed mainly of keratin, but the keratin is more closely compressed. The base of the nail—the root—is composed of living cells and is mostly covered by the cuticle. Part of the root, the lunula, is exposed and looks like a white crescent. The remainder of the nail is called the **nail body.** It appears pink because of the blood vessels lying immediately beneath it.

ASSESSMENT OF THE SKIN

INSPECTION AND PALPATION

A thorough assessment of the skin helps identify many diseases that result if the skin is penetrated by an outside organism. However, the beginning nurse should remember that recognizing skin conditions by inspection takes time and experience.

The nurse should begin the assessment by obtaining a careful health history from the patient. The nurse should ask the patient about the following: (1) recent skin lesions or rashes, (2) where the lesions first appeared, and (3) how long the lesions have been present.

The nurse should ask the patient about a personal or family history of asthma, seasonal rhinitis, or drug allergies. All complaints of pain, pruritus (the symptom of itching), tingling, or burning should be explored.

The patient should be asked about personal skin care. The nurse should ask about the following: (1) any recent skin color changes, (2) exposure in the sun with or without sunscreen, and (3) family history of skin cancer.

When assessing the skin, the nurse should have natural lighting and use the senses of sight, touch, and smell while inspecting and palpating the skin. The area to be assessed needs to be exposed for the nurse to view while maintaining privacy. It is important for the nurse to remember to wear gloves when inspecting the skin, mucous membranes, and any involved area. The morning bath provides an excellent opportunity for the nurse to assess the patient's skin without exposure or embarrassment.

Nurses should observe the skin for color. The color of the skin depends on many physiological factors, including the following:
- Amount of hemoglobin in the blood
- Oxygen saturation in the blood
- Amount of substances such as bilirubin, urea, or other chemicals in the blood
- Quality and quantity of blood circulating in the superficial blood vessels
- Amount of melanin in the epidermis

Assessment of specific skin lesions, their appearance, and location assists the dermatologist to diagnose skin disorders and the nurse to provide care. Most disorders have only one or two types of lesions.

Some of the typical clinical manifestations of skin disorders are shown in Table 3-1.

Assessment also includes the presence of rashes, scars, lesions, or ecchymoses and the distribution of hair. Temperature and texture should be assessed by touch using the palms of the hands to compare opposite body areas. For example, the nurse should feel both legs before stating that the left leg is cold. Using a cotton-tipped applicator to touch the sole of the foot provides a means to assess sensation. The nails should be inspected for normal development, color, shape, and thickness. Clubbing (broadening) of the fingertips indicates decreased oxygen (hypoxemia) and should be reported. The hair should be inspected for thickness, dryness, or dullness. Assessment also includes inspecting the mucous membranes for pallor or cyanosis. Profuse sweating or any sign of impaired skin integrity needs to be documented. The ceruminous and sebaceous glands should be inspected for overactivity or underactivity using appropriate questions, such as, "Tell me how often the physician has had to remove the wax from your ears."

Assessment of Dark Skin

The degree of color of the dark-skinned person is genetically determined. The dark skin color results from the reflection of light as it strikes the underlying skin pigment. Increased activity of melanocytes results in large amounts of melanin production and accounts for the darker skin color. This increased melanin forms a natural sun shield for dark skin and results in a decreased incidence of skin cancer in people with dark skin.

The structures of dark skin are no different from those of lighter skin, but they are more difficult to assess. Practice and comparison are necessary. Assessment of color is more easily made in areas where the epidermis is thin, such as the lips and mucous membranes. Rashes are often difficult to observe and may need to be palpated.

Dark skin is predisposed to certain skin conditions, including pseudofolliculitis, keloids, and mongolian spots. Because of the darkness of the skin of some individuals, color often cannot be used as an indicator of systemic conditions (e.g., flushed skin with fever) (Cultural and Ethnic Considerations box).

CHIEF COMPLAINT

When skin lesions are found accompanying a skin disorder, the exact location, length, width, general appearance, and name should be documented. The nurse should assess the chief complaint, including the (1) provocative and palliative factors (things that cause the condition), (2) quality or quantity (characteristics and size) of the skin problem, (3) specific region of the body, (4) severity of the signs and symptoms, and (5) length of time the patient has had the disorder. A

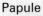 **Table 3-1** *Primary Skin Lesions*

DESCRIPTION	EXAMPLES		
Macule A flat, circumscribed area that is a change in the color of the skin; less than 1 cm in diameter	Freckles, flat moles (nevi), petechiae, measles, scarlet fever	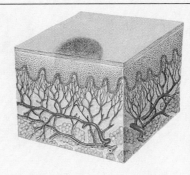	Measles[a]
Papule An elevated, firm, circumscribed area less than 1 cm in diameter	Wart (verruca), elevated moles, lichen planus	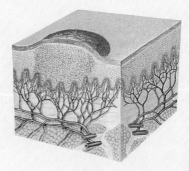	Lichen planus[b]
Patch A flat, nonpalpable, irregularly shaped macule more than 1 cm in diameter	Vitiligo, port-wine stains, mongolian spots, café-au-lait spot	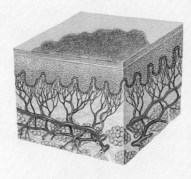	Vitiligo[b]
Plaque Elevated, firm, and rough lesion with flat top surface greater than 1 cm in diameter	Psoriasis, seborrheic and actinic keratoses	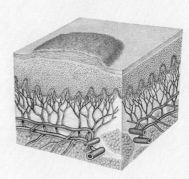 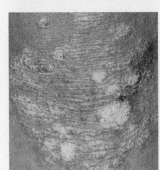	Plaque[a]

Modified from Thompson, J. & Wilson, S. (1995). *Health assessment for nursing practice.* St. Louis: Mosby.
Sources: [a]Habif, T.P. (1996). *Clinical dermatology.* (3rd ed.). St. Louis: Mosby; [b]Weston, W.L., et al. (1996). *Color textbook of pediatric dermatology.* St. Louis: Mosby.

Continued

Table 3-1 | *Primary Skin Lesions—cont'd*

DESCRIPTION	EXAMPLES		
Wheal Elevated irregularly shaped area of cutaneous edema; solid, transient; variable diameter	Insect bites, urticaria, allergic reaction	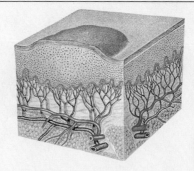	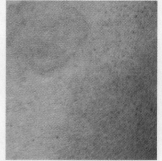 Wheal[c]
Nodule Elevated, firm, circumscribed lesion; deeper in dermis than a papule; 1 to 2 cm in diameter	Erythema nodosum, lipomas	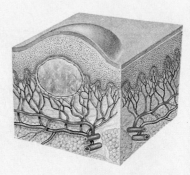	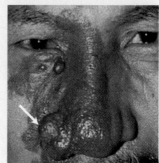 Hypertrophic nodule[d]
Tumor Elevated and solid lesion; may or may not be clearly demarcated; deeper in dermis; greater than 2 cm in diameter	Neoplasms, benign tumor, lipoma, hemangioma	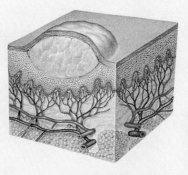	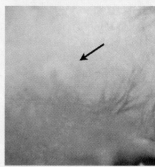 Hemangioma[b]
Vesicle Elevated, circumscribed, superficial, not into dermis; filled with serous fluid; less than 1 cm in diameter	Varicella (chickenpox), herpes zoster (shingles)	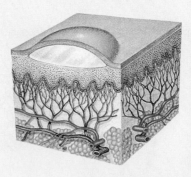	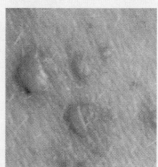 Vesicles caused by varicella[c]

Sources: [b]Weston, W.L., et al. (1996). *Color textbook of pediatric dermatology.* St. Louis: Mosby; [c]Farrar, W.E., et al. *Infectious diseases,* (2nd ed.). London: Gower; [d]Goldman, M.P. & Fitzpatrick, R.E. (1994). *Cutaneous laser surgery: the art and science of selective photo thermolysis.* St. Louis: Mosby.

Table 3-1 *Primary Skin Lesions—cont'd*

DESCRIPTION	EXAMPLES		
Bulla Vesicle greater than 1 cm in diameter	Blister, pemphigus vulgaris		Blister[e]
Pustule Elevated, superficial lesion; similar to a vesicle but filled with purulent fluid	Impetigo, acne		Acne[b]
Cyst Elevated, circumscribed, encapsulated lesion; in dermis or subcutaneous layer; filled with liquid or semisolid material	Sebaceous cyst, cystic acne		Sebaceous cyst[b]
Telangiectasia Fine, irregular red lines produced by capillary dilation	Telangiectasia in rosacea		Telangiectasia[d]

Sources: [b]Weston, W.L. et al. (1996). *Color textbook of pediatric dermatology.* St. Louis: Mosby; [d]Goldman, M.P. & Fitzpatrick, R.E. (1994). *Cutaneous laser surgery: the art and science of selective photo thermolysis.* St. Louis: Mosby; [e]White, G.M. (1994). *Color atlas of regional dermatology.* St. Louis: Mosby.

Continued

Table 3-1 *Primary Skin Lesions—cont'd*

DESCRIPTION	EXAMPLES		
Scale Heaped-up keratinized cells; flaky skin; irregular; thick or thin; dry or oily; variation in size	Flaking of skin with seborrheic dermatitis following scarlet fever, or flaking of skin following a drug reaction; dry skin	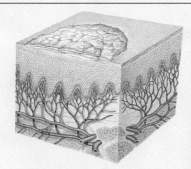	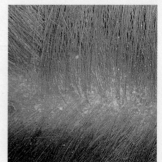 Fine scaling[f]
Lichenification Rough, thickened epidermis secondary to persistent rubbing, itching, or skin irritation; often involves flexor surface of extremity	Chronic dermatitis	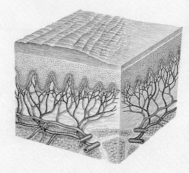	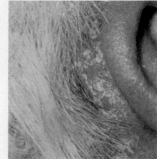 Stasis dermatitis in an early stage[g]
Keloid Irregularly shaped, elevated, progressively enlarging scar; grows beyond the boundaries of the wound; caused by excessive collagen formation during healing	Keloid formation following surgery	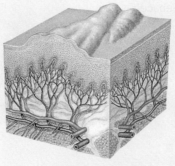	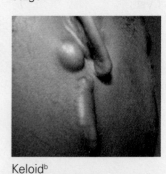 Keloid[b]
Scar Thin to thick fibrous tissue that replaces normal skin following injury or laceration to the dermis	Healed wound or surgical incision	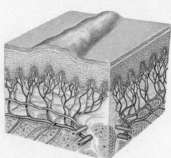	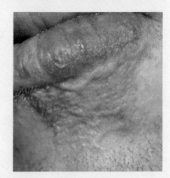 Hypertrophic scar[d]

Sources: [b]Weston, W.L., et al. (1996). *Color textbook of pediatric dermatology.* St. Louis: Mosby; [d]Goldman, M.P. & Fitzpatrick, R.E. (1994). *Cutaneous laser surgery: the art and science of selective photo thermolysis.* St. Louis: Mosby; [f]Baran, R. et al. (1991). *Color atlas of the hair, scalp, and nails.* St. Louis: Mosby; [g]Marks, J.G., Jr & DeLeo, V.A. (1991). *Contact and occupational dermatitis.* St. Louis: Mosby.

Table 3-1 *Primary Skin Lesions—cont'd*

DESCRIPTION	EXAMPLES		
Excoriation Loss of the epidermis; linear hollowed-out crusted area	Abrasion or scratch, scabies	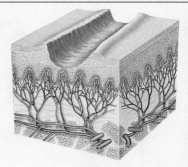	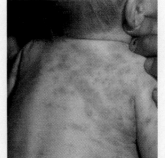Scabies[b]
Fissure Linear crack or break from the epidermis to the dermis; may be moist or dry	Athlete's foot, cracks at the corner of the mouth	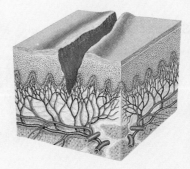	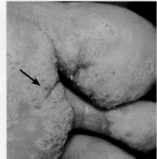Fissures[d]
Erosion Loss of part of the epidermis; depressed, moist, glistening; follows rupture of a vesicle or bulla	Varicella, variola after rupture	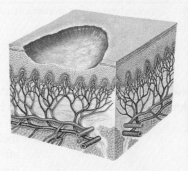	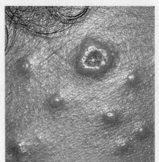Erosion[h]
Ulcer Loss of epidermis and dermis; concave; varies in size	Pressure sores, stasis ulcers	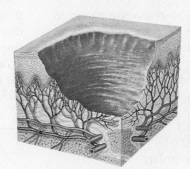	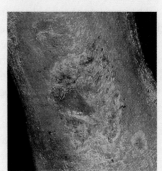Stasis ulcer[a]

Sources: [a]Habif, T.P. (1996). *Clinical dermatology.* (3rd ed.). St. Louis: Mosby; [b]Weston, W.L., et al. (1996). *Color textbook of pediatric dermatology.* St. Louis: Mosby; [d]Goldman, M.P. & Fitzpatrick, R.E. (1994). *Cutaneous laser surgery: the art and science of selective photo thermolysis.* St. Louis: Mosby; [h]Cohen, B.A. (1993). *Pediatric dermatology.* London: Wolfe.

Continued

Table 3-1 *Primary Skin Lesions—cont'd*

DESCRIPTION	EXAMPLES	
Crust Dried serum, blood, or purulent exudate; slightly elevated; size varies; brown, red, black, tan, or straw. Scab on abrasion; eczema	Scab on abrasion, eczema	 Scab[g]
Atrophy Thinning of skin surface and loss of skin markings; skin translucent and paperlike	Striae; aged skin	 Aged skin[g]

Source: [g]Marks, J.G., Jr & DeLeo, V.A. (1991). *Contact and occupational dermatitis.* St. Louis: Mosby.

helpful way to remember to assess the chief complaint is to remember the following letters:

P—Provocative/palliative

Q—Quality/quantity

R—Region

S—Severity

T—Time

An important objective in skin assessment is to identify possible malignancies. The three most common are melanoma, basal cell carcinoma, and squamous cell carcinoma. When assessing growths or changes in a mole, the nurse should ask the following questions, which can be recalled by using the mnemonic device **ABCDE:**

A: Is the mole **A**symmetrical?

B: Are the **B**orders irregular?

C: Is the **C**olor uneven or irregular?

D: Has the **D**iameter of the growth changed recently?

E: Has the surface area become **E**levated?

A positive finding of any of these characteristics should be promptly reported to a physician.

When the assessment is complete, the nurse should document the findings. Proper assessment and identification serve as a baseline for the nurse to make evaluations of nursing care and determine if changes need to be made.

Additionally, the nurse should acknowledge and include in the general assessment the psychological effect an integumentary disorder may have on the patient. In Western culture, well-cared-for skin is a psychological, physiological, and social asset. Every patient with an integumentary disorder has a potential threat to emotional security. Therefore the nurse should assess the interaction of the patient with family and others. Nonverbal behavior such as covering the involved area at all cost and poor eye contact may yield data to support a potential self-image problem.

PSYCHOSOCIAL ASSESSMENT

The person with an integumentary disorder may have a chronic or acute condition. Regardless of the severity, recovery may be lengthy because no outward improvement may be seen by the patient or others. A person's body image and self-esteem may be affected. Society's reaction to a skin condition has a significant effect on the patient. Personal appearance is a primary

Skin Care

- The darker the person's skin, the more difficult it is to assess for changes in color. A baseline needs to be established in natural lighting if possible or with at least a 60-watt lightbulb.
- Baseline skin color should be assessed in areas with the least pigmentation. Examples are palms of the hands, soles of the feet, underside of forearms, abdomen, and buttocks.
- All skin colors have an underlying red tone. Pallor in black-skinned individuals is seen as ashen or gray. Pallor in brown-skinned individuals appears as a yellowish color. Nurses need to assess pallor in mucous membranes, lips, nailbeds, and conjunctivae of the lower eyelids.
- To assess rashes and skin inflammation in dark-skinned individuals, the nurse should rely on *palpation* for warmth and *induration* rather than observation.
- Some folk remedies may be misdiagnosed as injuries. Three folk practices of Southeast Asia can leave marks on the body that can be mistaken for signs of abuse or violence. *Cao gio* is the rubbing of the skin with a coin to produce dark blood or ecchymotic strips; it is done to treat a thrombus or the symptoms of the flu. *Bat gio* is skin pinching on the temples to treat headaches or on the neck for a sore throat. The treatment is considered a success if petechiae or ecchymosis appears. *Paua* is the burning of the skin with the tip of a dried weedlike grass: It is believed the burning will cause the noxious element that causes the pain to leave the body.

concern to many individuals, and others may think the condition is infectious and may socially isolate the patient because of the condition's appearance. The effect of an integumentary disorder on a patient's self-concept can be detrimental because of the value society places on a person's physical characteristics.

The nurse needs to assess the patient's coping abilities by encouraging him or her to talk and ventilate feelings. Open-ended questions are used to facilitate communication. The nurse should validate or correct a patient's knowledge base. Rarely are skin diseases fatal, and few are contagious. Nurses need to have worked through their own feelings about a patient's skin appearance before they can be a source of encouragement. The nurse's attitude and interventions should be nonjudgmental, warm, and accepting. The nurse must be skilled and knowledgeable about skin care.

Anxiety may be a problem in a patient with a skin disorder. Nurses may decrease a patient's anxiety by implementing the following interventions:

- Provide patients with consistent information related to their plan of care.
- Include the family in the treatment plan. The family may be able to support instructions given, which helps to decrease anxiety.
- Provide positive feedback to the patient concerning the patient's efforts and progress no matter how large or small. Referral to a support group should be done as soon as possible if appropriate.

VIRAL DISORDERS OF THE SKIN

HERPES SIMPLEX
Etiology/Pathophysiology

The herpetovirus *Herpesvirus hominis* is the cause of the herpes simplex virus. Two types of the virus are known. Type 1, the most common, causes the common cold sore and is usually associated with febrile conditions. The virus is self-limiting with no cure.

Type 2 causes lesions in the genital area and is known as genital herpes. Type 2 is the same virus as type 1 and is discussed with sexually transmitted diseases in Chapter 12.

Transmissions of both types of virus may occur by direct contact with any open lesion. However, in type 2, the primary mode is through sexual contact. The lesions are usually present for 2 to 3 weeks and are the most painful during the first week. Complications may be severe if the disease spreads to other body areas.

Clinical Manifestations

Type 1 herpes simplex is characterized by a vesicle (circumscribed elevation of skin filled with serous fluid; smaller than 0.5 cm) at the corner of the mouth, on the lips, or on the nose. It is commonly known as a cold sore (Figure 3-2). The involved area is usually erythematous and edematous. The vesicle then appears, ulcerates, and encrusts. When the vesicle ruptures, a burning pain is felt. General malaise and fatigue are expressed by the patient. Usual occurrence is during an acute illness or infection.

Type 2, genital herpes, produces various types of vesicles that rupture and encrust, causing ulcerations. The cervix is the most common site in women, and the penis is the most common area in men. Flulike symptoms occur 3 to 4 days after the vesicles erupt. Headache, fatigue, myalgia, elevated temperature, and anorexia are common.

Assessment

Assessment primarily involves inspection of the skin. The nurse must obtain a complete health history to support assessment data. Collection of subjective data

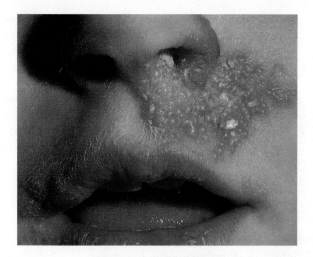

FIGURE **3-2** Herpes simplex.

will include complaints of fatigue, pruritus in the mouth for herpes simplex type 1 and in the genital area for herpes simplex type 2, and complaints of a burning pain in the involved area.

Collection of **objective data** for herpes simplex type 1 includes an edematous, erythematous area at the corner of the lip. In herpes simplex type 2, the labia, vulva, or penis will appear edematous and erythematous. The vesicular lesions may rupture and develop a dried exudate (fluid, cells, or other substances that have been slowly exuded, or discharged, from cells or blood vessels through small pores or breaks in cell membranes).

Diagnostic Tests
Diagnosis of herpesvirus is made by laboratory assessment of cultures from the lesion. Inspection and health history also support the diagnosis.

Medical Management
There is no cure for the herpesvirus, but treatment is aimed at relieving symptoms. Acyclovir (Zovirax) is an antiviral agent that can alter the course of the disease. Acyclovir can be administered orally, topically, or intravenously (Medications for the Integumentary System table).

Nursing Interventions and Patient Teaching
Nursing interventions are primarily directed toward treatment of symptoms and prevention of the spread of the disease. Warm compresses can be used to relieve pain and severe pruritus. The lesions should be kept dry and direct contact avoided. Analgesics such as acetaminophen (Tylenol) are effective in pain control. The specific nursing diagnoses for herpes are based on assessment data gathered.

Nursing diagnoses and interventions for the patient with herpes include but are not limited to the following:

NURSING DIAGNOSES	NURSING INTERVENTIONS
Pain, related to pruritus	Assess factors that precipitate pruritus. Apply local anesthetic, such as Orabase, for pain. Apply drying agent to lesions. Apply warm compresses. Have patient wear loose-fitting cotton clothing that will not constrict movement or occlude circulation.
Impaired skin integrity, related to open lesions	Inspect lesions for drainage, color, and location. Wash hands before and after contact. Keep area dry. Administer antiviral agents as ordered. In genital herpes, use of a hair dryer can promote drying of the lesions and patient comfort.
Risk for infection related to skin excoriation	Body substance precautions Teach patient proper skin care. Wash hands before and after care. Keep area dry. Administer antiviral drugs as ordered.

The prevention of infection remains the number one priority of care when caring for a patient with an open skin lesion. Patient teaching focuses on the principles of medical asepsis and includes specific measures to prevent spread of the disease. Using good hygiene in all areas of care is critical in preventing secondary infections. The complications and precipitating factors should be included in patient teaching as well as discharge planning.

Prognosis
There is no cure for the herpesvirus. Unfortunately, 75% of all patients have at least one recurrence, but it is milder and of shorter duration than the primary infection.
- **Type 1** Herpes simplex: Healing within 10 to 14 days. May recur with depression of the immune system.
- **Type 2** Genital herpes: Lesions usually present 7 to 14 days. Approximately two thirds of infected individuals will have one to five recurrences annually.

MEDICATIONS | *The Integumentary System*

MEDICATION	TRADE NAME	ACTION	SIDE EFFECTS	NURSING IMPLICATIONS
Acyclovir	Zovirax	Antiviral	Topical—burning, rash, pruritus, stinging	Topical—use glove to apply, cover lesion completely
			Systemic—headache, seizures, renal toxicity, phlebitis at IV site	Systemic—ensure adequate hydration to prevent crystallization in kidneys, administer IV dose for at least 1 hour
Alpha-Keri	Same	Emollient	Local irritation, allergic reactions	For external use only, exercise caution when using in tub to avoid slipping
Aluminum acetate solution	Burow's solution	Astringent	Local irritation, allergic reactions	For external use only, do not use with occlusive dressings
Antihistamines	Benadryl, Vistaril, Atarax, others	Blocks histamine at the H_1 receptor site, inhibiting many allergic reactions	Drowsiness, dizziness, confusion, dry mouth, urinary retention	If drowsiness occurs, avoid activities that require concentration, avoid using with alcohol or other CNS depressants
Benzoyl peroxide	Many	Antiacne agent	Excessive drying of skin, allergic reactions	Discontinue use if excessive drying or peeling occurs, avoid contact with hair or fabric
Chlorhexidine gluconate	Hibiclens	Antimicrobial skin cleanser	Irritation, dermatitis, allergic reactions	For external use only, do not use on broken skin unless directed by a physician
Calamine lotion	Many	Astringent	Local irritation	For external use only
Coal tar	Many	Treatment of pruritic dermatoses, including eczema and psoriasis	Photosensitivity, dermatitis, allergic reactions	Avoid exposure to sunlight for 72 hours after use, may stain clothes and bathtub, for external use only
Corticosteroids (topical)	Lidex, Kenalog, Valisone, many others	Antiinflammatory agent	Local irritation, maceration, superinfection, atrophy, itching, and drying of skin (more severe local reactions and systemic effects are possible with higher doses and potency or when used with occlusive dressings)	Do not use occlusive dressings unless directed by a physician, washing or soaking area before application increases drug penetration
Crotamiton	Eurax	Scabicidal and antipruritic	Local irritation, allergic reactions	For external use only, do not apply to severely irritated skin
Curel	Same	Emollient	Local irritation, allergic reactions	For external use only
Eucerin	Same	Emollient	Local irritation, allergic reactions	For external use only
Fluconazole	Diflucan	Antifungal	Headache, nausea vomiting, diarrhea	May elevate liver function test, monitor BUN, creatinine

Continued

MEDICATIONS | *The Integumentary System—cont'd*

MEDICATION	TRADE NAME	ACTION	SIDE EFFECTS	NURSING IMPLICATIONS
Griseofulvin	Fulvicin, Grisactin, Grifulvin, others	Antifungal agent	Hypersensitivity reactions, photosensitivity, nausea, fatigue, mental confusion	Avoid exposure to sunlight, drug absorption increased when given with meals, clinical response may appear only after full course of therapy
Isotretinoin	Accutane	Antiacne agent	Severe dryness of skin, mouth, eyes, mucous membranes, nose, and nails; skin fragility; epistaxis; joint and muscle pain; nausea; abdominal pain	Absolutely contraindicated in pregnant women or women contemplating pregnancy, female patients of childbearing age must practice contraception during therapy and 1 month before and after therapy, take drug with meals, do not take vitamin supplements containing vitamin A, avoid exposure to sunlight
Itraconazole	Sporanox	Antifungal	Hypertension, headache, nausea, anovexial	Give with food, check hepatic functions, can increase PT level
Lindane	Kwell	Scabicide, ovicide	Local irritation, dizziness, seizures (rare)	For external use only, avoid applying to open skin lesions
Lubriderm	Same	Emollient	Local irritation, allergic reactions	For external use only, exercise caution when using in tub to avoid slipping
Methoxsalen	Oxsoralen, Oxsoralen-Ultra, 8-MOP	Skin pigmenting agent	Severe photosensitivity, nausea, nervousness, insomnia, headache, hypopigmentation	Avoid all exposure to sunlight for 8 hours after oral ingestion and for several days after topical application, wear UVA-absorbing sunglasses for 24 hours after oral ingestion, sunscreens may be used to prevent exposure to sunlight, take agent with food or milk or in divided doses, clinical response may not appear until after several months
Povidone-iodine	Betadine	Topical antimicrobial agent	Local irritation	For external use only; may stain skin and clothing
Pyrethrin	RID, others	Pediculicide	Local irritation	For external use only; do not use for infestations of eyebrows or eyelashes
Salicylic acid	Numerous	Keratolytic agent	Local irritation, erythema, scaling	For external use only; may damage clothing, plastic, wood, and other materials on contact
Terbinafine	Lamisil	Antifungal	Pruritus, local burning, erythema	Should be applied only externally, do *not use* occlusive dressings unless by physician order

MEDICATIONS | *The Integumentary System—cont'd*

MEDICATION	TRADE NAME	ACTION	SIDE EFFECTS	NURSING IMPLICATIONS
Tetracycline	Numerous	Antibacterial agent	Topical—stinging, burning Systemic—nausea, diarrhea, photosensitivity	Topical—slight yellowing of skin may occur Systemic—take on empty stomach; avoid concomitant administration of dairy products, laxatives, antacids, and products containing iron; avoid contact with sunlight; may cause permanent tooth discoloration when used in children
Tolnaftate	Tinactin, Aftate, others	Antifungal agent	Local irritation	For external use only

HERPES ZOSTER (SHINGLES)
Etiology/Pathophysiology

Herpes zoster is caused by the same virus that causes chickenpox (herpes varicella). The lesions are located along the nerve fibers of spinal ganglia.

Herpes zoster is commonly known as **shingles.** The virus causes an inflammation of the spinal ganglia. It is believed that the virus responsible for shingles lies dormant in patients until their resistance to infections has been lowered. The virus then advances to the skin by way of the peripheral nerves. At the skin surface the virus multiplies and forms an erythematous rash of small vesicles along a spinal nerve pathway (Figure 3-3). Sometimes the virus may affect a single nerve such as the trigeminal nerve.

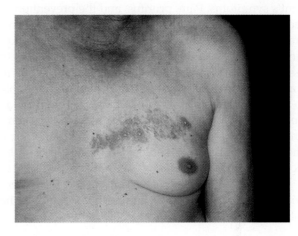

FIGURE **3-3** Herpes zoster.

Clinical Manifestations

The eruption of the vesicles is preceded by pain. The rash generally occurs in the thoracic region; the vesicles erupt in a line along the involved nerve. The vesicles rupture and form a crust, and the serous fluid in the vesicle may become purulent. The virus can also affect the lumbar, cervical, or cranial areas. The course of this painful condition is from 7 to 28 days.

The pain associated with herpes zoster is severe; most patients describe the pain as burning and knifelike. Extreme tenderness and pruritus in the affected area are noted. Patients with herpes zoster request analgesic medications at frequent intervals during the acute episode.

Herpes zoster is usually not permanently disabling to healthy adults. The greatest risk occurs to patients who have a lowered resistance to infection, such as those on chemotherapy or are taking large doses of prednisone, in whom the disease could be fatal due to the patient's compromised immune system.

Assessment

Assessment of the patient should include both the subjective and objective data. A good health history and thorough inspection skills are necessary to gather relevant data.

Collection of **subjective data** will include these symptoms: (1) sharp, burning pain, usually on one side only; (2) severe pruritus of the lesions; (3) general malaise; and (4) a history of chickenpox (varicella).

Collection of **objective data** includes (1) evidence of skin excoriation (injury to the surface layer of skin caused by scratching or abrasion) related to scratching, (2) patches of vesicles on erythematous skin following a peripheral nerve pathway, and (3) demonstration of tenderness to touch in the involved area. Other objective signs may include frequent requests for analgesics.

Diagnostic Tests

The diagnostic test for herpes zoster is a culture that isolates the virus. Other diagnostic measures are physical examinations and a thorough health history obtained upon admission to the health care facility.

Medical Management

Medical interventions are directed at controlling the pain and preventing secondary complications. Analgesics are given for the pain; many times the pain requires opioid analgesics. Steroids may be given to decrease inflammation and edema. Lotions may be used to relieve pruritus (Kenalog, Lidex), and corticosteroids may be used to relieve the pruritus and inflammation. Oral and intravenous acyclovir (Zovirax), when administered early, reduces the pain and duration of the virus. Recovery generally occurs in 2 to 3 weeks. Approximately 20% of patients experience some form of neuralgia following the episode.

Nursing Interventions and Patient Teaching

Nursing interventions are directed at relieving a patient's symptoms. Pain, pruritus, and the prevention of secondary complications are the primary concerns. Tranquilizers such as lorazepam (Ativan) and hydroxyzine HCl (Atarax) are prescribed to decrease the anxiety associated with severe pain. Analgesics are given to control pain. The nurse needs to understand and be able to apply the principles of pain management to provide nursing interventions. Medicated baths and warm compresses may be ordered to soothe the skin. The nurse should use aseptic technique when caring for open lesions (Nursing Care Plan box).

Nursing diagnoses and interventions for the patient with herpes zoster include but are not limited to the following:

NURSING DIAGNOSES	NURSING INTERVENTIONS
Acute pain, related to inflammation of the involved nerve pathways	Assess pain and pruritus for necessary relief measures. Administer medications for pain and pruritus. Stress relaxation techniques and diversional activities.
Risk for infection, related to tissue destruction	Assess factors that contribute to infection, such as a compromised patient (one who has decreased white blood cell [WBC] level). Monitor for signs of infection, such as pyrexia and leukocytosis. Stress aseptic handwashing technique. Maintain aseptic technique when providing care. Limit visitors. Don gloves when caring for lesions.

Patient teaching should begin with an assessment of the knowledge and readiness of the patient. Areas to cover include (1) methods for controlling

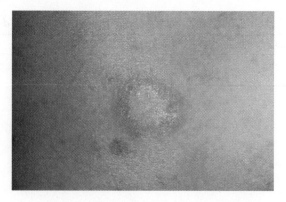
FIGURE **3-4** Pityriasis rosea herald patch.

pain, (2) application of medication and wet dressings, (3) methods for inhibiting the spread of disease, (4) techniques to prevent secondary infections, and (5) proper diet with vitamin C to promote healing.

Prognosis

The prognosis is generally good; however, older adult patients are more susceptible to complications such as posttherapy neuralgia, which may persist for several months after the skin lesions have cleared. Evidence indicates the herpes zoster virus remains latent in the body of a person once infected, and a person lacking varicella (chickenpox) immunity can acquire chickenpox from someone who has shingles.

PITYRIASIS ROSEA

Pityriasis rosea usually affects people between 6 and 30 years of age. This skin rash begins as a single pink, scaly patch that resembles a large ringworm. It ranges from 1 to 3 inches in diameter.

Etiology/Pathophysiology

Most sources note that pityriasis rosea results from a virus. The rash generally disappears without treatment.

Clinical Manifestations

Pityriasis rosea begins as a single lesion, known as a herald patch, that is scaly, has a raised border, and a pink center. Seven to 14 days after the initial eruption, smaller matching spots of the rash become widespread on both sides of the body. The rash consists of pink oval-shaped spots that are ¼ to ½ inch across. The rash appears mainly on the chest, abdomen, back, groin, and axillae (Figure 3-4).

Assessment

Assessment involves inspection of the skin and the gathering of a detailed health history. The nurse should ask questions related to the objective data.

NURSING CARE PLAN

The Patient with Herpes Zoster

Ms. L., a 28-year-old teacher, is admitted with herpes zoster located around her left orbital area. She has several vesicles that have crusted and several vesicles that are still intact. She is complaining of pruritus and pain. She keeps asking the nurse if the lesions will leave a scar.

NURSING DIAGNOSIS *Impaired tissue integrity related to the open lesions around the left eye*

Patient Goals/Expected Outcomes	Nursing Interventions	Evaluation
Patient's tissue integrity will improve as manifested by: • No signs of infection such as erythema, purulent drainage, and elevated WBC count during hospitalization. • Remaining skin showing no signs of skin impairment during hospitalization. • Decrease in the number of lesions within 72 hours. • Stating pain level has decreased from a "9" in degree of pain to a "4" within 24 hours.	Assess skin, especially eye area, for changes in color, texture, turgor, or increase in lesion size. Assess lesions for signs of infection shift. Monitor albumin and WBC levels as ordered. Use principles of aseptic technique. Administer or apply medications as ordered to decrease pain or pruritus. Teach patient importance of using medical asepsis in care of lesions.	The goal was met. The patient showed no signs of erythema or purulent drainage. The goal was met. The patient showed improvement of vesicles. The number of lesions increased during the first day of hospitalization but decreased during the next 48 hours. Continue plan of care as desired. Goal was met. Patient stated that pain was a "3" within 24 hours of medication administration.

NURSING DIAGNOSIS *Disturbed body image, related to location of lesions as manifested by continual remarks to the nurse, "Will these sores leave a scar?"*

Patient Goals/Expected Outcomes	Nursing Interventions	Evaluation
The patient will verbalize and demonstrate acceptance of appearance as manifested by: • Verbalizing positive feelings about body image. • Participation in normal activities.	Assess patient's feelings about personal appearance by encouraging patient to express her feelings. Encourage patient to ask questions about her health problem. Provide reliable information and reinforce the information already given. Clarify any misconceptions about the care the patient is receiving. Provide privacy and avoid criticism. Teach patient about the disease and the course of the disease.	The goal was met. The patient stated she felt that lesions would not be permanent. The patient returned to work after dismissal from the hospital before the lesions had completely healed. The goal was met.

? CRITICAL THINKING QUESTIONS

1. Ms. L. turns on her call light. She is crying and states she is in severe pain. She describes the pain as a burning, stabbing pain over her left forehead and eye. She rates her pain at a 7 on the pain scale of 0 to 10. She also complains of pruritus. What would be the most appropriate nursing interventions to provide comfort and pain control for Ms. L.?

2. Ms. L. tells the nurse that a friend told her she could not come visit because she has not had chickenpox. Her friend is afraid she might develop chickenpox from Ms. L.'s shingles. Give the accurate patient teaching in response to Ms. L.'s statements.

Diagnostic Tests

Diagnosis of rosea stems from inspection and subjective data from the patient. No specific laboratory tests support a definitive diagnosis.

Medical Management

Generally, rosea requires no treatment. Preventive interventions are often necessary to control secondary infections related to pruritus. If the skin becomes dry, moisturizing cream may be helpful. For pruritus, the patient should use 1% hydrocortisone cream two or three times a day.

Ultraviolet light shortens the course of pityriasis rosea. Sunbathing for 30 minutes shortens the course of the disease.

Nursing Interventions

The nursing interventions for pityriasis rosea include symptomatic relief of the presenting symptoms such as pruritus. Analgesics and Aveeno baths may be ordered as well to help decrease the pain and pruritus. Antihistamines and topical steroids may be used to control the pruritus. Sun exposure aids in the resolution of the lesions.

Prognosis

The disease is thought to be viral in nature; the nurse should teach the patient that the disease is self-limiting and resolves in a few weeks.

BACTERIAL DISORDERS OF THE SKIN

CELLULITIS
Etiology/Pathophysiology

Cellulitis, a potentially serious infection of the skin, involves the underlying tissues of the skin. Although it is not contagious, the bacteria that cause cellulitis can be spread by direct contact with an open area on a person that has an infection. The most common causes in adults are group A streptococci and *Staphylococcus aureus; Haemophilus influenzae* type B is more common in children. The following conditions increase the risk: venous insufficiency or stasis, diabetes mellitus, lymphedema, surgery, malnutrition, substance abuse, presence of another infection, compromised immune function due to human immunodeficiency virus (HIV), treatment with steroids or cancer chemotherapy, or autoimmune diseases, such as lupus erythematosus.

Cellulitis develops as an edematous, erythematous area of skin that feels hot and tender. It occurs when bacteria enter the body through a break in the skin, such as a cut, scratch, or insect bite that is not cleansed with soap and water. Skin on the lower extremities or face is most commonly affected by this infection, though cellulitis can occur on any part of the skin.

Generally occurring as a superficial infection, cellulitis may spread and become a life-threatening condition as the infection invades the deeper tissues and the blood, thus resulting in the lay term "blood poisoning." The infection can spread into the lymph nodes and bloodstream.

Clinical Manifestations

Cellulitis results in an infection of the skin and underlying subcutaneous tissues. The affected areas become erythematous, edematous, tender, and warm to the touch. The changes in the skin's appearance may be accompanied by a fever. The first signs and symptoms generally are erythema, pain, and tenderness over an area of skin. These signs and symptoms are caused by bacteria themselves and by the body's attempts to halt the infection. The infected skin may look slightly pitted, like an orange peel. Over time, the area of erythema spreads and small red spots may appear. Vesicles may form and burst or large bullae sometimes appear on the infected skin. As the infection spreads, nearby lymph nodes may become enlarged and tender (lymphadenitis). Erysipelas is one form of streptococcal cellulitis in which the skin is bright red and noticeably edematous and the edges of the infected area are raised. Edema occurs because the infection occludes the lymphatic vessels in the skin. Most patients with cellulitis feel only mildly ill, but some have fever, chills, tachycardia, headache, hypotension, and confusion.

Assessment

Assessment primarily involves inspection of the skin. The nurse collects a health history to support assessment data. **Subjective data** include complaints of fatigue, tenderness, pain, limited movement of the involved extremity, and a feeling of general malaise. **Objective data** include edema, erythema, and areas that are warm to touch. Vesicles may be present. An elevated temperature accompanied by tachycardia and leukocytosis often occurs.

Diagnostic Tests

The physician will diagnose cellulitis based on its appearance and signs and symptoms. If a patient is seriously ill, cultures may need to be conducted for laboratory identification of the bacteria from blood, purulent exudate, or tissue specimens. A complete blood count (CBC) would reveal leukocytosis. A Gram stain may be done to determine the appropriate antibiotic therapy. Occasionally the physician will perform tests to differentiate cellulitis from deep vein thrombosis of the lower extremity because the signs and symptoms of these disorders are similar. Occasionally, x-ray, ultrasound, computed tomography, or magnetic resonance imaging is used to determine the extent of inflammation and to identify abscess formation.

Medical Management

Prompt treatment with antibiotics can prevent cellulitis from spreading rapidly and reaching the blood and organs. Antibiotic therapy that is effective against both streptococci and staphylococci provides successful treatment for most cases. Patients with mild cellulitis may take oral antibiotics. If the patient has rapidly spreading cellulitis, high fever, or other evidence of a serious infection, the physician will order intravenous antibiotics.

Nursing Interventions and Patient Teaching

Nursing interventions involve treating signs and symptoms and preventing spread of the disease. The nursing interventions should be directed at administering the antibiotic, monitoring the patient's progress, assessing pain, administering an analgesic, changing dressings, and monitoring the nutrition and hydration status of the patient. The affected body part, when possible, remains immobile and is elevated to help reduce edema. Warm, moist dressings applied to the infected area may relieve discomfort.

Signs and symptoms of cellulitis usually disappear after a few days of antibiotic therapy. However, signs and symptoms often progress before they improve, probably because with the death of the bacteria, substances that cause tissue damage are released. When this occurs, the body continues to react even though the bacteria are dead. Antibiotics are continued for a minimum of 10 days. The nurse must teach patients the importance of taking the entire prescription of antibiotics and to monitor for signs and symptoms of secondary diseases such as yeast infections. The specific nursing diagnoses for cellulitis depend on the assessment data gathered and the extent of the infection. Analgesics such as acetaminophen (Tylenol) or oxycodone-acetaminophen (Percocet) help to control the pain and fever associated with cellulitis.

Prognosis

Cure is possible with 7 to 10 days of treatment. Cellulitis may be more severe in people with chronic diseases and those who are susceptible to infection such as the immunosuppressed. Complications from cellulitis may include the following: sepsis, meningitis, and lymphangitis.

IMPETIGO CONTAGIOSA
Etiology/Pathophysiology

Impetigo is caused by *Staphylococcus aureus,* streptococci, or a mixed bacterial invasion of the skin. The result is a highly contagious inflammatory disorder. Impetigo is seen at all ages but is particularly common in children.

The bacteria invade the skin. The lesions start as macules (small, flat blemishes that are flush with the skin surface) that develop into pustulant vesicles (small, circumscribed elevations of the skin that con-

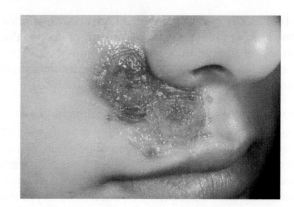

FIGURE **3-5** Impetigo and herpes simplex.

tain pus) that rupture and form a dried exudate. The crust is honey colored and easily removed. Under the dried exudate is smooth, red skin (Figure 3-5).

Clinical Manifestations

The exposed areas of the body most often affected are the face, hands, arms, and legs. The pustulant lesions are distributed randomly over the involved area. The honey-colored dried exudate ranges in size from pinpoint to the size of a nickel or larger. Impetigo is highly contagious to a person who directly contacts the exudate of a lesion. The disease may be spread by touching personal articles, linens, and clothing of the infected person.

Assessment

Collection of **subjective data** will include symptoms of (1) pruritus, (2) pain, (3) malaise, (4) spreading of the disease to different body parts, and (5) other diseases present.

Collection of **objective data** will reveal all or part of the following: (1) focal erythema, (2) pruritic areas, (3) honey-colored crust over dried lesions, (4) smooth, red skin under the crust, (5) low-grade fever, (6) leukocytosis, (7) positive culture for streptococcus or *S. aureus,* and (8) purulent exudate.

Diagnostic Tests

The diagnosis is made from a culture of the exudate. The specific bacterium is identified from this culture. Inspection and symptoms are the standard means to identify the condition.

Medical Management

The physician prescribes systemic antibiotics (such as erythromycin, dicloxacillin, or a cephalosporin) based on the culture and sensitivity test. Topical antibiotics such as mupirocin (Bactroban) have proven effective when started early in the treatment, but most physicians include a systemic antibiotic as well. Medical treatment may emphasize the use of antiseptic soaps to remove crusted exudate and cleansing agents to thoroughly clean the involved area before application of an antibiotic cream, ointment, or lotion. Prevention of glomerulonephritis (inflammation of the glomerulus of the kidney) that may occur after streptococcal infections becomes a primary goal.

Nursing Interventions and Patient Teaching

Interventions are aimed at disrupting the course of the disease and preventing the spread of infection. Antibiotics are used to arrest the disease process. Systemic parenteral penicillin is one of the most commonly used antibiotics, although ceftriaxone sodium (Rocephin) is being widely used as well. Other antibiotics such as cephalosporins may be used. The nurse should don gloves and administer special cleansing agents to wash the lesions. Antiseptics such as povidone-iodine solution (Betadine) and chlorhexidine gluconate (Hibiclens) are examples.

The lesions are usually soaked with an antiseptic solution, and the dried exudate is removed using special instruments. Topical antibiotics are applied several times a day using sterile technique.

Nursing diagnoses and interventions for the patient with impetigo include but are not limited to the following:

NURSING DIAGNOSES	NURSING INTERVENTIONS
Impaired skin integrity, related to crusted, open lesions	Inspect the lesions every day for drainage, size, and extent of body area covered. Keep area clean and dry. Don gloves when giving direct patient care.
Deficient knowledge, related to the cause and spread of the disease	Assess the patient's knowledge level and readiness to learn. Demonstrate appropriate care and application of topical medications. Stress importance of individual personal items, such as linens and towels. Involve family in patient teaching.

The patient and family members should be instructed in the principles of hygiene. The nurse assesses the patient's level of knowledge. When demonstrating home care techniques, reinforcement of correct information is recommended. It is imperative to stress the importance of preventing the spread of the disease by contact.

Prognosis

With proper treatment the prognosis is good. Emphasis should be given to taking all of the prescribed antibiotic.

FOLLICULITIS, FURUNCLES, CARBUNCLES, AND FELONS
Etiology/Pathophysiology

Folliculitis is an infection of a hair follicle, generally from *S. aureus* bacteria. The infection may involve one or several follicles. It often occurs after men or women shave. A stye is an example of folliculitis.

A **furuncle** (boil) is an inflammation that begins deep in the hair follicles and spreads to the surrounding skin. Irritation is a common predisposing factor to a furuncle. Common locations are the posterior area of the neck, the forearm, buttocks, and the axillae (Figure 3-6).

A **carbuncle** is a cluster of furuncles. It is an infection of several hair follicles that spreads to surrounding tissue. Obesity, poor nutrition, untreated diabetes mellitus, and poor hygiene contribute to the formation of carbuncles.

Felons occur when the soft tissue under and around an area such as the fingernail becomes infected. The involved finger becomes erythematous, edematous, and tender to touch.

Clinical Manifestations

The involved area is usually edematous, erythematous, and painful, commonly with pruritus. After several days the infected area will become localized. The exact area may get shiny, point up, and if it is a furuncle or carbuncle, the center will turn yellow. Carbuncles can have four to five cores with spontaneous rupture of the core. The pain stops immediately upon rupture of the core. A surgical incision and drainage (I&D) can be performed if the core does not rupture.

Assessment

Collection of **subjective data** includes asking questions to ascertain the patient's general symptoms. Common symptoms are tenderness and pain with movement. The nurse should question the patient about a family history of diabetes mellitus or the wearing of improperly fitting clothing.

Collection of **objective data** includes noting erythema and edema in the involved area. The patient is often overweight and may use poor body hygiene techniques.

Diagnostic Tests

Diagnosis is based primarily on a thorough physical examination, health history, and inspection of the area. A culture of the drainage may be done.

Medical Management

Medical treatment is aimed at preventing the spread of the infection. Patients in the hospital are isolated, using wound and secretion precautions. Surgical treatment may include draining the lesion and applying topical antibiotics.

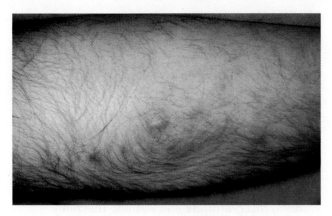

FIGURE **3-6** Furuncle of the forearm.

Nursing Interventions and Patient Teaching

Warm soaks, two or three times a day, can be used to speed the process of suppuration (production of purulent material). When the lesion ruptures, the hot soaks are discontinued to prevent damage of the surrounding skin and spread of the infection. The nurse must use good medical asepsis while caring for these patients. In the hospital, isolation procedures for drainage and secretion should be followed. If the lesion is incised and drained, sterile technique should be used to apply topical antibiotics. The affected part needs to be immobilized to prevent pain and elevated to decrease the edema.

Nursing diagnoses and interventions for the patient with bacterial disorders include but are not limited to the following:

NURSING DIAGNOSES	NURSING INTERVENTIONS
Impaired skin integrity, related to exudate from wound	Assess wound daily for exudate and excoriation.
	Don gloves when providing care; use correct isolation technique.
	Apply skin protectant to opening.
Pain, related to edema	Assess area for any edema and tenderness.
	Elevate involved body part above the level of the heart.
	Apply hot soaks, and immobilize affected part.

Patients should be taught not to touch the exudate. Meticulous handwashing is a must before and after contact with the lesions. Good hygiene practices should be demonstrated and return demonstrations done by the patient and family. The entire family needs individual toilet items and bath linens and should be encouraged to use bacteriostatic soap and shampoo. Proper disposal and cleaning of contaminated articles need to be demonstrated by the nurse.

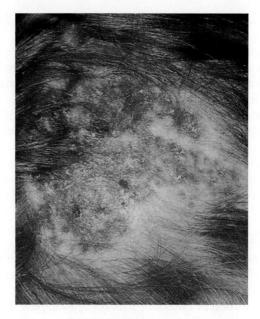

FIGURE **3-7** Tinea capitis.

Prognosis

Patients make full recovery when the treatment plan is followed. A follow-up examination with a physician may be needed to determine if any underlying disease process, such as diabetes mellitus, is apparent.

FUNGAL INFECTIONS OF THE SKIN

Fungal infections, which are known as **dermatophytoses,** are superficial infections of the skin. The most common types are tinea capitis, tinea corporis, tinea cruris, and tinea pedis.

Etiology/Pathophysiology

Tinea capitis is commonly known as ringworm of the scalp. *Microsporum audouinii* is the major fungal pathogen. The fungus is spread by contact with infected articles. Trauma or irritation breaks the skin and facilitates spread of the infection (Figure 3-7).

Tinea corporis is known as ringworm of the body. It occurs on parts of the body with little or no hair.

Tinea cruris is known as jock itch. It is found in the groin area.

Tinea pedis is the most common of all fungal infections. Commonly known as athlete's foot, it is seen between the toes of people whose feet perspire heavily. The fungus can also be spread from contaminated public bathroom facilities and swimming pools.

Clinical Manifestations

Tinea capitis (ringworm of the scalp) is usually an erythematous, round lesion with pustules around the edges (see Figure 3-7). Temporary alopecia occurs at the site, and infected hairs will turn blue-green under a Wood's light.

Tinea corporis (ringworm of the body) produces flat lesions that are clear in the center with erythematous borders. Scaliness may also be found, and pruritus is severe (Figure 3-8).

Tinea cruris (jock itch) has brownish red lesions that migrate out from the groin area. Pruritus and skin excoriation from scratching are found.

Tinea pedis (athlete's foot) produces more skin maceration than the others. Commonly seen are fissures and vesicles around and below the toes, with occasional discoloration of the infected area.

Assessment

The nurse's collection of the **subjective data** will include any symptoms of extreme pruritus and tenderness from excoriation of the area.

Collection of **objective data** for tinea capitis should include an inspection and location of a round, scaled lesion that has pustules around the edges of the scalp. The involved area is erythematous and has no hair. In tinea corporis the nurse will find flat lesions with clear centers and erythematous borders on non-hairy body parts. In tinea cruris the groin area reveals brown to red lesions that radiate outward, with skin excoriation from intense scratching. In tinea pedis the nurse will find fissures between the toes and soft skin accompanied by vesicular lesions and thick toenails.

Diagnostic Tests

The diagnosis is primarily by visual inspection. A Wood's light or Wood's lamp is an ultraviolet light used to diagnose tinea capitis. The light causes hairs infected by the fungus to become brilliantly fluorescent. No other tests are performed, but a thorough health history supports the diagnosis of all fungal infections of the skin.

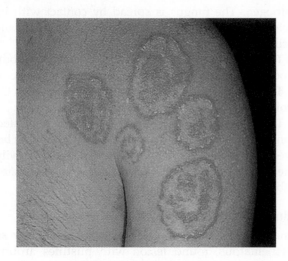

FIGURE **3-8** Tinea corporis.

Medical Management

Medical treatment involves the use of topical or oral antifungal drugs. Griseofulvin (Fulvicin, Grifulvin) is the most common oral drug given; topical drugs do not penetrate the hair bulb. Antifungal soaps and shampoos are recommended. Antifungal agents such as tolnaftate 1% (Tinactin), clotrimazole (Lotrimin AF), or Desenex can be applied directly. Treatment may last from 2 to 6 weeks. See the Medications table on page 77 for a list of drugs commonly used for fungal and other integumentary infections.

Nursing Interventions and Patient Teaching

Nursing interventions for fungal infections involve two primary principles. The first is to protect the involved area from trauma and irritation by keeping it clean and dry; the second is the proper application of medications and warm compresses to alleviate the fungus.

Tinea pedis should be treated with warm soaks using Burow's solution and topical antifungal agents. Excellent foot care is stressed. The feet should be cleaned and dried thoroughly, paying special attention to the toes. Wearing sandal-type shoes or going barefoot helps decrease foot moisture. Footwear, such as stockings, needs to be of an absorbent material.

Nursing diagnosis and interventions for the patient with fungal infections include but are not limited to the following:

NURSING DIAGNOSES	NURSING INTERVENTIONS
Impaired skin integrity, related to increased moisture and pruritus	Keep involved area clean and dry. Have patients wear loose-fitting clothing and shoes. Apply medications as directed.

Patient education involves teaching proper skin care and comfort measures to relieve pruritus. The nurse should review the medications to be taken and the procedures to be done at home by the patient, emphasizing that fungal skin disorders may take months to cure. General education about athlete's foot should be stressed and the many misconceptions clarified.

Prognosis

Prognosis for recovery is good. Few complications result when treatment is followed.

INFLAMMATORY DISORDERS OF THE SKIN

Superficial infection of the skin is known as **dermatitis.** It can be caused by numerous agents, such as drugs, plants, chemicals, metals, and food. Regardless of the precipitating factor, the lesions associated with dermatitis develop along the same pattern. The nurse first observes erythema and edema, followed by the eruption of vesicles that rupture and encrust. Pruritus is always present, which promotes further skin excoriation.

CONTACT DERMATITIS
Etiology/Pathophysiology

Contact dermatitis is caused by direct contact with agents in the environment to which a person is hypersensitive. The epidermis becomes inflamed and damaged by the repeated contact with the physical and chemical irritants. Common causes of dermatitis are detergents, soaps, industrial chemicals, and plants such as poison ivy.

Clinical Manifestations

Lesions appear first at the point of contact with the irritant. Usually the patient feels burning, pain, pruritus, and edema. The involved area is soon erythematous, with papules (small, raised, solid skin lesions less than 1 cm in diameter) and vesicles appearing most often on the dorsal surfaces.

Assessment

The nurse needs to thoroughly research the history of the patient's activities. The nurse may ask the patient to write a log of activities for the 48 hours before development of symptoms.

Collection of **subjective data** usually reveals that the patient has (1) tried a new soap, (2) been traveling and using different personal items, or (3) been working with plants or flowers; the patient may have (4) severe pruritus and (5) difficulty moving the involved area.

Collection of **objective data** by the nurse should find (1) erythema, (2) papules and vesicles that generally ooze and weep a clear fluid, (3) scratch marks resulting from intense pruritus, and (4) edema of the area.

Diagnostic Tests

The primary diagnostic test is accurate collection of a health history to identify the agent. Intradermal skin testing may be done to identify plants and environmental agents, and elimination diets are used to identify food allergies. Elevated serum IgE levels and eosinophilia support the diagnosis. It is thought that both tests relate to various abnormalities of T-cell function.

Medical Management

Medical intervention is directed at identifying the cause of the hypersensitive reaction. Symptomatic treatment for the inflammation, edema, and pruritus may include application of corticosteroids and the oral administration of antihistamines such as diphenhy-

dramine (Benadryl). If there is a history of asthma (reactive airway disease), the patient may have an acute asthmatic episode. Hydroxyzine (Atarax) and inhalation treatments provide prophylactic treatment for asthma.

Nursing Interventions and Patient Teaching

The primary goal is to identify the offensive agent so as to rest the involved skin and protect it from further damage. To help identify the cause, the nurse needs to describe the pattern of the reaction.

Wet dressings, using Burow's solution, help promote the healing process. To prevent infection, aseptic technique is used to apply the corticosteroids to the open lesions.

Pruritus is responsible for most of the discomfort. A cool environment with increased humidity decreases the pruritus. Cold compresses may be applied to decrease circulation to the area (vasoconstriction). Daily baths to cleanse the skin should be taken with an application of oil. Fingernails should be cut at the level of the fingertips to decrease excoriation from scratching. Clothing should be lightweight and loose to decrease trauma of the involved area.

Nursing diagnoses and interventions for the patient with inflammation of the skin include but are not limited to the following:

Nursing Diagnoses	Nursing Interventions
Impaired skin integrity, related to scratching	Assess for signs of scratching. Have patient keep fingernails short and wear mittens. Apply medications as directed.
Pain, related to pruritus	Assess degree of pruritus and discomfort every shift. Keep environment cool. Apply cold compresses.

The patient should be taught to keep an accurate history of possible predisposing offensive agents. As soon as the primary irritant has been identified, it should be avoided, as well as soaps, excessive heat, and rubbing of the area. Any time the skin is exposed to the primary irritant, the affected area should be washed thoroughly. Topical creams may be applied only as directed by a physician.

Prognosis

Removal of the offensive agent results in full recovery. Desensitizing the individual may be necessary if recurrences are frequent.

DERMATITIS VENENATA, EXFOLIATIVE DERMATITIS, AND DERMATITIS MEDICAMENTOSA

Etiology/Pathophysiology

Dermatitis venenata results from contact with certain plants, commonly **poison ivy** and poison oak. The signs and symptoms of this dermatitis include mild to severe erythema with pruritus. In this condition, on first exposure the body undergoes a sensitizing antigen formation. This results in an immunologic change in certain lymphocytes. Subsequent exposure to the antigen causes the lymphocytes to release irritating chemicals, leading to inflammation, edema, and vesiculation. The lesions are mainly found on the body part exposed to the sensitizing agent.

Exfoliative dermatitis may be caused by the infestation of certain heavy metals, such as arsenic or mercury, or by antibiotics, aspirin, codeine, gold, or iodine. The skin sloughs off, and the area becomes edematous and erythematous. Severe pruritus with fever occurs, and most patients require hospitalization. Treatment is individualized. If the cause can be determined, it should be removed or treated appropriately. Care is essential to prevent secondary infection, to avoid further irritation, and to maintain fluid balance.

Dermatitis medicamentosa occurs when people are given a medication to which they are hypersensitive. Any drug can cause a reaction, but the common agents are penicillin, codeine, and iron.

Clinical Manifestations

Clinical manifestations range from mild to severe erythema with vesicular eruptions. In severe reactions, respiratory distress may occur. Any type of lesion may be found.

Assessment

Collection of **subjective data** for dermatitis is pruritus and a burning pain in the involved area.

Collection of **objective data** reveals lesions that are white in the center and red on the periphery. Vesicles are common in dermatitis venenata. In dermatitis medicamentosa, severe dyspnea caused by respiratory distress may be noted.

Diagnostic Tests

A careful patient history is of prime importance in the diagnosis of dermatitis venenata, exfoliative dermatitis, and dermatitis medicamentosa. A laboratory examination for serum IgE and eosinophilia is ordered.

Medical Management

The medical treatment for dermatitis ranges from therapeutic baths to administration of corticosteroids. The medical treatment is directed at the cause.

Nursing Interventions and Patient Teaching

In dermatitis venenata the patient should wash the affected part immediately after contact with the offending allergen. After the lesions appear, only cool, open, wet dressings should be used. However, calamine lotion is a common over-the-counter medication used for pruritus.

Pruritus is the primary symptom in all dermatitis. Therapeutic baths using colloid solution, lotions, and ointments are used to help relieve the pruritus. Emotional support is necessary. The physical appearance of the patient is difficult for the patient and family members to accept.

In dermatitis medicamentosa, interventions revolve around identifying the drug and discontinuing its use. If the specific drug that is the offending allergen cannot be pinpointed, no drugs should be given. The physician must be notified. The lesions will disappear after the medication is discontinued. More specific nursing intervention is directed by individual patient symptoms.

Nursing diagnoses and interventions for the patient with dermatitis include but are not limited to the following:

NURSING DIAGNOSES	NURSING INTERVENTIONS
Impaired skin integrity, related to crusted, open lesions	Inspect the lesions every day for exudate, size, and specific body area involved. Keep area clean and dry. Don gloves when giving direct patient care.
Risk for infection, related to break in skin	Assess skin for signs of infection. Identify interventions to prevent or reduce the risk of infection. Monitor vital signs; assess for elevated temperature. Stress medical aseptic handwashing technique. Use aseptic technique, and keep involved areas dry when providing care.
Deficient knowledge, related to the cause and spread of the disease	Assess the patient's knowledge level and readiness to learn. Demonstrate appropriate care and application of topical medications. Stress importance of individual personal items, such as linens and towels. Involves patient and family teaching.

It is important to educate the patient to wear a medical alert bracelet or necklace showing the name of the allergen; the patient should be instructed to notify all health care personnel of the medication allergy.

Prognosis

Full recovery occurs when the offending agent is removed.

URTICARIA
Etiology/Pathophysiology

Urticaria is the term applied to the presence of wheals or hives in an allergic reaction commonly caused by drugs, food, insect bites, inhalants, emotional stress, or exposure to heat or cold. The wheals (round elevation of the skin; white in the center with a pale red periphery) (see Table 3-1) of urticaria appear suddenly.

Urticaria or hives is caused by the release of histamine in an antigen-antibody reaction.

Clinical Manifestations

The increased histamine causes the capillaries to dilate, resulting in increased permeability. Respiratory involvement may occur.

Assessment

Collection of subjective data includes pruritus, edema, and a burning pain. Dyspnea may be noted.

Collection of **objective data** will identify transient wheals of varying shapes and sizes with well-defined erythematous margins and pale centers. Intense scratching may be seen, and in some cases respiration may be compromised. Assessment of respiratory status provides a baseline for future assessments.

Diagnostic Tests

A detailed health history is the primary tool to identify the cause of hives. An allergy skin test may be performed using minute quantities of the antigen to identify the allergic substances. A serum examination for immunoglobulin E (IgE) elevation may be ordered.

Medical Management

Relief from urticaria can be achieved by administering an antihistamine and sometimes epinephrine. Identification of the cause of the urticaria is important to prevent recurrence.

Nursing Interventions and Patient Teaching

Nursing interventions are directed at helping the patient identify the cause and decreasing the discomfort from the pruritus.

The patient should be taught possible causes and prevention methods. Medications should be explained thoroughly and therapeutic baths demonstrated. The signs and symptoms of an anaphylactic reaction should be reviewed to include shortness of breath, wheezing, and cyanosis.

Prognosis

Patients recover fully when the offensive agent is determined and avoided. Compliance with the therapeutic treatment regimen influences the outcome.

ANGIOEDEMA
Etiology/Pathophysiology

Angioedema is a form of urticaria. It occurs in the subcutaneous tissue, whereas urticaria is a skin and mucous membrane lesion. Angioedema is caused by the same offenders that cause urticarial lesions.

Angioedema is characterized by local edema of an entire area, such as an eyelid, hands, feet, tongue, larynx, gastrointestinal (GI) tract, genitalia, or lips. Seldom does more than a single edematous area appear at one time.

Assessment

The collection of **subjective data** will include symptoms of burning, pruritus, acute pain if in the GI tract, or respiratory distress if in the larynx.

The collection of **objective data** will find lesions that have a normal appearance on the outer skin with edema.

Diagnostic Tests

A careful patient history is essential in the diagnosis of angioedema. Patients with a history of allergies are more likely to have angioedema.

Medical Management

Treatment to relieve angioedema may include the use of antihistamine drugs such as diphenhydramine (Benadryl). Epinephrine and corticosteroids such as methylprednisolone (Solu-Medrol) may be given.

Nursing Interventions

A cold pack or cold compress may be used. Continual respiratory assessment is essential to detect respiratory distress. Patients should be taught to wear a medical alert bracelet. Education is the key to preventing recurrent episodes.

Prognosis

With treatment, the prognosis is excellent.

ECZEMA (ATOPIC DERMATITIS)
Etiology/Pathophsiology

Eczema is primarily a disease of infants and is associated with allergies. The common allergies are to chocolate, eggs, wheat, and orange juice.

The allergen causes histamine to be released, and an antigen-antibody reaction occurs.

Clinical Manifestations

Papular and vesicular lesions appear and are surrounded by erythema. The vesicles generally rupture, discharging a yellow, tenacious exudate that dries and encrusts. If the lesions become infected, the skin may depigment and become shiny with dry scales.

Assessment

Collection of **subjective data** includes pruritus and scratching. Children are generally more fussy and irritable, and anorexia is commonly found. The skin is sensitive to touch. A family history of allergies supports the findings in many cases, and asthma may be associated with children who have eczema.

Collection of **objective data** will include vesicles and papules found on the scalp, forehead, cheeks, neck, and the surfaces of the extremities. The involved area is erythematous and dry. Tiny cracks in the epithelium allow fluid to escape and further promote dryness. The primary signs result from the scratching from pruritus. Scales accompanied by dryness in the involved area provides a distinguishing characteristic of eczema.

Diagnostic Tests

The diagnosis is generally made during a thorough health history that reveals a family history of eczema, because heredity is a prominent factor. Diet elimination and skin testing may be used to identify the specific substance to which the patient is hypersensitive. IgE serum tests provide data related to allergic response.

Medical Management

The medical treatment is concerned with reducing the amount of allergen exposure. The eruptions and pruritus can be relieved if the aggravating factor is identified and controlled. The primary goal is to break the inflammation cycle. Hydration of the skin is the key to treatment. The skin is dry because of tiny cracks that allow body fluids to escape.

The skin may be hydrated by soaking the affected area in warm water for 15 to 20 minutes and then applying an occlusive ointment to retain the water. Examples of occlusive preparations are petrolatum, corticosteroid ointments, and vegetable shortenings. The skin should be patted dry after the bath and the occlusive preparation applied immediately to the damp skin.

Nursing Interventions and Patient Teaching

Nursing interventions are directed toward treatment of symptoms for the eczematous patient. The nurse is responsible for administering the therapeutic bath and occlusive preparations as directed. Wet dressings may be used to maximize hydration of the skin. Topical steroids may be applied to relieve the discomfort of the lesions.

When the lesions begin to heal, a lotion such as Eucerin, Alpha Keri, Lubriderm, or Curel should be applied three or four times a day to add moisture to the skin. Wet wraps and occlusive preparations only hold water already present.

The emotional impact experienced by patients with eczema ranges from anger to depression. The nurse must provide an emotional outlet for these patients. Encouraging the patient to verbalize emotions becomes an important nursing consideration. Using effective listening skills and open-ended questions provides a means to establishing a therapeutic rapport with the patient.

Before the development of steroids, coal tar products were used to reduce the skin inflammation. Coal tar products do not decrease inflammation as quickly as steroids, but they last longer and have fewer side effects. Therefore coal tar preparations are recommended for chronic eczema. Coal tar preparations are applied once a day at bedtime with a moisturizer. Examples of coal tar preparations are Estar-Gel and Psori-Gel.

Nursing diagnoses and interventions for the patient with eczema include but are not limited to the following:

Nursing Diagnoses	Nursing Interventions
Impaired skin integrity, related to open lesions	Assess skin for signs of secondary infection. Monitor CBC for elevated white blood cell count. Apply ordered medications using medical aseptic techniques.
Risk for situational low self-esteem, related to change in body image	Assess mental status of patient. Observe interaction with family and staff members.
Risk for infection, related to open lesion	Report at once the signs of wound infection such as erythema, especially beyond the wound margins. Increasing edema, purulent exudate, change in the description of the pain or increased pain, and increased warmth in the involved area are signs and symptoms of infection.

ACNE VULGARIS
Etiology/Pathophysiology

Acne is an inflammatory papulopustular skin eruption that involves the sebaceous glands; it occurs primarily in adolescents. The exact cause is unknown. However, several factors that have been considered are diet, stress, heredity, and overactive hormones. Hygiene has not been found to be a significant factor in the development of acne.

Acne develops when the oil glands become occluded. At puberty, androgens secreted increase the size of the oil glands, causing the sebum to combine more readily with epithelial cells and bacteria. Sebum may then occlude a hair follicle, forming a comedo (plural, comedones). A comedo is a blackhead. It is dark because of the effect of oxygen on sebum, not because of the presence of dirt.

Clinical Manifestations

Acne is found most often on the face, neck, upper chest, shoulder, and back (Figure 3-9). The first symptom is usually tenderness and edema in the area, followed by the comedo. The skin is oily and shiny, and the lesions last up to 10 days. Scarring results from large lesions that are traumatized when the individual tries to rupture the comedo.

Assessment

Collection of **subjective data** includes asking the adolescent how acne affects lifestyle: Does it affect participation in activities or group communication? Most patients acknowledge that acne affects their self-image. Common locations are the face and chin. Lesions increase with emotional upsets and stress.

Collection of **objective data** will include noting the presence of edema in the involved area. Comedones (blackheads) are found on the face, back, or chest. The nurse will also observe that patients with acne do not take part in many group activities.

Diagnostic Tests

The medical diagnosis is primarily made by inspection of the lesions and a health history that supports the diagnosis. Sometimes blood samples are drawn to measure hormone levels.

Medical Management

The medical management can involve topical, systemic, or intralesional medications. Topical therapy peels away the superficial skin layer to prevent sebum occlusions. A common topical medication is benzoyl peroxide gel (such as Clearasil). Effective topical therapy requires the use of special cleansing agents followed by applications of vitamin A acids, antibiotics, and sulfur-zinc lotions.

Systemic antibiotic therapy, combined with topical therapy, provides one means to decrease the scarring associated with acne. Systemic antibiotics such as tetracycline are used. Isotretinoin (Accutane), a form of vitamin A, is used frequently. Isotretinoin (Accutane) reduces the sebum production and abnormal keratinization of gland ducts. Accutane must be prescribed with extreme caution in adolescent females because it is destructive to fetal development during pregnancy. Depression is a side effect of isotretinoin. Changes in behavior should be noted and referred for assistance. All patients taking isotretinoin must have monthly liver function tests to determine if the drug is hepatotoxic.

Nursing Interventions and Patient Teaching

In planning nursing interventions the nurse needs to be aware that most adolescents do not comply with long-term treatment regimens. The nurse must assess

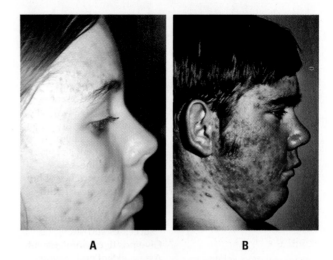

FIGURE 3-9 Acne vulgaris. **A,** Comedones with a few inflammatory pustules. **B,** Papulopustular acne.

and consider what acne means to them. The actual extent of the condition is not as important as the adolescent's feelings. When a patient's face constantly has ugly black and white lesions, it is hard for an adolescent to maintain a healthy self-esteem.

In addition to psychological concerns, the nurse should focus on preventive nursing interventions. The important areas are skin care, compliance, and emotional support. Prevention stresses identification of factors that directly increase acne. Although poor hygiene may not be a cause, cleanliness decreases infection and promotes healing. The patient's hands and hair should be kept away from the face. Clothes should not restrict affected areas, and hair should be washed daily. The skin should be washed two or three times a day with a medicated soap. Cosmetics need to be water based, and products that have wax esters should be avoided. Compliance is difficult because improvement is slow. Often 3 weeks of treatment are required before noticeable improvement is seen by the patient, the family, or friends (Health Promotion Considerations for Healthy Skin box).

Nursing diagnoses and interventions for the patient with acne vulgaris include but are not limited to the following:

Nursing Diagnoses	Nursing Interventions
Impaired skin integrity, related to occluded oil glands	Assess extent of occluded oil glands by inspecting lesions for size, color, and location. Monitor for signs of infection. Wash involved areas three or four times a day. Apply medications to decrease occlusion of oil glands.

Continued

Nursing Diagnoses	Nursing Interventions
Situational low self-esteem, related to physical appearance	Assess primary cause of low self-esteem and extent of feelings.
	Assess family support.
	Assess patient awareness and ways to deal with the situation.
	Note nonverbal language to discover patient's perception of the illness.
	Stress the importance of not comparing oneself with others.
	Have patient list current successes and strengths.
	Give positive reinforcement.
Social isolation, related to decreased self-esteem	Assess extent and feelings of isolation.
	Assess factors that contribute to sense of helplessness.
	Listen to and spend time with patient.
	Involve patient in support group.
	Focus on patient's strengths.

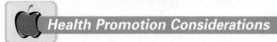

Health Promotion Considerations

Healthy Skin

- Adequate nutrition (especially fluids; protein; vitamins A, B complex, and C; iron; adequate calories; and unsaturated fatty acids) promotes healthy skin.
- Refrain from smoking to improve color of skin and to prevent circulation difficulties.
- Drink 8 glasses of water a day to help rid the skin of waste products.
- Exercise increases circulation and dilates blood vessels. In addition to the healthy glow produced by exercise, the psychological effects can also improve one's appearance and mental outlook. However, caution must be used to protect the exerciser from overexposure to heat, cold, and sun during outdoor exercise.
- In general, the skin and hair should be washed often enough to remove excess oil and excretions and to prevent odor.
- The use of neutral soaps, as well as avoiding hot water and vigorous rubbing, can noticeably decrease local irritation and inflammation.
- Older adults should avoid using harsh soaps and shampoos because of the increased dryness of their skin.
- Moisturizers should be used after bath or shower, while the skin is still damp, to seal in this moisture.
- Obesity has an adverse effect on the skin. Increased subcutaneous fat can lead to stretching and overheating. Overheating causes an increase in perspiring, which has an adverse effect on normal or inflamed skin.

Patient teaching should include the physical and emotional needs of the patient. The nurse should address diet, hygiene, stress reduction, makeup, and medications. Coping skills may need to be retaught and counseling referrals made. The extensive treatment time should be covered in minute detail because this disease is chronic and exacerbations will occur. Keeping the adolescent communicating about feelings will decrease any long-term affects that acne may have on his or her personality. Patients taking isotretinoin will develop dry skin. Nurses should teach patients to take measures to prevent dry skin.

Prognosis

Prognosis for acne is good. However, lasting psychological effects can occur from the scarring that may result. In extreme cases eczema may develop from taking medications for acne, such as isotretinoin.

PSORIASIS
Etiology/Pathophysiology

Psoriasis is a noninfectious skin disorder; it is a hereditary, chronic, proliferative disease involving the epidermis and can occur at any age. No specific predisposing factors are known. The skin cells divide much more rapidly than normal. The normal time for the entire skin to be replaced, through sloughing and generation of new cells, is 28 days; in psoriasis the time may decrease to 7 days. The severe scaling is a result of the rapid cell division.

Clinical Manifestations

The lesions appear as raised, erythematous, circumscribed, silvery scaling plaques. The primary lesion is papular. The papules become plaques located on the scalp, elbows, chin, and trunk (Figure 3-10). Based on severity, the disease may be classified as mild, moderate, or severe.

Assessment

Collection of **subjective data** initially will reveal only mild pruritus. Sometimes feelings of depression, frustration, and loneliness are expressed. Patients report that observers stare and avoid contact with them, increasing their awareness that their appearance differs from the norm.

Collection of **objective data** includes observing dull, erythematous, sharply outlined plaques covered with silvery scales on the elbows, knees, and scalp. Fingernails can be affected and will show pitting with yellowish discoloration.

Diagnostic Tests

No specific diagnostic tests exist for psoriasis. Primary diagnosis is made by observation of the patient and the symptoms displayed.

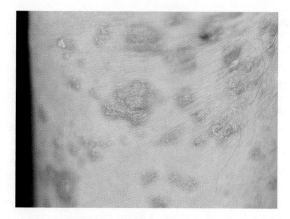

FIGURE **3-10** Psoriasis.

Medical Management

Medical management is aimed at slowing the proliferation of epithelial layers of the skin. Topical steroids and keratolytic agents are used in occlusive wet dressings to decrease inflammation. Keratolytic agents such as tar preparations and salicylic acid (Calicylic) decrease shedding of the outer layer of the skin. Topical steroids used are hydrocortisone and betamethasone valerate (Valisone).

Photochemotherapy may also be used. This treatment involves the use of a drug enhanced by exposure to light. PUVA therapy combines the use of methoxsalen (Psoralen), which is given orally, and the concurrent use of ultraviolet light A (UVA); hence, the acronym PUVA. Methotrexate as well as vitamin D reduce epidermal proliferation in some cases.

Nursing Interventions and Patient Teaching

Nursing interventions include proper administration of the treatment modality. Additional rest and measures to promote psychological well-being, such as counseling, are necessary. The emotional needs of this patient are as important as the physical needs. Because this disease is chronic, the patient should be encouraged to focus on positive attributes.

Nursing diagnoses and interventions for the patient with psoriasis include but are not limited to the following:

NURSING DIAGNOSES	NURSING INTERVENTIONS
Impaired skin integrity, related to proliferation of epithelial cells	Assess extent of the scaliness. Administer treatment method correctly. Use medical aseptic technique.
Situational low self-esteem, related to appearance	Assess patient's concept of body. Help patient to focus on positive aspects. Discuss with patient ways to conceal obvious lesions.

NURSING DIAGNOSES	NURSING INTERVENTIONS
Social isolation, related to decreased self-esteem	Assess activity pattern and social outlets. Demonstrate ways to conceal lesions with clothes. Involve patient in support group.

The primary points in patient teaching include the nature of the disease, correct application of the treatment modality, and compliance with medical care. It should be stressed that patients should not treat themselves. The patient should be informed that the disease is not curable.

Prognosis

Psoriasis is a chronic disease. The clinical course is variable, but less than half of the patients followed for a prolonged period will have a prolonged remission; severity may range from a minimal cosmetic problem to a life-threatening emergency.

SYSTEMIC LUPUS ERYTHEMATOSUS

Lupus is the Latin word for "wolf," used since AD 1230 to describe the cutaneous skin changes that resemble the zygomatic erythema of a red wolf (Figure 3-11). Lupus erythematosus affects the skin and may become systemic. An inflammatory condition with skin mani-

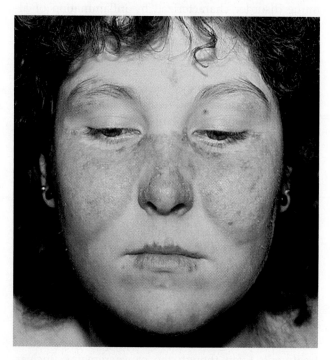

FIGURE **3-11** Systemic lupus erythematosus (SLE) flare. The classic butterfly rash occurs in 10% to 50% of patients with acute cutaneous lupus erythematosus. The rash appears over the nose and cheek area.

Box 3-2 *Pathogenic Occurrences and Clinical Manifestations in Body Systems of Persons with Systemic Lupus*

MUSCULOSKELETAL

Inflammation of vessels, tendons, and muscle tissue occurs because of deposits of fibrin. Polyarthralgia and polyarteritis occur in approximately 90% to 95% of patients.

GASTROINTESTINAL

Ulceration occurs on mucosal membranes because of degeneration of collagen tissue, with GI manifestations of hemorrhage, abdominal pain, pancreatitis, cholecystitis, and bowel infarction.

RENAL

Glomerular sclerosis and glomerulonephritis occur.

HEMATOLOGIC

Cells are destroyed, and interference with coagulation occurs because of circulating antibodies. Anemia, leukopenia, lymphopenia, thrombocytopenia, and elevated erythrocyte sedimentation rate result.

CARDIOVASCULAR

Pericarditis is the most common cardiac manifestation. It often is the first clinical problem the patient manifests.

Pericardial rub, commonly associated with pericarditis, can lead to dysrhythmias; vasculitis in the small vessels may occur.

PULMONARY

Pleurisy and pleural effusions resulting from inflammation of the pleura are relatively common.

CUTANEOUS

Classic characteristics include the erythematous butterfly rash over the bridge of the nose and on the cheeks and linear erythema along the eyelids (see Figure 3-11). Other features may include bullae, patchy areas of purpura, urticaria, and subcutaneous nodules.

NEUROLOGICAL

Mental and neurological signs and symptoms occur in 35% to 40% of patients with SLE. Signs and symptoms relate to the central nervous system, not to the peripheral nerves. Mental and behavioral changes may occur, as well as seizures, headaches, and strokes.

---

festation describes discoid lupus that can lead to the autoimmune systemic lupus erythematosus.

Etiology/Pathophysiology

Systemic lupus erythematosus (SLE) is an autoimmune disorder characterized by inflammation of almost any body part. A chronic, multisystem inflammatory disorder that affects women more than men, SLE occurs when the body produces antibodies against its own cells. Resulting antigen and antibody complexes damage connective tissues. Known as a disease of exacerbations and remissions that may be triggered by genetic, hormonal, and environmental factors, SLE is distinguished by an inflammatory lesion that affects several organ systems, specifically the skin, joints, kidneys, and serous membranes.

SLE is a chronic, incurable, and multicausal disease. Although the origin of the syndrome remains a mystery, increasing evidence suggests that immunologic, hormonal, genetic, and possibly viral factors may contribute to the onset of this disease, which is most prevalent in women of childbearing age. Nine times more women than men are affected by this disorder, and three times as many African-Americans as whites are affected. Survival rates have increased to longer than 15 years after diagnosis with this disorder.

SLE remains a serious illness despite advances in treatment. Even though the cause remains unclear, with more than one factor likely, genetic predisposition seems apparent in most instances, coupled with a precipitating agent or factor. T-suppressor cells de-

crease in the person with SLE. Those T-suppressor cells that remain function in a limited manner. Antibodies develop against other antigens.

Clinical Manifestations

Clinical manifestations include oral ulcers, arthralgias or arthritis, vasculitis, rash, nephritis, pericarditis, synovitis, organic brain syndromes, peripheral neuropathies, anemia, leukopenia, thrombocytopenia, coagulopathies, immunosuppression, and dermatitis. Anemia tends to be the most common complication (Box 3-2).

Diagnostic Tests

Diagnostic tests for SLE are given in Box 3-3. Many of these test results are positive in the presence of inflammatory disease. No single test is considered conclusive for diagnostic purposes. However, positive results of one or more diagnostic tests along with at least three other criteria lead to the diagnosis of SLE. Criteria for diagnosis include the following:

- Erythematous butterfly rash (see Figure 3-11) over the nose and cheeks and along the eyelids; alopecia (hair loss) with frontal alopecia, seen more frequently in women; other skin features including bullae, patchy areas of purpura, thickening of epidermis
- Photosensitivity
- Oral ulcers
- Polyarthralgias and polyarthritis
- Pleuritic pain, pleural effusion, pericarditis, and vasculitis

Box 3-3   *Diagnostic Tests for Systemic Lupus Erythematosus*

Antinuclear antibody (ANA)
DNA antibody
Complement
Complete blood count (CBC)
Erythrocyte sedimentation rate (ESR)
Sedimentation rate
Coagulation profile
Rheumatoid factor (RF)
Rapid plasma reagin (RPR)
Skin and renal biopsy
C-reactive protein (CRP)
Coombs' test
Lupus erythematosus cell preparation (LE cell prep)
Urinalysis
Chest radiographic study

- Renal disorders as evidenced by the presence of protein or cellular casts in the urine
- Neurological signs, such as seizures of unknown cause
- Hematologic disorders—such as hemolytic anemia, leukopenia, lymphopenia, or thrombocytopenia—in the absence of other diagnostic reasons
- Immunologic disorder identified with positive lupus erythematosus (LE) prep or antinuclear antibody (ANA) or double-stranded DNA (ds-DNA)
- Positive ANA in the absence of patient use of drugs known to cause drug-induced lupus erythematosus

Medical Management

SLE treatment goals include relief of the symptoms. The outcomes of the medical plan include relief of symptoms, attempts to induce remission of the disease, alleviation of exacerbations early, and prevention of untoward complications. Additional outcomes include therapeutic management of the signs and symptoms of the syndrome and suppression of inflammation.

Drug therapy includes nonsteroidal antiinflammatory agents, such as acetylsalicylic acid (ASA) and ibuprofen (Motrin); antimalarial drugs (hydroxychloroquine [Plaquenil] or chloroquine); and corticosteroids (such as prednisone) in low doses given several times a day. Methylprednisolone may be used intravenously in cases of exacerbation. Peak amounts of steroids help to achieve remission. The steroid doses are decreased slowly until a maintenance dose is reached. Topical corticosteroid creams are used for the rash of SLE. Antineoplastic drugs such as azathioprine (Imuran), cyclophosphamide (Cytoxan), or chlorambucil (Leukeran) may be used therapeutically to achieve remission or to control the signs and the symptoms of the patient's illness.

Antimalarial drugs (hydroxychloroquine) are used to control discoid and other skin lesions and rheumatic manifestations. Because retinal toxicity may occur at high doses, patients should receive pretreatment and annual ophthalmic examinations.

Antiinfective agents are used both to treat and to prevent infections in the patient with SLE. The specific antibiotic depends on the infection site. Urinary tract infections respond well to ciprofloxacin (Cipro).

Peritoneal dialysis or hemodialysis may be indicated in patients who have moderate to severe renal involvement. Laboratory tests such as assessing blood urea nitrogen (BUN) and serum creatinine provide information regarding kidney function. Analgesics and diuretics may be used to treat symptoms often found in individuals with SLE. Supportive therapy—such as balanced diet, a balance of rest and activity, and reduction of exposure to the sun—may also be indicated.

Nursing Interventions and Patient Teaching

Because SLE is a multisymptom disease, a thorough assessment is indicated. The plan of care should be individually tailored to include (1) skin care, including teaching avoidance of direct sunlight and use of protective clothing and sunscreen; (2) balancing rest and activity; (3) assisting the patient to recognize signs of exacerbation (i.e., fever, rash, cough, or increasing muscle and joint pain); (4) early recognition of signs and symptoms of infection; (5) stress reduction and management; and (6) balanced nutrition and reduction of sodium intake. Because the disease is one of exacerbation and remissions, each exacerbation will intensify the patient's stress and subsequently decrease the patient's ability to cope. The nurse should provide psychosocial, emotional, and spiritual support for the patient.

Patients with impaired immune system function must endure the consequences of chronic or incurable disease. A caring and gentle approach to patient care, as well as understanding, will help lessen the burden and stress of these illnesses (Nursing Care Plan: The Patient with Systemic Lupus Erythematosus).

The nurse's responsibilities in patient education are related to the information needed for the patient to live a normal life. The nurse should focus on activity level, prevention of infection, and potential complications.

Prognosis

There is no known cure for SLE. Management of the disease depends on the nature and severity of the manifestations and the organs affected. Earlier treatment modalities have contributed toward a better prognosis.

NURSING CARE PLAN
The Patient with Systemic Lupus Erythematosus

Ms. T., age 34, is suffering from an acute exacerbation of systemic lupus erythematosus. She is admitted to the medical unit with severe joint pain, butterfly rash, generalized edema, and Sjögren's syndrome.

NURSING DIAGNOSIS *Impaired skin integrity related to skin rash (butterfly across face), hair loss, skin atrophy, discoid lesions involving other parts of the body*

Patient Goals/Expected Outcomes	Nursing Interventions	Evaluation
Patient will verbalize understanding of skin care regimen and positioning schedule. Patient will demonstrate behaviors to promote skin healing. Patient will experience improved wound and lesion healing.	Assess and monitor skin and mucous membranes and describe lesions' size, characteristics, and changes noted. Monitor for signs of infection. Assess nutritional status and areas at risk for pressure. Measure I&O. Encourage oral hygiene. Develop positioning schedule. Use appropriate devices, such as air mattress, egg crate mattress, sheepskin, or foam padding, where indicated. Provide optimum nutrition. Encourage patient to keep sun exposure at minimal by wearing long-sleeved blouses or shirts and wide brim hats and by using sunscreens with a sun protection factor (SPF) of 15. Teach skin care maintenance.	Patient verbalizes she understands skin care regimen to promote skin healing. She verbalizes understanding of the purpose of changing positions q2h to prevent skin impairment. Patient's skin lesions are beginning to show signs of healing.

NURSING DIAGNOSIS *Disturbed body image, related to baldness, skin pattern pathologies*

Patient Goals/Expected Outcomes	Nursing Interventions	Evaluation
Patient will verbalize understanding of altered body image. Patient will have a positive, accepting, and realistic body image. Patient will perform self-care activities within level of own ability. Patient will identify personal community resources that can provide assistance.	Assess patient's perception of body image; investigate what aspects are not pleasing and how changes are perceived as deviating from social norms. Teach patient ways to improve body image (e.g., improved personal hygiene, wearing makeup, change in clothes, protecting self from sun). Encourage family members and significant others to maintain open communication with patient. Record emotional changes. Set limits on maladaptive behavior.	Patient states she understands that skin changes and hair loss are part of the disease process of systemic lupus erythematosus. Patient verbalizes importance of open communication with her family and significant other concerning her feelings of body image disturbance.

? CRITICAL THINKING QUESTIONS

1. Ms. T. has painful, edematous joints that greatly decrease her mobility. She has 4+ pitting edema to the lower extremities secondary to the loss of protein through her kidney. What are the most appropriate nursing interventions to decrease Ms. T.'s pain level and to increase her mobility?
2. On entering the room, the nurse notes Ms. T. crying. She verbalizes that her lifestyle is severely altered because she is unable to be in the sun to work in her beloved garden. What nursing interventions would be most beneficial?
3. Ms. T. confides that she fears that this severe increase in her symptoms will lead to an early death. What initial response to this statement would be of greatest assistance?

PARASITIC DISEASES OF THE SKIN

PEDICULOSIS

Etiology/Pathophysiology

Pediculosis (lice infestation) is a parasitic disorder of the skin that is usually associated with poor living conditions and poor personal hygiene. This is not always the case, however; pediculosis can occur in any lifestyle. Lice obtain their nutrition from the blood of their victims. They leave their eggs (nits) on the skin surface attached to the shaft of the hair (Figures 3-12 and 3-13).

Humans have three types of lice: the head louse, the body louse, and the pubic louse. In pediculosis capitis the head louse attaches itself to the hair shaft and lays 8 to 16 eggs per day. The eggs can be seen best at the back of the neck as gray, shiny, oval bodies.

In pediculosis corporis the body louse is found around the neck, waist, and thighs. The louse is generally found in the seams of clothing. Severe pruritus and pinpoint hemorrhages are caused from the bite of the louse.

The pubic louse, the parasite involved in pediculosis pubis, does not resemble the head or body louse. It looks like a crab with sharp pincers that attach to the pubic hair. Transmission can be through sexual contact, bed clothing, or bath towels.

Clinical Manifestations

Nits or lice can be seen on the body. Pinpoint raised red macules, pinpoint hemorrhages, and severe pruritus confirm the diagnosis. Excoriation is common because of the intense pruritus.

Assessment

Collection of **subjective data** will include complaints of pruritus in the area involved. Tenderness and difficulty wearing clothes are also noted.

Collection of **objective data** will reveal erythema, petechiae, and skin excoriation in the area.

Diagnostic Tests

The diagnostic test is a physical examination of the involved area. A health history supports the diagnosis. Removal of the parasite confirms the diagnosis.

Medical Management

The topical application of a pediculicide such as lindane (Kwell) or pyrethrins (RID) is used in any area the contaminated patient has contacted. The specific technique for applying these products varies and should be followed closely to control the lice.

Nursing Interventions and Patient Teaching

The primary nursing interventions involve the application of the medication to rid the patient of the lice. Every place the patient has had contact needs to be cleaned. Health teaching stresses the transmission of the disease by contact. Assessment of the patient's emotional needs is important. Having a lice infestation carries a negative implication by society that the patient has poor hygiene practices.

Nursing care focuses on identifying involved people and appropriate health teaching. The nature and transmission of the disease are stressed. Each family member should be assessed for nits and taught measures to reduce pruritus, such as cool compresses and corticosteroid ointments. Any furniture or nonwashable materials with which the patient has come in contact should be properly cleaned to prevent reinfection. Bed linens should all be washed in hot water and dried in a dryer.

Prognosis

The prognosis is good; proper treatment results in full recovery.

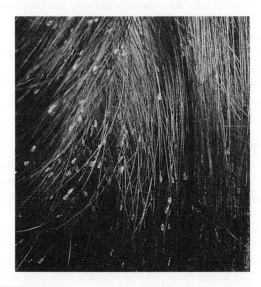

FIGURE **3-12** Eggs of *Pediculus* attached to shafts of hair.

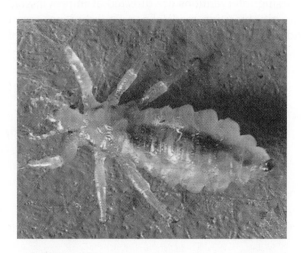

FIGURE **3-13** Lice have six legs and are wingless.

SCABIES

Etiology/Pathophysiology

The cause of scabies is the female itch mite *(Sarcoptes scabiei)*. The mite penetrates the skin and makes a burrow. Once under the skin, the mite lays eggs that mature and rise to the skin surface. Scabies is transmitted by prolonged contact with an infected area. Overcrowded living conditions, poverty, changing sexual behaviors, and world travel have increased the incidence of scabies. Scabies now occurs in all age groups and socioeconomic classes.

Clinical Manifestations

Scabies causes wavy, brown, threadlike lines on the body. Pruritus is severe and secondary infections are common from the excoriation caused by scratching. Locations for the threadlike lines are hands, arms, body folds, and genitalia (Figure 3-14).

Assessment

Collection of **subjective data** includes the severe pruritus associated with scabies and the skin excoriation resulting from scratching.

Collection of **objective data** includes finding the wavy brown lines on the body and severe erythema from the scratching.

Diagnostic Tests

Identification can be confirmed by microscopic examination of infected skin. A health history and characteristic signs and symptoms support the diagnosis.

Medical Management

Medical treatment attempts to eliminate the mite and prevent complications. Drug therapy is basically the same as for pediculosis. Two additional drugs used are crotamiton (Eurax) and a 4% to 8% solution of sulfur in petrolatum.

Nursing Interventions and Patient Teaching

Nursing interventions are directed at improving skin integrity by using medical aseptic techniques to provide hygiene and to apply medications. Proper application of medication is essential to destroy the parasite. The nurse must also consider the emotional well-being of the patient. Using open-ended questions and listening skills helps the nurse to support the emotional well-being of the patient.

The primary concern is to educate the family members about the transmission of scabies. Each family member needs to treat the whole body with a scabicide. Clothing, linens, and bath articles should be washed in hot water and dried in a dryer. If clothes are line dried, they should be ironed. Each member should realize the importance of compliance with the treatment. It is important that the nurse teach the family that scabies infestations can happen to anyone. The nurse must be able to use and convey a nonjudgmental attitude toward these patients.

Prognosis

The prognosis is good; with adequate treatment, full recovery will result.

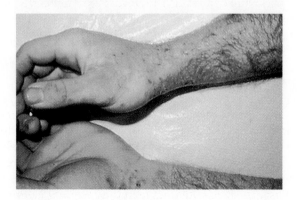

FIGURE **3-14** Scabies.

TUMORS OF THE SKIN

Overgrowth of the skin cells can develop from any layer or its appendages. The majority of skin tumors are benign. Many outgrowths or tumors can be predisposing factors for skin cancer.

Clinical Manifestations

The specific signs and symptoms of skin tumors relate to the type of tumor. Keloids, which originate in scars, are hard and shiny. Angiomas resemble birthmarks, and warts (verrucae) are located on the arms and hands. Nevi are considered to be predisposers of cancer and create anxiety in the patient when a color change is noted. Skin cancers may be life threatening and occur wherever exposure to the sun may have been the greatest.

Any changes in a skin lesion should be reported to a physician. These changes could be in the size, color, border, surface, or elevation of the lesion. The development of pain, bleeding, or pruritus should also be reported.

Assessment

Collection of **subjective data** includes a good health history. The patient's risk factors should be assessed first. Lifestyle, occupation, family history, and geographical location are important risk factors.

Collection of **objective data** includes describing the lesion in detail. The size, location, and any pain are significant factors in determining the type of skin tumor. The appearance of the lesions can take several forms.

Diagnostic Tests

The diagnostic test for tumors of the skin is biopsy of the lesion. A health history and visual inspection support the diagnosis.

Medical Management

The primary medical intervention for skin tumors is surgical removal. Other treatment modalities are radiation therapy to decrease the size of the tumor and application of topical medications such as corticosteroids to decrease the size and inflammation.

Nursing Interventions and Patient Teaching

The potential threat of malignancy causes great concern for the patient. Careful explanations of treatments, medications, and tests help decrease anxiety. If surgery is the treatment of choice, the patient will need to be prepared for surgery.

Nursing intervention revolves around preparing the patient for the treatment needed. Skin tumors may be a threat to the patient's self-concept. Emotional care is important; the nurse should encourage the patient to verbalize feelings of fear or anxiety.

Nursing diagnoses and interventions discussed with malignant melanoma are applicable to most skin cancers. Although the tumors previously mentioned are not all malignant, the problems posed are the same until a definite diagnosis is made.

Discharge instructions include skin care, dressing changes, and follow-up care. The nurse should involve the family in patient teaching to support the patient. The signs and symptoms of an infection should be covered for patients who have had tumors surgically removed.

KELOIDS

Keloids (an overgrowth of collagenous scar tissue at the site of a wound of the skin) are seen more often in African Americans than in whites. Collagen tissue becomes raised, hard, and shiny. Keloids usually originate from a scar and can be located anywhere on the body. The sternum, ears, neck, and arms are common locations. Keloids are usually surgically excised but may recur. Steroids and radiation therapy are two treatment measures (Figure 3-15).

ANGIOMAS

An angioma develops when a group of blood vessels dilate and form a tumorlike mass. A common angioma is a birthmark, such as the port-wine birthmark. This stain is not elevated and may be found on one side of the face or any part of the body. Treatment involves electrolysis or radiation.

A spider angioma or telangiectasis is associated with liver disease. A group of venous capillaries dilate and branch out like a spider. Spider angiomas will usually resolve as the disease improves.

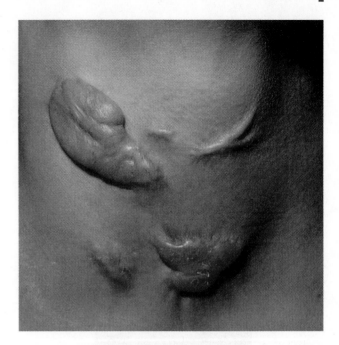

FIGURE **3-15** Keloids.

VERRUCA (WART)

A verruca is a benign, viral, warty skin lesion with a rough, papillomatous (nipplelike) growth occurring in many forms. Verrucae may occur singly or in groups and are thought to be contagious. Common locations are the hands, arms, and fingers, but warts can occur anywhere on the body. The plantar wart develops on the sole of the foot and is extremely painful. Treatment of a wart depends on the type, location, and number. Cauterization, solid carbon dioxide, liquid nitrogen, and preparations of salicylic acid are used to remove warts from the body.

NEVI (MOLES)

Nevi (singular, nevus; a pigmented, congenital skin blemish that is usually benign but may become cancerous) or moles are described as nonvascular tumors, also called **birthmarks.** There are many types of nevi, and several may become malignant, especially if traumatized. The raised, black nevus is considered one of the most threatening, and removal is recommended to prevent its becoming malignant. Any change in color, size, or texture or any bleeding or pruritus of a nevus deserves investigation.

BASAL CELL CARCINOMA

Basal cell carcinoma is one type of skin cancer. Related factors to the development of skin cancer include frequent contact with certain chemicals, overexposure to the sun, and radiation treatment. Fair-skinned people are more likely to develop skin cancer, possibly because less melanin is distributed on the skin surface.

Basal cell carcinomas arise in the basal cell layer of the epidermis. These are often found on the face and upper trunk and are not noticed by the patient. Metastasis is rare, but underlying tissue destruction can progress to include vital structures. Basal cell carcinoma is usually scaly in appearance. It may be a pearly papule with a central crater and waxy pearly border.

With early detection and complete removal, the outcome is favorable; however, this type of cancer recurs in 40% to 50% of patients treated (Figure 3-16).

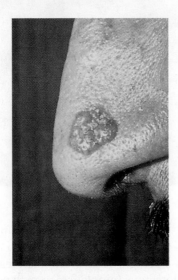

FIGURE **3-16** Basal cell carcinoma.

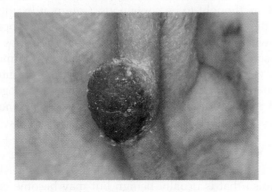

FIGURE **3-17** Squamous cell carcinoma.

SQUAMOUS CELL CARCINOMA

Squamous cell carcinoma arises in the epidermis. This cancerous neoplasm is a firm, nodular lesion topped with a crust or a central area of ulceration and indurated margins (Figure 3-17). Rapid invasion with metastasis by way of the lymphatic system occurs in 10% of the patients. Larger tumors are more likely to be prone to metastasis.

Sun-exposed areas, especially the head, neck, and lower lip, are common places of occurrence. Other sites of chronic irritation or injury (scars, irradiated skin, burns, and leg ulcers) are also places this cancer may occur.

Squamous cell carcinoma can metastasize quickly via the lymphatic system; therefore early detection and treatment are important.

MALIGNANT MELANOMA
Etiology/Pathophysiology

A malignant melanoma is a cancerous neoplasm in which pigment cells (melanocytes) invade the epidermis, dermis, and sometimes the subcutaneous tissue. Several types of melanoma are known, and they are categorized by location and description. Melanoma has the ability to metastasize to any organ, including the brain and heart. This is the most deadly skin cancer and its incidence is increasing worldwide, faster than any other cancer (Figure 3-18).

Most melanomas arise from melanocytes in the epidermis, but some may appear in preexisting moles. Heredity is a factor, and any person who has a large number of moles with a variety of sizes and colors should be monitored.

The occurrence of melanoma has doubled in the past two decades, a fact associated with increased recreational exposure to the sun. The person who has a history of skin cancer is at greater risk (Health Promotion Considerations box on prevention of skin cancer).

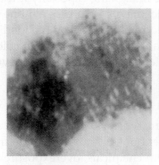
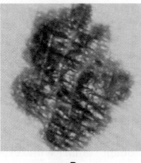
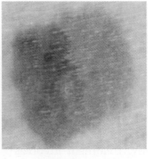
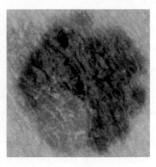

| A | B | C | D |

FIGURE **3-18** The ABCDs of melanoma. **A, A**symmetry (one half unlike the other). **B, B**order (irregularly scalloped or poorly circumscribed border). **C, C**olor varied from one area to another; shades of tan and brown, black, and sometimes white, red, or blue; change in shape, size, or color of mole. **D, D**iameter larger than 6 mm as a rule (diameter of a pencil eraser).

Health Promotion Considerations

Prevention of Skin Cancer

The American Academy of Dermatology (AAD) has recommended these three preventive steps for prevention of skin cancer:

Wear protective clothing, including a hat with a 4-inch brim.

Apply sunscreen all over the body and avoid sun from 10 AM to 3 PM.

Regularly use a broad-spectrum sunscreen with a skin protection factor (SPF) of 15 or higher, even on cloudy days.

The following six steps have been recommended by the AAD and the Skin Cancer Foundation to help reduce the risk of sunburn and skin cancer:

- Minimize exposure to the sun at midday—between 10 AM and 3 PM.
- Apply sunscreen, with at least an SPF-15 or higher that protects against both ultraviolet A (UVA) and ultraviolet B (UVB) rays, to all areas of the body that are exposed to the sun.
- Reapply sunscreen every 2 hours, even on cloudy days. Reapply after swimming or perspiring.
- Wear clothing that covers the body and shades the face. Hats should provide shade for both the face and back of the neck. Wearing sunglasses reduces the amount of rays reaching the eyes by filtering as much as 80% of the rays, and protecting the eyelids as well as the lenses.
- Avoid exposure to UV radiation from sunlamps and tanning parlors.
- Protect children. Keep them from excessive sun exposure when the sun is strongest (10 AM to 3 PM), and apply sunscreen liberally and frequently to children ages 6 months and older.

Clinical Manifestations

Basically, there are four types of malignant melanomas: (1) superficial spreading melanomas, (2) malignant lentigo melanomas, (3) nodular melanomas, and (4) acral lentiginous melanomas.

Superficial spreading melanomas are the most common and occur anywhere on the body. These melanomas are slightly elevated, irregularly shaped lesions in a varying combination of hues; common colors are tan, brown, black, blue, gray, and pink. The **lentigo melanomas** are usually found on the heads and necks of older adults. Characteristically these appear as tan, flat lesions that undergo changes in shape and size. The nodular melanoma grows and metastasizes faster than the other types. **Nodular melanomas** appear as a blueberry-type growth, varying from blue-black to pink. The patient often describes the lesion as a blood blister that fails to resolve. **Acral lentiginous melanomas** occur in areas not exposed to sunlight and where no hair follicles are present. Common locations are the hands, soles, and mucous membranes of dark-skinned people.

Assessment

The collection of **subjective data** should include a thorough health history related to skin cancer. Patients at greatest risk have fair complexions, blue eyes, red or blond hair, and freckles.

The collection of **objective data** includes the location, color, and appearance of the lesions.

Diagnostic Tests

Diagnosis primarily depends on the biopsy of the tissue. The patient is also examined thoroughly for suspicious lesions. Any lesion that is variegated in color, has an irregular border, or has an irregular surface should be monitored.

Medical Management

Medical management depends on the level of invasion and the thickness of the melanoma.

A wide, surgical excision of the primary lesion with a margin of normal skin is the treatment of choice. Skin grafts are sometimes needed.

Subsequent treatment modalities such as chemotherapy, nonspecific immunotherapy, chemoimmunotherapy, and radiation may be planned, depending on the stage of the disease. Gene therapy is currently being examined as another treatment option (Lewis et al, 2004).

Nursing Interventions and Patient Teaching

The major goals of nursing care include relief of pain, reduction of anxiety, and palliative treatment of the disease. The nurse needs to be aware that fear of the unknown is a major concern of the patient with a melanoma. Explaining procedures and diagnostic tests in terms that the patient can understand may help to decrease anxiety.

Nursing diagnoses and interventions for the patient with melanomas include but are not limited to the following:

Nursing Diagnoses	Nursing Interventions
Pain, related to lesion	Assess pain using the five PQRST variables of the chief complaint. Provide nursing comfort measures, such as back rubs, to decrease pain. Administer pain medication as needed. Teach relaxation techniques.
Anxiety, related to cancer, its treatment, and prognosis	Listen to and accept expression of anger, sadness, and helplessness.

Discharge instructions include wound care, medication, cleansing, and follow-up care. The nurse needs to assess the family's knowledge base about the seriousness and treatment of the disease.

Explain to the patient the need for regular physical examinations and regular skin self-assessment. Encourage the patient to protect skin from the sun by using sunscreens and protective clothing and limiting exposure. Medical aseptic techniques are stressed to prevent a secondary infection.

Prognosis

The key prognostic factor in malignant melanoma is the thickness of the lesion. Individuals with lesions less than 0.76 mm thick have a survival rate of almost 100%, whereas those with lesions 3 mm thick or thicker have survival rates of less than 50%. If spread to regional lymph nodes occurs, the patient has a 50% 5-year survival rate. The tumor may metastasize by vascular or lymphatic spread, with rapid movement of melanoma cells to other parts of the body. If metastasis occurs, treatment is largely palliative.

DISORDERS OF THE APPENDAGES

ALOPECIA

Alopecia is the loss of hair. The cause can be aging, drugs such as antineoplastics, anxiety, or disease processes. Alopecia is usually not permanent unless the loss is from aging; the hair will usually grow back but can take several months. Any time that a patient loses hair, the body image and self-esteem are threatened.

HYPERTRICHOSIS (HIRSUTISM)

Hypertrichosis is an excessive growth of hair in a masculine distribution. It can be hereditary or acquired as a result of hormone dysfunction and medications. The treatment is removal by dermabrasion, electrolysis, chemical depilation, shaving, plucking, or rubbing with pumice. Treatment of the specific cause will usually stop growth of additional hair.

HYPOTRICHOSIS

Hypotrichosis is the absence of hair or a decrease in hair growth. Skin disease, endocrine problems, and malnutrition are associated factors. Treatment involves identifying and removing the cause.

PARONYCHIA

Paronychia is a disorder of the nails. The nails get soft or brittle, and the shape can change as they grow into the soft tissue (ingrown nails). In paronychia an infection of the nail develops and spreads around the nail, thus giving it the nickname "runaround." Involved nails become painful as the nail loosens and separates from the tissue. Application of wet dressings or topical antibiotics may be used. Sometimes a surgical incision and drainage of the infected area are performed.

BURNS

Etiology/Pathophysiology

Each year more than 2.5 million people in the United States seek medical attention for burns. About 100,000 of them need to be hospitalized and 70,000 require extensive care services. An estimated 12,000 of these people die annually as a direct result of their burns. The incidence of burn injury dropped during the last 10 years and the number of deaths resulting from burn injury also decreased. This decrease stems from the creation of regional burn centers, a national focus on fire safety, the use of smoke detectors, and occupational safety mandates.

Burns may result from thermal or nonthermal causes. Thermal burns result from flames, scalds, and thermal energy (heat). Thermal burns provide the most common type of burn injury. Nonthermal burns result from electricity, chemicals, and radiation (Safety Considerations box on prevention of burns). Skin destruction depends on the burning agent, the temperature of the burning agent, condition of skin before injury, and the duration of the person's contact with the agent.

Burns cause dramatic changes in most physiologic functions of the body beginning in the first few min-

 Safety Considerations

Prevention of Burns

- The major cause of fires in the home is carelessness with cigarettes. Preventive education is imperative.
- Other causes of burns include hot water from water heaters set higher than 140° F (60° C), cooking accidents, space heaters, combustibles such as gasoline and charcoal lighter fluid, steam from radiators, and chemicals.
- Most burns can be prevented. The nurse as a citizen and health care provider is in a good position to conduct home safety assessments and to educate people about burn injuries before accidents occur. Home safety measures include using smoke alarms and fire extinguishers. Families should have fire drills, and each family member should know where to go and what to do in case of a fire.
- Local fire departments can inform the public of regional fire codes and perform home safety checks.
- Knowledge of potential sources for burn injury allows problem solving for burn prevention.
- Teaching people proper use of appliances (e.g., space heaters, electrical cords, wiring, outlets, outdoor grills, and water heaters) can prevent burn injury.

utes to the first 12 to 24 hours after the burn injury. The effect of the burn depends on two factors: the extent of the body surface burned and the depth of the burn injury. Documented as a percentage of body surface area burned, the extent of the total body surface area injured (TBSA) varies with the injury. Burns exceeding 20% TBSA result in massive evaporative water losses and fluid loss into the interstitial spaces. Depth depends on the layers of the skin involved.

With any burn injury, a pathophysiologic process ensues. In the damaged area the capillaries dilate, resulting in capillary hyperpermeability that lasts for about 24 hours. The increased cell permeability causes the fluid to shift from the capillaries into the surrounding tissues (interstitial spaces), resulting in edema and vesiculation (blistering). The larger the burned area involved, the greater is the shift of fluid, resulting in a rapid shift of fluid from the intravascular area into the interstitial area (sometimes known as third spacing). This shift causes the greatest threat to life because the cells become dehydrated. As a result, the body experiences hypovolemic shock and hyperviscosity. The blood pressure drops, and blood flow to the kidneys decreases, increasing the chances of acute renal failure. Symptoms of hypovolemic shock develop and acute renal failure may result.

The pathophysiology and care of burns may be divided into three stages. The emergent phase, stage 1, is from the onset of the injury until the patient stabilizes. In the emergent phase, hypovolemic shock becomes the major concern for up to 48 hours after a major burn. Stage 2, the intermediate or acute (or diuretic) phase, begins 48 to 72 hours after the burn injury. At this time the greatest concern is circulatory overload. Circulatory overload may result from the fluid shift back from the interstitial spaces into the capillaries. Progression into the acute phase begins when the kidneys excrete large volumes of urine (hence the name "diuretic stage"). Stage 3, the long-term rehabilitation phase, begins when the burn wound treatment begins. In the third stage the patient care outcome involves returning the patient to as normal a status as possible. A second outcome would include freedom from wound infection.

In a burn injury, usually the greatest fluid loss occurs within the first 12 hours. The proteins, plasma, and electrolytes shift from the vascular compartment to the interstitial compartment. Red blood cells tend to remain in the vascular system, causing increased viscosity of the blood and a falsely elevated hematocrit level. Acute dehydration is present, and renal perfusion is seriously compromised. This fluid shift and the loss of intravascular fluids may cause the person to develop burn shock. Hypotension; a decreased urine output; an increased pulse; rapid, shallow respirations; and restlessness develop, signifying the burn shock. This rapid loss of fluid places a strain on the heart because the blood volume diminishes and the heart can

no longer supply enough blood to perfuse the vital organs. The body responds by increasing the peripheral resistance. A decreased pulse pressure, an increased pulse (tachycardia), and an increased respiratory rate (tachypnea) exemplify burn shock. Most deaths from burns result directly from burn shock.

Fluids begin to shift back to the vascular compartment in approximately 48 to 72 hours. Fluid return denotes the end of the hypovolemic stage and the beginning of the diuretic stage. Reabsorption of the interstitial fluid back into the intravascular area causes an increased blood volume. As the blood volume increases, the cardiac output increases, resulting in increased renal perfusion. The result includes diuresis. However, a great risk for the patient includes fluid overload because of the rapid movement of fluid back into the intravascular space. The patient's vital signs, urinary output, and consciousness must be carefully monitored. Patients with preexisting cardiac problems as well as the very young and very old create the greatest risk for developing circulatory overload.

A burn victim may experience smoke inhalation. Inhalation damage results from breathing the chemicals produced by the burn. The fumes produce damage to the cilia and mucosa of the respiratory tract. Alveolar surfactant decreases and atelectasis can occur. Breathing difficulties may take several hours to occur. While assessing a patient who has sustained any burn to the upper chest, neck, and face, the nurse must consider the patient at high risk for respiratory distress. Signs that signify respiratory difficulty include a hoarse voice or a productive cough. Other physical findings suggesting an inhalation injury include the following:
- Singed nasal hairs
- Agitation, tachypnea, flaring nostrils, or intercostal retractions
- Brassy cough, grunting, or guttural respiratory sounds
- Erythema or edema of the oropharynx or nasopharynx
- Sooty sputum

Clinical Manifestations

Traditionally, burns have been classified as first, second, or third degree (Table 3-2). Using only the visual characteristics of the burn wound provides an inaccurate description of the burn. An accurate description includes superficial thickness injuries, partial-thickness injuries, and full-thickness injuries, which graphically describes the burn and indicates the depth and severity of the tissue injury (Figures 3-19, 3-20, and 3-21).

Assessment

The nursing assessment integrates (1) depth of the burn, (2) causative agent, (3) temperature and duration of contact, and (4) skin thickness. The patient's age and other disease processes present have an effect

Table 3-2 | *Causes and Factors Determining Depth of Burn Injury*

DEPTH	CAUSE	APPEARANCE	COLOR	SENSATION
Superficial (first degree)	Flash flame, ultraviolet light (sunburn)	Dry, no vesicles Minimal or no edema Blanches with fingertip pressure and refills when pressure removed	Increased erythema	Painful
Partial-thickness (second degree)	Contact with hot liquids or solids Flash flame to clothing Direct flame Chemicals Ultraviolet light	Large, moist vesicles that will increase in size Blanches with fingertip pressure and refills when pressure removed	Mottled with dull, white, tan, pink, or cherry red areas	Very painful
Full-thickness (third degree)	Contact with hot liquids or solids Flame Chemicals Electrical contact	Dry with leathery eschar Charred vessels visible under eschar Vesicles rare but thin-walled vesicles that do not increase in size may be present No blanching with pressure	White, charred, dark tan Black Red	Little or no pain Hair easily pulls out

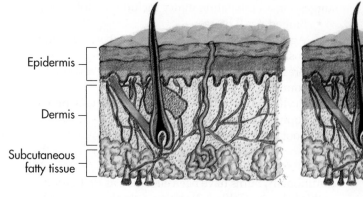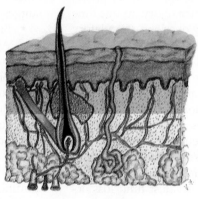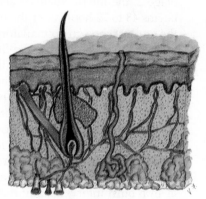

Epidermis

Dermis

Subcutaneous fatty tissue

	Superficial (first degree)	**Partial-thickness (second degree)**	**Full-thickness (third degree)**
Type of burn	Sunburn: low-intensity flash; brief scald	Scalds: flash flame	Fire: contact with hot objects
Appearance	Dry surface; red, blanches on pressure and refills	Blistered; moist; mottled pink or red, reddened; blanches on pressure and refills	Tough, leathery; brown, tan or red; doesn't blanch on pressure; dull, dry
Sensation	Painful	Very painful	Little pain

FIGURE **3-19** Classification of burn depth.

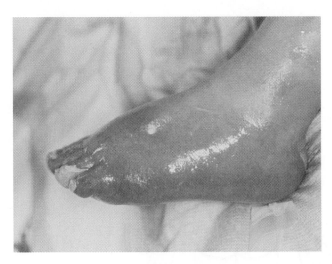

FIGURE **3-20** Superficial partial-thickness injury.

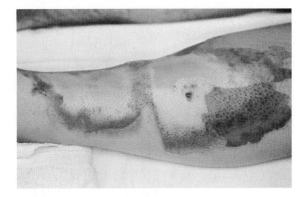

FIGURE **3-21** Full-thickness thermal injury.

on the outcome of the burn. The rule of nines determines the total body surface area (BSA) burned (Figure 3-22). The rule of nines divides the body into multiples of nine. The entire head is 9%; the anterior and posterior aspects of the arms are a total of 9% each; the legs are 9% anterior and 9% posterior; the chest and back are 18% each; and the perineum is 1%. The rule of nines does not take into account the different levels of growth and is not accurate for children.

The rule of nines for calculating percentage of body area burned for infants and children differs from that for adults because the surface area of the child's head is greater (relative to the body) than in an adult. The child's body part and percentage of total BSA are calculated as follows:

- Arm (shoulder to fingertips), 9% each
- Head to neck, 18%
- Anterior trunk, 18%
- Posterior trunk, 18%
- Leg (groin to toe), 14% each

Collection of **subjective data** will reveal the causative agent, other diseases present, the temperature and duration of contact, and the patient's age. The patient's complaints of pain are assessed. If able, the patient should be asked to rate the pain on a scale from 0 to 10.

Collection of **objective data** includes the depth of the burn, the skin thickness involved, the percentage of body surface area burned, the specific location, and any other injuries sustained. Any time a patient has a burn that involves the face, neck, or chest, the nurse needs to be observant for respiratory difficulty. It is important to identify whether the victim has had a tetanus booster in the past 5 years to prevent complications.

The severity of the burn depends on several factors. Major burns are those that require the most skilled nursing interventions. Moderate and minor burns require fewer nursing interventions. Factors determining a major, moderate, or minor burn are the (1) per-

centage of the body surface area burned, (2) age of the victim, (3) specific location of the burn, (4) cause of the burn, (5) other diseases present, (6) depth of the burn, and (7) injuries sustained during the burn (Box 3-4).

Diagnostic Tests

The primary diagnostic test is a physical examination to determine the amount of burned area. Blood assessments—such as those for electrolytes, complete blood count (CBC), serum chemistries, and arterial blood gases—may be done to establish the severity of the dehydration. In inhalation burns, carboxyhemoglobin level is evaluated. Most fatalities occur among survivors with severe asphyxiation or carbon monoxide intoxication. Carbon monoxide binds to hemoglobin with greater affinity than does oxygen, and therefore tissue hypoxia results.

Medical Management

The medical treatment of burns is divided into three phases. Priorities exist in each phase. It is important to remember that these phases are not always clearly defined and may overlap.

Emergent phase. The primary concern in the emergent phase is to stop the burning process using the "stop, drop, and roll" technique. Also, removing clothing and shoes from the victim may eliminate the source of the burn to arrest skin damage. Ice should not be applied to burns because it can cause rapid vasoconstriction, which may cause more trauma to the tissues by increasing the depth of the burn.

Step two is to provide an open airway and to control bleeding. Third, all nonadherent clothing and jewelry (rings, watches) should be removed. Fourth, the victim should be covered with a clean sheet or cloth. Fifth, the victim should be transported to the hospital. In the case of a chemical burn, it is important to rinse the skin generously with water to remove all chemicals. Electrical burns have an entry point and an exit point that need to be identified. Most electrical burns result in cardiac arrest, and the patient requires CPR or astute cardiac monitoring.

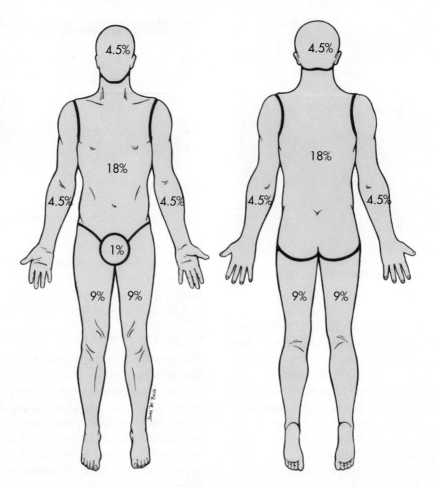

FIGURE **3-22** Rule of nines.

Box 3-4 *Classification of Severity of Burns*

MAJOR BURN INJURIES

Greater than 25% body surface area (BSA) (greater than 20% in children less than 10 years and adults more than 40 years of age)
Greater than 10% BSA, full-thickness
Involvement of face, eyes, ears, hands, feet, perineum
Electrical burns
Burns complicated by inhalation injury or major trauma
Burns in patients with preexisting disease (diabetes, heart failure, or chronic renal failure)

MODERATE BURN INJURIES

15% to 25% BSA in adults, partial-thickness (10% to 20% BSA in children less than 10 years and adults more than 40 years of age)
Less than 10% BSA, full-thickness
Burns with no concurrent injury
Burns in patients with no preexisting disease

MINOR BURN INJURIES

Less than 15% BSA in adults (10% in children or older adults)
Less than 2% BSA, full-thickness
Burns in patients with no preexisting disease

During the primary survey assessment, the nurse should quickly assess the ABCs (airway, breathing, and circulation) and look for life-threatening injuries, such as blunt chest trauma. Immediate assessment of the patient's airway becomes and remains the first priority of nursing care. The nurse suspects inhalation injury especially if the injury occurred in a closed or confined area. Signs and symptoms of inhalation injury include singed facial hair, black-tinged sputum, soot in the throat, hoarseness, and neck or face burns. Stridor is a life-threatening sign.

Carbon monoxide (CO) poisoning is likely if the patient has been in an enclosed area. CO displaces oxygen from hemoglobin. Do not rely on pulse oximetry to rule out carbon monoxide poisoning. Oximeters cannot distinguish between oxyhemoglobin and carboxyhemoglobin. Early signs of CO include headache, nausea, vomiting, and unsteady gait. Treatment includes administering 100% oxygen.

Once the patient is in the hospital, the severity of the burn dictates the care given. The nurse performs a thorough assessment every 30 minutes to 1 hour in the emergent phase. Patients with major burns generally are transferred to burn care centers or units for treatment but must be stabilized before

Initial Treatment of Major Burns in the Emergency Department

1. Establish airway.
2. Initiate fluid therapy by intravenous catheters.
3. Insert indwelling Foley catheter for hourly urine measurement.
4. Do circulatory assessment for circumferential occlusion resulting from eschar.
5. Insert nasogastric tube and connect to wall suction to remove stomach contents and prevent gastric distention.
6. Insert central intravenous catheter, if appropriate.
7. Manage pain by intravenous opioids in small, frequent doses.
8. Provide tetanus immunization prophylaxis.

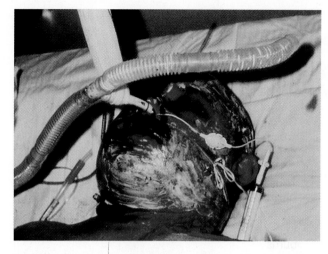

FIGURE **3-23** Endotracheal intubation for patient with severe edema 5 hours after a burn injury.

transfer. Patients with moderate to severe burns are treated using the following steps (Box 3-5):

1. Establish airway—administer oxygen as ordered. Often the physician will insert an endotracheal tube to ensure a patent airway (Figure 3-23).
2. The nurse will initiate fluid therapy; intravenous fluid therapy of Ringer's lactate is begun immediately. The amount of fluid given is in accordance with the percentage of body surface area burned. The patient is weighed so the physician can determine the amount of fluids needed.
3. Insert Foley catheter for hourly output. An hourly urine output of 30 to 50 mL is recommended. Intravenous fluids are given to maintain renal perfusion.
4. The nurse will insert a nasogastric tube to prevent aspiration. Patients with severe burns often develop a paralytic ileus as a result of trauma.
5. The nurse will administer intravenous analgesics in small, frequent doses for pain control. Morphine may be used. Any degree of hypovolemia can increase the effects of medications. Carefully assess the respiratory status of patients when administering morphine.
6. Maintain airway and fluid status, and monitor vital signs.
7. Give tetanus immunization prophylaxis as needed. Analgesics should be given intravenously rather than intramuscularly because of poor absorption. (Patients who have been immunized against tetanus do not need a tetanus toxoid booster unless the last injection was more than 5 years ago. If the patient has never had a tetanus immunization, tetanus serum and active immunization should be administered in the emergency department.)

The first 72 hours require diligent medical care to prevent death. Intravenous fluids are ordered to

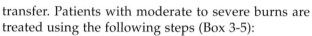

Indications for Fluid Resuscitation

- Burns greater than 20% body surface area (BSA) in adults
- Burns greater than 10% BSA in children
- Patient older than 55 or younger than 4 years of age
- Patient with preexisting disease that would reduce normal compensatory responses to minor hypovolemia (cardiac or pulmonary disease, diabetes)
- Electrical burns

maintain the urine output at 30 to 50 mL per hour (see Box 3-5; Box 3-6).

The primary goals in the emergent phase are to maintain respiratory integrity and to prevent hypovolemic shock, which may result in death (Box 3-7).

Acute phase. The acute phase begins when fluids shift back to the intravascular compartment, usually 72 hours after the burn. During the acute phase the patient's metabolism increases. Urinary output also increases as the fluid shifts back into the blood circulation. As the urinary output increases, the edema in the tissues begins to decrease. The acute phase may last from 10 days to months. The two primary treatment goals include treatment of the burn wound and the prevention and management of complications. Infection is the most common complication and cause of death after the first 72 hours. Other complications include heart failure, renal failure, **contractures** (shortening or tension of muscles that affects extension), paralytic ileus causing gastric dilation, and **Curling's ulcer** (a duodenal ulcer that develops 8 to 14 days after severe burns on the surface of the body; the first sign is usually vomiting of bright red blood).

Box 3-7 | *Nursing Diagnoses for the Emergent Phase of Burns*

- Ineffective airway clearance, related to edema of the respiratory passages
- Deficient fluid volume (dehydration), related to shift of body fluids
- Deficient fluid volume, related to capillary hyperpermeability with fluid moving out of the cells into the interstitial area
- Acute anxiety, related to injury
- Acute pain, related to loss of skin
- Risk for infection, related to impairment of skin integrity
- Impaired skin integrity, related to damage by the burns
- Decreased cardiac output, related to hypovolemia
- Risk for aspiration, related to decreased peristalsis
- Impaired swallowing, related to mucosal edema
- Impaired verbal communication, related to breathing difficulties
- Disturbed sleep pattern, related to hospital environment

Nursing interventions. Prioritizing nursing care using the ABCs remains the most important nursing intervention. Once the nurse completes the ABCs, then the data gathered should include (1) respiratory pattern, (2) vital signs, (3) circulation, (4) intake and output, (5) ambulation, (6) bowel sounds, (7) inspection of the wound itself, and (8) mental status in the head-to-toe assessment.

Fluid reshifting complications may also occur during the acute phase if renal damage has occurred. The patient must be monitored for signs of acute renal failure such as elevated serum creatinine and blood urea nitrogen (BUN). Heart failure may develop as a result of the rapid increase in blood volume from the return of fluid from the interstitial spaces into the intravascular vessels. The primary goals in the acute phase include maintaining respiratory integrity and preventing infection. Assessment for an infection of the burn wound includes observing the wound for increasing erythema, odor, or a green or yellow exudate. All of these may be signs of an infection and should be reported.

Once the patient's vital signs and urine output stabilize and the diuretic or acute phase begins, a nutritional assessment should be completed. Provision for adequate nutrition remains a cornerstone of burn care during the acute phase. Increased amounts of protein, calories, and vitamins help to repair the damaged tissue; oral intake of nutrients should be encouraged as soon as possible. The nutritional challenge includes providing enough nutrients to meet the increased metabolic requirement of the body. The nurse monitors nutritional improvement through daily measurement of weight, serum electrolytes, serum albumin levels, and urinalysis. Adequate nutrition decreases healing time. Skin grafts will not be successful unless nutrition is adequate. It is important that the burn patient not lose weight because this will increase healing time.

Nursing interventions include measures to control pain and to support the patient's psychological well-being. Intravenous opioids in small, frequent doses provide relief from pain, but the amount must not jeopardize respiratory integrity. Specific interventions include verbal support, unhurried care, truthful explanations, and effective listening. The nurse's communication skills must be excellent. A possible complication that should be addressed at the time of the burn is infection in the wound. Local and systemic infections complicate and increase recovery time (Figure 3-24). Wound cultures and sensitivities provide information as to the type of organism present and the most effective antibiotic for treatment.

Without an intact first line of defense—that is, the skin—the protective mechanisms function abnormally. As a result, the nurse uses protective isolation. Gowns, masks, caps, and gloves should be worn during each contact with a patient with major burns. Dressing changes require that strict surgical aseptic technique be followed. Use of proper equipment and cleaning procedures is imperative. Hydrotherapy (e.g., whirlpool) can be a source of infection.

The standard treatment for partial-thickness burns includes debriding the wound, applying topical antibiotics, and changing dressings twice a day. A new treatment for burns includes temporary skin substitutes. Made from a variety of materials, skin substitutes promote faster healing for burn wounds and can eliminate painful dressing changes and minimize scar-

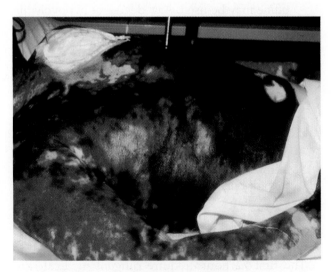

FIGURE **3-24** Postburn *Pseudomonas* infection.

ring. In 1997, TransCyte, a temporary skin substitute derived from human fibroblast cells, became the first bioengineered temporary skin substitute to be approved by the U.S. Food and Drug Administration (FDA) for the treatment of burns. TransCyte is designed as an alternative both to silver sulfadiazine for patients with partial-thickness burns and to cadaver skin for full-thickness burns and deep partial-thickness burns requiring surgical debridement. Made from neonatal human fibroblast cells, the fibroblasts secrete human derma, collagen, matrix proteins, and growth factors. All of these factors promote wound healing. TransCyte is typically applied only once, thus avoiding the frequent, painful dressing changes. Once applied to the burn wound, TransCyte provides a temporary covering that helps protect against fluid loss and reduces the risk of infection.

Traditional wound care involves the removal of the eschar that forms. Eschar is a black leathery crust (i.e., a slough) that the body forms over burned tissue; eschar can harbor microorganisms and cause infection. It may also compromise circulatory status. An escharotomy is often done to relieve the circulatory constriction (Figure 3-25). Daily debridement (removal of damaged tissue and cellular debris from a wound or burn to prevent infection and to promote healing) and special cleansing help to support regeneration of the tissues. Hydrotherapy softens the eschar with water to make removal less painful. It also promotes range of motion to decrease contractures.

The specific wound care method depends on the severity of the burn. The open or exposure method may be for burns of the face, neck, ears, and perineum. The area is cleaned and exposed to air. A hard crust forms, and the regeneration of tissue occurs.

Proper positioning and range-of-motion (ROM) exercises, which should be encouraged by the physical therapist and the nurse, are vital for the well-being of the burn patient. Special bed equipment is needed to prevent the burn from touching the linens. A bed cradle, a CircOlectric bed, or a Clinitron bed is recommended. Lights or heat lamps provide additional warmth.

Advantages to the open method include the following: (1) the wound can be observed more easily, (2) movement in bed is less restricted, (3) circulation of the body part is not restricted, and (4) exercises can be done more easily to prevent contractures. Disadvantages to the open method are (1) pain; (2) chilling; (3) contamination of wound by the health care provider; (4) unattractive appearance of the patient, which causes emotional distress; and (5) the need for protective isolation precautions for the immunocompromised patient.

The pain can be controlled with intravenously administered opioids in the early days of the acute phase. However, considering the long-term nature of a burn, addiction is a potential problem. Diazepam (Valium) has been found to be effective, but morphine remains a common drug used. Chilling may be controlled by keeping the room temperature at 85° F (24.4° C). Humidity should be between 40% and 50%.

The closed (or occlusive) method involves cleaning the burn, applying the prescribed medication, and dressing the wound as ordered. Advantages of the closed method are that (1) it protects the burn area from injury, and (2) it prevents contamination of the area by the health care provider. Circulation checks are important with pressure dressings to assess for adequate arterial perfusion to the involved areas.

The topical medications used to hasten healing and prevent infection vary. Topical administration is preferred because the capillaries are coagulated by the burn. Mafenide (Sulfamylon), silver sulfadiazine (Silvadene), and silver nitrate are common drugs used in burn care. Each drug has specific advantages and disadvantages (Topical Medications for Burn Therapy table).

Burn care essentials include a lightweight dressing. A single layer of gauze covered with medication and a single wrap of Kerlix provide adequate coverage. When applying gauze to the burn area, place gauze between skin areas that touch to prevent skin-to-skin contact.

Changing burn dressings is painful; therefore, the nurse should administer an analgesic 30 minutes before the procedure. This medication may be 5 to 10 mg of intravenous morphine sulfate or a sedative. Most dressings are changed after hydrotherapy. When changing dressings, the nurse removes all old medication and eschar before any new medication is applied. Failure to debride promotes infection, delays healing, and increases scarring.

Skin grafts are used as soon as possible to cover the full-thickness burns. Grafting promotes healing and

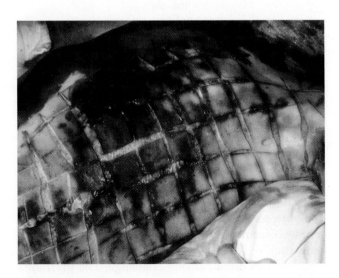

FIGURE **3-25** Grid escharotomy used to alleviate circulatory and pulmonary constriction.

MEDICATIONS | *Topical Medications Used in Burn Therapy*

TOPICAL MEDICATION	ADVANTAGES	DISADVANTAGES
Mafenide (Sulfamylon)	Bacteriostatic against gram-negative and gram-positive organisms Penetrates thick eschar	Metabolic acidosis Pain on application Allergic rash
Silver sulfadiazine (Silvadene)	Broad antimicrobial activity against gram-negative, gram-positive, and *Candida* organisms No electrolyte imbalances Painless and somewhat soothing Not nephrotoxic	Repeated application may develop slimy, grayish appearance, simulating an infection despite negative cultures Prolonged use may cause skin rash and depress granulocyte formation
Silver nitrate	Bacteriostatic effect Lessens pain and eliminates odor Reduces evaporative water loss from burns	Electrolyte imbalances Stains everything it comes into contact with Does not penetrate eschar Pain on application
Nitrofurazone (Furacin)	Inhibits enzymes necessary for bacterial metabolism Broad spectrum of activity Effective against *Staphylococcus aureus* Not absorbed systemically Low incidence of sensitivity	Contact dermatitis in unaffected skin Urine turns a reddish color
Gentamycin sulfate (Garamycin)	Broad antimicrobial activity Painless	Ototoxicity Nephrotoxicity Development of resistant bacterial strains
Neomycin	Broad antimicrobial activity Causes miscoding in the messenger RNA of bacterial cells	Serious toxic effects Ototoxicity Nephrotoxicity
Scarlet red	Nonantiseptic (applied to gauze soaked with oil-based red dye) Drying agent Applied to donor site Promotes epithelialization	No antimicrobial effects Stains and irritates skin Infection may develop beneath scarlet red gauze, which may have systemic effects
Xeroform	Nonantiseptic Debrides and protects donor site Protects graft	Removal may be painful, because it sometimes adheres to wound Neither antiseptic nor antimicrobial
Sodium hypochlorite (Dakin's solution)	Chlorine-based solution that is bactericidal Aids in debriding wounds Aids cleaning of copious drainage	Dissolves blood clots May inhibit clotting May irritate the skin
Sutilains ointment (Travase)	Topical enzymatic agent Dissolves necrotic tissue by proteolytic action Facilitates removal of eschar and purulent drainage	Mild, transient pain on application Paresthesia, bleeding, dermatitis Dressing must be kept moist at all times

prevents infection. Grafting generally occurs during the first 3 weeks of care. Four types of grafts may be used. An **autograft** (surgical transplantation of any tissue from one part of the body to another location in the same individual) comes from the burn victim. A **homograft (allograft)** (the transfer of tissue between two genetically dissimilar individuals of the same species, such as skin transplant between two humans who are not identical twins) comes from another person, such as a cadaver. A **heterograft (xenograft)** (tissue from another species; used as a temporary graft) comes from another species such as a pig or a cow. Fi-

nally, synthetic graft substitutes are now available. The autograft is permanent, whereas the other types are temporary.

Grafts are applied by either the **pedicle method** (the tissue is left partially attached to the donor site and the other portion of the tissue is attached to the burn site) or the **free-standing method** (the tissue is completely removed from the donor site and is attached to the burn site).

Graft sites are a nursing challenge. The graft area needs as little movement as possible so as not to dislodge the graft. Dressings are not changed until or-

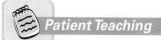
Patient Teaching

Skin Grafts

1. Do not remove dressing unless ordered.
2. Report changes in the graft (hematoma, fluid, collection) to physician.
3. Protect grafted skin from direct sunlight with a sunscreen lotion for at least 6 months.
4. Keep surface of healed graft moistened daily with skin lotion for 6 to 12 months. (Grafted skin does not perspire; it dries and cracks easily.)
5. Wear a strong elastic stocking for 4 to 6 months with grafts on lower extremities.

---

dered. Any movement that results in pulling the graft area can dislodge the graft. The donor site resembles a partial-thickness burn after the graft. Donor site care is as important as care of the burn site. Pain is a primary complaint after the graft and should be treated. The nurse should inspect the donor site for signs of infection, such as erythema and malodor (Patient Teaching box).

The nutritional aspect of burn care continues to be a nursing challenge. Destroyed body proteins and fluid loss present a challenge for the health care team. The body tries to compensate by increasing metabolism to meet the body's extra demands. Therefore the body requires enough energy to maintain homeostasis while meeting the increased need for repairing the injury.

Burn patients should eat by mouth as soon as their condition permits. Intake needs must meet the increased caloric and protein requirements. Protein requirements are greater than normal. Normal protein intake encompasses 0.8 g per kg of body weight. The burned patient requires 1.5 to 3.2 g per kg of body weight (a normal 150-pound person needs 55 g of protein a day; if burned, the same person needs 102 to 158 g of protein, depending on the extent of the burn). Daily caloric requirements range from 2000 calories to more than 6000 calories, depending on the burn. Meeting these enormous requirements requires diligent nursing interventions. Foods need to be concentrated, high-calorie foods that are offered frequently. The body also requires additional amounts of vitamins A, B, and C to promote digestion, absorption, and repair of tissue. Increased amounts of calcium, zinc, magnesium, and iron are needed. Vitamin C and zinc aid in wound healing, and added B complex vitamins aid metabolism of the extra protein and carbohydrate intake. Adding oral supplements such as Ensure, Sustacal, and Carnation Instant Breakfast can increase vitamin, mineral, and protein intake. Total parenteral nutrition provides an alternative to oral intake of proteins only if the patient is unable to take in adequate nutrients by mouth. The daily calorie requirement is

Box 3-8 | *Nursing Diagnoses for the Acute Phase of Burns*

- Acute anxiety, related to change in body image
- Fear, related to chronic illness
- Chronic pain, related to procedures performed
- Risk for infection, related to open skin wounds
- Imbalanced nutrition: less than body requirements, related to increased metabolic demands
- Social isolation related to perceived change in body image
- Impaired physical mobility, related to burns
- Self-care deficit, in activities of daily living (ADLs), related to area of burn involved
- Deficient knowledge, all areas, related to expected care
- Interrupted family processes, related to long-term hospitalization
- Disturbed body image, related to disfigurement from burns
- Deficient diversional activity, related to confinement during care
- Ineffective coping, related to seriousness of injury and perceived role changes
- Powerlessness related to prolonged recovery, loss of income, loss of physical attractiveness

---

estimated by the use of the formula (25 kcal × body weight in kg) + 40 kcal × %TBSA burned = kcal). Most burn victims have poor appetites; therefore getting the patient to eat is difficult. Small, frequent feedings of high-calorie, high-protein, low-volume foods provide the best solution to the nutritional needs of the patient. Some patients develop Curling's ulcer 8 to 14 days after the burn injury. The increased gastric acidity contributes to the development of the ulcer. The first sign is vomiting of bright, red blood. The prophylactic treatment involves intravenous or oral administration of cimetidine (Tagamet), ranitidine (Zantac), omeprazole (Prilosec), or famotidine (Pepcid) (Box 3-8).

Rehabilitation phase. Rehabilitation of the burn patient begins at admission. However, in terms of a burn, the third phase of burn care begins when 20% or less of the BSA remains burned. The goal becomes to return the patient to a productive life. Social and physical skills are addressed. The rehabilitation process may take years.

Mobility limitations constitute the major concerns. The patient requires a comprehensive physical therapy program for positioning, skin care, exercise, ambulation, and activities of daily living (ADLs). The complication of contractures remains an ever-present concern in the care of a burn patient. Although physical therapists provide most of the rehabilitative care, the nurse assists in determining whether the care has been provided and that continuity is maintained. When planning the care of the person with a burn, the nurse should set short-term goals. Setting realistic expected outcomes helps to motivate patients to try to achieve more.

Maintaining and/or restoring the patient's independence remains the primary rehabilitative goal. The psychological possibility of a changed body image requires that the nurse encourage the patient to verbalize fears and concerns. A holistic plan of care must be developed that includes members such as social workers or counselors to provide the comprehensive care needed. During visiting hours the nurse can assess family interactions. Helping the family to cope with the changes in their loved one becomes a major part of nursing interventions.

The nursing diagnoses that apply to burn victims are numerous. The family, patient, and social role of the patient are considered (Box 3-9).

Patient Teaching

Before discharge, the burn patient and family need education. Instructions should be written, complete, comprehensive, easy to understand, and realistic. Return demonstrations provide the best evaluation by

---

| Box 3-9 | *Nursing Diagnoses for the Rehabilitation Phase of Burns*

- Ineffective airway clearance, related to edema of the respiratory passages
- Impaired physical mobility, related to splinting, dressings, or pain
- Activity intolerance, related to prolonged bed rest
- Anxiety, acute to moderate, related to role change
- Disturbed body image, related to scarring
- Deficient knowledge, related to impaired home maintenance management
- Self-care deficit (ADLs), related to pain or fatigue
- Fear, related to impending surgery
- Risk for disuse syndrome, related to noncompliance
- Post-trauma syndrome, related to the cause of the burn
- Impaired adjustment, related to lack of ability to limited expectations of self
- Ineffective coping, related to long-term rehabilitation
- Disturbed personal identity, related to inability to return to previous lifestyle for prolonged period
- Care-giver role strain, related to prolonged recovery period
- Ineffective management of therapeutic regimen, related to complexity and chronicity of rehabilitation
- Anticipatory grieving, related to loss of wellness

Home Health Considerations

Burns

- Bathe twice a day with mild soap.
- Test the water temperature before getting into the shower because your skin is sensitive to extremes of hot and cold.
- Be sure to clean the tub well before each bath.
- If itching becomes severe, take a lukewarm bath with Alpha Keri lotion added to the bath water.
- Do not use lotions that contain lanolin or alcohol because they will cause blisters.
- Avoid direct sunlight. Wear light clothing to cover areas that have been burned because these areas burn easily.
- Discoloration and scarring are normal during healing. The color of the scar may remain red because of the healing process. Usually within 6 months to a year the scar loses its red color and becomes softer. Normal color to the area may take several months to return.
- Report to the physician:
  Any signs of infection
  Fever greater than 101° F
  Feeling of inability to cope

---

the nurse that learning has taken place. The major topics to cover should be (1) wound care, (2) signs and symptoms of complications, (3) dressings, (4) skin care for the burned area, (5) exercises, (6) clothing, (7) ADLs, and (8) social skills (Home Health Considerations box).

Evaluation

Evaluation depends on meeting the stated goals. In evaluating the burn patient, the nurse should ask the following questions:

- Can the patient take care of self?
- Can the patient ambulate without difficulty?
- Can the patient cope?
- Can the family cope?
- Does the patient have contractures?
- Does the patient understand the treatment process?

Burn care is extensive, and the exact nursing interventions for each patient are individualized. Many times the patient must change vocations, and family relationships change. The degree of scarring—emotionally and physically—cannot be predicted, and the acceptance by society cannot be ascertained.

Prognosis

The factors that determine the outcome for the patient with burns depend on the size of the burn; depth of the burn; age of the victim; body part involved; burning agent; and history of cardiac, pulmonary, endocrine, renal, or hepatic disease and other injuries sustained at the time of the burn.

NURSING PROCESS *for the Patient with an Integumentary Disorder*

The role of the licensed practical nurse/licensed vocational nurse (LPN/LVN) in the nursing process as stated is that the LPN/LVN will:

- Participate in planning care for patients based on patient needs
- Review patient plan of care and recommend revisions as needed
- Review and follow defined prioritzation for patient care
- Use Clinical pathways/care maps/care plans to guide and review patient care

Assessment

Assessment of the skin is an important aspect in the care of the patient. Skin changes can reflect specific skin disorders, but they may also alert the nurse to a systemic disorder. Skin assessment allows the nurse to identify obvious and subtle changes in the patient's state of health. Effective skin assessment takes a critical eye and knowledge of the expected normal findings.

The nurse should assess the skin in a private area that has sufficient light, preferably using natural light. Because assessment of the skin is done most often during the assessment of other body systems, nurses tend to discredit all the valuable information that can be obtained. Assessing the skin provides a baseline knowledge of the hygiene measures, nutritional status, circulatory status, and sensory perception of a patient. The skin is the first line of defense against infection. Therefore ongoing assessment of the skin is important in the maintenance of health and the prevention of infection.

Assessment of the older adult can be challenging for the health care professional. The normal changes that occur related to aging are important for the nurse to know. The older patient population is growing, as are the opportunities for the student to assess the older patient (Older Adult Considerations box).

Nursing Diagnosis

Assessment provides the data from which the nurse identifies the problems, strengths, potential complications, and learning needs of the patient. Once the diagnoses are defined, then the nurse can start forming a plan of care that meets the needs of the patient in a hierarchical manner. Being able to prioritize the nursing interventions needed helps contribute to a more predictable recovery for the patient. Possible nursing diagnoses that should be considered for the patient with a skin disorder are as follows:

NURSING DIAGNOSES	NURSING INTERVENTIONS
Anxiety, related to altered appearance	Assess anxiety level every shift. Observe verbal and nonverbal behavior. Encourage the patient to verbalize feelings. Teach relaxation techniques. Assess patient for pain.
Pain, related to loss of superficial skin layers	Initiate nursing measures to minimize or relieve pain.
Deficient knowledge, related to cause of skin disorder	Assess the patient for learning needs daily. Involve patient in setting goals. Use audiovisuals. Evaluate the patient's success.
Risk of infection, related to impaired skin integrity	Assess the patient for risk factors such as abrasions, elevated white blood cell (WBC) count, and temperature daily. Implement nursing measures to decrease risk factors such as using good handwashing and keeping patient's nails trimmed.

Older Adult Considerations

Effects of Aging on the Integumentary System

- Physiologic changes make the skin of the older adult more fragile and susceptible to impairment.
- Aging changes include decreases in tissue fluid, subcutaneous fat, and sebaceous secretions. This results in dryness, flaking, pruritus, loss of elasticity, altered turgor, and a wrinkled appearance.
- Hyperkeratotic changes are typically seen in the nails, which make them thick and caring for them difficult. Podiatric care is recommended for older adults, particularly those with circulatory impairment.
- Circulatory changes and decreased mobility increase the risk of senile purpura and decubitus ulcers.
- Significant hair and scalp changes can manifest with aging:
  - Loss of pigmentation leading to graying
  - Decreased thickness and increased incidence of balding
  - Increased incidence of seborrheic dermatitis of the scalp requiring special care
  - Growth of facial hair on women, which can be damaging to self-image
- Localized clusters of melanocytes surrounded by areas of decreased pigmentation result in "age spots."
- The incidence of basal and squamous cell carcinoma increases with age, particularly in individuals who have had a high level of sun exposure. Aging skin should be closely inspected for changes in the appearance of moles or warts.

NURSING DIAGNOSES	NURSING INTERVENTIONS
Deficient knowledge, related to treatment of pruritus	Assess causes of contributing factors of pruritus. Promote hydration of the skin by avoiding hot showers and applying emollients after bathing. Encourage adequate fluid intake. Implement nursing measures to decrease skin irritation, such as avoiding clothes made of rough weave. Encourage patient to stop scratching by rubbing or applying pressure to the area. Administer prescribed medications for pruritus such as corticosteroids and antihistamines as ordered.
Risk for trauma, related to excessive scratching	Assess onset and contributing factors of episodes of pruritus. Encourage patient to stop scratching by rubbing or apply pressure to the involved area.
Social isolation, related to anticipated of actual response of others to disfiguring skin disorders	Encourage patient to discuss feelings of loneliness. Identify available support systems to the patient.
Situational low self-esteem, related to disfiguring skin	Assess patient concerning feelings of self-worth by having disorder patient describe feelings about self. Implement nursing measures to assist patient to deal with body image. Accept feelings of anger or hostility from patient. Suggest clothing to conceal changes in skin integrity.

Expected Outcomes/Planning

When planning patient care, the nurse should look at the nursing diagnoses and establish the cause of the nursing problem. By determining the cause, the nurse can direct the plan of care to include nursing interventions to eliminate the cause if possible. The patient should be included in this planning. The nurse will want to ascertain the patient's preferences and capabilities. Including the patient is one way to promote compliance. Most skin problems are chronic, and progress is often slow. Also, many patients are older and require more time for healing.

Planning includes the development of realistic goals and outcomes that stem from the identified nursing diagnoses. Short- and long-term goals must be established.

Examples of measurable goals include the following:
- Patient shows no signs of infection in abdominal wound as evidenced by the wound remaining free of erythema, purulent drainage, odor, and localized tenderness.
- Patient will be able to change dressing correctly as evidenced by the patient following the written guidelines during demonstration.

Goals should have a date of when they will be evaluated. Failing to attain a goal means the nurse should reevaluate the chosen interventions and determine why the goals have not been met.

Implementation

When providing nursing interventions related to the skin, the nurse should (1) include ways to prevent skin problems, (2) provide education in home care management, and (3) provide safety tips for the patient. Patients with skin diseases are usually managed at home and need to be aware of the potential for infection secondary to skin that is not intact (see Box 3-1; Home Health Considerations box).

Nursing measures for the skin include a variety of simple or complex interventions. Nursing interventions include applying medications, dressings, and heat or cold and teaching the patient how to perform these measures at home. Using the principles of surgical and medical asepsis are important nursing interventions to follow when providing nursing interventions. The nurse should also incorporate nutritional guidelines for the patient to follow. Patients need extra

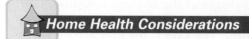

Home Health Considerations

Home Care Guidelines for Baths and Soaks
- The water temperature should be comfortable—usually 90° to 100° F (32° to 38° C).
- Medication should be completely dissolved while tub is filled.
- The soak should last 20 to 30 minutes.
- When oils are added, patients are assisted out of the water to prevent slipping.
- Skin is patted dry, not rubbed, to avoid skin irritation.
- Creams or ointments are applied immediately after the bath to retain moisture.
- Water should be drained from the tub before the patient gets out.
- The door should not be locked, and a helper should be within hearing distance.
- A bath mat should be used to prevent slipping.
- Hand rails may be needed in the shower or tub.
- A seat may be needed in the shower or tub.
- After a medicated bath, pour 1 cup of bleach into used tub water; let stand 5 minutes; wipe sides and bottom of tub; drain tub, and clean as usual.

Complementary & Alternative Therapies

Integumentary Disorders

- The management of integumentary disorders is often difficult. Nutritional and herbal approaches to the treatment of skin problems have been shown to be effective for some disorders, often with fewer side effects than with conventional methods.
- Chinese herbs have long been used in Asian countries for the treatment of skin diseases. A landmark study done in England showed the effectiveness of Chinese herbs in treating atopic dermatitis. This study was undertaken after dermatologists were impressed by the results in their patients who were also under the care of a Chinese herbalist. Participants in the study who received the active herbal formula reported decreases in the number of lesions and itching, as well as improved sleep.
- A traditional Australian plant remedy, tea tree oil (from *Melaleuca alternifolia*), has been effective in the treatment of acne.
- A topical mixture of the essential plant oils of thyme, rosemary, lavender, and cedarwood, in a carrier of jojoba and grapeseed oils, has been found to have significant effect in the treatment of alopecia areata.
- A published report from Taiwan states that acupuncture has been effective in the treatment of urticaria (hives).

Sheehan, M.P., et al: Efficacy of traditional Chinese herbal therapy in adult atopic dermatitis. *Lancet,* 340, 13-17, 1998.

nutrients, such as protein, for the building and repair of tissues.

The nurse should consider the cultural beliefs, personal values, and economic resources of the patient when selecting the appropriate care. There is currently an increase in the use of other forms of treatment for integumentary disorders besides traditional medical therapy (Complementary & Alternative Therapies box). To promote compliance with planned treatment, the patient's independence, dignity, privacy, and physical strengths and limitations should be considered.

Evaluation

During and after the planned nursing interventions, the nurse should determine the outcomes. This is an ongoing process whereby the nurse is continually trying to establish the most effective plan of care.

It is important to consider economic and home care implications. Today patients are being discharged from the health care facility more quickly, and insurance companies are more selective in how they pay for the care and supplies needed by the patient. Creativity and critical thinking are important skills for the nurse to use to meet the needs of today's patient.

Evaluation involves determining if the established goals have been met. The goals are evaluated by the nurse and patient to see if the criteria for measurement have been met. For example, the nurse established in the previously stated goal that the patient's wound would not become infected using the criterion that the wound would show no erythema, purulent drainage, or odor. If at the end of the designated time frame the wound showed no signs of infection, the goal would have been met.

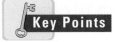

Key Points

- The skin, including nails, hair, and glands, makes up the integumentary system.
- The main functions of the integumentary system are protection, temperature regulation, and vitamin D synthesis.
- The two layers of true skin are the epidermis and dermis.
- The layer of tissue directly beneath the skin is the subcutaneous layer; it is composed of adipose tissue and loose connective tissue.
- The sudoriferous (sweat) glands release perspiration through the skin.
- The sebaceous (oil) glands secrete sebum, which lubricates the skin and prevents invasion of bacteria through the skin.
- Any injury to the skin poses a threat to a person's self-concept.
- It is important to establish a therapeutic relationship to meet the psychological needs of the patient.
- Most skin disorders are not contagious and are rarely fatal. They are often chronic in nature.
- Sterile technique and isolation techniques are required with any open, draining lesion.
- Wet dressings need to be checked frequently. Constant moisture softens the skin and contributes to skin maceration.
- Application of medications must be done to clean skin.
- The nursing interventions of a skin disorder depend on the cause; however, common problems are decreased skin integrity, risk for infection, lack of knowledge concerning the disease, and ineffective coping.
- A primary nursing intervention is patient teaching to alert the patient about the mode of transmission of the particular disease.
- The assessment of patients with skin disorders includes collection of both subjective and objective data.
- Wet dressings and baths may be done to soothe, vasoconstrict, debride, or decrease pruritus.
- Before initiating heat and cold therapy, the nurse must understand normal body responses to local temperature variations, assess the integrity of the body part, determine the patient's ability to sense temperature, and ensure proper operation of equipment.
- Malignant skin diseases need to be prevented by educating the public about causes.
- Burns can be classified by depth and body surface area involved.
- The pathophysiology and care of burns involve three stages: the hypovolemic or emergent phase, the diuretic

or acute phase, and the long-term or rehabilitation phase.

- The three phases of burn care are overlapping, with different goals and nursing interventions in each.
- A first priority in nursing intervention for the burn patient in the emergent phase is to establish and maintain an open airway.
- The treatment method of a burn patient depends on age, body surface area involved, location, depth, and other diseases present.
- The primary causes of death in burn victims are hypovolemic shock in the first 72 hours and infection during the acute phase.

- The nurse should suspect inhalation injury if the burn injury occurred in a closed or confined area.
- A treatment for burns is use of temporary skin substitutes derived from human fibroblast cells.

Go to your free CD-ROM for an Audio Glossary, animations, video clips, and Review Questions for the NCLEX-PN® Examination.

evolve   Be sure to visit the companion Evolve site at http://evolve.elsevier.com/Christensen/adult/ for WebLinks and additional online resources.

CHAPTER CHALLENGE

1. The physician has ordered oral griseofulvin for tinea capitis. The mother asks the nurse why an oral medication is used rather than a cream. The best reply for the nurse is that:
   1. topical creams do not reach the root of the hair to kill the fungus.
   2. oral medications are more economical.
   3. topical medications cause more pain when applied.
   4. it is more convenient to take the medication once a day rather than applying the cream once a day.

2. The most important nursing intervention for the patient with a skin disorder is:
   1. patient teaching.
   2. prevention of secondary infections.
   3. application of medications.
   4. referral for counseling.

3. The physician instructs the mother to take her child out in the sun for approximately an hour or until the skin turns red (not sunburned). This is a common medical treatment for:
   1. atopic dermatitis.
   2. acne vulgaris.
   3. pityriasis rosea.
   4. psoriasis.

4. Which of the following assessments should the nurse report to the physician immediately for an adult patient with partial-thickness burns over 25% of his body?
   1. Complaints of pain every 4 to 6 hours
   2. Decreasing appetite
   3. Hourly urine output of 10 to 15 mL
   4. Edema at the IV site

5. J. has a rash on her back that began as an identifying patch with a raised, scaly border and a pink center about 10 days ago. Now she has more on both sides of her back. From these signs, you would assess the rash to be:
   1. impetigo contagiosa.
   2. pityriasis rosea.

   3. contact dermatitis.
   4. infantile eczema.

6. A patient complains of a burning pain on his lower thoracic area. Upon inspection the area is found to be erythematous and edematous with a cluster of vesicles. You suspect the patient has:
   1. herpes zoster.
   2. herpes simplex.
   3. varicella.
   4. impetigo.

7. A patient complains that he has basal cell carcinoma and is going to die. As a nurse, you know that:
   1. basal cell carcinoma is rarely terminal.
   2. without proper medication it can result in melanoma.
   3. it is a heredity disorder caused by decreased melanin.
   4. treatment involves strong chemotherapeutic agents.

8. It is important to teach the patient the warning signs for skin cancer. Which of the following is a warning sign of skin cancer?
   1. Border irregularity
   2. Smooth surface
   3. Decreasing diameter
   4. Mole symmetry

9. A patient has an inhalation burn injury. Which of the following is a medical emergency?
   1. Singed facial hair
   2. Neck or face burns
   3. Pallor
   4. Respiratory stridor

10. Which method of assessing burn size applies only to adults?
    1. Lund-Browder
    2. Rule of nines
    3. Parkland method
    4. Primary survey

11. You have just finished performing an assessment for a patient with systemic lupus erythematosus. Which of the following clinical manifestations would you expect to find?

    1. Oral ulcers and erythematous rash over nose and cheeks
    2. Leukocytosis and urticaria
    3. Anemia and jaundice
    4. Diarrhea and hypokalemia

12. The physician has scheduled a debridement for a patient that has partial-thickness burns on his chest and right upper leg. Which of the following nursing interventions is most important for the nurse to accomplish?

    1. Ambulate the patient to increase the blood flow to the area.
    2. Administer an opioid analgesic intravenously prior to the debridement.
    3. Teach the patient to remove the old dressings using clean technique.
    4. Explain to the patient that the procedure will be painful.

13. A patient is admitted with partial- and full-thickness burns on his right lower extremity. From this observation, the nurse should plan for the patient to have a(n):

    1. closed dressing change every 3 hours.
    2. open dressing.
    3. temporary skin cover.
    4. incision and drainage of the wound.

14. A patient is admitted with partial-thickness burns on his upper chest and face. It would be most important for the nurse to initially monitor the patient for:

    1. respiratory problems.
    2. burn shock.
    3. infection of the wound.
    4. cellulitis of the affected area.

15. An electrical burn must be assessed for:

    1. infection.
    2. cardiac irregularities.
    3. burn depth.
    4. hypovolemic shock.

16. A patient is admitted with herpes zoster. The nurse should plan to administer which medication on a frequent basis?

    1. acyclovir (Zovirax)
    2. cefaclor (Ceclor)
    3. acetaminophen (Tylenol)
    4. cimetadine (Tagamet)

17. The most common symptom of patients with scabies is:

    1. nausea.
    2. nocturnal pruritus

    3. localized pain.
    4. skin paresthesia.

18. It is most important to assess the adolescent with acne for:

    1. suicidal tendencies.
    2. low self-esteem.
    3. increased intake of fatty foods.
    4. change in weight.

19. A patient with thermal burns over 30% of his body has been able to maintain urine output of 250 mL for the past 8 hours. From this information, the nurse might suspect that the:

    1. patient is not improving as expected.
    2. stage of hypovolemic burn shock is resolving.
    3. pain is decreasing.
    4. nutritional status is improving.

20. Ms. P. tells the nurse she has not gone out of the house for weeks because she hasn't been able to cover the lesions on her face with makeup. Based on this information, which of the following would be an appropriate nursing diagnosis?

    1. Disturbed body image, related to change in personal appearance
    2. Defensive coping, related to lack of social contact
    3. Anxiety, related to the fear of permanent disfigurement
    4. Activity intolerance, related to lack of exercise

21. When inspecting the skin, the nurse should remember that the skin provides a primary:

    1. source for vitamin D storage.
    2. protective device against microorganisms.
    3. means of preventing overhydration.
    4. defense against hyperthermia.

22. When teaching a patient to care for herpes zoster lesions at home, the most important instruction for the nurse to give is:

    1. how to clean the lesions with sterile saline daily.
    2. to wash his hands for at least 1 to 2 minutes before applying medication.
    3. to report to the physician when the lesions are crusted.
    4. to launder his clothes in vinegar.

23. A nurse is reviewing the history for a patient who has been admitted with cellulitis. Which of the following conditions would predispose the patient to cellulitis? Note: More than one answer may be correct.

    1. Malnutrition, substance abuse
    2. Treatment with steroids or chemotherapy
    3. Coronary artery disease
    4. Infectious tonsillitis

Continued

24. A parent tells the dermatologist that her daughter seems to be losing interest in school. If you believe this change is due to medication, which of the following patient's medication may cause changes in behavior?
    1. isotretinoin (Accutane)
    2. minocycline (Minocin)
    3. tazarotene (Tazoracp
    4. penicillin

25. An African-American patient presents with impending shock after an accident. How would the nurse expect the skin to appear during the assessment of the patient?
    1. Ruddy blue
    2. Generalized pallor
    3. Ashen, gray, or dull
    4. Whitish, blue, or bright

26. You assess that Mr. G. has a solid, elevated circumscribed lesion that is less than 1 cm in diameter. In your documentation you would chart this as a _____.

27. A 28-year-old electrical lineman is brought to the emergency department after coming in contact with a live overhead wire. He has two quarter-size burns on his right hand. He is admitted to the hospital. What is the most important rationale for admission to the hospital?
    1. The skin provides the least resistance to the flow of electricity.
    2. The evident skin injury seldom represents the full extent of the damage.
    3. Ventricular fibrillation may follow within 48 hours after the burns.
    4. Lethal arc burns may develop after a burn.

Care of the Patient with a Musculoskeletal Disorder

MARTHA E. SPRAY

After reading this chapter, the student should be able to do the following:

Anatomy and Physiology

1. List the five basic functions of the skeletal system.
2. List the two divisions of the skeleton.
3. Describe the location of major bones of the skeleton.
4. Describe three vital functions muscles perform when they contract.
5. Describe the location of the major muscles of the body.
6. List the types of body movements.

Medical-Surgical

7. Define the key terms as listed.
8. Describe the following conditions: lordosis, scoliosis, and kyphosis.
9. List diagnostic procedures pertinent to musculoskeletal function.
10. Compare methods for assessing circulation, nerve damage, and infection in a patient who has a traumatic insult to the musculoskeletal system.
11. Compare the medical regimens for patients suffering from gouty arthritis, rheumatoid arthritis, and osteoarthritis.
12. Discuss the nursing interventions appropriate for rheumatoid arthritis.
13. Describe the nursing interventions appropriate for degenerative joint disease (osteoarthritis and ankylosing spondylitis).
14. List at least four healthy lifestyle measures people can practice to reduce the risk of developing osteoporosis.
15. Describe the surgical intervention for arthritis of the hip and knee.
16. Describe the nursing interventions for the patient undergoing a total hip or knee replacement.
17. Discuss nursing interventions appropriate for a patient with a fractured hip after open reduction with internal fixation (ORIF) and bipolar hip prosthesis (hemiarthroplasty).
18. Discuss the physiology of fracture healing (hematoma, granulation tissue, and callus formation).
19. Describe the signs and symptoms of compartment syndrome.
20. List nursing interventions appropriate for a fat embolism.
21. List at least two types of skin and skeletal traction.
22. List four nursing interventions appropriate for bone cancer.
23. Describe the phenomenon of phantom pain.

Be sure to check out the bonus material on the free CD-ROM, including selected audio pronunciations.

ankylosis (ang-kĭ-LŌ-sĭs, p. 133)
arthrocentesis (ăr-thrō-sĕn-TĒ-sĭs, p. 130)
arthrodesis (ăr-thrō-DĒ-sĭs, p. 144)
arthroplasty (ĂR-thrō-plăs-tē, p. 144)
bipolar hip replacement (hemiarthroplasty) (hē-mĭ-ĂR-thrō-plăs-tē, p. 152)
blanching test (p. 189)
callus (p. 159)
Colles' fracture (KŌL-ēz FRĂK-shŭr, p. 158)
compartment syndrome (p. 164)
crepitus (KRĔP-ĭ-tŭs, p. 160)
fibromyalgia (fī-brō-mī-ĂL-jă, p. 143)
kyphosis (kĭ-FŌ-sĭs, p. 189)
lordosis (lŏr-DŌ-sĭs, p. 189)
open reduction with internal fixation (ORIF) (p. 161)
paresthesia (păr-ĕs-THĒ-zē-ă, p. 181)
scoliosis (skō-lē-Ō-sĭs, p. 189)
sequestrum (sĕ-KWĔS-trŭm, p. 143)
subluxations (sŭb-lŭk-SĀ-shŭn, p. 180)
tophi (TŌ-fī, p. 139)
Volkmann's contracture (VŌLK-mănz kŏn-TRĂK-shŭr, p. 165)

OVERVIEW OF ANATOMY AND PHYSIOLOGY

Bones and joints form the framework of the body, and the contraction and relaxation of the muscles allow movement. All movement of the body is orchestrated by the functioning of the bones, the joints, and the muscles attached to the bones. This chapter will discuss the structure and function of bones and muscles and how they serve the body.

FUNCTIONS OF THE SKELETAL SYSTEM

The skeletal system is composed of 206 bones. The skeletal system has five basic functions: support, protection, movement, mineral storage, and hematopoiesis.

Support

The skeleton provides the body framework that supports internal tissues and organs.

Protection

The skeleton forms a firm cagelike structure that protects many internal structures. The cranium (skull) protects the brain, the vertebrae protect the spinal cord, the ribs and sternum (breastbone) protect the lungs and heart, and the pelvis protects the digestive and reproductive organs.

Movement

Because the skeletal muscles are attached to the bones, the bones provide leverage for movement. As a muscle contracts, it exerts pull on the bone and movement occurs.

Mineral Storage

The bones serve as a storage area for various minerals, particularly calcium and phosphorus. When the body does not receive adequate intake of these minerals, the minerals are released by the bones.

Hematopoiesis

Hematopoiesis (blood cell formation) takes place in the red bone marrow. The red bone marrow is spongy bone found in the ends of the long bones. A child's bones contain a proportionally larger amount of red bone marrow than an adult's. As a person ages, much of the red bone marrow converts to yellow bone marrow, which is composed of fat cells.

STRUCTURE OF BONES

There are four classifications of bones, based on their form and shape: long, short, flat, and irregular. Long bones are found in the extremities, short bones are found in the hands and feet, flat bones are found in the skull and sternum, and irregular bones make up the vertebrae (backbone).

ARTICULATIONS (JOINTS)

Bones cannot bend without damage. To allow movement, individual bones articulate (move) at joint sites (Figure 4-1). Bones are held together by flexible connective tissue. The joint is the point of contact between the individual bones. The structure of the individual bones depends on the function of the area. Every bone in the body (except the hyoid bone, which anchors the tongue) connects or articulates with at least one other bone.

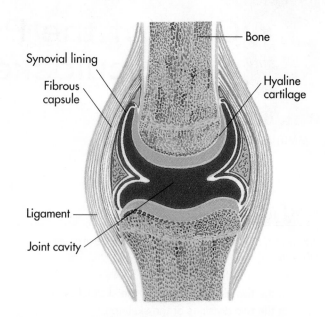

FIGURE **4-1** Structure of a freely movable (diarthrotic) joint. Note these typical features: joint capsule, joint cavity lined with synovial membrane, and articular (hyaline) cartilage covering the end surfaces of the bones within the joint capsule.

Joints perform two important functions: they hold the bones together to form the skeleton, and they allow movement and flexibility of the skeleton.

The most common way to classify joints is according to the degree of movement they permit. There are three types of joints:

1. Synarthrosis: No movement
2. Amphiarthrosis: Slight movement
3. Diarthrosis: Free movement

DIVISIONS OF THE SKELETON

The skeleton is divided into the axial and the appendicular skeletons (Box 4-1). The axial skeleton is composed of the skull, vertebral column, and the thorax (chest). The appendicular skeleton is composed of the upper extremities, lower extremities, shoulder girdle, and pelvic girdle (excluding the sacrum) (Figures 4-2 and 4-3).

| Box 4-1 | **Main Parts of the Skeleton** |

AXIAL SKELETON	APPENDICULAR SKELETON
SKULL	**UPPER EXTREMITIES**
Cranium	Shoulder (pectoral) girdle
Ear bones	Arms
Face	Wrists
	Hands
SPINE	
Vertebrae	**LOWER EXTREMITIES**
	Hip (pelvic) girdle
THORAX	Legs
Ribs	Ankles
Sternum	Feet

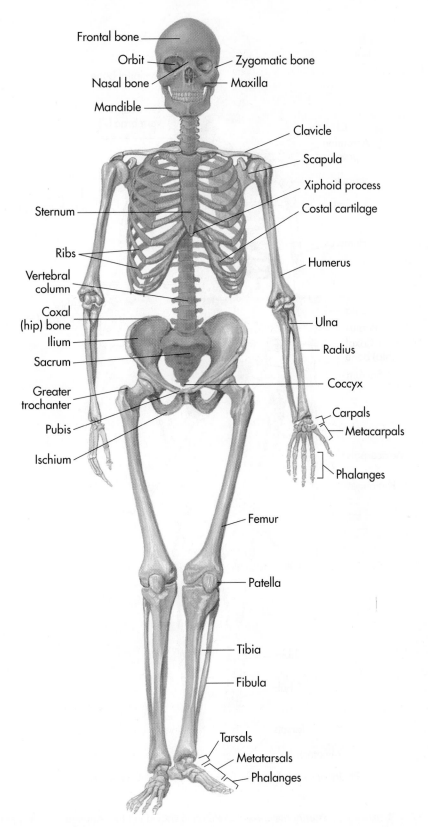

FIGURE **4-2** Skeleton, anterior view. Axial skeleton is shown in blue. Appendicular system is bone colored.

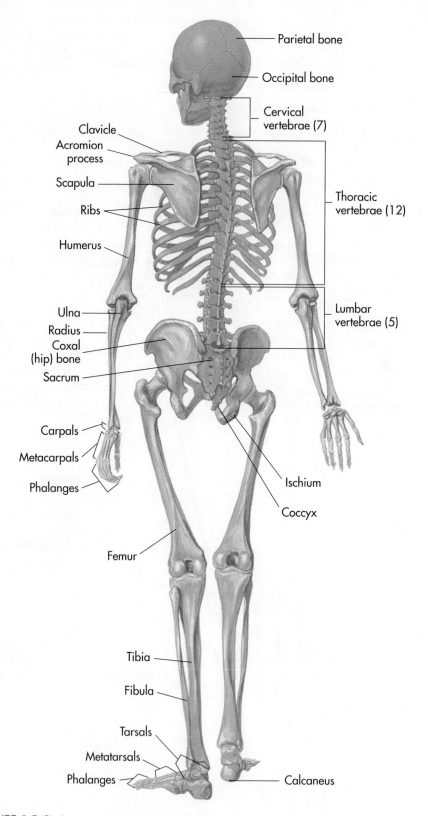

FIGURE **4-3** Skeleton, posterior view. Axial skeleton is shown in blue. Appendicular system is bone colored.

FUNCTIONS OF THE MUSCULAR SYSTEM

The bones and joints provide the framework of the body, but the muscles are necessary for movement. This motion results from contraction and relaxation of the individual muscles.

The body is composed of more than 600 muscles. They usually act in groups to execute a body movement. They make up approximately 40% to 50% of the total body weight.

As muscles contract, they perform three vital functions: motion, maintenance of posture, and production of heat. Contraction also assists in return of venous blood and lymph back to the right side of the heart.

All body movements rely on the integrated functioning of the bones, joints, and muscles. Certain involuntary kinds of motion include activities conducted by the internal organs, such as the heart beating, the gallbladder releasing bile, and the stomach churning food. Muscle tissue is under voluntary or involuntary control. Voluntary muscle is under conscious control, whereas involuntary muscle tissue responds to internal commands without any conscious control of it.

The contraction of certain skeletal muscles gives the body proper posture. These muscles exert a pull on various bones, which allows the body to maintain a sitting or standing position.

As skeletal muscles contract, they produce body heat. It is estimated that approximately 85% of all body heat is generated by the contraction of the skeletal muscles.

Skeletal Muscle Structure

A skeletal muscle is composed of hundreds of muscle fibers (cells). Each skeletal muscle is surrounded by a covering of connective tissue called the **epimysium.** The epimysium joins with two other inner coverings, the perimysium and the endomysium, to extend beyond the muscle to form a tough cord of connective tissue known as a **tendon.** Tendons anchor muscles to bones. As a muscle contracts, the tendon and bone corresponding to that particular muscle are pulled toward the muscle. This is how movement occurs. Tendons in the ankle and wrist are enclosed in sleeves or tubelike structures of connective tissue known as **tendon sheaths.** These tendon sheaths contain synovial fluid and permit the tendons to slide easily; the sheaths also keep the tendons in place. All the tendons, ligaments, and aponeuroses of the body are composed of various sizes, shapes, and densities of connective tissue. These are collectively known as **fasciae.**

Nerve and Blood Supply

Because of the physical demands placed on the skeletal muscles, they need a constant supply of oxygen and nutrition. They are well supplied with blood vessels that carry oxygen and nutrition to the area and remove the waste products of metabolism.

Because the skeletal muscles are voluntary, they need a constant source of information, which is supplied by nerve cells or fibers. These nerve cells continually send impulses that stimulate the muscle cells. These impulses enter at the neuromuscular junction, the point of contact between the nerve ending and the muscle fiber. As a nerve impulse passes through this junction, chemicals are released that cause the muscle to contract.

Usually one artery, two veins, and one nerve penetrate a particular muscle. Each muscle cell comes in contact with several capillaries and a portion of a nerve cell. The muscle cells, in union with the nerve cell that controls them, are called a **motor unit.**

The impulse from the nerve cell must travel across a small gap because the nerve cell and the muscle cell do not directly touch each other. This small gap is called a **synaptic cleft** and is filled with tissue fluid. A special chemical **(neurotransmitter)** travels through the fluid to stimulate the muscle fiber. Acetylcholine is the specific neurotransmitter for skeletal muscle tissue. An enzyme called **cholinesterase** breaks down the acetylcholine once it has transferred the message. This allows the muscle cell to relax between impulses.

Muscle Contraction

Muscle stimulus. Muscle cells are governed by the "all or none" law, which states that when a muscle cell is adequately stimulated or shocked, it will contract completely. Because each skeletal muscle is composed of thousands of muscle cells that react to many different nerve cells, the muscle as a whole contracts according to the principle of graded response. The strength of the contraction of the muscle, therefore, depends on the number of individual muscle cells responding. These muscle responses allow us to tenderly brush a baby's cheek or destroy an irritating mosquito.

Muscle tone. The skeletal muscles are in a constant state of readiness for action. At any given time, several muscle cells within a certain muscle are contracted; the remainder of the muscle cells are relaxed. The muscle tone provided is necessary for good posture but does not provide movement of the body. To understand the importance of muscle tone, one can observe an extremity that has become paralyzed—the muscles are flaccid, limp, or atrophied (wasted) and incapable of producing movement because the cells are no longer receiving stimuli from the nerve fibers.

Types of body movements. Some muscles can move some body parts in only two directions, whereas others can move certain body parts in several directions. Some of the more common movements that the body is capable of producing are flexion, extension, abduction, adduction, rotation, supination, pronation, dorsiflexion, and plantar flexion (Tables 4-1 and 4-2; Box 4-2; Figure 4-4).

| Table 4-1 | *Principal Muscles of the Body* | | |

MUSCLE	FUNCTION	INSERTION	ORIGIN
MUSCLES OF THE HEAD AND NECK			
Frontal	Raises eyebrow	Skin of eyebrow	Occipital bone
Orbicularis oculi	Closes eye	Maxilla and frontal bone	Maxilla and frontal bone (encircles eye)
Orbicularis oris	Draws lips together	Encircles lips	Encircles lips
Zygomaticus	Elevates corners of mouth and lips	Angle of mouth and upper lip	Zygomatic bone
Masseter	Closes jaw	Mandible	Zygomatic arch
Temporal	Closes jaw	Mandible	Temporal region of the skull
Sternocleidomastoid	Rotates and extends head	Mastoid process	Sternum and clavicle
Trapezius	Extends head and neck	Scapula	Skull and upper vertebrae
MUSCLES THAT MOVE THE UPPER EXTREMITIES			
Pectoralis major	Flexes and helps adduct upper arms	Humerus	Sternum, clavicle, and upper rib cartilages
Latissimus dorsi	Extends and helps adduct upper arm	Humerus	Vertebrae and ilium
Deltoid	Abducts upper arm	Humerus	Clavicle and scapula
Biceps brachii	Flexes lower arm	Radius	Ulna
Triceps brachii	Extends lower arm (called "boxer's muscle"—straightens the elbow when a blow is delivered)	Ulna	Scapula and humerus
MUSCLES OF THE TRUNK			
External oblique	Compresses abdomen	Midline of abdomen	Lower thoracic cage
Internal oblique	Compresses abdomen	Midline of abdomen	Pelvis
Transversus abdominis	Compresses abdomen	Midline of abdomen	Ribs, vertebrae, and pelvis
Rectus abdominis	Flexes trunk	Lower ribcage	Pubis
MUSCLES THAT MOVE THE LOWER EXTREMITIES			
Iliopsoas	Flexes thigh or trunk	Ilium and vertebrae	Femur
Sartorius	Flexes thigh and rotates lower leg	Tibia	Ilium
Gluteus maximus	Extends thigh	Femur	Ilium, sacrum, and coccyx
Gluteus medius	Abducts thigh	Femur	Ilium
Adductor group			
Adductor longus	Adducts thigh	Femur	Pubis
Gracilis	Adducts thigh	Tibia	Pubis
Pectineus	Adducts thigh	Femur	Pubis
Hamstring group			
Semimembranosus	Flexes lower leg	Tibia	Ischium
Semitendinosus	Flexes lower leg	Tibia	Ischium
Biceps femoris	Flexes lower leg	Fibula	Ischium and femur
Quadriceps group			
Rectus femoris	Extends lower leg	Tibia	Ischium
Vastus lateralis, intermedius, and medialis	Extends lower leg	Tibia	Femur
Tibialis anterior	Dorsiflexes foot	Metatarsals (foot)	Tibia
Gastrocnemius	Plantar flexes foot	Calcaneus (heel)	Femur
Soleus	Plantar flexes foot	Calcaneus (heel)	Tibia and fibula
Peroneus group			
Peroneus longus and brevis	Plantar flexes foot	Tarsals and metatarsals (ankle and foot)	Tibia and fibula

Table 4-2 | *Muscles Grouped According to Function*

PART MOVED	FLEXORS	EXTENSORS	ABDUCTORS	ADDUCTORS
Upper arm	Pectoralis major	Latissimus dorsi	Deltoid	Pectoralis major and latissimus dorsi contracting together
Lower arm	Biceps brachii	Triceps brachii	None	None
Thigh	Iliopsoas and sartorius	Gluteus maximus	Gluteus medius	Adductor group
Lower leg	Hamstrings	Quadriceps group	None	None
Foot	Tibialis anterior	Gastrocnemius and soleus	Peroneus longus	Tibialis anterior

Skeletal Muscle Groups

Skeletal muscles are usually classified into two broad categories: axial and appendicular. The axial muscle groups are those muscles located on the head, face, neck, and trunk. The appendicular muscle groups are all the muscles of the extremities. Figures 4-5 and 4-6 show the location of the muscles of the body.

LABORATORY AND DIAGNOSTIC EXAMINATIONS

RADIOGRAPHIC STUDIES

The diagnostic study most often used for determining musculoskeletal system integrity is the radiographic, roentgenographic, or (as it is more commonly known) x-ray examination or diagnostic imaging.

A radiographic examination of a joint reveals the presence of fluid, irregularity of the joint with spur formation, and changes in the size of the joint contour. Radiographic examination is used to determine presence of a skeletal fracture. It is important to ask women of childbearing age if there is any possibility that they are pregnant before performing radiographic examinations because pregnant women should not be exposed to radiographs unless in an emergency situation because of potential damage to the fetus.

Laminography or **planography** is also called **body section roentgenography.** This radiographic procedure is useful in locating small cavities, foreign bodies, and lesions that are overshadowed by opaque structures.

Scanography (a method of producing a radiograph of internal body organs by using a series of parallel beams that eliminate size distortion) is a radiographic procedure that allows accurate measurement of the bone's length.

Myelogram

Myelogram examination involves injection of a radiopaque dye into the subarachnoid space at the lumbar spine to determine the presence of herniated disk syndrome (herniated nucleus pulposus) or tumors. The test involves the same procedure as a lumbar puncture (spinal tap), which is discussed in Chapter 14. Radio-

Box 4-2 | *Types of Body Movement*

Flexion: A movement that is allowed by certain joints of the skeleton that decreases the angle between two adjoining bones. For example, if the arm is bent at the elbow, the angle between the humerus and the ulna is decreased.

Extension: (see Figure 4-4): A movement allowed by certain joints of the skeleton that increases the angle between two adjoining bones. For example, if the leg is extended, the angle between the femur and tibia is increased. If the extension angles more than 180 degrees, the extremity is **hyperextended.**

Abduction: A movement of an extremity away from the midline of the body.

Adduction: A movement of an extremity toward the axis of the body.

Rotation: A movement of the bone around its longitudinal axis (e.g., a pivot motion, such as shaking the head "no").

Supination: A movement of the hand and forearm that causes the palm to face upward or forward.

Pronation: A movement of the hand and forearm that causes the palm to face downward or backward.

Dorsiflexion: A movement that causes the top of the foot to elevate or tilt upward.

Plantar flexion: A movement that causes the bottom of the foot to be directed downward.

graphic dye will cause allergic reactions in patients with allergies to iodine and seafood. It is important that the physician be notified about such allergies so that a nonionic contrast agent can be used or medications such as steroids or antihistamines can be given before the examination to minimize any reaction to the radiographic dye. This examination may involve the entire spine or just the cervical or lumbar area. After the myelogram, oil-based dye is removed through the spinal needle to prevent meningeal irritation. Water-soluble dye is used most often and does not need to be removed; it will be absorbed by the body and excreted in the urine.

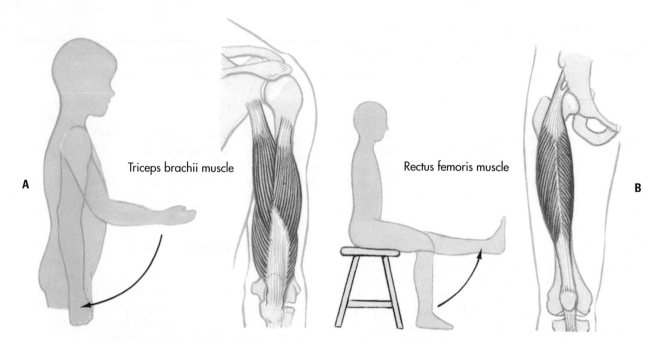

Triceps brachii muscle

A

Rectus femoris muscle

B

FIGURE **4-4** Extension of the lower arm and lower leg. **A,** When the triceps brachii muscle *(shown at right)* contracts, it extends the lower arm at the elbow joint *(shown at left)*. **B,** When the rectus femoris muscle (part of the quadriceps femoris muscle group) *(shown at right)* contracts, it extends the lower leg at the knee joint *(shown at left)*.

The most common discomfort after a myelogram is headache. If water-soluble dye is used, the patient should lie quietly in a semi-Fowler's position for approximately 8 hours. The positioning of the patient is important to keep the dye in the lower spine. During this time, encouraging fluids will help the body absorb the dye from the spinal column. If oil-based dye is used, the patient will need to rest in a flat position for as long as 12 hours. It is important to instruct the patient to inform the nurse if there is headache, stiff neck, leg weakness, or difficulty voiding. Rare complications include seizure, infection, drowsiness, severe headache, numbness, and paralysis.

Patients needing a myelogram fear the needle will be inserted into the spinal canal and damage the cord. It is important that the nurse inform the patient that the tap is done in the lumbar region of the spine at approximately the fourth or fifth lumbar (L4/L5) space. The spinal cord starts at the level of the foramen magnum and ends at the second lumbar (L2) space (lower border of ribcage).

Nuclear Scanning

Tests in which nuclear scanning is used are done in the nuclear medicine department, which has scanners or camera detectors that record the images on radiographic film. The dosages of radioactive isotopes are low for diagnostic tests; precautionary measures that are required for radium therapy are not necessary.

Nursing interventions required when patients are scheduled for nuclear scanning procedures involve (1) obtaining written consent from the patient, (2) informing the patient that the radioactive isotopes will not affect family or visitors, and (3) following instructions as outlined by the nuclear medicine department as to special preparations for specific scans.

Magnetic Resonance Imaging

Magnetic resonance imaging (MRI) is used to detect pathological conditions of the cerebrum and spinal cord. It is currently used to detect herniated nucleus pulposus. The test involves the use of magnetism and radio waves to make images of cross sections of the body. MRI can give much more detailed pictures of fluid-filled soft tissue and blood vessels than any other test.

Patient preparation involves having the patient remove any metal, such as jewelry, clothing with metal fasteners, glasses, and hair clips. Patients with metal prostheses such as heart valves, orthopedic screws, or cardiac pacemakers cannot undergo MRI.

The machine looks like a narrow tunnel, and patients are required to lie still in this machine for 45 to 60 minutes. The patient enters the tunnel head first. This may cause anxiety and a feeling of claustrophobia. The procedure is painless; however, if the patient is extremely anxious, a sedative is given. Patients should be encouraged to use relaxation techniques, such as imagery, during the test. Because the procedure requires the patient to be motionless, relaxation techniques that require flexing and relaxing of the muscles are not appropriate.

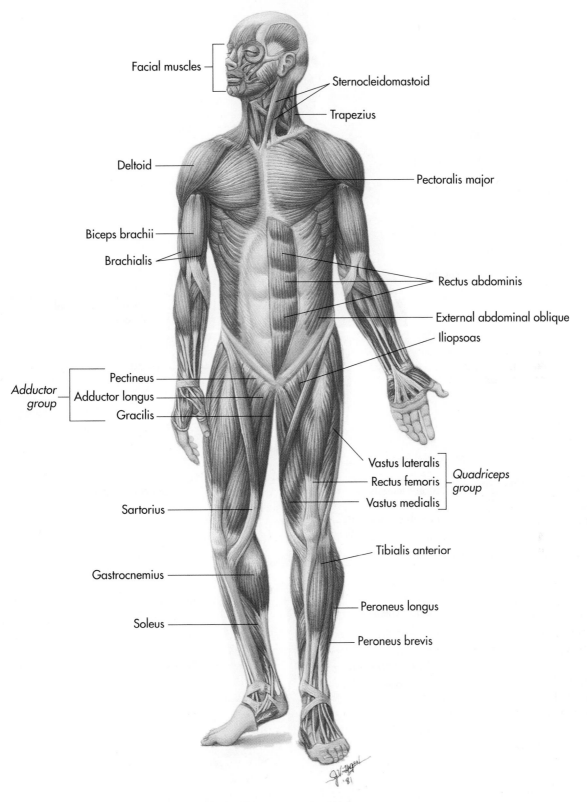

FIGURE 4-5 Anterior view of the body.

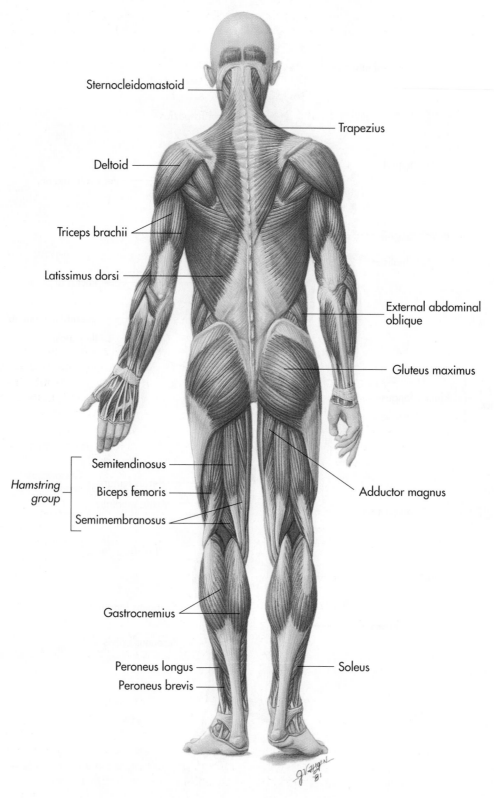

FIGURE **4-6** Posterior view of the body.

After the test, routine vital sign measurements are taken and pretest activities can be resumed. There are no adverse effects.

Computed Axial Tomography (CT or CAT Scan)

Body sections can be examined from many different angles using a CT scanner that produces a narrow x-ray beam. Consequently, a three-dimensional picture of the structure being studied is made. The CT scanner is approximately 100 times more sensitive than the radiograph machine and should not be used unnecessarily because of radiation exposure. Iodine contrast dye is sometimes used. CT scan is used for the head and body. It is useful in locating injuries to the ligaments or tendons and tumors of the soft tissue and in identifying fractures in areas difficult to define by other means. Patient preparation includes (1) having the patient sign a consent form authorizing the examination if not included on the initial hospital consent form, (2) questioning the patient regarding allergies (e.g., iodine and seafood), (3) keeping the patient on NPO (nothing by mouth) status 3 to 4 hours before the test (necessary in case contrast dye is used because the dye can cause nausea and vomiting), (4) measuring vital signs to be used as a baseline, (5) having the patient void before the test, (6) removing such articles as jewelry and hairpins, and (7) telling the patient that he must lie still during the test and may feel warm and slightly nauseated for a few minutes when dye is injected.

After the test the patient is observed for delayed allergic reactions (if contrast dye was used). Fluids are encouraged unless contraindicated. Pretest diet and activity can usually be resumed.

Bone Scan

The bone scan test is especially valuable in detecting metastatic and inflammatory bone disease (osteomyelitis). This test involves the intravenous administration of nuclides (atomic material) approximately 2 to 3 hours before the test is scheduled. There are no food or fluid restrictions, and patients are encouraged to drink water over the next 1 to 3 hours to aid renal clearance of any radioisotope not picked up by the bone. After the patient has voided, a scanning camera reveals the degree of radionuclide uptake; areas of concentrated nucleotide uptake may represent a tumor or other abnormality. These areas of concentration can be detected days or weeks before an ordinary radiograph can reveal a metastatic lesion. The test takes approximately 30 to 60 minutes and requires the patient to lie still.

ENDOSCOPIC EXAMINATION

For an endoscopy, a lighted tube is used to visualize inside a body cavity. Although some procedures require general anesthesia, most require only local anesthesia. Emotional support and complete explanations

help relieve the patient's anxiety. Preparation for an endoscopic examination is similar to surgical preparation: (1) a consent form is signed; (2) a preoperative checklist is completed with special attention to removing jewelry, dentures, and contact lenses; (3) NPO status is initiated 6 to 12 hours before the examination; (4) premedications may be given, such as atropine and a sedative; (5) the patient is encouraged to void; (6) vital signs are taken and recorded; and (7) bed rest with side rails up is maintained after the premedication is given.

Arthroscopy

Arthroscopy is an endoscopic examination that enables direct visualizing of a joint. The procedure is used to accomplish the following: (1) exploration of the joint to determine the presence of a disease process, (2) drainage of fluid from the joint cavity, and (3) removal of damaged tissue or foreign bodies from the joint.

This examination is most commonly done on the knee joint, with the synovium, articular surfaces, and meniscus (a curved, fibrous cartilage in the knee) visualized through the scope. The procedure involves insertion of a large-bore needle into the suprapatellar pouch and saline instillation into the joint. The patient may be given a general or local anesthetic agent. After the arthroscopic examination, the patient may be advised to limit activities for several days.

Endoscopic Spinal Microsurgery

Surgeons can perform spinal surgery with less damage to surrounding tissues by passing endoscopic equipment through small incisions. Special scopes enable surgeons to successfully treat spinal column disorders such as herniated disc, spinal stenosis, and spinal deformities such as scoliosis and kyphosis. Spinal microsurgery can be performed under local anesthesia and the patient dismissed from the hospital after a brief stay. Candidates for microsurgery procedures are evaluated on information obtained from x-rays, MRI scans, CT scans, bone scan, and discography.

ASPIRATION

An aspiration procedure is done to obtain a specimen of body fluid. A needle is inserted into a cavity after a local anesthetic agent is administered to the site. This procedure is performed using sterile technique. It is fairly common for the physician to take a biopsy of tissue at the same time the aspiration procedure is done. Nursing interventions are similar for all aspiration tests, with special emphasis on (1) having the consent form signed; (2) reinforcing the physician's explanation of the procedure; (3) encouraging the patient to remain immobile during the procedure; (4) having the patient void before the procedure; (5) maintaining sterile technique; (6) supporting the patient emotionally; (7) applying a sterile pressure dressing to the puncture site and maintaining the dressing until bleeding has stopped; (8) assisting with collecting, labeling, and transporting a specimen to the laboratory immediately; and (9) observing for emotional and physical distress after the procedure.

Synovial Fluid Aspiration

Arthrocentesis (the puncture of a patient's joint with a needle and the withdrawal of fluid, which is performed to obtain samples of synovial fluid for diagnostic purposes) is helpful in diagnosing trauma, systemic lupus erythematosus, gout, osteoarthritis, and rheumatoid arthritis. Normally a patient's synovial fluid is straw colored, clear, or slightly cloudy. If trauma or a disease process is present, the synovial fluid will appear cloudy, milky, sanguineous, yellow, green, or gray.

After the procedure, proper support should be given to the affected extremity. Placing the extremity on a pillow and maintaining joint rest for approximately 12 hours may be indicated. It may be necessary to apply ice to the affected joint for 24 to 48 hours unless otherwise ordered. The nurse will assess the patient for signs of infection. After the removal of the pressure dressing from the site, an adhesive bandage can be used.

ELECTROGRAPHIC PROCEDURE

For electrographic procedures, electrodes are used to measure electrical activity in specific areas of the body.

Electromyogram (EMG)

An electromyogram is a procedure that involves the insertion of needle electrodes into the skeletal muscles so that electrical activity can be heard, seen on an oscilloscope (an instrument that displays a graphic representation of electron beams on a screen), and recorded on paper at the same time. Muscles do not produce an electrical charge at rest, but with neuromuscular disorders unusual patterns can be observed. Nerves can be observed for neuropathy and muscles for myopathy with this procedure. Electromyography can be used to detect chronic low back pain based on muscle fatigue patterns.

LABORATORY TESTS

Specific laboratory tests are ordered when musculoskeletal disorders are suspected (Table 4-3).

EFFECTS OF BED REST ON MINERAL CONTENT IN BONE

Studies done on people confined to bed rest reveal a loss of body calcium. Men and women patients aged 18 to 80 years who were confined to bed rest for an

Table 4-3 *Laboratory Tests for Musculoskeletal Disorders*

NORMAL VALUE	POSSIBLE CAUSE FOR INCREASE/DECREASE
CALCIUM	
9.0-10.5 mg/dL	Increased in metastatic tumor to the bone, Addison's disease, Paget's disease of the bone, acromegaly, acute osteoporosis, hyperparathyroidism, vitamin D deficiency, renal failure, malabsorption, and rickets.
ERYTHROCYTE SEDIMENTATION RATE (ESR)	
Males: up to 15 mm/hr	Indicates the presence of inflammation as seen in rheumatoid arthritis and rheumatic fever.
Females: up to 20 mm/hr	One of the most objective measurements of rheumatoid arthritis severity. ESR increases as the disease worsens.
	The ESR is a nonspecific test used to detect inflammatory, neoplastic, infectious, and necrotic processes. Increased levels are seen in multiple myeloma, acute myocardial infarctions, toxemia, and bacterial infections. Decreased levels are seen in CHF, sickle-cell anemia, polycythemia vera, infectious mononucleosis, degenerative arthritis, and angina pectoris.
LUPUS ERYTHEMATOSUS (LE) PREPARATION	
No LE cells seen	Lupus erythematosus, rheumatoid arthritis, scleroderma, and drug sensitivities.
RHEUMATOID FACTOR (RF)	
<60 units/mL	An immunoglobulin found in approximately 80% of adults with rheumatoid arthritis; other diseases such as systemic lupus erythematosus (SLE) may cause a positive RF.
URIC ACID (BLOOD)	
Males: 2.1-8.5 mg/dL	Increased in patients with gout, kidney failure, alcoholism, leukemia, metastatic cancer, multiple myeloma, or dehydration.
Females: 2.0-6.6 mg/dL	

average of 27 days because of musculoskeletal disorders or lumbar disk protrusion averaged 0.9% loss in mineral content per week from the lumbar vertebrae. This rate of loss over several weeks is a serious concern for an older individual in terms of regaining mobility; it also increases the risk of fracture. Studies done on astronauts have shown that they experienced rates of bone loss similar to bed rest rates in a weightless environment.

DISORDERS OF THE MUSCULOSKELETAL SYSTEM

INFLAMMATORY DISORDERS
ARTHRITIS

Arthritis is a type of disease in which there is an inflammation of the joint. An estimated 50 million Americans are affected by arthritis, and 4 million of these are dependent and unable to work, attend school, or participate in social functions. There are many types of arthritis, but the most common are rheumatoid arthritis, rheumatoid spondylitis, osteoarthritis (degenerative joint disease), and gout (gouty arthritis). See Table 4-4 for a comparison of rheumatoid arthritis and osteoarthritis.

Rheumatoid Arthritis

Etiology/pathophysiology. Rheumatoid arthritis (RA) is the most serious form of the disease and leads to severe crippling. It is a chronic, systemic disease that affects 3% of the general population. RA can strike anyone; however, certain factors make some people more susceptible than others. Of the approximately 6 million Americans who have RA, 75% are women. Although RA can occur at any age, it most often occurs in women of childbearing age. Rheumatoid arthritis is thought to be an autoimmune disorder, although there is evidence of genetic predisposition.

RA can affect many organ systems (lungs, heart, blood vessels, muscles, eyes, and skin). RA is characterized by a chronic inflammation of the synovial membrane (synovitis) of the diarthrodial joints (also called synovial joints: freely movable joints in which continuous bony surfaces are covered by cartilage and connected by ligaments lined with synovial membrane).

Clinical manifestations. RA is believed to involve an immune reaction that will not shut off because of some failure in the immune system; agents that should protect the body attack joint tissues instead and cause a chronic inflammatory reaction in the synovial membrane. This in turn results in damage to the affected joint and surrounding tissue, possibly leading to gross deformity and loss of function (Figure 4-7).

RA is characterized by periods of remission and exacerbation. During remission the symptoms actively cease. The inflammation, pain, stiffness, and edema subside, and progression of tissue damage is halted. (The patient may experience residual joint dysfunction even with remission.)

Assessment. Collection of **subjective data** includes noting the patient's complaints of malaise, muscle weakness (especially grip strength), loss of appetite, and generalized aching.

Collection of **objective data** includes observing the joints for edema, tenderness, subcutaneous nodules, limitation in range of motion (morning stiffness especially), symmetrical joint involvement, and fever.

Diagnostic tests. There is no single, definitive test for RA. Diagnosis is based on patient history and findings during a physical examination. The four classic symptoms most frequently reported are morning stiffness, joint pain, muscle weakness, and fatigue. Radiographic studies reveal loss of articular cartilage and change in subchondral bone. Laboratory tests are often used in confirming a diagnosis and in ruling out the presence of other diseases. They are as follows:

- Erythrocyte sedimentation rate: An increase indicates the presence of inflammatory reaction somewhere in body
- Rheumatoid factor (RF): An elevation of this titer indicates abnormal serum protein concentration is present
- Latex agglutination test: Detects presence of IgM version of rheumatoid factor, the anti-IgG antibodies
- Red cell count: Detects anemia, often present during chronic infection
- Synovial fluid aspiration: Normal fluid is usually clear and highly viscous; however, when inflammation is present, fluid is cloudy, yellow, less viscous, and contains increased protein
- Synovial fluid biopsy: Shows changes in tissue

Medical management. Aggressive treatment given early in the course of the disease benefits the RA patient. The medical management of RA is directed toward achieving the following goals:

- Controlling the disease activity by administering disease-modifying and antiinflammatory drugs (see the Medications table)
- Pain relief (see the Medications table)
- Prolonging joint function (physical therapy, traction, and splints are often used)
- Slowing the progression of joint damage by promoting activities of daily living, exercise program, and weight management

Advances in cell and molecular biology has influenced the current treatment of RA with the development of medications that actually target the pathophysiology of the disease. Disease-modifying antirheumatoid medications offer wider treatment options for patients. These medications target an enzyme known as tumor necrosis factor (TNF). The tumor necrosis factor is a proinflam-

Table 4-4 *Comparison of Rheumatoid Arthritis and Osteoarthritis*

	RHEUMATOID ARTHRITIS (RA)	OSTEOARTHRITIS (OA)
PATHOPHYSIOLOGY	Inflammation of synovial membrane, destruction of bones, ligaments, tendons, cartilage, and joint capsule.	Degeneration of cartilage from wear and tear; bone spur formation.
JOINTS MOST COMMONLY AFFECTED	Symmetrical joint involvement noted in wrists, knees, and knuckles.	Often only one side of body affected with changes noted in hands, spine, knees, and hips.
CLINICAL SIGNS AND SYMPTOMS	Edema, erythema, heat, pain, tenderness, nodule formation, fatigue, stiffness, muscle aches, and fever. Systemic manifestations occur. Vasculitis (inflammation of blood vessels) may be responsible for a variety of systemic complications, including peripheral neuropathy, myopathy, cardiopulmonary involvement, and ischemic ulcerations of the skin. Potential complications include infection, osteoporosis, and Sjögren syndrome. Dry mouth and decreased tearing occur in Sjögren syndrome.	Localized pain, stiffness, bony knobs of end joints of fingers (Heberden's nodes), edema not as pronounced as in RA. No systemic involvement is present. Constitutional symptoms such as fatigue or fever are not present. Other organ involvement is absent as well, which is an important differentiation between OA and RA.
AGE AT ONSET	Children nearing adolescence. Adults between 20 and 50.	Ages 45 to 90. Most people have some features with increasing age.
SEX	Females affected more often than males, occurring 3:1 in females over males.	Males and females affected equally.
HEREDITY	Familial tendency.	The form with knobby fingers can be hereditary.
DIAGNOSTIC TESTS	Rheumatoid factor found in serum of about 85% of patients with RA. Erythrocyte sedimentation rate, C-reactive protein, complete blood count, x-rays, examination of joint fluid are helpful in diagnosing RA.	X-rays, no specific laboratory abnormalities are useful in diagnosing OA.
TREATMENT	Control inflammation and pain with medications. Balance exercise with rest. Provide joint protection; encourage weight control and stress reduction. Surgical replacement of joints.	Maintain activity level. Control pain with medication. Encourage exercise, joint protection, weight control, stress reduction. Surgical joint replacement may be necessary.

matory substance that is produced by the synovial cells and other cells of the body and has the ability to produce signs and symptoms of inflammation (Medications: Rheumatoid Arthritis table).

Nursing interventions and patient teaching. Nursing intervention is aimed at patient education to help the patient and family understand what is happening and what to expect as the disease progresses. Rest is important because fatigue is a major problem. Sleeping

8 to 10 hours a night and taking a 2-hour nap during the day are recommended. Exercise helps prevent the joints from "freezing" and the muscles from weakening. A typical exercise program calls for two or three 10- to 15-minute daily sessions of "quiet" exercise that puts joints gently through range of motion (ROM). Heat is often used to relax and soothe muscles. Hot packs, heat lamps, and applications of hot paraffin wax are helpful. Rehabilitation is aimed at helping the

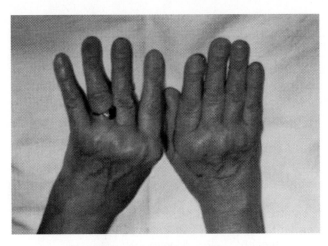

FIGURE **4-7** Rheumatoid arthritis of hands.

patient learn ways of adapting to physical limitations and promoting normal daily activities.

Nursing diagnoses and interventions for the patient with rheumatoid arthritis include but are not limited to the following:

NURSING DIAGNOSES	NURSING INTERVENTIONS
Pain, related to joint inflammation	Administer prescribed salicylate or NSAIDs.
	Assist patient with an exercise program prescribed by a physical therapist, including proper body mechanics and use of a walker or cane.
	During acute stages of disease, encourage patient to rest inflamed joints.
	Maintain bed rest as ordered; maintain proper body alignment.
	Assist and teach patient to extend joints as possible and to avoid external rotation of extremities; use sandbags or trochanter rolls.
	Avoid use of pillow under knees.
	Immobilize and/or support joints.
Chronic low self-esteem, related to negative self-evaluation about self or capabilities	Encourage the patient to express feelings about health problems, progress, and prognosis concerning diagnosis.
	Encourage the patient to explore ways to remain active while experiencing limited mobility (i.e., doing tasks that can be done while sitting as opposed to standing or walking).

As with any chronic illness, patient teaching is perhaps the most important aspect of nursing interventions of patients with rheumatoid arthritis. Patient teaching includes information about the following:

- Joint protection and energy conservation techniques
- Proper balance of rest and activity
- Proper use of medications—that is, names of drugs, dosages, precautions in administration, and side effects or toxic effects
- Plans for implementation of the exercise program prescribed by the physician or physical therapist
- Proper application of heat or cold packs
- Proper use of walking aids
- Safety measures to prevent injury
- Basics of good nutrition and importance of avoiding weight gain
- Danger of following programs that promise a "cure"

Prognosis. The course of the disease is variable but is most frequently marked by remissions and exacerbations. The prognosis is based on a variety of clinical and laboratory findings. Stage I represents early effects. Stage IV, the terminal category, includes marked joint deformity, extensive muscle atrophy, soft tissue lesions, bone and cartilage destruction, and fibrous or bony ankylosis.

Ankylosing Spondylitis

Etiology/pathophysiology. Ankylosing spondylitis (AKS) is a chronic, progressive disorder of the sacroiliac and hip joints, the synovial joints of the spine, and the adjacent soft tissues. It can affect both sexes but is seen more often in young men. There is a strong hereditary tendency. Women develop a milder form of AKS, and fusion of the spine is rarely seen. It is sometimes referred to as **rheumatoid spondylitis.**

Clinical manifestations. AKS involves inflammation of the spine. As a result, the bones of the spine grow together (ankylosis, fixation of a joint, often in abnormal position, usually results from destruction of articular cartilage and subchondral bone).

AKS involves inflammation in which the ligament or tendon attaches to the bone and does not affect the synovial membrane, as seen in rheumatoid arthritis. AKS can affect joints such as the neck, jaw, shoulders, knees, and hips. The disease process causes the ligaments to become ossified (hardened). The cardiovascular system can be involved, and heart enlargement and pericarditis can occur. If the costovertebral joints are affected, kyphosis can occur and alter respirations. The patient may have difficulty expanding the ribcage while breathing. Many patients with the disease also have inflammatory bowel disease. Vision loss occurs with chronic AKS, and blindness may result from the glaucoma and pupil damage.

MEDICATIONS | *Rheumatoid Arthritis*

MEDICATION	ACTION	SIDE EFFECTS/TOXIC EFFECTS	NURSING IMPLICATIONS
SALICYLATES			
Example: acetyl-salicylic acid	Analgesic, antipyretic, anti-inflammatory	Gastric irritation; dose-related salicylism; skin rash; hyper-sensitivity	Give with food, milk, or antacid; space q 4-6 hr to maintain an-tiinflammatory effect.
NONSTEROIDAL ANTIINFLAMMATORY DRUGS (NSAIDs)			
Indomethacin (Indocin)	Analgesic, antiinflammatory	Headache; vertigo; insomnia; confusion; GI irritation; can decrease effect of ACE in-hibitors	Give with food, milk, or antacid; discontinue if CNS symptoms develop and notify physician. Monitor BP.
Ibuprofen (Motrin)	Analgesic, antiinflammatory	Same as indomethacin but believed less irritating to GI tract; fluid retention; can cause hypertension.	Know that delayed absorption occurs if taken with food. Monitor BP.
Tolmetin sodium (Tolectin)	Analgesic, antiinflammatory	Same as ibuprofen	Give with food or milk.
Naproxen (Naprosyn)	Analgesic, antiinflammatory	Same as ibuprofen; also drowsiness	Give with food, milk, or antacid; tell patient to avoid driving until dosage effect is established.
Meloxicam (Mobic)	Antiinflammatory, anal-gesic, antipyretic	Dizziness, headache, insom-nia, seizures, dysrhyth-mias, heart failure, hemorrhage, diarrhea, indi-gestion, nausea, pancreati-tis, renal failure, leukopenia, thrombocy-topenia, asthma, bron-chospasm, angioedema. Drug is contraindicated in women who are pregnant or plan to become preg-nant.	Monitor blood pressure. Instruct patient to avoid using aspirin or products containing aspirin. Assess patient for history of al-lergic reactions to aspirin or other NSAIDs before starting drug. Tell patient the drug can be taken without regard to meals. Advise patient to report signs and symptoms of GI ulcers and bleeding. Advise patient to report any skin rash, weight gain, or edema. Alert patient with history of asthma that asthma may recur while taking the drug. Advise patient to avoid alcohol and tobacco products while taking the drug. NSAIDs can cause fluid reten-tion; closely monitor patients with hypertension, edema, or heart failure. Inform patient that consistent pain relief may take several days of drug administration.
Diflunisal (Dolobid)	Analgesic, antiinflammatory	Gastric irritation; headache; vertigo; skin rash; tinnitus; fluid retention	Give with food or milk; do not use with salicylates or other antiinflammatory medications.
Piroxicam (Feldene)	Analgesic, antiinflammatory	Gastric irritation; anemia; skin rash; fluid retention; vertigo; headache	Give with food or antacid.

MEDICATIONS | *Rheumatoid Arthritis—cont'd*

MEDICATION	ACTION	SIDE EFFECTS/TOXIC EFFECTS	NURSING IMPLICATIONS
Nabumetone (Relafen)	Analgesic, antiinflammatory	Dizziness, anxiety, depression, gastric irritation, edema, prolonged bleeding, rash	Give with meals or antacids. Advise patients to avoid the use of alcohol, aspirin, or aspirin products, or acetaminophen without physician's consent. Arthritic relief noted in 1-2 weeks.
Meclofenamate (Meclofen)	Analgesic, antiinflammatory	Gastric irritation, headache, dizziness, edema	Advise patients to avoid aspirin and aspirin products. Give 30 minutes before or 2 hours after eating.
COX-2 INHIBITOR			
Celecoxib (Celebrex)	Analgesic, antiinflammatory	Mild to moderate indigestion; risk of GI bleeding; diarrhea; abdominal pain Has been linked to an increased risk of cardiovascular events, such as MI or stroke (FDA Alert, April 7, 2005)	Medication is given po. Can be taken with or without food. Celebrex is indicated for the relief of the signs and symptoms of osteoarthritis and rheumatoid arthritis. Do not administer medication to patients who have asthma, urticaria, or allergic reactions to aspirin or other NSAIDs. Do not give Celebrex to patients who are allergic to sulfonamide. Celebrex should be used cautiously with ACE inhibitors, warfarin, lithium, and furosemide. Monitor patients for signs of GI bleeding.
POTENT ANTIINFLAMMATORY AGENTS			
Adrenocorticosteroids (example: prednisone)	Interfere with body's normal inflammatory responses	Fluid retention, sodium retention, potassium depletion; hypertension; decreased healing potential; increased susceptibility to infection; GI irritation; hirsutism; osteoporosis; fat deposits; diabetes mellitus; myopathy; adrenal insufficiency or adrenal crisis if abruptly withdrawn	Give with food, milk, or antacid; do not increase or decrease dosage without physician supervision; give in morning if given on once-a-day basis.
Phenylbutazone (Butazolidin)	Antiinflammatory; analgesic at subcortical site in brain	GI irritation; hematologic toxicity; hypertension; impaired renal function	Use for short term (7-10 days); give with food or milk.
SLOW-ACTING ANTIINFLAMMATORY AGENTS **Antimalarials**			
Hydroxychloroquine (Plaquenil)	Antiinflammatory (mechanism unknown); effect not expected to be noted for 6-12 months after beginning therapy	GI disturbances; retinal edema that may result in blindness	Instruct patient to obtain eye examination before beginning therapy and every 6 months thereafter.

Continued

MEDICATIONS | *Rheumatoid Arthritis—cont'd*

MEDICATION	ACTION	SIDE EFFECTS/TOXIC EFFECTS	NURSING IMPLICATIONS
Gold salts—IM			
Gold sodium thiomalate (Myochrysine)	Antiinflammatory; effect not noted for 3-6 months after beginning therapy	Renal and hepatic damage; corneal deposits; dermatitis; ulcerations in mouth; hematologic changes	Monitor urinalysis and CBC before each injection; report dermatitis, metallic taste in mouth, or lesions in mouth to physician.
Antineoplastic			
Methotrexate (Folex, Rheumatrex)	Alters the way the body uses folic acid, which is necessary for cell growth; decreases inflammation	Upset stomach, nausea, vomiting, anorexia, diarrhea, or sore mouth; headache, blurred vision, dizziness	Drug is taken po or injection. Monitor vital signs, WBCs, platelets, I&O, appetite. Advise patient to avoid pregnancy while on drug. Vaccinations must not be taken without physician's consent.
DISEASE-MODIFYING ANTIRHEUMATOID DRUGS (DMARDs)			
Etanercept (Enbrel)	Blocks the normal and inflammatory immune responses seen in rheumatoid arthritis (RA); binds tumor necrosis factor (TNF), which is involved in immune and inflammatory reactions	Pain at injection site, upper respiratory infections and sinusitis	Given twice weekly subcutaneously in the thigh, abdomen, or upper arm. Medication must be refrigerated and never frozen. Must be used with caution in patients with chronic infections. May cause or aggravate systemic lupus erythematosus.
Leflunomide (Arava)	Reduces the signs and symptoms of RA and retards structural bone damage	Diarrhea, elevated liver enzymes, alopecia, and rash	Medication is taken po. Urinary output must be monitored. Medication is not recommended for patients with hepatic impairment or positive for hepatitis B or C.
Infliximab (Remicade)	An antibody that binds specifically to proinflammatory enzymes that are produced by the synovial cells	Upper respiratory infections, headache, nausea, sinusitis, rash, and cough	Administered intravenously at 2 and 6 weeks initially, then every 8 weeks thereafter. Should not be given to patients with a clinically active infection.

Assessment. Collection of **subjective data** includes patient complaints of low backache, stiffness, and alternating or bilateral "sciatica pain" that lasts for a few days at a time and then subsides. Pain is more pronounced when an erect position is maintained. Inactivity exacerbates the pain, and exercise gives relief. Complaints of weight loss, abdominal distention, visual problems, and fatigue are common.

Collection of **objective data** includes assessment for tenderness over the spine and sacroiliac region. Peripheral joint edema and decreased ROM may be seen. Assessment of vital signs may indicate elevated temperature, tachycardia, and hyperpnea. Respiratory difficulties will arise if there is limited expansion of the chest, as is often seen in kyphosis.

Diagnostic tests. Patients with AKS will often have the following laboratory test results:
- Low hemoglobin and hematocrit, indicative of anemia
- Elevated erythrocyte sedimentation rate (ESR), common in chronic inflammatory disease
- Elevated serum alkaline phosphatase levels, seen in patients who are immobilized or have bone resorption

Radiographic examination often reveals sacroiliac joint and intervertebral disk inflammation with bony erosion and joint space fusion.

Medical management. The physician usually prescribes oral analgesics and nonsteroidal antiinflammatory drugs (NSAIDs). Exercise programs (swimming and walking) are important to prevent demineralization of bone.

Surgery may be necessary to replace fused joints (hip or knee is most common). Cervical or lumbar osteotomy can be done for severe kyphosis.

Endoscopic microsurgery can be performed on select candidates. Microsurgery allows the bone or tissue that is putting pressure on the spinal nerves to be removed by using endoscopic equipment placed through small incisions. Most patients are able to leave the hospital within 24 hours and start physical therapy within a few days.

Nursing interventions and patient teaching. Nursing intervention is aimed at maintaining alignment of the spine. Providing a firm mattress, bed board, and back brace helps provide support. Postural and breathing exercises help compensate for the possibility of impaired gas exchange caused by the changes in posture and chest cavity size. Encouraging the patient to lie on the abdomen at least 15 to 30 minutes four times daily (qid) helps to extend the spine. Turning and positioning every 2 hours helps to prevent pressure sores.

Nursing diagnosis and interventions for the patient with ankylosing spondylitis include but are not limited to the following:

NURSING DIAGNOSIS	NURSING INTERVENTIONS
Chronic low self-esteem, related to body image	Encourage verbalization about fears and anxiety of disease change process. Deal with behavior changes: denial, powerlessness, anxiety, and dependence. Be supportive and kind but firm in setting goals. Encourage independence and provide for tasks accomplished. Be aware of limitations and encourage discussion of feelings and concerns.

The patient should be taught the appropriate use of prescribed medications, prescribed postural exercises, and methods of applying heat to back and hips. Correct posture and prevention of complications should be promoted by the following:
- Encouraging use of a firm mattress
- Encouraging the patient to sleep without a pillow under the head
- Encouraging respiratory exercises

Prognosis. Ankylosing spondylitis is a chronic disease occurring younger than age 30 that generally burns itself out after a course of 20 years, leaving permanent, irreversible systemic involvement.

Box 4-3 | *Osteoarthritis*

- Osteoarthritis (OA) is the most common form of arthritis and the leading cause of disability in people older than age 65. Men and women younger than 55 years of age are affected equally. In older individuals, OA of the hip is more common in men and OA of interphalangeal joints and thumb is more common in women. Osteoarthritis occurs more frequently in people who are obese or who experience repetitive stress to the joints.
- More than 70% of total hip and knee replacements are for osteoarthritis.
- Overweight people have a higher risk of knee and hip osteoarthritis.
- Weight-loss programs for overweight older adults lessen symptoms in those with the disease.
- Acetaminophen is recommended by the American College of Rheumatology for OA pain because of fewer gastrointestinal and renal side effects compared with other drugs.
- Bicycling and swimming are considered good exercises for people with OA of the knee; walking should be done on level ground.
- People with OA of the knee or hip should avoid climbing stairs, bending, stooping, or squatting.

Osteoarthritis (Degenerative Joint Disease)

Etiology/pathophysiology. Degenerative joint disease (DJD) is also known as osteoarthritis, hypertrophic arthritis, osteoarthrosis, or senescent arthritis. Almost everyone past 40 years of age has hypertrophic changes in the joints (Box 4-3). The disease is an almost inevitable consequence of aging and is a major cause of severe chronic disability. There are two forms of osteoarthritis: primary (cause is unknown) and secondary (caused by trauma, infections, previous fractures, rheumatoid arthritis, stress on weight-bearing joints from obesity, or such occupations as coal mining or boxing). A comparison of rheumatoid and osteoarthritis is found in Table 4-4.

Osteoarthritis is a nonsystemic, noninflammatory disorder that progressively causes bones and joints to degenerate.

Clinical manifestations. This disorder affects the joints of the hand, knee, hip, and cervical and lumbar vertebrae. Osteoarthritis appears to be related to aging, but researchers are unclear as to the cause. Nearly all people older than 60 years will show osteoarthritic changes, with women being affected more often than men. The disease affects the hands in women more often, whereas in men the hips are affected.

Assessment. Collection of **subjective data** involves questioning the patient about complaints of pain and stiffness (rest usually relieves pain in the early stages).

Past illnesses, surgical procedures, or trauma may be relative, and information about excessive weight gain and occupation may be significant. Complaints of muscle spasms and reduced grip strength are common.

Collection of **objective data** includes assessment for joint edema, tenderness, instability, and deformity. **Heberden's** nodes appear on the sides of the distal joints of fingers (Figure 4-8), and **Bouchard's nodes** appear on the proximal joints of fingers—these are hard, bony, and cartilaginous enlargements. The patient's gait will reveal a limp, especially if the hips or legs are affected (Figure 4-9).

Diagnostic tests. There is no specific test to diagnose osteoarthritis. However, radiographic studies, arthroscopy, synovial fluid examination, and bone scans are used to provide information.

Medical management. The physician will order an exercise plan that is balanced with rest periods. Physical therapy using heat application helps reduce stiffness, pain, and muscle spasms. Gait enhancers—such as canes, walkers, and shoe inserts—help relieve discomfort while weight-bearing joints are used. Drug therapy involves using large dosages (10 to 15 g tid to qid after meals) of salicylates (aspirin) or NSAIDs (such as Motrin 400 mg qid). Steroids (cortisone) are sometimes used in low dosages or injected into joints to produce immediate pain relief and temporarily halt the destructive process. Patients with hypertension must be screened carefully while taking NSAIDs because certain NSAIDs are known to elevate blood pressure. Patients need to inform their physician so that a safe and effective combination of drugs can be chosen. Indomethacin can decrease the effect of enalapril (an angiotensin-converting enzyme [ACE] inhibitor used for hypertension; e.g., Vasotec) and the combination of ibuprofen and lisinopril (Prinivil, Zestril) can trigger a hypertensive response. Acetaminophen is commonly used as an analgesic and does not affect the blood pressure. Tramadol hydrochloride (Ultram) is a synthetic analgesic used for moderate to severe pain and can be used for patients taking antihypertensives.

Alternatives to NSAIDs. The discomfort associated with acute or chronic rheumatoid arthritis, osteoarthritis, gouty arthritis, and ankylosing spondylitis may also be decreased through the use of nonpharmacologic measures. Measures such as relaxation techniques, massage therapy, imagery, and therapeutic touch have proven to be effective in reducing discomfort and decreasing the need for NSAIDs.

Glucosamine is found in the body as a lubricant and shock absorber necessary for repairing and maintaining healthy joint function. By supplementing natural glucosamine, the patient's body is able to promote the manufacture of collagen and proteoglycans and resupply lubricant found in the synovial fluid necessary for restoring healthy cartilage (Complementary & Alternative Therapies box). Supplemental glucosamine acts like the glucosamine found naturally in cartilage. The aging process has been linked to the loss of glucosamine and other substances in the cartilage. Glucosamine supplements have been linked with reduced articular pain, joint tenderness, and restricted joint movement in people suffering from arthritis. People

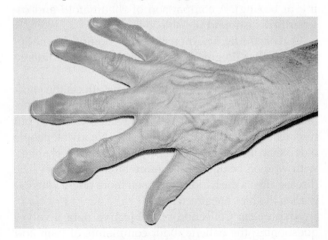

FIGURE **4-8** Heberden's nodes.

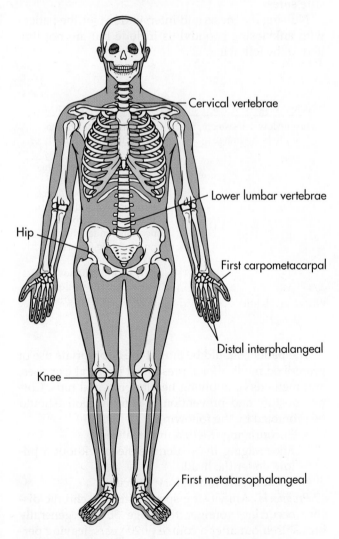

FIGURE **4-9** Joints most frequently involved in osteoarthritis.

allergic to shellfish should not take glucosamine supplements without consulting their physician.

Surgical intervention, such as osteotomy, may help correct malalignment. Joint replacement may be necessary to replace all or part of the joint's articulating surface. Arthroplasty of the hip and knee is the most common surgical intervention.

Nursing interventions and patient teaching. Nursing intervention involves encouraging the patient to maintain activities of daily living (ADLs) and adapt to limitations of the disease. Encouraging the patient to alternate sitting, walking, and standing with periods of rest can help reduce joint discomfort and deterioration. Older patients may be physically capable of turning and moving in bed but may forget to do so because of alteration in their level of orientation. Assisting the patient with a weight-reduction plan may be necessary if obesity is a problem. If splints are needed to support a painful joint, the nurse needs to assess for neurovascular impairment above and below the site of application. Gait enhancers should be checked for safety considerations, such as rubber tips on ends, proper size, and patient knowledge about use. If the patient has been taking aspirin over a period of time, GI bleeding may occur. It may be necessary for the nurse to perform a guaiac test on stool and emesis to determine the presence of occult blood.

As with rheumatoid arthritis, teaching the person with osteoarthritis about the disease process and the steps to control that process is the most important aspect of nursing interventions. Patient teaching should include the same information as for rheumatoid arthritis.

Prognosis. Degenerative joint disease (osteoarthritis) is a chronic disease that ultimately causes permanent destruction of affected cartilage and underlying bone with variable pain and disability.

Gout (Gouty Arthritis)

Etiology/pathophysiology. Gout is a metabolic disease resulting from an accumulation of uric acid in the blood. It is an acute inflammatory condition associated with ineffective metabolism of purines. Gout can be primary (linked with hereditary factors), secondary (resulting from use of certain medications or complication of another disease), or idiopathic (unknown origin). It affects men approximately eight times more frequently than women and usually occurs in middle life. It does not occur before puberty in the male or before menopause in the female. It takes approximately 20 years for sufficient urates to accumulate in the body before causing signs and symptoms when the disease is primary. Of all people with gout, 85% have a genetic tendency to develop the disease. Tophi (calculi containing sodium urate deposits that develop in periarticular fibrous tissue, typically in patients with gout) result in inflammation of the joint; it is unclear why this occurs. Typically the big toes are involved, but other joints can also be affected.

Clinical manifestations. Onset occurs at night, with excruciating pain, edema, and inflammation in the affected joint. The pain may be of short duration, returning at intervals, or it may be severe and continuous for 5 to 10 days. The patient may have repeated attacks or only one attack in a lifetime. Tophi are seen around the rim of the ear and can disfigure the ear. Surgical removal may be necessary.

Assessment. Collection of **subjective data** involves noting a complaint of pain occurring at night involving the great toe. Data collection involves a dietary history, with specific questions concerning consumption of alcohol and foods high in purine, such as organ meats (brain, kidney, liver, and heart), anchovies, yeast, herring, mackerel, and scallops.

Collection of **objective data** includes assessment of joints (especially the great toe) for signs of edema, heat, discoloration (may appear erythematous or purple), and limited movement. Vital sign data may reveal an elevated temperature and hypertension, tachycardia, and tachypnea. Careful assessment of urinary output is necessary because tophi can form in the kidneys and alter kidney function. The patient should be assessed for the presence of tophi (typically seen on the earlobes, fingers, hands, and toes).

Diagnostic tests. Laboratory tests used to diagnose gout include serum (see Table 4-3) and urinary uric

---

✿ Complementary & Alternative Therapies

Musculoskeletal Disorders

- Compounds are being considered as alternative therapies in the treatment of osteoarthritis. Glucosamine and chondroitin appear to provide pain relief, perhaps even slowing the disease process. Glucosamine apparently stimulates cartilage cells to manufacture proteoglycans, whereas chondroitin inhibits enzymes that break down cartilage. Recent research examines only the short-term effects of these compounds. It is difficult to determine whether patients with osteoarthritis will benefit over the long term or if they will experience adverse effects.
- Chiropractic adjustment has been effective in patients with some types of back pain. Many insurance companies allow for this form of therapy.
- Other manual healing methods—therapy that includes touch and manipulation of soft tissues or realignment of body parts to correct a dysfunction that affects the function of other body parts include:
  Massage and other physical healing methods
  Acupuncture
  Reflexology
  Rolfing (a technique of deep massage intended to help in realignment of the body by altering the length and tone of myofascial tissues).

acid levels (elevation is significant), complete blood count (leukocytosis and anemia may be present), and elevated ESR. Radiographic studies reveal cysts and toe bone pockets. Synovial fluid will contain urate crystals.

Medical management. Several drugs are used in the treatment of the disease. For acute attacks, colchicine is administered orally or may be given intravenously. When administered orally, 0.5 mg may be given hourly for 12 doses. The drug is discontinued if GI symptoms develop or the patient has not been relieved of pain. Phenylbutazone (Butazolidin) and indomethacin (Indocin) are affective antiinflammatory drugs in treating gout. Corticosteroids can be administered orally, intravenously, or intraarticularly and will relieve signs and symptoms within 12 hours. The physician may order allopurinol (Zyloprim) to decrease the production of uric acid; probenecid (Benemid) to increase secretion of uric acid by the kidneys; and sulfinpyrazone (Anturane) to prevent the development of tophi in various parts of the body, including the kidneys.

Nursing interventions and patient teaching. Nursing intervention is aimed at giving medications prescribed by the physician for relief of pain and inflammation. When giving colchicine it is important to observe for side effects, such as diarrhea, nausea, and vomiting. Increasing the patient's fluid intake to at least 2000 mL daily helps eliminate the excess urinary urates. Approximately 10% to 20% of patients with gouty arthritis have uric acid kidney stones. Careful documentation of intake and output (I&O) is necessary. Bed rest and joint immobilization are maintained during the time the patient is symptomatic. Bed cradles prevent pressure from bed linens on the affected great toe.

Nursing diagnoses and interventions for the patient with gout include but are not limited to the following:

NURSING DIAGNOSES	NURSING INTERVENTIONS
Pain, related to disease process	Maintain patient in position of comfort with foot supported and in alignment; place bed cradle over foot; no weight bearing.
	Apply cold packs as ordered, keeping pressure off joint.
	Administer analgesics and anti-gout and antiinflammatory agents as ordered; observe for side effects.
Deficient knowledge, related to lack of information concerning medications and home care management	Provide medication schedule, including name, dosage, purpose, and side effects.
	Discuss importance of diet, exercise, and rest program.
	Encourage follow-up visits with physician.

Patient teaching is aimed at giving information about the disease and stressing the importance of keeping the serum uric acid levels within normal range by taking the prescribed medications; following the prescribed diet; and avoiding infections, lack of sleep, and stress. Colchicine, probenecid, allopurinol, and sulfinpyrazone are drugs that the patient may need to take for several years, even when the signs and symptoms are not present.

Prognosis. The signs and symptoms are recurrent; episodes become longer each year. The disorder is disabling and, if untreated, can progress to the development of tophi and destructive joint changes.

OTHER MUSCULOSKELETAL DISORDERS

OSTEOPOROSIS
Etiology/Pathophysiology

Osteoporosis is a disorder that results in reduction in the mass of bone per unit of volume. This reduction is sufficient to interfere with the mechanical support function of the bone. The cause of osteoporosis has not been completely identified. Women between the ages of 55 and 65 years are identified as a high-risk group for postmenopausal osteoporosis, and many researchers believe that this is related to the loss of the female hormone estrogen. Studies of postmenopausal osteoporosis suggest estrogen deficiency is connected with increased bone reabsorption and sensitivity to parathyroid hormone (substance that weakens bone by increasing calcium movement from bone into extracellular fluid). Senile osteoporosis is seen in people between ages 70 and 85 years and affects twice as many women as men. Other factors that may contribute to the condition include immobilization, use of steroids, anticonvulsants or heparin, and high intake of caffeine. Genetic (small bone structure) and environmental (limited exercise) factors can contribute to the rate of bone loss. Osteoporosis affects the vertebrae, neck of the femur, pelvis, hands, and wrists. Individuals most at risk to develop osteoporosis are small-framed, nonobese, menopausal, white females who smoke. Contributing factors are diets low in calcium throughout life, smoking, excessive coffee intake, too much protein in the diet, and a sedentary lifestyle (Cultural and Ethnic Considerations box).

Clinical Manifestations

The disorder develops slowly. The first symptom is a complaint of backache. As the disease progresses, the bones become porous and brittle, which is caused by a lack of calcium.

Assessment

Collection of **subjective data** includes questioning the patient about lifestyle practices and complaints of pain (low thoracic and lumbar) that worsens with sitting, standing, coughing, sneezing, and straining.

Cultural and Ethnic Considerations

Osteoporosis

- White and Asian women have a higher incidence of osteoporosis than African-American women.
- African-American women have 10% more bone mass than white women.
- Postmenopausal women are at the highest risk regardless of cultural background or ethnic group.
- African-American men have dense bones and a low incidence of osteoporosis.

Collection of **objective data** involves assessing the patient for dowager's hump (spinal deformity and height loss that develop from repeated spinal vertebral fractures) and increased lordosis, scoliosis, and kyphosis (Figure 4-10). Assessment should be done for gait impairment associated with inability to maintain erect posture.

Diagnostic Tests

The physician will order a complete blood count, serum calcium, phosphorus, and alkaline phosphatase, blood urea nitrogen, creatinine level, urinalysis, liver and thyroid function tests, and radiographic studies. A bone density (densitometry) test is recommended for women around the time of menopause. Bone densitometry is performed by a dual energy x-ray absorptiometry (DEXA). The measured sites are most often the hip and spine. The test takes about 10 minutes and has very low amounts of radiation. The World Health Organization has defined criteria for adult women as follows:

- Normal bones have a bone mineral density (BMD) within 1 standard deviation of the young adult average.
- Low bone mass (osteopenia) is 1 standard deviation below the young adult average.
- Osteoporosis is 2.5 standard deviations below the young adult average.

Medical Management

The physician will order a treatment regimen aimed at promoting the increase of bone density and the retardation of bone loss. Calcium supplements that bring the total calcium intake to 1000 mg for men and 1500 mg for postmenopausal women are recommended (vitamin D, 50,000 international units once or twice per week). Weight-bearing exercise programs to improve muscle tone, such as walking, have been effective in preventing further bone loss and stimulating new bone formation. Treatment may include adequate doses of estrogen. Estrogen will not correct the condition but will help to prevent fractures and may be approved for women at significant risk.

Alendronate (Fosamax) is classified as a bone resorption inhibitor. The drug absorbs calcium phosphate crystal in bone and is given orally to treat symptoms of osteoporosis. It is important to administer alendronate first thing in the morning with 6 to 8 ounces of water at least 30 minutes before other medications, beverages, or food. Caution patient to remain upright for 30 minutes following dose to facilitate passage to stomach and minimize risk of esophageal irritation.

Risedronate (Actonel) is another bone resorption inhibitor. The drug absorbs calcium phosphate crystal in bone and inhibits bone resorption without inhibiting bone formation or mineralization. It is given orally. The patient should sit upright for 30 minutes after dose to prevent esophageal irritation.

Teriparatide (Forteo) is the most recent drug recommended for treating osteoporosis. It is a form of parathyroid hormone and is approved for postmenopausal women who are at increased risk for osteoporosis fractures or who cannot use other treatments. The drug prevents osteoblast (a bone cell that forms new bone) sloughing in porous or spongy bones and increases bone mass in the spine and hip. Teriparatide treatment requires a daily subcutaneous injection of the drug and is limited to a 24-month period. The drug must be kept refrigerated. The most common

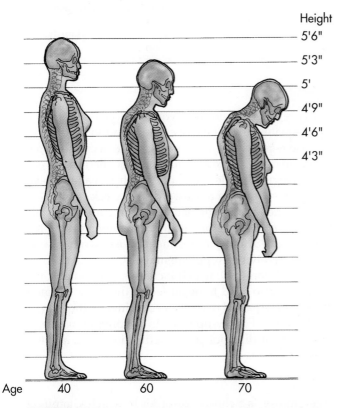

			Height
			5'6"
			5'3"
			5'
			4'9"
			4'6"
			4'3"
Age	40	60	70

FIGURE **4-10** A normal spine at age 40 years and osteoporotic changes at ages 60 and 70 years. These changes can cause a loss of as much as 6 inches in height and can result in the so-called dowager's hump *(far right)* in the upper thoracic vertebrae.

side effects are nausea, dizziness, leg cramps, hypercalcemia, and orthostatic hypotension. The drug is not recommended for patients with an increased risk of osteosarcoma.

Surgical interventions for osteoporosis. Women with severe osteoporosis who are unresponsive to an analgesic may be candidates for a surgical procedure to relieve the pain. Vertebroplasty and kyphoplasty are 90% successful in relieving pain from compression fractures of the spine. Vertebroplasty (plastic surgery on a vertebra) involves high-pressure injection of a polymethyl methacrylate cement into the spine, which pushes the vertebrae apart. The procedure is done under a general or local anesthetic, and the major complications involve the damage to the posterior vertebral walls from the high pressure used to inject the cement and movement of the cement out of vertebral spaces into the spinal canal.

Kyphoplasty (plastic surgery on dowager's hump that causes an abnormal curvature of the spine) involves the use of a balloon that is inserted into the center of the collapsed vertebrae, which restores the position of the vertebrae so that polymethyl methacrylate cement can be injected into the space created by the balloon. Porous bone is packed around the outside edge. This procedure is less risky than vertebroplasty because the balloon removes the need to use high pressure for the cement placement.

Nursing considerations. Patients are admitted to the hospital and required to stay up to 23 hours following the procedure. Flat bed rest is ordered for the first 4 hours postoperatively, then patients are allowed to ambulate as able. A small dressing is used to cover the operative site, and antibiotics and steroids are typically ordered for three doses following the procedure.

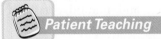

Patient Teaching

Dietary Needs in Osteoporosis

- Calcium is a mineral that can slow bone loss and may decrease fractures.
- A total of 1500 mg of calcium is needed daily in the diet or through supplements.
- Food sources of calcium include milk products, many green vegetables, calcium-fortified orange juice, and soy milk.
- Vitamin D helps calcium absorption and stimulates bone formation.
- A diet low in sodium, animal protein, and caffeine is recommended.
- Foods that are high in calcium include whole and skim milk, yogurt, turnip greens, cottage cheese, ice cream, sardines, and spinach.

Nursing Interventions and Patient Teaching

Nursing interventions are aimed at preventing further bone loss and fractures. A diet rich in milk and dairy products provides most of the calcium in the diet (Patient Teaching box). Food and beverages that contain caffeine also contain phosphorus, which contributes to bone loss. Teaching patients relaxation techniques and encouraging them to stop smoking are recommended. Estrogen therapy is not without risk, and patients who take estrogen need information about the higher risk for thromboembolism, endometrial cancer, and possibly breast cancer. Hormone replacement must be prescribed at the lowest dose possible and for a short duration. Safety measures, such as side rails, hand rails, bedside commodes with seat elevators, and rubber mats in showers can prevent falls in the older patient. Efforts are made to keep patients with osteoporosis ambulatory to prevent further loss of bone substance as a result of immobility. The nurse should encourage weight-bearing exercise to increase bone density.

Nursing diagnosis and interventions for the patient with osteoporosis include but are not limited to the following:

NURSING DIAGNOSIS	NURSING INTERVENTIONS
Deficient knowledge, related to issues of home care	Stress importance of activity and rest; provide aerobic management exercise schedule; caution patient to avoid jogging. Take recommended medications. Maintain healthy diet.

To prevent osteoporosis, women are advised to have an adequate daily intake of calcium and vitamin D; to exercise regularly; to avoid smoking; to decrease coffee intake; to decrease excess protein in the diet; and to engage in regular moderate activity such as walking, bike riding, or swimming at least 3 days a week.

After menopause the usual recommended daily allowance of 1000 mg of calcium in women taking estrogen and 1500 mg in postmenopausal women who are not receiving supplemental estrogen is recommended. Vitamin D, which increases calcium absorption, may also need to be added to the daily regimen of postmenopausal women according to the physician's orders. Follow-up visits to the physician are encouraged for direction as to medication, diet, and exercise regimen.

Prognosis

Osteoporosis is a chronic disorder in which vitamin D and calcium may help stop the rate of bone loss. In postmenopausal women, therapy with estrogen decreases the rate of bone resorption, but bone formation does not increase. Prevention of osteoporosis should begin before bone loss has occurred.

OSTEOMYELITIS
Etiology/Pathophysiology
Osteomyelitis (local or generalized infection of bone and bone marrow) can occur from bacteria introduced through trauma, as in the case of a compound fracture or surgery. Also, bacteria may travel by the bloodstream from another site in the body to a bone, causing the bone to become infected. Staphylococci are the most common causative agents.

Bacteria invade the bone, and degeneration of bone tissue occurs. If osteomyelitis becomes chronic, the bone tissue affected often will be weakened and predisposed to spontaneous fractures.

Clinical Manifestations
The patient with osteomyelitis is subject to contractures in the affected extremity if positioned incorrectly. It is not unusual for a new focus of infection to develop months and sometimes years after the initial infection is diagnosed.

Assessment
Collection of **subjective data** includes a complete history of injuries, surgical procedures, and diseases. An assessment includes patient's complaints of persistent, severe, and increasing bone pain and tenderness, as well as regional muscle spasm. An assessment of allergies should be done, especially to medications, because antibiotics are given long term.

Collection of **objective data** includes careful inspection of any wounds. The drainage is assessed for color, amount, and presence of odor. Vital signs are assessed for signs of infection (temperature elevation, tachycardia, and tachypnea). Assessment for edema is noted, especially in joints with limited mobility.

Diagnostic Tests
A complete history is taken, along with physical examination. The physician will order radiographic studies and bone scan, complete blood count (leukocytosis may be present), ESR, and cultures of blood and drainage (if present).

Medical Management
Intravenous antibiotic therapy is ordered; a broad-spectrum antibiotic, such as cephalothin (Keflin) is used. Parenteral antibiotics are usually necessary for several weeks. Bed rest is usually prescribed.

For some patients, surgery may be performed to remove a fragment of necrotic bone that is partially or entirely detached from the surrounding or adjacent healthy bone (sequestrum).

Nursing Interventions and Patient Teaching
Nursing intervention includes gentleness in moving the diseased extremity. Absolute rest of the affected part may be necessary, with careful positioning using pillows and sandbags for good alignment. During the early phase of infection, pain is extremely severe and extraordinary gentleness in moving and manipulating the infected part is essential. Often wounds are irrigated with hydrogen peroxide or other antiseptic or antibiotic solution and then covered with a sterile dressing, using strict surgical asepsis. Patients are placed on drainage and secretion precautions. Dietary planning is done with emphasis on a diet high in calories, protein, and vitamins.

Teaching includes information about the signs of infection, such as elevated temperature. Because chronic osteomyelitis may last a lifetime, it is important for the patient to be aware of the recurrence of signs and symptoms. Patients must avoid trauma to the affected bone because pathological fractures are common.

Prognosis
Acute osteomyelitis may respond to treatment after several weeks. Chronic osteomyelitis may persist for years with exacerbations and remissions.

FIBROMYALGIA SYNDROME (FMS)
Etiology/Pathophysiology
Fibromyalgia is a musculoskeletal chronic pain syndrome of unknown etiology that causes pain in the muscles, bones, or joints. It is associated with soft tissue tenderness at multiple characteristic sites. It contributes to poor sleep, headaches, altered thought processes, and stiffness or muscle aches. Fibromyalgia affects more women than men, with up to 5% of the population affected. The disorder is more common in people between ages 20 and 50. Fibromyalgia has been referred to as **fibrositis, fibromyositis, myofascial pain syndrome,** and **psychogenic rheumatism.** The cause of FMS is unknown. It is not considered life threatening and does not cause permanent damage.

Clinical Manifestations
Patients with FMS frequently complain of a generalized achiness typically in axial locations, such as the neck and lower back, accompanied by stiffness that is worse in the morning. Factors that aggravate the condition include cold or humid weather, physical or mental fatigue, excess physical activity, and anxiety or stress.

Additional problems experienced by patients with FMS include irritable bowel syndrome, tension headaches beginning with neck discomfort, paresthesia (sensation of numbness or tingling) of the upper extremities with normal nerve conduction studies, and the sensation of edematous hands with no visible signs of edema. Complaints of fatigue are often associated with dysfunctional sleep. Patients complain of non-restorative or nonrefreshing sleep.

Assessment

Collection of **subjective data** includes questioning the patient about muscle pain, often described as muscle ache, the occurrence of tension or migraine headaches, premenstrual tension, jaw pain, excessive fatigue, anxiety, and depression. It is important to include questions about sensations of numbness, tingling, and perception of insects crawling on or under the skin. Complaints of being forgetful and unable to recall recent information—such as appointments, location of parked car, or getting lost while driving to familiar places—are significant.

Objective data include noting periodic limb movement, especially at night, or a persistent need to move the lower extremities day and night. Assessment of sleep deprivation and the patient's ability to complete self-care activities is important.

Diagnostic Tests

No specific laboratory and radiographic tests diagnose FMS. Blood chemistry screening, a complete blood count, and erythrocyte sedimentation rate (ESR) will be normal in patients with FMS. A sleep study may be ordered in patients with a history suggestive of particular types of sleep disturbances; however, sleep study findings are typically normal in FMS patients.

Medical Management

The primary treatment approach includes patient education and reassurance. The FMS patient is informed that this is not a psychiatric disturbance and that symptoms are not uncommon in the general population. Although there is no single treatment for FMS, combining pharmacologic agents has been helpful.

Tricyclic antidepressants are used in the treatment of uncontrollable pain disorders. Benefits of these agents include (1) antidepressant results, (2) antiinflammatory features, (3) central skeletal muscle relaxation effects, and (4) pain inhibition through suppressing serotonergic and noradrenergic pathways (Medications for Fibromyalgia table).

MEDICATIONS | *Fibromyalgia Syndrome*

DRUG	EFFECT
Amitriptyline (Elavil, Endep)	Diminishes local pain and stiffness, improves sleep pattern
Cyclobenzaprine (Flexeril)	Diminishes local pain, improves sleep pattern, and decreases number of tender points
Clonazepam (Klonopin)	Decreases symptoms of constant leg movement, especially at night

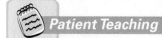

Sleep Hygiene

- Maintain regular sleep patterns by going to bed and awaking the same time each day; avoid long naps; take a hot bath within 2 hours of bedtime
- Control environmental factors by avoiding large meals 2 to 3 hours before bedtime and keeping sleep environment dark, quiet, and comfortable
- Exercise regularly each day
- Recognize the effects of drugs on sleep such as nicotine, alcohol, and caffeine

Nursing Interventions

Nursing interventions are individualized, holistic, and goal oriented. Management of FMS must focus on functional goals that empower the patient. Treatment programs include education, exercise, and relaxation techniques. Patients are taught the basic principles of good sleep hygiene (Patient Teaching: Sleep Hygiene box).

Exercise programs consist of gentle, progressive stretching. A warm-up of muscles is important before stretching and can be accomplished by either gentle exercise or warm baths. Stretching helps release tight muscles. Nonimpact exercise such as swimming, walking, or stationary cycling is helpful.

Prognosis

Prognosis is generally excellent.

SURGICAL INTERVENTIONS FOR TOTAL KNEE OR TOTAL HIP REPLACEMENT

Surgical procedures can prevent progressive deformities; relieve pain; improve function; and correct deformities resulting from rheumatoid arthritis, osteoarthritis, and other disorders. Tendon transplants can be done to replace damaged muscles. Patients with rheumatoid arthritis may need a synovectomy (excision of synovial membrane) to maintain joint function. An osteotomy (cutting into bone to correct bone or joint deformities) can help to improve function and relieve pain. Arthrodesis (surgical fusion of a joint) can be performed when severe joint destruction has occurred. Total joint replacement arthroplasty (refers to repair or refashioning of one or both sides, parts, or specific tissue within a joint) is often required on the elbow, hip, knee, or shoulder joint to restore or increase mobility.

KNEE ARTHROPLASTY (TOTAL KNEE REPLACEMENT)

Replacement of the knee joint may be necessary to restore motion of the joint, relieve pain, or correct deformity. Figures 4-11 and 4-12 show the tibial and femoral

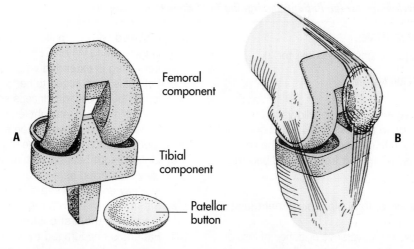

FIGURE **4-11 A,** Tibial and femoral components of total knee prosthesis. Patellar button, made of polyethylene, protects the posterior surface of the patella from friction against the femoral component when the knee is moved through flexion and extension. **B,** Total knee prosthesis in place.

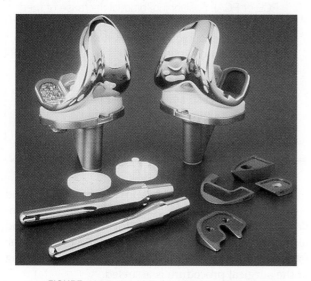

FIGURE **4-12** Total joint replacements: knee.

components of a knee prosthesis. Nursing interventions for the patient undergoing total knee replacement are shown in Box 4-4 (Figure 4-13).

UNICOMPARTMENTAL KNEE ARTHROPLASTY

Unicompartmental knee replacement is also referred to as partial knee replacement. This modified surgical procedure is performed on patients who do not need a total knee replacement because only one of the compartments of the knee is affected by arthritic changes. If both sides of the bones in the knee, including the underside of the patella, are damaged a total knee replacement is necessary (see Figure 4-13).

The knee has three compartments: (1) media or inside compartment (2) lateral or outside compartment, and (3) patello-femoral compartment, which is where

the kneecap rests. The minimally invasive knee surgery removes only the most damaged areas of cartilage and a small plastic disk replaces the worn cartilage, providing a new cushion between the bones.

The surgery is recommended for select patients ages 50 and older. Patients with rheumatoid arthritis or lupus erythematosus arthritis are not candidates for the surgery. The long-term benefits of the surgery will last from 5 to 15 years compared with a total knee procedure, which lasts from 20 to 30 years. Patients undergoing a unicompartment knee replacement may eventually need a total knee replacement. A total knee replacement may be more difficult in patients after having a unicompartmental knee replacement.

The partial knee surgery involves making a small incision over the knee and exposing the worn-out cartilage. The rough edges of the distal area of the femur and superior area of the tibia are cut flat and cleaned, and the unicompartmental device is put into place. Some of the devices are cemented in place.

Because there is no disruption of the kneecap, the patient can resume walking 3 to 4 hours after the operation. There is minimal blood loss and reduced risk of deep vein thrombosis. The surgery is performed in the hospital under a spinal block or general anesthetic and takes approximately 60 to 90 minutes.

Assessment

Collection of **subjective data** includes a medical history of home medications, allergies, past surgeries, and significant medical problems such as rheumatoid arthritis, or lupus erythematosus arthritis. Patients with these conditions are not candidates for the surgery. The patient should be assessed for complaints of pain on one side of the knee with weight bearing,

Box 4-4 | *Nursing Interventions for the Patient Undergoing Total Knee Replacement*

PREOPERATIVE INTERVENTIONS

Same as for any major surgery (see Chapter 2).

POSTOPERATIVE INTERVENTIONS

1. Positioning
   a. The operative leg is elevated on pillows to enhance venous return for the first 24 hours only. Pillows are placed with caution not to flex the knee.
   b. The patient may be turned from side to back to side.
2. Wound care
   a. Care of drains as for total hip replacement (usually Hemovac).
   b. Patient is assessed for systemic evidence of loss of blood (hypotension, tachycardia) if bulky compression dressing is used because it may hold large quantities of drainage before drainage is visible.
   c. Bulky dressings are removed before the patient begins continuous passive motion (CPM) flexion greater than 20 degrees.
3. Activity
   a. Passive flexion in a CPM machine within prescribed flexion-extension limits may be started in the postanesthesia care (PAC) unit (see Figure 4-13). Patient's leg should remain in machine as much as tolerated (up to 22 hours per day) to facilitate even healing of tissue. The physical therapist will increase extension on CPM as patient tolerates. (Once the large bulky dressing is replaced with a smaller dressing, flexion degree is increased.) When CPM is not occurring, patient's leg is extended with no pillow under leg.
   b. Patient is encouraged to perform active dorsiflexion of the ankles; quadriceps setting; and, after the drain is removed, straight leg raising exercises.
   c. Patient begins active flexion exercises three or four times a day about the fifth postoperative day.
   d. Light weight bearing with an assistive device may be started as early as the first postoperative day and increased as the patient tolerates.
   e. Sitting in a chair with the leg elevated may be started on the first postoperative day.
   f. Patient is encouraged to wear a resting knee extension splint (immobilizer) on the operated leg until able to demonstrate quadriceps control (independent straight leg raising).
4. Pain control
   a. Initial control of pain with opioids (usually with a PCE or PCA), positioning, gradual decrease of medication to nonopioid analgesics as patient tolerates.
   b. Patient is encouraged to use K-Kooler at 40° F continuously on knee.
5. Discharge instructions
   a. Patient must observe partial weight-bearing restriction and use ambulatory aid for approximately 2 months following discharge.
   b. Patient should continue active flexion and straight leg–raising exercises at home.

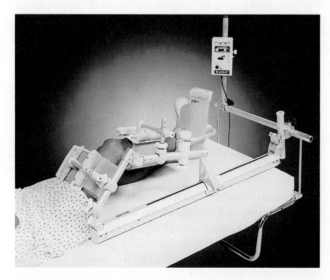

FIGURE **4-13** Example of CPM machine.

data concerning the effectiveness of conservative treatments such as medications, cortisone injections, strengthening exercises, weight loss, and use of gait enhancers. The surgery is recommended for patients 50 years and older.

Collection of **objective data** involves vital signs and weight. Patients who are obese or have significant inflammation are not candidates for the surgery. Blood tests, (ECG), and chest x-ray are done to evaluate the patient's state of health. The patient's understanding of the surgical procedure is assessed.

Diagnostic Tests

An x-ray of the knee shows a narrowing on the affected side of the joint.

Nursing Interventions and Patient Teaching

Nursing intervention is aimed at promoting healing and facilitating mobility. The typical postoperative stay for patients having unicompartmental knee surgery is one or two nights.

- Monitor pain and administer analgesics as needed.
- Help patient do deep breathing and coughing every 2 hours.
- Encourage use of an incentive spirometer.
- Begin clear liquids and advance to regular diet as tolerated.
- Monitor intravenous fluids and antibiotics.
- Resume weight bearing 3 to 5 hours postoperatively.

- Change dressing as needed.
- Assess patient's ability to use gait enhancer such as crutches.
- Begin physical therapy the first day after surgery (patient must practice going up and down stairs before being discharged). Basic postoperative exercises are taught by a physical therapist.
- Instruct patient that prophylactic antibiotics are recommended before routine dental cleaning or any dental procedure up to 2 years following the surgery.

HIP ARTHROPLASTY (TOTAL HIP REPLACEMENT)

A hip arthroplasty, or total hip replacement, is a commonly performed procedure when arthritis involves the head of the femur and acetabulum. A Vitallium cup is cemented into the arthritic acetabulum to receive the head of the femur. Total hip replacement was originally developed by John Charnley, a British orthopedic surgeon. There are several variations, but each type uses similar equipment. The Bechtol total hip system involves the use of a white plastic cup cemented in place to replace the damaged acetabulum. A stainless steel or Vitallium ball on a stem replaces the head of the femur, which is surgically removed. The stem is cemented into the femoral canal, and the new head fits precisely into the plastic acetabulum, providing friction-free movement in the joint. The cement used is a soft, surgical bone cement that hardens quickly and stabilizes the prosthesis to prevent future erosion of surrounding bone (Figure 4-14).

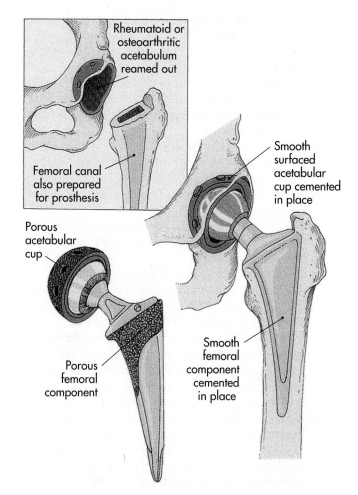

FIGURE **4-14** Hip arthroplasty (total hip replacement).

Assessment

Collection of **subjective data** involves assessing the patient's level of orientation because disorientation can be present in the older adult resulting from a change in the environment (home to hospital setting). Complaints of pain and numbness, tingling, or paresthesia indicate neurovascular impairment.

Collection of **objective data** includes assessment of the patient's compliance with nursing interventions to promote circulation, prevent impairment of skin integrity, and prevent hypostatic pneumonia by such means as coughing, turning (to the unaffected side; additional pillows are used to keep the affected leg abducted), deep breathing every 2 hours and use of incentive spirometer. Assessment of vital signs for evidence of excessive bleeding includes hypotension, tachycardia, and tachypnea. Decreased urinary output is indicative of hypovolemia. A careful assessment of the surgical wound for drainage is made at least every 4 hours. Hemovacs or other suction devices are placed in the wound during surgery to provide closed-wound suction. Assessing approximation of incision line and signs of inflammation (erythema, edema, fever, and pain) is necessary. Also included is assessing traction (if used) for correct amount of weight and proper alignment; maintaining the affected leg in an abducted position; and carefully observing for any reaction to the cement, signs of phlebitis (edema, erythema, and pain), and urinary retention (indwelling catheters may be used for the first 24 to 48 postoperative hours).

Nursing Interventions and Patient Teaching

Nursing intervention is aimed at promoting healing and facilitating mobility. The patient is taught to do isometric exercises on the quadriceps and gluteal muscles of the affected extremity by keeping the toes pointed up, flexing the ankles, and flexing and extending the knee of the unaffected extremity. Careful documentation of the patient's I&O is needed. Thigh-high antiembolism stockings are applied before or during surgery. A plan of weight bearing and physical therapy will be ordered by the physician and must be explained to the patient.

- Empty and record Hemovac drainage every 4 hours, if ordered; otherwise, empty and record as needed.
- Give oxygen at 1 to 2 L per nasal cannula as needed.

- Instruct patient in use of incentive spirometer every 2 to 4 hours.
- Help patient do deep breathing and coughing every 2 hours.
- Record intake and output (I&O).
- Maintain bed rest for 24 to 48 hours (varies with the security of the replacement prostheses and physician's choice).
- Change dressing using surgical asepsis after 24 to 48 hours as ordered; may reinforce dressing if necessary.
- Begin clear liquids and advance to regular diet as tolerated.
- Perform neurovascular checks every hour for 24 hours, then every 2 hours for 24 hours, and then every 4 hours.
- Check vital signs every 4 hours.
- Maintain position of operative area with splint, abduction pillow (Figure 4-15), immobilizer, and brace; turn patient to the unoperated side.
- Patient should be up but bearing no weight on operative limb after bed rest order expires (24 to 48 hours, depending on whether cemented or noncemented replacement was done); some physicians may permit touch-down weight bearing.
- Begin physical therapy exercises on second postoperative day; exercises and schedule vary; exercises are either active or passive to all joints, excluding the operated joint, and include quadriceps setting, straight leg raising, flexion and extension, or other individually prescribed exercises for the particular joint replaced.
- Patient should be up with walker or crutches four times daily; ambulation should increase as patient is able with up to 25 pounds weight to operative limb, gradually increasing to full weight bearing with crutches or walker.
- Patient should sit in chair for 10 to 15 minutes only, two or three times daily for first week, then may sit in chair 20 or 30 minutes four times daily.

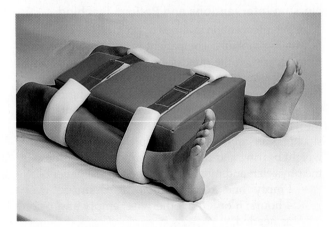

FIGURE **4-15** Maintaining postoperative abduction following total hip replacement.

- Encourage fluid intake and high-fiber foods (if tolerated) to prevent constipation; administer rectal suppository if needed to empty rectum.
- Patient should wear antiembolism hose or a pneumatic stocking pump system.
- Patient should use toilet riser (prevents hyperflexion of hip after total replacement).

Nursing diagnoses and interventions for the patient with a total hip replacement include but are not limited to the following:

NURSING DIAGNOSES	NURSING INTERVENTIONS
Pain, related to preoperative arthritic pain necessitating surgery and postoperative hip incisional pain secondary to bone and soft tissue trauma of surgery	Explain analgesic therapy, including medication, dose, and schedule. If patient is candidate for patient-controlled analgesia (PCA) or patient-controlled epidural (PCE), explain concept and routine. Respond quickly to pain complaints. Obtain pain scale rating from patient. Instruct patient to request analgesic before pain is severe. Administer analgesics as ordered and per hospital policy or procedure. Encourage use of analgesics 30 to 45 minutes before therapy. Unrelieved pain hinders rehabilitation progress. Provide eggcrate mattress. Change position (within hip precautions) every 2 hours. Document all responses to analgesics.
Impaired physical mobility, related to surgical procedure and discomfort	Allow patient to dangle feet at bedside several minutes before getting out of bed. Reinforce physical therapist's instructions for exercises and ambulation techniques and devices. Maintain weight-bearing status on affected extremity as prescribed. Consistent instructions from interdisciplinary team members promote safe, secure rehabilitation environment. Keep abduction pillow between legs while turning in bed (see Figure 4-15). No side lying on operative side. Leg is maintained in abduction when lying supine or on the nonoperative side. Use trapeze in bed to assist in mobility.

Discharge instructions include the following:

- Patient must use ambulatory aid, avoid adduction, and limit hip flexion to 90 degrees for approximately 2 to 3 months.
- A raised toilet seat is to be obtained and used at home until flexion restrictions are removed.
- Patient may need a long-handled shoehorn and reacher to facilitate ADLs within flexion restriction.
- Patient must be made aware of the lifelong need for antibiotic prophylaxis to protect the prosthesis from bacterial infection during dental work, intrusive procedures, or surgery.

FRACTURE OF THE HIP
Etiology/Pathophysiology

Hip fractures are the most common type of fracture treated in the hospital (Older Adult Considerations, and Health Promotion Considerations boxes). Women may be at a higher risk because of the potential for developing osteoporosis and because they have a longer life expectancy than men. Fractures of the hip include intracapsular fracture, when the femur is broken inside the joint, and include those of the femoral head or neck that are contained within the hip capsule (Figure 4-16, *A* to *C*). Intracapsular fractures may disrupt the blood supply to the head of the femur, with subsequent development of avascular necrosis of the head of the femur (Figures 4-17 and 4-18). Therefore fractures of the head or proximal femoral neck may be treated with insertion of a femoral prosthesis (Figure 4-19). The more common type of hip fracture is an extracapsular fracture, one that occurs outside the hip joint capsule. These are referred to as intertrochanteric or subtrochanteric fractures (see Figure 4-16, *D*). These fractures heal well without vascular necrosis with the use of compression screws or nails because the blood supply to the fracture site comes from the surrounding vessels outside the capsule (see Figures 4-17 and 4-18). Side plates attached to the nails help maintain a stable reduction while healing progresses (Figure 4-20). An intertrochanteric fracture occurs below the lesser trochanter and is frequently seen in younger patients suffering from hip trauma (see Figure 4-16, *D*).

Health Promotion Considerations

Hip Fracture

- Factors that contribute to the occurrence of a hip fracture in older adults include a propensity to fall, inability to correct a postural imbalance, inadequacy of local tissue shock absorbers (e.g., fat, muscle bulk), and underlying skeletal strength.
- Several factors have been identified in older adults that increase their risk of falling. These include gait and balance problems, decreased vision and hearing, diminished reflexes, orthostatic hypotension, and medication use.
- Leading hazards of falls are loose rugs and slippery or uneven surfaces.
- Many falls are associated with getting in or out of a chair or bed.
- Falls to the side, the most common type in the frail elderly, are more likely to result in a hip fracture than a forward fall.
- Two important factors influencing the amount of force imposed on the hip are the presence of energy-absorbing soft tissue over the greater trochanter and the state of leg muscle contraction at the time of the fall.
- Because many older adults have poor muscle tone, these are important factors in the severity of a fall.
- Older women often have osteoporosis and accompanying low bone density, which increases the risk of hip fracture.
- Targeted interventions to reduce hip fractures in the elderly include a variety of strategies. Calcium and vitamin D supplementation, estrogen replacement, and drug therapy have been shown to decrease bone loss or increase bone density and decrease the likelihood of fracture. Nurses must be vigilant in planning interventions for the older adult that are known to reduce the incidence of hip fracture.

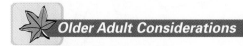

Older Adult Considerations

Musculoskeletal Disorder

- Physiologic changes of aging result in decreased joint flexibility and muscular strength.
- Changes in bone mass, particularly in older women, increase the risk of fractures. Hip fractures and compression fractures of the spine are most common.
- Degenerative joint disease related to "wear and tear" on joints is common. Joint replacement is increasingly common and has done much to improve mobility and the quality of life.
- Changes in the foot can occur from a lifetime of use, poorly fitted shoes, or heredity. Bunions and hammer toe are commonly seen in older adults. These may cause pain and lead to decreased mobility. Older adults should be encouraged to wear properly fitted shoes to reduce discomfort. If discomfort is severe, surgical correction may be necessary.
- The homes of older adults should be checked for safety hazards such as rugs that could cause falls.
- Climbing unsteady or uneven surfaces should be avoided because coordination and balance change with age and falls may result.
- Older adults should be instructed in the correct use of assistive devices such as canes or walkers. They should be encouraged to use these regularly to prevent injury.

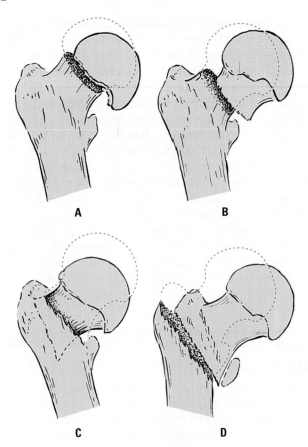

FIGURE **4-16** Fractures of the hip. **A,** Subcapital fracture.
B, Transcervical fracture. **C,** Impacted fracture of the base of
the neck. **D,** Intertrochanteric fracture.

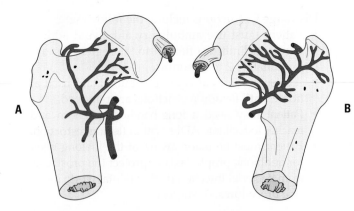

FIGURE **4-18 A,** Anterior arterial blood supply to hip joint.
B, Posterior arterial blood supply to hip joint.

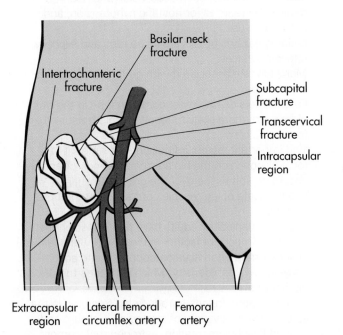

FIGURE **4-17** Femur with location of various types of fractures.

Clinical Manifestations

Signs and symptoms of hip fracture are severe pain at
the fracture site, inability to move the leg voluntarily,
and shortening or external rotation of the leg.

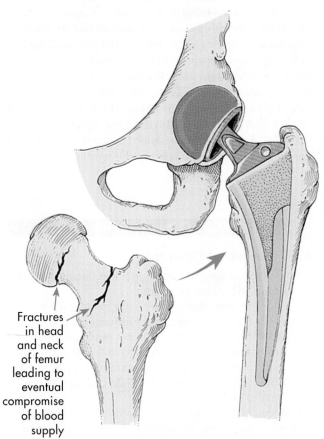

FIGURE **4-19** Bipolar hip replacement (hemiarthroplasty).

Assessment

Collection of **subjective data** includes an accurate history of the events before the injury. It is important to
assess the patient's level of orientation. Disorientation
can occur, especially in older adults when they are in
pain and anxious or are placed in an unfamiliar environment. The patient's medical and surgical history is
significant, as well as any family history of bone disease. Signs and symptoms of a fracture will vary with
the type and location of the break. There is usually
some degree of discomfort that may be more pro-

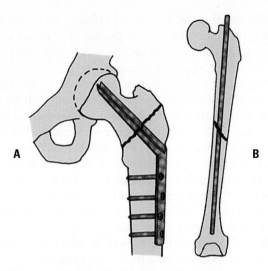

FIGURE **4-20** **A,** Neufeld nail and screws in repair of intertrochanteric fracture. **B,** Küntscher nail (intramedullary rod) used in repair of midshaft femoral fracture.

Box 4-5 | *Circulation Check (Neurovascular Assessment)*

- Circulation check is also known as a neurovascular assessment. CMS checks circulation, motion, and sensation. The assessment is made on patients following musculoskeletal trauma; post-operatively if damage to nerves and blood vessels is at risk; and following casting, splinting, or bandaging.
- The assessment is made every 15 minutes to 30 minutes for several hours and every 3 to 4 hours thereafter, with proper documentation of the findings.
- **Subjective data** include complaints of numbness or tingling not relieved by flexing the fingers and toes and repositioning the extremity. **Objective data** include cool, pale, or cyanotic skin above or below the altered site, edema, greater than 2 seconds capillary refill time, and absent or diminished pulses.
- Remember the 7 Ps when completing assessment:
    1. Pulselessness
    2. Paresthesia (numbness or tingling sensation)
    3. Paralysis or paresis
    4. Polar temperature
    5. Pallor
    6. Puffiness (edema)
    7. Pain
- Verbal complaints of numbness or tingling may result from general decreased mobility and may be relieved by flexing the fingers and toes and repositioning the extremity. However, if the numbness and tingling are not relieved by these measures and the extremity feels cool to the touch, is slow in capillary refill, has diminished or absent pulses, and appears pale or cyanotic, these are significant symptoms of neurovascular impairment and the findings must be reported immediately.

nounced with slight movement of the affected part. Most patients will complain of pain in the affected leg after sustaining a fractured hip, although patients suffering from an impacted intracapsular fracture have little pain, if any, immediately after the fracture. The nurse assesses edema, tenderness, muscle spasms, deformity, and loss of function. Patients may say they heard a "snap" or "pop" at the time the bone was injured. Impaired sensation may indicate nerve damage from the bone fragments "pinching" or severing the nerve.

Collection of **objective data** includes assessment for soft tissue injury with erythema or ecchymosis noted. When the injured limb is compared with the uninjured limb, obvious differences may be apparent. A change in the curvature or length of bone may indicate fracture. The nurse notes that the affected leg is shorter, usually externally rotated approximately 90 degrees, and slightly flexed after an extracapsular hip fracture. With an intracapsular fracture the nurse notes that the upper thigh is more edematous than the area below and the affected leg is shortened with external rotation. Subtrochanteric fractures cause excessive bleeding into the soft tissue, and the affected leg is shortened and rotated anteriorly. Crepitus may be felt or heard as the broken bone ends rub together. Neurovascular status of the extremity is assessed (Box 4-5).

It is most important that the nurse keep the injured part at rest because movement of a fractured bone can cause additional damage and may cause a closed fracture to become an open fracture. Data should also include an assessment of the patient's nutritional status. Both thin and obese patients are at risk for impaired skin integrity if bed rest is ordered. After the fracture is reduced, regular inspection of skin areas in contact with cast edges or traction apparatus to assess for signs of neurovascular compromise is necessary. It is also important for the nurse to note that patients suffering from any trauma are at risk for shock. Treating the shock takes precedence over treating the fracture.

Diagnostic Tests

Diagnosis is confirmed by radiographic examination of the injured part. Blood tests, such as hemoglobin determination, often show decreased laboratory values because of bleeding at the fracture site; the blood glucose level may be elevated because of the stress of the trauma.

Medical Management

Surgical repair is the preferred method of managing intracapsular and extracapsular hip fractures. Surgical treatment permits the patient to be out of bed sooner and decreases the major complications associated with immobility.

Initially the affected extremity may be temporarily immobilized by either Buck's or Russell's traction until the patient's physical condition is stabilized and surgery can be scheduled.

The choice of fixation device depends on the location of the fracture and the potential for avascular necrosis of the femoral head and neck. The use of these devices is called internal fixation. Prosthetic implants, such as the bipolar hip replacement (hemiarthroplasty) (see Figure 4-19) are used to replace the femoral head and neck in fractures when the vascular supply to the femoral head may be compromised. A Neufeld nail and screws are used in the repair of intertrochanteric fractures (see Figure 4-20, *A*). A Küntscher nail (intramedullary rod) is used to repair midshaft femoral fractures (see Figure 4-20, *B*). Sliding nails are used in repair of intertrochanteric fractures. Sliding nails usually permit the patient to bear weight to some degree because they "give" slightly when subjected to weight-bearing forces without shifting their placement or penetrating the femur. Bone grafts, either autograft (patient's bone) or allograft (cadaver bone), may be used with internal fixation devices when excessive bone is lost at the fracture site. If a stable reduction cannot be achieved, the physician may do an arthroplasty (surgical reconstruction of a joint). Immobilization devices, such as casts or splints, may also be used with open reduction.

Nursing Interventions

Nursing intervention specific for fractured hip is concerned with prevention of shock and further complications. A major emphasis is placed on maintaining proper alignment through traction and abduction of the hip when turning a patient with a fractured hip from side to side. Some physicians do not want patients turned onto their sides for several days after surgery; others may order the patient to be turned only on the unoperated side. It is important to know what has been ordered. Educating patients about activity restrictions is most important. Patients who have had an internal fixation for a fractured hip should avoid elevating the affected extremity when sitting. The head of the bed is elevated a maximum of 45 degrees to avoid acute flexion of the hip and strain on the fixation device. Instructing the patient *not* to cross the legs is important because crossing the legs can adduct the affected extremity and dislocate the hip.

Postoperative interventions for a patient with hip fracture repair include wound assessment with special attention to color, amount, and odor of exudate. Vital signs are assessed, as well as the suture line for approximation of skin edges and intact sutures or staples at least every 8 hours. Jackson-Pratt drainage tubes or Hemovacs are often used and must be assessed for amount and color of wound drainage at least every 4 hours. Accurate I&O findings are documented to help the physician establish the need for intravenous fluid therapy. The use of incentive spirometers is valu-

able in assisting the patient to perform adequate respiratory ventilation to prevent pneumonia. Turning and moving the patient on schedule will maintain skin integrity and promote circulation.

Leg manipulation during surgery and immobility afterward place the patient at risk for deep vein thrombosis and pulmonary embolism. Antiembolic stockings, Ace wraps, or pneumatic compression stockings and foot and leg exercises increase venous flow to the heart. The stockings are removed once each shift to assess for compression points and skin integrity. Anticoagulation therapy with enoxaparin (Lovenox), aspirin, or warfarin (Coumadin) is often prescribed (Clinical Pathway for Hip Fracture box).

Special consideration should be taken in regard to patients who have had a prosthetic implant or bipolar hip replacement (Figure 4-21). Isometric exercises are done on the quadriceps and gluteal muscles to strengthen the muscles used for walking (Patient Teaching: Quadriceps Setting Exercises box).

Nursing interventions also involve postoperative maintenance of leg abduction by using an abduction splint (a wedge-shaped foam bolster or pillow) for 7 to 10 days to prevent dislocation of the prosthesis. The abductor splint is placed between the patient's legs when in a supine position. Patients are turned with the extremities maintained in proper alignment. This can be accomplished by using the log-rolling procedure with the assistance of at least two nurses. A pillow is placed between the legs when turning the patient to maintain abduction of the legs and reduce the risk of dislocating the prosthesis. Most physicians order the patient to be turned toward the unoperated side; the nurse should check each order by the physician. The patient is transferred from bed to chair on the unoperated side by pivoting on the unaffected leg. The injured leg is kept extended forward to avoid extreme hip flexion and possible dislocation of the pros-

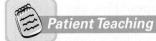

Patient Teaching

Quadriceps Setting Exercises

Quadriceps and gluteal muscles must be strong for ambulation. The quadriceps muscles stabilize the knee joint. The patient is taught to do the following exercises 10 to 15 times hourly:

- Quadriceps muscle strengthening involves pushing the knee down against the mattress while raising the heel of the foot off the bed; contraction is maintained for a count of five and relaxed for a count of five.
- Gluteal setting exercises are accomplished by contracting, or "pinching," the buttocks together until the count of five, then relaxing for a count of five.
- It is important to have the patient strengthen the unaffected leg by pushing down against the footboard, holding for a count of five, releasing for a count of five, and repeating.

CLINICAL PATHWAY | *Hip Fracture*

Genesis Healthcare System **Good Samaritan Medical Center** Zanesville, Ohio HIP FRACTURE CLINICAL PATHWAY – 209	ADMISSION DATE _____ DRG: 209 _____ DIAGNOSIS: Hip Fracture c̄ Hemiarthroplasty _____ ATTENDING PHYS. _____ CONSULTING PHYS. _____ CASE MANAGER _____

EXPECTED OUTCOMES BY DC

1. The pt. will verbalize pain less than 4 on scale of 0-10.

2. The pt. will be free of S/S of complications: pneumonia, atelectasis, pulmonary emboli, DVT, neurovascular compromise, hemorrhage.

3. The pt. will demonstrate self-care by amb. at least 40 feet with walker—maintaining WB as ordered and transfer with CG or SBA.

4. Pt.'s IV site and incision will remain free of S/S infection.

5. Pt. will return to preop pattern of elimination.

6. Pt. will demonstrate: use of walks _____ WB; therapeutic exercises; understanding of meds and food and drug interactions; S/S requiring medical care.

KEY:
√ = Met   0 = Not met   * = Ancillary documentation
If expected outcome not achieved, document follow-up action.

CAUSE CODE*   **VARIANCE ANALYSIS**

DATE	VARIANCE	CAUSE	ACTION	SIGNATURE

*P = Patient   S = System   D = Doctor   N = Staff

Continued

NURSING DIAGNOSES

1. Acute pain
2. Impaired physical mobility
3. Deficient knowledge
4. Impaired home maintenance
5. Risk for ineffective peripheral tissue perfusion
6. Risk for infection

ND	INTERVENTION CATEGORIES	DAY 1 DATE _____ PREOP PHASE	D	E	N	DAY 2 DATE _____ SURGERY	D	E	N	DAY 3 DATE _____ POD 1	D	E	N
	Assessment	—VS WNL —Alert/oriented —Skin W/D —Pain controlled (q4°) —Abdomen soft —Bowel sounds present —Negative for: 　—Fever 　—Chills 　—Dyspnea 　—Chest pain —Distal pulses palpable —Toes symmetrical/WB & pink —Sensation and mobility intact —Affected leg shortened & externally rotated				—VS WNL —Alert/oriented —Skin W/D —Pain controlled (q4°) —IV access negative for erythema & edema —Abdomen soft —Bowel sounds present —Negative for: 　—Fever 　—Chills 　—Dyspnea 　—Chest pain —Distal pulses palpable —Toes symmetrical/WD & pink —Sensation and mobility intact —Alignment anatomically correct —Dressing dry and intact				—VS WNL —Alert/oriented —Skin W/D —Pain controlled (q4°) —IV access negative for erythema & edema —Abdomen soft —Bowel sounds present —Negative for: 　—Fever 　—Chills 　—Dyspnea 　—Chest pain —Distal pulses palpable —Toes symmetrical/WD & pink —Sensation and mobility intact —Alignment anatomically correct —Dressing dry and intact			
	Activity	—BR c̄ Buck's traction _____ # Maintained —Turn q2Hc̄ pillow				—BR - Turn q2h c̄ abduction pillow				—Up in chair at BS. WB as ordered —Up to BSC *—Transfer max of 1 *—Maintains precautions			
	Diet	—NPO p MN				—Clear liq → Home diet				—Home diet *Initial nutrition screen completed			
	Treatment	—Apply TED & ICD to unoperative leg —Send other to OR c̄ patient —Povidone-iodine (Betadine) scrub to affected hip @ bedtime —Ice to affected hip —I&O q 8° —S & cath if unable to vd. —C&DB & ankle pumps q2° —IS				—TED & ICD bilat —Ice or cool temp. maintained —Reinforce dsg. prn —Straight cathed prn —Abduction pillow maintained				—TED & ICD bilat —IS, C&DB q1° WA —Ice or cool temp. maintained —I&O q8°—drainage included —Dressing reinforced prn —I&O q8°—drainage included —Straight cath or Foley prn —C&DB, IS, & AP q1° WA —Fleet enema prn —Abduction pillow maintained			
	Diagnostic Testing	—CBC, UA, SMA, Lytes, PT, INR, PTT —Results on chart —Chest x-ray, EKG								—CBC, Lytes —Daily Protime and INR if on coumadin —Guaiac stool if on Lovenox			
	Medication	—√ c̄ anesthesia about giving home meds preoperatively				—Preop IV atb —IV atb & IV fluids administered p̄ op —Parenteral or epidural pain med.				—IV atb - IV cont'd to Int. —Parenteral or epidural analgesic			
	Education	—Preop teaching & packet given —C&DB, IS, TED, ICD —Permit signed —Expected LOS —What to expect on nursing unit p̄ op				—Reinforce T, C&DB, IS, AP q1° WA. —Post-op care understood —Hip precautions understood				*—PT eval. & teach transfers: precautions & exercises in room —Nursing reinforces			
	Consults	—DC assessment done —Medical clearance —Anesthesia to see —Case management —Dietary if NDB indicated				—Medical Dr. to follow postop —Absence of D/C needs				—Pt. consulted —Absence of D/C needs			

Date	Time	Signature and Title	Date	Time	Signature and Title

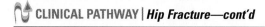

NURSING DIAGNOSES

7. Risk for impaired gas exchange
8. Risk for constipation

VS Parameters
T <100.5   P 60–100
R 12–20   B/P 90/60–140/90

DAY 4 DATE ____ POD 2	D	E	N	DAY 5 DATE ____ POD 3	D	E	N	DAY 6 DATE ____ POD 4	D	E	N	DATE:	D	E	N
—VS WNL —Alert/oriented —Skin W/D —Pain controlled (q4°) —IV access negative for erythema & edema —Abdomen soft —Bowel sounds present —Negative for: —Fever —Chills —Dyspnea —Chest pain —Distal pulses palpable —Toes symmetrical/WD & pink —Sensation and mobility intact —Alignment anatomically correct —Dressing dry and intact —Incision s̄ erythema/purulent drainage —Staples intact				—VS WNL —Alert/oriented —Skin W/D —Pain controlled (q4°) —IV access negative for erythema & edema —Abdomen soft —Bowel sounds present —Negative for: —Fever —Chills —Dyspnea —Chest pain —Distal pulses palpable —Toes symmetrical/WD & pink —Sensation and mobility intact —Alignment anatomically correct —Incision s̄ erythema/purulent drainage —Staples intact				—VS WNL —Alert/oriented —Skin W/D —Pain controlled (q4°) —Abdomen soft —Bowel sounds present —Negative for: —Fever —Chills —Dyspnea —Chest pain —Distal pulses palpable —Toes symmetrical/WD & pink —Sensation and mobility intact —Alignment anatomically correct —Dressing dry and intact —Incision s̄ erythema/purulent drainage —Staples intact							
—Up in chair and up to BR WB as ordered *Amb. 10'-20' *Transfer c̄ min → mod 1 Maintains precautions				—Ambulate to BR. ↑ toilet set *Amb. 20'-30' *Transfer c̄ min → CG Maintains precautions				—Ambulate to BR. ↑ toilet set *Amb. 30'-40' *Transfer CG → SBA Maintains precautions							
—Home diet				—Home diet				—Home diet							
—TED & ICD bilat —IS, C&DB q1° WA —Ice or cool temp. maintained —Dressing changed—drain DC'd —IV site changed or discontinued —I&O q8°—drainage included —Straight cath or Foley PRN —C&DB, IS & AP q1° WA —Fleet enema prn —Abduction pillow maintained				—TED & ICD bilat —IS, C&DB q1° WA —Ice prn comfort —Dressing changed —I&O q8° —DC Foley cath of used CK Vd —Fleet enema PRN —Abduction pillow @ bedtime —Bed pillow during the day				—TED & ICD bilat —IS, C&DB q1° WA —Ice prn comfort —Dressing changed —I&O q8° —DC foley cath of used CK Vd —Fleet enema prn —Abduction pillow @ bedtime —Bed pillow during the day							
—CBC —Guaiac store if on warfarin —PT and INR if on warfarin				—CBC, lytes —PT and INR if on warfarin (Coumadin)				—Guaiac stool if on enoxaparin (Lovenox) —PT and INR if on warfarin							
—IV atb completed —IV DC'd if Hgb > 8.5 —po pain med				—po analgesic				—DC c̄ script —po analgesic							
*—Pt in dept for ambulation c̄ walker, exercises, transfers & precautions bid —Nursing reinforces				*—Pt. return demonstrates: —Amb. c̄ walker —Exercises —Transfers —Precautions				—Verbalizes understanding of DC instructions and home care —DC home c̄ HH or transferred to rehab, SNF/SAR PRN							
—Absence of D/C needs				—OT consulted PRN *PT Rec. —Absence of D/C needs				—DC home c̄ HH or transferred to rehab, SNF/SAR prn.							

Date	Time	Signature and Title	Date	Time	Signature and Title

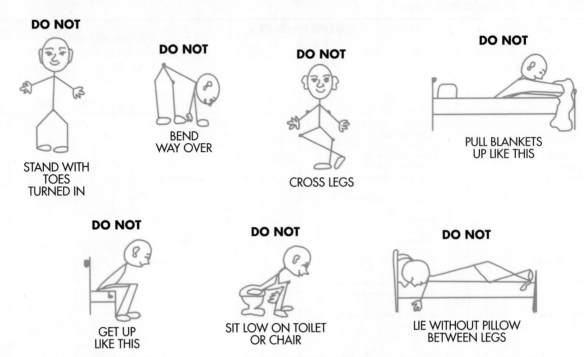

FIGURE **4-21** Instruction sheet for patient with a bipolar hip replacement (hip prosthetic implant).

thesis. Limit weight bearing on the hip by providing walking assists such as a walker or crutches. Provide a chair with a firm, nonreclining seat and arms; elevate the sitting surfaces as necessary with pillows or foam cushions to keep the angle of the hip within the prescribed limits when the patient is sitting.

In general, patients who have had *any* kind of internal fixation for a fractured hip should avoid elevation of the operated leg when sitting in a chair, since this puts excessive strain on the fixation device.

See Nursing Care Plan: The Patient with a Fractured Hip.

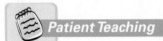 *Patient Teaching*

Open Reduction Internal Fixation

Special considerations that should be taken in regard to patients who have **internal fixation** with hip nails or pins related to hip modification in weight bearing follow:

- Assess ability to understand instructions and limitations.
- Assist to dangle feet at bedside on first postoperative day, then to pivot to chair with no weight on operative leg, or touch-down weight if allowed.
- Stress that operative foot should be placed on floor but weight should be borne on the unoperative leg (refer to limb as either left or right leg so patient has a clear understanding) to maintain safety in care.
- Turn every 2 hours; prop with pillows between legs or back to maintain position.
- Assist with ROM exercises to maintain muscle strength.
- Help physical therapist walk patient with walker and limited weight to operative limb (if assistance is needed) for comfort and safety.
- Encourage patient and family members to walk together for patient's safety. Instruct family about weight-bearing techniques for clarity and safety.

- If a stable plate and screw fixation is used to repair the fractured hip, the patient should not bear weight for 6 weeks to 3 months to protect the fracture site.
- A telescoping nail fixation allows minimal to partial weight bearing during the first 6 weeks to 3 months.

Hip Prosthetic Implant

Activity is restricted according to the fractured hip fixation device used. If a patient has a **hip prosthetic implant**, teaching includes the following (see Figure 4-21):

- Avoid hip flexion beyond 60 degrees for approximately 10 days.
- Avoid hip flexion beyond 90 degrees for 2 to 3 months.
- Avoid adduction of the affected leg beyond midline for 2 to 3 months.
- Maintain partial weight-bearing status for approximately 2 to 3 months.
- Avoid positioning on the operative side in bed.
- Maintain abduction of the hip by using a wedge-shaped foam bolster or pillows arranged in a wedge; this will require nursing assistance.

NURSING CARE PLAN
The Patient with a Fractured Hip

Ms. D., age 72, fell in her kitchen while removing cookies from the oven. She sustained a subcapital fracture of the right hip. Ms. D. is scheduled in the morning for a bipolar (hemiarthroplasty) prosthesis.

NURSING DIAGNOSIS *Ineffective tissue perfusion, related to vascular injury or interruption of arterial/venous flow secondary to edema*

Patient Goals/Expected Outcomes	Nursing Interventions	Evaluation
Patient's circulation will be maintained to fulfill body requirements.	Palpate site for warmth. Observe site for color. Apply moderate pressure to nailbed and subsequently observe speed of capillary refill. Assess pedal pulse bilaterally every 4 hours. Question patient regarding pain and paresthesia in injured part. Assist and teach patient to turn and cough every 2 hours and deep breathe every hour. Apply antiembolic stockings as ordered. Monitor vital signs every 2 to 4 hours.	Distal pulses palpable; toes symmetrical, warm, dry, and pink; sensation and mobility intact

NURSING DIAGNOSIS *Deficient knowledge, related to home care management*

Patient Goals/Expected Outcomes	Nursing Interventions	Evaluation
Patient and/or significant other will demonstrate understanding of home care and follow-up instructions through interactive discussion and actual return demonstration.	Stress importance of prescribed rehabilitation plan of activity, rest, and exercise. Provide diet instructions as to type and amount, and teach to avoid weight gain if applicable. Discuss medications: name, purpose, schedule, dosage, and side effects. Discuss signs and symptoms to report to physician: severe pain, changes in temperature, color, or sensation in extremity, malodorous drainage from wound. Stress home safety factors such as throw rugs, use of safety bars on the bathtub, elevated toilet seats. Encourage follow-up visits with physician.	Patient demonstrates ambulation with walker, exercises, transfers, and precautions, verbalizes understanding of discharge instructions and home care

? CRITICAL THINKING QUESTIONS

1. The first postoperative evening, Ms. D. is restless and disoriented. What nursing interventions are needed to prevent dislocation of her bipolar hip prosthesis?
2. Ms. D. is in her third postoperative day, and the nurse notes an erythematous area on her coccyx. What are the therapeutic measures to prevent skin impairment?
3. On Ms. D.'s third postoperative day, she complains of pain in her right calf when the nurse performs dorsiflexion. What is the most appropriate immediate action by the nurse?

Prognosis

Complications of hip fractures are the most common cause of death after the age of 75. Hip fractures in older adults are often complicated by the presence of other medical conditions such as diabetes mellitus, cardiac problems (e.g., heart failure), and neurological disorders (e.g., stroke).

A large bone such as the hip heals slowly in older patients, and this predisposes them to various complications. They are at high risk for pneumonia, deep vein thrombosis, fat embolus, pulmonary embolus, pressure sores, urinary retention, constipation, mental disorientation, and depression.

OTHER FRACTURES

Etiology/Pathophysiology

A fracture is a traumatic injury to a bone in which the continuity of the tissue of the bone is broken. Most fractures result from an insult to the bone, such as a forceful blow (twisting or crushing), which places more stress on the bone than it can absorb. Fractures that occur without trauma are referred to as pathological or spontaneous fractures and can be caused by a weakening of the bone because of osteoporosis, metastatic cancer and tumors of the bone, Cushing syndrome, malnutrition, and complications of long-term steroid therapy.

Fractures may result from (1) direct force, which results in a fracture at the site of the trauma; (2) torsion, which is seen in a twisting injury in which the fracture occurs at a point remote from the trauma (e.g., a forceful twisting of the wrist may cause a fracture of the arm); or (3) violent contractions involving highly developed muscles (e.g., severe muscle spasms may cause a fracture in a paraplegic patient).

The more than 150 types of fractures can be classified in various ways. First, they are described as either open (compound) or closed (simple) (Figure 4-22), meaning that the fracture has occurred with protrusion of the bone through the skin or the fractured bone has not protruded through the skin. Open fractures are more serious because they involve more soft tissue damage, require surgical treatment to repair, and are prone to infections. A bullet wound (injury is directed inward) that has fractured a bone is another example of an open fracture. A closed fracture does not involve a break in the skin. These fractures can sometimes be realigned by external manipulation, which does not require invasive surgery.

A description of a fracture can be given in terms of appearance (Figure 4-23), such as greenstick, complete, comminuted, impacted, transverse, oblique, and spiral. They are briefly described as follows:

- **Greenstick fracture:** Incomplete fracture in which the fracture line extends only partially through the bone. The bone is broken and bent but still secured at one side. This fracture is common in children because their bones are softer and more flexible than those of adults.
- **Complete fracture:** Fracture line extends entirely through the bone, with the periosteum disrupted on both sides of the bone.
- **Comminuted fracture:** Bone is splintered into three or more fragments at the site of the break. There is more than one fracture line.
- **Impacted fracture:** Sometimes called a *telescoped* fracture because one bone fragment is forcibly wedged into another bone fragment. In long bones this can create a shortening of the extremity.
- **Transverse fracture:** Break runs directly across the bone; it is at a right angle of the bone's axis.
- **Oblique fracture:** Break runs along a slant to the length of the bone; it is at approximately a 45-degree angle to the shaft of the bone.
- **Spiral fracture:** Break coils around the bone. It is sometimes called a torsion fracture and will result from a twisting force.

Fractures are described according to their location on the bone—for example, proximal, midshaft, or distal. Fractures can also be classified according to the force that caused the break. An example of this is the marching fracture, which can occur in the metatarsals as a result of a long march.

Physicians who have been the first to describe a type of fracture have given their names to fractures. Examples of these include the following:

- **Colles' fracture:** Fracture of the distal portion of the radius within 1 inch of the joint of the wrist that commonly occurs when a person attempts to break a fall by putting the hands down.
- **Pott's fracture:** Occurs at the distal end of the fibula and is characterized by chipping off of a piece of the medial malleolus with a displacement of the foot outward

Fractures are sometimes referred to as joint fractures if they involve or are close to a joint. Articulation fracture involves the surface of a joint. Extra-

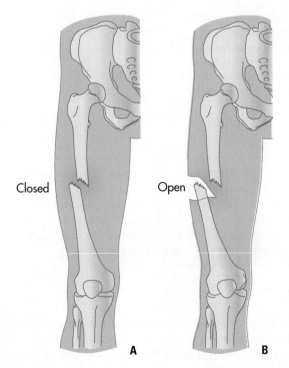

FIGURE **4-22 A,** Closed fracture. **B,** Open fracture with bone protruding through skin.

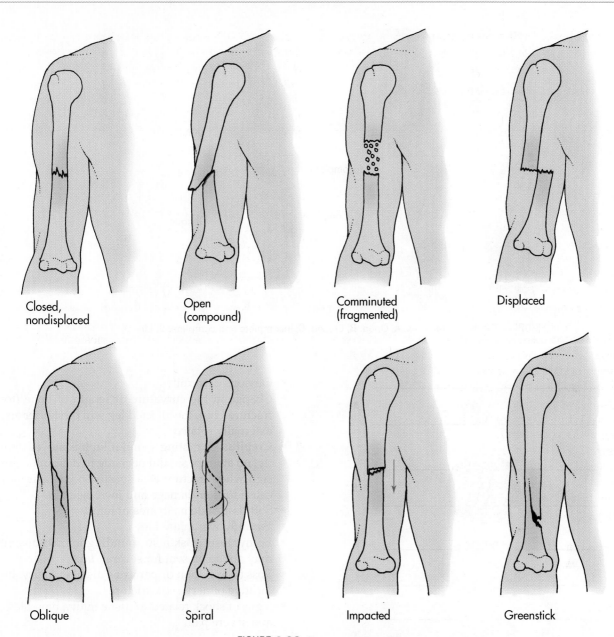

FIGURE **4-23** Common types of fractures.

Closed,
nondisplaced

Open
(compound)

Comminuted
(fragmented)

Displaced

Oblique

Spiral

Impacted

Greenstick

capsular fracture involves a fracture near the joint but one that has not entered the joint capsule. Intracapsular fracture is a fracture within the joint capsule.

Fractures can also be described according to their displacement. Figure 4-24 shows that fragments may be displaced sideways, can override the opposite fractured surface, may angulate or create a bend in the bone, and may rotate away from the fracture site. When a bone is displaced, the bone fragments can cause soft tissue damage. The patient will consequently experience severe pain, edema, and muscle spasms in the early stages of healing.

Bone is vascular; therefore, when a fracture occurs, there is bleeding at the site of the fracture, as well as in surrounding tissue. A clot will form at the ends of the fractured bone (Figure 4-25). The next phase of healing occurs when the hematoma becomes organized as fibroblasts invade the area and a fibrin meshwork is formed. Inflammation is localized as the white cells wall off the area. Osteoblasts enter the fibrous area to help hold the union firm. Blood vessels develop, and collagen strands start to incorporate calcium deposits. Callus (bony deposits formed between and around the broken ends of a fractured bone during healing) formation occurs when the osteoblasts continue to lay the network for bone buildup and osteoclasts destroy dead bone. The collagen strengthens and continues to incorporate calcium deposits. Remodeling is the final step and occurs when the excess callus is reabsorbed and trabecular bone is laid down along the lines of stress.

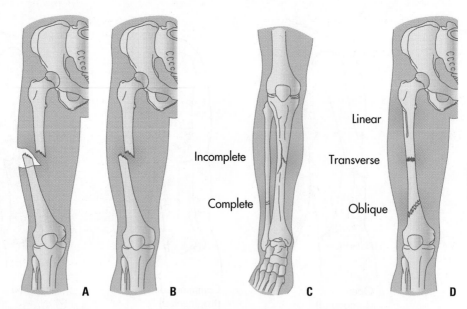

FIGURE **4-24** Bone fractures. **A,** Open. **B,** Closed. **C,** Incomplete and complete. **D,** Linear, transverse, and oblique.

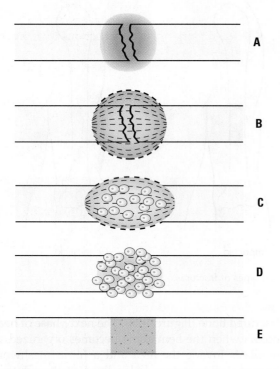

FIGURE **4-25** Bone healing (schematic representation).

Clinical Manifestations

The signs and symptoms of fractures vary according to the location and function of the involved bone, the strength of its muscle attachment, the type of fracture sustained, and the amount of related damage. Signs and symptoms are as follows:

- Pain
- Loss of normal function: The injured part may be incapable of voluntary movements

- Obvious deformity
- Change in the curvature or length of bone (for fractured hip, the affected leg will be shorter and externally rotated)
- Crepitus, or grating sound if limb is moved gently; no attempt should be made to determine this sign when fracture is suspected because it may cause further damage and increase pain
- Soft tissue edema in area of injury
- Warmth over injured area
- Ecchymosis of skin surrounding injured area; it may not be present for several days
- Loss of sensation or paralysis distal to injury: Indicative of nerve constricture
- Signs of shock related to tissue injury, blood loss, and severe pain

Assessment

Rapid orthopedic and peripheral vascular assessment. **The seven Ps of orthopedic assessment** are performed for a baseline and to monitor changes in the patient's muscular function, bone integrity, distal circulation, and sensation:

- Pain: Does it seem out of proportion to the patient's injury? Does the pain increase on active or passive motion?
- Pallor
- Paresthesia or numbness
- Paralysis
- Polar temperature: Is the extremity cold compared with the opposite extremity?
- Puffiness from edema or a hematoma
- Pulselessness: A Doppler ultrasound device may be useful to determine the presence or absence of blood flow if unable to palpate distal pulses

Collection of **subjective data** includes the following:
- Pain at site of injury
- Loss of sensation or movement of affected part
- Determine cause of injury

Collection of **objective data** includes the following:
- Warmth, edema, and ecchymosis
- Obvious deformity
- Loss of normal function in the injured part
- Signs of systemic shock
- Signs of any circulatory, motor, or sensory impairment

Diagnostic Tests

An accurate diagnosis of the fracture is made by radiographic examination or fluoroscopy.

Medical Management

Immediate management includes the following:
1. Splinting to prevent edema of the affected part
2. Preservation of body alignment
3. Elevation of body part to limit edema
4. Application of cold packs (during first 24 hours) to reduce hemorrhage, edema, and pain
5. Administration of analgesics
6. Observation for change in color, sensation, or temperature
7. Observation for signs of shock

Secondary management includes the following:
I. Simple fracture—optimal reduction: replacing bone fragments in their correct anatomical position
   a. Closed reduction: manual manipulations, moving bony fragments into position by applying traction and pressure to distal fragments
   b. Traction
   c. Open reduction with internal fixation (ORIF) is a surgical procedure allowing fracture alignment under direct visualization while using various internal fixation devices applied to the bone
   d. Immobilization
      1. External fixation: cast or splint
      2. Traction
      3. Internal fixation devices such as pins, plates, screws, wires, and prostheses (see Figure 4-20)
      4. Combination of the above
II. **Compound fracture**—additional measures taken:
   a. Surgical debridement of wound to remove dirt, foreign materials, devitalized tissue, and necrotic bone
   b. Administration of tetanus toxoid
   c. Culture of wound
   d. Treatment with antibiotics
   e. Observation for signs of osteomyelitis, tetanus, or gangrene
   f. Closure of wound when there is no sign of infection

g. Reduction of fracture
h. Immobilization of fracture
i. Treatment of complications

Nursing Interventions and Patient Teaching

The nursing intervention of patients with fractures is essentially that given any surgical patient. The care of the patient in traction and in a cast will be discussed later in this chapter. The patient needs a well-balanced diet, but opinions differ on the value of vitamin and mineral supplements in hastening bone repair. Fluids should be encouraged. Exercise of the unaffected joints, muscle-setting exercises, skin care, and elimination are important considerations in patient care. Internal fixation has simplified nursing intervention for many patients with fractures and shortened the period of hospitalization, but many patients will require longer periods of hospitalization. If activity is restricted, the complications that result from immobility must be anticipated and prevented.

Patient teaching should include the following:
- How to move comfortably in bed
- How to transfer safely in and out of bed
- What weight-bearing restrictions to observe and for how long
- What activity limitations to observe and for how long
- How to properly use ambulatory assistive devices
- How to avoid edema in the affected part by proper elevation
- How to control pain or discomfort in the affected part
- What exercises to perform to maintain strength and enhance circulation
- Proper method of cleansing pins, using surgical asepsis per physician's protocol
- How to perform muscle toning (isometric) exercises on a regular basis

Prognosis

Bone production and fracture healing depend on the age and general health of the patient. Presence of other systemic diseases complicates the healing process.

FRACTURE OF THE VERTEBRAE
Etiology/Pathophysiology

Injuries such as diving accidents or blows to the head or body can result in fractures of the vertebrae. Patients with osteoporosis and metastatic cancer are at risk for vertebral fractures. Motorcycle and car accidents (especially head-on collisions) occur more frequently with young men (ages 16 to 30 years).

Fractures of the vertebrae may involve the vertebral body, lamina, and articulating processes and may occur with or without displacement. If the fracture has displaced the vertebral structures, pressure may be placed on spinal nerves. The sharp bone fragments may also sever the spinal cord nerves, causing permanent paralysis from the point of injury downward.

Clinical Manifestations

Signs and symptoms of vertebral fracture include the following:

- Pain at site of injury
- Partial or complete loss of mobility or sensation below level of injury
- Evidence of fracture/fracture dislocation on routine radiographic examination, myelography, or CT scans.

Assessment

Collection of **subjective data** includes assessment for pain (if fracture has altered the spinal cord, pain may not be present), numbness, tingling, and inability to move extremities from below the level of the trauma site.

Collection of **objective data** involves careful assessment of neurological function, such as pupillary reaction to light, hand grip, ability to move extremities, level of orientation, vital signs, and reaction to painful stimulation (see Chapter 14). The nurse should observe for fecal and urinary retention. The nurse should observe for signs of hemorrhage such as hypotension, tachycardia, tachypnea, and decreased renal functioning. The continuity of traction (e.g., weights hanging free and ropes not twisted) and skin integrity (e.g., erythema, tenderness, and edema), as well as surrounding traction equipment, should be assessed.

Diagnostic Tests

Radiographic studies are done to determine whether there is compression of the vertebral bodies. A spinal cord injury may result from a fracture or dislocation of a vertebra, and if this is suspected, the physician performs a spinal tap for evaluation of the spinal fluid (presence of blood indicates trauma). Spinal fluid is normally clear in color (see Chapter 14).

Medical Management

Stable injuries to the vertebrae that are not a threat to spinal cord integrity are treated with pain medication and muscle relaxants. Anticoagulant therapy may be ordered as a prophylaxis for thromboembolic complications. Maintaining erect posture can be enhanced by the use of a back support, corset brace, or a cast. The patient may be allowed to ambulate with assistance (gait enhancers) when discomfort subsides.

Unstable fractures that involve a degree of displacement are more serious, and treatment is aimed at fracture reduction. The fracture may be reduced by postural positioning and traction. Cranial skeletal traction is used with cervical spine fractures (see Chapter 14). A halo brace (Figure 4-26), an external immobilization device in which a plaster or plastic brace that incorporates metal struts attached to pins is inserted into bone,

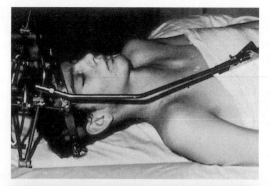

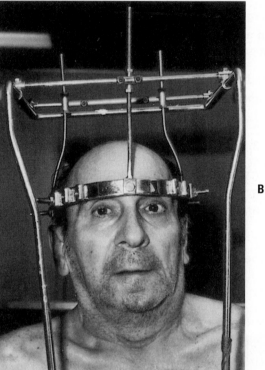

FIGURE **4-26 A,** Halo attached to body cast. Metal strut will be anchored firmly into body cast with additional plaster. **B,** Metal ring, or halo, that attaches to skull.

is used to allow mobility of the patient. Pelvic traction is used for lumbar spinal fractures. An open reduction may be necessary with internal fixation using a Harrington rod. After this surgical procedure the patient is placed in a body cast.

Nursing Interventions and Patient Teaching

Nursing intervention is aimed at maintaining the stability of the fracture fixation by (1) log-rolling the patient for position changes; (2) following the correct procedure for turning a patient in a special bed, such as a Stryker frame or Foster bed; (3) elevating the head of the bed no more than 30 degrees; and (4) using stabilization devices for the head and back.

Nursing diagnoses and interventions for the patient with a vertebral fracture include but are not limited to the following:

NURSING DIAGNOSES	NURSING INTERVENTIONS
Powerlessness, related to decreased mobility/pain	Use active listening, and permit verbalization of anger and helplessness. Assist patient with identifying coping mechanisms that will reduce feeling of powerlessness; use those that have been successful in past. Offer positive recognition for increased activity level. Assist patients in identifying areas over which they have control. Involve patients in decision-making process for their own care.
Risk for infection, related to immobility and/or surgical intervention	Monitor patient for signs and symptoms of infection (elevated temperature, increased pulse rate, malodorous exudate, erythema, cloudy urine, diminished breath sounds, and presence of crackles and wheezes). Monitor laboratory values (such as complete blood count [CBC]) and blood and wound cultures. Protect patient from cross-contamination by practicing good handwashing techniques, maintaining surgical asepsis when changing dressings, and using strict surgical asepsis with catheter care. Encourage coughing, deep breathing, and leg exercises. Encourage use of incentive spirometer. Prevent people with infectious processes from coming in contact with patient.
Impaired physical mobility, related to neuromuscular/skeletal impairment, pain, and discomfort	Maintain bed rest in correct body alignment; avoid lifting or twisting body. Place patient in immobilization device as ordered, such as cervical head halter, skeletal traction, Stryker frame, or CircOlectric bed; maintain cervical spine in extension. Assess neurovascular status every 2 hours; monitor pulse, color, temperature, sensation, and mobility of all extremities. Perform passive or assist with and teach active ROM exercises for all extremities every 2 hours.

NURSING DIAGNOSES	NURSING INTERVENTIONS
	As fracture heals, traction is replaced with cast. Ambulate with assistance when ordered; monitor for vertigo and weakness; progress slowly.

Patient teaching involves teaching the patient to support the back by (1) using a firm mattress; (2) sitting in straight, firm chairs (for no longer than 20 to 30 minutes), when allowed; (3) using proper lifting techniques (using the leg muscles, not the back); and (4) doing back exercises to strengthen spinal extensor muscles.

Prognosis

Stable injuries to the vertebrae that are not a threat to spinal cord integrity have an excellent prognosis with full recovery. Unstable fractures are more serious, and prognosis is guarded when spinal cord injury is involved.

FRACTURE OF THE PELVIS
Etiology/Pathophysiology

Most pelvic fractures result from trauma involving great force, such as falls from extreme heights, automobile accidents, or crushing accidents.

When trauma is severe enough to fracture the pelvis, vital abdominal organs may also be damaged, such as the bladder, vagina, uterus, liver, spleen, intestines, or kidneys. Because the pelvis has a rich blood supply, a fracture of the pelvis can result in extensive blood loss (as much as 1 to 4 L).

Clinical Manifestations

The patient with a fractured pelvis will be unable to bear weight without discomfort. Local tenderness and edema are common at the trauma site. Hematuria (blood in the urine) may result from trauma to the bladder. Hemorrhage is by far the most life-threatening complication to a patient with a pelvic fracture.

Assessment

Collection of **subjective data** involves complaints of pelvic pain or tenderness and backache. Complaints of restlessness, anxiety, and progressive disorientation may indicate signs of shock.

Collection of **objective data** involves assessment of muscle spasms in the pelvic region; ecchymosis over the pelvis, perineum, groin, or suprapubic area; inability to raise the legs when supine; and external foot rotation on the affected side with noticeable shortening of one leg. Vital sign assessment may indicate shock (hypotension, tachycardia, tachypnea, oliguria, and diaphoresis). Careful observation for fat embolism syndrome (FES) is especially pertinent for patients with pelvic fractures. Assessing bowel sounds in all four quadrants and documenting the findings is important; large bowel and rectal lacerations are possible in patients with pelvic fractures. Assessing color and amount of urine output is necessary because of the possibility of laceration of the bladder.

Diagnostic Tests

Abdominal radiographic studies are done in the supine and lateral positions. Computed tomography provides an evaluation of both the bony pelvis and intraabdominal contents. Intravenous pyelogram is performed to determine kidney damage. Interpretation of laboratory values for hemoglobin, hematocrit, urinalysis, and stool for occult blood helps determine whether the patient is bleeding and whether anemia is present.

Medical Management

The patient often remains on bed rest for 3 weeks and then walks with crutches for approximately 6 weeks. If the patient has a symphysis pubis fracture and an iliac fracture on the same side, the physician will perform surgery. After surgery, skeletal traction is applied for approximately 6 weeks to maintain the leg's position. When traction is released, the patient may ambulate without bearing weight for approximately 3 months. For a bilateral fracture of the pelvis, the physician may order a pelvic sling to support the fracture. To treat severe fractures that totally disrupt the pelvic ring and dislocate the sacroiliac joints, the physician may apply an external skeletal fixation device. He or she may also apply a spica or body cast to support the fracture.

Nursing Interventions and Patient Teaching

Nursing intervention involves monitoring the patient for signs of progressive shock (hypotension, tachycardia, tachypnea, and decreased urinary output). Measuring the abdominal girth for signs of increased abdominal pressure that could result from internal hemorrhaging is done at least every 8 hours. I&O are accurately monitored for signs of hypovolemia, laceration of the bladder, and potential kidney trauma. A Foley catheter is inserted for monitoring of urine output and color. Nursing interventions appropriate for impaired mobility, impaired skin integrity, fluid volume deficit, and pain management are implemented.

Nursing diagnosis and interventions for the patient with a pelvic fracture include but are not limited to the following:

NURSING DIAGNOSIS	NURSING INTERVENTIONS
Risk for ineffective tissue perfusion, related to hemorrhage, hypovolemia, and/or shock	Assess for ecchymosis over pelvis and perineum. Monitor vital signs every 15 minutes for evidence of shock until stable.
	Insert Foley catheter per physician's order to monitor color and amount of urine output. Monitor parenteral fluids per physician's order. Provide quiet, therapeutic environment. Administer oxygen per physician's order. Maintain bed rest per physician's order. Monitor bowel sounds and measure abdominal girth to ascertain possible lacerated bowel.

The nurse reinforces the reasons for immobility and not bearing full weight; anxiety may prevent the patient from hearing or understanding initial explanations. The nurse also explains measures for dealing with acute pain and changes in using medications as pain decreases. In addition, turning and moving techniques to prevent skin impairment are explained.

Prognosis

Hemorrhage is by far the most life-threatening complication. The long-term prognosis depends on the severity of the fracture, the age of the patient, and the presence of other systemic disorders.

COMPLICATIONS OF FRACTURES
COMPARTMENT SYNDROME

Compartment syndrome is a pathologic condition caused by the progressive development of arterial vessel compression and reduced blood supply to an extremity. Fractures of the forearm or tibia usually precede the onset of muscle edema within the fasciae, which form compartments for the muscles of the forearm and lower leg. When there is severe trauma, such as fractures or compression of blood vessels as a result of a tight cast or dressing, muscle ischemia (decreased blood supply to the muscles) can occur. Irreversible muscle ischemia can occur within 6 hours as a result of compression of the arteries, nerves, and tendons entering the compartment. Paralysis and sensory loss follow, with contracture and permanent disability of the extremity seen within 24 to 48 hours.

Assessment

Collection of **subjective data** includes pain assessment. Usually the patient will complain of sharp pain that increases with passive movement of the hand or foot. The patient experiences deep, unrelenting, progressive, and poorly localized pain unrelieved by analgesics or elevation of the extremity. Numbness or tingling in the affected extremity is common.

Collection of **objective data** involves assessment of the patient's inability to flex the fingers or toes, coolness of the extremity, and absence of pulsation in the affected extremity. Assessment of skin color for signs of pallor or cyanosis is made. Gentle palpation of the extremity will reveal slowing of the capillary refilling time (blanching). Close monitoring and proper documentation of vital signs are essential (especially temperature to detect signs of tissue necrosis) (see Box 4-5).

Medical Management

The majority of these cases require a fasciotomy (incision into the fascia) to relieve pressure and allow return of normal blood flow to the area. This will be done immediately (within 30 minutes). The incision is often left open to heal by granulation (healing by second intention) (Figure 4-27).

Nursing Interventions

Nursing intervention includes administration of analgesics with careful documentation of relief obtained. To slow further circulatory compromise, the affected limb can be elevated, no higher than heart level, to maintain arterial pressure. Application of cold packs and removal of any constricting material, such as an elastic bandage, are necessary. The most common complication when decompression is delayed is infection as a result of tissue necrosis. Purulent drainage from the dressing is a sign of infection and must be reported immediately. If drainage and secretion isolation are required, careful instructions should be given to the patient, who may feel isolated. Patients are encouraged to express their fears and emotional needs to the nurse. Volkmann's contracture is a permanent contracture (with clawhand, flexion of wrist and fingers, and atrophy of the forearm) that can occur as a result of compartment syndrome. Proper positioning and alignment can reduce the risk of this complication.

Prognosis

Compartment syndrome can result in a permanent contracture deformity of the hand or foot.

SHOCK

Shock can occur as a result of blood loss from a fractured bone (bone is vascular) or from severed blood vessels, seen especially in compound fractures. Pain and fear can also cause shock.

Assessment

Collection of **subjective data** includes monitoring the patient's level of consciousness. Restlessness or complaints of anxiety may suggest a decrease in cerebral perfusion, resulting in brain hypoxia. Complaints of weakness and lethargy are common.

Collection of **objective data** includes monitoring vital signs. Typical shock signs include hypotension, tachycardia, and tachypnea. As shock progresses, hypothermia will occur. There may be pallor and cool, moist skin. Oliguria (diminished urinary output) is present with shock.

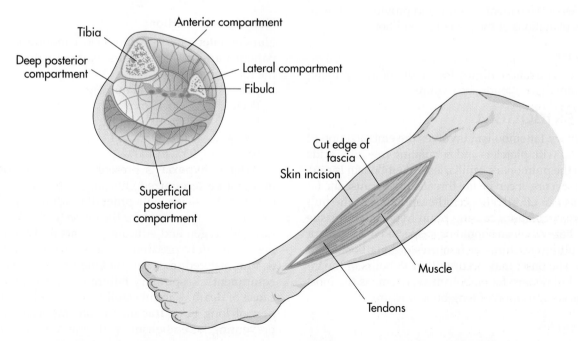

FIGURE **4-27** Compartment syndrome. Often more than one compartment is involved, and anterior compartment is especially vulnerable. Causes include trauma, severe burn, or excessive exercise. A single incision may open more than one compartment.

Medical Management

The physician's main concern will be to restore blood volume so that there can be a rapid return of oxygen to the tissues. Blood volume can be expanded with intravenous (IV) fluids (lactated Ringer's solution, 5% dextrose in normal saline). Whole blood, plasma, and plasma substitutes may also be given. Respiratory assistance may be given by administering oxygen. A central venous catheter may be inserted for accurate monitoring of vital signs to prevent pulmonary edema. Shock trousers may be applied. These are pneumatic trousers designed to counteract hypotension associated with internal or external bleeding and hypovolemia.

Nursing Interventions

Nursing intervention includes the nurse's responsibilities in IV fluid administration. These include checking (1) the contents and IV flow rate against the physician's orders, and (2) the infusion site for signs of infiltration (erythema, edema, pain, and induration [hardening of tissue]). The patient's vital signs are monitored every 15 minutes until stable. Urinary output is monitored every hour. Less than 30 mL of urine per hour is indicative of decreased renal perfusion. The patient should remain flat in bed. If there are no head injuries, the lower extremities can be raised slightly to improve venous return. The Trendelenburg position should be avoided because it tends to push the abdominal organs against the diaphragm, reducing the effectiveness of heart and lung functions. The patient must be kept warm, but external heat should be avoided. Nothing should be given by mouth, and sedatives, tranquilizers, and narcotics should be avoided. The nurse should be aware of the anxieties of the patient's family and provide them with brief explanations of the patient's condition.

Prognosis

Shock can be fatal within a few hours of injury, therefore immediate attention is required.

FAT EMBOLISM

Pulmonary fat embolism involves the embolization of tissue fat with platelets and circulating free fatty acids within the pulmonary capillaries. Fat embolism is rare, but if it occurs, it can be life threatening because the fat droplets can effectively occlude capillaries of the pulmonary circulation, causing brain hypoxia and tissue death. Fat embolism should be suspected if the patient has multiple fractures or fractures of long bones and pelvis. The onset may occur within 48 hours of the injuries. Pulmonary fat embolism syndrome is the most serious complication of long bone fractures.

Assessment

Collection of **subjective data** includes assessment of mental disturbances, such as irritability, restlessness, disorientation, stupor, and coma. These symptoms can result from effects of severe hypoxemia. There may be complaints of chest pain, especially on inspiration, and complaints of localized muscle weakness, spasticity, and rigidity.

Collection of **objective data** includes assessing for tachypnea, dyspnea, hypoxemia, and auditory crackles and wheezes in the lung field. As the lung filters and traps embolic material, ventilation is disturbed. Assessment of the apical pulse is performed to detect dysrhythmias. Patients will be placed on cardiac monitoring for observation of dysrhythmias and cardiovascular collapse. The nurse assesses the patient for petechiae (especially in the buccal membranes, conjunctival sacs, hard palate, chest, and anterior axillary folds) caused by occlusion of capillaries.

Diagnostic Tests

The diagnosis is made on clinical signs and symptoms. These occur within 24 to 48 hours of injury. Blood gases are indicative of hypoxemia. Hemoglobin and hematocrit laboratory values are decreased. Fat will be present in the blood and urine. The sedimentation rate is increased, and the platelet count is decreased.

Medical Management

The physician will order the administration of intravenous fluids to prevent shock and dilute free fatty acids. Steroid therapy is recommended to counteract the inflammatory response to the free fatty acids. Digoxin is often ordered to increase the patient's cardiac output. Oxygen will be administered if the P_{O_2} is less than 70 mm Hg. Incentive spirometry is ordered to improve lung expansion and oxygenation.

Nursing Interventions

Nursing intervention includes close monitoring of the patient's arterial blood gases. Normal values include the following:

pH	7.35 to 7.45 mm Hg
P_{CO_2}	35 to 45 mm Hg
P_{O_2}	80 to 100 mm Hg
HCO_3	21 to 28 mEq/L
Sa_{O_2}	95% to 100%

Arterial hypoxia is present with fat emboli and may not be recognized clinically. If hypoxia is present, the physician will order the administration of oxygen. It is important for the nurse to check the liter flow of oxygen and educate patients and their families as to safety precautions necessary when oxygen is administered (e.g., no smoking or use of electrical equipment). Respiratory failure is the most common cause of death. Careful stabilization and immobilization of long bone fractures is an important step in preventing fat embolism syndrome. Careful support when turning and positioning the patient can prevent the manipulation of the fracture and reduce the risk of fat embolism syndrome. An accurate record of intake, output, and daily weights is essential to monitor fluid balance.

Prognosis

Fat embolism can be life threatening.

GAS GANGRENE

Gas gangrene is a severe infection of the skeletal muscle caused by gram-positive *Clostridium* bacteria, particularly *Clostridium perfringens,* which may occur in the presence of compound fractures and lacerated wounds. These injuries can produce exotoxins that destroy tissue. The onset is usually sudden and may occur 1 to 14 days after injury. These organisms are anaerobic (grow and function without oxygen) and spore formers. They are normally found in soil and the intestinal tract of humans. As the clostridia bacteria invade devitalized tissue (especially where blood supply is diminished), they multiply and produce toxins that cause (1) hemolysis (breakdown of red blood cells and release of hemoglobin); (2) vessel thrombosis; and (3) damage to the myocardium, liver, kidneys, and brain.

Assessment

Collection of **subjective data** includes observation of pain, which is usually sudden and severe at the site of the injury. A characteristic finding is toxic delirium.

Collection of **objective data** includes careful inspection of the skin for gas bubbles, which may be seen at the site of the wound. The various species of clostridia produce a characteristic cellulitis in which gas is present under the skin. This causes a crepitation (crackling sensation when the skin is touched). Signs of infection may be apparent with elevated temperature, tachycardia, tachypnea, and edema around the wound. The skin around the wound becomes necrotic and ruptures, revealing necrotic muscle. There will be a foul odor from the wound discharge, which is thin and watery. Careful documentation of the patient's progress relative to antibiotic therapy is made (e.g., decline in temperature and decrease in amount of wound drainage).

Medical Management

Treatment of gas gangrene involves establishing a larger wound opening to admit air and promote drainage. Antibiotics, such as penicillin G or cephalothin, will be ordered intravenously and must be administered as scheduled. The patient should be observed for adverse reactions.

Nursing Interventions

Nursing intervention includes wound care using strict medical asepsis. Spore-forming bacteria are not destroyed by ordinary disinfecting methods. Therefore all contaminated equipment and linens must be autoclaved. Drainage and secretion isolation procedures are necessary to prevent the spread of the infection to other patients.

Prognosis

If left untreated, gas gangrene is rapidly fatal. Prompt treatment, including excision of gangrenous tissue and administration of penicillin G intravenously, saves 80% of patients. If massive gangrene develops, amputation is necessary.

THROMBOEMBOLUS
Etiology/Pathophysiology

Thromboembolus is a condition in which a blood vessel is occluded by an embolus carried in the bloodstream from the site of formation of the clot. It is associated with reduced skeletal muscle contractions and bed rest. The person suffering from pelvic and hip fractures is at high risk for this complication.

Clinical Manifestations

The area supplied by an obstructed artery may tingle and become cold, numb, and cyanotic. An embolus in the lungs causes a sudden, sharp thoracic or upper abdominal pain, dyspnea, cough, fever, and hemoptysis.

Assessment

Collection of **subjective data** includes careful investigation of the patient's complaints of pain in the lower extremities (especially the calf of the leg). A complaint of tenderness over the area is common. The patient may complain of a sharp pain in the thoracic area when an embolus is in the lung.

Collection of **objective data** includes assessing for a positive Homans' sign, which is indicative of thromboembolus. Homans' sign is pain in the calf of the affected leg upon dorsiflexion of the foot. The affected area may be erythematous, warm to touch, and edematous. The nurse should assess for differences in leg size (circumference) bilaterally from thigh to ankle. The nurse will assess the patient for dyspnea and presence of blood in the sputum if pulmonary embolus is present. When anticoagulant therapy is ordered, the nurse will assess for signs of bleeding, such as petechiae, epistaxis, hematuria, hematemesis, and occult or gross blood in the stool.

Diagnostic Tests

A complete history is taken and a physical examination is performed. In addition to checking Homans' sign, a prothrombin time, INR, D-dimer, and complete blood count are obtained. Diagnostic tests for deep vein thrombosis may include Doppler ultrasonography or duplex scanning.

A spiral computed tomography (CT) scan of the lung, a ventilation/perfusion (V/Q) scan, or a pulmonary arteriogram may be ordered to rule out pulmonary embolism.

Medical Management

Treatment will include administration of anticoagulants, such as heparin, enoxaparin (Lovenox) or warfarin (Coumadin). A surgical procedure known as thrombectomy (removal of a thrombus from a blood vessel) may be done.

Nursing Interventions

Nursing intervention involves caring for the patient on activity restriction. Many times this involves bed rest with the foot of the bed elevated to aid venous return. The nurse should teach the patient to do active exercise, such as dorsiflexion (pointing backward) and plantar flexion (pointing forward) of the toes, several times each hour. This exercise is effective in stimulating circulation to the legs. Continuous hot, moist compresses are usually ordered. Antiembolic stockings and the use of intermittent pneumatic compression devices are ordered while the patient is on bed rest and are maintained even after the patient is ambulatory. Assessment of lung sounds every 4 hours is indicated. It is important that the nurse adhere to the activity ordered. If the patient is receiving anticoagulants, close monitoring of prothrombin (PT), International Normalized Ratio (INR), and partial thromboplastin times (PTT) is necessary (Safety Considerations box).

Prognosis

Obstruction of the pulmonary artery or one of its branches may be fatal. A thrombus in an extremity usually resolves with treatment, and a favorable prognosis is noted.

DELAYED FRACTURE HEALING

Delayed complications deal with fracture healing. A **delayed union** is a fracture that fails to heal within the usual time for fracture healing. The healing is impaired but has not completely stopped and will eventually repair itself. **Nonunion** is failure of the ends of the fractured bone to unite. A nonunion fracture fails to unite and produce a stable union after 6 to 9 months. The calcification of cartilage and bone formation do not occur. Bone grafting, prosthetic implant, internal fixation, external fixation, or a combination of these methods can be used to correct the problem of delayed or nonunion bone fractures.

Electrical stimulation is being used by physicians as a new method of treatment in promoting healing of nonunion fractures. The use of electrical probes on bone stimulates bone production.

Prognosis

Bone production and fracture healing depend on the age and general health of the patient. Presence of other systemic diseases complicates the healing process.

SKELETAL FIXATION DEVICES

EXTERNAL FIXATION DEVICES

External fixation devices are used to hold bone fragments in normal position. Casts, skeletal and skin traction, braces, and metal pins are examples of these devices.

Skeletal Pin External Fixation

One external fixation technique immobilizes fractures by the use of pins inserted through the bone and attached to a rigid external metal frame (Figure 4-28). This technique is becoming more popular because it provides rigid support of comminuted open fractures, infected nonunions, and infected unstable joints. However, an advantage to having the fracture open to air is the visibility of the area and accessibility for wound care. The patient can use the muscles and joints above and below the fixation and experiences less discomfort.

This procedure is performed with the patient under general anesthesia. Patients need to be reassured that the pain after the insertion of the pins is minimal. Immediately after the procedure, the extremity is placed in balanced suspension traction to help relieve the edema. Pins that are inserted through the bone are assessed at least every 8 hours, with careful observation for signs of infection and loose pins. Removing dried exudate from around the pins is done once or twice daily with hydrogen peroxide or alcohol, using surgical asepsis. Patients are permitted to ambulate on crutches when soft tissue edema is relieved. They are permitted to shower when the wounds have healed but must avoid salt or chlorinated water to prevent fixator corrosion.

NONSURGICAL INTERVENTIONS FOR MUSCULOSKELETAL DISORDERS

CASTS

Casts are immobilization devices made up of layers of plaster of paris, fiberglass, or plastic roller bandages. The application is similar to that for an elastic bandage. Types of casts are indicative of the part of the body immobilized. Examples include (1) short arm cast, which extends from below the elbow to the prox-

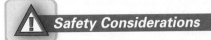

⚠ Safety Considerations

Thromboembolus

Never massage a patient's lower extremities. Thromboembolus can be present without clinical signs and symptoms.

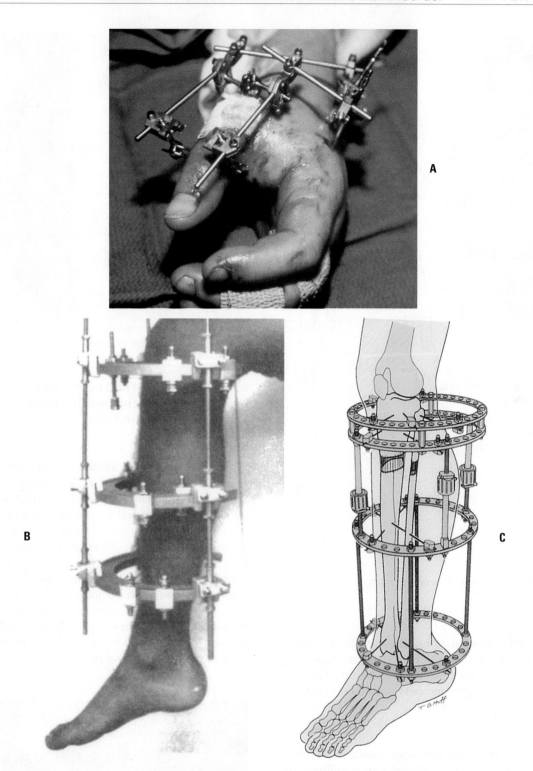

FIGURE **4-28** External fixation apparatuses. **A,** Hoffman. **B,** The Monticello-Spinelli Circular Fixator. **C,** Ilizarov apparatus with corticotomies for lengthening lower leg.

imal palmar crease; (2) long leg cast, which extends from the upper thigh to the base of the toes; (3) spica cast or body cast, which covers the trunk of the patient and one or both extremities (Figure 4-29).

Casts are applied after the physician has properly aligned the bone through either external or internal fixation. Cast application is relatively painless except

for the manipulation of the traumatized extremity. The casting procedure involves the application of a piece of stockinette that covers the length of the extremity and area to be casted, followed by sheet wadding (pressed cotton that comes in rolled bandages), followed by the casting material. Most physicians will bring the stockinette up and over the distal and proximal edge of the

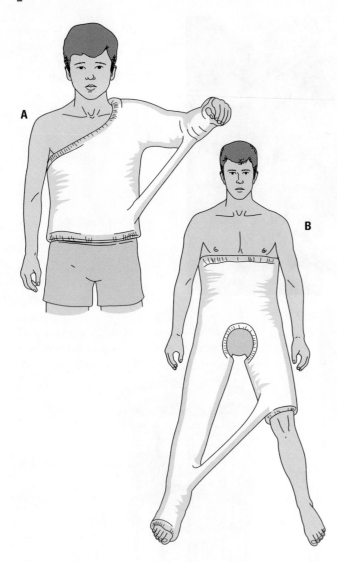

FIGURE **4-29** Spica casts. **A,** Shoulder spica. **B,** One and one-half leg-hip spica.

cast. It is important to assess these edges for rough pieces of casting that may irritate the skin. Superficial burns can occur as the cast begins to set up, especially if the patient is not appropriately padded or too much fiberglass material is used.

CAST BRACE

The cast brace is an alternative appliance to the traditional leg cast. It provides support and stability of the plaster cast, with additional support and mobility provided by a hinged brace. The appliance is most effective for fractures of the shaft of the femur and permits early ambulation and weight bearing. It is used approximately 2 to 6 weeks after fracture reduction.

Cast bracing is based on the concept that limited weight bearing helps promote the formation of bone. A problem encountered frequently with cast bracing is edema around the knee. Patients are instructed to elevate the leg when sitting to promote venous return. A

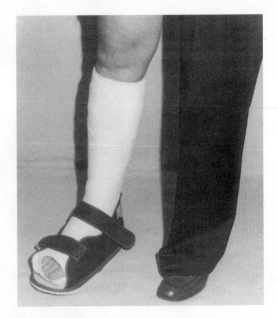

FIGURE **4-30** Short-leg walking cast with cast shoe.

cast shoe or walking heel incorporated into a lower extremity cast will permit weight bearing without damaging the cast (Figure 4-30).

Assessment

Nursing assessment is similar regardless of what kind of casting material is used. A neurovascular assessment including capillary refill is done every 15 to 30 minutes for several hours after casting and every 4 hours the first few days (see Box 4-5). Capillary filling time (capillary refill) is an assessment of arterial flow to the extremities; the patient's nailbeds are squeezed to produce blanching and observed for the return of color. With normal arterial capillary perfusion, the color will return to normal within 2 seconds (Figure 4-31). The skin at the cast edges is observed for erythema and irritation. It is important to note any odor or drainage coming from under the cast and doc-

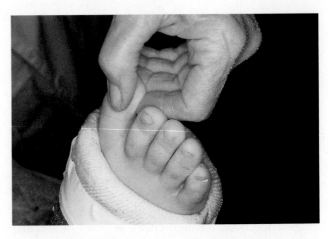

FIGURE **4-31** Capillary refill assessment.

ument the findings. Both of these signs indicate infection. The nurse should assess the patient's ability to use crutches using a three-point gait to establish normal gait and rhythm and should assess crutches for safety concerning proper fit and presence of large, rubber, suction tips on the ends.

Nursing Interventions and Patient Teaching

Nursing intervention for the patient in a cast (Skill 4-1) includes patient education concerning the prevention of infection, irritation, neurovascular pressure, and misalignment of bone ends. A wet cast must be handled gently and supported with the flat of the hand or on pillows to avoid indentations that will cause pressure on the skin and lead to skin impairment. Never use the bar in a spica cast as support when turning patient. Turning the patient frequently will aid the drying process. If a cast dryer is used, the setting should be on warm—never hot (drying a plaster of paris cast too quickly from the outside may weaken the cast). Elevating the casted extremity will reduce edema (usually elevation is recommended for 24 to 48 hours). Patients using crutches should be instructed to support

their weight on their hands; weight borne on the axillae can damage the brachial plexus nerves (crutch paralysis).

Cast syndrome can occur after the application of a spica (body) cast (see Figure 4-29) and involves acute obstruction of the duodenum. If symptoms of nausea occur, place the patient prone to relieve pressure symptoms and alert the charge nurse. Gastric decompression may be necessary, and if conventional measures fail, surgical intervention (duodenojejunostomy—making an opening into the small intestine) may be necessary.

Patient teaching includes information about cleaning around the cast site with a mild soap and rinsing excessive soap so that it does not accumulate around the cast and impair the skin. A synthetic cast can be flushed with water if it becomes soiled. It must be dried afterward to prevent skin impairment and maceration (softening of the skin). Drying a synthetic cast can be accomplished by blotting it with a towel and then using a blow dryer on cool or warm setting in a sweeping motion across the cast. Proper drying may take as long as 1 hour.

Skill 4-1   Care of the Patient in a Cast

1. Patient teaching. (**Ensures patient cooperation; reduces patient anxiety.**)
   a. Explain why the cast is being applied and how it will be applied. (**Sudden movement during procedure could cause injury.**)
   b. Advise the patient that the plaster cast will feel warm as it dries.
   c. Explain the extent of immobilization.
   d. Explain care of the cast and expectations after discharge.
   e. Instruct patient not to insert sharp objects (coat hangers or pencils) under the cast. (**These may abrade the skin and lead to infection.**)

2. Handling the new cast.
   (A fiberglass cast dries immediately after application; a plaster extremity cast dries in approximately 24 to 48 hours; a plaster spica or body cast dries in 48 to 72 hours [see Figure 4-29].)
   a. Support wet cast with the flat of the hands or on pillows. (**Avoids indentations that will cause pressure on underlying skin.**)
   b. Place cotton blankets or other absorbent material under the cast. (**Aids drying of cast.**)
   c. Expose the cast to air as much as possible. (**Aids drying of cast.**)

   d. Turn the patient frequently. (**Aids drying of cast.**)
   e. Use a cast dryer or hair dryer on a warm (not hot) setting. (**Circulates air over the cast.**)
   f. Do not apply paint, varnish, or shellac to the cast. (**Plaster is a porous material that allows air to circulate to the skin.**)

3. Skin care. (**Decreases the chance of skin irritation or tissue injury.**)
   a. Inspect skin at edges of cast and underlying cast for erythema or skin impairment.
   b. Remove plaster crumbs from skin with a washcloth moistened with warm water.
   c. Use creams and lotions sparingly. (**They may soften the skin and cause the cast to stick to the skin.**)
   d. Apply waterproof material around perineal area. (**Prevents soiling of and damage to cast and prevents skin impairment.**)
   e. Attend to patient's complaint of pain under the cast, particularly over bony prominences. (**This may indicate pressure on the skin.**); if discomfort is not relieved by repositioning, report to physician (**Cast pressure may need to be relieved by windowing or bivalving [cutting into halves].**)

Continued

Skill 4-1 | Care of the Patient in a Cast—cont'd

4. Turning—turning to any position is generally permitted as long as the integrity of the cast is not compromised and the patient is comfortable; do not turn by grasping the abductor bar. **(Is not safe transport.)**

5. Toileting—for a long leg or hip spica cast.
   a. Use a fracture pan with blanket roll or padding. **(Provides support under the small of the back.)**
   b. Elevate the head of the bed, if permitted, or place the bed in reverse Trendelenburg's position. **(Eases procedure.)**

6. Abdominal discomfort—cast may be "windowed" (an opening cut into it). **(Provides relief of abdominal distention or a port for checking bladder distention.)**

7. Mobilization.
   a. Weight bearing is at the discretion of the physician, and the amount of weight bearing will be prescribed.
   b. A cast shoe or a walking heel incorporated into a lower extremity cast (see Figure 4-30). **(Permits weight bearing without damaging the cast.)**

8. Prevention of neurovascular problems—establish baseline measurements and assess neurovascular status before cast application; palpate distal pulses; assess color, temperature, and capillary refill of the appropriate fingers or toes; assess neurological function, including sensation and motion in the affected and unaffected extremity. **(Changes in neurovascular status may occur after casting, possibly further compromising already injured tissues. It is important to note the baseline neurovascular status so that those changes, if they occur, can be readily assessed.)**
   a. Perform neurovascular checks every hour for at least 24 hours after cast application to detect difficulty from edema or pressure of cast on nerves or vessels; notify physician of color changes, alterations in sensation, or motion unrelieved by position change; cast may need to be bivalved (cut in two) to relieve pressure (see illustration below).
   b. Elevate affected extremity on pillows. **(Danger of edema is usually 24 to 48 hours.)**
   c. After mobilization of patient with lower extremity or upper extremity cast, avoid keeping extremity in dependent position for prolonged periods. **(Prevents edema.)**
   d. After lower extremity cast is removed, encourage patient to wear elastic stocking and elevate affected leg at rest until full mobility is regained. **(After immobilization, the involved joints and muscles will be weak and ROM may be limited. Activity must be resumed slowly. Elastic stockings enhance deep vein circulation.)**

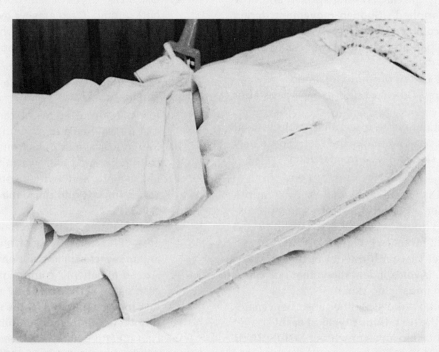

Step **8a**

Patients often complain of pruritus (itching) of the skin that is covered by a cast (especially after having the cast for a few weeks). The nurse can recommend diversional activities when the pruritus begins in addition to having the patient gently rub the area below and above the cast to retard the desire to scratch. It is important to warn patients not to stick sharp objects underneath the cast to relieve the pruritus. This may cause impairment of the skin, and serious complications can occur.

CAST REMOVAL

Cast removal is done with an electric vibrating saw rather than a cutting saw. Bivalving a cast may be done to relieve cast pressure. This involves splitting the cast down both sides and securing the cast pieces so that the extremity is supported (see Skill 4-1, step 8a). Patients should be reassured that the saw poses little risk to injuring the skin beneath the cast, even though it is noisy and has the appearance of a cutting saw. Cutting the cast can cause a very fine powder or dust to escape into the air. If this powder is inhaled over a period of time, the plaster deposits can build up in the lungs' small air sacs and cause respiratory distress. It is a safe practice for the nurse, physician, and patient to wear a mask when casts are removed with a cast cutter.

After removal of a cast, the buildup of secretions and dead skin on the affected extremity can be removed by gently washing and applying lotion or cream to the area. This may take several days, but the patient should be cautioned against trying to remove the devitalized material rapidly for fear of causing skin impairment. Muscle atrophy is common, especially if the extremity has been casted for several weeks. Patients should be reassured that the muscle will regain strength and size with proper exercise through either physical therapy or home exercise programs.

TRACTION

Traction is the process of putting an extremity, bone, or group of muscles under tension by means of weights and pulleys to (1) align and stabilize a fracture site by reducing the fractured part, (2) relieve pressure on nerves as in the case of herniated disk syndrome, (3) maintain correct positioning, (4) prevent deformities, and (5) relieve muscle spasms. The two general types of traction are skeletal and skin. Traction applied for the purpose of stabilizing a fracture will be continuous traction and must not be disconnected unless ordered by the physician. It will be easier to make the patient's bed from top to bottom when bed rest is maintained. Cervical and pelvic traction is sometimes ordered as intermittent traction to be applied as ordered by the physician.

Skeletal Traction

Skeletal traction (Figure 4-32) is applied directly to a bone. Wires and surgical pins are inserted through the bone distal to the fracture site while the patient is under local or general anesthesia. The pin protrudes through the skin on both sides of the extremity, and weights are attached to a rope that is tied to a spreader bar for the purpose of traction. Skeletal traction can be used for fractures of the femur (see Figure 4-32, *A*), tibia (see Figure 4-32, *B*), humerus, and cervical spine (see Chapter 14).

Skin Traction

Skin traction is accomplished by using weight that pulls on sponge rubber, moleskin, elastic bandage with adherent, or plastic materials attached to the skin below the site of the fracture, with the pull exerted on the limb. Buck's, Russell's, and Bryant's are types of skin traction.

Buck's traction. Buck's traction (Figure 4-33, *C*) is a form of traction used as a temporary measure to provide support and comfort to a fractured extremity until a more definite treatment is initiated. Traction (pull) is in a horizontal plane with affected extremity. This traction is frequently used to maintain the reduction of a hip fracture before surgery. It can also be used to treat muscle spasms and minor fractures of the lower spine.

Russell's traction. Russell traction (see Figure 4-33, *B*) is set up similar to Buck's traction. However, a knee sling is used to provide support of the affected leg. It allows more movement in bed and permits flexion of the knee joint. Russell traction is commonly used to treat hip and knee fractures.

Bryant's traction. Bryant's traction is used in pediatrics for small children with fractured femurs. Both legs are suspended at a 90-degree angle to the trunk of the body, and the weight of the lower body pulls the bone fragments of the fractured leg into alignment.

Nursing Interventions

Nursing intervention of patients in traction includes measures to maintain the body in proper alignment and careful assessment of traction equipment. Care of a patient in skeletal traction involves assessment of the pin sites and application of hydrogen peroxide or normal saline per physician's order. Traction care is summarized in Box 4-6.

ORTHOPEDIC DEVICES

Frames can be used for orthopedic patients to assist with turning and positioning while maintaining proper alignment. The **Balkan frame** is a wooden or steel attachment to the hospital bed. The frame has adjustable pulleys and a trapeze bar attached to an overhead bar.

The **Bradford frame** is made of rectangular steel with two pieces of canvas stretched tightly and laced to the frame. A space is left in the buttocks area for toileting and hygiene.

The **Stryker wedge turning frame** and **Foster bed** are similar and assist in changing the patient's position from supine to prone. Patients may become apprehensive when turned on a frame for fear of falling, so thorough explanations and reassurances are helpful.

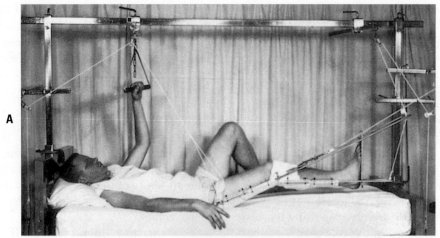

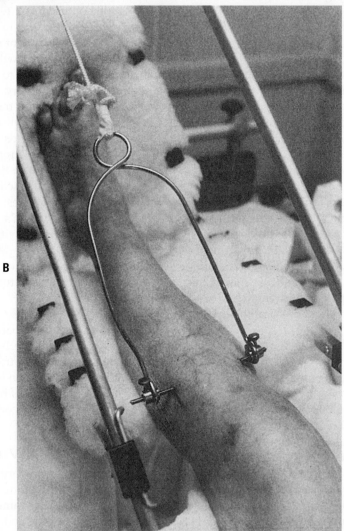

FIGURE **4-32 A,** Balanced suspension skeletal traction to the femur. **B,** Tibial pin traction with Steinmann pin used in treatment of distal femoral fracture. The bow attached to the pin provides a place of attachment for the rope that holds the traction weights. The pull exerted by the weight keeps the fracture fragments aligned. Pin sites must be inspected at least daily to detect signs of pin reaction or infection.

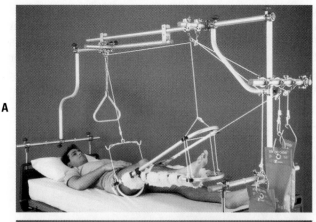

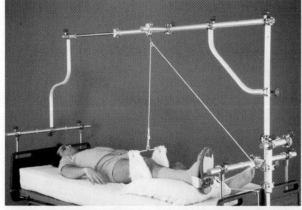

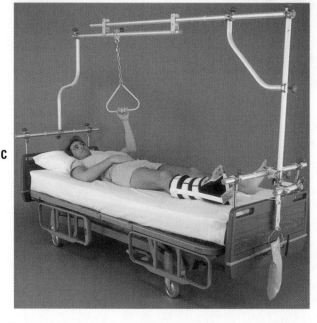

FIGURE **4-33 A,** Balanced traction with a Thomas ring and a Pearson attachment. **B,** Russell's traction. **C,** Buck's traction.

The **CircOlectric bed** is a vertical turning bed that can be operated electrically by one person and placed in a variety of positions. Side-to-side movement can be accomplished while maintaining proper positioning if traction is ordered.

The **RotoRest bed** can rock a patient as much as 62 degrees, 17 times an hour. The electric-powered bed can promote pressure ulcer healing, prevent ve-

| Box 4-6 | *Nursing Interventions for the Patient in Traction* |

- Maintain the patient's body in proper alignment. The force or pull on the extremities should be in alignment with the long axis of the bone.
- Ensure that weights hang freely from the bed and are never removed without a physician's order.
- Question patients as to their understanding of the purpose of the traction, and assess their ability to use a trapeze bar for self-movement. Elevate the foot of the bed to help prevent the patient from sliding down toward the foot of the bed (counter-traction).
- Observe the condition of the traction cords, making sure they are not weakened or frayed. All knots used on the rope or cord are to be square knots.
- Center the ropes on the traction pulley.
- Assess, document, and report neurovascular impairment.
- Ensure that weight used is the correct weight as ordered by the physician.
- Carefully observe the skin for signs of skin impairment. Use sheepskin heel protectors and bed pads to reduce impairment.
- If skeletal traction is used, assess the pin site for signs of infection. Cleanse the pin site q8h with hydrogen peroxide or normal saline, as ordered.
- Assess the distal pulses bilaterally for circulatory integrity of the extremities.
- Inspect for loss of sensation in the dorsal area of the foot with weakness and inversion of the foot (inside surface turned outward).

nous thrombosis, and reduce kidney stone formation. Orthopedic traction can be attached to the bed, as well as a television set for diversional activity.

Splints, crutches, and **braces** are used to immobilize and assist with ambulation. There are numerous types of splints and braces, and it is important that the nurse understand the procedure for proper application for each one.

Safety is the first concern when ambulatory devices such as crutches are used. Crutch safety is outlined in the Safety Considerations box. The nurse should encourage the patient to do push-ups by pressing the

Safety Considerations

Crutch Safety

Crutch safety involves:
- Proper measurement (weight must be on hands, not axillae, to avoid brachial plexus paralysis), and proper measurement involves a 2-inch width between the axillary fold and the armpiece on the crutches.
- Rubber tips on the ends of the crutches to prevent slippage.
- Adequate muscle strength in the upper extremities to support the patient's weight.

hands against the mattress and lifting the upper body to gain muscle strength.

Types of **crutch walking** depend on the number of points making contact with the floor (Figure 4-34). For example, a three-point gait involves two crutch points plus one leg making contact with the floor (patient must have strong arms to support body weight). In addition to three-point gait, there are the four-point gait (slower, but stable) and two-point gait (faster; requires balance). Another type of crutch walking is swing-to or swing-through gait. This involves the patient swinging the body up to or beyond the two points of the crutch

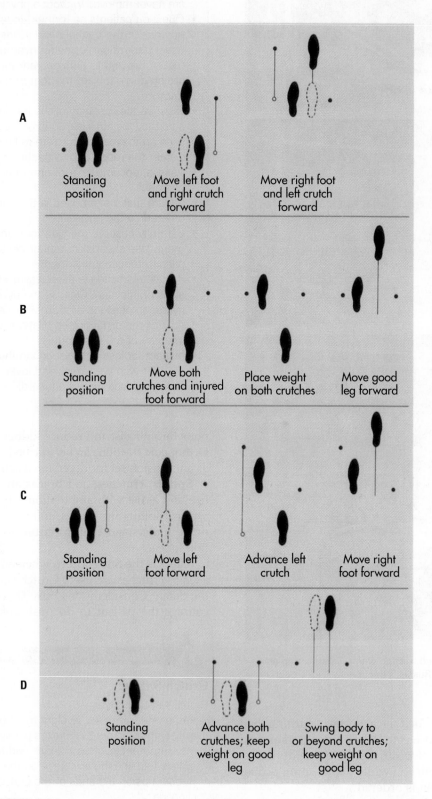

FIGURE **4-34** Crutch walking. **A,** Two-point gait. **B,** Three-point gait. **C,** Four-point gait. **D,** Swing-through.

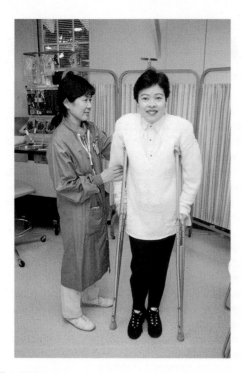

FIGURE **4-35** Assisting the patient with crutch walking. Note how the therapist guards the patient and how the patient's elbows are at no more than 30 degrees of flexion.

tips. Most crutch walking is taught by a physical therapist (Figure 4-35). However, it is important for the nurse to monitor the patient's progress (Figure 4-36).

Cane walking is more popular with older patients and is used for balance and support. The patient is instructed to hold the cane in the opposite hand of the affected extremity and advance the cane at the same time the affected leg is advanced forward. An effective rubber tip on the point will help prevent any slippage (Figure 4-37). Walkers are also used by the older adult and will assist the patient in maintaining balance. Safety concerns are the same as those for the cane (Figure 4-38).

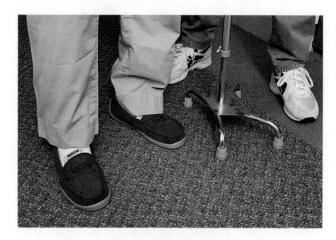

FIGURE **4-37** Quad cane.

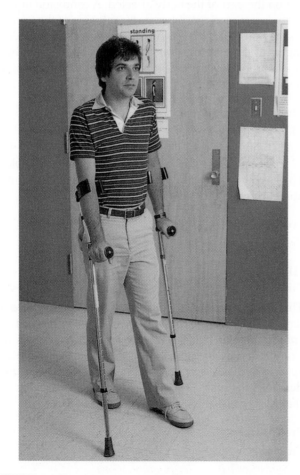

FIGURE **4-36** Double adjustable Lofstrand or forearm crutches.

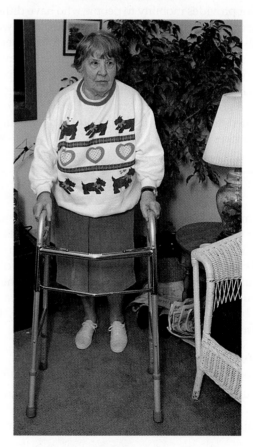

FIGURE **4-38** Patient using a walker.

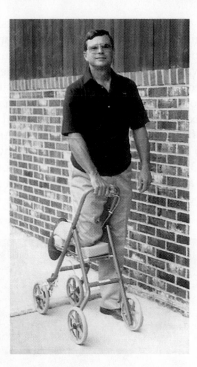

FIGURE **4-39** The Roll-A-Bout walker.

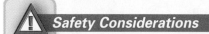

Safety Considerations

Preventing Musculoskeletal Trauma

- The public should be taught to take appropriate safety precautions to prevent injuries while at home, at work, when driving, or when participating in sports.
- Nurses should be vocal advocates for personal actions known to reduce injuries such as regular use of seat belts, driving within posted speed limits, stretching before exercise, use of protective athletic equipment (helmets and knee, wrist, and elbow pads), and not combining drinking and driving.
- Older adults should be encouraged to participate in moderate exercise to aid in the maintenance of muscle strength and balance.
- To reduce falls, older adults' living environment should be examined to rule out the use of scatter rugs, to ensure adequate footwear and lighting, and to clear paths to bathrooms for nighttime use.
- The nurse should also stress the importance of adequate calcium and vitamin D intake.

The Roll-A-Bout walker is a new gait enhancer designed for patients who have an injury below the knee such as a fractured tibia, fibula, ankle, or foot. The Roll-A-Bout provides mobility to people who have difficulty using crutches. It allows the patient to distribute weight evenly by resting half of the weight on the walker. The knee of the injured leg is placed on the knee pad and the ankle is supported on the rear support while the patient propels the Roll-A-Bout with the unaffected leg. It is lightweight, compact, and folds for easy storage. It is designed for strength and stability and is equipped with brakes for easy control and safety (Figure 4-39).

TRAUMATIC INJURIES

Traumatic injuries to the musculoskeletal system can occur in all age groups. However, older adults may have disorders that predispose them to musculoskeletal injuries. The more serious injuries involving fractures are treated in a hospital, whereas the less serious—such as contusions, sprains, or strains—may be treated in an outpatient facility (Safety Considerations box).

CONTUSIONS
Etiology/Pathophysiology/Clinical Manifestations

Contusions are the most common soft tissue injury. An injury from a blow or blunt force will cause local bleeding under the skin and possibly a hematoma (sac filled with blood). Contusions can be serious, depending on the part of the body affected. A contusion of the brain is very serious, whereas a contusion of the arm is less serious. Large areas affected by soft tissue bleeding with slow absorption of the blood have a higher potential of developing into cellulitis (an infection of the subcutaneous tissue).

Medical Management

Most contusions are treated by applying ice bags or cold compresses for 15 to 20 minutes intermittently for 12 to 36 hours for the vasoconstricting effects of cold. The involved extremity is elevated to reduce edema and suppress pain.

Prognosis

Prognosis is excellent.

SPRAINS
Etiology/Pathophysiology/Clinical Manifestations

This injury can result from a wrenching or hyperextension of a joint, tearing the capsule and ligaments. A sprain can involve bleeding into a joint (hemarthrosis). Common sites include the knee, ankle, and cervical spine (whiplash). Sprains are often the result of a sudden, twisting injury. Medical management is similar to that for contusions.

Prognosis

Prognosis is excellent.

WHIPLASH
Etiology/Pathophysiology/Clinical Manifestations

Injury at the cervical spine is known as whiplash and is classified under cervical disk syndrome.

Whiplash is caused by an injury that involves hyperextension, which results in compression of the anatomical structures. This type of injury usually occurs as a result of sudden acceleration or deceleration, such as rear-end car collisions that cause violent back-and-forth movements of the head and neck. Symptoms of a whiplash may not be obvious for a few days or even a week after the injury. Cervical fractures can accompany a whiplash injury.

Assessment

Collection of **subjective data** includes the patient's complaint of pain (the most common symptom), which usually begins in the cervical area but may radiate down the arm to the fingers and increase with cervical motion. The pain may increase sharply with coughing, sneezing, or any radical movement. Other signs and symptoms may be paresthesia (numbness or tingling), headache, blurred vision, decreased skeletal function, and weakened hand grip.

Collection of **objective data** includes edema in the cervical spine region with tightening of the muscles. Vital signs are usually within normal ranges. However, if the assessment findings indicate hypertension with widened pulse pressure and bradycardia, increased intracranial pressure (IICP) should be suspected; the findings should be reported and documented immediately. A neurological assessment is done every 15 to 30 minutes to rule out IICP.

Diagnostic Tests

Physical examination and radiographic studies are used to confirm the physician's diagnosis.

Medical Management

Recurrence of symptoms is common. A medical approach is most often used for treatment of whiplash. Analgesics and muscle relaxants are prescribed, along with intermittent cervical traction. Surgery may be necessary if cervical fracture with displacement occurs. (See the discussion of herniated nucleus pulposus.)

Nursing Interventions

Nursing intervention involves care of the patient with restricted activity to immobilize the cervical vertebrae to decrease irritation and provide rest for the traumatized area. This is accomplished with cervical traction.

Other treatments include special exercises, heat therapy, and administration of mild analgesics as ordered by the physician to control the pain. A soft foam rubber neck brace collar may be used for whiplash injuries to limit head movement. Careful inspection of the skin around the neck and chin is made for signs of excoriation.

Prognosis

Prognosis depends on the extent of neurological involvement. Prognosis is excellent with minor trauma, but because the spinal canal is full of neural tissue in the cervical area, more extensive injury can produce profound disability.

ANKLE SPRAINS
Etiology/Pathophysiology

An ankle sprain is often referred to as a twisted ankle and is caused by a wrenching or twisting of the foot and ankle (Safety box).

Clinical Manifestations

The ankle area will become edematous quickly, with spasms of the muscles and pain on passive movement of the joint.

Assessment

Collection of **subjective data** includes assessment of pain and tenderness in the affected ankle that intensifies with movement of the foot or ankle.

Collection of **objective data** includes assessment of the traumatized ankle for signs of edema, limited movement and function of the joint, and ecchymosis of the soft tissue around the ankle.

Diagnostic Tests

A radiographic examination of the injured area is the only accurate way to ensure that there is no bone injury.

Medical Management

Surgery may be indicated for severe sprains. The physician will suture torn ligament fibers together. If the ligaments have been torn from the bone, the surgeon will reattach them by drilling small holes in the medial malleolus (rounded bony protrusion on the medial area of the ankle).

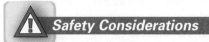

Safety Considerations

Strains and Sprains

A strain and a sprain are not the same. Strains are produced by minute muscle tears and overstretching of tendons, whereas sprains are caused by a twisting of the joint.

Nursing Interventions

The injured area must be elevated and kept at rest. Application of ice for 15 to 20 minutes intermittently for 12 to 36 hours—followed after 24 hours with the application of mild heat for 15 to 30 minutes, four times daily—will promote absorption of blood and fluid from the area. Compressive dressings and splinting are used to help support the injured area. A neurovascular assessment is necessary to detect impaired tissue perfusion.

Prognosis

Prognosis is generally excellent.

STRAINS
Etiology/Pathophysiology/Clinical Manifestations

This injury is characterized by microscopic muscle tears as a result of overstretching muscles and tendons. An acute strain results when the muscles and tendons are overstretched in a forceful movement, such as unaccustomed vigorous exercise.

Assessment

Collection of **subjective data** involves noting the patient's complaint of sudden and severe pain away from the joint, which increases with activity. Chronic muscle strain can occur from repeated muscle overuse, and the pain may not appear for several hours after the patient has used the muscles. The patient typically complains of soreness, stiffness, and tenderness in the area.

Collection of **objective data** includes observation of stiffness, ecchymosis, and slight edema over the injury site. The most common sites are calf muscles, hamstrings, quadriceps, and the lumbosacral area. Edema can occur rapidly in the muscle and tendon area.

Diagnostic Tests

A radiographic study is necessary to rule out bone trauma.

Medical Management

It is important to encourage exercises of the legs to prevent development of thrombosis.

Surgical repair will be necessary if the muscle is completely ruptured. Analgesics and muscle relaxants are ordered by the physician. An exercise program is almost always prescribed if the strain is in the lumbosacral region. The exercises are aimed at strengthening the lower abdominal muscles.

Nursing Interventions

Nursing intervention for a strain is similar to that for a sprain. Ice application helps relieve pain, but some physicians prefer heat application rather than ice.

Back strains are among the most common strains, and during exacerbation of symptoms the patient is advised to avoid strenuous activities, use a firm chair with rigid back support, avoid wearing high heels, use a firm mattress for sleep, never sleep on the abdomen, and place a pillow under the knees to take pressure off the back.

Prognosis

Prognosis is usually favorable.

DISLOCATIONS
Etiology/Pathophysiology

Dislocations usually involve tearing of the joint capsule; subluxations (partial or incomplete dislocations) involve stretching of the joint capsule. Both are temporary displacements of bones from their normal position within joints. A dislocation may be (1) congenital (e.g., congenital hip displacement), (2) caused by a disease process, or (3) caused by trauma. Stretching and tearing of ligaments and tendons, as well as fractures, can accompany a dislocation or subluxation. The displaced bone may rupture blood vessels. When subluxation occurs, the joint's articulating (movable) surfaces are partially separated.

Clinical Manifestations

Dislocation may or may not be visible. Sometimes a dislocation will change the length of an affected extremity. Pain and loss of function may be similar to that occurring with a fracture. However, dislocation partially immobilizes a joint, whereas a fracture site typically has abnormal free movement. Common dislocation sites include the shoulder, hip, and knee.

Assessment

Collection of **subjective data** includes the patient's description of the injury and pain. When the dislocation is of the shoulder, the nurse should assess for complaints of sensation loss and paresthesia.

Collection of **objective data** includes the assessment of any erythema, discoloration, edema, pain, tenderness, limitation of movement, and deformity or shortening of the extremity. The nurse should compare both sides for validation. Neurovascular assessment is important to determine whether vascular or nerve injury is present in the affected area. For shoulder dislocation, the nurse should assess for an absent radial pulse, hypothermia of the hand, and wrist drop.

Diagnostic Tests

The diagnosis is based on the present complaints of discomfort, physical examination, and diagnostic radiographic examination of the injured site.

Medical Management

The physician may perform a closed reduction, which corrects the deformity through manipulation of the extremity. Surgical intervention to restore joint articulation is sometimes required.

Nursing Interventions and Patient Teaching

Nursing intervention includes measures for (1) reduction of edema and discomfort, (2) immobilization of the injured part to promote healing, and (3) patient education. Ice application is recommended for the first 24 hours after trauma. After 24 hours, heat may be used if there are no indications of bleeding. Elevation of the injured extremity on pillows and the application of elastic bandages help relieve edema. Immobilization of joints may involve application of a splint, sling, or elastic bandage. The air cast or air splint brace is an immobilization device. It is inflatable, lightweight, and conforms to the extremity's size and shape. When immobilization devices are used, a neurovascular assessment is done frequently (see Box 4-3 and Nursing Diagnoses box below). Analgesics should be administered as prescribed by the physician as needed. Asking the patient to rate the pain on a scale from 0 to 10 is helpful in determining pain severity. For control of extreme pain, the physician may order an opioid, such as morphine. For moderate to mild pain, ibuprofen (Motrin) or acetaminophen (Tylenol) may be prescribed. Positioning and repositioning the injured part can help reduce discomfort.

Nursing diagnoses and interventions for the patient for neurovascular integrity include but are not limited to the following:

NURSING DIAGNOSES	NURSING INTERVENTIONS
Ineffective peripheral tissue perfusion, related to injury/treatment	Position extremities in alignment; elevate affected extremity. Carefully monitor distal pulses, capillary refill, and temperature of involved area.
Risk for injury, related to neurovascular impairment	Compare affected extremity with unaffected extremity, using same hand for palpation. Test capillary refill (blanching test). Check each digit for sensation and motion. Document location and characteristics of pain. Palpate pedal, tibial, or radial pulses and compare with unaffected extremity. Assess for edema with pallor, cyanosis, and coldness. Elicit description of sensations from patient. Document all findings.

Promoting an accident-free environment is essential. The nurse can explore areas of preventive medicine with patients. They are as follows:

- Environmental safety can include grab bars mounted in the bathroom near the toilet or tub and rubber mats or slip guards in the tub and shower.
- Removing throw rugs and obstacles from the floor can prevent falls.
- If the patient is using a gait enhancer, such as a cane, crutches, or a walker, it is important that it be used correctly.
- Safety precautions, such as using rubber tips on the points that make contact with the floor to prevent slippage, should be taken.
- Patients in the hospital are at risk of falling out of bed if their disease, condition, or medication results in disorientation. These patients need a careful assessment of their level of orientation, side rails applied to their beds, and safety reminder devices to prevent self-injury.
- Using a safe ladder when climbing can help prevent a fall.
- Wearing protective clothing while engaging in dangerous work or contact sports is recommended.
- Appropriate health teaching should be targeted for people at risk for musculoskeletal diseases, such as osteoporosis, which can predispose to pathologic or nontraumatic fractures.

Prognosis

Prognosis is generally excellent.

AIRBAG INJURIES

Airbag deployment injuries include chemical burns, ocular trauma, cervical injury, soft tissue injury, and upper extremity and chest trauma. Orthopedic injuries tend to involve the upper extremities, especially the wrist, hand, and elbow. Injuries from airbag deployment can be life threatening in the very young. People at increased risk include the older adult and small children. Airbag-induced injuries are associated with a rapid, forceful inflation, lasting less than 1 second from inflation to deflation. Research is continuing to develop safer airbag deployment.

CARPAL TUNNEL SYNDROME
Etiology/Pathophysiology

Carpal tunnel syndrome is a painful disorder of the wrist and hand, induced by compression on the median nerve between the inelastic carpal ligament and other structures in the carpal tunnel.

Carpal tunnel syndrome results from pressure on the median nerve of the wrist (Figure 4-40). The symptoms of paresthesia (any subjective sensation as of

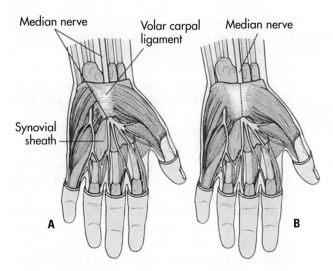

FIGURE **4-40 A,** Wrist structures involved in carpal tunnel syndrome. **B,** Decompression of median nerve.

pricks of pins and needles) and **hypoesthesia** (a decrease in sensation in response to stimulation of the sensory nerves), of the thumb, index, and middle fingers may develop spontaneously or occur as a result of disease or injury. There is a higher incidence of this condition in obese, middle-aged women and individuals employed in occupations involving repetitive motions of the fingers and hands (e.g., computer usage, basket weaving, meat carving, and typing). Carpal tunnel syndrome has become one of the three most common industrial or work-related conditions and is related to increased computer usage in all industries and departments in industries and government. Edema of the tendon sheaths caused by rheumatoid arthritis can predispose to carpal tunnel syndrome. Curiously, pregnant women may develop the syndrome during their last trimester. The reasons for this have not yet been determined, although fluid retention and edema may be contributing factors.

Clinical Manifestations

Anatomically the median nerve passes through a tunnel surrounded by the carpal bones and ligaments. When inflammation and edema of the synovial lining of the tendon sheaths occur, the tunnel space is narrowed, resulting in compression of the median nerve. The affected hand has altered ability to grasp or hold small objects. Atrophy of the thenar eminence (the padded area of the palm below the base of the thumb) is noted as the disease progresses.

Assessment

Collection of **subjective data** includes the patient's description of discomfort, such as complaints of burning pain or tingling in the hands relieved with vigorous shaking or exercising of the hands (pain may be inter-

mittent or constant and is often more intense at night), numbness (hypesthesia) of the thumb, index, and ring fingers, especially after prolonged flexion of the wrist; and inability to grasp or hold small objects.

Collection of **objective data** includes assessment of the hand, wrist, or fingers for edema; muscle atrophy; or a depressed appearance of the soft tissue at the base of the thumb on the palmar surface.

Diagnostic Tests

The following diagnostic tests are used to diagnose carpal tunnel syndrome:
- **Physical examination:** Deficits in sensory mapping along median nerve innervation pathways; positive Tinel's sign; increased tingling with gentle tap over tendon sheath on ventral surface of central wrist; edema of fingers noted; thenar surfaces of palm thinner than normal (wasting); holding wrists against each other in forced palmar flexion for 1 minute can elicit sensory changes of numbness and tingling, which is a positive Phalen's maneuver test, one indication of carpal tunnel syndrome.
- **Electromyogram:** Weakened muscle response to stimulation.
- **MRI:** Shows compression and flattening of the median nerve, increased signal intensity within the median nerve, abrupt changes in diameter of the median nerve.
- **Handheld electroneurometer:** Used if emergency medical personnel not available; predicts motor latency of median nerve diagnostic of carpal tunnel syndrome.

Medical Management

If the symptoms are mild and surgery is not a desirable option, an immobilizer such as a splint can be used. Hydrocortisone acetate suspension injections can be given into the carpal tunnel for relief of mild symptoms. Surgery is indicated for severe symptoms with the occurrence of muscle atrophy. The standard surgical treatment is decompression of the median nerve by section of the transverse carpal ligament.

Nursing Interventions and Patient Teaching

If surgery is not required, the nurse will be involved with the application of an immobilizer to promote comfort. Use of a wrist cock-up splint to relieve pressure and to lessen wrist flexion, elevation to relieve edema, range-of-motion (ROM) exercises to lessen sense of clumsiness, and restriction of twisting and turning activities of the wrist are general nursing interventions that are helpful. If surgery is required, the postoperative interventions will include the following: (1) elevating the hand and arm for 24 hours;

(2) implementing and evaluating active thumb and finger motion within limits imposed by the dressing; (3) administering prescribed analgesics as needed; (4) monitoring vital signs (temperature elevation could indicate infection); and (5) checking fingers for circulation, sensation, and movement every 1 to 2 hours for 24 hours.

Patients are encouraged to use the affected hand in normal activities as soon as 2 to 3 days after surgery.

Prognosis

Mild symptoms of carpal tunnel syndrome are relieved by nonsurgical treatment; severe symptoms require surgical intervention with excellent prognosis. If the patient is pregnant, relief of symptoms usually occurs after delivery.

HERNIATION OF INTERVERTEBRAL DISK (HERNIATED NUCLEUS PULPOSUS)
Etiology/Pathophysiology

Herniated nucleus pulposus is a rupture of the fibrocartilage surrounding an intervertebral disk, releasing the nucleus pulposus that cushions the vertebrae above and below. This displacement puts pressure on nerve roots. Lumbar and cervical herniations are most common (Figure 4-41). Herniated nucleus pulposus can occur suddenly (from lifting, twisting, or trauma) or gradually (from degenerative changes [as seen with degenerative joint disease, osteoporosis, aging, and chronic diseases affected bones]). Herniations of the lumbar spine usually affect people 20 to 45 years old; cervical herniations are seen most in people 45 years old and older. Men are more prone to this disorder than women.

Clinical Manifestations

Low back pain that occurs with the slightest movement is the most common symptom of lumbar herniations. The pain radiates over the buttock and down the leg, following the sciatic nerve pathway **(radicular pain)**, causing numbness and tingling in the affected leg. Neck pain, headache, and neck rigidity are common symptoms of cervical herniations. Complaints of pain in the back radiating down the leg (sciatica) are common. Complaints about activity intolerance and alteration in bowel and bladder elimination (constipation and urinary retention) are significant.

Assessment

Collection of **subjective data** involves pain assessment and patient-stated relief measures. Pain is often exacerbated with activity. Complaints of pain in the back radiating down the leg (sciatica) are common. Complaints about activity intolerance and alteration in bowel and bladder elimination (constipation and urinary retention) are significant.

Collection of **objective data** includes observing for signs of limited spinal flexibility (limited forward bending) and gait alteration (patient may favor supporting weight on one extremity). An ineffective breathing pattern may be present and result from pain and decreased mobility. Assessment includes determination of bowel and bladder elimination and maintenance of traction equipment.

Diagnostic Tests

Complete history and physical examination is obtained. The physician will order radiographic studies, computed tomography, myelography, and electromyelography (to determine nerve involvement).

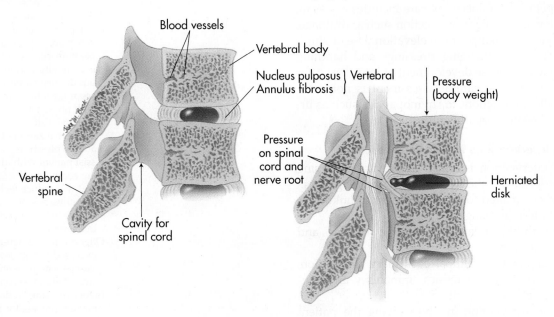

FIGURE **4-41** Sagittal section of vertebrae showing both normal and herniated disks.

Medical Management

The physician will order bed rest, pain control, physical therapy (aimed at muscle strengthening and comfort), and skin traction (may be pelvic or cervical). If the patient demonstrates neurological deterioration or continued pain, a surgical procedure may be required, such as the following:

- **Laminectomy:** Surgical removal of the bony arches or one or more vertebrae performed to relieve compression of the spinal cord caused by bone displacement from an injury or degeneration of a disk or to remove a displaced vertebral disk.
- **Spinal fusion** (arthrodesis; the surgical immobilization of a joint; artificial ankylosis): Removal of the lamina and several herniated nuclei pulposi. A portion of bone taken from the patient's iliac crest or from a bone bank is used as a bone graft in the vertebral spaces.
- **Diskectomy:** Often done with a microscope. Only the extruded disk material is removed. Percutaneous lateral diskectomy is performed under local anesthesia with the surgeon cutting a window around the anulus fibrosus.
- **Endoscopic spinal microsurgery:** Can be performed under local anesthesia. Special scopes enable the surgeon to successfully remove herniated discs with minimal damage to surrounding tissues.
- **Chemonucleolysis:** Can be done on patients who have no nerve involvement. The procedure involves administering a local anesthetic agent and then guiding a needle into the nucleus pulposus to inject chymopapain (a drug that dissolves the nucleus pulposus).

Postoperative laminectomy care includes assessing the incision site for signs of infection such as drainage, edema, odor, and temperature elevation. Use of surgical asepsis when changing dressings and handling drainage will decrease development of infection. After a chemonucleolysis, careful assessment is noted for signs of allergic reactions to chymopapain, such as urticaria and respiratory difficulties.

Nursing Interventions and Patient Teaching

Nursing intervention is aimed at providing nursing care appropriate for the following nursing diagnoses:

- Anxiety, related to discomfort, fear of unknown, and lifestyle changes
- Pain (back), related to muscle spasms and painful diagnostic tests
- Constipation and impaired urinary elimination, related to pain, analgesics, immobility, and neurological involvement

Nursing intervention involves giving the patient and the family information about procedures and hospital protocol to help reduce their anxiety. It is important to administer the medications prescribed on schedule and document the effectiveness of the medication. Distraction, heat or ice application (if ordered), and moving (by log-rolling) and positioning the patient every 2 hours (if not contraindicated because of maintaining traction) can help promote patient comfort. Dietary monitoring is important to ensure that the patient maintains a high-protein, iron- and vitamin-enriched diet.

Observe dressing for bleeding or cerebrospinal fluid leakage. Apply antiembolic stockings if ordered. Careful documentation of I&O provides information about bowel and bladder function. Ensure that the patient has voided in the first 8 hours, and use nursing measures to promote voiding before resorting to catheterization. The nurse should encourage the patient to sit in a straight, firm chair for no longer than 30 minutes at one time. It is important to monitor the patient for evidence of respiratory distress and paralytic ileus as complications that may occur in laminectomy patients.

Nursing diagnoses and interventions for the patient with herniated disk include but are not limited to the following:

NURSING DIAGNOSES	NURSING INTERVENTIONS
Deficient knowledge, related to home care management	Stress importance of rehabilitation plan of activity, rest, and exercise. Provide diet instructions as to type and amount, and weight maintenance (no gain) if applicable. Discuss medications: name, purpose, schedule, dosage, and side effects. Discuss signs and symptoms to report to physician: severe pain; changes in temperature, color, or sensation in extremity; and malodorous drainage from wound. Encourage follow-up visits with physician.
Powerlessness, related to decreased mobility/pain	Use active listening and permit verbalization of anger and helplessness. Assist patient with identifying coping mechanisms that will reduce feeling of powerlessness; use those that have been successful in the past. Offer positive recognition for increased activity level. Assist patient in identifying areas that can be controlled. Involve patients in decision-making process for their own care.

Activity out of bed may begin as early as 1 day after a simple laminectomy or 2 to 4 days after a laminectomy and fusion. The nurse should transfer the patient out of bed with as little time spent in the sitting position as possible. The patient may be permitted to walk as much as tolerated, with assistance if necessary. Braces or corsets, if prescribed, are applied before the patient gets out of bed. The nurse should encourage the patient to participate in activities of daily living (ADLs) within prescribed limits of mobility.

The patient should be instructed not to lift or carry anything heavier than 5 pounds (2.25 kg) for at least 8 weeks, not to drive a car until permitted by the surgeon, and to avoid twisting motions of the trunk. Reinforce importance of follow-up visit to physician.

Prognosis

With conservative treatment, some patients will receive relief of symptoms; if neurological pathology develops, surgical intervention is needed. The prognosis is usually quite favorable.

TUMORS OF THE BONE
Etiology/Pathophysiology

Tumors of the bone may be primary or secondary and may be benign or malignant. As with other types of tumors, the cause of bone tumors is not always known. Carcinoma of the prostate, lung, breast, thyroid, and kidney may metastasize to the bones. **Osteogenic sarcoma** is a primary malignant bone tumor that is seen most often in young people. Osteogenic sarcoma can metastasize to the lungs and to the rest of the body via the bloodstream. Osteochondroma is a type of benign tumor.

Osteogenic sarcoma is a fast-growing and aggressive tumor that affects the long bones of the body, particularly in the regions of the distal femur, proximal tibia, and proximal humerus. This affects males between the ages of 10 and 25 more often than females.

Osteochondroma is the most common benign osteogenic tumor. This tumor is seen more often in males between 10 and 30 years of age. Osteochondromas can occur as a single tumor or as multiple tumors. They usually affect the humerus, tibia, and femur.

Clinical Manifestations

When healthy bone cells are replaced by cancer cells, the strength of the bone is altered and spontaneous fractures can occur. Anemia occurs when cancer invades the long bones and interrupts the manufacturing of red blood cells in the bone marrow. Cancerous bone tumors metastasize and invade other bones and lung tissue.

Benign bone tumors can grow large enough to put pressure on blood vessels and nerves. Benign tumors do not spread. However, they may undergo cancerous changes and become malignant.

Assessment

Collection of **subjective data** includes an awareness that malignant and benign bone tumors will cause pain in the affected bone site. Complaints of pain, especially with weight bearing, are common. The pain may result from a spontaneous fracture. The patient may also complain of tenderness at the affected site.

Collection of **objective data** includes assessment of the painful part, which may reveal edema and discoloration of the skin.

Diagnostic Tests

Diagnosis is confirmed with radiographic studies, bone scan, bone biopsy, and laboratory studies, such as complete blood cell count and platelet count (relative to bone marrow involvement), serum protein levels (elevated in multiple myeloma), and serum alkaline phosphatase level (elevation may indicate osteogenic sarcoma).

Medical Management

The physician will evaluate the tumor type, size, and location and plan the treatment accordingly.

Larger, symptomatic, benign tumors and malignant tumors require surgical intervention. The surgical procedure depends on the tumor size, location, and extent of tissue involvement. The surgery may involve (1) wide excision or resection, (2) bone curettage, or (3) leg or arm amputation.

Treatment is aimed at destroying or removing the malignant lesion. Amputation of the affected extremity may be necessary. Radiation and chemotherapy may be used before surgery to decrease tumor size or tissue involvement. Limb-salvage surgical procedures in combination with radiation and chemotherapy are being used more frequently for treatment of malignant bone tumors.

Chemotherapy is aimed at destroying cancer cells at both primary and metastatic sites. Patients usually receive chemotherapy in cycles of 3- or 4-week intervals. Radiation therapy may be given internally and externally. It is important for the nurse to know the safety precautions and side effects of both chemotherapy and radiation therapy. See Chapter 17 for a discussion of care of the patient with cancer.

Nursing Interventions

Preoperatively the patient and family need complete and concise information about procedures and postoperative expectations.

Postoperative nursing interventions will include the following:
- Performing a neurovascular assessment (see Box 4-5)
- Monitoring vital signs

- Administering analgesics and evaluating the effectiveness
- Providing cast care or dressing changes with careful documentation of drainage, odors, and signs of circulation impairment
- Cooperating with physical and occupational therapists to promote mobility and ADLs
- Educating the patient and family about home health care and early detection of tumor recurrence

Nursing diagnosis and interventions for the patient with a tumor of the bone include but are not limited to the following:

NURSING DIAGNOSES	NURSING INTERVENTIONS
Anxiety, related to fear of cancer, body image change, lifestyle change, and possible death	Establish therapeutic relationship: acknowledge fear, encourage patient to acknowledge and express feelings. Give accurate information about condition and therapies. Refer to resources when necessary (e.g., social worker and religious counselor).

Prognosis

The prognosis for bone tumors has been improved in recent years by the combination of local surgery, chemotherapy, and radiation. Disease-free survival rates for patients whose osteogenic sarcoma is treated with surgery, chemotherapy, and radiation appear to be greater than 50% at 5 years.

AMPUTATION

The amputation of a portion of or an entire extremity may be necessary because of malignant tumors, injuries, impaired circulation (caused by diabetes mellitus or arteriosclerosis), congenital deformities, and infections. Most amputations are elective surgery unless the amputation is necessary because of trauma. Advances in microsurgery techniques have made it possible for surgeons to reattach severed extremities. Therefore traumatic amputations can sometimes be reversed by replantation of the part if the severed limb is kept sterile and moist in a plastic bag filled with ice water. (The part should be protected from direct contact with ice, and dry ice should not be used.)

Amputation of long bones can result in postoperative anemia. A traumatic or surgical amputation of an extremity can cause serious blood loss. Malignant bone tumors can metastasize via the bloodstream to other body systems.

Preoperative Assessment

Collection of **subjective data** includes questioning to determine the patient's understanding of the nature of the injury or disease process. Assessment of complaints of pain and symptoms of neurovascular impairment is made and documented. Assessment of the patient's level of orientation is important because many amputations occur in the older population as a result of medical conditions that impair circulation.

Collection of **objective data** includes assessment of vital signs (temperature elevation, tachycardia, and tachypnea indicate infection). Arterial blood flow is assessed by palpation of bilateral pedal pulses and Doppler pressure measurements. Assessment is done of wound drainage for color, amount, and presence of odor. Evaluation of upper body muscle strength and nutritional status is important.

Diagnostic Tests

A complete blood count is done to determine blood dyscrasias, such as anemia and bleeding tendencies, which would influence the surgical outcome and increase postoperative complications (such as hemorrhage, delayed wound healing, and disorientation). Laboratory studies—such as blood urea nitrogen (BUN), potassium levels, and routine urinalysis—are ordered. An electrocardiogram (ECG) is ordered to detect cardiac dysrhythmias, which are often present in the older patient.

Medical Management

When the amputation results from traumatic injury to an extremity, the physician's interventions will include measures to restore circulating blood volume, control pain, prevent infection in the wound, perform a plastic surgical repair at the amputation site to facilitate the use of a prosthesis, and maintain adequate urinary output.

If the amputation is an elective surgical procedure, the physician makes an assessment of the patient's physiologic, psychological, and emotional status. If any infection is present in the body (gangrene may occur in the presence of impaired circulation), treatment should include administration of antibiotics, and every attempt must be made to control the infection before any surgery is performed. The physician will discuss the possibility of the patient using a prosthesis. Much of the preoperative preparation will focus on the patient attaining a physical and emotional status conducive to wearing a prosthesis or achieving mobility through the use of a wheelchair or a gait enhancer such as crutches or a walker.

Postoperative Assessment, Nursing Interventions, and Patient Teaching

Collection of **subjective data** involves careful assessment of pain. **Phantom pain** (pain felt in the missing extremity as if it were still present) may occur and be frightening to the patient. Phantom pain occurs because the nerve tracks that register pain in the amputated area continue to send a message to the brain—this is normal.

Collection of **objective data** includes observing for signs of hemorrhage, such as hypotension, tachycardia, tachypnea, pallor, decreased urinary output, restlessness, and progressive loss of consciousness. Monitoring suction drainage and documenting it is important, as are assessing and protecting the remaining extremity. The nurse should observe for neurovascular impairment (done hourly in the immediate postoperative period) from tightly applied elastic wraps, dressings, or casts (see Box 4-5).

Nursing intervention is aimed at prevention of deformities (contractures, especially in the joint above the amputation, or abduction deformities are common). Flexion hip contractures can be prevented postoperatively by raising the foot of the bed slightly to elevate the residual extremity (care should be taken not to flex the patient's hips by elevating the stump on a pillow), encouraging movement from side to side, and placing the patient in a prone position at least twice a day. This will stretch the flexor muscles. The nurse will be involved with teaching the patient how to strengthen remaining muscles to facilitate mobility and prevent muscle atrophy (push-ups from a prone position and sit-ups from a seated position). The application of elastic wraps to shrink and reshape the residual extremity into a cone is necessary to facilitate the proper fit and subsequent use of a prosthesis (Figure 4-42). A prosthesis may be fitted as early as 2 or 3 weeks postoperatively. Because many amputations are performed in people between 60 and 70 years of age, the patient must be observed carefully for pulmonary complications (such as pulmonary embolus) and cardiovascular collapse. Suction equipment and oxygen should be at the bedside. Patient education concerning the phenomenon of phantom-limb sensation can help relieve patient fears if patients know it is a normal physiologic response. The response may be one of pain or other sensations, such as burning, tingling, throbbing, or pruritus in the amputated extremity. These sensations can last for months or decades on a consistent or intermittent basis. It is recommended that patients gently rub the residual extremity for relief. Analgesics may be necessary.

The patient should be encouraged to ventilate feelings over the loss of the extremity. The loss of an extremity results in a grieving process. The patient should be taught the importance of allowing the grieving process to occur.

For persistent, severe phantom pain, the following measures may be employed:

- Stump revision with reamputation at a higher level
- Local infiltration of the stump with procaine
- Mechanical percussion by striking the sensitive digital stump against a solid object—believed to shrink neuromas (small tumors that form in the scar tissue of the stump)
- Sympathetic nerve block

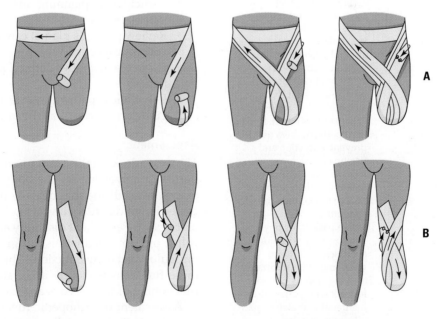

FIGURE **4-42** Correct method of bandaging amputation stump. **A,** It is important to anchor bandage around patient's waist. **B,** Method of bandaging midcalf stump, where bandage need not be anchored around waist.

Nursing diagnoses and interventions for the patient undergoing an amputation include but are not limited to the following:

NURSING DIAGNOSES	NURSING INTERVENTIONS
Disturbed body image, related to loss of limb	Assess effects of amputation on body image.
	Allow and encourage patient to express feelings of mutilation grief anger, and loss to aid adaptation processes.
	Encourage patient to help with dressing changes and wrapping of stump as able. Teach family member wrapping techniques if necessary to increase competence and independence.
	Encourage family members to walk with patient to maintain strength and social contacts.
	Encourage grooming and wearing of personal clothing to maintain individuality and personality.
	Encourage activities for self-care and ambulation to maintain positive outlook and maximum strength.
	Encourage or arrange for social services consultation for economic and employment aid.
	Arrange for follow-up care referral to aid rehabilitation.
Impaired physical mobility, related to loss of limb	Assess ability to use remaining limbs.
	Turn and position on side, back, and abdomen (after 24 hours) to maintain muscle and joint ROM.
	Teach adduction and extension exercises and help patient perform them q4h to prevent abduction and flexion contractures.
	Assist with sitting in chair and ambulation with aid as able to maintain muscle strength.
	Prepare patient for physical therapy, transportation for exercises, and stump wrapping, if appropriate.
	Encourage family members to walk with patient during initial ambulation periods, accompanied by health professionals, to increase independence.

NURSING DIAGNOSES	NURSING INTERVENTIONS
	Teach purposes of prone and extension positions to prevent contractures.
	Assist prosthetist with prosthesis measurements and fitting as needed to aid rehabilitation.

Discharge teaching is as follows:
- Teach the patient and family proper positions, exercises, and ambulation techniques.
- Demonstrate stump-wrapping techniques to the patient and family (see Figure 4-42).
- Explain to the patient and family that prolonged phantom pain experiences are unusual and should receive medical attention.
- Discuss skin care with the patient and family to prevent stump irritation or impairment.
- List signs of a wound infection, and discuss these with the patient and family.

Prognosis

The prognosis for successful adaptation to an amputation is dependent upon the patient's age, the condition that resulted in amputation, other systemic disorders, emotional health, and support system.

NURSING PROCESS *for the Patient with a Musculoskeletal Disorder*

The role of the licensed practical nurse/licensed vocational nurse (LPN/LVN) in the nursing process as stated is that the LPN/LVN will:
- Participate in planning care for patients based on patient needs
- Review patient's plan of care and recommend revisions as needed
- Review and follow defined prioritzation for patient care
- Use clinical pathways/care maps/care plans to guide and review patient care

Assessment

The musculoskeletal system provides protection, support, and movement for the body. Orthopedics is the branch of medicine that deals with the prevention or correction of disorders involving locomotor structures of the body. Permanent disability and crippling will result if prompt treatment is not given to patients with musculoskeletal dysfunction. The ability to perform these functions is closely associated with the proper functioning of the nervous and circulatory systems.

Assessment of orthopedic function is necessary on all patients, but especially on those individuals who are (1) having difficulty with gait; (2) experiencing muscle weakness; (3) suffering from trauma of soft tissue and bone; (4) unable to produce movement that will enable activities for personal, economic, and social fulfillment; (5) experiencing diseases of the musculoskeletal system; or (6) chronically ill.

Assessment of a patient's mobility includes bone integrity, posture, joint function, muscle strength, gait, pain, and neurovascular disturbances related to pressure. It is important to compare body symmetry. For example, assess both legs for same length and diameter size and for comparable muscle strength. Observation of the patient's gait provides the nurse with information about unsteadiness or irregular movements. Difficult ambulation associated with shortness of breath can indicate cardiovascular or respiratory system difficulties.

Assessment of posture and gait is made easily by observing the patient walking. Common posture deformities include lateral (or S) curvature of the spine, known as scoliosis; a rounding of the thoracic spine (hump-backed appearance), known as kyphosis; and an increase in the curve at the lumbar space region that throws the shoulders back, making the "lordly or kingly" appearance that is known as lordosis (Figure 4-43). Rigidity of the spine can result from ankylosing spondylitis, whereby the vertebrae are fused with loss of mobility, producing a rigid gait or "poker spine" appearance.

Assessment of neurological and circulatory function is important if the patient has experienced a traumatic injury; damaged blood vessels and nerves can cause permanent disabilities.

Assessing the skin for signs of coolness, pallor, sensation, or cyanosis can help the nurse determine the patient's circulatory status. A faint or absent pulse in an extremity indicates impaired circulation. Palpating the femoral, popliteal, and dorsalis pedis pulses on both extremities provides data pertinent to the lower extremities. If the pulse is not readily palpated with a light touch of the finger, a Doppler instrument can be used, which will enable the listener to hear a magnified sound of the pulsation. The absence of a pulse is serious and must be reported to the charge nurse immediately. The brachial and radial pulses are assessed to determine circulation in the upper extremities. It may be difficult to palpate a pulse when a cast or bandage makes the extremity inaccessible. It is important to reach under the cast or bandage if possible. An assessment of the pulse in the unaffected extremity is made for a comparison.

Blanching test (meaning to whiten or pale) is a test of the rate of capillary refill, which signals circulation status. This is also referred to as a **capillary nail refill test.** The nurse compresses each fingernail or toenail of the affected extremity (noting the white color as pressure is applied), releases the pressure, and notes how quickly the pink color returns to the nailbed. The nailbed color should return to normal within 2 or 3 seconds. If the color is slow to return, this indicates that circulation is impaired, and prompt attention is needed to improve circulation (see Box 4-5).

Neurovascular assessments are made on patients with musculoskeletal trauma or damage to nerves and blood vessels resulting from surgery, tight bandages, splints, or casts. Impaired circulation resulting in alteration of nerve function can cause loss of the use of an extremity; this impairment is generally seen in the extremities. See Box 4-5 for information concerning neurovascular (circulation) assessment.

Nursing Diagnosis

Nursing assessment establishes the patient's needs regarding mobility. Care of the patient is based on the following nursing diagnoses:

- Impaired physical mobility, related to musculoskeletal impairment
- Impaired bed mobility
- Activity intolerance, related to musculoskeletal impairment
- Ineffective coping
- Anxiety, related to changes in body integrity
- Pain, related to musculoskeletal disorder
- Deficient knowledge regarding therapeutic regimen
- Risk for disuse syndrome

Expected Outcomes/Planning

The plan for facilitating mobility must center on improving and restoring performance and preventing deterioration. Nursing interventions focus on helping the patient regain, adapt, reduce, or eliminate activities that cause pain.

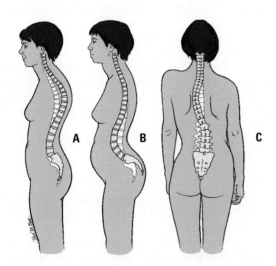

FIGURE **4-43** Abnormal spinal curvatures. **A,** Kyphosis. **B,** Lordosis. **C,** Scoliosis.

It is important to consider the amount of assistance needed for ambulation. Assessment of range of motion and muscle strength helps decide whether the patient is able to ambulate safely. Ambulation following surgery often requires physical assistance in addition to the use of mobility aids such as walkers, canes, and crutches.

The plan of care focuses on accomplishing individual goals and outcomes that relate to the identified nursing diagnoses. Examples of these include the following:

Goal #1: Patient will demonstrate the use of adaptive devices to increase mobility.

Outcome: Patient demonstrates more independence in mobility by meeting self-care needs.

Goal #2: Patient will demonstrate ambulation and verbalize safety precautions before discharge from health care facility.

Outcome: Patient demonstrates ambulation skills and verbalizes correct safety precautions before discharge.

Implementation

Improving the patient's mobility includes an awareness of physician's orders specific to ambulation. Nursing measures involve checking mobility aids for correct size. Patient education includes safety measures. The presence and condition of rubber tips are necessary to ensure safety. Shoes that are easy to get on, have nonslip soles, and provide foot and ankle support are safer than bedroom slippers or stockings.

Activities need to be alternated with rest periods. Administering analgesics at least 30 minutes before ambulation may be necessary for patients experiencing pain. Patients are encouraged to pace themselves. Patient assistance may be necessary to complete activities of daily living such as ambulating to the bathroom or to a bedside commode.

Specific principles are involved with mobility:

- Bone loss occurs when patients are confined to bed rest.
- The activities of the human body depend on effective interaction between normal joints and the neuromuscular parts that pilot them.
- Muscles, tendons, ligaments, cartilage, and bones all do their share to ensure smooth function.

Nurses working with patient mobility needs must be supportive of physical therapy department activities and goals. Assessment of a patient's perceptions helps the nurse determine motivation for mobility independence. For example, when older adults perceive themselves to be too fragile to walk, they may be fearful of trying. A safety belt can be used when a patient's stability is questioned. The belt encircles the patient's waist; the nurse grasps the belt in the middle of the back, helping the patient stand, gain balance, and ambulate.

Patients may have difficulty coping with mobility aids and perceive them as a visible sign of weakness. It is important to point out that devices to help mobility are not dissimilar to using glasses to help eyesight. Mobility aids increase proficiency of activities and promote joint rest and protection.

Evaluation

During and after mobility, the nurse evaluates the success of interventions by noting patient progress based on stated goals and outcomes. For example, if the patient is not able to ambulate the distance to use the bathroom for elimination purposes, a shorter distance may be more practical. Mobility may be accomplished by encouraging the use of a bedside commode. When patients are unable to meet expected outcomes, the nurse must be ready to revise the care plan to promote outcome success. Examples of goals and their corresponding outcomes include the following:

Goal #1: Patient will demonstrate the use of adaptive devices to increase mobility.

Outcome: The patient ambulates within physical environment.

Goal #2: Patient will understand safety precautions concerning use of mobility aids.

Outcome: The patient checks rubber tips on mobility aid and uses equipment correctly.

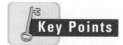
Key Points

- The skeletal system has five basic functions: support of the body, protection of internal organs, movement of the body, storage of minerals, and blood cell formation.
- The skeleton is composed of two main divisions:
    The axial skeleton, containing the skull, vertebrae, and thorax
    The appendicular skeleton, containing the upper and lower extremities
- The skeleton is divided into the axial and the appendicular skeletons. The axial skeleton is composed of the skull, vertebral column, and thorax. The appendicular skeleton is composed of the upper extremities, lower extremities, shoulder girdle, and pelvic girdle.
- The three types of joints and their movement are:
    Synarthrosis: no movement
    Amphiarthrosis: slight movement
    Diarthrosis: free movement
- Joints hold the bones together and allow movement and flexibility. Differences in the structure determine the amount of flexibility.
- Some of the more common movements that the body is capable of producing are flexion, extension, abduction, adduction, rotation, supination, pronation, dorsiflexion, and plantar flexion.

- The bones and joints provide the framework of the body, but the muscles are necessary for movement. Movement results from contraction and relaxation of the individual muscles.
- An erythrocyte sedimentation rate (ESR) is the most objective laboratory test for determining the severity of rheumatoid arthritis.
- Rheumatoid arthritis affects a young population (ages 30 to 55) with crippling changes in the synovial membrane of the joints.
- Salicylates and nonsteroidal antiinflammatory drugs (NSAIDs) are used to treat rheumatoid arthritis and osteoarthritis.
- Osteoarthritis is a degenerative joint disease (DJD) that affects the population older than 40 years of age and causes articular cartilage degeneration.
- Porous and brittle bones caused by a lack of calcium is one of the physiologic changes noted in osteoporosis.
- Vertebroplasty and kyphoplasty are surgical procedures used to relieve pain in women with osteoporosis who do not respond to other pain management programs.
- Arthroplasty procedures (such as hip and knee arthroplasty) are commonly performed on patients suffering from severe arthritis.
- Unicompartmental knee arthroplasty is also referred to as partial knee replacement and is performed on patients who have only one of the compartments of the knee affected by arthritis.
- Nursing intervention specific to the care of a patient suffering from a fractured hip involves maintaining abduction of the affected leg.
- Fractured hip fixation devices—such as hip prosthetic implant, plate and screw fixation, and telescoping nail fixation—require some degree of non–weight bearing for 6 weeks to 3 months.
- A significant postoperative nursing intervention for a patient with an amputation is proper care of the stump to facilitate the use of a prosthetic device.

- Herniated nucleus pulposus is seen most often in the cervical and lumbar spinal regions and can be treated surgically (laminectomy and spinal fusion) or medically (medication, traction, and physical therapy).
- Osteogenic sarcoma is a common primary malignant tumor seen in young people; it can metastasize to the lungs.
- Compartment syndrome, shock, fat embolism, gas gangrene, thromboembolus, and osteomyelitis are complications resulting from a fractured bone.
- External fixation devices such as casts, braces, metal pins, and skeletal and skin traction are used to hold bone fragments in normal position.
- Regardless of whether the casting material is plaster of paris or a synthetic material, proper drying, cleansing, handling, and assessing are required to prevent patient complications.
- The nurse caring for a patient in traction is responsible for knowing (1) the purpose of the traction (traction applied for fractures must be continuous); (2) the equipment needed and appropriate safety measures; (3) the amount of weight ordered; and (4) the patient's knowledge regarding the traction.
- Crutches, canes, walkers, and the Roll-A-Bout are used as gait enhancers for patients with altered mobility.
- Crutch walking involving the three-point gait is most commonly used for patients wearing leg casts.

Go to your free CD-ROM for an Audio Glossary, animations, video clips, and Review Questions for the NCLEX-PN® Examination.

evolve   Be sure to visit the companion Evolve site at http://evolve.elsevier.com/Christensen/adult/ for WebLinks and additional online resources.

CHAPTER CHALLENGE

1. The bones serve as storage specifically for which two minerals?

    1. Sodium and potassium
    2. Calcium and phosphorus
    3. Copper and iodine
    4. Magnesium and chloride

2. Hematopoiesis takes place in:

    1. the lymph nodes.
    2. the spleen.
    3. the yellow bone marrow.
    4. the red bone marrow.

3. Movement of an extremity away from the midline of the body is called:

    1. adduction.
    2. pronation.
    3. flexion.
    4. abduction.

4. Mr. A., 65 years of age, has been diagnosed with rheumatoid arthritis (RA). A diagnostic test used to assist in the confirmation of RA is:

    1. complete blood count.
    2. erythrocyte sedimentation rate.
    3. prothrombin time.
    4. urinary uric acid level.

Continued

CHAPTER CHALLENGE—cont'd

5. A clinical sign of gouty arthritis is:
   1. Heberden's nodes.
   2. pathologic fractures.
   3. tophi deposits.
   4. Homans' sign.

6. Ms. P., 55 years old, reveals a postmenopausal history of three previous fractures and daily consumption of caffeine. According to her history, she is at increased risk for:
   1. osteomyelitis.
   2. osteoarthritis.
   3. osteogenic sarcoma.
   4. osteoporosis.

7. An appropriate nursing intervention specific for a patient suffering from a fractured hip with bipolar hip repair is:
   1. release traction weight every 4 to 6 hours.
   2. maintain abduction of the affected extremity.
   3. maintain adduction of the affected extremity.
   4. encourage active range of motion in the affected extremity.

8. Ms. G. is being discharged following a prosthetic hip implant. She asks when she can begin to bear weight on the affected leg. Select the most appropriate response:
   1. You must not bear weight on your affected leg for 6 to 12 months."
   2. Most patients bear weight in 5 days."
   3. You must learn to use a gait enhancer and keep the majority of weight off the unaffected leg."
   4. Most patients require some degree of non–weight bearing for 6 weeks to 3 months."

9. A significant postoperative nursing intervention for a patient with an amputation is:
   1. maintaining abduction of the stump.
   2. elevating the stump with no more than two pillows.
   3. proper stump care to facilitate prosthetic use.
   4. leaving the stump open to air to assess suture site.

10. Mr. J. is a 75-year-old retired construction worker. He has been seeing the physician for complaints of osteoarthritis. Today he is discussing concerns over his condition and asks what has caused his osteoarthritis. An appropriate response would be:
    1. "You have osteoarthritis because of the difficult construction work you did for so many years."
    2. "Everyone your age has arthritis; you are fortunate you are still able to walk."

3. "The cause of osteoarthritis is unknown. However, almost everyone older than 40 years of age has some changes in their joints."
4. "You probably did not exercise as much as you should have, and you should start vigorous exercising now to prevent further complications."

11. An appropriate nursing intervention for Mr. S., a 32-year-old patient in skeletal traction, would be:
    1. provide cast care.
    2. cleanse pin sites daily with hydrogen peroxide and observe for signs of infection.
    3. place patient on drainage and secretion precautions.
    4. encourage the patient to sit in a straight, firm chair for no longer than 20 minutes each time.

12. Following a fracture of the forearm or tibia, complaints of sharp, deep, unrelenting pain in the hand or foot unrelieved by analgesics or elevation of the extremity indicate which complication?
    1. Fat embolism
    2. Compartment syndrome
    3. Gas gangrene
    4. Cast syndrome

13. Mr. L. is a 45-year-old who suffered a knee injury while playing football with his son. He is scheduled for an arthroscopic examination and asks the nurse to explain the procedure. The most appropriate nursing response would be:
    1. "Your physician will insert a small scope into your knee joint to visualize the joint for damaged tissue."
    2. "The test involves the use of magnetism and radio waves to make images of cross-sections of the body."
    3. "The radiographic technician will inject your knee joint with an atomic material and take a radiograph of your affected knee."
    4. "The physician will insert needle electrodes into the knee muscle so that electrical activity of the knee can be documented."

14. Mr. C., 51 years of age, is suffering from rheumatoid arthritis. He asks if there is a cure for RA. The most appropriate response is:
    1. "Yes, new drugs being developed offer a cure."
    2. "No, but new drugs being developed can interfere with the body's reaction to inflammation and better control the disease process."
    3. "Yes, but the patient must take medication for at least 10 years."
    4. "No, most patients with RA also develop osteoarthritis."

15. Mr. A. is scheduled for endoscopic spinal microsurgery to correct a herniated disk. Select the most accurate statement concerning this type of surgery.
    1. Endoscopic spinal microsurgery requires a general anesthetic.
    2. Special scopes are placed through small incisions, causing minimal damage to surrounding tissue.
    3. Patients older than 80 years of age are always candidates for endoscopic spinal microsurgery.
    4. Endoscopic spinal microsurgery is limited to the repair of herniated disks.

16. Ms. C. is a 45-year-old patient with a history of lactose intolerance, excessive caffeine intake, and excessive cigarette smoking. The physician orders a bone density index test for Ms. C. Select the most appropriate statement that would provide the patient with information about the test.
    1. The test is also called DEXA and is considered an invasive procedure.
    2. The test involves drawing a small amount of blood to determine your blood calcium level.
    3. The test takes about 10 minutes and involves very low amounts of radiation.
    4. A bone density test is always recommended for women more than 30 years of age.

17. Ms. M., a 62-year-old patient with osteoarthritis of the knee, is seeking information from the nurse about glucosamine supplements. The most appropriate response would be:
    1. "Glucosamine is a natural substance in the body and it is not necessary to take a supplement."
    2. "Glucosamine supplements are relatively safe in people younger than 40 years of age."
    3. "Studies suggest that glucosamine supplements are helpful in maintaining healthy joint function, with minimal side effects unless you are allergic to shellfish."
    4. "A healthy lifestyle with high-impact exercise is more important than taking a supplement."

18. Select the most appropriate nursing assessment for the nursing diagnosis of ineffective tissue perfusion, secondary to fractured hip.
    1. Assess for ecchymosis over pelvis and perineum.
    2. Protect patient from cross contamination.
    3. Assess for adventitious lung sounds.
    4. Assess distal pulses.

19. Ms. R. is 72 years of age and has just undergone total hip replacement. She asks why she cannot cross her legs when sitting but is supposed to do straight leg raising exercises. The most appropriate response would be:
    1. "Straight leg–raising exercises help strengthen the leg muscles; crossing your legs puts pressure on the joints and could cause damage to the hip prosthesis."
    2. "Straight leg–raising exercises keep you from getting too tired while you sit; when you want to cross your legs, it is time to rest."
    3. "Straight leg–raising exercises strengthen the muscles in your upper legs to help you walk."
    4. "The doctor ordered straight leg–raising exercises and did not order you to cross your legs."

20. Which of the following objective information is seen in patients with compartment syndrome?
    1. Hypotension, tachycardia, and tachypnea
    2. Gas bubbles under the skin
    3. Positive Homans' sign
    4. Absence of pulsation in the affected extremity

21. Ms. F., 77 years old, has persistent complaints of severe back pain related to osteoporosis. She walks with a stooped posture and has a noticeable kyphosis. She has been unresponsive to a traditional pain management program. Based on this information, Ms. F. may be a candidate for:
    1. unicompartmental arthroplasty.
    2. complete bed rest.
    3. kyphoplasty.
    4. injections of Forteo.

Continued

CHAPTER CHALLENGE—cont'd

22. Ms. E. is a 47-year-old patient experiencing signs and symptoms of menopause. She recently fell and fractured her wrist. After doing a bone density test, her physician gave her a diagnosis of osteoporosis. She asks about the benefits of taking estrogen. Select the most accurate response.

    1. "Estrogen will not help bone density."
    2. "Estrogen can cause cancer of the breast."
    3. "Estrogen will not correct the condition but will help to prevent fractures and is approved for women at significant risk."
    4. "Forteo is a type of estrogen."

23. Mr. H. is a 51-year-old active patient who exercises routinely. He has been noticing pain on the lateral area of his knee for the past 6 months during and after exercise. He is scheduled for a unicompartmental knee arthroplasty. He asks you to explain the surgery. Select the most accurate response.

    1. "The procedure involves the replacement of the entire knee joint."
    2. "You will need to be in the hospital for approximately 5 days."
    3. "You will not need an anesthetic."
    4. "The minimally invasive knee surgery removes only the most damaged areas of cartilage and a small plastic disk replaces the worn cartilage, providing a new cushion between the bones."

Care of the Patient with a Gastrointestinal Disorder

BARBARA LAURITSEN CHRISTENSEN

OVERVIEW OF ANATOMY AND PHYSIOLOGY

DIGESTIVE SYSTEM

Although it is understood that food is necessary for existence, not everyone understands (1) what happens to food once it is chewed and swallowed; (2) how food is prepared for its trip to each individual cell; and (3) the many changes that food undergoes, both chemically and physically. This chapter will review these changes and their effect on the body.

The digestive tract, or alimentary canal, is a musculomembranous tube extending from the mouth to the anus and is approximately 30 feet long (Figure 5-1). It consists of the mouth, pharynx, esophagus, small intestine, large intestine, and anus. Peristalsis is the coordinated, rhythmic, serial contraction of smooth muscle that forces food through the digestive tract, bile through the bile duct, and urine through the ureter. During peristalsis the tract shortens to approximately 15 feet.

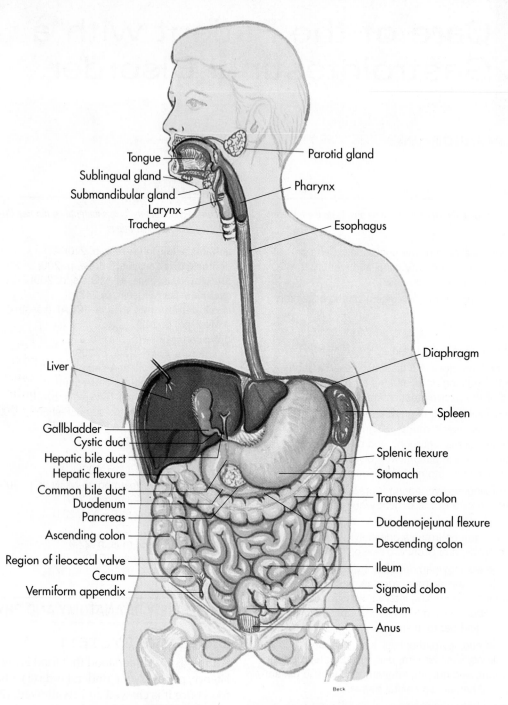

FIGURE **5-1** Location of digestive organs.

Accessory organs aid in the digestive process but are not considered part of the digestive tract. They release chemicals into the system through a series of ducts. The teeth, tongue, salivary glands, liver, gallbladder, and pancreas are considered accessory organs. These will be discussed in the chapter.

Organs of the Digestive System and Their Functions (Box 5-1)

Mouth. The mouth marks the entrance to the digestive system. The floor of the mouth contains a muscular appendage, the tongue. The tongue is involved in chewing, swallowing, and the formation of speech. Tiny elevations, called **papillae** contain the taste buds. They differentiate between bitter, sweet, sour, and salty sensations.

Digestion begins in the mouth. Here the teeth mechanically shred and grind the food and the enzymes begin the chemical breakdown of carbohydrates.

Teeth. Each tooth is designed to carry out a specific task. Immediately to the center of the mouth lie the incisors, which are structured for biting and cutting. Posterior to the incisors are the canines, pointed teeth used for tearing and shredding food. The molars are to the rear of the jaw. These teeth have four cusps (points) and are used for mastication (to crush and grind food).

Box 5-1 | *Organs of the Digestive System*

ORGANS OF THE ALIMENTARY CANAL

- Mouth
- Pharynx (throat)
- Esophagus (food pipe)
- Stomach
- Small intestine
  Duodenum
  Jejunum
  Ileum
- Large intestine

- Cecum
- Colon
  Ascending colon
  Transverse colon
  Descending colon
  Sigmoid colon
- Rectum
- Anal canal

ACCESSORY ORGANS

- Teeth and gums
- Tongue
- Liver
- Gallbladder
- Pancreas

- Salivary glands
  Parotid
  Submandibular
  Sublingual

Salivary glands. There are three pairs of salivary glands (see Figure 5-1). They are the parotid glands, submandibular glands, and sublingual glands. They secrete a fluid called saliva, which is approximately 99% water with enzymes and mucus. Normally these glands secrete enough saliva to keep the mucous membranes of the mouth moist. Once food enters the mouth, the secretion increases to lubricate and dissolve the food and to begin the chemical process of digestion. The salivary glands secrete about 1000 to 1500 mL of saliva daily. The major enzyme is salivary amylase (ptyalin), which is responsible for the initiation of carbohydrate metabolism. Another enzyme, lysozyme, destroys bacteria, which protects the mucous membrane from infections and protects the teeth from decay. After food has been ingested, the salivary glands continue to secrete saliva, which cleanses the mouth.

Esophagus. The esophagus is a muscular, collapsible tube that is approximately 10 inches long, extending from the mouth through the thoracic cavity and the esophageal hiatus to the stomach. No digestion takes place here. Peristalsis moves the bolus (food broken down and mixed with saliva, ready to pass to the stomach) through the esophagus to the stomach in 5 or 6 seconds.

Stomach. The stomach is located in the left upper quadrant of the abdomen, directly inferior to the diaphragm (Figure 5-2). When the stomach is filled, it is the size of a football and holds approximately 1 L. The entrance to the stomach is the cardiac sphincter (so named because of the proximity to the heart); the exit is the pyloric sphincter. As food leaves the esophagus, it enters the stomach through the relaxed cardiac

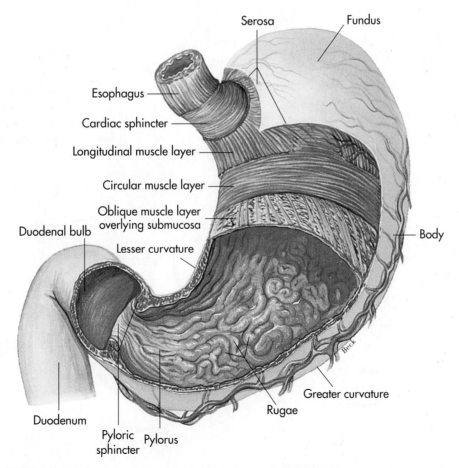

FIGURE **5-2** Stomach. Cut-away sections show muscle layers and interior mucosa thrown into folds called **rugae**.

sphincter. The sphincter then contracts, preventing reflux (splashing or return flow), which can be irritating.

Once the bolus has entered the stomach, the muscular layers of the stomach churn and contract to mix and compress the contents with the gastric juices and water. The gastric juices are a group of secretions that are released by the gastric glands. Digestion of protein begins in the stomach. Hydrochloric acid softens the connective tissue of meats, kills bacteria, and activates pepsin (the chief enzyme of gastric juices that converts proteins into proteoses and peptones). Mucin is released to protect the stomach lining. Intrinsic factor (a substance secreted by the gastric mucosa) is produced to allow absorption of vitamin B_{12}. After the stomach has completed its work, the food has been broken down into a viscous semiliquid substance called chyme. The chyme is sent through the pyloric sphincter into the duodenum for the next phase of digestion.

Small intestine. The small intestine is a 20-foot-long tube; it is 1 inch in diameter. It begins at the pyloric sphincter and ends at the ileocecal valve. It is divided into three major sections: **duodenum, jejunum,** and **ileum.** Most digestion takes place here—as much as 90%. The intestinal juices finish the metabolism of carbohydrates and proteins. Bile and pancreatic juices enter the duodenum. Bile from the liver breaks molecules into smaller droplets, which enables the digestive juices to complete their process. Pancreatic juices contain water, protein, inorganic salts, and enzymes. Pancreatic juices are essential in breaking down proteins into their amino acid components, in reducing dietary fats to glycerol and fatty acids, and in converting starch to simple sugars.

The inner surface of the small intestine contains millions of tiny fingerlike projections called **villi,** which are clustered over the entire mucous surface. They are responsible for absorbing the products of digestion into the blood stream. They increase the absorption area of the small intestine 600 times. Inside each villus is a rich capillary bed, along with modified lymph capillaries called lacteals. The lacteals are responsible for the absorption of metabolized fats.

Large intestine. Once the small intestine has finished with its specific tasks, the ileocecal valve opens and re-

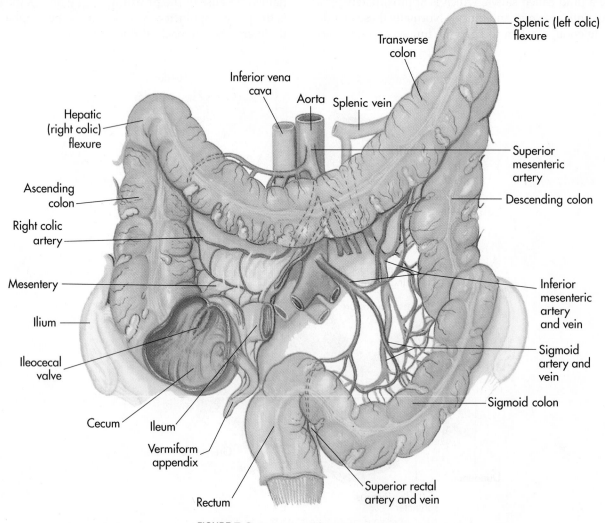

FIGURE **5-3** Divisions of the large intestine.

leases the contents into the large intestine. The tube is larger in diameter (2 inches) but shorter (5 feet) than the small intestine. It is composed of the cecum; appendix; ascending, transverse, descending, and sigmoid colons; rectum; and anus (Figure 5-3). The process of digestion is completed here in the terminal portion of the digestive tract. Basically the large intestine has four major functions: (1) completion of absorption, (2) manufacture of certain vitamins, (3) formation of feces, and (4) expulsion of feces.

Just inferior to the ileocecal valve is the cecum, a blind pouch approximately 2 to 3 inches long. Dangling from the cecum is a small wormlike, tubular structure: the vermiform appendix. To date, no function for the appendix is known. The open end of the cecum connects to the ascending colon; continues upward on the right side of the abdomen to the inferior area of the liver; becomes the transverse colon; and crosses to the left side of the abdomen, where it becomes the descending colon to the level of the iliac crest. The sigmoid colon begins here and continues toward the midline to the level of the third sacral vertebra.

Bacteria in the large intestine change the chyme into fecal material by releasing the remaining nutrients. The bacteria are also responsible for the synthesis of vitamin K, needed for normal blood clotting, and the production of some of the B-complex vitamins. As the fecal material continues its journey, the remaining water and vitamins are absorbed into the blood stream by osmosis.

Rectum. The last 8 inches of the intestine form the rectum, where the fecal material is expelled.

ACCESSORY ORGANS OF DIGESTION
Liver
The liver is the largest glandular organ in the body and one of the most complex. In the adult it weighs 3 pounds. It is located just inferior to the diaphragm, covering most of the upper right quadrant and extending into the left epigastrium. It is divided into two lobes. Approximately 1500 mL of blood is delivered to the liver every minute by the portal vein and the hepatic artery. The cells of the liver produce a product called bile, a yellow-brown or green-brown liquid. Bile is necessary for the metabolism of fats. The liver releases 500 to 1000 mL of bile per day. Bile travels to the gallbladder through hepatic ducts. The gallbladder is a sac about 3 to 4 inches long located on the right inferior surface of the liver. Here bile is stored until needed for fat digestion (Figure 5-4).

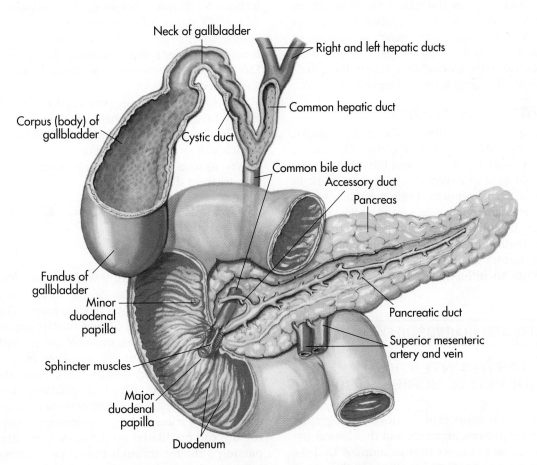

FIGURE **5-4** Gallbladder and bile ducts. Obstruction of the hepatic or common bile duct by stone or spasm occludes the exit of the bile from being ejected into the duodenum.

In addition to producing bile, the liver has many other functions: managing blood coagulation; manufacturing cholesterol; manufacturing albumin to maintain normal blood volume; filtering out old red blood cells and bacteria; detoxifying poisons (alcohol, nicotine, drugs); converting ammonia to urea; providing the main source of body heat; storing glycogen for later use; activating vitamin D; and breaking down nitrogenous waste (from protein metabolism) to urea, which the kidneys can excrete as waste from the body.

Pancreas

The pancreas is an elongated gland that lies posterior to the stomach (see Figure 5-4). It is an active organ that is involved in both endocrine and exocrine duties. In this chapter, discussion of the pancreas is limited to its exocrine activities.

Each day the pancreas produces 1000 to 1500 mL of pancreatic juice to aid in digestion. This pancreatic juice contains the digestive enzymes protease (trypsin), lipase (steapsin), and amylase (amylopsin), which are important because of their ability to digest the three major components of chyme—proteins, fats, and carbohydrates. These enzymes are transported through an excretory duct to the duodenum. This pancreatic duct connects to the common bile duct from the liver and gallbladder and empties through a small orifice in the duodenum called the major duodenal papilla or **papilla of Vater.** In addition, the pancreas contains an alkaline substance, sodium bicarbonate, that has the ability to neutralize the hydrochloric acid in the gastric juices that enter the small intestine from the stomach.

REGULATION OF FOOD INTAKE

The hypothalamus, a portion of the brain, contains two centers that have an effect on eating. One center stimulates the individual to eat and the other signals the individual to stop eating. These centers work in conjunction with the rest of the brain to balance eating habits. However, many other factors also affect eating. For example, distention decreases appetite. Other controls in our bodies, lifestyle, eating habits, emotions, and genetic factors all influence intake of food and blend together to influence each individual's body build.

LABORATORY AND DIAGNOSTIC EXAMINATIONS

UPPER GASTROINTESTINAL STUDY (UPPER GI SERIES, UGI)
Rationale

The upper GI study consists of a series of radiographs of the lower esophagus, stomach, and duodenum using barium sulfate as the contrast medium. A UGI series will detect any abnormal conditions of the upper GI tract, any tumors, or other ulcerative lesions.

Nursing Interventions

The patient should maintain nothing by mouth (NPO) status after midnight. Tell the patient to avoid smoking after midnight the night before the study. The nurse should explain to the patient the importance of rectally expelling all the barium after the examination. Stools will be light colored until all the barium is expelled up to 72 hours after the test. Eventual absorption of fecal water may cause a hardened barium impaction. Increasing fluid intake is usually effective. Milk of magnesia (60 mL) is commonly given after the examination unless contraindicated.

TUBE GASTRIC ANALYSIS
Rationale

The contents of the stomach are aspirated to determine the amount of acid produced by the parietal cells in the stomach. The analysis is done to determine the completeness of a vagotomy, confirm hypersecretion or achlorhydria (an abnormal condition characterized by the absence of hydrochloric acid in the gastric juice), estimate acid secretory capacity, or assay for intrinsic factor.

Nursing Interventions

The patient should receive no anticholinergic medications for 24 hours before the test and should maintain NPO status after midnight so the gastric acid secretion will not be altered. The nurse should inform the patient that smoking is prohibited before the test because nicotine stimulates the flow of gastric secretions.

The nurse or radiology personnel will insert a nasogastric tube into the stomach to aspirate gastric content. Specimens should be labeled properly and sent to the laboratory immediately. The nasogastric tube is removed as soon as specimens are collected. The patient may then eat if indicated.

ESOPHAGOGASTRODUODENOSCOPY (EGD, UGI ENDOSCOPY, GASTROSCOPY)
Rationale

Endoscopy (*endo*, within, inward; *scope*, to look) enables direct visualization of the upper GI tract by means of a long, fiberoptic flexible scope. The esophagus, stomach (Figure 5-5), and duodenum are examined for tumors, varices, mucosal inflammations, hiatal hernias, polyps, ulcers, presence of *Helicobacter pylori*, strictures, and obstructions. Also, the endoscopist can remove polyps, coagulate sources of active GI bleeding, and perform sclerotherapy of esophageal varices through endoscopy. Areas of narrowing can be dilated by the endoscope itself or by passing a dilator through the scope. Camera equipment may be attached to the viewing lens, and the existing pathologic condition can be photographed. The

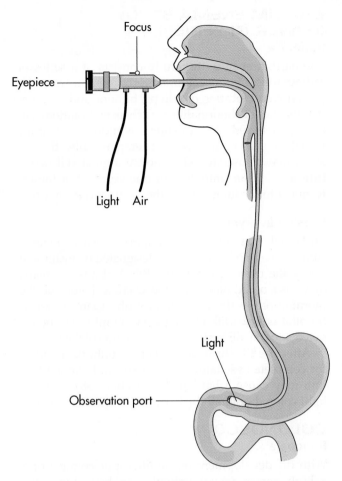

FIGURE **5-5** Fiberoptic endoscopy of the stomach.

endoscope can also be used in obtaining tissue specimens for biopsy or culture to determine presence of *H. pylori.*

Endoscopy enables evaluation of the esophagus, stomach, and duodenum; by using a longer fiberoptic scope, the upper small intestine can be evaluated. This is referred to as enteroscopy.

Nursing Interventions

The nurse should explain the procedure to the patient. The patient should maintain NPO status after midnight. The nurse must obtain the patient's signature on a consent form and complete a preoperative checklist for the endoscopic examination. The patient is usually given a preprocedure intravenous sedative such as midazolam (Versed). Because the patient's pharynx has been anesthetized (by spraying) with lidocaine HCl (Xylocaine), the nurse should not allow the patient to eat or drink until the gag reflex returns (usually about 2 to 4 hours). The nurse should assess for any signs and symptoms of perforation, including abdominal pain and tenderness, guarding, oral bleeding, melena, and hypovolemic shock.

BARIUM SWALLOW/ GASTROGRAFIN STUDIES
Rationale

This barium contrast study is a more thorough study of the esophagus than that provided by most UGI examinations. As in most barium contrast studies, defects in luminal filling and narrowing of the barium column indicate tumor, scarred stricture, or esophageal varices. With a barium swallow, anatomical abnormalities, such as hiatal hernia, are easily recognized. Left atrial dilation, aortic aneurysm, and paraesophageal tumors (such as bronchial or mediastinal tumors) may cause extrinsic compression of the barium column within the esophagus.

A product called Gastrografin is now used in place of barium for patients in whom bleeding from the GI system may occur and surgery is being considered. Gastrografin is water soluble and rapidly absorbed, so it is preferable when a perforation is suspected. Gastrografin facilitates imaging through radiographs, but if the product escapes from the GI tract, unlike barium, it is absorbed by the surrounding tissue. Complications can occur if barium leaks from the GI tract.

Nursing Interventions

The patient should maintain NPO status after midnight. Food and fluid in the stomach will prevent the barium from accurately outlining the GI tract, and the radiographic results may be misleading. The nurse should explain to the patient the importance of rectally expelling all barium. Stools will be light colored until this occurs. Eventual absorption of fecal water may cause a hardened barium impaction. Increasing fluid intake is usually effective. Milk of magnesia (60 mL) is usually given after the barium swallow examination unless contraindicated.

ESOPHAGEAL FUNCTION STUDIES (BERNSTEIN TEST)
Rationale

The Bernstein test, an acid-perfusion test, is an attempt to reproduce the symptoms of gastroesophageal reflux. It aids in differentiating esophageal pain caused by esophageal reflux from that caused by angina pectoris. If the patient suffers pain with the instillation of hydrochloric acid into the esophagus, the test is positive and indicates reflux esophagitis.

Nursing Interventions

The nurse should avoid sedating the patient, because the patient's participation is essential for swallowing the tubes, swallowing during acid clearance, and describing any discomfort during the instillation of hydrochloric acid. The patient is NPO for 8 hours before the examination, and any medications that may interfere with the production of acid, such as antacids and analgesics, are withheld.

EXAMINATION OF STOOL FOR OCCULT BLOOD
Rationale

Tumors of the large intestine grow into the lumen (the cavity or channel within a tube or tubular organ) and are subjected to repeated trauma by the fecal stream. Eventually the tumor ulcerates and bleeding occurs. Usually the bleeding is so slight that gross blood is not seen in the stool. If this occult blood (blood that is obscure or hidden from view) is detected in the stool, a benign or malignant GI tumor should be suspected. Tests for occult blood are also called guaiac, Hemoccult, and Hematest.

Occult blood in the stool may occur also in ulceration and inflammation of the upper or lower GI system. Other causes include swallowing blood of oral or nasopharyngeal origin.

Stool may be obtained by digital retrieval by the nurse or physician. However, the patient is usually asked to collect stool in an appropriate container. A specimen for occult blood must be obtained before barium studies are done.

Nursing Interventions

The nurse should instruct the patient to keep the stool specimen free of urine or toilet paper, because either can contaminate the specimen and alter the test results. The nurse or patient should don gloves and use tongue blades to transfer the stool to the proper receptacle. Keep diet free of red meat for 24 to 48 hours before a guaiac test.

SIGMOIDOSCOPY (LOWER GI ENDOSCOPY)
Rationale

Endoscopy of the lower GI tract allows visualization and, if indicated, access to obtain biopsy specimens of tumors, polyps, or ulcerations of the anus, rectum, and sigmoid colon. Because the lower GI tract is difficult to visualize radiographically, the direct visualization afforded through sigmoidoscopy is beneficial. Microscopic review of tissue specimens obtained using this procedure can provide the diagnoses of many lower bowel disorders.

Nursing Interventions

The nurse should explain the procedure to the patient. The patient should sign a consent form for the procedure. The nurse administers enemas as ordered on the evening before and/or the morning of the examination to ensure optimum visualization of the lower GI tract. After the examination, the nurse observes the patient for evidence of bowel perforation (abdominal pain, tenderness, distention, and bleeding).

BARIUM ENEMA STUDY (LOWER GI SERIES)
Rationale

The barium enema (BE) study consists of a series of radiographs of the colon used to demonstrate the presence and location of polyps, tumors, and diverticula. Positional abnormalities (such as malrotation) can also be detected. Barium sulfate is more effective for visualizing mucosal detail. Therapeutically, the BE study may be used to reduce nonstrangulated ileocolic intussusception (infolding of one segment of the intestine into the lumen of another segment) in children.

Nursing Interventions

The nurse may administer cathartics such as magnesium citrate or other cathartics designated by institution policy the evening before the BE. A cleansing enema may also be administered the evening before or the morning of the BE if directed by physician's order or hospital policy. Milk of magnesia (60 mL) may be ordered after the BE to stimulate evacuation of the barium.

After the BE study, the patient should be assessed for complete evacuation of the barium. Retained barium may cause a hardened impaction. Stool will be light colored until all the barium has been expelled.

COLONOSCOPY
Rationale

With the development of the fiberoptic colonoscope, a high percentage of patients can have the entire colon—from anus to cecum—examined. Therefore, with colonoscopy, the detection of lesions in the proximal colon—which would otherwise be undetected by sigmoidoscopy—is possible. Benign and malignant neoplasms, mucosal inflammation or ulceration, and sites of active hemorrhage can also be visualized. Biopsy specimens can be obtained and small tumors removed through the scope with the use of cable-activated instruments. Actively bleeding vessels can be coagulated.

Patients who have had cancer of the colon are at high risk for developing a subsequent colon cancer; patients who have a family history of colon cancer are at high risk. For these patients, colonoscopy allows early detection of any primary or secondary tumors.

Nursing Interventions

The patient signs a consent form. The nurse explains the procedure to the patient. The patient is instructed regarding dietary restrictions: usually a clear liquid diet is permitted 1 to 3 days before the procedure to decrease the residue in the bowel, and then NPO status is maintained for 8 hours before the procedure. The nurse administers a cathartic, enemas, and pre-

Box 5-2 **GoLYTELY Bowel Preparation**

1. Give patient one metoclopramide (Reglan) 10-mg tablet, as prescribed, orally 30 minutes before proceeding with step 2.
2. Administer the GoLYTELY solution* (prepared by pharmacy) per physician's orders:
   a. 240 mL orally every 15 minutes *or*
   b. 30 mL/min via NG tube. Use a Travasorb enteral feeding container and a size 10 feeding tube. Administer until stools are clear yellow.
   c. Keep patient warm with heated blankets; they often become chilled after consuming copious amounts of GoLYTELY solution.
   d. Provide a bedside commode if patient is an older adult or weak.

*Administer a minimum of 1 gallon of solution over a 2-hour period.

medication as ordered to decrease the residue in the bowel. GoLYTELY (Box 5-2), an oral or nasogastric (NG) colonic lavage, is an osmotic electrolyte solution that is now commonly used as a cathartic. It is a polyethylene glycol solution. If taken orally, instruct the patient to drink the solution rapidly: 8 ounces (240 mL) every 15 minutes until enough solution has been consumed to make the colonic contents a light yellow liquid. Powdered lemonade may be added to make the oral solution more palatable. If it is given per lavage, it must be given rapidly. Taking the solution slowly will not clean the colon efficiently. Provide warm blankets during the procedure. Many patients experience hypothermia during the GoLYTELY procedure. Provide a commode at the bedside for older adults and frail patients.

A preprocedure IV sedative such as midazolam is often given.

After colonoscopy, the nurse checks for evidence of bowel perforation (abdominal pain, guarding, distention, tenderness, excessive rectal bleeding, or blood clots) and examines stools for gross blood. Assess for hypovolemic shock.

STOOL CULTURE
Rationale
The feces (stool) can be examined for the presence of bacteria, ova, and parasites (a plant or animal that lives upon or within another living organism at whose expense it obtains some advantage). The physician may order a stool for culture of bacteria or for ova and parasites (O&P). Many bacteria (such as *Escherichia coli*) are indigenous in the bowel. Bacterial cultures are usually done to detect enteropathogens (such as *Staphylococcus aureus*, *Salmonella*, *Shigella*, *E. coli* 0157:H7, or *Clostridium difficile*).

When a patient is suspected of having a parasitic infection, the stool is examined for O&P. Usually at least three stool specimens are collected on subsequent days. Because culture results will not be available for several days, they will not influence initial treatment, but they will guide subsequent treatment if bacterial infection is present.

Nursing Interventions
If an enema must be administered to collect specimens, only normal saline or tap water should be used. Soapsuds or any other substance could affect the viability of the organisms collected.

Stool samples for O&P are obtained before barium examinations. The patient is instructed not to mix urine with feces. The nurse dons gloves to collect the specimen. The specimen should be taken to the laboratory within 30 minutes of collection in specified container.

OBSTRUCTION SERIES (FLAT PLATE OF THE ABDOMEN)
Rationale
The obstruction series is a group of radiographic studies performed on the abdomen of patients who have suspected bowel obstruction, paralytic ileus, perforated viscus (any large interior organ in any of the great body cavities), or abdominal abscess. This series usually consists of at least two radiographic studies. The first is an erect abdominal radiographic study that should include visualization of the diaphragm. Radiographs are examined for evidence of free air under the diaphragm, which is pathognomonic (signs or symptoms specific to a disease condition) of a perforated viscus. This radiographic study is used also to detect air-fluid levels within the intestine.

Nursing Interventions
For adequate visualization, the nurse should ensure that this study is scheduled before any barium studies.

DISORDERS OF THE MOUTH

Common disorders of the mouth and esophagus that interfere with adequate nutrition include poor dental hygiene, infections, inflammation, and cancer.

DENTAL PLAQUE AND CARIES
Etiology/Pathophysiology
Dental decay is an erosive process that results from the action of bacteria on carbohydrates in the mouth, which in turn produces acids that dissolve tooth enamel. Most Americans (95%) experience tooth decay

at some time in their life. Dental decay can be caused by one of several factors, among which are the following:

- The presence of dental plaque, a thin film on the teeth made of mucin and colloidal material found in saliva and often secondarily invaded by bacteria
- The strength of acids and the ability of the saliva to neutralize them
- The length of time the acids are in contact with the teeth
- Susceptibility of the teeth to decay

Medical Management

Interventions include treatment of dental caries by removal of affected areas of the tooth and replacement with some form of dental material. Treatment of periodontal disease centers on removal of plaque from the teeth. If the disease has advanced, surgical interventions of the gingivae and alveolar bone may be necessary.

Nursing Interventions and Patient Teaching

Proper technique for brushing and flossing the teeth at least twice a day is the nurse's primary focus of teaching for these patients. Plaque forms continuously and must be removed periodically through regular visits to the dentist. The patient must understand the importance of prevention through continual care. Because carbohydrates create an environment in which caries develops and plaque accumulates more easily, proper nutrition is included in patient teaching. When the patient is ill, the normal cleansing action of the mouth is impaired. Illnesses, drugs, and irradiation all interfere with the normal action of saliva. If the patient is unable to manage oral hygiene, the nurse must assume this responsibility.

Nursing diagnoses and interventions for the patient with dental plaque and caries include but are not limited to the following:

NURSING DIAGNOSES	NURSING INTERVENTIONS
Deficient knowledge, related to inability to prevent dental caries and periodontal disease	Assess and observe the oral cavity for moisture, color, and cleanliness. Stress importance of meticulous oral hygiene. Explain need to see dentist at least yearly for examination.
Noncompliance, related to hygiene and dietary restrictions	Brush teeth twice daily (bid) and as needed (prn) with toothpaste or powder, baking soda, or mouthwash. Rinse with water or mouthwash. Cleanse mouth with equal parts of hydrogen peroxide and water prn for halitosis. Teach oral hygiene to patient.

Prognosis

The prevention and elimination of dental plaque and caries are directly related to oral hygiene, dental care, nutrition, and heredity. All but heredity are controllable characteristics. The prognosis is more favorable for people who brush, floss, regularly visit the dentist for removal of affected areas, eat low-carbohydrate foods, and drink fluoridated water.

CANDIDIASIS
Etiology/Pathophysiology

This condition is any infection caused by a species of *Candida,* usually *C. albicans. Candida* is a fungal organism normally present in the mucous membranes of the mouth, intestinal tract, and vagina and is also found on the skin of healthy people. This infection is also referred to as **thrush** and **moniliasis.**

This disease appears more commonly in the newborn infant, who becomes infected while passing through the birth canal. In the older individual, candidiasis may be found in patients with leukemia, diabetes mellitus, or alcoholism, and in the person who has been taking antibiotics (chlortetracycline or tetracycline) or steroids for long periods or who is in a general weakened state. It is often seen in patients receiving chemotherapy and/or radiation therapy.

Clinical Manifestations

Candidiasis appears as pearly, bluish white "milk-curd" membranous lesions on the mucous membranes of the mouth, tongue, and larynx. One or more lesions may be on the mucosa, depending on the duration of the infection. If the patch or plaque is removed, painful bleeding can occur.

Medical Management

Treatment may include 1 to 4 mL of nystatin (Mycostatin) dropped in the infected infant's mouth several times a day. For the adult, nystatin or amphotericin B (an oral suspension) or buccal tablets and half-strength hydrogen peroxide/saline mouth rinses may provide some relief. For treatment of adult *Candida* vaginal infection, nystatin vaginal tablets (100,000 units dissolved) inserted into the vagina twice a day is effective. Ketoconazole taken systemically appears to be equally effective.

Nursing Interventions

The nurse must use meticulous handwashing to prevent spread of infection. The infection may be spread in the nursery by carelessness of nursing personnel. Handwashing, care of feeding equipment, and cleanliness of the mother's nipples are important to prevent spread. The nurse should cleanse the infant's mouth of any foreign material, rinsing the mouth and lubricating the lips. The mouth should be inspected using a flashlight and tongue blade.

For adults, instruct the patient to use a soft-bristled toothbrush and administer a topical anesthetic (lidocaine or benzocaine) to the mouth 1 hour before meals. Give soft or pureed foods and avoid hot, cold, spicy, fried, or citrus foods.

Prognosis

If the host has a strong defense system and medical treatment is initiated early in the course of the disease, the prognosis is good.

CARCINOMA OF THE ORAL CAVITY
Etiology/Pathophysiology

The lips, the oral cavity, the tongue, and the pharynx are prone to develop malignant lesions. The tonsils occasionally may be involved. The largest number of these tumors are squamous cell epitheliomas that grow rapidly and metastasize to adjacent structures more quickly than do most malignant tumors of the skin. In the United States, oral cancer accounts for 4% of the cancers in men and 2% in women. An estimated 28,260 new cases are expected in 2004. An estimated 7230 deaths from oral cavity and pharynx cancer are expected in 2004. Death rates have been decreasing since the 1970s, with rates declining faster in the 2000s.

Tumors of the salivary glands occur primarily in the parotid gland and are usually benign. Tumors of the submaxillary gland have a high incidence of malignancy. These malignant tumors grow rapidly and may be accompanied by pain and impaired facial function.

Kaposi's sarcoma is a malignant skin tumor that occurs primarily on the legs of men between 50 and 70 years of age. Recently it has been seen with increased frequency as a nonsquamous tumor of the oral cavity in patients with acquired immunodeficiency syndrome (AIDS). The lesions are purple and nonulcerated. Irradiation is the treatment of choice.

Cancer or neoplasm is characterized by the uncontrolled growth of anaplastic cells that tend to invade surrounding tissue and to metastasize to distant body sites.

The tumor seen with cancer of the lip is usually called an **epithelioma.** It occurs most frequently as a chronic ulcer of the lower lip in men. The cure rate for cancer of the lips is high because the lesion is easily apparent to the patient and to others. Metastasis to regional lymph nodes has occurred in only 10% of people when diagnosed. In some instances a lesion may spread rapidly and involve the mandible and the floor of the mouth by direct extension. Occasionally the tumor may be a basal cell lesion that starts in the skin and spreads to the lip.

Cancer of the anterior tongue and floor of the mouth may seem to occur together because their spread to adjacent tissues is so rapid. Metastasis to the neck has already occurred in more than 60% of patients when the diagnosis is made because of the tongue's abundant vascular and lymphatic drainage. Recent investigation has revealed a higher incidence of cancers of the mouth and throat among people who are heavy drinkers and smokers. Also, data show that the mortality for young men between the ages of 10 and 20 has doubled over the past 30 years as a result of the use of smokeless tobacco (snuff). This combination of high alcohol consumption and smoking or chewing tobacco causes an apparent breakdown in the body's defense mechanism. Predisposing factors include exposure to the sun and wind, but more important is the progression of leukoplakia to an epidermoid lip cancer.

Clinical Manifestations

Leukoplakia (a white, firmly attached patch on the mouth or tongue mucosa) may appear on the lips and buccal mucosa. These nonsloughing lesions cannot be rubbed off by simple mechanical force. They can be benign or malignant. A small percentage develop into squamous cell carcinomas, and biopsy is recommended if the lesions persist for longer than 2 weeks. They occur most frequently between the ages of 50 and 70 years and appear more commonly in men.

Assessment

Collection of **subjective data** includes understanding that malignant lesions of the mouth are usually asymptomatic. The patient may feel only a roughened area with the tongue. As the disease progresses, the first complaints may be (1) difficulty in chewing, swallowing, or speaking; (2) edema, numbness, or loss of feeling in any part of the mouth; and (3) earache, facial pain, and toothache, which may become constant. Cancer of the lip is associated with discomfort and irritation caused by the presence of a nonhealing lesion that may be raised or ulcerated. Malignancy at the base of the tongue produces less obvious symptoms: slight dysphagia, sore throat, and salivation.

Collection of **objective data** includes observing for premalignant lesions, including leukoplakia (white patches). Unusual bleeding in the mouth, some blood-tinged sputum, lumps or edema in the neck, and hoarseness may be observed.

Diagnostic Tests

Indirect laryngoscopy is an important diagnostic test for examination of the soft tissue. This procedure is especially important for men 40 years of age or older who have dysphagia and a history of smoking and alcohol ingestion. Radiographic evaluation of the mandibular structures is also an essential part of the head and neck examination to rule out the presence of cancer. Excisional biopsy is the most accurate method for a definitive diagnosis. Oral exfoliative cytology is a means of screening intraoral lesions. A scraping of the lesion provides cells for cytologic examination. The chance for a false-negative finding is about 26%.

Medical Management

Treatment depends on the location and staging of the malignant tumor. Stage I oral cancers are treated by surgery or radiation. Stages II and III cancers require both surgery and radiation. Treatment for stage IV cancer is usually palliative. The survival rate for patients with oral cancers averages less than 50%.

Small, accessible tumors can be excised surgically and include a glossectomy, removal of the tongue; hemiglossectomy, removal of part of the tongue; mandibulectomy, removal of the mandible; and total or supraglottic laryngectomy, removal of the entire larynx or the portion above the true vocal cords.

Large tumors usually require more extensive and traumatic surgery. In a functional neck dissection of neck cancer with no growth in the lymph nodes, the lymph nodes are removed, but the jugular vein, sternocleidomastoid muscle, and spinal accessory nerve are preserved. In radical neck dissection, all these structures are removed and reconstructive surgery is necessary after tissue resection. These patients may have drains in the incision sites that are connected to suction to aid healing and reduce hematomas. A tracheostomy may also be performed, depending on the degree of tumor invasion.

Because of the location of the surgery, complications can occur. These include airway obstruction, hemorrhage, tracheal aspiration, facial edema, fistula formation, and necrosis of the skin flaps. Neurological complications can occur because of nerves being severed and manipulated during surgery.

Radiation may be in the form of external radiation by use of roentgenograms or other radioactive substances or in the form of internal radiation by means of needles or seeds. The purpose of radiation therapy is to shrink the tumor. It can be given preoperatively or postoperatively, depending on the physician's preference and the patient's disease process. In more advanced cases, chemotherapy may be combined with radiation postoperatively to make the patient more comfortable. Other treatment options include laser excision.

Nursing Interventions and Patient Teaching

It is important that the nurse have a holistic approach to the patient. This includes being aware of the patient's level of knowledge regarding the disease, the emotional response and coping abilities, and the spiritual needs. The nursing interventions must be individualized to the patient—beginning with the preoperative stage, continuing through the postoperative stage, and ending after the patient's rehabilitation in the home environment. Family members, hospice members, close friends, social workers, and pastoral care staff may be necessary for information and support during this potentially fatal disease.

Nursing diagnoses and interventions for the patient with oral cancer include but are not limited to the following:

Nursing Diagnoses	Nursing Interventions
Imbalanced nutrition, less than body requirements, related to oral pain or postoperative tissue loss (mucous membranes).	Monitor the patient for changes in the character and quantity of mucus after radiation therapy. Provide meticulous oral hygiene. Observe for temporary or permanent loss of taste and the need for alternative routes for nutrition by monitoring daily weights.
Disturbed body image and personal identity, related to disfiguring appearance of an oral lesion or reconstructive surgery	Provide alternative methods for communication if dysarthria (difficult, poorly articulated speech, resulting from interference in the control over muscles of speech) results from radiation treatment. Provide information to the patient and family to help with difficult decisions related to surgery, radiation, or chemotherapy. Be a support person to the patient and family.

Prevention centers on avoidance of predisposing factors: excess exposure to sun and wind on the lips, elimination of smoking or chewing tobacco, and maintenance of good oral and dental care. There is a high correlation between the incidence of cancer of the mouth and cirrhosis of the liver associated with alcohol intake. Early detection of oral cancer can help increase the patient's chance of survival. Any person with a mouth lesion that does not heal within 2 to 3 weeks is urged to seek immediate medical care. Preoperative and postoperative care must be taught to the surgical patient, with full explanations regarding speech loss and alternate methods of nutritional intake. Explanation of tracheostomy care and other tubes the patient may be discharged with will relieve anxiety and encourage the patient's control over the situation.

Prognosis

Staging and biologic characterization of the neoplasm provide prognostic information. The prognosis of carcinoma in the oral cavity is directly related to the size of the primary tumor, the involvement of regional nodes, and the presence or absence of metastasis. The patient's immunologic response and general condition also influence the prognosis and the choice of therapy.

Carcinomas of the lip can be detected early by the person, the physician, or the dentist during examination, and the prognosis for cure is good. If the carcinoma is difficult to detect, as on the anterior tongue and floor of the mouth, it will be in the more advanced stage when detected and the prognosis will be bleak. The 5-year survival rate for cancer of the oral cavity and pharynx is 53% for whites and 34% for African Americans.

DISORDERS OF THE ESOPHAGUS

GASTROESOPHAGEAL REFLUX DISEASE
Etiology/Pathophysiology

Gastroesophageal reflux disease (GERD) is a backward flow of stomach acid up into the esophagus. Symptoms typically include burning and pressure behind the sternum. Most cases are attributed to the inappropriate relaxation of the lower esophageal sphincter in response to an unknown stimulus. Reflux allows gastric contents to move back into the distal esophagus. Symptoms of GERD develop when the lower esophageal sphincter (LES) is weak or experiences prolonged or frequent transient relaxation, conditions that allow gastric acids and enzymes to flow into the esophagus. Reflux is much more common in the postprandial state (after meals); more than 60% of reflux sufferers have delayed gastric emptying. Gastroesophageal reflux disease occurs in all age groups and is estimated to affect up to 45% of the population to some degree, which translates to more than 60 million people.

Clinical Manifestations

The clinical manifestations of GERD are consistent in their nature, but they vary substantially in severity. The irritation of chronic reflux produces the primary symptom, which is heartburn **(pyrosis).** The pain is described as a substernal or retrosternal burning sensation that tends to radiate upward and may involve the neck, jaw, or back. The pain typically occurs 20 minutes to 2 hours after eating. An atypical pain pattern that closely mimics angina may also occur and needs to be carefully differentiated from true cardiac disease. The second major symptom of GERD is regurgitation, which is not associated with either eructation or nausea. The individual experiences a feeling of warm fluid moving up the throat. If it reaches the pharynx, a sour or bitter taste is perceived. Water brash, a reflux salivary hypersecretion that does not have a bitter taste, occurs less commonly.

In severe cases, GERD can produce dysphagia or odynophagia (painful swallowing). Eructation and a feeling of flatulence are other common complaints. Nocturnal cough, wheezing, or hoarseness all may occur with reflux, and it is estimated that greater than 80% of adult asthmatics may have reflux. The frequency and severity of reflux episodes usually determine the severity of the symptoms.

Assessment

Collection of **subjective data** includes heartburn, a substernal or retrosternal burning sensation that may radiate to the back or jaw (in some cases the pain may mimic angina); and regurgitation (not associated with nausea or eructation), in which a sour or bitter taste is perceived in the pharynx. Frequent eructation, flatulence, and dysphagia or odynophagia usually occurs only in severe cases.

Collection of **objective data** may include nocturnal cough, wheezing, and hoarseness.

Diagnostic Tests

Mild cases of GERD are diagnosed from the classic symptoms, and treatment is initiated based on the presumptive diagnosis. More involved cases may require other screening tools. The gold standard for diagnosis is 24-hour pH monitoring, which accurately records the number, duration, and severity of reflux episodes and is considered to be 85% sensitive. The esophageal motility and Bernstein tests can be performed in conjunction with pH monitoring to evaluate lower esophageal sphincter competence and the response of the esophagus to acid infusion. The barium swallow with fluoroscopy is widely used to document the presence of hiatal hernia. Endoscopy is routinely performed to evaluate the presence and severity of esophagitis and to rule out malignancy.

Medical Management

In its simplest form, GERD produces mild symptoms that occur only infrequently (twice a week or less). In these cases, avoiding problem foods or beverages, stopping smoking, or losing weight if needed may solve the problem. Additional treatment with antacids or acid-blocking medications called H_2 receptor antagonists—such as cimetidine (Tagamet), ranitidine (Zantac), famotidine (Pepcid), or nizatidine (Axid)—may also be used. More severe and frequent episodes of GERD can trigger asthma attacks, cause severe chest pain, result in bleeding, or promote a narrowing (stricture) or chronic irritation of the esophagus. In these cases, more powerful inhibitors of stomach acid production called proton pump inhibitors, such as omeprazole (Prilosec), esomeprazole (Nexium), pantoprazole (Protonix), rabeprazole (Aciphex), and lansoprazole (Prevacid), may be added to the treatment prescribed. Metoclopramide (Reglan) is used in moderate to severe cases of GERD. It is an example of a class of drugs called promotility agents that increase peristalsis without stimulating secretions. As a last resort, a surgical procedure called **fundoplication** is performed to strengthen the sphincter. The procedure involves wrapping a layer of the upper stomach wall around the sphincter and terminal esophagus to lessen the possibility of acid reflux (see Figure 5-16). If GERD is left untreated, serious pathologic (precancerous) changes in the esophageal lining may develop—a condition called **Barrett's esophagus.** In Barrett's esophagus there is replacement of the normal squamous epithelium of the esophagus with columnar epithelium. Because patients with Barrett's esophagus are at higher risk for adenocarcinoma, they may need to be monitored on a regular basis (every 1 to 3 years) by endoscopy and biopsy.

Nursing Interventions and Patient Teaching

Nursing intervention involves educating the patient about diet and lifestyle modifications that may alleviate symptoms of GERD:

- Diet
  Eat four to six small meals daily.
  Follow a low-fat, adequate-protein diet.
  Reduce intake of chocolate, tea, and all foods and beverages that contain caffeine.
  Limit or eliminate alcohol intake.
  Eat slowly, and chew food thoroughly.
  Avoid evening snacking, and do not eat for 2 to 3 hours before bedtime.
  Remain upright for 1 to 2 hours after meals when possible, and never eat in bed.
  Avoid any food that directly produces heartburn.
  Reduce overall body weight if indicated.
- Lifestyle
  Eliminate or drastically reduce smoking.
  Patients who smoke are encouraged to stop.
  Avoid constrictive clothing over the abdomen.

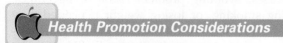
Health Promotion Considerations

Prevention or Early Detection of Esophageal Cancer

- Patients with diagnosed GERD and hiatal hernia need to be counseled regarding regular follow-up evaluation.
- Health considerations should focus on elimination of smoking and excessive alcohol intake.
- Maintenance of good oral hygiene and dietary habits (intake of fresh fruits and vegetables) may be helpful.
- Patients diagnosed with Barrett's esophagus need to be monitored because this is considered a premalignant condition. Regular endoscopic screening with biopsy may be needed.
- Patients are encouraged to seek medical attention for any esophageal problems, especially dysphagia.

Avoid activities that involve straining, heavy lifting, or working in a bent-over position.
Elevate the head of the bed at least 6 to 8 inches for sleep, using wooden blocks or a thick foam wedge.
Never sleep flat in bed.

Prognosis

If GERD is not successfully controlled, it can progress to serious and even life-threatening problems. Esophageal ulceration and hemorrhage may result from severe erosion, and chronic nighttime reflux is accompanied by a significant risk of aspiration. Adenocarcinoma can develop from the premalignant tissue (termed Barrett's epithelium). Gradual or repeated scarring can permanently damage esophageal tissue and produce stricture.

CARCINOMA OF THE ESOPHAGUS
Etiology/Pathophysiology

Carcinoma of the esophagus is a malignant epithelial neoplasm that has invaded the esophagus and has been diagnosed as the presence of a squamous cell carcinoma or an adenocarcinoma.

Estimates of the percentage of esophageal cancer that are adenocarcinomas range from 30% to 70%, with the remainder being squamous cell. The incidence of squamous cell esophageal cancer is currently decreasing in the United States, whereas the incidence of adenocarcinoma of the distal esophagus is increasing (Lewis et al, 2004). Risk factors for esophageal cancer include alcohol intake and tobacco use and possibly long-standing achalasia (an abnormal condition characterized by the inability of a muscle to relax, particularly the cardiac sphincter of the stomach). Environmental carcinogens, nutritional deficiencies, chronic irritation, and mucosal damage have all been considered as causes of esophageal cancer. Another risk factor is Barrett's esophagus. It is estimated that 1 of 200 cases of Barrett's esophagus will progress to esophageal adenocarcinoma (Health Considerations box). Unfortunately, because of the location, esophageal cancer is usually at a late stage when discovered and treatment is aimed toward comfort and control rather than cure. Carcinoma of the bronchus, stomach, or breast may metastasize to the esophagus. The prevalent age group for esophageal cancer is 55 to 70 years. It occurs more commonly in men.

Clinical Manifestations

The most common clinical symptom is progressive dysphagia (difficulty in swallowing) over a 6-month period, and may be expressed as a substernal feeling as if food is not passing.

Assessment

Collection of **subjective data** includes noting that initially the patient may have difficulty in swallowing when bulky foods are eaten; later it occurs with soft foods and finally with liquids and even saliva. Another symptom is odynophagia (painful swallowing). Pain is a late symptom and indicates local extension of the malignancy.

Collection of **objective data** includes the nurse observing the patient for regurgitation (a backward flowing or the casting up of undigested food), vomiting, hoarseness, chronic cough, and iron deficiency anemia. Weight loss may be directly related to the tumor or a side effect of treatment or the inability to swallow.

Diagnostic Tests

A barium swallow examination with fluoroscopy and endoscopy is used to detect esophageal cancer. A biopsy and cytologic examination provide a high degree of accuracy in the final diagnosis. Computed tomography (CT) and magnetic resonance imaging (MRI) also are used to assess the extent of the disease.

Medical Management

Tumor staging must be addressed to determine tumor size and patient management. In advanced cases, surgery is offered for palliative purposes to relieve dysphagia and restore continuity of the alimentary tract. An aggressive approach provides excellent palliation (therapy designed to relieve or reduce intensity of uncomfortable symptoms but not to produce a cure), increased longevity, and a chance for a cure. Standard resection seems to give as good a result as a radical procedure.

Radiation therapy may be curative or palliative. Special problems associated with radiation therapy include the development of an esophagotracheal fistula (an abnormal passage between two internal organs). Aspiration from the fistula and edema from the radiation must be anticipated. Chemotherapeutic agents cisplatin (Platinol), paclitaxel (Taxol), and 5-FU in combination with radiation before and/or after surgery are currently used. If the tumor is in the upper third of the esophagus, radiation is indicated. A tumor in the lower third is usually resected surgically. Because of the extreme toxicity of these drugs, side effects of respiratory and liver dysfunction, nausea and vomiting, leukopenia, and sepsis can be anticipated. The following four types of surgical procedures can be performed:

1. **Esophagogastrectomy:** resection of a lower esophageal section with a proximal portion of the stomach, followed by anastomosis (a surgical joining of two ducts or blood vessels to allow flow from one to the other) of the remaining portions of esophagus and stomach
2. **Esophagogastrostomy:** resection of a portion of the esophagus with anastomosis to the stomach
3. **Esophagoenterostomy:** resection of the esophagus and anastomosis to a portion of the colon
4. **Gastrostomy:** insertion of a catheter into the stomach and suture to the abdominal wall; performed when it is assumed that the patient will not be able to take food orally because of inoperable cancer of the esophagus interfering with swallowing

Nursing Interventions and Patient Teaching

Nursing diagnoses and interventions for the patient with esophageal carcinoma include but are not limited to the following:

Nursing Diagnoses	Nursing Interventions
Ineffective breathing pattern, related to incisional pain and proximity to the diaphragm	Monitor respirations carefully because of proximity of incision to diaphragm and patient's difficulty in carrying out breathing exercises.
Imbalanced nutrition: less than body requirements, related to dysphagia, decreased stomach capacity, anorexia	Monitor I&O and daily weights to determine adequate nutritional intake. Assess patient to determine which foods patient can and cannot swallow to select and prepare edible foods. Administer gastrostomy tube feedings, if present.

The nurse should discuss with the patient and family all aspects of care, including surgery, radiation, and chemotherapy if necessary. Psychological adjustment of the patient who cannot ingest food orally, whether temporary or permanent, is difficult. Step-by-step explanations of all diagnostic tests, medications, procedures, and the treatment plan will help decrease the patient's anxiety. The nurse should support the patient with this serious diagnosis by allowing time for questions.

Prognosis

In carcinoma of the esophagus, the disease is usually well advanced by the time symptoms exist. The delay between the onset of early symptoms and the time when the patient seeks medical advice is often 12 to 18 months. High mortality rates among these patients are affected by the following issues: (1) the patient is generally older, (2) the tumor has usually invaded surrounding structures, (3) the malignancy tends to spread to nearby lymph nodes, and (4) the location of the esophagus in relation to the heart and lungs makes these organs accessible to the extension of the tumor.

The esophagus, with its extensive lymphatic network, facilitates the rapid spread of malignant cells to varying local and distant sites. Carcinoma of the esophagus has a 5-year survival rate of 12%. The only prognostic variable is the stage of disease (an indication of the importance of early diagnosis).

ACHALASIA
Etiology/Pathophysiology

Achalasia, also called **cardiospasm,** is an abnormal condition characterized by the inability of a muscle to relax, particularly the cardiac sphincter of the stomach.

Although the cause is unknown, nerve degeneration, esophageal dilation, and hypertrophy are thought to contribute to the disruption of the normal neuromuscular activity of the esophagus. This results in decreased motility of the lower portion of the esophagus, absence of peristalsis, and dilation of the lower portion. Thus little or no food can enter the stomach, and in extreme cases, the dilated portion of the esophagus can hold as much as a liter or more of fluid. This disease may occur in people of any age, but it is more prevalent in those between 20 and 50 years.

Clinical Manifestations

The primary symptom of achalasia is dysphagia. The patient has a sensation of food sticking in the lower portion of the esophagus. As the condition progresses, the patient complains of regurgitation of food, which relieves prolonged distention of the esophagus. There may be some occurrence of substernal chest pain.

Assessment

The nurse should observe for loss of weight, poor skin turgor, and weakness.

Diagnostic Tests

Radiologic studies show esophageal dilation above the narrowing at the cardioesophageal junction. The diagnosis is confirmed by manometry, which shows the absence of primary peristalsis. Esophagoscopy is also used to confirm the diagnosis.

Medical Management

The conservative treatment of achalasia includes drug therapy and forceful dilation of the narrowed area of the esophagus. Anticholinergics, nitrates, and calcium channel blockers reduce pressure in the lower esophageal sphincter.

Dilation is done by first emptying the esophagus. Then a dilator with a deflated balloon is passed down to the sphincter. The balloon is inflated and remains so for 1 minute; it may need to be reinflated once or twice.

A cardiomyotomy is the preferred surgical approach. In this procedure the muscular layer is incised longitudinally down to but not through the mucosa. Two thirds of the incision is in the esophagus, and the remaining one third is in the stomach; this permits the mucosa to expand so that food can pass easily into the stomach.

Nursing Interventions and Patient Teaching

Nursing interventions for esophageal surgery are presented in Box 5-3.

Box 5-3 *Nursing Interventions for the Person Experiencing Esophageal Surgery*

PREOPERATIVE NURSING INTERVENTIONS
1. Encourage improved nutritional status.
   a. High-protein, high-calorie diet if oral diet is possible.
   b. Total parenteral nutrition may be necessary for severe dysphagia or obstruction.
   c. Gastroscopy tube feedings if indicated.
2. Give meticulous oral hygiene; breath may be malodorous.
3. Give preoperative preparation appropriate for thoracic surgery.
4. Give prescribed antibiotics before esophageal resection or bypass, as ordered.

POSTOPERATIVE NURSING INTERVENTIONS
1. Promote good pulmonary ventilation.
2. Maintain chest drainage system as prescribed.
3. Maintain gastric drainage system.
   a. Small amounts of blood may drain from nasogastric tube for 6 to 12 hours after surgery.
   b. Do not disturb nasogastric tube (to prevent traction on suture line).
4. Maintain nutrition.
   a. Start clear fluids at frequent intervals when oral intake is permitted.
   b. Introduce soft foods gradually to several small meals of bland foods.
   c. Have patient maintain semi-Fowler's position for 2 hours after eating and while sleeping if heartburn (pyrosis) occurs.

Nursing diagnoses and interventions for the patient with achalasia include but are not limited to the following:

NURSING DIAGNOSES	NURSING INTERVENTIONS
Imbalanced nutrition: less than body requirements, related to difficulty swallowing both liquids and solids	Encourage fluids with meals to increase lower esophageal sphincter pressure and push food into stomach. Monitor liquid diet for 24 hours after dilation procedure.
Anxiety, related to continuous dilation process with threat of complications	Monitor for signs of esophageal perforation (chest pain, shock, dyspnea, fever) after dilation. Provide calm, nonstressful environment. Reinforce physician's explanation of disease process. Encourage verbalization of fears; assist patient with identifying stressors and positive coping behaviors.

Home care and follow-up care should be discussed in preparation for dismissal. A family member or support person should be included if possible, and patient should be an active participant in the planning. The following teaching should be included:

- Explain need for high-calorie, high-protein diet, and provide printed material describing same.
- Explain need to elevate head while sleeping and to avoid bending and stooping.
- Discuss medications if prescribed: name, dosage, time of administration, purpose, and side effects.
- Discuss methods of avoiding constipation by using high-fiber foods if tolerated and natural laxatives.
- Explain importance of follow-up care with physician.
- Discuss symptoms of recurrence or progression of disease and need to report these to physician.

Prognosis

Esophageal motility is not restored by dilation procedure, but the open sphincter relieves the dysphagia in about 80% of cases, and the esophageal lumen is reduced in size. Surgical separation, in addition to bag dilation, permits normal peristalsis to return in approximately 10% of patients with achalasia.

DISORDERS OF THE STOMACH

GASTRITIS (ACUTE)
Etiology/Pathophysiology

Gastritis is an inflammation of the lining of the stomach. Acute gastritis refers to a temporary inflammation associated with alcoholism, smoking, and stressful physical problems, such as burns; major surgery; food allergens; presence of viral, bacterial, or chemical toxins; chemotherapy; or radiation therapy. Changes in the mucosal lining interfere with acid and pepsin secretion. Acute gastritis is often a single occurrence that resolves when the offending agent is removed.

Clinical Manifestations

If the condition is acute, fever, epigastric pain, nausea, vomiting, headache, coating of the tongue, and loss of appetite may occur. If the condition results from ingestion of contaminated food, the intestines are usually affected and diarrhea may occur.

Assessment

Collection of **subjective data** involves observing for anorexia, nausea, discomfort after eating, and pain, although some patients with gastritis have no symptoms.

Collection of **objective data** includes observing for vomiting, hematemesis, and melena caused by gastric bleeding.

Diagnostic Tests

Testing the stools for occult blood, noting WBC differential increases related to certain bacteria, evaluating serum electrolytes, and observing for elevated hematocrit related to dehydration all aid in the diagnosis.

Medical Management

If medical treatment is required, antiemetic—such as prochlorperazine (Compazine) or trimethobenzamide (Tigan)—may be prescribed. Antacids and cimetidine (Tagamet) or ranitidine (Zantac) may be given in combination. Antibiotics are given if the cause is a bacterial agent. Intravenous fluids are used to correct fluid and electrolyte imbalances. Patients who experience GI bleeding from hemorrhagic gastritis require fluid and blood replacement and nasogastric lavage.

Nursing Interventions and Patient Teaching

The nurse records the patient's I&O. Foods and fluids are withheld orally as prescribed until the signs and symptoms subside. The nurse should monitor the patient's tolerance to oral feedings. The nurse will monitor the intravenous feedings as prescribed.

Nursing diagnosis and interventions for the patient with gastritis include but are not limited to the following:

NURSING DIAGNOSIS	NURSING INTERVENTIONS
Deficient fluid volume, related to vomiting, diarrhea, and blood loss	Keep patient NPO or on restricted food and fluids as ordered, and advance as tolerated. Monitor laboratory data for fluid and electrolyte imbalance (potassium, magnesium, sodium, and chloride). Maintain intravenous feedings. Record I&O.

Patient education should include an explanation of (1) the effects of stress on the mucosal lining of the stomach; (2) how salicylates, nonsteroidal antiinflammatory medications, and particular foods may be irritating; and (3) how lifestyles that include alcohol and tobacco may be harmful. The nurse should be able to assist the patient in locating self-help groups in the community to deal with these stressful behaviors.

Prognosis

Because of the many classifications and causes of gastritis, prognosis is variable. Generally, prognosis is good in individuals who are willing to change their lifestyles and follow a medical regimen.

PEPTIC ULCERS

Peptic ulcers are ulcerations of the mucous membrane or deeper structures of the GI tract. They most commonly occur in the stomach and duodenum. The term peptic ulcer refers to ulcers that are the result of acid and pepsin imbalances.

Peptic ulcer disease remains a major health problem and affects more men than women. The older adult reflects an increase in this disease, perhaps as a result of the use of nonsteroidal antiinflammatory drugs. Symptoms are common between the ages of 25 to 50, with the peak occurrence at age 40. Peptic ulcers require the presence of gastric acid and result from four major causes: (1) an excess of gastric acid (duodenal ulcers), (2) decrease in the natural ability of the GI mucosa to protect itself from acid and pepsin (gastric ulcers), (3) infection with spiral-shaped bacteria *Helicobacter pylori,* and (4) gastric injury from NSAIDs, aspirin, and corticosteroids.

The understanding of the factors that contribute to ulcer formation is developing rapidly at the present time. The discovery of the bacterium *H. pylori* provides a new understanding of ulcer formation. *H. pylori* is thought to be a dominant factor in the promotion of peptic ulcer formation. *H. pylori* has been identified in more than 70% of gastric ulcer patients and 95% of those with duodenal ulcers. In Western cultures, half of all people older than age 50 harbor *H. pylori,* yet most do not develop peptic ulcer disease. Scientists still have to determine what triggers ulcers in those with *H. pylori.*

A common belief is that people exhibiting certain traits such as tenseness or a striving for perfection or success are more likely to develop peptic ulcers. Conclusive evidence to support this belief is lacking.

GASTRIC ULCERS
Etiology/Pathophysiology

The most common site of a gastric ulcer is in the distal half of the stomach. The cause of gastric ulcer is not clear. There are relationships between factors such as diet, genetic predisposition, ingestion of excessive amounts of salicylates, NSAIDs, the use of tobacco, and *H. pylori* with increased incidence of gastric ulcers. Once the gastric mucosal barrier is damaged, acid secretion is stimulated. Without intervention, the cells die, erosion occurs, and ulcers develop. Gastric mucosal damage can occur in some individuals within 1 hour after the ingestion of acetylsalicylic acid. Reflux of duodenal contents (bile acids) also causes severe gastric mucosal damage. Gastric ulcers may occur on the surface of a gastric tumor because of interference with the blood supply.

PHYSIOLOGIC STRESS ULCERS

Physiologic stress ulcers are acute ulcers that develop following a major physiologic insult such as trauma or surgery. A stress ulcer is a form of erosive gastritis. It is believed that the gastric mucosa of the body of the stomach undergoes a period of transient ischemia in association with hypotension, severe injury, extensive burns, and complicated surgery. The ischemia is due to decreased capillary blood flow or shunting of blood away from the GI tract so that blood flow bypasses the gastric mucosa. This occurs as a compensatory mechanism in hypotension or shock. The decrease in blood flow produces an imbalance between the destructive properties of hydrochloric acid and pepsin and protective factors of the stomach's mucosal barrier, especially in the fundus portion, resulting in ulceration. Multiple superficial erosions result, and these may bleed.

DUODENAL ULCERS
Etiology/Pathophysiology

The term *duodenal ulcer* is given to a group of disorders that may or may not be caused by hypersecretion. Excessive production or excessive release of gastrin or increased sensitivity to gastrin is found in 40% of people with these ulcers. In the other 60%, the amount of acid produced is normal but perhaps the buffering ability is lacking in the duodenum. Risk factors include *H. pylori* infection, NSAIDs, cigarette smoking, and coffee. The organism *H. pylori* is implicated in the development of duodenal ulcers. Ulceration occurs when the acid secretion exceeds the buffering factors.

Clinical Manifestations

Both gastric and duodenal ulcers may have similar symptoms but differ in timing, degree, or factors that worsen or alleviate the symptoms. Pain is the characteristic symptom and is described as dull, burning, boring, or gnawing; it is located in the midline of the epigastric region.

Assessment

Collection of **subjective data** requires an awareness that, in gastric ulcer patients, the pain is closely associated with food intake and usually does not awaken the patient at night like the pain experienced by those with duodenal ulcers. Nausea, eructation, and distention are common complaints, termed **dyspepsia.** All these subjective symptoms intensify if the complications of perforation and obstruction are manifested.

Collection of **objective data** includes observing for hemorrhage, a common complication with gastric ulcers; more gastric ulcers bleed than do duodenal ulcers. Duodenal ulcers are more apt to have chronic bleeding and are more prone to perforate than gastric ulcers.

When GI bleeding occurs, one sign is vomiting blood (**hematemesis**) that has a "coffee grounds" appearance as a result of action of the gastric acid on the hemoglobin molecule. There may be presence of **melena** (tarlike, fetid-smelling stool containing undigested blood) when the blood becomes black and tarry as it passes through the digestive tract. In extreme cases, bright red blood may be passed rectally. Both salicylates and alcohol aggravate bleeding in patients with a history of peptic ulcers.

Bleeding from a gastric ulcer is more difficult to control than bleeding from a duodenal ulcer. Hemorrhage, with accompanying symptoms of shock, occurs when the ulcer erodes into a blood vessel. Surgical intervention is indicated if the patient remains unstable after receiving blood over several hours.

Perforation occurs when the ulcer crater penetrates the entire thickness of the wall of the stomach or duodenum. The release of gastric acid, pancreatic enzymes, or bile causes signs and symptoms of pain, emesis, fever, hypotension, and hematemesis. Perforation is considered the most lethal complication of peptic ulcer.

Gastric outlet obstruction is a complication of peptic ulcer disease that can occur at any time. Gastric outlet obstruction occurs more often in the patient whose ulcer is located close to the pylorus. Relief of symptoms may be achieved by constant NG aspiration of stomach contents. This allows edema and inflammation to subside and then permits normal flow of gastric contents through the pylorus.

Diagnostic Tests

Fiberoptic endoscopy can detect both gastric and duodenal ulcers. This is called **esophagogastroduodenoscopy.**

Fiberoptic endoscopy is the procedure most often used. It is more reliable than barium contrast studies because of the maneuverability of fiberoptic scopes for viewing the entire esophagus and gastric and duodenal mucosa. This procedure also can be used to determine the degree of ulcer healing after treatment. During endoscopy, specimens can be obtained for identification of *H. pylori*. When gastric malignancy is a possibility, the endoscope can be used in obtaining tissue specimens for biopsy. The patient is sedated but remains conscious throughout the endoscopy procedure. Local anesthetics are used to anesthetize the throat, decrease the gag reflex, and minimize pain during the procedure. No liquids or food are allowed for 1 to 2 hours or until the patient can swallow.

In September 1996 the U.S. Food and Drug Administration (FDA) approved a breath test to detect *H. pylori*. The test calls for the patient to drink a solution containing 13 carbon–enriched urea, a natural, nonradioactive substance. If *H. pylori* is present, it breaks down the compound and releases 13 carbon dioxide ($13\ CO_2$). Thirty minutes after drinking the solution, the patient exhales into a collection bag, which is sent to the manufacturer for analysis. A finding of $13\ CO_2$ confirms *H. pylori* infection. The test may prove especially useful after a patient receives antibiotic therapy, to determine whether the *H. pylori* infection has been eradicated. A serum test for *H. pylori* antibodies and breath testing are reliable, noninvasive methods if the patient has mild or occasional symptoms. Another noninvasive test to confirm *H. pylori* infection includes serum or whole blood antibody test, in particular, immunoglobulin G (IgG). This test is approximately 90% to 95% sensitive for *H. pylori* infection. This test cannot distinguish active from recently treated disease.

Radiologic studies (UGI) are not as specific for small lesions but are still commonly used. Hematest of feces for detecting occult blood in the intestinal tract may also be used for diagnosis.

Medical Management

The physician may order a nasogastric tube to be inserted to remove gastric content and blood. Surgery is indicated usually for complications: perforation, penetration, obstruction, or intractability (no longer responding to medical management).

Scar tissue builds up with repeat episodes of ulceration and healing, causing obstruction, particularly at the pylorus. The patient may present with gastric dilation, vomiting, and distention. When fluid and electrolyte balance is achieved, surgical intervention is possible.

The primary treatment for peptic ulcers is to reduce signs and symptoms by decreasing or neutralizing normal gastric acidity with drug therapy. The types of drugs most commonly used include the following (see the Medications table).

- **Antacids:** neutralize or reduce the acidity of the stomach contents; these are Maalox, Gaviscon, Rolaids, Tums, Mylanta, and Riopan.
- **Histamine H$_2$ receptor blockers:** decrease acid secretions by blocking the histamine H$_2$ receptors; these include cimetidine (Tagamet), ranitidine (Zantac), famotidine (Pepcid), and nizatidine (Axid). Do not give histamine receptor antagonists within 2 hours of antacids.
- **Proton pump inhibitor:** antisecretory agent to inhibit secretion of gastrin by the parietal cells of the stomach; this includes omeprazole (Prilosec), lansoprazole (Prevacid), and pantoprazole (Protonix), and esomeprazole (Nexium).
- **Mucosal healing agents:** heal ulcers without antisecretory properties, possibly by adhering to the proteins in the ulcer base; this includes sucralfate (Carafate).
- **Antisecretory and cytoprotective:** inhibits gastric acid secretion and protects gastric mucosa; this includes misoprostol (Cytotec). Cytotec is the only drug approved in the United States for the prevention of gastric ulcers induced by NSAIDs and aspirin.

Text continued on p. 217

MEDICATIONS | *Gastrointestinal Disorders*

MEDICATION	TRADE NAME	ACTION	SIDE EFFECTS	NURSING IMPLICATIONS
Antacids (aluminum, calcium, and magnesium salts and sodium bicarbonate are all used)	Maalox, Mylanta, Titralac, Alternagel, others	Neutralizes gastric acid; aluminum and calcium antacids also bind phosphates in renal failure patients	Aluminum—constipation, hypophosphatemia; calcium—constipation, rebound hyperacidity, hypercalcemia; magnesium—diarrhea, hypermagnesemia; sodium bicarbonate—sodium and water retention, alkalosis, rebound hyperacidity	Monitor serum electrolytes with long-term use; do not give antacid simultaneously with other medications because absorption of the other medication may be affected; best to separate administration by 2 hours.
Antispasmodics (includes atropine, scopolamine, hyoscyamine, dicyclomine, clidinium, others)	Donnatal, Bentyl, others	Anticholinergic agents that decrease GI motility by relaxing GI smooth muscle	Dry mouth and skin, constipation, paralytic ileus, urinary retention, tachycardia, drowsiness, dizziness, confusion, altered vision	Avoid using other CNS depressants or alcohol concomitantly; avoid driving or other potentially hazardous tasks until accustomed to sedating effects.
Bismuth subsalicylate	Pepto-Bismol	Antidiarrheal agent, also used in peptic ulcer disease due to *Helicobacter pylori*	Fecal impaction, tinnitus	May turn stools dark gray-black; avoid use with aspirin; consult physician if diarrhea is accompanied by high fever or lasts more than 2 days.
Cimetidine	Tagamet	H$_2$ receptor antagonist; inhibits gastric acid secretion	Confusion, headache, gynecomastia, bone marrow suppression (rare)	Increases serum levels and clinical effects of oral anticoagulants, theophylline, phenytoin, some benzodiazepines, and propranolol (these medications may require dosage reduction).
Dimenhydrinate	Dramamine, others	Antiemetic agent; blocks central vomiting center	Drowsiness, dry mouth, constipation	Avoid use with other CNS depressants and alcohol; avoid driving or other hazardous activities until accustomed to sedating effects.
Diphenoxylate/atropine	Lomotil	Antidiarrheal agent (diphenoxylate—narcotic, atropine—anticholinergic)	Drowsiness, sedation, constipation, dry mouth, urinary retention	Avoid use with other CNS depressants and alcohol; avoid driving or other hazardous activities until accustomed to sedating effects; do not use in infectious diarrhea.

MEDICATIONS | *Gastrointestinal Disorders—cont'd*

MEDICATION	TRADE NAME	ACTION	SIDE EFFECTS	NURSING IMPLICATIONS
Famotidine	Pepcid	H₂ receptor antagonist; inhibits gastric acid secretion	Headache, dizziness, constipation thrombocytopenia (rare)	Unlike cimetidine, does not affect serum levels of hepatically metabolized drugs (warfarin, phenytoin, theophylline).
Kaolin-pectin	Kaopectate	Antidiarrheal agent	Constipation	Shake well before using.
Ketoconazole	Nizoral	Antifungal agent	Gynecomastia, impotence, hepatotoxicity, abdominal pain	Requires acid environment for absorption; do not use with antacids, H₂ receptor blockers, or omeprazole; do not use with terfenadine, astemizole, or loratadine—has caused dysrhythmias and death; monitor liver function tests often; monitor serum levels and clinical effects of warfarin, cyclosporine, and theophylline.
Lansoprazole	Prevacid	Binds to an enzyme in the presence of acid gastric pH, preventing the final transport of hydrogen ions into the gastric lumen	Drowsiness, abdominal pain, diarrhea, nausea	Sucralfate (Carafate) decreases absorption of Prevacid (take 30 min before Carafate); administer before meals. Assess patient routinely for epigastric or abdominal pain. May cause abnormal liver function tests.
Loperamide	Imodium	Antidiarrheal agent	Drowsiness, dry mouth, constipation	Monitor for dehydration; do not use in infectious diarrhea.
Mesalamine	Rowasa, Asachol	GI antiinflammatory agent	Abdominal cramps and gas, rash, headache, dizziness	Swallow tablets whole; give enema at bedtime, retain 10-15 min.
Misoprostol	Cytotec	Prostaglandin analogue that acts as gastric mucosal protectant, protects against NSAID-induced ulcers	Diarrhea, nausea, vomiting, flatulence, uterine cramping	Absolutely contraindicated in pregnant women; women of childbearing age must use reliable contraception.

Continued

MEDICATIONS | *Gastrointestinal Disorders—cont'd*

MEDICATION	TRADE NAME	ACTION	SIDE EFFECTS	NURSING IMPLICATIONS
Nizatidine	Axid	H_2 receptor antagonist, inhibits gastric acid secretion	Drowsiness, headache, dizziness, sweating, thrombocytopenia (rare)	Does not affect serum levels of hepatically metabolized drugs (warfarin, phenytoin, theophylline).
Nystatin	Mycostatin, Nilstat, others	Antifungal agent, available as oral suspension and topical product	Oral: nausea, vomiting, diarrhea; topical: local irritation	Long-term therapy may be needed to clear infection; use for entire course.
Olsalazine	Dipentum	GI antiinflammatory agent	Diarrhea, abdominal pain and cramps, nausea, allergic reactions, arthralgia, rash, anaphylaxis	Take with food; notify physician if severe diarrhea occurs.
Omeprazole	Prilosec	Proton pump inhibitor, totally eradicates gastric acid production	Headache, dizziness, abdominal pain, nausea, vomiting, rare bone marrow suppression	Inhibits hepatic metabolism of warfarin, phenytoin, benzodiazepines, and other drugs metabolized by liver; do not crush or chew capsule contents.
Ranitidine	Zantac	H_2 receptor antagonist; inhibits gastric acid secretion	Headache, abdominal discomfort, granulocytopenia and thrombocytopenia (both rare)	Minimal effect on serum levels of hepatically metabolized drugs (phenytoin, warfarin, theophylline).
Sucralfate	Carafate	Gastric mucosal protectant agent; adheres to site of ulcer	Constipation, hypophosphatemia	Do not give with other drugs; coating action may interfere with the absorption of other drugs—separate by 2 hours.
Sulfasalazine	Azulfidine	GI antiinflammatory agent	Nausea, vomiting, abdominal pain, photosensitivity, rash, Stevens-Johnson syndrome (rare), renal failure, bone marrow suppression (rare), allergic reactions, anaphylaxis	Ensure adequate hydration to prevent crystallization in kidneys; avoid exposure to sunlight; women on oral contraceptives need to use alternative methods because of decreased effectiveness of oral contraceptives, may increase effect; monitor CBC, renal function; take with meals.

Antibiotic therapy eradicates *H. pylori*. This includes metronidazole (Flagyl), tetracycline, amoxicillin, and clarithromycin (Biaxin). Treatment is typically combined in therapeutic regimen with other medications, such as bismuth or omeprazole (Prilosec). Another drug combination has entered the battle against *H. pylori*. It is a combination of bismuth, metronidazol (Flagyl), and tetracycline. Marketed under the brand name Helidac, the medication kit contains a 14-day supply of the three drugs, with each daily dose packaged on a blister card to improve patient compliance.

Among patients whose *H. pylori* is treated with antibiotics, the peptic ulcer recurrence may be as low as 2%. Patients who do not receive antibiotics have a relapse rate of 75% to 90%.

Dietary modification may be necessary so that foods and beverages irritating to the patient can be avoided or eliminated. There is considerable controversy over the actual therapeutic benefits derived from a bland diet, because the rationale is not supported by scientific evidence. Therefore it is recommended that smaller meals be taken more frequently throughout the day to decrease the degree of gastric motor activity.

Smoking has an irritating effect on the mucosa, increases gastric motility, and delays mucosal healing. Smoking should be eliminated completely or severely reduced. The combination of adequate rest and cessation of smoking accelerates ulcer healing. Because caffeinated and decaffeinated coffee, tobacco, alcohol, and aspirin aggravate the mucosal lining of the stomach and duodenum, an effort should be made to change the lifestyle of the patient with ulcers.

Surgery is usually indicated for complications. Surgical intervention has decreased drastically with more effective diagnosis and medical treatment. Approximately 20% of patients with ulcers require surgical intervention. Types of surgical procedures include the following:

- **Antrectomy:** removal of the entire antrum, the gastric-producing portion of the lower stomach, to eliminate the main stimuli to acid production.
- **Gastroduodenostomy (Billroth I)** (Figure 5-6, *A*): fundus of the stomach is directly anastomosed to the duodenum; used to remove ulcers or cancer located in the antrum of the stomach.
- **Gastrojejunostomy (Billroth II)** (see Figure 5-6, *B*): duodenum is closed, and the fundus of the stomach is anastomosed into the jejunum; used to remove ulcers or cancer located in the body of the fundus.
- **Total gastrectomy:** removal of the entire stomach; rarely used for patients with gastric cancer.
- **Vagotomy:** removal of the vagal innervation to the fundus, decreasing acid produced by the parietal cells of the stomach. Vagotomy is usually done with a Billroth I or II procedure (Figure 5-7).
- **Pyloroplasty:** surgical enlargement of the pylorus to provide drainage of the gastric contents.

The decision as to which procedure to use is difficult; the choice depends on physician preference and results of diagnostic testing. Regardless of the procedure selected, postoperative complications can occur.

Bleeding may occur up to 7 days after gastric surgery. Abdominal rigidity, abdominal pain, restless-

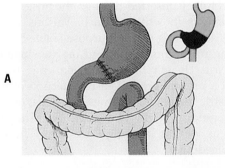
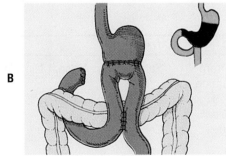

FIGURE **5-6** Types of gastric resections with anastomoses. **A,** Billroth I. **B,** Billroth II.

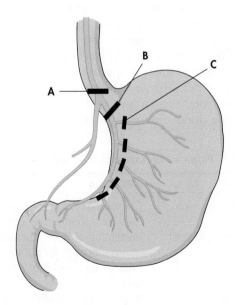

FIGURE **5-7** Types of vagotomies. *A,* Truncal. *B,* Selective. *C,* Proximal or parietal cell.

ness, an elevated temperature, increase in pulse, decrease in blood pressure, and leukocytosis are all possible indications of postoperative bleeding. The amount and type of drainage from the incision must be noted. Surgical intervention may be necessary to correct the bleeding.

Dumping syndrome is a rapid gastric emptying causing distention of the duodenum or jejunum produced by a bolus of hypertonic food. Increased intestinal motility and peristalsis and changes in blood glucose levels occur. Diaphoresis, nausea, vomiting, epigastric pain, explosive diarrhea, borborygmi (noises made from gas passing through the liquid of the small intestine), and dyspepsia may be reported by patients. Dumping syndrome can occur after gastric resection procedures. Approximately one third to one half of patients experience dumping syndrome after peptic ulcer surgery. Treatment includes eating six small meals daily that are high in protein and fat and low in carbohydrates, eating slowly, and avoiding fluids during meals. Treatment also includes (1) anticholinergic agents to decrease stomach motility, and (2) reclining for approximately 1 hour after meals.

Several other complications after gastric surgery present serious health threats. Diarrhea is common and usually responds to conservative treatment of controlled diet and antidiarrheal agents. Diphenoxylate (Lomotil), Imodium, paregoric, or codeine is often used. Reflux esophagitis and nutritional deficits—including weight loss, malabsorption, anemia, and vitamin deficiency—can also be life threatening.

Pernicious anemia is a serious potential complication in any patient who has had a total gastrectomy or extensive resections. This is caused by a deficiency of the intrinsic factor, produced exclusively by the stomach, that aids intestinal absorption of vitamin B_{12}. It is recommended that all patients with a partial gastrectomy have a blood serum vitamin B_{12} level measured every 1 to 2 years so that replacement therapy can be instituted before anemia appears. The most common cause of anemia after gastric surgery is iron deficiency. Iron-deficiency anemia is caused by impaired absorption in the duodenum and proximal jejunum as a re-

sult of rapid gastric emptying. Replacement therapy consists of oral iron in the ferrous form.

Nursing Interventions and Patient Teaching

Nasogastric (NG) tube insertion, irrigation, and GI suctioning are often performed while a patient is feeling ill and uncomfortable. In addition to being skilled and knowledgeable in performing these procedures, the nurse is responsible for allaying the patient's fears and anxieties. Eliciting patient cooperation not only makes the procedures easier but also helps reduce patient discomfort.

An understanding of the following points will enable the nurse to help patients through the experience of GI intubation:

- For most patients, GI intubation is a new and frightening experience.
- Inability to chew, taste, and swallow food and liquids may contribute to patient anxieties during GI intubation.
- A patient with an NG or intestinal tube is usually on NPO status. Occasionally ice chips are allowed.
- An NG tube is connected to either continuous or intermittent suctioning, usually at 100 mm Hg.
- The presence of an NG or intestinal tube is a constant irritant to the nasopharynx and nares, requiring frequent care to the mouth and nose.
- A patient with a GI tube may be afraid that moving will dislodge the tube. The nurse must implement frequent position changes to enhance tube functioning and prevent complications of immobility.

An NG tube is inserted through the nose, pharynx, and esophagus into the stomach. Various tubes are available, depending on the purpose (Table 5-1).

Nursing interventions depend on the stage of the ulcer disease. The emphasis on patient care should always be on prevention and early detection of pain in the epigastric region, hematemesis, melena, or tenderness and rigidity of the abdomen. (See Therapeutic Dialogue as well as Nursing Care Plan: The Patient with GI Bleeding.)

Table 5-1 *Purposes of Nasogastric Intubation*

PURPOSE	DESCRIPTION	TYPE OF TUBE
Decompression	Removal of secretions and gaseous substances from GI tract; prevention or relief of abdominal distention	Salem sump, Levin, Miller-Abbott
Feeding (gavage)	Instillation of liquid nutritional supplements or feedings into stomach for patients unable to swallow fluid	Duo, Dubhoff, Levin
Compression	Internal application of pressure by means of inflated balloon to prevent internal GI hemorrhage	Sengstaken-Blakemore
Lavage	Irrigation of stomach in cases of active bleeding, poisoning, or gastric dilation	Levin, Ewald, Salem sump

Nursing diagnoses and interventions for the specific stages of ulcer care include but are not limited to the following:

NURSING DIAGNOSES	NURSING INTERVENTIONS
Peptic ulcer disease	
Deficient knowledge, related to medications, diet, and signs and symptoms of bleeding, perforation, or gastric outlet obstruction	Provide verbal and written instructions on exact dosage and time intervals for medications and if medication is taken with or without food. Have dietitian provide instructions on therapeutic diet. Explain that repeat episodes are not uncommon; listen carefully for aggravating factors.
Pain, related to gastric acid on ulceration of gastric or duodenal mucosa	Give prescribed histamine H₂ receptor antagonists—cimetidine (Tagamet), ranitidine (Zantac), famotidine (Pepcid), or nizatidine (Axid)—with meals and at bedtime. Give prescribed antacid 1 and 3 hours after meals. Teach relaxation measures as appropriate. Instruct patient on side effects of antacid drugs (constipation or diarrhea) and importance of contacting physician if this occurs.
Noncompliance, related to risk behaviors (use of tobacco/alcohol) and dietary patterns	Assess patient's level of knowledge regarding food and other irritants to mucosal lining. Teach preventive measures, such as quitting smoking. Explain need for small and frequent meals. Caution patient to avoid high-fiber foods, sugar, salt, caffeine, and alcohol, as well as milk. Remind to take fluids between meals, not with meals. Explain to eat slowly and chew food well. Discuss importance of adequate rest and exercise.
Imbalanced nutrition: less than body requirements, related to preoperative food and fluid restrictions	Maintain NPO status. Connect NG tube to intermittent suction apparatus. Note color and amount of gastric output every 4 hours. Do not reposition tube. Maintain patency of tube by irrigation with measured amounts of saline *only* if ordered; Note: After gastrectomy, output will be minimal.

NURSING DIAGNOSES	NURSING INTERVENTIONS
	Monitor parenteral fluids with electrolyte additives as ordered. Measure intake and output. When bowel sounds return, administer clear liquids as ordered. Progress to small, frequent meals of soft food as ordered. Avoid milk because it may cause dumping syndrome.

It is necessary for the nurse to form a trusting relationship with the patient because of the severity of the condition and the long-term treatment of the patient with an ulcer. The family should be included with the patient for understanding and support, and the patient should be involved in goal setting if compliance is to be obtained (Home Health Considerations box).

The patient should be aware that if severe and sudden pain occurs, medical attention should be sought

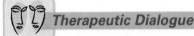 **Therapeutic Dialogue**

NURSE: *You look like you are resting better, Mrs. S. How have you been feeling? (Reaffirming a relationship that was begun yesterday.)*

PATIENT: *Hello, Mrs. F. My stomach pain is much better. The medicine helped.*

NURSE: *If you are comfortable, perhaps you and your husband have some questions about why you are here. (Trying to determine whether the patient is receptive to patient teaching. A knowledge deficit was suspected on admission.)*

PATIENT: *I was scared when I started to vomit blood. It has happened before but not this much. Where does the blood come from?*

NURSE: *You have a diagnosis of GI bleeding with questionable duodenal ulcer. That means you have bleeding in the gastrointestinal system, either in the stomach or in some part of the intestine. (The nurse begins with the admitting diagnosis and explains one thing at a time, making sure the patient verbalizes understanding before continuing.) Do you understand what I have said so far?*

PATIENT: *Well, I understand where the bleeding is coming from, but why am I bleeding there?*

NURSE: *We are not sure yet, Mrs. S., but you are scheduled for a procedure that will allow the doctor to actually look at the surface of the stomach and a portion of the intestine. It is called an endoscopy, and it will be done tomorrow morning. Did someone explain this to you? (The nurse answers the patient's question openly and honestly and uses her answer to lead into further patient education.)*

NURSING CARE PLAN

The Patient with Gastrointestinal Bleeding

Mr. D., a 33-year-old stockbroker, is admitted with pain in the epigastric region and copious hematemesis. He appears anxious; his skin is pale, cool, and clammy, and he is breathing rapidly. This patient has a history of recurrent episodes of vomiting blood that has a coffee-grounds appearance. He denies the presence of passing blood rectally but admits his stools have changed in consistency.

NURSING DIAGNOSIS *Risk for deficient fluid volume, related to hemorrhage, vomiting, and diarrhea*

Patient Goals/Expected Outcomes	Nursing Interventions	Evaluation
Patient will have normal fluid balance as evidence by balanced I&O within 24 hours, including stable weight.	Monitor IV and blood transfusion therapy as ordered.	Patient has urine output of 1500 mL for prior 24-hour period.
Blood pressure, pulse, and respiratory rate will be within normal limits.	Accurately record I&O every hour until stable: emesis, urine, and stool.	Patient's blood pressure, pulse, and respiratory rate are within patient's pregastrointestinal bleeding baseline levels.
Patient will have normal tissue turgor within 24 hours.	Document fluid losses for possible imbalance; urine output less than 30 mL/hr may indicate hypovolemia.	Patient's tissue turgor is normal.
	Monitor for signs and symptoms of dehydration and fluid electrolyte imbalance (dry mucous membranes poor skin turgor, thirst, decreased urinary output, and changes in behavior) every 15 minutes until stable, then every 2 hours.	
	Document characteristics of output.	
	Test all emesis and fecal output for presence of blood as ordered.	
	Prepare to assist with inserting an NG tube and connect to wall suction.	
	Irrigate NG tube with saline as ordered to promote clotting; irrigation removes old blood from the stomach.	

NURSING DIAGNOSIS *Anxiety, related to hospitalization and illness*

Patient Goals/Expected Outcomes	Nursing Interventions	Evaluation
Patient will demonstrate decrease in anxiety as evidenced by ability to sleep and/or rest at frequent intervals, verbalization of feelings, and blood pressure and pulse within normal limits.	Assess physiologic components of anxiety: restlessness, increased pulse and respirations, diaphoresis, and elevated blood pressure at least every 8 hours.	Patient is sleeping 5 to 6 hours during the night and resting at intervals during the day.
	Provide concise explanations for all procedures; prepare patient for surgery if indicated.	Patient verbalizes a feeling of less stress and anxiety.
	Develop rapport with patient and family members with each contact.	Therapeutic rapport with nurse, patient, and family members is noted.

? CRITICAL THINKING QUESTIONS

1. Mr. D. has a nasogastric tube connected to wall suction that is draining sanguineous fluid. He complains of severe fatigue and epigastric pain. He is pale and drawn, with a hemoglobin level of 5.1 g/dL. Mr. D. puts his light on and requests the nurse to assist him to the bathroom for a bowel movement. What are the appropriate interventions to ensure Mr. D.'s safety?

2. During assessment of Mr. D., what signs and symptoms would indicate deficient fluid volume?

3. Mr. D. verbalizes to the nurse that he fears he may die. He appears anxious and tremulous. What is the most therapeutic approach to help decrease his fears?

immediately. Assistance should be given to the patient in describing signs and symptoms of weakness, anorexia, nausea, diarrhea, constipation, anxiety, or restlessness. When medications are prescribed, the patient must fully understand (1) the purpose of taking antibiotic therapy to eradicate *H. pylori;* (2) the importance of taking all prescribed medications such as H$_2$ receptor antagonists, antiulcer drugs, prostaglandin E analog, and proton pump inhibitors as prescribed; (3) why the antacids are taken in large doses (30 mL) seven times daily (1 and 3 hours after a meal and at bedtime) or at the specific times ordered; and (4) the side effects that are known (diarrhea and constipation). Preventive teaching includes identifying risk behaviors in the patient's lifestyle, such as the use of tobacco, caffeine, and alcohol. Dietary needs should emphasize six smaller meals daily and avoidance of any foods that cause noticeable stomach discomfort.

If surgery is required, procedures should be explained thoroughly, including the reasons for them. The nurse should explain immediate postoperative care, including deep breathing; coughing; position changes; the need for frequently monitoring vital signs; intravenous tubing, NG tubing, catheters, and other drainage tubes; and the use of patient-controlled analgesia or other medications for pain relief. The ability of the patient to eat normally after healing will depend on the type of surgery and when peristalsis returns.

turns. The nurse should help the patient to realize that repeat episodes of symptoms are not unusual and to seek medical care if they recur.

Prognosis for Peptic Ulcers

Recurrence of an ulcer is possible and may happen within 2 years in about one third of all patients. Among patients whose *H. pylori* is treated with antibiotics, the peptic ulcer recurrence drops to 2%. Patients who do not receive antibiotics have a relapse of close to 75% to 90%. The likelihood of recurrence is lessened by eliminating foods that aggravate the condition. If symptoms recur, the prognosis is better in patients who resume antacid medications hourly and seek further medical treatment.

CANCER OF THE STOMACH
Etiology/Pathophysiology

The incidence of gastric cancer has declined significantly in western Europe and the United States. In the 1940s gastric cancer was the most common malignant disease in the United States. The most common neoplasm or malignant growth in the stomach is adenocarcinoma. The primary location is in the pyloric area, but the incidence of proximal tumors appears to be rising (Figure 5-8). Because of the location, the tumor may metastasize to lymph nodes, liver, spleen, pancreas, or esophagus. Gastric cancer is more common in people 50 to 70 years of age.

The cause is not known, but numerous factors are associated with the disease. These include history of polyps, pernicious anemia, hypochlorhydria (deficiency of hydrochloride in the stomach's gastric juice), gastrectomy, chronic atrophic gastritis, and gastric ulcer. Because the stomach has prolonged contact with food, an association exists between cancer in this part

---

🏠 Home Health Considerations

Peptic Ulcer Disease

- The patient who has recurrence of ulcer disease following initial healing must learn to live with a disease that is chronic.
- The patient may be angry and frustrated, especially if the prescribed mode of therapy has been faithfully followed yet has failed to prevent the recurrence or extension of the disease process.
- Unfortunately, many patients do not comply with the plan of care originally designed, and experience repeated exacerbation.
- Changes in lifestyle are difficult for most people and may be met with resistance.
- If the patient has been instructed to stop smoking or to avoid the use of alcohol, this request may be met with resistance.
- The goal should be adhering to the prescribed therapeutic regimen, including drug therapy, nutritional management, cessation of smoking, and decreased use of alcohol and caffeine.
- A patient with chronic ulcers needs to be aware of the complications that may result from the disease, the clinical manifestations indicating their presence, and what to do until the physician can be seen.

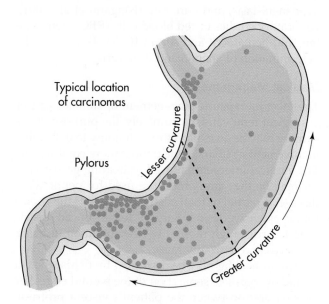

FIGURE **5-8** Typical sites of gastric cancer.

of the body and diets high in salt, smoked and preserved foods (which contain nitrites and nitrates), and carbohydrates and low in fresh fruits and vegetables. Infection with *H. pylori*, especially at an early age, is considered a definite risk factor for gastric cancer.

Clinical Manifestations

The patient may be asymptomatic in early stages of the disease. With more advanced disease, the physical examination may reveal that the patient is pale and lethargic if anemia is present. When the appetite has been poor and weight loss has been considerate, the patient may appear cachectic.

Assessment

Collection of **subjective data** may include complaints of vague epigastric discomfort or indigestion and postprandial (meal) fullness; 10% of patients have complaints of an ulcerlike pain that does not respond to therapy. Anorexia and weakness are also common.

Collection of **objective data** may include weight loss, bleeding in the stools, hematemesis, and vomiting after drinking fluids or eating meals. Anemia is a common occurrence. It is caused by chronic blood loss as the lesion erodes through the mucosa or as a direct result of pernicious anemia, which develops when intrinsic factor is lost. The presence of ascites is a poor prognostic sign.

Diagnostic Tests

The tumor is diagnosed by radiographic barium studies (GI series). Endoscopic/gastroscopic examinations with biopsy remain the best diagnostic tool. Stool examination provides evidence of occult or gross bleeding. Carcinoembryonic antigen (CEA) and carbohydrate antigen (CA) 19-9 tumor markers are usually elevated in advanced gastric cancer. Serum tumor markers are correlated with the degree of invasion, liver metastasis, and cure rate (Ishigami et al., 2001). Laboratory studies of red blood cells (RBC), hemoglobin, and hematocrit and serum B_{12} levels assist in the determination of anemia and its severity.

Medical Management

The most therapeutic management of stomach cancer is surgical removal. Unfortunately, the purpose of the surgery may be an exploratory celiotomy to determine involvement or to make the patient more comfortable. The surgical intervention used in treating gastric cancer may be the same procedure used for peptic ulcer disease. A partial or total gastric resection is the choice for an extensive lesion. Surgery for advanced gastric cancer carries high morbidity (the condition of being diseased) and mortality rates.

Wound healing may be disrupted by dehiscence (a partial or complete separation of the wound edges) or by evisceration (when the patient's viscera protrude

through the disrupted wound). Dehiscence and evisceration may be caused by problems in suturing the wound or by poor tissue integrity. Some of the factors that may predispose a wound to dehiscence are excessive coughing, straining, malnutrition, obesity, and infection. Nursing interventions for the patient who has experienced dehiscence include instructing the patient to remain quiet and to avoid coughing or straining. The patient should be positioned to remove further stress on the wound. If evisceration occurs, the patient is kept on bed rest and the protruding viscera are loosely covered with a warm sterile saline dressing. The surgeon should be notified immediately because treatment consists of reapproximating the wound edges.

Chemotherapy has greater response and longer survival rates than radiation. Radiation combined with chemotherapy has been more effective. These treatment modalities are often used with surgery.

Nursing Interventions and Patient Teaching

The nurse should provide further clarification of the disease and the surgical intervention to the patient and family. The preoperative preparation includes improving the patient's nutritional status by monitoring total parenteral nutrition and providing supplemental diet feedings. Postoperative teaching is necessary to relieve anxiety and promote understanding of drainage tubes, feeding tubes, dressing changes, weakness, medications, and other routine care.

Nursing diagnoses and interventions for the patient with cancer of the stomach include but are not limited to the following:

Nursing Diagnoses	Nursing Interventions
Ineffective breathing pattern, related to pain, exploration of chest and abdominal cavities, and abdominal distention	Place patient in semi-Fowler's position to aid ventilation. Encourage and assist with gentle turning and repositioning. Encourage patient to turn, breathe deeply, and cough at least every 2 hours until patient is ambulating well; splint incision before patient coughs; encourage use of incentive spirometer; encourage ambulation.
Risk for injury, related to aspiration, infection, hemorrhage, anastomotic leak into abdominal cavity, and anemia/vitamin deficiency	Monitor closely for elevated temperature, bleeding from incision, pallor, dyspnea, cyanosis, tachycardia, increased respirations, and chest pain. Monitor laboratory results and activity tolerance because of possible anemia. Change dressings using sterile technique.

Because care encompasses so many areas, instruction should be (1) planned according to the patient's needs and level of understanding, (2) given when the patient is free of pain and rested, and (3) communicated both verbally and in print. Surgery, chemotherapy, radiation therapy, continued nutritional needs, pain relief, and support groups for psychosocial needs should be explained.

Weight loss will indicate the need for additional caloric intake and can be measured by monitoring weights compared with the patient's normal weight before illness. Prevention of skin excoriation around the feeding tube is important. Hypermotility or diarrhea that follows radiation therapy can be treated with medication. Alternative methods of care for the debilitated patient and family may include referral for hospice care.

Prognosis

The prognosis for patients with gastric cancer is poor. About 60% have clinical findings at the time of diagnosis, resulting in a low cure rate. Only 10% to 20% of patients develop disease confined to the stomach. The 5-year survival rate is 75% in patients with early stages of gastric cancer and less than 30% in those with advanced disease.

DISORDERS OF THE INTESTINES

INFECTIONS
Etiology/Pathophysiology

Intestinal infections are the invasion of the alimentary canal (both the small and large intestine) by pathogenic microorganisms that reproduce and multiply. The infectious agent can enter the body by several routes. The most common entry is through the mouth by contaminated food or water. Some intestinal infections occur as a result of person-to-person contact. Fecal-oral transmission occurs through poor handwashing after elimination. In active homosexual males, "gay bowel syndrome" is introduced by single-cell protozoal infections.

Bacterial flora grow naturally in the intestinal tract and help the immune system combat infection. Their presence can be altered through long-term antibiotic therapy. The impaired immune response in some individuals delays the body's attempt to destroy invading pathogens.

Infectious diarrhea causes secretion of fluid into the intestinal lumen. *Clostridia, Salmonella, Shigella,* and *Campylobacter* bacteria are associated with intestinal infections. These bacteria produce toxic substances, and the mucosal cells respond by secreting water and electrolytes, causing an imbalance. The amount of fluid secreted exceeds the ability of the large intestine to reabsorb the fluid into the vascular system.

One strain of *E. coli*—serotype 0157:H7—often has a virulent course. Unlike other strains of *E. coli*, serotype 0157:H7 is not part of the normal flora of the human intestine. Found in the intestines of approximately 1% of food cattle, this strain can, even in small amounts, contaminate a large amount of meat, especially ground beef. It is transmitted in contaminated, undercooked meats such as hamburger, roast beef, ham, and turkey; in produce that has been rinsed with water contaminated by animal or human feces; or by a person who has been handling contaminated food. The bacterium has also been cultured in unpasteurized milk, cheese, and apple juice and can be found in lakes and pools that have been contaminated by fecal matter. Bloody diarrhea and severe cramping accompanied by diffuse abdominal tenderness develop between the second and fourth days. Antidiarrheals should not be given because these medications prevent the intestines from getting rid of the *E. coli* pathogen. Antimotility drugs such as diphenoxylate HCl with atropine (Lomotil) or antibiotic therapy are not recommended because they increase the likelihood of developing the dreaded complication of kidney pathology—hemolytic-uremic syndrome (HUS) (MacKenzie, 1999).

Sigmoidoscopic or colonoscopic examination and stool specimens are used in the diagnosis of a specific type of inflammation or colitis called **antibiotic-associated pseudomembranous colitis** (AAPMC). This type of colitis is a complication of treatment with a wide variety of antibiotics, including lincomycin, clindamycin, ampicillin, erythromycin, tetracycline, cephalosporins, and aminoglycosides. A *C. difficile* test is ordered on the stool specimen to aid in the diagnosis of AAPMC in both inpatients and outpatients. The identification of characteristic lesions of AAPMC is done on tissues obtained through endoscopic examination.

Treatment with antibiotics (especially clindamycin, ampicillin, amoxicillin, and the cephalosporins) results in the inhibition of normal bacterial growth in the intestine. This inhibition of normal flora can lead to the overgrowth of other bacteria such as *C. difficile*. Under the right conditions, *C. difficile* produces two toxins, A and B. The literature states that both toxin A and toxin B are produced by *C. difficile* at the same time and that these two toxins cause the tissue damage seen in AAPMC disease. The incidence of *C. difficile* toxin found in the stool has ranged from 1% to 2% in a normal population to 10% in hospital inpatients and up to 85% to 90% in patients with proven AAPMC. The *C. difficile* test used alone is not conclusive but does aid in the diagnosis of AAPMC.

Because the level of *C. difficile* antigens associated with the disease state may vary, a negative *C. difficile* test result alone may not rule out the possibility of *C. difficile*–associated colitis. The nurse must monitor signs and symptoms of the disease such as the duration of antibiotic treatment and duration and severity of diarrhea. These observations, along with the presence of colitis or pseudomembranes, are all factors the physician must consider when diagnosing AAPMC disease.

The physician will treat a mild case of antibiotic-related *C. difficile*–associated diarrhea by simply discontinuing the antibiotic and providing fluid and electrolyte replacement. In more severe cases the physician will need to both discontinue the antibiotic and start antimicrobial therapy; the drugs of choice are either metronidazole (Flagyl) or vancomycin. Current practice is to start with metronidazole and then use vancomycin if treatment fails.

Clinical Manifestations

Diarrhea is the most common manifestation of an intestinal infection. The fecal output has increased water content, and if the intestinal mucosa is directly invaded, the feces may contain blood and mucus.

Assessment

Collection of **subjective data** includes noting complaints of diarrhea, rectal urgency, tenesmus (ineffective and painful straining with defecation), nausea, and abdominal cramping.

Collection of **objective data** may include a fever greater than 102° F (38.8° C) and vomiting. History taking will provide useful information regarding number and consistency of bowel movements, recent use of antibiotics, recent travel, food intake, and exposure to noninfectious causes of diarrhea. Noninfectious diarrhea may be caused by heavy metal poisoning, shellfish allergy, and ingestion of toxic mushrooms and fish toxins. Diarrhea from noninfectious causes is usually characterized by a short incubation period (minutes to hours after exposure).

Diagnostic Tests

The key laboratory test for patients with intestinal infections is a stool culture. Another laboratory test that may be included is a blood chemistry study to monitor changes in the patient's fluid and electrolyte status.

Medical Management

Usually the treatment of intestinal infections is conservative, letting the body limit the infection. Antibiotics may be given in cases of prolonged or severe diarrhea with a stool positive for leukocytes. If fluid and electrolyte replacement is necessary to offset the losses from diarrhea, the oral route is usually sufficient. The intravenous route is indicated if the patient cannot take sufficient fluids orally.

The use of antidiarrheals and antispasmodic agents may actually increase the severity of the infection by prolonging the contact time of the microbe with the intestinal wall. Kaolin and pectin (Kaopectate) may be used to increase stool consistency. Bismuth subsalicylate (Pepto-Bismol) can effectively decrease intestinal secretions and decrease the diarrhea volume. These medications require large doses to be effective (30 to 60 mL every 30 minutes to 1 hour), and their use remains controversial.

Nursing Interventions and Patient Teaching

The nurse must do a thorough assessment to determine the seriousness of the intestinal infection. Determining the onset of the disease and the number of people exposed is important, because the majority of GI infections are communicable and represent a community health problem. The nurse must also assess for fluid imbalance. This assessment should include measurement of postural changes in blood pressure, skin turgor, mucous membrane hydration, and urine output.

Nursing diagnoses and interventions for the patient with intestinal infections include but are not limited to the following:

NURSING DIAGNOSES	NURSING INTERVENTIONS
Deficient fluid volume, related to excessive losses from diarrhea and vomiting	If oral intake can be tolerated, apple juice, clear carbonated beverages, clear broth, plain gelatin, and water should be offered.
	If intravenous feedings are required to maintain intravascular volume, these fluids should have electrolytes added.
	Maintain accurate I&O.
Imbalanced nutrition: less than body requirements, related to decreased intake and decreased absorption	Monitor for decreasing episodes of diarrhea.
	Monitor blood pressure, tissue turgor, mucous membranes, and urinary output.
	Monitor weight loss if symptoms are severe.

The nurse should instruct the patient to report the number, color, and consistency of bowel movements; abdominal cramping; and pain. The patient and family should understand the importance of handwashing after bowel movements to interrupt the fecal-oral route of transmission. Those family members responsible for food preparation should be made aware of the importance of proper methods of food preparation and storage to reduce the growth of infecting organisms.

Prognosis

Intestinal infections. The body may be able to successfully defend against the infection without intervention. In severe cases, medications and fluid replacement assist the body and the cure rate is good.

Antibiotic-associated pseudomembranous colitis. The prognosis of AAPMC is better when the disease is diagnosed early and the antibiotics are changed. This allows the normal growth of bacteria in the intestine to resume.

IRRITABLE BOWEL SYNDROME
Etiology/Pathophysiology

Irritable bowel syndrome (IBS) is a disorder with episodes of alterations in bowel function. The American Gastroenterological Association defines IBS as a combination of chronic and recurrent gastrointestinal symptoms—mainly intestinal pain and disturbed defecation or abdominal distention—that are not explained by structural or biochemical abnormalities; it is a dysfunction of the intestinal muscles. The syndrome is now thought to result from hypersensitivity of the bowel wall, which leads to disruption of the normal functioning of the intestinal muscles (Heitkemper & Jarrett, 2001).

IBS is extremely common, occurring in about 20% of community populations. A small number of these people (5%) have severe symptoms that are difficult to manage. The cause of IBS may be a low pain threshold to intestinal distention caused by abnormal intestinal sensory neural circuitry.

The patient with IBS may have associated psychological problems. In patients without psychological problems, the symptoms are attributed to spastic and uncoordinated muscle contractions of the colon, usually related to ingestion of excessively coarse or highly seasoned foods. However, there is also (1) a correlation of panic attacks in patients with IBS, and (2) an association of chronic low abdominal (pelvic) pain and a history of childhood sexual abuse.

Clinical Manifestations

Alterations of bowel function include abdominal pain relieved after a bowel movement; more frequent bowel movements with pain onset; a sense of incomplete evacuation; flatulence; and constipation, diarrhea, or both. Functional diarrhea is increased by stress; usually weight loss does not occur. The physical examination is generally normal, and nocturnal symptoms are rarely present. The symptoms of IBS are deceptive in nature and are frustrating to manage.

Assessment

Collection of **subjective data** for the patient with IBS includes complaints of abdominal distress, pain at onset of bowel movements, abdominal pain relieved by defecation, and feelings of incomplete emptying after defecation. Collection of **objective data** includes mucus in stools, visible abdominal distention, and frequent or unformed stools.

Diagnostic Tests

The key to accurate diagnosis of IBS is a thorough history and physical examination. Emphasis should be on symptoms, health history (including psychosocial aspects such as physical or sexual abuse), family history, and drug and dietary history.

Diagnosis of IBS occurs by exclusion. Patients who present with symptoms of intermittent or chronic abdominal pain and altered bowel motility are screened for pathology such as Crohn's disease, ulcerative colitis, cancer of colon, diverticulitis, and infections such as *Salmonella*. When no pathology or structural abnormality is detected and when symptoms and signs include abdominal pain and altered motility, IBS is a probable diagnosis.

Medical Management

Diet and bulking agents. Increasing dietary fiber increases stool bulk and frequency of passage and also bloating. Adequate fiber is more reliably provided with bulking agents (e.g., Metamucil) than with diet unless the patient is a strict vegetarian. The bulking agents seem to be most effective in the treatment of constipation-predominant IBS, although they may alleviate mild diarrhea. If a patient consistently has exacerbation of symptoms after certain foods, those should be avoided.

Medication. Anticholinergic drugs relieve abdominal cramps. Milk of magnesia may be prescribed if constipation does not respond to augmented fiber or if the patient cannot tolerate it. Mineral oil, in sufficient doses, is cheaper, "gasless," and generally effective. Opioids can be quite effective in diarrhea-predominant IBS. Antianxiety drugs may help patients suffering from panic attacks associated with IBS. Antidepressants may be used sparingly for diarrhea-predominant IBS in patients with severe pain who have not responded to other measures. New drug therapies are in development. Drugs that affect serotonin receptors hold promise in the treatment of IBS.

Patients with IBS often report higher levels of psychological distress, including anxiety, panic, and depression, which can amplify symptoms and affect treatment response. Psychological nonpharmacologic treatment may include counseling and cognitive-behavioral interventions such as hypnotherapy and progressive muscle relaxation techniques that are aimed at stress reduction. Studies have shown that a significant proportion of patients with IBS had fewer or less severe symptoms after stress-reduction treatment.

Some patients have reported benefits derived from the use of complementary therapies such as acupuncture, Chinese herbal therapy, chiropractic techniques, and hatha yoga; patients with IBS are significantly more likely (11%) to use alternative remedies such as herbs than are patients with Crohn's disease (4%) (Complementary & Alternative Therapies box).

Complementary & Alternative Therapies

Irritable Bowel Syndrome

- Traditional Chinese medicine has long been used to treat a variety of gastrointestinal complaints. Herbal formulas are generally administered and are chosen according to the specifics of the diagnostic patterns of traditional Chinese medicine. Most of the literature about such usage appears in either Chinese or Japanese journals or in textbooks of Chinese medicine, some of which are now available in English translations.*

- Peppermint oil, an herbal extract, has also been studied for its use in irritable bowel syndrome. There was a significant improvement in irritable bowel syndrome manifestations with peppermint oil preparations, but the researchers cautioned that study design flaws make a fully positive conclusion difficult.

- Another area of research that has good results in the treatment of irritable bowel syndrome is biofeedback. Also called "psychophysiologic self-regulation," biofeedback is a relaxation training method that gives individuals a greater degree of awareness and control of physiologic function. Usually, computer-based biofeedback equipment is used, which gives immediate feedback to the patient as to progress in influencing certain parameters, such as muscle electrical activity and skin temperature.

- Other similar interventions have used various psychotherapy, stress management, and relaxation exercises, often in combination.

- Herbs that can cause GI upset include milk thistle (silybun), goldenseal (*Hydrastus canadensis*), ginger (*Zingiber officinale*), kelp (*Fucus vesiculosus*), comfrey (*Symphytum officinale*), chaparral (*Larrea divaricata*), cayenne (capsicum), and alfalfa (*Medicago sativa*).

- Some people have found that nausea and vomiting may be relieved with acupuncture or acupressure. Special wristbands that apply gentle pressure have been used to prevent motion sickness.

- Some people have found that chiropractic adjustment has improved blood flow to digestive organs and improved digestion.

- Anise has been used to decrease bloating and flatulence and as an antispasmodic. (Do not confuse with Chinese star anise.)

- Comfrey is used to treat gastritis.

- Fennel is used to treat mild, spastic disorders of the GI tract, feelings of fullness, and flatulence.

- Queen Anne's lace seeds are used for flatulence, colic, singultus, and dysentery.

---

*From Bensoussan, A., et al. Treatment of irritable syndrome with Chinese herbal medicine—a randomized controlled trial, *JAMA*, 280:1585.
Modified from Black, J.M., et al. (2005). *Medical-surgical nursing.* (7th ed.). Saunders.

Although some studies have examined the use of such therapies in the treatment of IBS, clinical trial data are inadequate to determine their efficacy or to recommend any one as the sole therapy in the treatment of the syndrome. However, Bensoussan and colleagues (2001) found that both individualized and standardized Chinese herbal medicine significantly decreased the severity of IBS patients' symptoms and improved their quality of life; patients whose herbal formulations had been individualized had sustained the improvement at a 3-month follow-up (Heitkemper & Jarrett, 2001).

Nursing Interventions and Patient Teaching

Most patients with IBS learn to cope with their symptoms sufficiently well to live with reasonable comfort. It is the nurse's role to assist in identifying the 5% of patients with IBS who need management. Nurses skilled in history taking, listening skills, nutrition planning, and understanding the relationship of psychological effects on the body can assist the patient in setting goals to manage the disease. The nurse should emphasize the importance of keeping a daily log showing diet; number and type of stools; presence, severity, and duration of pain; side effects of medication; and life stressors that aggravate the disorder. This information will assist in the diagnosis and treatment of IBS.

Nursing diagnoses and interventions for the patient with an irritable bowel include but are not limited to the following:

NURSING DIAGNOSES	NURSING INTERVENTIONS
Pain, related to diet consumed and bowel evacuation	Logging the type of food for fiber content, consistency of stool, degree of pain.
Deficient knowledge, related to the effect of fiber content on spastic bowel	Patient teaching regarding the relationship of fiber to both constipation and diarrhea.
	Patient teaching regarding the use of bulking agents.

IBS involves many personal feelings that the patient must recognize and be comfortable with before a plan of care can be established. Therefore it is important to establish a strong relationship with the patient before patient teaching begins. Patient teaching includes diet management and ways to control anxiety in daily living. The goal of patient teaching is to empower the patient to help control the disorder. Community resources for counseling should be provided to the patient if the nurse has observed a relationship of psychological problems to increased or decreased elimination accompanied by pain and discomfort.

Prognosis

Approximately 95% of these patients are successfully managed. Compliance with a diet low in residue and nonstressful daily regimen contribute significantly to a good prognosis.

CHRONIC INFLAMMATORY BOWEL DISEASE

Ulcerative colitis and Crohn's disease are chronic, episodic, inflammatory diseases. These disorders afflict young adults with education, careers, and the raising of families ahead of them. Ulcerative colitis and Crohn's disease appear more often in women, in the Jewish population, and in the nonwhite population; there seems to be a familial tendency.

The causes of ulcerative colitis and Crohn's disease are unknown, although theories exist. These include both genetic and environmental factors, including viral infection, allergies to certain foods, immunological factors, and psychosomatic disorders. Inflammatory bowel diseases are characterized by exacerbations (increase in the severity of the disease or any of its symptoms) and remissions (a decrease in the severity of the disease or any of its symptoms).

The two diseases require similar nursing interventions but different surgical interventions. Other similarities and differences exist (Table 5-2). Patients have been known to have features of both diseases, making a definite diagnosis difficult.

ULCERATIVE COLITIS
Etiology/Pathophysiology

The incidence of ulcerative colitis is twice that of Crohn's disease. The common enteric bacterium *E. coli* may play a role. Psychosomatic factors may cause, aggravate, or be a result of inflammatory bowel disease. The social isolation and frustration that accompany this chronic illness cause difficulties in effectively coping with daily life.

Ulcerative colitis is confined to the mucosa and submucosa of the colon. The disease can affect segments of the entire colon, depending on the staging (phases or periods in the course of the disease). This disease usually starts on the left side of the colon and progresses to the right side. Tiny abscesses form, which grow and produce purulent drainage, sloughing of the mucosa, and subsequent ulceration. Capillaries become friable and bleed, causing the characteristic diarrhea containing pus and blood. Pseudopolyps are common in chronic ulcerative disease and may become cancerous. With healing and the natural formation of scar tissue, the colon may lose elasticity and absorptive capability.

Table 5-2 | *Comparison of Ulcerative Colitis and Crohn's Disease*

FACTOR	ULCERATIVE COLITIS	CROHN'S DISEASE
Cause of disorder	Unknown; possible cause is enteric bacterium *E. coli*	Unknown; possible cause is an altered immune state
Area of involvement	Confined to mucosa or submucosa of the colon	Can occur anywhere along the gastrointestinal tract Most common site is terminal ileum
Area of inflammation	Mostly mucosal	Transmural (pertaining to the entire thickness of the wall of an organ)
Characteristics of inflammation	Tends to be continuous, starting at the rectum and extending proximally; limited to the mucosal lining	May be continuous or interspersed between areas of normal tissue; may extend through all layers of the bowel
Character of stools	Blood present No fat 15 to 20 liquid stools daily	No blood present Steatorrhea (fat in stool) 3 or 4 semisoft stools daily
Major complication	Toxic megacolon	Malabsorption
Major complaint	Rectal bleeding Abdominal cramping	Right lower abdominal pain with mass present
Reason for surgery	Poor response to medical therapy	Complications
Response to surgery	Removal of the colon cures the intestinal disease, but not extraintestinal symptoms, such as inflammation of joints and liver disease	Indicated to remove diseased areas that don't respond to aggressive medical therapy. Surgery doesn't cure the disease
Cancer potential	Increased risk	Risk increases with age
Biopsy findings	Architectural changes consistent with chronic inflammation, including crypt abscesses	Architectural changes consistent with chronic inflammation; may show granulomas

Clinical Manifestations

Pathologic findings differ in particular individuals, but diarrhea is a predominant sign. It is not uncommon for a patient with ulcerative colitis to have as many as 15 to 20 liquid stools a day, containing blood, mucus, and pus. With severe diarrhea there may be losses of sodium, potassium, bicarbonate, and calcium ions. Abdominal cramps may occur before the bowel movement. The feeling of the urge to defecate lessens as scarring within the bowel progresses. This results in involuntary leakage of stool.

Complications of ulcerative colitis include toxic megacolon (toxic dilation of the large bowel). This life-threatening complication occurs in less than 5% of patients. The bowel becomes distended and so thin that perforation could happen at any time. Clinical manifestations of toxic megacolon include a temperature of 104° F (40° C) or more and abdominal distention. In those who have had chronic ulcerative colitis for 10 to 15 years, carcinoma of the colon occurs in 40% to 50% of cases with total colonic involvement. Surgical interventions for treatment of this complication are usually necessary.

Assessment

Collection of **subjective data** for the patient with ulcerative colitis includes complaints of rectal bleeding and abdominal cramping. Lethargy, a sense of frustration, and loss of control result from painful abdominal cramping and the unpredictable bowel movements.

Collection of **objective data** for the patient with ulcerative colitis includes weight loss, abdominal distention, fever, tachycardia, leukocytosis, and observation of frequency and characteristics of stools.

Diagnostic Tests

Barium studies of the intestine, sigmoidoscopy and colonoscopy with possible biopsy, and checking the stool for melena aid the physician in diagnosis. Additional studies include radiologic examination of the abdomen, determination of serum electrolytes and albumin levels and liver function, and other hematological studies.

Medical Management

The medical interventions chosen depend on the phase of the disease and the individual response to therapy. Common treatment modalities include medication, diet intervention, and stress reduction.

Drug therapy. The four major categories of drugs used are (1) those that affect the inflammatory response, (2) antibacterial drugs, (3) drugs that affect the immune system, and (4) antidiarrheal preparations.

- Sulfasalazine (Azulfidine): a combination of sulfapyridine and 5-aminosalicylic acid (5-ASA). containing acetylsalicylic acid is the drug of choice for mild chronic ulcerative colitis. It affects the in-

flammatory response and provides some antibacterial activity. It is effective in maintaining clinical remission and in treating mild to moderately severe attacks.

- Nonsulfa drugs include olsalazine (Dipentum), given orally, and mesalamine (Rowasa), given by retention enema.
- Corticosteroids are antiinflammatory drugs effective in relieving symptoms of moderate and severe colitis; they can be given systemically or topically.
- Antidiarrheal agents are recommended over anticholinergic agents because anticholinergic drugs can mask obstruction or contribute to toxic colonic dilation. Loperamide (Imodium) may be used to treat cramping and diarrhea of chronic ulcerative colitis. Azathioprine (Imuran) is also beneficial.

Diet therapy. Diet therapy that excludes milk products and highly spiced foods has been effective in approximately 20% of patients. A high-protein, high-calorie diet is recommended for people who are nutritionally deficient. Total parenteral nutrition may be used for nutrition, fluid, and electrolyte replacement in severe cases.

Stress control. Ulcerative colitis is aggravated by stress. Identifying the factors that cause stress is the first step in controlling the disease. Working with the patient to find healthful coping mechanisms is part of the holistic approach in nursing interventions.

Surgical intervention. If an acute episode does not respond to treatment, if complications occur, or if the risk of cancer becomes greater because of the presence of chronic ulcerative colitis, surgical intervention is indicated (Box 5-4). Most surgeons prefer a conservative approach, removing only the diseased portion of the colon. The operations of choice may be a single-stage

---

Box 5-4 *Surgical Interventions*

Colon resection: Removal of a portion of the large intestine and anastomosis of the remaining segment

Ileostomy: Surgical formation of an opening of the ileum onto the surface of the abdomen, through which fecal matter is emptied

Ileoanal anastomosis: Removal of the colon and rectum but the anus is left intact along with the anal sphincter; anastomosis is formed between the lower end of the small intestine and the anus

Proctocolectomy: Removal of anus, rectum, and colon; ileostomy is established for the removal of digestive tract wastes

Kock pouch (Kock continent ileostomy): Surgical removal of the rectum and colon (proctocolectomy) with formation of a reservoir by suturing loops of adjacent ileum together to form a pouchlike structure, nipple valve, and stoma

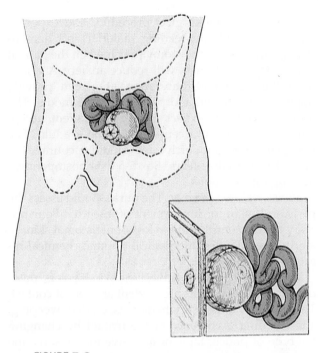

FIGURE **5-9** Kock pouch (Kock continent ileostomy).

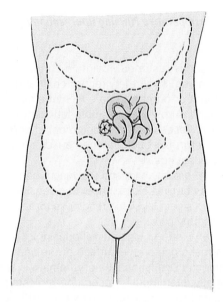

FIGURE **5-10** Ileostomy with absence of resected bowel.

total proctocolectomy with construction of internal reservoir and valve (Kock pouch, or Kock continent ileostomy) (Figure 5-9), total proctocolectomy with ileoanal anastomosis (surgical joining of two areas to allow flow from one area to the other) with or without construction of an internal reservoir, and temporary ileostomy. In the case of a poor-risk patient, a subtotal colectomy may be performed with ileostomy (Figure 5-10). After the patient's recovery (approximately 2 to 4 months), removal of the rectum or construction of an internal reservoir can be done.

Today some patients view a permanent ileostomy as more forbidding than the disease itself. These surgical procedures are not without risk, and the patient may want to live with the disease and long-term risk of cancer rather than undergo the procedure.

Nursing Interventions

Areas of nursing intervention include a thorough assessment of the patient's bowel elimination, knowledge level, support systems, coping abilities, nutritional status, pain, and ability to understand the disease process and treatment required. Patients need a complete understanding of the plan of care so that they can make informed choices. Prevention of future episodes is a goal for the ulcerative colitis patient.

Preoperative care for these patients includes (1) selection of stoma site, (2) performing additional diagnostic tests if cancer is suspected, (3) allocation of time to accept that previous treatments were unsuccessful in curing the disease, and (4) preparation of the bowel for surgery. The bowel is prepared 2 or 3 days preoperatively. A bland to clear liquid diet is ordered, and a

bowel prep of laxatives, GoLYTELY (an oral or NG colonic lavage/electrolyte solution), and enemas is ordered (see Box 5-2). Antibiotics, such an erythromycin and neomycin, are given to decrease the number of bacteria in the bowel.

Postoperative nursing interventions depend on the type of procedure performed and the individual's response. Areas of concern are bowel and urinary elimination; fluid and electrolyte balance; tissue perfusion; comfort/pain, nutrition; gas exchange; infection; and in the case of ostomy construction, assessment of the ileostomy and peristomal skin integrity.

Nursing diagnoses and interventions for the patient with chronic inflammatory bowel disease include but are not limited to the following:

Nursing Diagnoses	Nursing Interventions
Imbalanced nutrition: less than body requirements, related to bowel hypermotility and decreased absorption	Provide small frequent meals, which will help patients with poor appetite or intolerance to larger amounts. Eliminate foods that aggravate condition.
Powerlessness, related to loss of control of body function	Assist weakened patient with activities of daily living (bathing, oral hygiene, shaving, and other grooming needs). Offer choices to patient, when possible, to facilitate patient control.

Nursing diagnoses for the surgical patient may be focused on risk for ineffective coping, situational low self-esteem, and disturbed body image. Nursing interventions include reinforcement of the physician's

Box 5-5 | *Postoperative Nursing Interventions*

1. Monitor NG suction for patency until bowel function is resumed. Maintain correct wall suctioning. Accurately record color and amount of output. Irrigate NG tube as needed. Apply water-soluble lubricant to nares. Assess bowel sounds, being certain to turn off NG suction when auscultating bowel sounds.
2. Initiate ostomy care and teaching when bowel activity begins. Nurse should be sensitive to patient's pain level and readiness for teaching of ostomy care.
3. Observe stoma (an artificial opening of an internal organ on the surface of the body) for color and size (should be erythematous and slightly edematous). Document assessment of stoma (example, "stoma pink and viable").
4. Select pouch that has skin-protective barrier, accordion flange to ease pressure applied to new incisional site, adhesive backing, and pouch opening no more that 1/16 inch larger than the stoma. Stomas change in size over time and should be measured before new supplies are ordered.
5. Empty pouch when it is approximately one third full to prevent breaking seal, resulting in pouch leakage.
6. Explain that initial dark green liquid will change to yellow-brown as patient is allowed to eat.
7. Teach patient to care for the stoma; this includes having patient look at stoma and gradually assist with emptying, cleaning, and changing pouch; teach patient that normal grieving occurs after loss of rectal function. Be supportive of patient's concerns.
8. Promote independence and self-care to decrease state of denial.
9. Instruct on follow-up home care, including changing pouch every 5 to 7 days. Using antacids, skin protective paste, and liquid skin barrier may be appropriate if skin excoriation is observed.
10. Patient may shower or bathe with or without pouch on.
11. Patient should avoid lifting objects heavier than 10 pounds until physician instructs differently.
12. A special diet is not necessary, but fluids should include 8 to 10 glasses of water a day, food should be chewed well, and certain gas-forming foods should be limited or avoided.
13. Sexual relationships can be resumed when physician feels it is not harmful to the surgical area. Counseling may be appropriate if patient has fear of resuming this activity.

explanation of the surgical procedure and expected outcomes. Providing reading material and demonstrating the care of an ostomy pouch when the patient demonstrates readiness will reduce anxiety. A visitor from the United Ostomy Association can provide hope, as a recovered and productive role model. The nurse should not expect immediate patient acceptance of the stoma; acceptance will be gradual. The nurse should be supportive and should encourage the patient to verbalize fears. Box 5-5 lists postoperative nursing interventions.

Peristomal area integrity. The nurse should assess the peristomal skin for impairment of integrity. Four primary factors contributing to loss of peristomal skin integrity are allergies, mechanical trauma, chemical reactions, and infection.

Allergies to pouches, adhesives, skin barriers, powders and paste, or belts are evident at areas of contact. The skin may appear erythematous, eroded, weeping, and bleeding. Avoidance of the irritant by changing the type of pouch, tape, or adhesive may resolve the problem.

Mechanical trauma caused by pressure, friction, or stripping of adhesives and skin barriers can be avoided by less frequent changes of the pouch, using adhesive tape sparingly, and wearing a belt only when the patient feels it is necessary. The skin must be protected when the pouch is removed.

The most common chemical irritant is the stool from the stoma. The skin must be protected from these digestive enzymes by using skin barriers before applying the pouch. Skin barriers include adhesives (Stomahesive), powders (Stomahesive power), liquid skin barriers (Skin Prep), and caulking paste (Stomahesive paste).

A common cause of infection of the peristomal skin is *Candida albicans.* People who have been on antibiotics for 5 or more days may be prone to this problem. Treatment is application of nystatin powder or cream, by physician order. A skin barrier should be applied over the medicated area to ensure adherence of the adhesive.

Patient Teaching

The patient or significant other must be taught the appropriate care of the ileostomy or colostomy to foster independence. This includes pouch change, cleansing, irrigation, and skin care. A list of foods that are known to commonly cause problems of constipation, diarrhea, blockage, odors, and flatus is helpful. A list of resource people, phone numbers, where to obtain supplies, and what to ask for should be sent home with the patient.

Prognosis

The prognosis in patients with chronic ulcerative colitis is directly related to the number of years they have had the disease. This is due to the increased incidence of carcinoma when the colon is extensively involved over a length of time. The disease carries a higher mortality rate in patients who have the disease 15 to 20 years.

CROHN'S DISEASE
Etiology/Pathophysiology

Crohn's disease, although not as prevalent as ulcerative colitis, is increasing in incidence. Crohn's disease is characterized by inflammation of segments of the GI tract. It can affect any part of the GI tract, from the mouth to the anus. It was once thought to be a disease specific to the small intestine and was called regional enteritis. The cause of the disease is not known, but there seems to be a strong association between Crohn's disease and altered immune mechanisms. It most often affects people 15 to 30 years of age. Only one segment of the bowel may be involved, or segments of healthy tissue may alternate with multiple segments of diseased tissue. In the early stages of Crohn's disease, tiny ulcers form on various parts of the intestinal wall. Over time, horizontal rows of these ulcers fuse with vertical rows, causing the mucosa to take on a cobblestone appearance (Klonowski & Masoodi, 1999). The inflammation, fibrosis, scarring, and transmural (pertaining to the entire thickness of the wall of an organ) characteristics of Crohn's disease primarily occur in the small intestine (jejunum and terminal ileum). Involvement of the esophagus, stomach, and duodenum is rare. In some patients the disease may involve the colon without any changes in the small intestine.

Malabsorption is the major problem when the small intestine is involved. Megaloblastic (pernicious) anemia results from decreased absorption of vitamin B_{12} in the small intestine. Fluid and electrolyte disturbances with acid-base imbalances can occur, particularly with a depletion of sodium or potassium associated with diarrhea or with excessive small intestine drainage through fistulas that may be associated with the pathologic process.

Clinical Manifestations

The manifestations depend largely on the anatomical site of involvement, extent of the disease process, and presence or absence of complications. The onset of Crohn's disease is usually insidious, with nonspecific complaints such as diarrhea, fatigue, abdominal pain, weight loss, and fever. As the disease progresses, there is increased weight loss, malnutrition, dehydration, electrolyte imbalance, anemia, and increased peristalsis.

Assessment

Collection of **subjective data** for the patient with Crohn's disease includes noting the patient's list of vague complaints, including weakness, loss of appetite, abdominal pain and cramps, intermittent low-grade fever, sleeplessness caused by diarrhea, and

stress. Right-lower-quadrant abdominal pain is characteristic of the disease and may be accompanied in the same area by a tender mass of thickened intestines.

Collection of **objective data** for the patient with Crohn's disease includes complaints of diarrhea—three or four semisolid stools daily, containing mucus and pus but no blood. Steatorrhea (excess fat in the feces) may also be present if the ulceration extends high in the small intestine. Scar tissue from the inflammation narrows the lumen of the intestine and may cause strictures and obstruction, a frequent complication. Intestinal fistulas are a cardinal feature and may develop between segments of bowel. Cutaneous fistulas, common in the perianal area, and rectovaginal fistulas may occur. Fistulas communicating with the urinary tract may cause urinary tract infections. Poor absorption of bile salts by the ileum may cause stools to become watery. Fever and unexplained anemia may also occur.

Diagnostic Tests

A small bowel barium enema is preferred over an upper GI roentgenographic series with small bowel follow-through for detecting defining mucosal abnormalities such as cobblestoning of the mucosa, fistulas, and stricturing of the ileum. The most definitive test to differentiate Crohn's disease from ulcerative colitis is colonoscopy with multiple biopsies of the colon and terminal ileum. The appearance of the mucosa in Crohn's disease can range from normal to severely inflamed, and areas of inflammation may be continuous or interspersed with areas that appear normal. Granulomas in the biopsy specimen confirm the diagnosis of Crohn's disease, but their absence does not rule it out. In contrast, biopsies from a patient with ulcerative colitis show chronic inflammatory changes with no granulomas Blood tests for anemia may also be ordered.

Medical Management

Treatment of the patient must be individualized depending on the age of the patient, the location and severity of the disease, and the type of complications that may be present. Once Crohn's has been diagnosed, the patient is started on drug therapy to try to get the disease in remission. Those with mild to moderate disease are usually put on antiinflammatory agents such as sulfasalazine or mesalamine (Asacol, Pentasa, Rowasa). When inflammation is severe, corticosteroids such as prednisone may be prescribed. Patients are weaned off steroids as soon as possible to avoid dependency and prevent long-term complications. Multivitamins and B_{12} injections are often recommended to correct deficiencies.

If first-line therapy fails, treatment with more toxic, second-line drugs becomes necessary. These include immunosuppressive agents such as azathioprine (Imuran), cyclosporine (Neoral, Sandimmune), methotrexate or MTX (Folex, Mexate, Rheumatrex), and IV immunoglobin. In August 1998 the FDA approved the use of infliximab (Remicade) for Crohn's disease. It is a monoclonal antibody drug given as a single IV infusion except to those with fistulizing disease, in which the patient will need two additional infusions. Infliximab works by neutralizing tumor necrosis factor, a protein that causes much of the intestinal inflammation. Infliximab is the only medication specifically indicated for the treatment of Crohn's disease (Klonowski & Masoodi, 1999).

Diet intervention, stress reduction, and surgery are also used to manage Crohn's disease.

Diet. Bowel symptoms and diarrhea are minimized by excluding from the diet (1) lactose-containing foods in patients suspected of having lactose intolerance; (2) brassica vegetables (cauliflower, broccoli, asparagus, cabbage, and brussels sprouts); (3) caffeine, beer, monosodium glutamate, and sugarless (sorbitol-containing) gum and mints; and (4) highly seasoned foods, concentrated fruit juices, carbonated beverages, and fatty foods.

Diets high in protein (100 g/day) are recommended for patients with hypoproteinemia caused by mucosal loss, malabsorption, maldigestion, or malnutrition. Elemental diets have been shown to induce remission in 90% of patients with Crohn's disease. Free elemental diets may help patients with diarrhea because they require minimal digestion and reduce stool volume. Such elemental dietary preparations include Criticare, Travasorb-HN, and Precision High Nitrogen. Total parenteral nutrition has been shown to be more effective in patients with Crohn's disease than in those with ulcerative colitis.

Medications. Corticosteroids continue to be the preferred medical treatment of active Crohn's disease when there is small intestinal involvement. Sulfasalazine (Azulfidine) is effective in active Crohn's disease, especially when there is colonic involvement. Antibiotics have been used for treating microabscess formation as a complication of Crohn's disease, rather than in treating the actual disease process. Antidiarrheal agents (Lomotil and Imodium) and antispasmodics (Donnatal and Bentyl) have proven effective but are used with caution because of side effects. Enteric-coated fish oil capsules can help prevent relapses in patients with Crohn's disease; however, their palatability has been low. Biologic drug therapies of Crohn's disease include monoclonal antibodies to tumor necrosis factor–alpha (TNF-α) (infliximab [Remicade]) and to a leukocyte adhesion molecule (natalizumab [Antegren]). Infliximab has been shown to reduce the degree of inflammation; however, not all patients with Crohn's disease respond to infliximab. Natalizumab (Antegren), however, works by interrupting the movement of lymphocytes into the endothelial layer of the gut wall. By reducing the migra-

tion of lymphocytes, the inflammatory process can be decreased. Particular problems with inadequate vitamin B_{12} absorption result when the terminal ileum is resected; lifelong replacement of vitamin B_{12} is then necessary.

Complications of inflammation with fibrous scarring, obstruction, fistula formation in the small intestine, abscesses, and perforation are indications for surgical excision and anastomosis. If surgery is performed, resection is preferred because bypass has a greater failure rate.

Two types of surgery used in Crohn's disease are (1) segmental resection of diseased bowel with anastomosis of ileum with the remaining ascending or transverse colon and; (2) bypass of the diseased bowel by anastomosis of ileum to the colonic area free of disease, leaving the diseased bowel intact. Complications of malabsorption occur with both types of surgery. Surgery is performed only in selected instances for Crohn's disease because of a high rate of recurrence.

Nursing Interventions

Nutrition, fluid balance, elimination, medications, psychological aspects, and sexuality must be considered in caring for the patient with Crohn's disease. Total parenteral nutrition may be ordered in cases of severe disease and marked weight loss. Tube feedings that allow rapid absorption in the upper GI tract are begun, and then oral intake of a low-residue, high-protein, high-calorie diet is gradually introduced. Vitamin supplements are frequently necessary, and vitamin B_{12} is given when there is a marked loss of ileum. When anemia is present, iron dextran (DexFerrum) is given by Z-track injection because oral intake of iron is ineffective due to intestinal ulceration.

Oral diets of 2500 mL per day to replace loss of fluids and electrolytes caused from diarrhea are not uncommon. Weight is monitored for losses or gains. The condition of the skin and all fluid I&O are monitored daily. A urinary output of at least 1500 mL per day is desired.

When a person is hospitalized, a bedside commode or a bedpan must be accessible at all times because of the urgency and frequency of stools. Emptying the bedpan immediately and deodorizing the room maintain an aesthetic environment. The anal region may become excoriated from frequency of stools. The anal area should be examined regularly and kept clean using medicated wipes (Tucks) and sitz baths. These nursing interventions will promote comfort and hygiene for the patient.

Instructions and information for the patient related to medications include the following:
- Take sulfasalazine in equally divided doses.
- Take medication with a full glass (240 mL) of water.

- If gastric upset occurs, take medication after meals or with food.
- Report side effects to physician (headache, photosensitivity, rash or peeling of skin, aching of joints, unusual bleeding or ecchymosis, jaundice, continuous nausea, vomiting).
- Male infertility may be a side effect but is completely reversed on discontinuation of the medication.

Most patients with Crohn's disease require emotional support from nurses, physicians, aides, stomal therapists, and others. The support groups sponsored by the Crohn's and Colitis Foundation of America (formerly the National Foundation of Ileitis and Colitis) have played a major part in helping these patients. Tranquilizers, antidepressants, and psychology or psychiatry services may be required when managing the disease. Current evidence suggests that Crohn's disease is not caused by psychological stress but that psychiatric disturbances are the result of the nature of the symptoms and chronicity of the disease.

Nursing diagnoses and interventions for patients with Crohn's disease include but are not limited to the following:

Nursing Diagnoses	Nursing Interventions
Powerlessness, related to exacerbations and remissions	Explore with the patient factors that aggravate the disease.
	Assist the patient in listing factors that can be controlled: diet, stressors, medication compliance, self-monitoring of symptoms.
Imbalanced nutrition: less than body requirements, related to bowel hypermotility and decreased absorption	Emphasize the importance of weighing daily, following special diets, and assessing energy levels.

Patient Teaching

The patient must understand the effects of diarrhea and rapid emptying of the small intestine on the nutritional needs of the body. This will lead to acceptance of special diets and the ability to retain some personal control of the disease.

The patient must also understand the relationship of emotional feelings to Crohn's disease. Identifying resources for emotional support in the family and community and among health professionals will promote coping skills and mental hygiene.

Prognosis

Crohn's disease is a chronic disorder; it has a high rate of recurrence, especially in patients under 25 years of age. The rate of recurrence after surgery is 50% for the first 5 years and 75% in 10 years. Prognosis depends on the extent of involvement, duration of illness, and success of medical interventions. No known therapy will maintain a patient with Crohn's disease in remission.

ACUTE ABDOMINAL INFLAMMATIONS
APPENDICITIS
Etiology/Pathophysiology

Appendicitis is the inflammation of the vermiform appendix, usually acute, which if undiagnosed leads rapidly to perforation and peritonitis.

Appendicitis is most apt to occur in teenagers and young adults and is more common in men.

The vermiform appendix is a small tube in the right lower quadrant of the abdomen. The lumen of the proximal end is shared with that of the cecum, whereas the distal end is closed. The appendix fills and empties regularly in the same way as the cecum. However, the lumen is tiny and is easily obstructed. The most common causes of appendicitis are obstruction of the lumen by a fecalith (accumulated feces), foreign bodies, and tumor of the cecum or appendix. If it becomes obstructed and inflammation occurs, pathogenic bacteria (*E. coli*) begin to multiply in the appendix and infection develops with the formation of pus. If distention and infection are severe enough, the appendix may rupture, releasing its contents into the abdomen. The infection may be contained within an appendiceal abscess or may spread to the abdominal cavity, causing generalized peritonitis.

Clinical Manifestations

Light palpation of the abdomen will elicit rebound tenderness. The abdomen musculature overlying the right lower quadrant may feel tense as a result of voluntary rigidity. The patient will often be lying on the back or side with knees flexed in an attempt to decrease muscular strain on the abdominal wall.

Assessment

Collection of **subjective data** includes the most common complaint of constant pain in the right lower quadrant of the abdomen around McBurney's point (exactly halfway between the umbilicus and the crest of the right ileum). The pain may be accompanied by nausea and anorexia.

Collection of **objective data** includes vomiting, a low-grade fever (99° to 102° F [37.2° to 38.8° C]), an elevated white blood cell (WBC) count, rebound tenderness, a rigid abdomen, and decreased or absent bowel sounds.

Diagnostic Tests

A WBC count with differential will be ordered. Approximately 90% of people have a WBC level above 10,000/mm³, and approximately 75% have a neutrophil count greater than 75%. An abdominal CT scan is helpful for diagnosis. When diagnosis is difficult, Hypaque contrast studies, ultrasound, and laparoscopy may be used.

Medical Management

Emergency surgical intervention is the treatment of choice for acute appendicitis (Safety Considerations box). It may be performed as an incidental procedure when a patient is having another abdominal surgical procedure. Because mortality correlates with perforation and perforation correlates with duration of symptoms, early diagnosis and appendectomy are essential for the lowest acceptable morbidity and mortality. Antibiotic therapy is given both prophylactically and when perforation is likely. Complications that can occur include infection, intraabdominal abscess, and mechanical small bowel obstruction.

Nursing Interventions and Patient Teaching

The nursing interventions of the patient include following general preoperative procedure. The nurse should explain diagnostic tests and possible surgical procedures to relieve anxiety. Other interventions include bed rest, NPO status, comfort measures for pain relief so that symptoms will not be masked by medication, and fluid and electrolyte replacement. The temperature, blood pressure, pulse, and respirations are monitored and documented every hour because of the threat of perforation with peritonitis.

Usually no opioids are given during diagnosis to prevent masking of symptoms; sedatives may be given if necessary. In some cases an ice bag to relieve pain is given; no heat is applied because this may increase circulation to the appendix and lead to rupture. A cleansing enema is not ordered because of the danger of rupture. General postoperative care is performed.

Nursing diagnoses and interventions for the patient with appendicitis include but are not limited to the following:

NURSING DIAGNOSES	NURSING INTERVENTIONS
Deficient fluid volume, related to vomiting	Monitor patient for signs of dehydration and fluid and electrolyte imbalance (poor skin turgor, flushed dry skin, coated tongue, oliguria, confusion, and abnormal sodium, potassium, and chloride levels).
Pain, related to inflammation	Provide support to patient and family through listening and explanation of tests and procedures; explain need to withhold medications.
	Monitor increase in amount of pain experienced, rebound tenderness, and abdominal rigidity.
	Take vital signs frequently (every 15 minutes).

Patient teaching may include the reason for intravenous fluids with gradual advancement of diet from clear liquids to general as peristalsis returns. If antibiotics or oral medications are continued postoperatively, the patient should understand the name, purpose, and side effects of each medication. If complications occur, necessitating an NG tube or drainage tubes, the nurse should ensure that the patient understands the reason for these interventions.

Prognosis

The rate of cure through surgical intervention is high in patients with appendicitis. The patient's prognosis is altered if peritonitis complicates this diagnosis.

DIVERTICULAR DISEASE OF THE COLON
Etiology/Pathophysiology

Diverticular disease has two clinical forms, **diverticulosis** and **diverticulitis**. Diverticulosis is the presence of pouchlike herniations through the muscular layer of the colon, particularly the sigmoid colon (Figure 5-11). Diverticulitis is the inflammation of one or more diverticula.

Diverticulosis affects increasing numbers of people older than 50 years of age and may be the result of the modern, highly refined, low-residue diet. The penetration of fecal matter through the thin-walled diverticula causes inflammation and abscess formation in the tis-

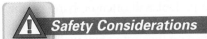

Safety Considerations

Appendicitis

- The patient with abdominal pain is encouraged to see a health care provider and to avoid self-treatment, particularly the use of laxatives and enemas.
- The increased peristalsis of laxatives and enemas may cause perforation of the appendix.
- Until the patient is seen by a health care provider, nothing should be taken by mouth (NPO) to ensure that the stomach is empty in the event that surgery is needed.
- An ice bag may be applied to the right lower quadrant to decrease the flow of blood to the area and impede the inflammatory process.
- Heat is *never* used because it may cause the appendix to rupture.
- Surgery is usually performed as soon as a diagnosis is made.

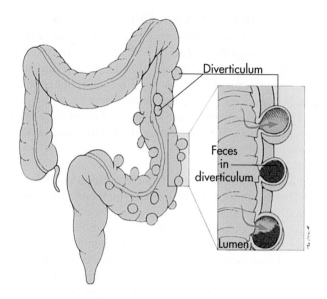

FIGURE **5-11** Diverticulosis.

sues surrounding the colon. With repeated inflammation, the lumen of the colon narrows and may become obstructed. When one or more diverticula become inflamed, diverticulitis results, which is a complication of diverticulosis. This inflammation can lead to perforation, abscess, peritonitis, obstruction, and hemorrhage.

Clinical Manifestations

When diverticula perforate and diverticulitis develops, the patient will complain of mild to severe pain in the lower-left quadrant of the abdomen and will have fever and an elevated white blood cell count and sedimentation rate. If the condition goes untreated, septicemia and septic shock can develop. This patient will be hypotensive and have a rapid pulse. Intestinal obstruction can occur, and the patient will experience abdominal distention, nausea, and vomiting.

Assessment

Collection of **subjective data** includes an awareness that the patient with diverticulosis may not display any problematic symptoms. Subjective complaints of constipation and diarrhea accompanied by pain in the lower-left quadrant are common to some. Other common symptoms include increased flatus and chronic constipation alternating with diarrhea, anorexia, and nausea.

Collection of **objective data** may include abdominal distention, low-grade fever, vomiting, and blood in the stool.

Diagnostic Tests

A CT scan with oral contrast is the test of choice for diverticulitis. A CBC, urinalysis, and fecal occult blood test should be performed. A barium enema is used to determine narrowing or obstruction of the colonic lumen. Colonoscopy may be beneficial in diagnosing

certain cases and is especially helpful in ruling out carcinoma. A patient with acute diverticulitis should not have a barium enema or colonoscopy because of the possibility of perforation and peritonitis.

Medical Management

The treatment of diverticulosis depends on the cause. If muscle atrophy is responsible for the disease, a low-residue diet, stool softeners, and bed rest are traditional interventions. When increased intracolonic pressure and muscle thickening are causes, a high-fiber diet of bran, fruits, and vegetables is recommended. Sulfa drugs have been used to treat uncomplicated signs of inflammation. Microperforation resulting in localized abscess is treated with a combination of antimicrobials effective against gram-negative, gram-positive, and anaerobic organisms. Analgesics are given per patient-controlled analgesia (PCA) for pain. Patients with acute attacks of diverticulitis that do not respond to antibiotics and bed rest may require hospitalization with NG drainage, parenteral fluids, and intravenous antibiotics.

Surgical treatment is advised if long-term problems do not respond to medical management and is mandatory if complications (e.g., hemorrhage, obstruction, abscesses, or perforation) occur. In elective surgery a thorough bowel preparation is most important. Laxatives, enemas, or intestinal lavage by GoLYTELY (see Box 5-2), as discussed, are given to cleanse the bowel, depending on the surgeon's preference. Antibiotics are given orally and parenterally.

In cases of perforation, abscess, peritonitis, or fistula, resection of the bowel with a temporary colostomy is needed. Either the one-stage procedure (resection of the affected bowel with anastomosis and no diverting colostomy) or the two-stage procedure (resection of the diseased bowel with diverting colostomy) is performed.

The bowel diversion can be accomplished by Hartmann's procedure (Figure 5-12), in which the descending colon is resected, the proximal end is brought to

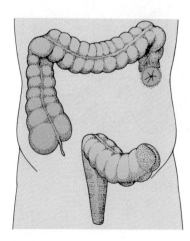

FIGURE **5-12** Hartmann's pouch.

the abdominal wall surface, and the distal bowel is sealed off for later anastomosis. The second procedure is the double-barrel colostomy, in which the bowel is brought up through the abdominal surface, or loop colostomy (Figures 5-13 and 5-14). The bowel can be opened at the time of surgery or postoperatively. Removal of the affected bowel segment and reanastomosis of the bowel are done during the initial procedure.

Closure of the temporary colostomy is the desired goal in the case of diverticular disease. Usually this is done from 6 weeks to 3 months after the initial surgical procedure. Again, the bowel must be prepared for closure by a liquid diet; laxatives; antibiotics; intestinal lavage as mentioned; and a cleansing colostomy irrigation of the proximal and, in the case of the loop or double-barrel colostomy, distal end of the stoma.

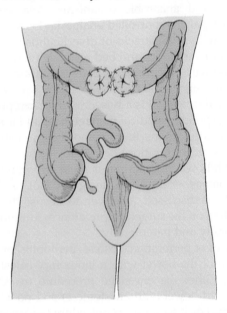

FIGURE **5-13** Double-barrel transverse colostomy.

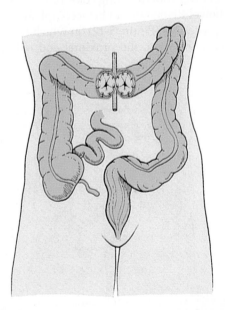

FIGURE **5-14** Transverse loop colostomy with rod or butterfly.

Nursing Interventions and Patient Teaching

Nurses should remember that when the distal loop is irrigated, irrigating solution and bowel contents will usually return from both the distal opening and rectum, so placement of the patient on the toilet or bedpan is important during the procedure.

The return of bowel activity after closure may take several days. The patient will again have intravenous fluids and an NG tube for the first few days postoperatively.

Nursing interventions include patient teaching of the disease process and surgery, if planned. The nutritional status must be assessed and discussion and reinforcement given as needed. The nurse should determine the nature of the pain the patient is having so that interventions of comfort measures or medication can be administered to provide relief. The patient and family should be included in the goals of the teaching plan.

Nursing diagnoses and interventions for the patient with diverticular disease include but are not limited to the following:

NURSING DIAGNOSES	NURSING INTERVENTIONS
Deficient knowledge, related to disease process and treatment	Instruct patient and significant others in disease process and signs and symptoms and acute diverticulitis attack.
Imbalanced nutrition: less than body requirements, related to decreased oral intake	Instruct in dietary roughage (for prevention) or bland, low-residue diet (for inflammatory phase). Assess daily weights, calorie counts, I&O. Monitor serum protein and albumin.

When a colostomy is performed, the patient or significant other should be able to verbalize and demonstrate understanding of the ostomy care to the nurse. The teaching of colostomy care should not be rushed and must be done when the patient is free of pain and receptive to learning. A family member may be taught to help until the patient is able to assume self-care, keeping in mind that the ultimate goal is patient independence. A home care referral may be needed so that the teaching process can continue after discharge.

Prognosis

With diverticulosis, the prognosis is good. Most patients have few symptoms except for occasional bleeding from the rectum. Diverticulitis has a good prognosis, with 30% of patients needing bowel resection of the affected part in acute cases to reduce mortality and morbidity.

PERITONITIS
Etiology/Pathophysiology

Peritonitis is an inflammation of the abdominal peritoneum. This condition occurs after fecal matter seeps from the rupture site, causing bacterial contamination of the peritoneal cavity. Some examples may be diverticular abscess and rupture, acute appendicitis with rupture, and strangulated hernia. Chemical irritation can also cause peritonitis. Blood, bile, necrotic tissue, pancreatic enzymes, and foreign bodies are examples of these chemical irritants.

Clinical Manifestations

Generalized peritonitis is an extremely serious condition characterized by severe abdominal pain. The patient usually lies on the back with the knees flexed to relax the abdominal muscles; any movement is painful. The abdomen is usually tympanic and extremely tender to the touch.

Assessment

Collection of **subjective data** includes observing for severe abdominal pain; any movement is painful. Nausea and vomiting occur, and as peristalsis ceases, constipation occurs with no passage of flatus. Chills, weakness, and abdominal tenderness (local and diffuse, often rebound) are also manifested.

Collection of **objective data** includes noting a weak and rapid pulse, fever, and lowered blood pressure. Leukocytosis and marked dehydration occur, and the patient can collapse and die.

Diagnostic Tests

A fat plate of the abdomen is ordered to ascertain if free air is present under the diaphragm as a result of visceral perforation. A CBC with differential is ordered to determine the degree of leukocytosis present. A blood chemistry profile to determine renal perfusion and electrolyte balance is done.

Medical Management

Aggressive therapy includes correction of the contamination or removal of the chemical irritant by surgery, and parenteral antibiotics. Nasogastric intubation is ordered to prevent GI distention. Intravenous fluids and electrolytes will prevent or correct imbalances. The patient may be placed on total parenteral nutrition because of increased nutritional requirements. Early treatment to prevent severe shock from the loss of fluid into the peritoneal space is essential.

Nursing Interventions and Patient Teaching

Nursing interventions for the patient with peritonitis include the following:

- Place patient on bed rest in semi-Fowler's position to help localize purulent exudate in lower abdomen or pelvis.
- Give oral hygiene to prevent drying of mucous membranes and cracking of lips from dehydration.
- Monitor fluid and electrolyte replacement.
- Encourage deep breathing exercises; patient tends to have shallow respirations as a result of abdominal pain or distention.
- Use measures to reduce anxiety.
- Use meticulous surgical asepsis for wound care.

The nurse should instruct the patient of the importance of ambulation, coughing, deep breathing, and leg exercises. If the patient has a draining wound at discharge, surgical asepsis should be taught for dressing changes. A nutritious diet is encouraged. The patient should be instructed not to lift more than 10 pounds until instructed by the physician to do so. The importance of the patient's keeping physician follow-up appointments is stressed.

Prognosis

The mortality rate of generalized peritonitis is 40% with the use of antibiotics and intensive support systems. Age, type of contamination, and ineffective tissue perfusion negatively affect the prognosis.

HERNIAS
EXTERNAL HERNIAS
Etiology/Pathophysiology

A hernia is a protrusion of a viscus through an abnormal opening or a weakened area in the wall of the cavity in which it is normally contained. Most hernias result from congenital or acquired weakness of the abdominal wall or postoperative defect, coupled with increased intraabdominal pressure from coughing, straining, or an enlarging lesion within the abdomen.

The various types of hernias include ventral (or incisional), femoral, inguinal, and umbilical. Ventral, or incisional, hernia is due to weakness of the abdominal wall at the site of a previous incision. It is found most commonly in patients who are obese, who have had multiple surgical procedures in the same area, and who have inadequate wound healing because of poor nutrition or infection. A femoral, or inguinal, hernia is caused by a weakness in the lower abdominal wall opening through which the spermatic cord emerges in men and the round ligament emerges in women.

A hernia may be reducible (can be returned to its original position by manipulation) or irreducible (or incarcerated: cannot be returned to its body cavity). When the hernia is irreducible or incarcerated, the intestinal flow may be obstructed. The hernia is strangulated when the blood supply and intestinal flow are occluded. Immediate surgical intervention is performed when a hernia strangulates, to prevent anaerobic infection in this affected area.

Factors such as age, wound infection, malnutrition, obesity, increased intraabdominal pressure, or abdominal distention affect formation of hernias after surgical incisions. Fewer hernias occur with transverse incisions than with longitudinal incisions. Also, upper abdominal incisions are associated with fewer hernias than lower abdominal incisions.

Assessment

Collection of **subjective data** includes palpation of the hernia area, revealing the contents of the sac as soft and nodular (omentum) or smooth and fluctuant (bowel). At no time should the nurse attempt to reduce the sac in the ring because this can lead to complications such as rupture of the strangulated contents.

Both subjective and objective signs and symptoms depend on where the hernia occurs. With an inguinal hernia, the patient may complain of pain, urgency, and the presence of a mass in the groin region.

Collection of **objective data** includes visibility of a protruding mass or bulge around the umbilicus, in the inguinal area, or near an incision; this is the most common objective sign. If complications such as incarceration or strangulation follow, there may be bowel obstruction, vomiting, and abdominal distention.

Diagnostic Tests

The diagnosis is aided by palpation of the weakened wall. Radiographs of the suspected area are diagnostic tests that may be ordered.

Medical Management

Hernias that cause no discomfort can be left unrepaired unless strangulation or obstruction follows. The patient should be taught to seek medical advice promptly if abdominal pain, distention, changing bowel habits, temperature elevation, nausea, or vomiting occurs. If the hernia can be reduced manually, a truss or firm pad placed over the patient's hernia site and held in place with a belt prevents the hernia from protruding and holds the abdominal contents in place.

Elective surgery for hernia repair may be done because of the inconvenience to the patient or constant risk of strangulation. A procedure to close the hernia defect by approximating adjacent muscles or using a synthetic mesh is done on either an inpatient or outpatient basis.

Nursing Interventions and Patient Teaching

The nursing interventions of the patient with an external hernia require observation of the hernia's location and size; the patient may be limited in activity and the type of clothing worn. Tissue perfusion to the area should be observed.

Open abdominal surgery may be necessary for the patient with a strangulated hernia. The patient should be prepared for a long hospitalization, which may include NG suctioning, intravenous antibiotics, fluid and electrolyte replacement, and parenteral analgesics until peristalsis returns.

Postoperatively the patient should be monitored for urinary retention; wound infection at the incision site; and, with inguinal hernia repair, scrotal edema. If scrotal edema is present, it may be decreased by elevating the scrotum on a rolled pad, applying an ice pack, and providing a supportive garment (jockstrap or briefs). The patient should deep breathe every 2 hours, but many physicians discourage coughing. The nurse should verify the postoperative orders. The patient should be taught support of the incision by splinting the area with pillow or pad. This support, along with analgesics, will help relieve pain.

Nursing diagnoses and interventions for the patient with a hernia include but are not limited to the following:

NURSING DIAGNOSES	NURSING INTERVENTIONS
Deficient knowledge, related to disease process	Instruct patient to observe and report hernias that become irreducible, begin to become edematous, or produce increased pain. Abdominal distention and change in bowel habits should be reported also. Explain reason to avoid prolonged standing, lifting, or straining. Instruct patient to support weakened area by use of truss or manually as needed (as when coughing).
Ineffective tissue perfusion, related to strangulation/incarceration of hernia	Monitor patient for increased pain, distention, changing bowel habits, abnormal bowel sounds, temperature elevation, nausea, and vomiting. Report changes in appearance and signs and symptoms to physician.

Follow-up care includes teaching the patient to limit activities and avoid lifting heavy objects or straining with bowel movements for 5 to 6 weeks. Also the patient should immediately report to the physician any erythema or edema of the surgical area or increased pain or drainage.

HIATAL HERNIA

A hiatal hernia (esophageal hernia or diaphragmatic hernia) results from a weakness of the diaphragm. Hiatal hernia is a protrusion of the stomach and other abdominal viscera through an opening in the membrane

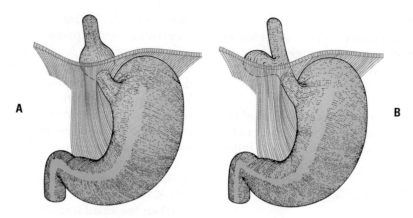

FIGURE **5-15** Hiatal hernia. **A,** Sliding hernia. **B,** Rolling hernia.

or tissue of the diaphragm (Figure 5-15). A hiatal hernia is the most common problem of the diaphragm that affects the alimentary tract. A hiatal hernia is an anatomical condition and not a disease. This condition occurs in about 40% of the population, and most people display few, if any, symptoms. The major difficulty in sympto-

matic patients is gastroesophageal reflux, and these patients complain of pyrosis (heartburn) after overeating. Complications of strangulation, infarction, or ulceration of the herniated stomach are serious and require surgical intervention. Factors contributing to the development of these hernias include obesity, trauma, and a general weakening of the supporting structures as a result of aging (Older Adult Considerations box).

Medical Management

The physician may select one of the following procedures:

- A posterior gastropexy, in which the stomach is returned to the abdomen and sutured in place.
- Transabdominal or transthoracic fundoplication, in which the fundus is wrapped around the lower part of the esophagus and sutured in place (Figure 5-16). The use of laparoscopic techniques has reduced the overall morbidity associated with abdominal surgery. A thoracic or open abdominal approach may also be used.

✤ *Older Adult Considerations*

Gastrointestinal Disorder

- Loss of teeth and resultant use of dentures can interfere with chewing and lead to digestive complaints.
- Dysphagia is commonly seen in the older adult population and may be caused by changes in the esophageal musculature or by neurological conditions.
- Hiatal hernias and esophageal diverticuli are significantly increased with aging because of changes in musculature of diaphragm and esophagus.
- There is decreased secretion of hydrochloric acid (hypochlorhydria and achlorhydria) from the parietal cells of the stomach. This results in an increased incidence of pernicious anemia and gastritis in the older adult population.
- Peptic ulcers are common, but often the symptoms are vague and go unrecognized until there is a bleeding episode. Medications such as aspirin, NSAIDs, and steroids that are taken for the chronic degenerative joint conditions common with aging should be used with caution because they can contribute to ulcer formation.
- Frequency of diverticulosis and diverticulitis increases dramatically with aging and can contribute to malabsorption of nutrients.
- Constipation is a problem for many older adults. Inactivity, changes in diet and fluid intake, and medications can contribute to this problem. Bowel elimination should be monitored and a bowel regimen established to prevent bowel impaction.

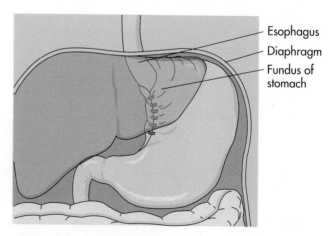

Esophagus
Diaphragm
Fundus of stomach

FIGURE **5-16** Nissen fundoplication for hiatal hernia showing fundus of stomach wrapped around distal esophagus and sutured to itself.

Nursing Interventions

Nursing care of the patient after surgery is similar to that after gastric surgery or thoracic surgery, depending on the procedure performed.

Prognosis

The prognosis for hernias is good because surgical intervention is usually successful. This, of course, can be altered if the patient is a poor surgical risk or if other complications exist.

INTESTINAL OBSTRUCTION
Etiology/Pathophysiology

Intestinal obstruction occurs when intestinal contents cannot pass through the GI tract; it requires prompt treatment (Figure 5-17). The obstruction may be partial or complete. The causes of intestinal obstruction may be classified as mechanical or nonmechanical.

Mechanical obstruction. Mechanical obstructions may be caused by an occlusion of the lumen of the intestinal tract. Most obstructions occur in the ileum, which is the narrowest segment of the small intestine. Mechanical obstructions account for 90% of all intestinal obstructions. Mechanical obstructions include adhesions (see Figure 5-17, *A*) or incarcerated hernias. Adhesions can develop after abdominal surgery. Other causes include impacted feces, tumor of the bowel, intussusception (prolapse of one segment of bowel into the lumen of another segment), volvulus (see Figure 5-17, *B*) (a twisting of bowel onto itself), or the strictures of inflammatory bowel disease. Residues from foods high in fiber, such as raw coconut or fruit pulp, can also obstruct the small bowel.

Nonmechanical obstruction. A nonmechanical obstruction may result from a neuromuscular or vascular disorder. **Paralytic (adynamic) ileus** is the most common form of nonmechanical obstruction. It occurs to some degree after any abdominal surgery. Other causes include inflammatory responses (e.g., acute pancreatitis, acute appendicitis), electrolyte abnormalities, and thoracic or lumbar spinal trauma from either fractures or surgical intervention. Vascular obstructions are rare and are due to an interference with the blood supply to a portion of the intestines. The most common causes are emboli and atherosclerosis of the mesenteric arteries. The celiac, inferior, and superior mesenteric arteries supply blood to the bowel. Emboli may originate from thrombi in patients with chronic atrial fibrillation, diseased heart valves, and prosthetic valves.

When the small intestine becomes obstructed, the normal process of secretion and reabsorption of 6 to 8 L of electrolyte-rich fluid is interrupted. Large amounts of fluid, bacteria, and swallowed air build up in the bowel proximal to the obstruction. Water and salts shift from the circulatory system to the intestinal lumen, causing distention and further interference with absorption. As the fluid increases, so does the pressure in the lumen of the bowel. The increased pressure leads to an increase in capillary permeability and extravasation of fluids and electrolytes into the peritoneal cavity. Edema, congestion, and necrosis from impaired blood supply and possible rupture of the bowel may occur. The retention of fluid in the intestine and peritoneal cavity can lead to a severe reduction in circulating blood volume and result in hypotension and hypovolemic shock.

Clinical Manifestations

The signs and symptoms of intestinal obstruction vary with the site and degree of obstruction. During partial or early phases of mechanical obstruction, auscultation of the abdomen will reveal loud, frequent, high-pitched sounds, but when smooth muscle atony (weak, lacking normal tone) occurs, bowel sounds will be absent.

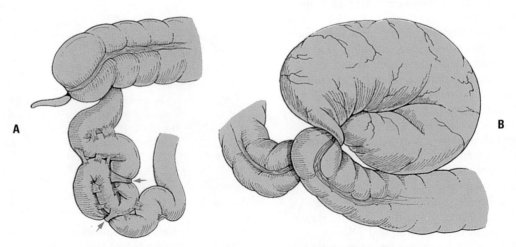

FIGURE **5-17** Intestinal obstructions. **A,** Adhesions. **B,** Volvulus.

Assessment

Collection of **subjective data** should include information about the pattern of the patient's pain, including onset, frequency, and characteristics. Nausea and the inability to pass flatus are common symptoms. Complaints of early intestinal obstruction of the small intestine include spasms of cramping abdominal pain as peristaltic activity increases proximal to the obstruction. As the obstruction progresses, the intestine becomes fatigued, and there may be periods of decreased or absent bowel sounds and complaints of increased abdominal pain. Any history of previous bowel disorders or abdominal surgeries and changes in bowel elimination should be noted.

Collection of **objective data** begins with assessment of the patient's abdomen. The abdominal surface is inspected for evidence of distention, hernias, scars indicating previous surgeries, or visible peristaltic waves. The increased peristaltic activity produces an increase in auscultated bowel sounds. Other objective data include vomiting, signs of dehydration caused by the fluid shift, abdominal tenderness and muscle guarding, and decreased blood pressure.

Obstruction of the colon causes less severe pain than obstruction of the small intestine, marked abdominal distention, and constipation. The patient may continue to have bowel movements. The colon distal to the obstruction continues to empty.

Diagnostic Tests

Abdominal x-rays are the most useful diagnostic aids. Upright and lateral x-rays show the presence of gas and fluid in the intestines. The presence of intraperitoneal air indicates perforation (it is sometimes referred to as free air under the diaphragm). Radiographic examination reveals the level of obstruction and its cause. The fluid and electrolyte balance can be monitored through laboratory test results. Elevated blood urea nitrogen (BUN) and decreased serum sodium, chloride, potassium, and magnesium are common. The patient's hemoglobin and hematocrit levels may be increased because of hemoconcentration associated with the fluid volume deficit.

Medical Management

Treatment is directed toward decompression of the intestine by removal of gas and fluid, correction and maintenance of fluid and electrolyte balance, and relief or removal of the obstruction. Treatment includes the evacuation of intestinal contents by means of an intestinal tube. An NG or nasojejunal tube is inserted and connected to wall suction to decompress the intestine. Surgical repair is necessary to relieve mechanical obstructions caused by adhesions, volvulus, and strangulated hernias. Fluid and electrolyte balances are restored by carefully monitored intravenous infusion. Nonopioid analgesics are usually prescribed to avoid the decrease in intestinal motility that often accompanies the administration of opioid analgesics.

Nursing Interventions and Patient Teaching

Unless surgery is indicated, the nursing intervention consists of careful monitoring of fluids and electrolytes, observation of the function of tubes used to decompress and relieve distention, and the administration of analgesics.

For the patient with intestinal obstruction undergoing surgery, the preoperative preparation will include explanations of the procedure at a level the patient can understand. Emotional support for the patient will be important because the patient is experiencing not only the stressors of pain and vomiting but also the added stressor of emergency surgery.

The postoperative nursing interventions are similar to those for any patient who has had abdominal surgery. The nurse should place the patient in Fowler's position for greater diaphragm expansion and should encourage the patient to breathe through the nose and not swallow air, which would increase distention and discomfort. She should encourage deep breathing and coughing. Nasointestinal suctioning will be continued until bowel activity returns. The nurse should assess for bowel sounds and abdominal girth to help to determine the return of peristalsis. Some patients may require temporary bowel diversion via a double-barrel or loop colostomy to manage the obstruction.

Nursing diagnoses and interventions for the patient with an intestinal obstruction include but are not limited to the following:

NURSING DIAGNOSES	NURSING INTERVENTIONS
Acute pain, related to increased peristalsis	Reposition patient frequently to help intestinal tube advance. Irrigate suction tubing with 30 mL sterile saline to keep tube patent. Explain purpose of all procedures. Provide comfort measures. Administer analgesics as ordered.
Deficient fluid volume, related to increased losses from vomiting and decrease in intestinal fluid absorption	Monitor for signs of dehydration, decreased blood pressure, change in laboratory values, and decreased urine output. Serum electrolyte levels should be monitored closely. Record and report frequency, amount, and nature of emesis. Strict intake and output record should be included.

Follow-up teaching focuses on prevention and includes dietary management, prevention of constipation, and recognition of early symptoms of recurrence and the need to seek prompt medical care. For the patient with a temporary ostomy, follow-up care will be necessary as plans are made for closure of the stoma.

Prognosis

The prognosis depends on early detection of the obstruction and the type and cause of the obstruction, as well as the success of medical interventions. The prognosis is poorer in patients who develop complications such as hypovolemic shock.

COLORECTAL CANCER
Etiology/Pathophysiology

Malignant neoplasms that invade the epithelium and surrounding tissue of the colon and rectum are the third most prevalent internal cancers in the United States and the second leading cause of cancer deaths.

In the colon, 45% of growths are seen in the sigmoid and rectal areas; 25% in the cecum and ascending colon; and the remaining 30% in the transverse splenic flexure, hepatic flexure, and descending colon. Cancer occurs with the same frequency in men and women, with the highest incidence in people 60 years and older.

The cause of colorectal cancer remains unknown, but certain conditions appear to be more prone to malignant changes. These conditions are termed predisposing or risk factors. Particular diseases over time, including ulcerative colitis and diverticulosis, increase the risk of colorectal cancer. Neoplastic polyps or adenomas may undergo malignant change and become frank carcinomas. Recent research has isolated a gene that causes colon cancer in certain families. History taking and regular checkups are important preventive measures. Other factors implicated in colorectal cancer include lack of bulk in the diet, high fat intake, and high bacterial counts in the colon. It is theorized that carcinogens are formed from degraded bile salts, and the stool that remains in the large bowel for a longer period as a result of too little fiber to stimulate its passage may overexpose the bowel to these carcinogens. There is also a theory that the increased transit time for low-fiber foods to pass through the intestine is related to malignancy. These factors have encouraged diet changes; decreased animal fat and increased high dietary fiber found in fruits, vegetables, and bran may have a protective effect and act as a primary preventive measure. Cruciferous vegetables such as cauliflower, broccoli, brussels sprouts, and cabbage may help protect against the malignancy.

Clinical Manifestations

Signs and symptoms of cancer of the colon vary with the location of the growth. During the early stages, most patients are asymptomatic.

Assessment

Collection of **subjective data** includes complaints of a change in bowel habits alternating between constipation and diarrhea, excessive flatus, and cramps. Constipation is more likely produced by descending colon cancer, while ascending colon cancer may occur with no change in bowel habits. The other complaint may be rectal bleeding, with the color varying from dark to bright red, depending on the location of the neoplasm. Later stages of colon cancer may include subjective symptoms of abdominal pain, nausea, and cachexia (weakness and emaciation associated with general ill health and malnutrition).

Collection of **objective data** includes observing for vomiting, weight loss, abdominal distention or ascites and test results that are compatible with the diagnosis. The most common clinical manifestations are chronic blood loss and anemia.

Diagnostic Tests

Early diagnosis of the tumor, including identifying the type of cells involved, is the most important factor in treating the disease. Digital examination can identify 15% of colorectal cancers. Proctosigmoidoscopy with biopsy can enable detection of 66% of these tumors.

Colonoscopy is the procedure of choice if a questionable lesion is seen on barium enema visualization or sigmoidoscopy. Other procedures include endorectal ultrasonography and CT scan of the abdomen and pelvis to localize the lesions or determine its size.

A baseline colonoscopy before age 50 should be performed on those who have a family history of colon cancer. The colonoscopy should be repeated every 4 years if one family member is affected or every 3 years if two first-degree relatives are affected.

The fecal occult blood examination followed by proctosigmoidoscopy remains the most reliable tool for screening (Health Promotions Considerations box). Other laboratory and diagnostic studies include an upper GI series, radiological abdominal series, and barium enema. Hemoglobin, hematocrit, and electrolyte levels are examined, and the blood test for carcinoembryonic antigen (CEA) (an oncofetal glycoprotein found in colonic adenocarcinoma and other cancers and in nonmalignant conditions) is done. Active malignancy growth within the body can be assayed by CEA when cancer and metastasis are suspected. The CEA is a glycoprotein antigen in adenocarcinomas of the GI tract. Antibodies to this antigen are measured. Because the CEA level can be elevated in benign and malignant diseases, it is not considered a specific test for colorectal cancer. Its use is limited to determining the prognosis and monitoring the patient's response to antineoplastic therapy.

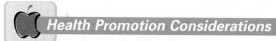

Health Promotion Considerations

Screening for Colorectal Cancer

Current recommendations from the American Cancer Society for colorectal cancer screening are as follows:

- Annual digital rectal examination beginning at age 50 years.
- Starting at the age of 50 years, fecal testing for occult blood should be done every year.
- Flexible sigmoidoscopy should be performed every 5 years.
- Positive findings should be followed with colonoscopy or double-contrast barium enema.
- Screening for high-risk patients should begin before age 50, usually beginning with colonoscopy.

Medical Management

Medical treatment includes radiation, chemotherapy, and surgery. Radiation therapy is often used before surgery to decrease the chance of cancer cell implantation at the time of resection. Radiation can both reduce the size of the tumor and decrease the rate of lymphatic involvement. There are few side effects from radiation before surgery, but there are complications.

Postoperatively those patients at high risk for recurrence or people whose disease has progressed may receive radiation administered over 4 to 6 weeks.

Chemotherapy is given (1) to patients with systemic disease that is incurable by surgery or radiation alone; (2) to patients in whom undetectable metastasis is suspected (e.g., when a patient has positive lymph node involvement at the time of surgery); or (3) for palliative therapy to reduce tumor size or relieve symptoms of the disease, such as obstruction or pain. Physician opinion and individual patient response vary regarding use of chemotherapy for colorectal cancer.

Surgical interventions for treatment depend on the location of the tumor, presence of obstruction or perforation of the bowel, possible metastasis, the patient's health status, and the surgeon's preferences. When obstruction has not occurred, a portion of the bowel on either side of the tumor is removed and an end-to-end anastomosis is done between the divided ends. When obstruction of the bowel occurs, the commonly used procedures are as follows:

- One-stage resection with anastomosis.
- Two-stage resection with (1) resection by bringing the ends of the bowel to the surface and creating a temporary colostomy and mucus fistula or Hartmann's pouch (see Figure 5-12); (2) a double-barrel colostomy (see Figure 5-13); or (3) a temporary loop colostomy (see Figure 5-14), for closure later.

Surgical procedures for colorectal cancer include the following:

- Right hemicolectomy: resection of ascending colon and hepatic flexure (Figure 5-18, *A*); ileum anastomosed to transverse colon.
- Left hemicolectomy: resection of splenic flexure, descending colon, and sigmoid colon (see Figure 5-18, *B*); transverse colon anastomosed to rectum.
- Anterior rectosigmoid resection: resection of part of descending colon, the sigmoid colon, and upper rectum (see Figure 5-18, *C*); descending colon anastomosed to remaining rectum.

In carcinoma of the rectum, every effort is made by the surgeon to preserve the sphincter. An end-to-end anastomosis is often used. The use of EEA (end-to-end anastomosis) staplers has allowed lower and more secure anastomosis. The stapler is passed through the anus, where the colon is stapled to the rectum. This technique has made it possible to resect lesions as low

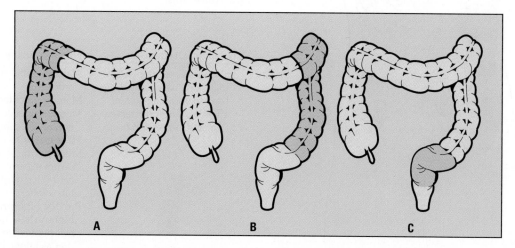

FIGURE **5-18** Bowel resection. **A,** Right hemicolectomy. **B,** Left hemicolectomy. **C,** Anterior rectosigmoid resection.

as 5 cm from the anus. If the surgeon is unable to do an anastomosis, an abdominoperineal resection may be done.

In the abdominoperineal resection, an abdominal incision is made and the proximal sigmoid is brought through the abdominal wall in a permanent colostomy. The distal sigmoid, rectum, and anus are removed through a perineal incision. The perineal wound may be closed around a drain or left open with packing to allow healing by granulation. Complications that can occur are delayed wound healing, hemorrhage, persistent perineal sinus tracts, infections, and urinary tract and sexual dysfunction (Figure 5-19).

Nutritional status is important because of the threat of infection and postoperative healing process that may follow a compromised state as a result of constipation, diarrhea, nausea, vomiting, and possible obstruction.

Nursing Interventions and Patient Teaching

The assessment of bowel and urinary elimination, fluid and electrolyte balance, tissue perfusion, nutrition, pain, gas exchange, infection, and peristomal skin integrity was discussed previously.

Preoperative care. The patient will have some type of bowel preparation, which usually includes 2 or 3 days of liquid diets; a combination of laxatives, GoLYTELY, or enemas; and oral antibiotics to sterilize the bowel. The antibiotic of choice may be neomycin, kanamycin, or erythromycin; each suppresses anaerobic and aerobic organisms in the colon.

Other aspects of preoperative care include instruction in turning, coughing, and deep breathing; wound splinting; and leg exercises. The patient should know that he will have intravenous lines, a Foley catheter, possibly an NG tube, and abdominal dressings after surgery.

If a stoma is to be created, the enterostomal therapist should be notified so that the stoma site can be marked before surgery. The stoma should be placed at the best site for the patient.

Postoperative care. The patient should be assessed for stable vital signs and return of bowel sounds. The dressings should be checked for drainage or bleeding and changed as needed per the physician's order. The NG tube and Foley catheter should be monitored for flow and amount and color of output. Accurate I&O records must be kept to maintain the fluid and electrolyte balance. Other postoperative care includes coughing, deep breathing, early ambulation, adequate nutrition, pain control, and meticulous wound and stoma care.

Paralytic ileus, a common complication of abdominal surgery, produces the classic signs of increased abdominal girth, distention, nausea, and vomiting. Interventions include decompression of the bowel with an NG tube connected to wall suction, NPO status, and increased patient activity.

Long-term complications of abdominal resection with permanent colostomy are urinary retention or incontinence, pelvic abscess, failure of perineal wound healing or wound infection, and sexual dysfunction.

In addition to monitoring the stoma for color, size, location, and the condition of the peristomal skin, the nurse must watch for possible complications. Common stoma complications in the immediate postoperative period are necrosis and abscess. Necrosis results from a compromised blood flow to the stoma, causing the stoma to appear pale and dusky to black. Abscess caused by stoma placement too close to the wound, retention sutures, and drains must be assessed promptly. All complications must be reported promptly to the surgeon and documented in the medical record.

Nursing diagnoses and interventions for the patient with cancer of the colon include but are not limited to the following:

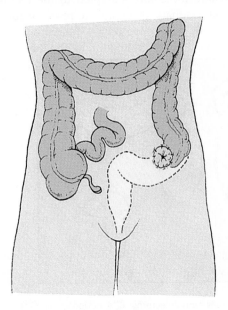

FIGURE **5-19** Descending or sigmoid colostomy.

NURSING DIAGNOSES	NURSING INTERVENTIONS
Imbalanced nutrition: less than body requirements, related to vomiting and/or anorexia, surgical intervention, and depression	Maintain NPO status as ordered. Monitor parenteral fluids. Monitor patency and function of NG tube. Measure I&O. Monitor vital signs and serum electrolytes, hematocrit (Hct), and hemoglobin (Hgb). Provide high-protein, high-carbohydrate, high-calorie, low-residue diet as allowed and tolerated.

NURSING DIAGNOSES	NURSING INTERVENTIONS
Disturbed body image, related to loss of normal body function (colostomy)	Allow time for grieving. Assist patient and significant other in accepting ostomy. Allow time for and encourage verbalization. Answer all questions, and explain treatment and procedure. Provide care in positive manner; always avoid facial expressions connoting distaste. Observe for signs of denial, grief, or anger. Provide privacy and safe environment. Encourage self-care and independence when patient demonstrates readiness.

The patient with a permanent end colostomy can be taught two forms of colostomy management: (1) emptying and cleansing the pouch as needed, and (2) managing colostomy irrigation. Factors to consider in planning patient teaching are past bowel habits, location of colostomy, age of the patient, general health of the patient, and the patient's personal preference.

Nerves that control the bladder may be damaged when a large amount of tissue is removed in the abdominoperineal resection. When the Foley catheter is removed after surgery, the patient may be unable to void or empty the bladder completely. If the problem does not resolve, the patient may need a Foley catheter and a urology consultation.

When a large amount of tissue is removed, as in the abdominoperineal resection, and a cavity is left as sanctuary for bacteria, there is increased risk of infection. The drain site is monitored for increased pain, erythema, and purulent drainage, and body temperature is monitored for elevation. The perineal wound may be closed in one of three ways. The closed wound with a drain to suction has a high risk for abscess formation. The semiclosed wound is partially closed with either a Davol or Penrose drain that is left in place longer, with the drain shortened over time by the physician or nurse. The open wound (in which packing is used and later removed) may need irrigating, and sitz baths may be required to facilitate healing. Changes in exudate color and odor and temperature elevation should be reported to the physician.

Sexual dysfunction of both men and women is related to removal of the rectum. Contributing factors may be partial to complete disruption of the nerve's supply to the genital organs, psychological factors, or decreased activity associated with age. When a comfortable relationship exists between the nurse and the patient, the topic of sex can be introduced more effectively. Exploring the patient's and the partner's fears and providing information on penile prosthesis surgery and simple suggestions to both partners will help decrease anxiety concerning intercourse. Counseling may be necessary if the patient's and partner's perceptions of body image have been altered. Support groups are available to the cancer patient in most communities. Above all, the nurse's silent communication of touch and eye contact can give the patient a message that he or she is accepted and valued.

Prognosis

The 5-year survival rate for patients with early localized colorectal cancer is 90% and 64% for cancer that has spread to adjacent organs and lymph nodes. Only distant metastases prevent the possibility of a cure.

HEMORRHOIDS
Etiology/Pathophysiology

Hemorrhoids are varicosities (dilated veins) that may occur outside the anal sphincter as external hemorrhoids or inside the sphincter as internal hemorrhoids. This condition is one of the most common health problems seen in humans, with the greatest incidence from ages 20 to 50 years. Etiologic factors include straining at stool with increased intraabdominal and hemorrhoidal venous pressures. With repeated increased pressure and obstructed blood flow, permanent dilation occurs. Factors causing hemorrhoids are constipation, diarrhea, pregnancy, congestive heart failure, portal hypertension, and prolonged sitting and standing.

Clinical Manifestations

The most common symptoms associated with enlarged, abnormal hemorrhoids are prolapse and bleeding. The bright red bleeding and prolapse usually occur at time of defecation.

Assessment

Collection of **subjective data** includes noting the patient's complaints of constipation, pruritus, severe pain when dilated veins become thrombosed, and bleeding from the rectum that is not mixed with feces.

Collection of **objective data** includes observing external hemorrhoids and palpating internal hemorrhoids on examination. Because bleeding and constipation are signs of cancer of the rectum, all patients with these symptoms should have a thorough examination to rule out cancer.

Medical Management

Conservative interventions include the use of bulk stool softeners—such as Metamucil, bran, and natural food fibers—to relieve straining. Topical creams with hydrocortisone relieve pruritus and inflammation, and analgesic ointments, such as dibucaine (Nupercainal), relieve pain. Sitz baths are usually given to relieve pain and edema and promote healing.

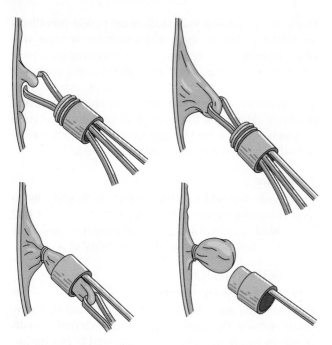

FIGURE **5-20** Rubber band ligation of an internal hemorrhoid.

Rubber-band ligation is a popular and easy method of treatment (Figure 5-20). Tight bands are applied with a special instrument in the physician's office, causing constriction and necrosis. The destroyed tissue sloughs off in about 1 week, and discomfort is minimal. Sclerotherapy (a needle is inserted at the apex of the hemorrhoid column and a sclerosing agent is injected), cryotherapy (tissue destruction by freezing), infrared photocoagulation (destruction of tissue by creation of a small burn), laser excision, and operative hemorrhoidectomy are additional interventions.

Hemorrhoidectomy, the surgical removal of hemorrhoids, can be performed if other interventions fail to relieve the distressing signs and symptoms. Surgery is indicated when there is prolapse, excessive pain or bleeding, or large hemorrhoids. In general, hemorrhoidectomy is reserved for patients with severe symptoms related to multiple thrombosed hemorrhoids or marked protrusion. Surgical removal may be done by cautery, clamp, or excision. After removal of the hemorrhoid, wounds can be left open or closed, although closed wounds are reported to heal faster. Although this surgery is not considered a major procedure, pain may be acute, requiring opioids and analgesic ointments. Complications of hemorrhoidectomy include hemorrhage, local infection, pain, urinary retention, and abscess.

Nursing Interventions and Patient Teaching

Rectal conditions can be embarrassing to the patient, and the nurse's direct but concerned attitude can decrease this embarrassment. The nurse can assess the knowledge level by asking patients about their con-

dition, what they have been told about treatment, and what treatments have been done before surgery and why.

The nurse should assess the patient with a prolapsed hemorrhoid for edema, thrombosis, and ischemia. Ischemic tissue will be dark red to necrotic (black). A low-bulk diet can produce chronic constipation, and this should be explained to the patient.

For the surgical patient, vital signs should be taken frequently for the first 24 hours to rule out internal bleeding. Sitz baths are given several times daily. Early ambulation and a soft diet facilitate bowel elimination. The patient may have a great deal of anxiety concerning the first defecation, and this should be discussed. An analgesic may be given before the bowel movement to reduce discomfort. A stool softener such as docusate (Colace) is usually ordered for the first few postoperative days.

Nursing diagnoses and interventions for the patient with hemorrhoids include but are not limited to the following:

NURSING DIAGNOSES	NURSING INTERVENTIONS
Pain, related to edema, prolapse, and surgical intervention	Instruct patient to wash anal area after defecation and pat dry. Sitz baths or local heat applied to site may be soothing. Use of local anesthetics (Nupercainal ointment or Tucks pads) may give relief. Reinforce need for high-residue diet. Instruct patient on manual reduction of external hemorrhoids. Apply ice packs to hemorrhoids if thrombosed to prevent edema and pain. Use a cushion for sitting postoperatively.
Anxiety, related to previous experiences, fear of first bowel movement postoperatively, and lack of knowledge regarding diet	Establish a supportive relationship with patient. Explain need for high-residue diet. Administer laxatives and oil-retention enema as ordered. Give analgesic before first bowel movement and a sitz bath after for pain relief.

The patient is advised to include in the diet bulk-forming foods, such as fresh fruits, vegetables, and bran cereals, as well as 8 to 10 glasses of fluid a day unless contraindicated. If the patient is anemic, discussion of foods high in iron—such as red meats, liver, and dark green leafy vegetables—can be included. Sitz baths are recommended for 1 to 2 weeks postoperatively. Moderate exercise and establishing a routine time for a daily bowel movement should be emphasized. The patient should also be instructed to report any signs of infection or delayed healing.

Prognosis

There are several preferred methods of treatment for hemorrhoids. Both conservative modes of treatment and surgical intervention for hemorrhoids have good prognostic rates.

ANAL FISSURE AND FISTULA

Anal fissure is a linear ulceration or laceration of the skin of the anus. Usually it is the result of trauma caused by hard stool that overstretches the anal lining. The fissure is aggravated by defecation, which initiates spasm of the anal sphincter; pain; and, at times, slight bleeding. If the lesion does not heal spontaneously, the tract is excised surgically.

An anal fistula is an abnormal opening on the cutaneous surface near the anus. Usually this is from a local crypt abscess and also is common in Crohn's disease. A perianal fistula may or may not communicate with the rectum. It results from rupture or drainage of an anal abscess. This chronic condition is treated by a fistulectomy (removal) or fistulotomy (opening of the fistula tract).

The postoperative care required for repair of an anal fissure or fistula is similar to that for the patient who has had a hemorrhoidectomy.

Prognosis

The prognosis for anal fissures and fistulas is good. This favorable prognosis is found in patients treated with conservative measures as well as in those who have surgical intervention.

FECAL INCONTINENCE
Etiology/Pathophysiology

Fecal incontinence is a complex problem that has a variety of causes. The external anal sphincter may be relaxed, the voluntary control of defecation may be interrupted in the central nervous system, or messages may not be transmitted to the brain because of a lesion within or external pressure on the spinal cord. The disorders that cause breakdown of conscious control of defecation include cortical clouding or lesions, spinal cord lesions or trauma, and trauma to the anal sphincter (e.g., from fistula, abscess, or surgery). Perineal relaxation and actual damage to the anal sphincter are often caused by injury from perineal surgery, childbirth, or anal intercourse. Relaxation of the sphincter usually increases with the general loss of muscle tone in aging. The normal changes that occur with aging are not of sufficient significance to cause incontinence, however, unless concurrent health problems predispose the patient to the disorder.

Normally the contents of the bowel are moved by mass movements toward the rectum. The rectum then stores the stool until defecation occurs. Distention of the rectum initiates nerve signals that are transmitted to the spinal cord and then back to the descending colon, initiating peristaltic waves that force more feces into the rectum. The internal anal sphincter relaxes, and if the external sphincter is also relaxed, defecation results. Defecation occurs as a reflex response to the distention of the rectal musculature, but this reflex can be voluntary inhibited. Voluntary inhibition of defecation is learned in early childhood, and control typically lasts throughout life. Emptying of the rectum occurs when the external anal sphincter (under cortical control) relaxes, and the abdominal and pelvic muscles contract.

Reflex defecation continues to occur even in the presence of most upper or lower motor neuron lesions, because the musculature of the bowel contains its own nerve centers that respond to distention through peristalsis. Reflex defecation therefore often persists or can be stimulated even when motor paralysis is present. Defecation occurs primarily in response to mass peristaltic movements that follow meals or whenever the rectum becomes distended. Any physical, mental, or social problem that disrupts any aspect of this complex learned behavior can result in incontinence.

Medical Management and Nursing Interventions

Biofeedback training is the cornerstone of therapy for patients who have motility disorders or sphincter damage that causes fecal incontinence. The patient learns to tighten the external sphincter in response to manometric measurement of responses to rectal distention. This technique has demonstrated effectiveness with alert motivated patients.

Bowel training is the major approach used with patients who have cognitive and neurological problems resulting from stroke or other chronic diseases. If a person can sit on a toilet, it may be possible to achieve automatic defecation when a pattern of consistent timing, familiar surroundings, and controlled diet and fluid intake can be achieved. This approach allows many patients to defecate predictably and remain continent throughout the day. Surgical correction is possible for a small group of patients whose incontinence is related to structural problems of the rectum and anus.

Patient Teaching

Bowel training requires significant amounts of time and effort on the part of the nursing staff, family, and patient. The nurse teaches the family about the training program and how they can assist and support the effort. Incontinence is a major issue in home care and frequently is cited as the most common reason for older adults to be admitted to nursing homes.

To plan the most effective approach, the nurse gathers specific information concerning the person's general physical and cognitive condition, ability to contract the abdominal and perineal muscles on command, and awareness of the need or urge to defecate. Data are also collected about the nature and frequency of the incontinence problem, particularly its relationship to meals or other regular activities.

The nurse teaches the family about the importance of a high-fiber diet and ensuring that the patient consumes at least 2500 mL of fluid daily. The need for a regular stool softener or bulk former is evaluated. When an optimal time for defecation has been established, usually after breakfast, a glycerin suppository may be inserted to stimulate defecation.

Despite honest efforts by family members, staff, and patient, the fecal incontinence may remain uncontrolled. Efforts will then shift toward odor control, preventing skin impairment, and supporting the patient's psychological integrity. Commercially available protective briefs are expensive, but they can substantially reduce the burden of care for the family and provide the patient with a sense of security and dignity.

NURSING PROCESS *for the Patient with a Gastrointestinal Disorder*

The role of the licensed practical nurse/licensed vocational nurse (LPN/LVN) in the nursing process as stated is that the LPN/LVN will:

- Participate in planning for patients based on patient needs.
- Review patient's plan of care and recommend revisions as needed.
- Review and follow defined prioritization for patient care.
- Use clinical pathways/care maps/care plans to guide and review patient care.

Assessment

As the nurse begins care of the patient admitted with a gastrointestinal disorder, a thorough, immediate, and accurate nursing assessment is an essential first step. The assessment should include the patient's level of consciousness; vital signs; skin color; edema; appetite; weight loss; nausea; vomiting; and bowel habits, including color and consistency of stools. The abdomen should be assessed for distention, guarding, and peristalsis. The assessment should include a past history of smoking or alcohol use, medications, epigastric or abdominal pain, and acute or chronic stressors and coping-stress tolerance.

Nursing Diagnosis

Assessment provides the data from which the nurse identifies the patient's problems, strengths, and potential complications, as well as learning needs of the patient. Once the diagnoses are defined, the nurse can assist in formulating a plan of care that meets the needs of the patient. Being able to prioritize the nursing interventions needed by the patient helps con-

tribute to a patient's well-being. Possible nursing diagnoses that should be considered for the patient with a gastrointestinal disorder include but are not limited to the following:

- Activity intolerance
- Anxiety
- Disturbed body image
- Constipation
- Ineffective coping
- Diarrhea
- Fear
- Risk for deficient fluid volume
- Impaired home maintenance
- Ineffective management of therapeutic regimen
- Imbalanced nutrition: less than body requirements
- Pain
- Risk for impaired skin integrity
- Disturbed sleep pattern
- Social isolation
- Ineffective tissue perfusion

Expected Outcomes/Planning

When planning the care of the patient with a gastrointestinal disorder, the nurse should note the nursing diagnoses and assist in a plan of care based on the patient's health care needs. By establishing the patient's needs the nurse can then assist in the plan of care to include nursing interventions to assist in eliminating the problems. The patient must be included in the planning to promote compliance with the nursing interventions.

The plan of care may be based on one or more of the following goals:

Goal #1: Patient will have no evidence of excoriation around stomal area.

Goal #2: Patient will begin to adjust to disturbed body image.

Implementation

Nursing interventions for the patient with a gastrointestinal disorder include a variety of interventions that may be simple to complex. Interventions include assessment, monitoring nutritional status, administering medications, promoting health, relieving pain, maintaining skin integrity, managing fluid and electrolyte imbalance, promoting normal bowel elimination patterns, preventing wound infection, health counseling to focus on elimination of smoking and excessive alcohol intake, and patient teaching for enterostomal therapy. Cultural considerations are a vital part of nursing interventions for the patient with a gastrointestinal disorder (Cultural and Ethnic Considerations box).

Evaluation

During and after the planned nursing interventions, the nurse should determine the outcomes of the nursing interventions. This is an ongoing process whereby the nurse is continuously endeavoring to establish the most effective plan of care.

Cultural and Ethnic Considerations

Gastrointestinal Disorder

- Inflammatory bowel disease (Crohn's disease and ulcerative colitis) is more common among whites than African-Americans and Asian-Americans.
- Inflammatory bowel disease is more common among Jewish people and those of middle European origin.
- Colorectal cancer is higher in the United States and Canada than in Japan, Finland, or Africa.
- Incidence of colorectal cancer is declining in the United States except among African-American men.

Evaluation involves determining whether the established goals have been met. The goals are evaluated by the nurse and patient to see whether the criteria for assessment have been met.

Evaluation for Goal #1: There is no impairment of skin integrity around stoma.

Evaluation for Goal #2: Patient is demonstrating adjustment to disturbed body image by expressing feelings about stoma and is beginning to assume some stoma and pouch care.

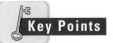

Key Points

- The digestive tract begins with the mouth, extends through the thoracic and abdominal cavities, and ends with the anus.
- The major processes of digestion and absorption take place in the small intestine.
- The large intestine is responsible for the preparation and evacuation of the waste products—feces.
- Diet therapy has an important role in the treatment of GI disorders.

- Treatment of esophageal disorders often involves providing the patient with a means of eating, in addition to treating the disorder.
- Common causes of gastric disorders are alcohol, tobacco, aspirin, and antiinflammatory agents.
- Duodenal ulcers are the most common type of peptic ulcer disease.
- Surgical procedures are available as alternatives to the traditional ileostomy and colostomy.
- A nursing goal for the patient with an ileostomy or colostomy is fostering patient independence in daily care when the patient demonstrates readiness.
- Keeping the surgical area free of contamination is of primary importance after rectal surgery.
- The approximate location of GI bleeding may be determined by the characteristics of the emesis or fecal material.
- The nurse explains the purpose of any diagnostic procedure, how the procedure is performed, and the preparation necessary for the procedure and assists in the patient's understanding of the results.
- *H. pylori* has been identified in more than 70% of gastric ulcer patients and 95% of those with duodenal ulcers.
- Individuals with inflammatory bowel disease have a greater risk of developing cancer of the bowel.
- Early detection of cancer in the GI system facilitates early treatment and a better prognosis.
- An NG tube is inserted to keep the stomach empty until peristalsis is resumed after a general anesthetic or any condition that interferes with peristalsis.
- Effective postoperative care begins with patient teaching during the preoperative period.

 Go to your free CD-ROM for an Audio Glossary, animations, video clips, and Review Questions for the NCLEX-PN® Examination.

evolve   Be sure to visit the companion Evolve site at http://evolve.elsevier.com/Christensen/adult/ for WebLinks and additional online resources.

CHAPTER CHALLENGE

1. Because the small intestine needs bile only a few times a day, bile is stored and concentrated in the:

   1. pancreas.
   2. gallbladder.
   3. liver.
   4. small intestine.

2. Although food is digested throughout the alimentary canal, up to 90% of digestion is accomplished in the:

   1. gallbladder.
   2. mouth.
   3. small intestine.
   4. large intestine.

3. The exit from the stomach is called the:

   1. cardiac sphincter.
   2. pyloric sphincter.
   3. lesser curvature.
   4. greater curvature.

4. The intrinsic factor is a gastric secretion necessary for the intestinal absorption of vitamin:

   1. B_1.
   2. B_{12}.
   3. C.
   4. K.

Continued

CHAPTER CHALLENGE—cont'd

5. Which organ manufactures heparin, prothrombin, and fibrinogen?

    1. Gallbladder
    2. Liver
    3. Pancreas
    4. Salivary gland

6. The digestive enzyme present in saliva is called:

    1. ptyalin.
    2. sucrase.
    3. lipase.
    4. trypsin.

7. In preparing the patient for endoscopic examination of the upper GI tract, the patient's pharynx is anesthetized with lidocaine (Xylocaine). Nursing interventions for postendoscopic examination include:

    1. allowing fluids up to 4 hours before examination.
    2. withholding anticholinergic medications.
    3. prohibiting smoking before the test.
    4. keeping patient NPO until gag reflex returns.

8. Mr. S., a 35-year-old patient, has been admitted with a diagnosis of peptic ulcers. The nurse recognizes which drugs as those most commonly used in these patients to decrease acid secretions?

    1. Maalox and Kayexalate
    2. Tagamet and Zantac
    3. erythromycin and Flagyl
    4. Dyazide and Carafate

9. Ms. P. is scheduled in the morning for a hemicolectomy for removal of a cancerous tumor of the ascending colon. The physician has ordered intestinal antibiotics for her preoperatively to:

    1. decrease the bulk of colon contents.
    2. reduce the bacteria content of the colon.
    3. soften the stool.
    4. prevent pneumonia.

10. Ms. B. is 78 years old and was admitted during the evening shift with a tentative diagnosis of cancer of the esophagus. The nurse in her initial assessment finds the patient's major complaint is:

    1. dysphagia.
    2. malnutrition.
    3. pain.
    4. regurgitation of food.

11. Deficient knowledge is a commonly used nursing diagnosis when patients need information regarding their conditions and diagnostic tests. Before a gastroscopy, the nurse should inform the patient that:

    1. fasting for 6 to 8 hours is necessary before the examination.
    2. a general anesthetic will be used.

    3. after gastroscopy, the patient may eat or drink immediately.
    4. it is necessary to be an inpatient in the hospital.

12. In evaluating the care of Ms. K., a young executive admitted with bleeding peptic ulcer, the nurse focuses on nursing interventions. A nursing intervention associated with this type of patient is:

    1. checking the blood pressure and pulse rates each shift.
    2. frequently monitoring arterial blood levels.
    3. observing vomitus for color, consistency, and volume.
    4. checking the patient's low-residue diet.

13. Mr. L., the staff nurse on the surgical floor, is aware of pulmonary complications that frequently follow upper abdominal incisions. These are most frequently related to:

    1. aspiration.
    2. pneumothorax if the chest cavity has been entered.
    3. shallow respirations to minimize pain.
    4. not forcing fluids.

14. Which of the following tests can distinguish between peptic ulcer disease and gastric malignancy?

    1. Radiographic GI series
    2. Breath test for *H. pylori*
    3. Serum test for *H. pylori* antibodies
    4. Endoscopy with biopsy

15. A recently approved medication for the treatment of Crohn's disease, infliximab, (Remicade) is classified as which type of drug?

    1. Enzyme
    2. Antimetabolite
    3. Alkylating agent
    4. Monoclonal antibody

16. During assessment of the patient with esophageal achalasia, the nurse would expect the patient to report:

    1. a history of alcohol use.
    2. a sore throat and hoarseness.
    3. dysphagia, especially with liquids.
    4. relief of pyrosis with the use of antacids.

17. A nursing intervention that is most appropriate to decrease postoperative edema and pain in the male patient following an inguinal herniorrhaphy is:

    1. applying a truss to the hernial site.
    2. allowing the patient to stand to void.
    3. elevation of the scrotum with a support or small pillow.
    4. supporting the incision during routine coughing and deep breathing.

18. The use of nonabsorbable antibiotics as preparation for bowel surgery is done primarily to:
    1. reduce the bacterial flora in the colon.
    2. prevent additional formation of ammonia.
    3. prevent postoperative formation of intestinal gas.
    4. stimulate bowel bacteria to increase production of vitamin K.

19. In planning care for the patient with ulcerative colitis, the nurse recognizes that a major difference between ulcerative colitis and Crohn's disease is that ulcerative colitis:
    1. causes more nutritional deficiencies than does Crohn's disease.
    2. causes more abdominal pain and cramping than does Crohn's disease.
    3. is curable with a colectomy, whereas Crohn's disease often recurs after surgery.
    4. is more highly associated with a familial relationship than is Crohn's disease.

20. Which group of medications should be avoided in patients with *E. coli* 0157:H7?
    1. Antiemetics
    2. Antimotility drugs
    3. Antilipidemic agents
    4. Beta blockers

21. Which of the following should a patient be taught after a hemorrhoidectomy?
    1. Do not use the Valsalva maneuver.
    2. Eat a low-fiber diet to rest the colon.
    3. Administer oil-retention enema to empty the colon.
    4. Use prescribed analgesic before a bowel movement.

6 Care of the Patient with a Gallbladder, Liver, Biliary Tract, or Exocrine Pancreatic Disorder

BARBARA LAURITSEN CHRISTENSEN

Objectives

After reading this chapter, the student should be able to do the following:

1. Define the key terms as listed.
2. Discuss nursing interventions for the diagnostic examinations of patients with disorders of the gallbladder, liver, biliary tract, and exocrine pancreas.
3. Explain the etiology, pathophysiology, clinical manifestations, assessment, diagnostic tests, medical management, and nursing interventions for the patient with cirrhosis of the liver, carcinoma of the liver, hepatitis, liver abscesses, cholecystitis, cholelithiasis, pancreatitis, and cancer of the pancreas.
4. Define jaundice and describe signs and symptoms that may occur with jaundice.
5. State the six types of viral hepatitis, including their modes of transmission.
6. List the subjective and objective data for the patient with viral hepatitis.
7. Discuss the indicators for liver transplantation and the immunosuppressant drugs to reduce rejection.
8. Discuss specific complications and teaching content for the patient with cirrhosis of the liver.
9. Discuss the two methods of surgical treatment for cholecystitis/cholelithiasis.

Key Terms

Be sure to check out the bonus material on the free CD-ROM, including selected audio pronunciations.

ascites (ă-SĪ-tēz, p. 258)
asterixis (ăs-tĕr-ĬK-sĭs, p. 262)
esophageal varices (ĕ-sŏf-ă-JĒ-ăl VĂR-ĭ-sēz, p. 260)
flatulence (FLĂT-ū-lĕns, p. 271)
hepatic encephalopathy (hĕ-PĂT-ĭk ĕn-sĕf-ĕ-LŎP-ĕ-thē, p. 261)
hepatitis (hĕ-pă-TĪ-tĭs, p. 255)
jaundice (JAWN-dĭs, p. 258)
occlusion (ŏ-KLOO-zhŭn, p. 278)
paracentesis (păr-ă-sĕn-TĒ-sĭs, p. 258)
parenchyma (pă-rĕng-KĪ-mă, p. 257)
spider telangiectases (SPĪ-dĕr tĕl-ăn-jĕ-ĔK-tĕ-sēz, p. 258)
steatorrhea (stē-ă-tō-RĒ-ă, p. 271)

This chapter discusses disorders of the accessory organs of digestion—namely the liver, gallbladder, and exocrine pancreas. These organs assist in digestion in various ways. See Chapter 5 for a review of the anatomy and physiology of the liver, biliary tract, gallbladder, and pancreas.

LABORATORY AND DIAGNOSTIC EXAMINATIONS IN THE ASSESSMENT OF THE HEPATOBILIARY AND PANCREATIC SYSTEMS

SERUM BILIRUBIN TEST

Normal values are as follows:
   Direct bilirubin: 0.1 to 0.3 mg/dL
   Indirect bilirubin: 0.2 to 0.8 mg/dL
   Total bilirubin: 0.3 to 1 mg/dL
   Total bilirubin in newborns: 1 to 12 mg/dL

Rationale

Total serum bilirubin determination measures both direct, or conjugated (water-soluble), and indirect, or unconjugated (water-insoluble), bilirubin. Total serum bilirubin level is the sum of the direct and indirect bilirubin levels. Testing for bilirubin in the blood provides valuable information for diagnosis and evaluation of liver disease, biliary obstruction, erythroblastosis fetalis, and hemolytic anemia. Jaundice is the discoloration of body tissues caused by abnormally high blood levels of bilirubin. This yellow discoloration is recognized when the total serum bilirubin exceeds 2.5 mg/dL.

Nursing Interventions

The nurse should keep the patient on nothing per mouth (NPO) status until after the blood specimen is drawn.

LIVER ENZYME TESTS

The normal values are as follows:
   AST (aspartate aminotransferase; formerly serum glutamic-oxaloacetic transaminase [SGOT]): Adult 0 to 35 units/L. (AST level is elevated in

myocardial infarctions, hepatitis, cirrhosis, hepatic necrosis, hepatic tumor, acute pancreatitis, and acute hemolytic anemia.)

ALT (alanine aminotransferase; formerly serum glutamate pyruvate transaminase [SGPT]): Adult/child 4 to 36 units/L. (ALT level is elevated in hepatitis, cirrhosis, hepatic necrosis, and hepatic tumors and by hepatotoxic drugs.)

LDH (lactic dehydrogenase): Adult 100 to 190 units/L. (Values are increased in myocardial infarction, pulmonary infarction, hepatic disease [e.g., hepatitis, active cirrhosis, neoplasm], pancreatitis, and skeletal muscle disease.)

Alkaline phosphatase: Adult 30 to 120 units/L. (Alkaline phosphatase level is elevated in obstructive disorders of the biliary tract, hepatic tumors, cirrhosis, hepatitis, primary and metastatic tumors, hyperparathyroidism, metastatic tumor in bones, and healing fractures.)

Gamma GT (gamma glutamyltransferase): Male and female older than age 45: 8 to 38 units/L; female younger than age 45: 5 to 27 units/L. (Levels are elevated in liver cell dysfunction such as hepatitis and cirrhosis; hepatic tumors; with the use of hepatotoxic drugs; jaundice; and in myocardial infarction [MI] [4 to 10 days after], heart failure, alcohol ingestion, pancreatitis, and cancer of the pancreas.)

Rationale

The liver is a storehouse of many enzymes. Injury or diseases affecting the liver will cause release of these intracellular enzymes into the bloodstream, and their levels will be elevated. Some of these enzymes are produced also in other organs, and injury or disease affecting these other organs will also cause an elevated serum level. Therefore, although elevation of these serum enzymes is found in pathologic liver conditions, the test is not specific for liver diseases alone.

Nursing Interventions

The nurse should assess the venipuncture site for bleeding.

SERUM PROTEIN TEST

The normal values are as follows:

Total protein: 6.4 to 8.3 g/dL
Albumin: 3.5 to 5 g/dL
Globulin: 2.3 to 3.4 g/dL
Albumin globulin (A/G ratio): 1.2 to 2.2 g/dL

Rationale

One way to assess the functional status of the liver is to measure the products that are synthesized there. One of these products is protein, especially albumin.

When disease affects the liver cell, the hepatocyte loses its ability to synthesize albumin and the serum albumin level is markedly decreased.

Low serum albumin levels may result also from excessive loss of albumin into urine (as in nephrotic syndrome) or into third-space volumes (as in ascites), liver disease, increased capillary permeability, or protein-caloric malnutrition.

Nursing Interventions

The nurse should assess the venipuncture site for bleeding.

ORAL CHOLECYSTOGRAPHY (OCG) (GALLBLADDER SERIES, GB SERIES, CHOLECYSTOGRAM)

Rationale

The oral cholecystogram provides roentgenographic visualization of the gallbladder after the oral ingestion of a radiopaque, iodinated dye. Adequate visualization of the gallbladder requires concentration of the dye within the gallbladder. An oral cholecystogram is less accurate than a gallbladder ultrasound and is less commonly used for visualizing the biliary tree. OCG will not visualize the biliary tree in the jaundiced patient. The following factors are necessary for adequate dye concentration:

- Ingestion by the patient of the correct number of dye tablets the evening before the examination
- Adequate absorption of the dye from the gastrointestinal (GI) tract; vomiting or diarrhea will preclude absorption of the dye
- Abstinence from food (especially a fatty meal) on the morning of the test
- Uptake from the portal system and excretion of the dye by the liver
- Patency of the cystic duct
- Concentration of the dye within the gallbladder

Nursing Interventions

Before administration of the dye, the nurse should make certain the patient is not allergic to iodine to prevent adverse or allergic reaction. This rarely occurs because the dye is not administered intravenously. If no allergy to iodine is present, the nurse administers six iopanoic acid (e.g., Telepaque, Priodax, Oragrafin) tablets orally, one every 5 minutes, beginning after the evening meal. The patient is on NPO status from midnight. The patient may be given a high-fat meal or beverage to stimulate emptying of the gallbladder after the test has begun. No other food or fluids will be allowed until the examination is complete.

INTRAVENOUS CHOLANGIOGRAPHY (INTRAVENOUS CHOLANGIOGRAM, IVC)

Rationale

In this study, intravenously administered radiographic dye is concentrated by the liver and secreted into the bile duct. IVC allows visualization of the hepatic and common bile ducts and also the gallbladder if the cystic duct is patent. IVC is used to demonstrate stones, stricture, or tumor of the hepatic duct, common bile duct, and gallbladder. IVC is a less commonly used method of visualizing the biliary tree. IVC will not visualize the biliary tree in a jaundiced patient.

OPERATIVE CHOLANGIOGRAPHY

In operative cholangiography the common bile duct is directly injected with radiopaque dye. Stones appear as radiolucent shadows, and tumors cause partial or total obstruction of the flow of dye into the duodenum. By visualization of the biliary duct structures, the surgeon is provided with a "road map" of a commonly difficult anatomic area. This reduces the possibility of inadvertently injuring the common duct.

If common duct stones are suspected, a cholecystectomy as well as a common duct exploration (CDE) must be performed. When intraoperative cholangiography is used routinely, CDE is performed only on those with positive cholangiography.

T-TUBE CHOLANGIOGRAPHY (POSTOPERATIVE CHOLANGIOGRAPHY)

Rationale

T-tube cholangiography is performed to diagnose retained ductal stones postoperatively in the patient who has had a cholecystectomy and a common bile duct exploration and to demonstrate good flow of contrast of bile into the duodenum. The test is performed through the use of a T-shaped rubber tube that the surgeon places in the bile duct during the operation. Through the end of the T-tube that exits through the abdominal wall, dye can be injected and radiographic films taken.

Nursing Interventions

The nurse should protect the patient from sepsis by connecting the T-tube (if left in place) to a sterile closed-drainage system. If the T-tube is removed, the T-tube tract site should be kept covered with a sterile dressing to prevent bacteria from entering the ductal system.

Before the administration of the dye, the nurse should ensure that the patient is not allergic to iodine. Preparation of the patient also includes NPO after midnight and until the examination is completed. The nurse administers a cleansing enema on the morning of the examination, if ordered.

ULTRASONOGRAPHY (ECHOGRAM) OF THE LIVER, GALLBLADDER, AND BILIARY SYSTEM

Rationale

Ultrasonography (ultrasound) is an imaging technique in which deep structures of the body are visualized by recording the reflections (echoes) of ultrasonic waves directed into the tissues. This diagnostic test is not effective in examining all tissue because ultrasound waves do not pass through structures that contain air, such as the lungs, colon, or stomach. Although fasting is preferred, it is not necessary for ultrasonography. Because this study requires no contrast material and has no associated radiation, it is especially useful for patients who are allergic to contrast media and for pregnant patients. Ultrasound is used with increasing frequency to corroborate data already obtained by "questionable positive" cholangiograms, liver scans, and oral cholecystograms.

Nursing Interventions

The patient is NPO from midnight. If the patient has had recent barium contrast studies, the nurse should request an order for cathartics. Ultrasound cannot penetrate barium, and the study will not be adequate.

GALLBLADDER SCANNING (HEPATOBILIARY SCINTIGRAPHY IMAGING, HIDA SCANNING)

Rationale

Through the use of IV injection of technetium (Tc) (technetium 99m), and positioned under camera to record distribution of tracer in the liver, biliary tree, gallbladder, and proximal small bowel, the biliary tract can be evaluated safely, accurately, and noninvasively. The primary use of this study is in the diagnosis of acute cholecystitis. This procedure is superior to oral cholecystography, ultrasonography, and CT scanning of the abdomen for the detection of acute cholecystitis. HIDA scanning is also useful for identifying diffuse hepatic disease (such as cirrhosis or neoplasm).

Nursing Interventions

The nurse should assure the patient that exposure to radioactivity is minimal because only a trace dose of the radioisotope is used. The patient is NPO from midnight until the examination is complete.

NEEDLE LIVER BIOPSY

Rationale

Needle liver biopsy is a safe, simple, and valuable method of diagnosing pathologic liver conditions. For this study a specially designed needle is inserted through the skin, between the sixth and seventh or eighth and ninth intercostal spaces, and into the liver. The patient lies supine with the right arm over the head. The patient should be instructed to exhale fully and not breathe while the needle is inserted. This procedure is often done using ultrasound or CT guidance. A piece of hepatic tissue is removed for microscopic examination. The tissue sample is placed into a correctly labeled specimen bottle containing formalin and sent to the pathology department. Percutaneous liver biopsy is used in the diagnosis of various liver disorders, such as cirrhosis, hepatitis, drug-related reactions, granuloma, and tumor.

Nursing Interventions

The nurse should explain the procedure to the patient and obtain the patient's signature on a consent form. The nurse ensures that platelet, clotting or bleeding time, and prothrombin time and International Normalized Ratio (INR) have been ordered and any abnormal values are reported to the physician. After the procedure the nurse observes the patient for symptoms of bleeding. Vital signs are monitored every 15 minutes (two times), then every 30 minutes (four times), and then every hour (four times).

Some pain is common. When leakage involves a large quantity of blood or bile, the peritoneal reaction is great and the resulting pain is severe. The nurse assesses for pneumothorax (collapsed lung) caused by improper placement of the biopsy needle into the adjacent chest cavity or for bile peritonitis. The nurse should report these signs and symptoms immediately to the physician. Keep the patient lying on the right side for a minimum of 2 hours to splint the puncture site. In this position, the liver capsule is compressed against the chest wall, thereby decreasing the risk of hemorrhage or bile leak.

RADIOISOTOPE LIVER SCANNING
Rationale

This radionuclide procedure is used to outline and detect structural changes of the liver. A radionuclide is given intravenously. Later, a gamma-ray detecting device (Geiger counter) is passed over the patient's abdomen. This records the distribution of the radioactive particles in the liver. The spleen can also be visualized by the detector when technetium 99m sulfur is used.

Nursing Interventions

The patient should be NPO from midnight. The nurse should assure patients that they will not be exposed to a large amount of radioactivity, because only trace doses of isotopes are used.

SERUM AMMONIA TEST
Normal value is 10 to 80 mcg/dL.

Rationale

Ammonia is a byproduct of protein metabolism. Most of the ammonia is made by bacteria acting on proteins present in the intestine. By way of the portal vein, ammonia goes to the liver, where it is normally converted into urea and then excreted by the kidneys. With severe liver dysfunction or when the blood flow to the liver is altered, ammonia cannot be catabolized and the serum ammonia level rises and the BUN level decreases. The serum ammonia level is primarily used as an aid in diagnosing hepatic encephalopathy and hepatic coma. Elevated serum ammonia levels suggest liver dysfunction as the cause of these signs and symptoms.

Nursing Interventions

The nurse should list on the laboratory requisition any antibiotics the patient is currently taking. Certain broad-spectrum antibiotics such as neomycin can cause a decreased ammonia level, thus giving inaccurate test results.

HEPATITIS VIRUS STUDIES (HEPATITIS-ASSOCIATED ANTIGEN [HAA])

A normal laboratory test result will be negative for the presence of the antigen.

Rationale

Hepatitis is an inflammation of the liver caused by viruses, bacteria, and noninfectious causes of liver inflammation. Six viruses are now recognized that can cause this disease: hepatitis A virus, hepatitis B virus, hepatitis C virus, hepatitis D virus, hepatitis E virus, and hepatitis G virus. Hepatitis A and B have been recognized for years, but hepatitis C, D, E, and G were identified more recently. The individual hepatitis viruses can be detected by different antigen and antibody levels, and different incubation periods must be considered. What happened to hepatitis F? Over time, researchers could not substantiate hepatitis F as a separate illness. They realized that some of the so-called cases of hepatitis F were really mutations of hepatitis C virus (Durston, 2004).

Nursing Interventions

The nurse should use standard precautions and should handle the serum specimen as if it were capable of transmitting viral hepatitis. Health care personnel must don gloves when handling any blood or body fluids and wash hands carefully after handling all equipment.

SERUM AMYLASE TEST
Normal value is 60 to 120 Somogyi units/dL, or 30 to 220 units/L (SI units).

Rationale

The serum amylase test is an easily and rapidly performed test for pancreatitis. Damage to pancreatic cells (as in pancreatitis) or obstruction to the pancreatic ductal flow (as in pancreatic carcinoma) will cause an outpouring of this enzyme into the intrapancreatic lymph system as well as into the free peritoneum. Blood vessels draining the free peritoneum and absorbing the lymph pick up this excess amylase. An abnormal rise in the serum level of amylase is the result, and it will occur within 12 hours of the onset of pancreatic disease. Because amylase is rapidly cleared by the kidney, serum levels may return to normal within 48 to 72 hours. Persistent pancreatitis, duct obstruction, or pancreatic duct leak (e.g., pseudocysts) will cause persistent elevated serum levels.

Nursing Interventions

The nurse should note on the laboratory requisition whether the patient is receiving intravenous (IV) dextrose or any medications, because these can cause a false-negative result.

URINE AMYLASE TEST

The normal value for this study is up to 5000 Somogyi units/24 hr or 6.5 to 48.1 units/hour.

Rationale

Because the kidney rapidly clears amylase, disorders affecting the pancreas will cause elevated amylase levels in the urine. Levels of amylase in the urine remain elevated for 7 to 10 days after the onset of disease. Urine amylase is particularly useful in detecting pancreatitis late in the disease course. This fact is important if the diagnosis of pancreatitis is to be made in patients who have had symptoms for 3 days or longer.

Nursing Interventions

The nurse should record the exact times of the beginning and end of the collection period. A 2-hour spot urine or 6-hour, 12-hour, or 24-hour collection can be performed, depending on the physician's order. The collection begins after the patient empties the bladder and discards that specimen. All subsequent urine is collected, including the voiding at the end of the collection period. The specimen should be kept on ice or refrigerated until it is sent to the laboratory.

SERUM LIPASE TEST

The normal value is 0 to 160 units/L.

Rationale

Serum lipase is also elevated in acute pancreatitis and is a helpful complementary test because other disorders (e.g., mumps, cerebral trauma, renal transplantation) may also cause an increase in serum amylase. As with amylase, lipase appears in the bloodstream following damage to the pancreas. The lipase levels usually rise a little later than amylase (24 to 48 hours after the onset of pancreatitis) and remain elevated for 5 to 7 days. Because lipase peaks later and remains elevated longer than serum amylase, it is more useful in the diagnosis of acute pancreatitis later in the course of the disease.

Nursing Interventions

Instruct the patient to remain NPO after midnight, except for water.

ULTRASONOGRAPHY OF THE PANCREAS
Rationale

Through the use of reflected sound waves, ultrasonography of the pancreas provides diagnostic information of this rather inaccessible abdominal organ. Ultrasound examination of the pancreas is mainly used to establish the diagnosis of carcinoma, pseudocyst, pancreatitis, and pancreatic abscess. Because ultrasound abnormalities persist from several days to weeks, the diagnosis of pancreatitis can be supported by this study even after the serum amylase and lipase levels have returned to normal. Furthermore, follow-up ultrasound study can be used to monitor the resolution of pancreatic inflammation and the response of a tumor to therapy.

Nursing Interventions

Fluids and foods are withheld for 8 hours before the examination, but fasting is not mandatory to obtain accurate results. If the patient's abdomen is distended with gas or if the patient has had a recent barium examination, this study should be postponed, because gas or barium will interfere with sound wave transmission.

COMPUTED TOMOGRAPHY (CT) OF THE ABDOMEN
Rationale

CT scan of the abdomen is a noninvasive, accurate radiographic procedure used to diagnose pathologic pancreatic conditions such as inflammation, tumor, cyst formation, ascites, aneurysm, and cirrhosis of the liver. The recognizable cross-sectional image produced by a CT scan is especially important for studying the pancreas, because this organ is retroperitoneal and well hidden by the overlying peritoneal organs.

Nursing Interventions

Fluids and food are withheld from midnight until the examination is complete; however, this test can be performed on an emergency basis on patients who have recently eaten. If possible, the nurse should show the patient a picture of the machine and encourage the patient to verbalize fears because some patients suffer claustrophobia when enclosed in the machine.

ENDOSCOPIC RETROGRADE CHOLANGIOPANCREATOGRAPHY (ERCP) OF THE PANCREATIC DUCT
Rationale

Not only can the biliary system be visualized by ERCP; the pancreatic duct also can be seen. During the test a fiberoptic duodenoscope is inserted through the oral pharynx, through the esophagus and stomach, and into the duodenum (Figure 6-1). Dye is injected for radiographic visualization of the common bile duct and pancreatic duct. ERCP of the pancreas is a sensitive and reliable procedure for detecting clinically significant degrees of pancreatic dysfunction. It can also be used to evaluate obstructive jaundice, remove common bile duct stones, and place biliary and pancreatic duct stents to bypass obstruction. Localized pancreatic duct narrowing indicates tumor. Chronic pancreatitis is demonstrated by multiple areas of ductal narrowing, which can be visualized by ERCP.

Nursing Interventions

Food and fluids are withheld for 8 hours before the examination, and the patient's signature on a consent form is obtained. The nurse should tell patients that the test takes approximately 1 to 2 hours, during which time they must lie completely motionless on a hard x-ray table, which may be uncomfortable for the patient. After the procedure, keep the patient NPO until gag reflex returns; assess for abdominal pain, tenderness, and guarding. Assess for signs and symptoms of pancreatitis, which is the most common ERCP complication. These signs and symptoms include increasingly intense abdominal pain, nausea, vomiting, and diminished or absent bowel sounds. Assess for hypovolemic shock.

DISORDERS OF THE LIVER, BILIARY TRACT, GALLBLADDER, AND EXOCRINE PANCREAS

The liver, gallbladder, and exocrine pancreas are all organs that assist with digestion. Review anatomy and physiology of accessory organs of digestion (see Chapter 5) and hepatic portal circulation.

CIRRHOSIS
Etiology/Pathophysiology

Cirrhosis is a chronic, degenerative disease of the liver in which the lobes are covered with fibrous tissue, the parenchyma (tissue of an organ as distinguished from supporting or connective tissue) degenerates, and the lobules are infiltrated with fat. The fibrous (scar) tissue restricts the flow of blood to the organ, which contributes to its destruction. Hepatomegaly (enlargement of the liver) and, later, liver contraction cause loss of the organ's function.

Cirrhosis is ranked as the ninth leading cause of death in the United States and fourth leading cause of death in people between the ages of 40 and 60.

There are several forms of cirrhosis, caused by different factors. Alcoholic cirrhosis, previously called Laënnec's cirrhosis, most commonly found in the Western world, affects more men than women and is found in patients with a history of chronic ingestion of alcohol. Postnecrotic cirrhosis, found worldwide, is caused by viral hepatitis, exposure to hepatotoxins (e.g., industrial chemicals), or infection. Primary biliary cirrhosis is found more often in women and results from destruction of the bile ducts. Secondary biliary cirrhosis is caused by chronic biliary tree obstruction caused by gallstones, a tumor, or biliary atresia in children. Cardiac cirrhosis results from longstanding, severe right-sided heart failure in patients with cor pulmonale, constrictive pericarditis, and tricuspid insufficiency.

With repeated insults, the liver can progress through the following stages: destruction, inflammation, fibrotic regeneration, and hepatic insufficiency. Although liver cells have a great potential for regeneration, repeated scarring decreases their ability to be replaced. As the blood supply continues to be diminished and the scar tissue increases, the organ atrophies.

Functions of the liver are altered in several ways. The liver's ability to synthesize albumin is reduced as a result of liver cell damage. The obstruction of the portal vein as it enters the liver results in portal hypertension, or increased pressure in the veins that drain the GI tract.

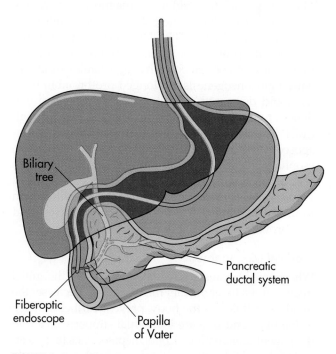

FIGURE **6-1** Endoscopic retrograde cholangiopancreatography (ERCP).

Portal hypertension is an increased venous pressure in the portal circulation caused by compression or by occlusion in the portal or hepatic vascular system. In most instances, portal hypertension that develops from cirrhosis is irreversible.

This increased pressure causes ascites (an accumulation of fluid and albumin in the peritoneal cavity). The damaged liver cannot metabolize protein in the usual manner; therefore protein intake may result in an elevation of blood ammonia levels. Reduced synthesis of protein and the leaking of existing protein result in hypoalbuminemia (reduced protein or albumin level in the blood), which reduces the blood's ability to regain fluids through osmosis. Protein must be present in adequate amounts to create colloidal osmotic pressure and "attract" the fluid to pass back into the blood vessels after it escapes in the capillaries. As fluid leaves the blood and the circulating volume decreases, the receptors in the brain signal the adrenal cortex to increase secretion of aldosterone to stimulate the kidneys to retain sodium and water. The normal liver inactivates the hormone aldosterone, but the damaged liver allows its effect to continue (hyperaldosteronism). Retention of fluid and sodium results in increased pressure in blood vessels and lymphatic channels, resulting in portal hypertension. Ascites is thus a result of portal hypertension, hypoalbuminemia, and hyperaldosteronism.

Hepatic insufficiency gradually causes veins in the upper part of the body to distend, including the esophageal vein. Esophageal varicosities develop and may rupture, causing severe hemorrhage.

Clinical Manifestations

Clinical manifestations of cirrhosis of the liver differ, depending on whether the patient is in the early or the later stages of disease. In the early stages, the liver is firm and therefore easier to palpate, and abdominal pain may be present because of rapid enlargement that produces tension on the fibrous covering of the organ. Later stages of the disease present manifestations of dyspepsia, changes in bowel habits, gradual weight loss, ascites, enlarged spleen, and spider telangiectases (small, dilated blood vessels with a bright red center point and spiderlike branches). Spider telangiectases occur on the nose, cheeks, upper trunk, neck, and shoulders. These later manifestations are the result of scarring of liver tissue that produces chronic failure of liver function and also fibrotic changes that cause obstruction of the portal circulation.

When enough cells of the liver become involved to interfere with its function and obstruct its circulation, the GI organs and the spleen become congested and cannot function properly. Anemia occurs because of the body's decreased ability to produce RBCs. The cirrhotic liver cannot absorb vitamin K or produce the clotting factors VII, IX, and X. This causes the patient with cirrhosis to have bleeding tendencies.

Assessment

Collection of **subjective data** in the **early stages** may include the patient describing symptoms as flulike, including loss of appetite, nausea and vomiting, general weakness, fatigue, indigestion, abnormal bowel function (either constipation or diarrhea), flatulence, and abdominal discomfort. The anatomic area most commonly affected is in the epigastric region or the right upper quadrant of the abdomen.

Collection of **subjective data** in the **later stages** includes noting those subjective symptoms listed under early stages, although they are more intense in later stages. The patient may complain of dyspnea, pruritus, and severe fatigue that interfere with the ability to carry out routine activities. Pruritus is due to an accumulation of bile salts under the skin from the jaundice.

Collection of **objective data** in the **early stages** may include observing low hemoglobin, fever, jaundice (yellow discoloration of the skin, mucous membranes, and sclerae of the eyes (scleral icterus), caused by greater than normal amounts of bilirubin in the serum), and weight loss.

Collection of **objective data** in the **later stages** may include noting epistaxis, purpura, hematuria, spider hemangiomas, and bleeding gums. Late symptoms are ascites, hematologic disorders, splenic enlargement, and hemorrhage from esophageal varices or other distended GI veins. The patient may also appear mentally disoriented and display abnormal behaviors and speech patterns. Any prolonged interference with gas exchange leads to hypoxia, coma, and ultimately death.

Diagnostic Tests

Many diagnostic tests aid in the diagnosis of cirrhosis. Abnormal electrolyte values; elevated serum bilirubin, AST (SGOT), ALT (SGPT), LDH, and gamma GT; decreased total protein and serum albumin; elevated ammonia; low blood glucose (hypoglycemia) from impaired gluconeogenesis; prolonged prothrombin time; INR; and decreased cholesterol levels may give evidence of poor liver functioning. Visualization through ERCP (to detect common bile duct obstruction), esophagoscopy with barium esophagography to visualize esophageal varices, scans and biopsy of the liver, and ultrasonography are used to diagnose cirrhosis. Paracentesis (a procedure in which fluid is withdrawn from the abdominal cavity) will relieve ascites and also provide fluid for laboratory examination.

Medical Management

When possible causes have been identified, the initial treatment is to eliminate these causes, decrease the buildup of fluids in the body, prevent further damage to the liver, and provide individual supportive care to the patient. Eliminating alcohol, hepatotoxins (e.g., acetaminophen [Tylenol]), or environmental exposure to harmful chemicals is essential to prevent further damage to the liver. Diet therapy is aimed at correcting malnutrition, promoting the regeneration of functional liver tissue, and compensating for the liver's inability to store vitamins, while avoiding fluid retention and hepatic encephalopathy. A diet that is well balanced, high in calorie (2500 to 3000 calories/day), moderately high in protein (75 g of high-quality protein/day), low in fat, low in sodium (1000 to 2000 mg/day), and with additional vitamins and folic acid will usually meet the needs of the patient with cirrhosis and improve deficiencies (with impending liver failure, restrict protein and fluids).

Antiemetics may be prescribed to control nausea or vomiting. The patient must be monitored closely for toxicity that develops quickly when the poorly functioning liver cannot clear these drugs from the system. Diphenhydramine (Benadryl) or dimenhydrinate (Dramamine) may be given, whereas prochlorperazine maleate (Compazine), hydroxyzine pamoate (Vistaril), or hydroxyzine HCl (Atarax) are contraindicated in severe liver dysfunction.

Later manifestations may be severe and result from liver failure and portal hypertension. Jaundice, peripheral edema, portal hypertension, esophageal varices, hepatic encephalopathy, and ascites develop gradually (Figure 6-2).

Complications and treatment. Ascites are the presence of excessive fluid in the peritoneal cavity. The severity of fluid retention will determine the treatment. Initially the patient will be placed on bed rest with accurate monitoring of intake and output (I&O). The patient's diet will be restricted for amount of fluid (500 to 1000 mL) and sodium (1000 to 2000 mg). Diuretic therapy may be added if the diet does not control the ascites and edema. Spironolactone (Aldactone) 300 to 1000 mg/day may be used to obtain the desired diuresis. Other diuretics may be added, including furosemide (Lasix) or hydrochlorothiazide (HydroDIURIL). Vitamin supplements may include vitamin K, vitamin C, and folic acid. Salt-poor albumin may be administered in an attempt to restore plasma volume if the intravascular volume is decreased significantly. Complications of diuretic therapy include plasma volume deficit, decreased renal function, and electrolyte imbalance.

Another method of treatment for ascites and edema is the LeVeen continuous peritoneal jugular shunt (Figure 6-3). This procedure allows the continuous shunting of ascitic fluid from the abdominal cavity through a one-way, pressure-sensitive valve into a silicone tube that empties into the superior vena cava. The patient with this shunt must be monitored care-

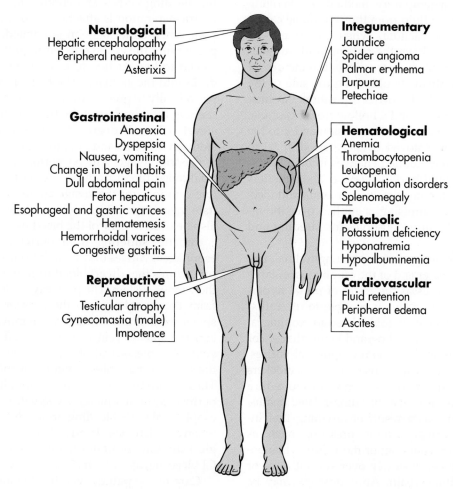

Neurological
Hepatic encephalopathy
Peripheral neuropathy
Asterixis

Gastrointestinal
Anorexia
Dyspepsia
Nausea, vomiting
Change in bowel habits
Dull abdominal pain
Fetor hepaticus
Esophageal and gastric varices
Hematemesis
Hemorrhoidal varices
Congestive gastritis

Reproductive
Amenorrhea
Testicular atrophy
Gynecomastia (male)
Impotence

Integumentary
Jaundice
Spider angioma
Palmar erythema
Purpura
Petechiae

Hematological
Anemia
Thrombocytopenia
Leukopenia
Coagulation disorders
Splenomegaly

Metabolic
Potassium deficiency
Hyponatremia
Hypoalbuminemia

Cardiovascular
Fluid retention
Peripheral edema
Ascites

FIGURE **6-2** Systemic clinical manifestations of liver cirrhosis.

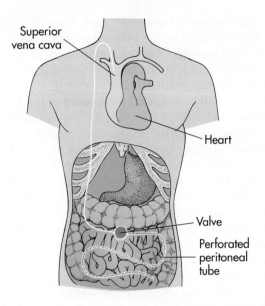

FIGURE **6-3** LeVeen continuous peritoneal jugular shunt.

fully for complications, which include congestive heart failure, leakage of the ascitic fluid, infection at the insertion sites, peritonitis, septicemia, and shunt thrombosis.

Paracentesis is a temporary method of removing fluid by withdrawing fluid from the abdominal cavity by either gravity or vacuum. When paracentesis is done the nurse must have the patient void immediately before the procedure to prevent puncture of the bladder. The patient should sit on the side of the bed or be placed in high Fowler's position. An incision is made in the skin, and a hollow trocar, cannula, or catheter is passed through the incision and into the cavity. The fluid is removed over a period of 30 to 90 minutes to prevent sudden changes in blood pressure (BP), which could lead to syncope. The patient is monitored closely for signs of hypovolemia and electrolyte imbalances. A dressing is applied over the insertion site, and the nurse observes for bleeding and drainage.

Esophageal varices (a complex of longitudinal, tortuous veins at the lower end of the esophagus) enlarge and become edematous as the result of portal hypertension. They are especially susceptible to ulceration and hemorrhage. The main goal related to esophageal varices is avoidance of bleeding and hemorrhage. For patients who have not bled from esophageal varices, prophylactic treatment with nonselective beta blockers (e.g., propranolol [Inderal]) has been shown to reduce the risk of bleeding, as well as bleeding-related deaths. Varices can rupture as a result of anything that increases the abdominal venous pressure, such as coughing, sneezing, vomiting, or the Valsalva maneuver. Rupture may occur slowly over several days or suddenly and without pain. An endoscopy may be performed to identify the varices or to rule out bleed-

ing from other sources. Endoscopic therapies include sclerotherapy and ligation of varices.

Therapeutic management of a ruptured esophageal varix is a medical emergency. The patient's airway must be maintained, the bleeding varix controlled, and IV lines established for fluids and blood replacement as needed. The hormone vasopressin, administered intravenously or directly into the superior vena cava, is used to decrease or stop the hemorrhaging. Vasopressin (VP) produces vasoconstriction of the vessels, decreases portal blood flow, and decreases portal hypertension. Current drug therapy in some institutions is a combination of VP and nitroglycerin (NTG). The NTG reduces the detrimental effects of VP, which are decreased coronary blood flow and increased blood pressure. VP should be avoided or used cautiously in the older adult because of the risk of cardiac ischemia. If the VP drip does not stop or control bleeding, a Sengstaken-Blakemore tube with openings at the tip may be inserted. This triple-lumen tube has a lumen for inflating the esophageal balloon, one for inflating the gastric balloon, and one for gastric lavage (Figure 6-4). The tube is passed through the nose, and when it is in place, the balloon in the stomach, the one in the esophagus, or both are inflated to press against the bleeding vessels and control the hemorrhage. The gastric aspiration is attached to low, intermittent suction. When either balloon is inflated, a Levin tube is passed into the esophagus through the mouth and attached to low suction to drain the saliva that cannot drain into the stomach. The balloon must be deflated periodically to prevent necrosis. The patient is allowed nothing by mouth, and the head of the bed should be elevated 30 to 45 degrees to help prevent aspiration of stomach contents and help the patient breathe.

Gastric lavage will be performed to remove any swallowed blood from the stomach. Iced isotonic saline solutions for the lavage are used by some to facilitate vasoconstriction. Endoscopic sclerotherapy may also be used to control the bleeding.

Patients suffering from portal hypertension and esophageal varices may benefit from surgical shunting procedures that divert blood from the portal system to the venous system. The portacaval shunt diverts blood from the portal vein to the inferior vena cava. The splenorenal shunt requires the removal of the spleen, and the splenic vein is anastomosed to the left renal vein. The mesocaval shunt involves anastomosis of the superior mesenteric vein to the inferior vena cava. These procedures have a high mortality. They may be performed in an emergency situation to control acute esophageal varix bleeding or in a therapeutic situation when a patient has already bled. Complications of surgical shunting procedures are hepatic encephalopathy, GI bleeding, ascites, and liver failure.

Care of the patient who has hemorrhaged from an esophageal varix includes maintenance of oxygen con-

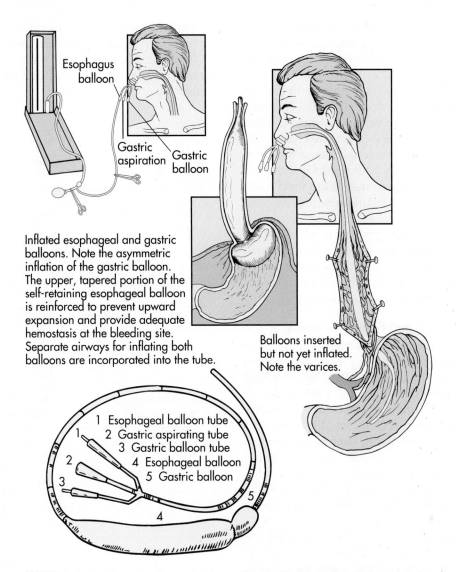

Esophagus balloon

Gastric aspiration   Gastric balloon

Inflated esophageal and gastric balloons. Note the asymmetric inflation of the gastric balloon. The upper, tapered portion of the self-retaining esophageal balloon is reinforced to prevent upward expansion and provide adequate hemostasis at the bleeding site. Separate airways for inflating both balloons are incorporated into the tube.

Balloons inserted but not yet inflated. Note the varices.

1 Esophageal balloon tube
2 Gastric aspirating tube
3 Gastric balloon tube
4 Esophageal balloon
5 Gastric balloon

FIGURE **6-4** Esophageal tamponade accomplished with Sengstaken-Blakemore tube.

tent levels within the blood, administration of fresh frozen plasma and packed red blood cells (RBCs), vitamin K (AquaMEPHYTON), and histamine (H_2) receptor blockers such as cimetidine (Tagamet), and electrolyte replacements as needed without fluid overload. Ammonia buildup can be avoided with the use of cathartics (e.g., lactulose [Chronulac]) and neomycin. Preventing ammonia buildup will keep hepatic encephalopathy from breaking down blood and releasing ammonia in the intestine.

Hepatic encephalopathy is a type of brain damage caused by liver disease and consequent ammonia intoxication. It is thought to be the result of a damaged liver being unable to metabolize substances that can be toxic to the brain, such as ammonia. The patient's signs and symptoms progress from inappropriate behavior, disorientation, flapping tremors, and twitching of the extremities to stupor and coma. Treatment of the patient with hepatic encephalopathy is to give supportive care that will prevent further damage to the liver.

The patient with hepatic encephalopathy is on a very-low-protein to no-protein diet. The goal of management of hepatic encephalopathy is the reduction of ammonia formation. This consists mainly of protein restriction and reduction of ammonia formation in the intestines. The degree of protein restriction is determined by the severity of mental change. The protein restriction may range from 0 to 40 g per day. With improvement of mental function, dietary protein content is increased gradually over days. Foods allowed include toast, cereal, rice, tea, fruit juice, and hard candies. Sufficient carbohydrate intake must be provided to maintain an intake of 1500 to 2000 calories to prevent hypoglycemia. Glucose polymer (Polycose) is protein free and can be used as a source of calories. It can be given orally or via NG tube.

Drugs that are normally detoxified by the liver are avoided until the liver regains adequate function. Medications may be given to cleanse the bowel and help decrease the serum ammonia. Lactulose (Chronulac) decreases the bowel's pH from 7 to 5, thus decreasing the production of ammonia by bacteria within the bowel. Lactulose may be administered orally or as a retention enema or via NG tube. It also functions as a cathartic. The lactulose traps the ammonia in the gut, and the laxative effect of the drug expels the ammonia from the colon. Antibiotics such as neomycin, which are poorly absorbed from the GI tract, are given orally or rectally. They reduce the bacterial flora of the colon. Bacterial action on protein in feces results in ammonia production. Because neomycin may cause renal toxicity and hearing impairment, lactulose is frequently the preferred drug.

Asterixis is a hand-flapping tremor in which the patient stretches out an arm and hyperextends the wrist with the fingers separated, relaxed, and extended. A rapid, irregular flexion and extension (flapping) of the wrist will occur in the patient who is acutely ill.

Nursing Interventions and Patient Teaching

The nurse should check vital signs every 4 hours, more often if evidence of hemorrhage is present. The patient should be observed for GI hemorrhage as evidenced by hematemesis, melena, anxiety, and restlessness.

Most patients will require a well-balanced, moderate, high-protein, high-carbohydrate diet with adequate vitamins. With impending liver failure, protein and fluids will be restricted. Sodium restriction is frequently necessary, which can make providing a palatable diet more difficult. Frequent oral hygiene and a pleasant environment should be provided to help the patient increase food intake.

A major nursing focus for many patients is helping them deal with alcoholism. This requires establishing trust that the health team is interested in the patient's well-being. Patients must admit that they have drinking problems. Confrontation may sometimes be used to help patients accept the problem. The nurse should provide information regarding community support programs, such as Alcoholics Anonymous (AA) for help with alcohol abuse.

Because of pruritus, malnutrition, and edema, the patient with cirrhosis is prone to skin lesions and pressure sores. Preventive nursing interventions to avoid impairment of skin integrity, such as eggcrate mattresses, alternating–air pressure mattress, frequent turning, and back rubs should be initiated. The nurse should apply soothing lotion to relieve pruritus.

The nurse should observe the patient's mental status and report changes such as disorientation, headache, or lethargy. It is important for the nurse to assist in activities of daily living (ADLs) as needed to promote good hygiene while conserving energy. The nurse observes for edema by measuring ankles daily and observes for ascites by measuring abdominal girth. An accurate I&O is recorded, as well as daily weight. Nursing intervention with concern and

warmth regardless of physical changes is essential in helping the patient maintain self-esteem.

Nursing diagnoses and interventions for the patient with cirrhosis include but are not limited to the following:

Nursing Diagnoses	Nursing Interventions
Ineffective tissue perfusion, gastrointestinal, related to impaired blood coagulation or hemorrhage from gastric or esophageal varices	Monitor patient for signs of bleeding: gums, injection sites, decrease in BP, increase in pulse, hematemesis, and melena. Monitor hemoglobin (Hgb) hematocrit (Hct), prothrombin time, and INR. Monitor parenteral fluids and blood transfusions. Administer vitamin K and neomycin as ordered. Instruct patient to avoid straining with stools and to avoid vigorous tooth brushing. Monitor gastric output—color and consistency.
Disturbed thought processes, related to potential increase of serum ammonia and hepatic coma	Observe frequently for changes in mental status; lethargy, drowsiness, and confusion. Monitor neurologic status for decreased motor ability. Encourage fluids (if not restricted). Give lactulose as ordered to decrease production of ammonia. Provide safe environment: side rails up, bed in low position, and safety reminder devices if necessary. Avoid use of sedatives, tranquilizers, and opioids. Provide low-protein or no-protein diet as ordered because ammonia (a breakdown product of protein) is responsible for mental changes.

The patient with cirrhosis must understand the need for adequate rest and avoiding infections. Activity must be planned around complete bed rest until strength is regained. Turning the patient at least every 2 hours and providing range-of-motion exercises will help avoid infection and prevent thrombophlebitis. The nurse should instruct the patient to use a soft-bristled toothbrush, use an electric razor, blow nose cautiously, and avoid straining at stools to prevent bleeding as a result of a lack of vitamin K and certain clotting factors. Soap, perfumed lotion, and rubbing alcohol should be avoided because they will cause further drying of the skin. If pruritus

Cirrhosis of the Liver

- The patient and the family need to understand the importance of continual health care and medical supervision.
- Measures to achieve and maintain a remission should be encouraged. These include proper diet, rest, avoidance of potentially hepatotoxic over-the-counter drugs (e.g., acetaminophen [Tylenol]), and abstinence from alcohol.
- The nurse should provide information regarding community support programs, such as Alcoholics Anonymous, for help with alcohol abuse.
- The emphasis on home care for the patient with cirrhosis should be on helping the patient maintain the highest level of wellness possible and initiate and maintain necessary lifestyle changes.

and dryness of skin are present, diphenhydramine (Benadryl) may be administered. The nurse should explain the relationship of the therapeutic diet to the diagnosis and ability of the liver to function.

Community resources for home health care and detoxification programs may help the patient and family deal with problems that arise after discharge. Help the patient and family identify community resources available for alcohol rehabilitation. Because of the seriousness of the disease, the patient and family need understanding and support throughout the treatment. See Home Health Considerations for a patient with cirrhosis of the liver.

Prognosis

The prognosis for cirrhosis of the liver is related to the cause of the disease, the susceptibility of the individual, and the extent of the involvement. Fibrosis of the cirrhotic liver cannot be cured, but its progression may be halted or slowed by proper management by the physician, nurse, patient, and significant others (Nursing Care Plan box).

CARCINOMA OF THE LIVER
Etiology/Pathophysiology

Primary carcinoma (originating in the liver) is rare. Metastatic carcinoma of the liver is more common. A high percentage of patients with primary cell carcinoma have cirrhosis of the liver. Some cases of hepatic carcinoma are associated with chronic hepatitis B or C. Men have a higher incidence of primary liver cancer than women.

The liver is a common site of metastatic growth because of its high rate of blood flow and extensive capillary network. Cancer cells in other parts of the body are commonly carried to the liver via the portal circulation.

The malignant cells cause the liver to be enlarged and misshapen. Hemorrhage and necrosis in the liver are common. Tumors may be singular or numerous and nodular or diffusely spread over the entire liver. Primary liver tumors commonly metastasize to the lung.

Clinical Manifestation/Diagnostic Tests

It is difficult to diagnose carcinoma of the liver. It is difficult to differentiate it from cirrhosis in its early stages because many of the clinical manifestations (e.g., hepatomegaly, weight loss, peripheral edema, ascites, portal hypertension) are similar. Other common manifestations include dull abdominal pain in the epigastric or right upper quadrant region, jaundice, anorexia, nausea and vomiting, and extreme weakness. Patients frequently have pulmonary emboli. Tests used to assist in the diagnosis are a liver scan, hepatic arteriography, endoscopic retrograde cholangiopancreatography (ERCP), and a liver biopsy. The test for alpha fetoprotein (AFP) may be positive in hepatocellular carcinoma. AFP helps distinguish primary cancer from metastatic cancer.

Medical Management and Nursing Interventions

Treatment of cancer of the liver is largely palliative. Surgical excision (lobectomy) is sometimes performed if the tumor is localized to one portion of the liver. Only 30% to 40% of patients have surgically resectable disease. Usually surgery is not possible because the cancer is too far advanced when it is detected. Surgical excision offers the only chance for cure of liver cancer. Medical management is similar to that for cirrhosis of the liver. Chemotherapy may be used, but there is usually a poor response. Portal vein or hepatic artery perfusion with 5-fluorouracil (5-FU) may be attempted.

Nursing intervention for the patient with liver carcinoma focuses on keeping the patient as comfortable as possible. Because this patient manifests the same problems as any patient with advanced liver disease, the nursing interventions discussed for cirrhosis of the liver apply.

Prognosis

The prognosis for cancer of the liver is poor. The cancer grows rapidly and death may occur within 4 to 7 months as a result of hepatic encephalopathy or massive blood loss from GI bleeding.

HEPATITIS
Etiology/Pathophysiology

Hepatitis is an inflammation of the liver resulting from several types of viral agents or exposure to toxic substances. Rarely, hepatitis is caused by bacteria, such as streptococci, salmonellae, and *Escherichia coli*.

NURSING CARE PLAN

The Patient with Cirrhosis of the Liver

Mr. K., a 49-year-old rancher, is admitted with loss of appetite, generalized edema, pruritus, flappy tremors of the hands, ascites, and lethargy. He appears disoriented. His skin has areas of excoriation caused by scratching and a sallow appearance. His wife states that he has been unable to concentrate, appears confused and listless, and has been eating poorly. Mr. K. has been an alcoholic for the past 18 years. His total bilirubin is 4.5 mg/dL, gamma GT 65 units/L, total protein 4.8 g/dL, albumin is 2.8 g/dL, and blood ammonia is 160 mcg/dL. He is demonstrating signs and symptoms of hepatic encephalopathy.

NURSING DIAGNOSIS *Imbalanced nutrition: less than body requirements, related to anorexia, nausea, and impaired utilization and storage of nutrients, as manifested by lack of interest in food, aversion to eating, inadequate food intake*

Patient Goals/Expected Outcomes	Nursing Interventions	Evaluation
Patient will eat 50% of meal. Patient will maintain baseline body weight.	Monitor weight to determine whether weight loss occurs. Provide oral care before meals to remove foul taste and improve taste of food. Administer antiemetics as ordered to relieve nausea and vomiting. Provide small, frequent meals at times the patient can best tolerate them to prevent feeling of fullness and to maintain nutritional status. Determine food preferences and allow these whenever possible to increase nutritional appeal for patient, because a low-protein diet is often unpalatable.	Patient is eating 50% to 75% of his meals. Patient has no weight loss.

NURSING DIAGNOSIS *Disturbed thought process, related to increased formation of ammonia as manifested by inability to concentrate, lethargy, disorientation, and flappy tremors of the hands*

Patient Goals/Expected Outcomes	Nursing Interventions	Evaluation
Patient will be oriented to person, place, time, and purpose.	Monitor for hepatic encephalopathy by assessing patient's general behavior, orientation to time and place, speech, and ammonia levels, because liver is unable to convert accumulating ammonia to urea for renal excretion. Encourage fluids (if not restricted) and give laxatives and enemas as ordered to decrease production of ammonia. Provide low-protein or no-protein diet as ordered because ammonia (a breakdown product of protein) is responsible for mental changes. Administer lactulose (Chronulac) or neomycin (Mycifradin) as prescribed. Limit physical activity because exercise produces ammonia as a by-product of metabolism. Control factors known to precipitate hepatic coma.	Patient responds appropriately to assessment of person, place, time, and purpose.

? CRITICAL THINKING QUESTIONS

1. Mr. K. is thrashing about in his bed and has attempted to climb over the side rails. He is disoriented to time and place. The appropriate nursing intervention to ensure the safety of Mr. K. would be:

2. Mrs. K. notes that her husband has a low-protein diet. She confides to the nurse that she feels he needs more meat, eggs, and cottage cheese to improve his nutrition. The most appropriate response by the nurse would be:

The six types of viral hepatitis are caused by distinct but similar viruses that produce almost identical signs and symptoms but vary in their incubation period, mode of transmission, and prognosis. Hepatitis A, formerly called infectious hepatitis, is the most common form today and is a short-incubation virus (10 to 40 days). Hepatitis B, formerly called serum hepatitis, is a long-incubation virus (28 to 160 days). A third virus, known as hepatitis C, has an incubation period of 2 weeks to 6 months, commonly 6 to 9 weeks. Hepatitis D, also called delta virus, causes hepatitis as a coinfection with hepatitis B and may progress to cirrhosis and chronic hepatitis. The incubation period is 2 to 10 weeks. Hepatitis E, also called enteric non-A–non-B hepatitis, is transmitted through fecal contamination of water, primarily in developing countries. It is rare in the United States. The incubation period is 15 to 64 days. Recently hepatitis G virus has been discovered. Hepatitis virus G has been found in blood donors and can be transmitted by transfusion. It frequently coexists with other hepatitis viruses, such as hepatitis C. Health officials are required by law to report all cases of viral hepatitis to the Centers for Disease Control and Prevention (CDC) in Atlanta. Modes of transmission for the different types of hepatitis are listed in Box 6-1. See Safety Considerations for prevention of acute viral hepatitis.

The basic pathologic findings in the six forms of viral hepatitis are identical. A diffuse inflammatory reaction occurs, and liver cells begin to degenerate and die. As the liver cells degenerate, the normal functions of the liver slow down. The outcome of the disease may be affected by the virulence of the virus, the preexisting condition of the liver, and the health care given when the disease is diagnosed.

Clinical Manifestations

The clinical manifestations for viral hepatitis vary greatly; some patients are asymptomatic, whereas others develop hepatic failure or hepatic encephalopathy.

Assessment

Collection of **subjective data** includes patients' reports of general malaise, aching muscles, photophobia, lassitude, headaches, and chills. Abdominal pain, dyspepsia, nausea, diarrhea, and constipation are reported also. The patient may complain of pruritus from the presence of bile on the skin. The patient will complain of tenderness in the liver and will remain fatigued for several weeks.

Collection of **objective data** includes observing hepatomegaly (enlarged liver), enlarged lymph nodes, weight loss, and rhinitis. Jaundice appears because of the damaged liver's inability to metabolize bilirubin; the resultant signs noted are yellowish skin, discoloration of the sclera (scleral icterus) and mucous mem-

---

Box 6-1 *Modes of Transmission of the Six Types of Viral Hepatitis*

- Hepatitis A (HAV) spreads by direct contact through the oral-fecal route, usually by food or water contaminated with feces. Up to 50% of all people in the United States have been infected by the time they reach adulthood, most of them suffering minimal symptoms or no symptoms at all. Two or more weeks before symptoms, the virus can be found in the bile, blood, and stool. Patients are rarely infectious once they develop jaundice (Durston, 2004).
- Hepatitis B (HBV) is transmitted by contaminated serum via blood transfusion, the use of contaminated needles and instruments, needlesticks, illicit IV drug use, and dialysis, and by direct contact with body fluids from infected people, such as breast milk and sexual contact. An ever-increasing risk comes from improper disposal of used needles and syringes. Sharing toothbrushes, razor blades, or personal items with an infected person may also lead to exposure.
- Hepatitis C (HCV) is transmitted through needlesticks, blood transfusions, and illicit IV drug use and by unidentified means. Hepatitis C virus can also be transmitted by sharing contaminated straws used for snorting cocaine. In the past, hepatitis C could not be detected in banked blood, so it was more easily transmitted through transfusion. The advent of routine blood screening in 1992 has greatly reduced the number of cases of transfusion-related hepatitis C.
- Hepatitis D is transmitted the same way as hepatitis B; it appears as a coinfection of hepatitis B.
- Hepatitis E is transmitted by the oral-fecal route; it spreads through the fecal contamination of water.
- Hepatitis G is frequently seen as a coinfection with hepatitis C; it spreads through bloodborne exposure. Hepatitis G has been found in some blood donors and can be transmitted by transfusion. Transmission occurs when contaminated injectable drugs are used; contaminated blood, organs, or tissues are received; through hemodialysis; or with unsafe methods of tattooing or body piercing.

---

brane (Figure 6-5), dark tea-colored urine, and clay-colored stools. It is not uncommon for relapses to occur in the convalescent stage.

Diagnostic Tests

Changes in the liver caused by viral hepatitis cause elevated direct bilirubin, gamma GT, AST (SGOT), ALT (SGPT), LDH, and alkaline phosphatase levels;

⚠ Safety Considerations

Prevention of Acute Viral Hepatitis

HEPATITIS A

- Wash your hands. Hepatitis A virus (HAV) is transmitted when people put something in their mouths that is contaminated with fecal material (called "fecal-oral transmission"). Teach patients the importance of good handwashing after using the bathroom or changing a diaper, as well as proper food preparation, to prevent the spread of HAV. The best protection against HAV transmission is the two-dose HAV vaccine.

HEPATITIS B

- One of the best preventive measures against hepatitis B virus is the HBV vaccine.
- Children younger than the age of 18 years are routinely vaccinated today.
- Individuals who are at risk for the virus, such as health care workers, should be vaccinated.
- People who play or work in inner-city parks and playgrounds are at risk for exposure to HBV from litter containers and used needles and syringes should be vaccinated, as should men who have sex with men, individuals who use illicit IV drugs, and those who travel to areas with a high infection rate.
- Those positive for HBV should not donate blood, organs, or tissue.

HEPATITIS C

- Hepatitis C is transmitted by needle sharing among illicit IV drug users.
- Other significant risk factors at work include receipt of clotting factor made before 1987, hemodialysis, receipt of blood or solid organs before 1992, maternal-fetal transmission, and multiple or infected sex partners.

HEPATITIS D

- Modes of HDV transmission are similar to those of HBV. Sexual transmission of HDV is less efficient than for HBV. Educate patients regarding risky behavior.

HEPATITIS E

- To help prevent HEV infection, educate patients to avoid drinking water or beverages with ice in areas with uncertain water quality. They should refrain from eating raw shellfish and avoid raw produce unless it is prepared with purified water. Hepatitis E is most often seen in southeastern and central Asia, the Middle East, Africa, and Mexico.

HEPATITIS G

- Hepatitis G has been detected in blood samples in Europe, Asia, and Australia.
- Transmission of HGV occurs when tainted injectable drugs are used; tainted blood, organs, or tissues are received through hemodialysis; or with unsafe methods of tattooing or body piercing (Durston, 2004).

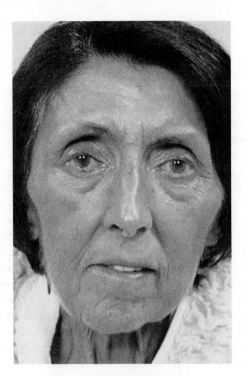

FIGURE **6-5** Severe jaundice.

a prolonged prothrombin time and INR; and, in severe hepatitis, a decreased serum albumin. Leukopenia is common in these patients, with a transient neutropenia and lymphopenia, followed by lymphocytosis. Hypoglycemia is present in approximately 50% of the patients with hepatitis. Serum is examined for the presence of HAA (hepatitis-associated antigen) A, B, C, D, or G.

Medical Management

Supportive therapy for existing signs and symptoms and preventing the transmission of the disease are important in the treatment of the patient with viral hepatitis. The patient's care can be in the hospital when bilirubin concentrations in the blood are more than 10 mg/dL and for those with a prolonged prothrombin time and INR, but usually the patient is cared for at home. Bed rest for several weeks is commonly prescribed.

Drug therapy for chronic hepatitis B is focused on decreasing the viral load, decreasing the rate of disease progression, and decreasing the rate of drug-resistant HBV. At present, several drugs are useful in suppressing viral activity and decreased viral load in patients with HBV. However, the percentage of patients seroconverting (developing antibodies against the virus) remains relatively low. Lamivudine (Epivir, 3TC), α-interferon, and adefovir dipivoxil (Hepsera) are three drugs being used in the treatment of chronic hepatitis B. In chronic hepatitis C, drug therapy is directed also at reducing the viral load, decreasing progression of the disease, and promoting seroconversion. Treatment options for HCV are interferon alfa-2b (Intron A) and ribavirin (Rebetol) and PEG-interferon alfa-2a (Pegasys). This combination therapy eradicates the virus more often than monotherapy. Another treatment option, liver transplantation, is available. In fact half of all liver recipients are HCV positive. Most transplanted livers will eventually become infected with HCV. But recipients can increase both quantity and quality of life by altering their lifestyle to avoid risky behaviors (Durston, 2004).

Alcohol in the diet is not allowed for at least 1 year, and the patient may need supportive care from the community to facilitate compliance. Most patients will tolerate small, frequent meals of a low-fat, high-carbohydrate diet. If the patient is dehydrated, intravenous fluids will be given with addition of vitamin C for healing, vitamin B complex to assist the damaged liver's inability to absorb fat-soluble vitamins, and vitamin K to combat prolonged coagulation time. Avoid all unnecessary medications, particularly sedatives. Gamma globulin or immune serum globulin should be given as soon as possible to people who have been in direct contact with a person with hepatitis A during the infectious period (2 weeks before and 1 week after onset of symptoms). The dosage of 0.02 mL per kg of body weight, given intramuscularly, is effective in preventing hepatitis A in 80% to 90% of the cases. There are currently three vaccines used to prevent hepatitis A: Havrix, Vaqta, and Avaxim.

Primary immunization consists of a single dose administered intramuscularly in the deltoid. A booster is recommended any time between 6 and 12 months after the initiation of the primary dose to ensure adequate antibody titers and long-term protection. However, a primary immunization provides immunity within 30 days after a single dose.

It is recommended that until routine vaccination of children is feasible, the following people who are at risk for infection be vaccinated for hepatitis A: people traveling to countries where hepatitis A is endemic; sexually active homosexual and bisexual men; patients with chronic liver disease; injecting drug users; and people at risk for occupational infection, such as those who work with hepatitis A in research laboratory settings.

Individuals who have been exposed to hepatitis B virus via a needle puncture or sexual contact should be protected with hepatitis B immune globulin (HBIG). A dose of 0.06 mL per kg of body weight is administered intramuscularly as quickly after exposure as possible. This dose is repeated 1 month later.

People identified as being at high risk for developing hepatitis B should be vaccinated if they are not already immune. These people include the following:

- All health care personnel (personnel at highest risk are emergency department, operating room, intensive care unit (ICU), and dialysis personnel, phlebotomists, and laboratory technicians)
- People with high-risk lifestyles (drug users, tattoo recipients, homosexual men, and prostitutes)
- Infants born to mothers who are hepatitis B surface antigen (HBsAg) positive
- Hemodialysis patients
- Individuals sharing a household with an infected person

Recommendations of the Centers for Disease Control and Prevention (CDC) Immunization Practices Advisory Committee include making hepatitis B vaccine a part of routine vaccination schedules for all newborns and adolescents. The protection program consists of three vaccinations: an initial vaccination, a vaccination 1 month later, and a third vaccination 6 months after the first injection. The hepatitis B vaccine has been shown to provide protection for 3 to 5 years in approximately 90% of the people treated. It is hoped that universal vaccination will lead to eventual prevention and control of hepatitis B.

Hepatitis B, C, D, and G are spread through blood transfusions. The blood used should be screened for elevated ALT (SGPT) and anti–hepatitis B core (anti-HBc), anti–hepatitis C, anti–hepatitis D, and anti–hepatitis G.

Liver transplantation. The first human liver transplant was performed in 1963. Liver transplantation has become a practical therapeutic option for many people with irreversible liver disease. It improves the quality of life for end-stage liver patients and is an accepted treatment modality for these patients. Indications for liver transplantation include congenital biliary abnormalities, inborn errors of metabolism, hepatic malignancy (confined to the liver), sclerosing cholangitis, and chronic end-stage liver disease. Liver disease related to chronic viral hepatitis is the leading indication for liver transplantation. Liver transplants are not recommended for the patient with widespread malignant disease.

The major postoperative complications are rejection and infection. Rejection is not as major a problem as it is in kidney transplants. The liver seems to be less susceptible to rejection than the kidney. Cyclosporine is an effective immunosuppressant drug. The use of cyclosporine has been a major factor in the success rates of liver transplantation. It does not cause bone marrow suppression and does not impede wound healing. Other immunosuppressants used include azathioprine (Imuran), corticosteroids, tacrolimus (Prograf), and the monoclonal antibody OKT3. New agents, including the interleukin-2 receptor antagonists basiliximab (Simulect) and daclizumab (Zenapax), are being used in combination with other immunosuppressive agents to reduce rejection. Other factors in the improved success rate are advances in surgical techniques, better selection of potential recipients, and improved management of the underlying liver disease before surgery.

Patients who have liver disease secondary to viral hepatitis often experience reinfection of the transplanted liver with hepatitis B or C. HCV recurrence as evidenced by histologic damage is almost universal after transplant. Approximately 20% to 30% of patients will develop cirrhosis of the transplanted liver by the fifth year posttransplant. Antiviral therapy for HCV-initiated posttransplant, even before the development of histologic evidence of recurrence, has failed to alter this recurrence pattern.

The patient who has had a liver transplant requires competent and highly skilled nursing interventions, either in an ICU or in some other specialized unit. Postoperative nursing care includes assessing neurological status; monitoring for signs of hemorrhage; preventing pulmonary complications; monitoring drainage, electrolyte levels, and urinary output; and monitoring for signs and symptoms of infection and rejection. Common respiratory problems are pneumonia, atelectasis, and pleural effusions. The nurse should have the patient use measures such as coughing, deep breathing, incentive spirometry, and repositioning to prevent these complications. Drainage from the Jackson-Pratt drain, nasogastric tube suctioning, and T-tube should be measured and recorded, and the color and consistency of drainage noted. A critical aspect of nursing interventions following liver transplantation is monitoring for infection. The first 2 months after the surgery are critical. Infection can be viral, fungal, or bacterial. Fever may be the only sign of infection. Emotional support and teaching the patient and family are essential (Lewis et al, 2004).

Nursing Interventions and Patient Teaching

The care of the patient with viral hepatitis includes ensuring rest, maintaining adequate nutrition, providing adequate fluids, and caring for the skin. The care of the patient with hepatitis continues over time, and support and patient education are necessary throughout the entire illness.

Preventing the transmission of the disease is of primary importance in caring for the patient with viral hepatitis. The patient, family, and health care providers must be knowledgeable about routes of transmission of the virus and take steps to avoid such transmission. Proper personal hygiene and good sanitation, as well as hepatitis A vaccine, will help prevent the spread of hepatitis A. Patients should be given a thorough explanation of the reasons for the precautions and should be instructed in the proper handling of their own secretions and body wastes and in thorough methods of handwashing. Gown and gloves should be worn when handling excreta, giving enemas, taking rectal temperatures, handling food wastes, handling needles, disposing of urine, or carrying out any other procedure or hygiene measure that involves direct contact with the patient's body fluids.

When the patient has hepatitis B, utmost care must be taken in handling syringes, needles, and other instruments that are contaminated with the patient's serum. Disposable equipment and dishes should be used and isolation precautions taken. Special handling of blood and body fluids such as saliva, semen, and vaginal secretions is essential to prevent the transmission of hepatitis B. Use enteric precautions for 7 days after onset of hepatitis A. Use standard precautions for all patients.

Nursing diagnoses and interventions for the patient with hepatitis include but are not limited to the following:

NURSING DIAGNOSES	NURSING INTERVENTIONS
Risk for injury, related to poor nutrition and prolonged clotting times	Pad side rails if necessary. Assist weakened patient with activities. Encourage use of electric razor and soft toothbrush.
Imbalanced nutrition: less than body requirements, related to inadequate intake associated with current anorexia, nausea, vomiting, and altered metabolism of nutrients by the liver	Provide diet high in carbohydrates and low in fats, and encourage total fluid intake of 2500 to 3000 mL daily. Monitor I&O. Monitor daily weight. Note color and consistency of stool and color and amount of urine. Administer antiemetics as ordered. Offer support and understanding. Promote adequate rest.

When the patient with viral hepatitis can be cared for at home, the family will need to be taught necessary precautions. Sexual activity should be avoided during the acute stage of hepatitis B, C, and D. Patients with hepatitis must wash hands thoroughly following toileting, must disinfect articles soiled with feces (boil 1 minute), and must not prepare foods for others during symptomatic disease.

If possible, separate bathroom facilities should be used by the patient. Personal care items and drinking glasses should not be shared. The patient's clothes should be laundered separately in hot water. Contaminated items should be disposed of properly.

The patient and family should be aware of signs and symptoms associated with hepatitis, including light-colored stools, dark-colored urine, jaundice, fever, GI disturbances, unusual bleeding that might be indicative of a prolonged prothrombin time and INR, and tenderness or pain in the abdomen. The danger of alcohol use and its effect on the liver should be clearly understood.

Prognosis

The prognosis of hepatitis differs with the causative agent. Recovery from hepatitis A is high, with a mortality rate of 0.5%.

Mortality from hepatitis B has been reported to be as high as 10%. Hepatitis B is a very serious form of hepatitis, often progressing to cirrhosis, chronic hepatitis, liver cancer, and death. Hepatitis C often progresses to chronic hepatitis, cirrhosis, liver cancer, and death. There is a greater risk for hepatitis C infection to become chronic compared with hepatitis B. Approximately 75% to 80% of patients who acquire hepatitis C virus go on to develop chronic infection and 20% develop liver failure. The prognosis of chronic hepatitis C virus has greatly increased the demand for liver transplants. Hepatitis D may progress to cirrhosis and chronic hepatitis. It has a high mortality rate. Hepatitis E has a 10% mortality rate in pregnant women; otherwise it is not believed to be fatal. Hepatitis G infections frequently coexist with other hepatitis infections, such as that of hepatitis C. However, most hepatitis G infections are not associated with chronic hepatitis, thus hepatitis G virus's association with liver disease is, at this time, uncertain.

Recovery from acute toxic hepatitis is rapid if the hepatotoxin is identified early and removed or if exposure to the agent has been limited. However, the prognosis is poor if the period between exposure and the onset of signs and symptoms is prolonged, because there are no effective antidotes.

LIVER ABSCESSES

If an infection develops anywhere along the GI tract, there is danger that the infecting organisms may reach the liver through the biliary system, portal venous system, or hepatic arterial or lymphatic systems. Most bacteria are promptly destroyed, but occasionally some gain a foothold. If the disease progresses, it can become life threatening. In the past the mortality rate was 100% because of the vague clinical symptoms, inadequate diagnostic tools, and inadequate surgical drainage of the abscess. Today medical management is more successful.

Etiology/Pathophysiology

If the body is not successful in destroying bacteria, the bacterial toxins attack neighboring liver cells, and the necrotic tissue produced serves as a protective wall for the organism. Meanwhile, leukocytes migrate into the infected area. The result is an abscess cavity full of a liquid containing living and dead leukocytes, liquefied liver cells, and bacteria. Pyogenic (pus-producing) abscesses of this type may be single or multiple.

Clinical Manifestations

Patients with liver abscess present vague signs and symptoms. Fever accompanied by chills, abdominal pain, and tenderness in the right upper quadrant of the abdomen are common complaints.

Assessment

Collection of **subjective data** includes chills, complaints of dull abdominal pain, abdominal tenderness, and discomfort.

Collection of **objective data** includes fever, hepatomegaly (abnormal enlargement of the liver), jaundice, and anemia.

Diagnostic Tests

The diagnosis is established by demonstrating a space-occupying lesion in the liver radiographically (radiograph, ultrasound, CT, and liver scan). Amebic (microscopic, single-celled parasite) liver abscess can also be confirmed by amebic serologic examination (laboratory examination of antigen-antibody reaction of amebae in serum).

Medical Management

Usually liver abscess can be managed by medical therapy. Treatment includes intravenous antibiotic therapy that is specific to the organism identified.

Percutaneous (performed through the skin) drainage of liver abscess is reserved for patients who are not responding to medical therapy or are at high risk for rupture. Open surgical drainage has been the standard in patients whose liver abscesses have ruptured into the peritoneal space, but some of these patients are now being managed with percutaneous drainage. All patients will require a full course of antibiotic therapy.

Nursing Interventions and Patient Teaching

Continuous monitoring and supportive care are indicated because of the seriousness of the patient's condition. Monitoring objective and subjective symptoms is important. If signs and symptoms increase in depth and severity, the physician should be notified.

The patient's individualized response to drug therapy is determined by a decrease in fever, tenderness and rigidity of the abdomen, chills, and discomfort. If percutaneous or open surgical drainage is instituted, the nurse must observe the drainage for amount, color, and consistency.

Nursing diagnoses and interventions for the patient with a liver abscess include but are not limited to the following:

Nursing Diagnoses	Nursing Interventions
Risk for imbalanced body temperature, related to infectious state	Check temperature as ordered by physician or as indicated by the patient's worsening condition and report findings to physician.
	Encourage fluids to prevent dehydration. Monitor intravenous (IV) fluids. Explain how fever and drainage can deplete fluids in the body. Record I&O. Monitor oral mucous membranes and skin turgor during assessment.

NURSING DIAGNOSES	NURSING INTERVENTIONS
Deficient knowledge, related to relationship of infection to nutritional needs	Explain the body's need for added calories and protein to fight infection.
	Weigh patient daily for weight gain or loss to determine adequate nutritional intake.

In addition to the relationship of infection and nutrition, the nurse may need to teach preoperative and postoperative procedures if the patient requires percutaneous or open surgical drainage. A thorough explanation and assessment for the patient's understanding are necessary to determine adequacy of teaching skills. Anxiety in the seriously ill patient decreases as the knowledge base increases and the patient feels more in control of the situation.

Prognosis

The prognosis for patients with liver abscesses was very poor in the past, with a mortality rate of 100%. The prognosis today is much improved because of advanced diagnostic tests, including the CT and liver scans, and aggressive medical and nursing interventions.

CHOLECYSTITIS AND CHOLELITHIASIS
Etiology/Pathophysiology

Disorders of the biliary system are common in the United States and are responsible for the hospitalization of more than a half million people a year. The two most common conditions are cholecystitis and cholelithiasis (Box 6-2). These two diseases are seen more commonly in women than men, in American Indians and whites than in Asian-Americans and African-

Americans, and in obese people, pregnant women, multiparous women, women who use birth control pills, and people with diabetes.

Cholecystitis can be caused by an obstruction, a gallstone, or a tumor. More than 90% of the cases of cholecystitis are caused by gallstones. The exact cause of stone formation in the gallbladder and the common bile duct is not known. However, an alteration in lipid metabolism and the role of female sex hormones are related to the disease. The stones most frequently occur in multiples but can occur singularly (Figure 6-6).

When an obstruction, gallstone, or tumor prevents bile from leaving the gallbladder, the trapped bile acts as an irritant, causing cellular infiltration of the gallbladder wall after 3 to 4 days. A typical inflammatory response occurs, and the gallbladder becomes enlarged and edematous. The vascular occlusion along with bile stasis causes the mucosal lining of the gallbladder to become necrotic. Initially the bile in the gallbladder is sterile. The bacterial growth is caused by the ischemia and occurs usually within a few days. There is danger of rupture of the gallbladder and spread of infection to the hepatic duct and liver. When the disease is severe enough to interfere with the blood supply, the gallbladder wall may become gangrenous.

Clinical Manifestations

The condition may be acute, with a sudden onset of nausea and vomiting and severe, colicky pain in the right upper quadrant of the abdomen, or chronic, evidenced by several milder attacks of pain and a history

---

Box 6-2 *Definitions*

chole pertaining to bile
cholang pertaining to bile ducts
cholangiography radiographic examination of bile ducts
cholangitis inflammation of bile duct
cholecyst pertaining to gallbladder
cholecystectomy removal of gallbladder
cholecystitis inflammation of gallbladder
cholecystography radiographic examination of gallbladder
cholecystostomy incision and drainage of gallbladder
choledocho pertaining to common bile duct
choledocholithiasis stones in common bile duct
choledochostomy exploration of common bile duct
cholelith gallstone
cholelithiasis presence of gallstones

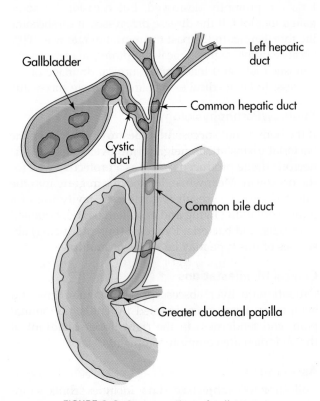

FIGURE **6-6** Common sites of gallstones.

of fat intolerance. Many patients with gallstones are asymptomatic, and the gallstones are discovered only during an examination for another problem.

Assessment

Collection of **subjective data** includes complaints of indigestion after eating foods high in fat. The pain of acute cholecystitis is abrupt in onset, reaches a peak intensity quickly, and remains at that level for 2 to 4 hours. It localizes in the right-upper-quadrant epigastric region. The pain radiates around the midtorso to the right scapular area. Anorexia, nausea, vomiting, and *flatulence* (excess formation of gases in the stomach or intestine) are also noted. The patient may experience increased heart and respiratory rates and become diaphoretic, leading the individual to think he or she is having a heart attack. These symptoms are decreased or absent in the patient with chronic cholecystitis.

Collection of **objective data** may include a low-grade fever and an elevated leukocyte count, as well as mild jaundice, stools that contain fat *(steatorrhea)*, and clay-colored stools caused by a lack of bile in the intestinal tract. The urine may be dark amber- to tea-colored and contain urobilinogen as the kidneys try to remove the excess bilirubin from the bloodstream.

Diagnostic Tests

A number of diagnostic studies are performed to confirm a diagnosis of cholecystitis and cholelithiasis. Fecal studies, serum bilirubin tests, ultrasound of the gallbladder and biliary system, HIDA scan, and oral cholecystogram may be done. Operative cholangiography—in which the common bile duct is directly injected with radiopaque dye—is most commonly done at the time of gallbladder surgery.

Medical Management

If the attack of cholelithiasis is mild, the patient is treated conservatively. Bed rest is prescribed, an NG tube is inserted and connected to low suction, and the patient is placed on no fluids by mouth (NPO). This allows the GI tract and thus the gallbladder to rest. Intravenous fluids are given to rehydrate the patient and replace drainage from the NG tube.

Antispasmodic and analgesic drugs may be given to decrease the patient's pain. Meperidine (Demerol) is commonly used, because there is decreased incidence of spasms of the sphincter of Oddi with this drug. Antibiotics may be given (1) prophylactically to prevent infection; (2) to treat an already present infection; and (3) after perforation, should it occur. A diet that is low in fat and cholesterol may be prescribed. Avoidance of spicy foods is also suggested. (Also see Complementary & Alternative Therapies.)

Lithotripsy. Extracorporeal shock wave lithotripsy (ESWL) is used to treat a patient who has mild or moderate symptoms caused by a few stones. The patient is

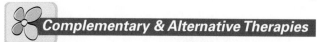
Complementary & Alternative Therapies

Gallbladder, Biliary, and Pancreatic Disorders

- Black root (fresh and dried): The fresh root is used as an emetic. The dried root has a gentler action and is used to treat constipation and liver and gallbladder disease and to increase bile flow. Caution patients with gallstones or bile duct obstruction to avoid using it because it may worsen these diseases.
- Blessed thistle is used orally to treat digestive problems such as liver and gallbladder diseases.
- Dandelion is traditionally used as a bile stimulator to treat gallbladder ailments.
- Onion is used as a gallbladder stimulant. It does increase risk of hypoglycemia, so monitor diabetic patients closely.
- Autumn crocus (colchicine, active ingredient) has been used to treat hepatic cirrhosis and primary biliary cirrhosis. Because of the plant's toxicity, internal use is not recommended.
- Papaya (pawpaw) is used to treat pancreatic insufficiency. Patients with a history of Crohn's disease and chronic gastritis should avoid this herb.
- Royal jelly (bee pollen complex) is used in treating liver disease and pancreatitis. Do not confuse royal jelly with bee pollen and honeybee venom. (Royal jelly should be used with extreme caution by patients with asthma because allergic reactions to royal jelly have led to asthma, anaphylaxis, and death.)

treated by a machine that discharges a series of shock waves through water or a cushion that breaks the stone into fragments. The natural flow of bile carries the stone fragments out of the gallbladder into the intestine for eventual excretion. Nursing intervention after the procedure is similar to that for patients undergoing liver biopsy.

Surgical intervention. A cholecystectomy (removal of the gallbladder) is usually the treatment of choice. The gallbladder is removed, and the cystic duct, vein, and artery are ligated. A laparoscopic cholecystectomy and open abdominal cholecystectomy are the two surgical procedures. (See Figure 6-7 for stone retrieval.) A Jackson-Pratt or Penrose drain or Davol (which promotes drainage and prevents pressure and fluid accumulation under the diaphragm) may be inserted if an open cholecystectomy is performed. If the stones are in the common bile duct and edema is present, a biliary drainage tube, or T-tube, will be inserted to keep the duct open and allow drainage of the bile until the edema resolves. The short end of the tube is placed in the common bile duct, and the longer end is brought to the surface through a stab wound (Figure 6-8). The long end is attached to a closed drainage system (bile bag) that is placed below the level of the common bile duct.

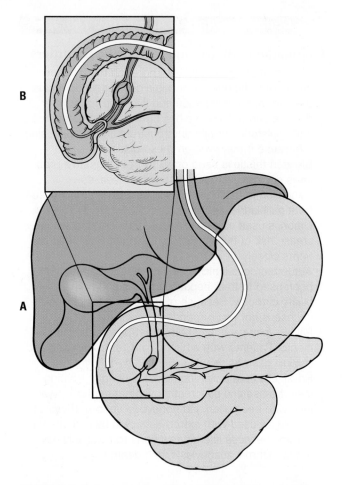

FIGURE **6-7 A,** During endoscopic sphincterotomy, a flexible endoscope is advanced through the mouth and stomach until its tip sits in the duodenum opposite the common bile duct. **B,** After widening the duct mouth by incising the sphincter muscle, the physician advances a basket attachment into the duct and retrieves the stone.

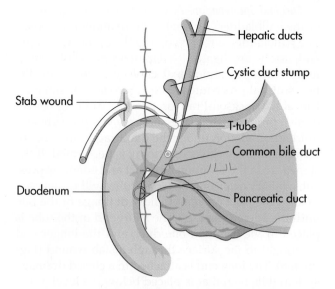

FIGURE **6-8** T-tube in common bile duct.

The T-tube also provides a route for postoperative cholangiography if desired (T-tube cholangiogram). The cholangiogram assesses the patency of the common bile duct. The T-tube will be removed 24 hours after the cholangiogram if the edema is resolved and the common bile duct appears normal. The 24-hour period allows the dye to drain out of the common bile duct. If the edema does not resolve in this time, the patient may be discharged with the T-tube in place.

The most recently developed operative procedure, which is now the most common treatment for cholecystitis and cholelithiasis, is done by way of endoscopy. It is called a **laparoscopic cholecystectomy** and uses a laser or cautery to remove the gallbladder.

This procedure is done instead of the open surgical procedure 80% to 85% of the time. It involves removing the gallbladder through one of four small punctures in the abdomen; this is a relatively minor procedure compared with the standard surgical treatment. The first laparoscopic cholecystectomy was performed in the United States in 1988. Laparoscopic cholecystectomy offers several advantages over the common open abdominal cholecystectomy, including the following:

- It is less invasive (and thus there is less chance of wound infection or respiratory impairment) and has a shorter healing time and a shorter recuperative time.
- There is no unsightly scar.
- There is less pain and thus more rapid return to normal activities.

When a medical history, physical examination, and blood studies are complete, an ultrasound is done to locate gallstones and detect any dilation of the hepatic bile ducts. If **choledocholithiasis** (stones in common bile duct) is confirmed, a sphincterotomy and stone extraction (see Figure 6-7) are performed before laparoscopic surgery (Clinical Pathway for Laparoscopic Surgery box).

It is important to obtain informed consent for endoscopic and open cholecystectomy in case converting from one procedure to the other is necessary. The conversion may be necessary if extensive adhesions, gallstones within the common bile duct, unusual vascular or ductal anatomy, unsuspected pathology of the abdomen, or excessive bleeding complicates the endoscopic procedure.

During surgery, the abdominal cavity is inflated with 3 to 4 L of carbon dioxide to improve visibility. The surgeon removes the deflated gallbladder through a laparoscope. If the organ contains excessive amounts of bile or gallstones, which can prevent it from collapsing, its contents will be aspirated first.

Postoperative care for laparoscopic cholecystectomy. A small number of patients report minor discomfort at the laparoscopic insertion site or mild shoulder pain resulting from diaphragmatic irritation

CLINICAL PATHWAY | *Laparoscopic Surgery*

Laparoscopic Surgery CareMap
Lakes Region General Hospital
Women and Children's Health Services
Ad Hoc Committee/
General Surgery Committee
Reviewed with Patient:_____

Procedure: _____

MD: _____

Patient Profile: _____

_____

_____

Initials/Date

Date Initiated:_____

NOTE: Acceptable medical practice generally does include a variety of responses to a particular clinical problem.

Addressograph

INTERVENTIONS	PREADMISSION (IF APPLICABLE) DATE:	AM ADMISSION VIA ODS DATE:	OPERATIVE DAY— POST PACU DATE:	POSTOP DAY 1 TO DISCHARGE DATE:	DISCHARGE DAY DATE:
Assessment	Preop interview as indicated by MD	Nursing assessment completed Operative consent signed and on chart Patient able to verbalize postop expectations and plan of care for hospital course Reassurance/ emotional support given	On admission and q4°: Patient easily aroused, oriented Skin color pale pink to pink, temperature warm and dry Vital signs Lungs clear without signs or symptoms of respiratory distress Pain controlled with prescribed analgesics If nausea/ vomiting— controlled with prescribed antiemetics Bowel sounds present Dressing/ bandages dry and intact Voiding spontaneously within 8° postop I&O q8° notify MD if <30 mL/hr (adult); <15 mL/hr (pediatric)	Assessment q shift: Patient alert, oriented Skin color pink, warm and dry Vital signs q4° Lungs clear Pain controlled with prescribed analgesics If nausea/ vomiting— controlled with prescribed antiemetics Bowel sounds positive Passing flatus Dressing off, may cover if patient desires Incisions without signs or symptoms of infection Voiding spontaneously I&O WNL Coping mechanisms effective If applicable— parents attentive, assist in care	Condition stable Patient alert, oriented Skin pink, warm, and dry Vital signs stable Lungs clear Pain controlled with oral analgesic No nausea, vomiting Bowel sounds present; passing flatus Incision healing without signs or symptoms of infection Voiding q shift Coping well If applicable— parents able to care for child

From Lewis, S. et al. (2004). *Medical-surgical nursing: assessment and management of clinical problems.* (6th ed.) St Louis: Mosby. (Courtesy Lakes Region General Hospital, Laconia, NH.)

Continued

CLINICAL PATHWAY | *Laparoscopic Surgery—cont'd*

INTERVENTIONS	PREADMISSION (IF APPLICABLE) DATE:	AM ADMISSION VIA ODS DATE:	OPERATIVE DAY— POST PACU DATE:	POSTOP DAY 1 TO DISCHARGE DATE:	DISCHARGE DAY DATE:
Assessment —cont'd			Coping mechanisms effective If applicable— parents attentive, assist in care		
Treatments and interventions		Preop meds given as ordered IVs as ordered	Provide comfort measures: turning, relaxing, breathing technique, splinting abdomen when C + DB Skin care q shift Mouth care q2° while NPO IV as ordered	Assist with general comfort measures Skin care q shift IV discontinued as ordered	
Diet	Dietary teaching appropriate to procedure	NPO after midnight except clear liquids until 3 hours before admission	Ice chips and clear liquids as tolerated	Clear to full liquids tolerated well Regular diet after flatus passed	Tolerating regular diet
Activity		Side rails up on stretcher after preop meds Call bell in reach To OR via stretcher	T, C, DB q2° × 8, then q4° Assist as necessary Call bell in reach; side rails as per standard OOB with assistance Personal hygiene with assistance	C + DB q4° Call bell in reach; side rails as per standard. Ambulate with minimal assist or ad lib Self-care/shower independently	Up ad lib Patient up to ADLs/self-care
Lab tests/other	Preop labs as ordered ECG if age ≥45 (male) ≥55 (female)	Preop testing done as ordered and results on chart			

🖐 CLINICAL PATHWAY | *Laparoscopic Surgery—cont'd*

INTERVENTIONS	PREADMISSION (IF APPLICABLE) DATE:	AM ADMISSION VIA ODS DATE:	OPERATIVE DAY— POST PACU DATE:	POSTOP DAY 1 TO DISCHARGE DATE:	DISCHARGE DAY DATE:
Teaching and discharge planning	Preop teaching initiated Questions answered	Preop teaching reviewed/ completed Questions answered	Orient to room/ unit and plan of care Reinforce preop and postop teaching Review needs identified on admission/ ongoing assessment Begin discharge teaching: Activity, restrictions Diet Symptoms to notify MD Medications Follow-up appointment Care of incision	Review plan of care Review needs identified on admission/ ongoing assessment Continue/ complete discharge teaching: Activity, restrictions Diet Symptoms to notify MD Medications Follow-up appointment Care of incision	Discharge teaching completed and patient verbalizes good understanding of all discharge instructions

Check, initial, and sign. Note detours (deviations from normal)	Signatures	Time	Date	Signatures	Time	Date	Signatures	Time	Date	Signatures	Time	Date	Signatures	Time	Date

From Lewis S et al: *Medical-surgical nursing: assessment and management of clinical problems,* ed 6, St Louis, 2003, Mosby. (Courtesy Lakes Region General Hospital, Laconia, NH.)

secondary to abdominal stretching or residual carbon dioxide. Oral analgesics or antiinflammatory agents relieve these symptoms.

Oral liquids and a light meal are given the first night after surgery. There will be four bandages at the puncture site on the abdomen. Vital signs are routinely assessed. The patient is ambulatory the first postoperative night.

Out of six patients, one is discharged the day of surgery. Most patients are discharged the next day. Patients are usually able to resume moderate activity within 48 to 72 hours.

Patient teaching. Before discharge, patients should be able to eat without difficulty and walk and should have no abdominal distention, evidence of bleeding, or bile leakage. They are instructed to report immediately any severe pain, tenderness in the right upper quadrant, increase in abdominal girth, leakage of bile-colored drainage from the puncture sites, increase in pulse, or symptoms of low BP. Patients are instructed

that they usually can return to work in 3 days and can resume full activity after 1 week.

Although there are contraindications for endoscopic cholecystectomies, most patients are able to choose this less painful, less expensive procedure.

Nursing Interventions and Patient Teaching

Nursing interventions begin with careful assessment of the characteristics of pain (if it is present) and any signs of jaundice of the skin, sclera, and mucous membrane. The patient's urine and stool should be observed for alterations in the presence of bilirubin.

When the patient is treated conservatively, the nursing interventions center on keeping the patient comfortable by carefully administering the medications prescribed and monitoring the patient's response to the medication. The patient on NPO status because of the presence of an NG tube must be monitored closely for amount, color, and consistency of output. The NG tube should be connected to low suction, and the nasal area should be inspected for irritation and necrosis from the tube. Antiemetics may be administered if nausea persists.

IV infusions are observed for patency, correct rates, and entry sites that are free from erythema and edema. I&O are measured and described carefully.

Preoperative care includes teaching the patient to turn, cough, and deep breathe and to use an incentive spirometer to facilitate air movement in and out of the lungs to prevent pneumonia. The patient will be able to follow postoperative instructions more easily by understanding how to splint the abdomen with the hands, small pillow, or rolled bath blanket before attempting a cough; practicing repositioning in the hospital bed; and assuming a sitting position from a standing or lying position. If an open cholecystectomy is anticipated, explaining the NG tube, intravenous tubing, and urinary catheter and their functions will help relieve patient anxiety. The patient should be familiar with any medications that may be used to relieve pain and nausea and should understand that vitamin K and antibiotics are given preoperatively to prevent hemorrhage and infection.

Postoperative care for open cholecystectomy includes monitoring vital signs and observing dressings frequently and carefully for exudate or hemorrhage. The dressings will usually require reinforcement at the drain site. The patient is placed in semi-Fowler's position to facilitate drainage. A Jackson-Pratt or Penrose drain or Davol must be monitored for patency. Initially there should be less than 50 mL of serosanguineous exudate during an 8-hour period. The surgeon should be notified if the drainage is excessive, contains bile, or is bright red.

The patient will need encouragement to perform deep breathing and coughing because of the location of the incision. Analgesics should be given frequently in the early postoperative period to facilitate movement and deep breathing. The patient is usually dangled the night of surgery and ambulated the first postoperative day. The patient's neurological status is monitored by checking ability to be aroused easily, orientation to the environment and family, and ability to move extremities equally on command.

Fluid balance is maintained with intravenous therapy; potassium is usually added to compensate for loss from surgery. The nurse should check the NG tube for proper drainage and may irrigate with physiological saline solution. Usually 30 mL of solution is sufficient to determine the tube's patency. The patient is given nothing by mouth while the NG tube is in place, although sips of water or ice chips may be allowed to keep the mouth moist. The nurse should check the physician's order before giving ice or fluids to the patient, and the patient should be allowed to rinse the mouth frequently. Glycerin or petroleum jelly should be applied to the lips, and the naris through which the tube is passed should be cleansed and lubricated. A tube guard is placed on the nose and to the NG tube to maintain tube placement.

The nurse will be responsible for the care of the T-tube if one is placed. The drainage bag for the T-tube is placed below the level of the common bile duct to prevent the reflux of bile. The bag must be positioned so the tube is not kinked or bile cannot drain from the liver. The position of the bag and tube and the color and amount of exudate must be checked frequently during the first 24 hours and recorded. A gauze roll should be placed under the tube, anchoring it to the patient's abdomen and preventing tension and pull on the tube caused by the weight of the bag. The tube will drain as much as 500 mL during the first 24 hours. The amount should decrease as the edema resolves and bile begins flowing through the common bile duct. The nurse must be careful not to dislodge the T-tube when the patient's dressings are changed as prescribed by the physician.

After oral intake is resumed, the physician may order the tube clamped for 1 to 2 hours before meals and unclamped 1 to 2 hours after the patient eats, to aid in the digestion of fat. While the tube is clamped, the patient may show signs of distress, which include abdominal pain, nausea, vomiting, light brown urine, and clay-colored stools. If distress occurs, the tube should be unclamped immediately. The time that the T-tube remains clamped will be increased as the patient tolerates the procedure. The tube may be left in place for as long as 10 days. The physician will remove the tube when the common bile duct is patent for drainage of bile.

Bowel sounds should be checked every 8 hours to determine the return of peristalsis. A clear liquid diet is usually ordered 24 to 48 hours postoperatively and increased as tolerated. When solid food is started, it will usually be low in fat. Flatulence or nausea after eating certain foods may persist after surgery, and the patient should be instructed to experiment with different foods.

The patient who undergoes a cholecystectomy must be observed for complications. These include jaundice (from an occluded common duct) and hemorrhage (indicated by a decrease in BP, a rise in pulse, and increased exudate at the dressing site). An elevated temperature could indicate peritonitis or wound infection. Pancreatitis may occur after cholecystectomy.

Patients at high risk of not surviving a cholecystectomy may need a cholecystostomy (forming an opening into the gallbladder through the abdominal wall). This can be done using a local anesthetic. The opening will provide a means of removing purulent exudate and possibly the stone. It also allows drainage of bile.

Nursing diagnoses and interventions for the patient with open cholecystectomy or cholecystostomy include but are not limited to the following:

NURSING DIAGNOSES	NURSING INTERVENTIONS
Ineffective breathing pattern, related to pain of high abdominal incision and failure to splint area with coughing and movement	Encourage use of incentive spirometer Assist patient to cough and to take 10 deep breaths hourly. Instruct patient on splinting techniques. Turn q2h. Administer analgesics as ordered to facilitate deep breathing and movement. Ambulate as early as possible.
Risk for impaired skin integrity, related to wound drainage and accidental obstruction of bile drainage	If T-tube is present: Maintain patency and prevent tension on tube. Promote drainage by placing patient in low to semi-Fowler's position. Observe, describe, and record amount and character of exudate at least q8h. Empty bag when half full. Clamp tube as ordered by physician 3 to 4 days postoperatively. Reinforce primary dressing and observe exudate; change and apply sterile, dry dressing as ordered; use Montgomery straps to secure if drainage is profuse. Cleanse skin thoroughly at insertion site before applying sterile dressing. Apply skin barriers as needed for added protection.

Dietary teaching is necessary for the patient who is treated conservatively for cholecystitis, as well as the patient who undergoes surgery. The patient who is treated conservatively must remain on continuous dietary restrictions of fatty foods. Foods to avoid include fried foods, cream, whole milk, butter, margarine, peanut butter, nuts, chocolate, pastries, and gravies. For the postsurgical patient, instruction is given to try small amounts of foods that previously caused discomfort and gradually eliminate those that continue to do so. The patient can usually resume a normal diet without difficulty.

The patient should understand that stones may recur elsewhere in the biliary system. The patient should be able to identify the signs of complications that should be reported. These include jaundice caused by occlusion or stricture of a duct, hemorrhage and/or leakage of bile, elevated temperature, pain, and dietary intolerance associated with another attack. The patient should also be able to demonstrate care of the T-tube, if present on discharge; identify activity restrictions; and identify a date for a return visit to the physician.

Prognosis

With prompt treatment of cholecystitis and cholelithiasis, the prognosis is excellent. Laparoscopic surgery has further decreased the number of complications. The prognosis is not as favorable in patients who develop pancreatitis. See Older Adult Considerations for information about the patient with gallbladder, liver, biliary tract, and exocrine pancreatic organ disorders.

PANCREATITIS
Etiology/Pathophysiology

Pancreatitis is an inflammatory condition of the pancreas that may be acute or chronic. Although the exact cause of pancreatitis remains unknown, many predisposing factors have been identified. Acute or chronic pancreatitis is generally the result of damage to the biliary tract, as by alcohol, trauma, infectious disease, or certain drugs. Alcoholism and biliary tract disease are the two factors most commonly associated with pancreatitis.

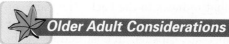

Older Adult Considerations

Gallbladder, Liver, Biliary Tract, or Exocrine Pancreatic Disorder

- Cholelithiasis increases with aging. Older individuals with histories of this should be observed closely for changes in the color of urine and stool or other signs and symptoms of problems of the gallbladder.
- As the body ages, a decrease occurs in the number and size of hepatic cells, which results in the overall decrease in the size and weight of the liver.
- In the older adult there is a decrease in protein synthesis in the liver and possible changes in the production of enzymes that assist in the metabolism of drugs, particularly anticonvulsants, psychotropics, and oral anticoagulants.
- The nurse should be alert to the signs and symptoms of drug toxicity, even when the drugs are administered in normal doses, because the decreased metabolism in the liver can cause an accumulation of the drug.
- The pancreas exhibits ductal hyperplasia and fibrosis with aging, but these changes are not necessarily associated with altered functioning. The output of pancreatic secretions steadily declines after age 40, but related problems with absorption cannot be documented.

In the pathophysiologic process of pancreatitis, the enzymes cannot flow out of the pancreas because of occlusion (an obstruction or closing off) of the pancreatic duct (duct of Wirsung) by edema, stones, or scar tissue. The pancreatic enzymes build up and increase pressure within the duct. The duct ruptures, releasing enzymes that begin digesting the pancreas (autodigestion). In chronic pancreatitis, atrophy of the acinar tissue allows replacement of fibrotic tissue, and necrosis of the pancreas occurs.

The development of pseudocysts or abscesses in pancreatic tissue is a serious complication. After autodigestion occurs, the pancreas and occasionally surrounding organs form walls around cystic fluid, including pancreatic enzymes, and necrotic debris. These pseudocysts can develop into an abscess.

Clinical Manifestations

Manifestations include severe abdominal pain radiating to the back. The pain is sometimes relieved by assuming a forward position, taking the stomach weight off the pancreas. Jaundice may be noted if the common bile duct is obstructed.

Assessment

Collection of **subjective data** may include noting that patients exhibit extreme symptoms or none at all. When symptoms are evident, it is difficult to distinguish the symptoms of pancreatitis from other abdominal disorders. The most specific complaint is abdominal pain that radiates to the back. The pain can be excruciating. This pain is caused by the enlargement of the pancreatic capsule, an obstruction, or the chemical irritation from the enzymes. The pain is usually decreased by flexing the trunk, leaning forward from a sitting position, or by assuming the fetal position. It is increased by eating or lying down. Other complaints include anorexia, nausea, malaise, and restlessness.

Collection of **objective data** may include noting the presence of low-grade fever, vomiting in 70% to 90% of patients, jaundice if the common bile duct is obstructed, weight loss, steatorrhea, and tachycardia.

Diagnostic Tests

Both acute and chronic pancreatitis are diagnosed by radiologic studies (abdominal CT scan and ultrasound of the pancreas), endoscopy, and laboratory analysis of the amount of pancreatic enzymes in the serum and urine. Laboratory tests will reveal an increased serum amylase and lipase during the first few days and then increased urine amylase thereafter. Leukocytosis, an elevated hematocrit level, hypocalcemia, hypoalbuminemia, and hyperglycemia may also be present. Pancreatic insulin production may be diminished if the islets of Langerhans become infected, and some patients develop diabetes mellitus.

Medical Management

Treatment is medical unless the precipitating cause is biliary tract disease; then surgery may be indicated. Food and fluids are withheld to avoid stimulating pancreatic activity, and IV fluids are administered. The patient is on NPO status, and an NG tube is inserted to decrease pancreatic stimulation, treat or prevent nausea and vomiting, and decrease abdominal distention. A common complaint is constant, severe pain; in such cases, meperidine (Demerol) via patient-controlled analgesia (PCA) is often administered. Morphine may cause spasms of the sphincter of Oddi. However, IV morphine may be used because of its longer half-life. Analgesics may be combined with an antispasmodic.

Parenteral anticholinergic medication, such as atropine or propantheline (Pro-Banthine), will help decrease pancreatic activity. Antacids or antihistamine H_2 receptor antagonists, such as cimetidine (Tagamet), may be given to prevent stress ulcers caused by decreased gastric pH. Antibiotics are prescribed by some physicians to counteract secondary infections.

If the patient has severe acute pancreatitis, peripheral or total parenteral nutrition may be required to maintain an adequate state of nutrition. As the patient improves, further attacks may be prevented by maintaining a bland, low-fat, high-protein, high-carbohydrate diet. The diet must be free of alcohol and gastric stimulants, such as coffee. Oral hypoglycemic agents or insulin may be needed if there is destruction of the islets of Langerhans.

Nursing Interventions and Patient Teaching

The presence and location of pain are important to determine, as well as what aggravates or relieves the pain. Keeping the patient as comfortable as possible involves proper administration of analgesic medications. The patient is usually on bed rest with bathroom privileges to decrease the flow of pancreatic enzymes. Nutritional needs are met by intravenous feedings as long as necessary. The patient who is addicted to alcohol may go through withdrawal while in the hospital. The nurse must be prepared to protect the patient from injury and provide supportive care to the patient and family. All replacement fluids and medications must be monitored carefully for proper administration.

Nursing diagnoses and interventions for the patient with pancreatitis include but are not limited to the following:

NURSING DIAGNOSES	NURSING INTERVENTIONS
Pain, related to stimulation of nerve endings caused by enlargement of pancreatic capsule, obstruction, or chemical irritation from enzymes	Administer medications as prescribed and monitor relief. Restrict diet as necessary to prevent aggravation of pain (free from fats, alcohol, caffeine).

NURSING DIAGNOSES	NURSING INTERVENTIONS
	Use alternative comfort measures: repositioning, positive imagery, and providing time for listening.
	Monitor nasogastric (NG) tube to wall suction for functioning to prevent abdominal distention.
Imbalanced nutrition: less than body requirements, related to inadequate intake associated with current anorexia, nausea, vomiting, and loss of enzymes necessary for the digestive process	Administer IV fluids or peripheral or total parenteral nutrition as ordered.
	Weigh patient daily at same time and using same scale.
	Record I&O, including NG tube suctioning output.
	Administer antacids and antiemetics as prescribed.
	Instruct patient in a diet that is bland, low in fat, and high in protein and carbohydrates.
Deficient fluid volume, related to decreased oral intake, vomiting, diarrhea, NG suctioning, and hemorrhage	Monitor I&O; weigh patient daily.
	Assess hemodynamic stability: pulse, BP.
	Assess patient for signs and symptoms of fluid volume deficit: decreased level of consciousness, poor skin turgor, cool, dry, or clammy skin, and weak peripheral pulses.
	Assess for signs and symptoms of hemorrhage; assess abdominal girth; monitor NG aspirate for occult or frank bleeding.
	Monitor for the administration of fluid volume replacement.

The patient will remain on a bland, low-fat, high-calorie, high-carbohydrate diet after discharge. Alcohol and beverages or foods containing caffeine will not be allowed if full recovery is desired. The patient should also understand the disease process and the severity of the disease and related complications.

Prognosis

The prognosis of pancreatitis depends on the course and complications of the disease. Two significant complications of acute pancreatitis are pseudocysts and abscess. In most patients, acute pancreatitis is mild, requiring less than 1 week of hospitalization. However, 5% to 25% of patients have a more complicated course. Interestingly, complications can occur with mild, acute, chronic, or severe pancreatitis. Mor-

tality rates for acute necrotizing pancreatitis range from 10% to 50%. See the Medications table for treatment of disorders of the gallbladder, liver, biliary tract, and exocrine pancreas.

CANCER OF THE PANCREAS

Although once considered relatively rare, pancreatic cancer is now the fourth leading cause of cancer death in the United States and Canada. A major factor in the high death rate from pancreatic cancer is the difficulty in diagnosing it at an early curable stage. This disease usually occurs after middle age. The risk increases with age, with the peak incidence occurring between 65 and 80 years of age.

Etiology/Pathophysiology

The cause of cancer of the pancreas is unknown, but it is diagnosed more often in cigarette smokers, people exposed to chemical carcinogens, and people with diabetes mellitus and pancreatitis. Diets high in meat, fat, and coffee consumption are also linked to pancreatic cancer.

The cancer may originate in the pancreas or be the result of metastasis from cancer of the lung, stomach, duodenum, or common bile duct. Most often the head of the pancreas is involved and causes jaundice by compressing and obstructing the common bile duct. As the cancer spreads, the posterior wall of the stomach, the duodenal wall, the colon, and the common bile duct may be invaded. Biliary obstruction and gallbladder dilation are subsequent complications. It is not uncommon for the tumor to grow rapidly and invade the vascular and lymphatic systems. Many patients live only 4 to 8 months after diagnosis is confirmed.

Clinical Manifestations

The insidious onset of the disease with initially vague symptoms generally accounts for delays in diagnosis. Pain occurs in about 85% of the patients. About half of the patients develop diabetes mellitus if islet cells are involved.

Assessment

A psychosocial history during patient assessment may reveal at-risk populations such as engineers, coal- and gas-plant employees, chemists, and workers exposed to betanaphthol and benzidine. Collection of **subjective data** includes anorexia; fatigue; nausea; flatulence; a change in stools; and steady, dull, and aching pain in the epigastrium or referred to the back. The pain is usually worse at night.

Collection of **objective data** includes weight loss, often gradual and progressive, which is one of the earliest signs. Jaundice usually is progressive and may occur late. Pruritus accompanies the jaundice. Many patients have recent onset of diabetes mellitus.

MEDICATIONS | *Disorders of the Gallbladder, Liver, Biliary Tract, and Exocrine Pancreas*

MEDICATION	TRADE NAME	ACTION	SIDE EFFECTS	NURSING IMPLICATIONS
Gemcitabine HCl	Gemzar	Exhibits antitumor activity. Is indicated as first-line treatment of locally advanced or metastatic adenocarcinoma of the pancreas	Myelosuppression; nausea and vomiting, macular papular pruritic rash	Monitor CBC. Provide an antiemetic to control nausea and vomiting. Provide relief measures to control pruritus.
Lactulose	Chronulac, Cephulac	Acidifies colonic contents, thus decreasing absorption of ammonia from gut; also has cathartic laxative properties; primarily used in hepatic encephalopathy	Nausea, vomiting, diarrhea	Titrate dose to 3 or 4 loose stools per day; monitor for dehydration; monitor for serum ammonia levels and improved mental status.
Spironolactone	Aldactone	Competes with aldosterone at receptor sites in distal tubule, resulting in excretion of sodium chloride, water, retention of potassium, phosphate (used in cirrhosis of the liver with ascites)	Headache, confusion, diarrhea, bleeding, dysrhythmias, impotence, hypokalemia	Assess electrolytes, Na, Cl, K, BUN, serum creatinine. Weigh daily, monitor I&O. Administer in AM to avoid interference with sleep.
Meperidine	Demerol	Binds to opiate receptors in CNS. Alters the perception of and response to painful stimuli, while producing generalized CNS depression (Used in biliary pain because morphine may cause spasms of the sphincter of Oddi)	Sedation, confusion, respiratory depression, hypotension, bradycardia, nausea, vomiting, urinary retention	Assess type, location, intensity of pain before and 1 hour after administration. If respiratory rate is less than 10/min, assess level of sedation.
Propantheline	Pro-Banthine	Antisecretory and antispasmodic agent; slows GI motility through anticholinergic activity Decreases pancreatic activity	Drowsiness, confusion, dry mouth, constipation, urinary retention, tachycardia, blurred vision	Avoid use with other CNS depressants or alcohol, avoid driving or other activities until accustomed to effects; may cause hypotension when given IV; do not use in patients with Parkinson's disease.
Vasopressin	Pitressin	Synthetic pituitary antidiuretic effects on kidney, a potent vasoconstrictor (used to treat bleeding esophageal varices)	Hypertension; ischemia to heart, mesenteric organs, and kidneys; angina, myocardial infarction, water retention, hyponatremia	Use with caution in older patients or patients with known coronary artery disease; use caution in patients with known CHF; discontinue if chest pain develops; monitor urine output and serum sodium.
Neomycin	Mycifradin, Myciguent	Inhibits protein synthesis in bacteria at the level of the 30S ribosome; used to decrease the number of ammonia-producing bacteria in the gut as part of management of hepatic encephalopathy	Ototoxicity, local stinging, burning, nephrotoxicity	Monitor neurologic status; monitor renal function.

MEDICATIONS | *Disorders of the Gallbladder, Liver, Biliary Tract, and Exocrine Pancreas—cont'd*

MEDICATION	TRADE NAME	ACTION	SIDE EFFECTS	NURSING IMPLICATIONS
Cholestyramine	Questran	Bind bile acids in the GI tract, forming an insoluble complex; relief of pruritus associated with elevated levels of bile acids	Nausea, constipation, abdominal discomfort	Assess severity of pruritus and skin integrity.
Pancrelipase	Pancrease, Cotazym	Increased digestion of fats, CHO, and proteins in the GI tract; treatment of pancreatic insufficiency associated with chronic pancreatitis, pancreatectomy	Diarrhea, nausea, stomach cramps, abdominal pain	Assess patient's nutritional status; monitor stools for high fat content; assess patient for allergy to pork; administer immediately before meals or with meals.

Diagnostic Tests

Better diagnostic measures are needed for detection of pancreatic cancer because most of the current methods detect only advanced stages. Diagnosis at the early stages of cancer of the pancreas is attempted by radioimmunoassay for circulating carcinoembryonic antigen (CEA) and tumor-associated antigen. Other diagnostic studies include transabdominal ultrasound and CT, duodenal endoscopy to obtain specimens for cytological examination, ERCP, and pancreatic scans. ERCP is the gold standard for visualization of the pancreatic duct and biliary system. When ERCP is used, pancreatic secretions as well as tissues can be collected for analysis of different tumor markers (see Figure 6-1).

Medical Management

Often, malignant tumors of the pancreas are inoperable by the time diagnosis is made. Treatment of pancreatic cancer is primarily surgical and has been associated with a high mortality rate. Cancer of the head of the pancreas is usually treated by pancreatoduodenectomy; the Whipple procedure involves resection of the antrum of the stomach, duodenum, and varying amounts of the pancreas. Anastomoses are constructed between the stomach, common bile duct and pancreatic ducts, and the jejunum (Figure 6-9).

Another procedure is total pancreatectomy with resection of parts of the GI tract. Subtotal pancreatic resection has complications of postoperative pancreatic fistulas and is not recommended.

Combinations of drugs such as 5-FU and gemcitabine (Gemzar) may produce a better response than single chemotherapeutic agents. Gemcitabine is a main treatment for pancreatic cancer that has metastasized. The current role of chemotherapy in pancreatic cancer is limited. Radiation therapy alters survival rate little but is effective for pain relief. Adjuvant therapy—which

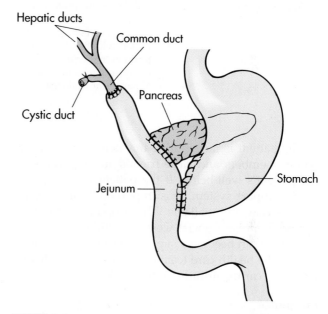

FIGURE **6-9** Whipple's procedure, or radical pancreaticoduodenectomy. This surgical procedure involves resection of the proximal pancreas, adjoining duodenum, distal portion of the stomach, and distal portion of the common bile duct. An anastomosis of the pancreatic duct, common bile ducts, and stomach to the jejunum is done.

uses surgical resection, radiation, and chemotherapy—is believed by some to be the most effective way to manage the almost always fatal cancer of the pancreas.

Nursing Interventions and Patient Teaching

Pancreatic surgery is radical surgery that requires critical care nursing. The major aspects of postoperative care are focused on maintaining fluid and electrolyte balance, preventing hemorrhage, preventing respiratory complications, and monitoring endocrine and exocrine functions of the pancreas.

Nursing diagnoses and interventions for patients with cancer of the pancreas include but are not limited to the following:

NURSING DIAGNOSES	NURSING INTERVENTIONS
Risk for deficient fluid volume, related to possible hemorrhage and drainage	Maintain patency of GI tubes to relieve distention and compression at the surgical site. Measure I&O and weigh daily. Monitor intravenous fluid replacement. Assess for signs and symptoms of dehydration (dry mucous membranes, poor tissue turgor, oliguria).
Risk for impaired skin integrity, related to drainage from wound	Monitor for excoriation and infection; use skin barriers and disposable postoperative pouches and appliances to prevent enzymatic contact with the skin and to aid in the accurate collection and measurement of pancreatic drainage.

The patient is facing a life-threatening illness, and family members and close friends are important for the patient's well-being. If the patient has an inadequate support system, it is important to use the resources that are available. The hospital chaplain or personal minister, social worker, dietitian, physician, and nurse can become a support system. These members of the health care team can provide active listening and a caring attitude for this patient.

Prognosis

The prognosis for patients with cancer of the pancreas is very poor. Median survival after diagnosis is only 5 to 12 months. The 5-year survival rate remains less than 10%. Resection of the tumor improves median survival to 17 to 20 months. Prognosis is related to the location of the tumor.

NURSING PROCESS *for the Patient with Gallbladder, Liver, Biliary Tract, or Exocrine Pancreatic Disorder*

The role of the licensed practical nurse/licensed vocational nurse (LPN/LVN) in the nursing process as stated is that the LPN/LVN will:
- Participate in planning care for patients based on patient needs.
- Review patients plan of care and recommend revisions as needed.
- Review and follow defined prioritization for patient care.

- Use clinical pathways/care maps/care plans to guide and review patient care.

Assessment

1. Nursing assessment of the patient with a gallbladder, liver, biliary tract, or exocrine pancreatic disorder must be performed accurately.
2. A head-to-toe assessment is performed.
3. The nurse assesses the patient for knowledge of the disease process, nutritional status, pain, discomfort, current health problems, and signs and symptoms. Changes in appetite and weight should also be noted.
4. The patient's vital signs are measured, noting any alterations from normal, such as hyperthermia, hypotension, hypertension, tachycardia, or tachypnea.
5. The skin, sclera, mucous membranes, urine, and stool are observed for alterations in the presence of bilirubin. The abdomen is inspected, auscultated, and palpated. Any abdominal tenderness, pain, or abnormal bowel sounds are documented.

Nursing Diagnosis

Assessment provides the data from which the nurse identifies the patient's problems, strengths, potential complications, and learning needs. Nursing diagnoses for patients with disorders of the liver, biliary tract, or exocrine pancreas include but are not limited to the following:
- Activity intolerance
- Ineffective breathing pattern
- Deficient fluid volume
- Impaired home maintenance
- Risk for injury
- Deficient knowledge
- Noncompliance
- Imbalanced nutrition: less than body requirements
- Acute pain
- Chronic pain
- Powerlessness
- Impaired skin integrity
- Disturbed thought processes

Expected Outcomes/Planning

When planning the care for the patient, the nurse should look at the nursing diagnosis and establish the cause of the nursing problem. The overall goals for the patient with disorders of the gallbladder, liver, biliary tract, and exocrine pancreas include (1) the relief of pain and discomfort; (2) the stabilization of fluid and electrolyte balance; (3) having minimal to no complications; (4) the ability to resume normal activities; (5) a return, if possible, to normal pancreatic and liver function without complications; and (6) a return to as normal a lifestyle as possible.

Planning includes the development of realistic goals and outcomes from the identified nursing diagnoses. Short- and long-term measurable goals must be established. Examples of measurable goals are:

- Patient will feel rested enough to assist in ADLs; have increased activity tolerance by walking 100 feet.
- Patient will report pain control less than a 4 on a scale of 0 to 10.

Implementation

Maintaining the patient's optimal level of health is important in reducing biliary and pancreatic symptoms. Nursing interventions may include nutritional management, pharmacologic management, and health promotion and maintenance to prevent complications. The nurse should encourage the early diagnosis and treatment of liver, biliary tract, and pancreatic disease. Nursing interventions involve supportive care with special attention to nutrition, hydration, skin care, and pain relief.

Evaluation

The nurse evaluates the expected outcomes. During and after the planned nursing interventions, the nurse should determine the outcomes of the interventions. This is an ongoing process whereby the nurse is continually trying to establish the most effective plan of care.

Evaluation involves determining whether the established goals have been met. The goals are evaluated by the nurse and patient to see whether the criteria for measurement have been met. Goals and evaluative measures for disorders of the liver, biliary tract, and exocrine pancreas may include the following:

Goal #1: Patient achieves improved activity tolerance.
Evaluative measure: Observe patient exercise.
Goal #2: Patient remains free of bodily injury.
Evaluative measure: Ask patient to list factors that increase the risk of injury.
See Cultural and Ethnic Considerations box.

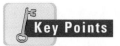

Key Points

- Cholecystectomy (removal of the gallbladder by means of laparoscopic or open abdominal procedure) is one of the most commonly performed surgical procedures.
- Clinical manifestations of acute pancreatitis include severe abdominal pain radiating to the back; the pain is sometimes relieved when the patient assumes a forward position, taking the weight of the stomach off the pancreas.
- The most common cause of cirrhosis of the liver is alcohol ingestion.
- Clinical manifestations of cirrhosis of the liver differ, depending on whether the patient is in the early or later stages of the disease.
- Pancreatic disorders may cause diabetes mellitus because of interference with insulin production.
- Planned nursing interventions must be individualized according to each patient's and family's unique needs.
- Prevention of the spread of viral hepatitis is a primary concern of health care professionals.
- Vaccine is now available to prevent the development of hepatitis A and hepatitis B.
- If an infection develops anywhere along the GI tract, there is danger that the infecting organism may reach the liver through the biliary system, portal venous system, or hepatic arterial or lymphatic system.
- An important aspect of nursing interventions in patients with hepatitis and cirrhosis of the liver is the relief of pruritus.

Go to your free CD-ROM for an Audio Glossary, animations, video clips, and Review Questions for the NCLEX-PN® Examination.

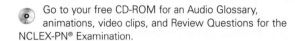 Be sure to visit the companion Evolve site at http://evolve.elsevier.com/Christensen/adult/ for WebLinks and additional online resources.

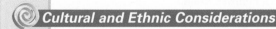 *Cultural and Ethnic Considerations*

Gallbladder, Liver, Biliary Tract, or Exocrine Pancreatic Disorder

- Mortality from cirrhosis occurs more frequently among African Americans than in other ethnic groups.
- Primary hepatic cancer has a higher incidence among African Americans, Asian Americans, and Inuit (Eskimos) than among whites.

- Pancreatic cancer occurs more frequently among African Americans and Asian Americans than among whites.
- Whites and American Indians have a higher incidence of gallbladder disease than African Americans and Asian Americans.

CHAPTER CHALLENGE

1. Nurses, as well as other health care providers, are at risk for hepatitis B. For prophylaxis to be most effective in these workers:

   1. prophylaxis must be instituted before exposure.
   2. prophylaxis can be instituted either before or after exposure.
   3. prophylaxis must be instituted after exposure.
   4. prophylaxis instituted before or after exposure is effective forever.

2. Liver needle biopsy is a safe, simple, and valuable method of diagnosing pathologic liver conditions. However, the nurse must anticipate possible complications, including which of the following nursing diagnoses?

   1. Pain, related to leakage of blood and bile into the peritoneal cavity
   2. Noncompliance, of medications, related to testing procedure
   3. Social isolation, related to tissue sample being removed for biopsy
   4. Disturbed sleep pattern, related to lack of information on hospital protocol

3. Mr. B., a 78-year-old patient, is admitted with common bile duct obstruction related to cancer of the pancreas. Choose all of the clinical manifestations the nurse would expect to assess.

   1. Brown feces
   2. Scleral icterus
   3. Dark, tea-colored urine
   4. Jaundice

4. It is especially important for the patient to cough and deep breathe postoperatively following an open cholecystectomy because:

   1. the patients are often obese.
   2. the patients usually smoke.
   3. the patient is on bed rest for a more prolonged period.
   4. the patient tends to take shallow breaths due to the placement of the incision.

5. In hepatic encephalopathy, when the nurse requests that the patient stretch out the arm and hyperextend the wrist with the fingers separated, relaxed, and extended to see whether rapid, irregular flexion and extension (flapping) of the wrist occur, the nurse is assessing for the presence of:

   1. varices.
   2. asterixis.
   3. pruritus.
   4. bacterial toxins.

6. Mr. E. has advanced cirrhosis of the liver. What type of food might you expect to find limited in his diet?

   1. Fruits
   2. Vegetables
   3. Meats
   4. Carbohydrates

7. Patients with liver abscess present with vague signs and symptoms, which are often:

   1. asterixis, ascites, esophageal varices.
   2. fever accompanied by chills, abdominal pain, and tenderness in right upper quadrant.
   3. enlarged spleen, spider telangiectases.
   4. constipation, left quadrant abdominal cramping, and loud, high-pitched abdominal sounds upon auscultation.

8. A small number of patients who have had a laparoscopic cholecystectomy report mild shoulder pain resulting from:

   1. paralytic ileus with mesenteric irritation.
   2. incision along the rectus abdominis muscle.
   3. diaphragmatic irritation secondary to residual carbon dioxide.
   4. spasm of the duct of Wirsung.

9. Ms. F. has been admitted with right upper quadrant pain and has been placed on a low-fat diet. Which of the following trays would be acceptable for her?

   1. Whole milk, veal, rice, and pastry
   2. Liver, fried potatoes, gelatin, and avocado
   3. Skim milk, lean fish, tapioca pudding, and fruit
   4. Ham, mashed potatoes, creamed peas, and gelatin

10. Hepatitis types B, C, D, and G are spread mainly through all of the following *except:*

    1. blood transfusions.
    2. contaminated needles and instruments.
    3. direct contact with body fluids from infected people, such as through breast milk and sexual contact.
    4. oral-fecal route.

11. In patients with acute pancreatitis, the administration of the analgesic morphine may cause:

    1. paralytic ileus.
    2. addiction.
    3. urinary retention.
    4. spasms of the sphincter of Oddi.

12. A patient is scheduled for surgery for a common bile exploration. The nurse would expect the patient to return from surgery with:

    1. an underwater-seal drainage.
    2. a T-tube connected to gravity drainage.
    3. a Penrose drain.
    4. a nephrostomy tube.

13. Which types of hepatitis now have vaccines for prevention?

    1. B only
    2. B and D
    3. A and B
    4. A, B, C, D, E, and G

14. The nursing intervention of the patient with cholecystitis associated with cholelithiasis is based on the knowledge that:

    1. the disorder can be successfully treated with oral bile salts that dissolve gallstones.
    2. morphine is the drug of choice to relieve the pain of bile duct spasms during an acute attack.
    3. a heavy meal with a high fat content may precipitate the signs and symptoms of the disease.

4. a low-cholesterol diet is indicated to reduce the availability of cholesterol for gallstone formation.

15. Teaching in relation to home management following a laparoscopic cholecystectomy should include:

1. keeping the bandages on the puncture sites for 48 hours.
2. reporting any bile-colored drainage or pus from any incision.
3. using over-the-counter antiemetics if nausea and vomiting occur.
4. emptying and measuring the contents of the bile bag from the T-tube every day.

16. A patient with advanced cirrhosis asks the nurse why his abdomen is so swollen. The nurse's response to the patient is based on the knowledge that:

1. a lack of clotting factors promotes the collection of blood in the abdominal cavity.
2. portal hypertension and hypoalbuminemia cause a fluid shift into the peritoneal space.
3. decreased peristalsis in the GI tract contributes to gas formation and bowel distention.
4. bile salts in the blood irritate the peritoneal membranes, causing edema and pocketing of fluid.

17. When caring for a patient with hepatic encephalopathy the nurse may give enemas, provide a low-protein diet, and limit physical activity. These measures are done to:

1. promote fluid loss.
2. eliminate potassium ions.
3. decrease portal pressure.
4. decrease the production ammonia.

18. In planning care for a patient with metastatic cancer of the liver, the nurse includes interventions that:

1. focus primarily on symptomatic and comfort measures.
2. reassure the patient that chemotherapy offers a good prognosis for recovery.
3. promote the patient's confidence that surgical excision of the tumor will be successful.
4. provide information necessary for the patient to make decisions regarding liver transplantation.

19. Patients who receive a liver transplant secondary to viral B or C hepatitis often experience _____ or _____ of the transplanted liver.

CHAPTER 7

Care of the Patient with a Blood or Lymphatic Disorder

BARBARA LAURITSEN CHRISTENSEN and ELAINE ODEN KOCKROW

Key Terms

Be sure to check out the bonus material on the free CD-ROM, including selected audio pronunciations.

anemia (ă-NĒ-mē-ă, p. 295)
aplasia (ă-PLĀ-zhă, p. 298)
disseminated intravascular coagulation (dĭ-SĔM-ĭ-nāt-ĕd, p. 314)
erythrocytosis (ĕ-rīth-rō-sī-TŌ-sĭs, p. 304)
erythropoiesis (ĕ-rīth-rō-pō-Ē-sĭs, p. 287)
hemarthrosis (hē-măr-THRŌ-sĭs, p. 312)
hemophilia A (hē-mō-FĒL-ē-ă, p. 312)
heterozygous (hĕt-ĕr-ō-ZĪ-gŭs, p. 302)
homozygous (hō-mō-ZĪ-gŭs, p. 302)
idiopathic (ĭd-ē-ō-PĂTH-ĭk, p. 311)
leukemia (loo-kĒ-mē-ă, p. 307)
leukopenia (loo-kō-PĒ-nē-ă, p. 305)
lymphangitis (lĭm-făn-GĪ-tĭs, p. 317)
lymphedema (lĭm-fĕ-DĒ-mă, p. 318)
multiple myeloma (MŬL-tĭ-pŭl mī-ĕ-LŌ-mă, p. 316)
myeloproliferative (mī-ĕ-lō-prō-LĬF-ĕr-ă-tĭv, p. 304)
pancytopenic (păn-sī-tō-PĔN-ĭc, p. 298)
pernicious (pĕr-NĬSH-ŭs, p. 297)
Reed-Sternberg cell (rēd-STĔRN-bĕrg sĕl, p. 318)
thrombocytopenia (thrŏm-bō-sīt-ō-PĒ-nē-ă, p. 311)

OVERVIEW OF ANATOMY AND PHYSIOLOGY

This chapter presents transportation and protection, two of the body's most important functions. Without transportation and protection for the cells, the homeostasis of the body would be threatened. The systems that provide these vital services for the body are the circulatory and lymphatic systems. This chapter discusses the primary transportation fluid—blood—and presents an overview of the lymphatic system. Blood not only performs vital transportation services, but also provides much of the protection necessary to withstand foreign invaders. The lymphatic system helps maintain fluid balance, and lymphoid tissues help protect the internal environment.

We live in a hostile and dangerous environment. Each day we are faced with potentially harmful toxins, disease-causing bacteria, viruses, and even cells from our own bodies that have been transformed into cancerous invaders. Fortunately, we are protected from this staggering variety of biologic enemies by a remarkable set of defense mechanisms.

CHARACTERISTICS OF BLOOD

In ancient times, blood was referred to as the "river of life" or "fluid of life." Some even believed it had magical properties. All knew it was necessary to maintain life.

Blood is a viscous (thick), red fluid that contains red blood cells, white blood cells, and platelets, which are suspended in a light yellow fluid called **plasma.** Plasma constitutes 55% of the blood's volume; the remaining 45% is composed of the blood cells and platelets (Figure 7-1). Blood is slightly alkaline, with a pH range of 7.35 to 7.45. It has a sodium chloride (NaCl) concentration of 0.9%. The average adult blood volume is 5 to 6 liters), or 10 to 12 pints.

The blood performs three critical functions. First, it transports oxygen and nutrition to the cells and waste products away from the cells and transports hormones from endocrine glands to tissues and cells. Second, it regulates the acid-base balance (pH) with buffers, aids with body temperature because of its water content, and controls the water content of its cells as a result of dissolved sodium ions. Third,

it protects the body against infection with special cells and prevents blood loss with special clotting mechanisms.

The individual components of the blood are discussed in the following sections.

Red Blood Cells

Erythrocytes (red blood cells [RBCs]) give blood its rich color. In men, red blood cells average approximately 5.5 million per cubic millimeter (mm³) of blood, and in women, they average approximately 4.8 million per mm³. A mature RBC contains cytoplasm and the red pigment hemoglobin (Hgb), a compound in the blood that carries oxygen to the cells from the lungs and carbon dioxide away from the cells to the lungs. The normal hemoglobin level is 14 to 18 g/dL for men and 12 to 16 g/dL for women. The average life span of an RBC is 120 days. An erythrocyte is the major cellular element of the circulating blood; its principal function is to transport oxygen and carbon dioxide. Erythrocytes are continuously produced in the red bone marrow, principally in the vertebrae, ribs, sternum, and proximal ends of the humerus and femur.

Erythropoiesis (the process of RBC production) depends on several factors, among them healthy condi-

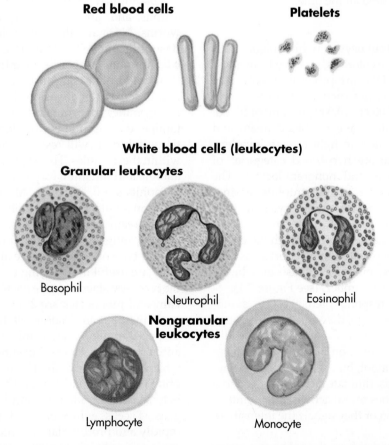

Red blood cells

Platelets

White blood cells (leukocytes)

Granular leukocytes

Basophil

Neutrophil

Eosinophil

Nongranular leukocytes

Lymphocyte

Monocyte

FIGURE **7-1** Human blood cells. There are approximately 30 trillion blood cells in an adult. Each cubic millimeter of blood contains from 4.5 to 5 million RBCs; 5000 to 10,000 WBCs; and 150,000 to 400,000 platelets.

tions of the bone marrow; dietary substances such as iron and copper, plus essential amino acids; and certain vitamins, especially vitamin B_{12}, folic acid, riboflavin (vitamin B_2), and pyridoxine (vitamin B_6). A feedback mechanism is energized when the amount of oxygen delivered to the tissues by RBCs is decreased. The decreased oxygen triggers the release of an enzyme, the renal erythropoietic factor, in the kidneys. Erythropoietin is carried to the bone marrow, where it initiates the development of mature RBCs. The increased number of RBCs allows more oxygen to be delivered to the tissues, and as a result, the signal to increase RBC production is shut off.

A common laboratory test called the **hematocrit** (a measure of the packed cell volume of red blood cells, expressed as a percentage of the total blood volume) can tell a physician a great deal about the volume of RBCs in a blood sample. Normally about 42% to 52% of the blood volume in men and 37% to 47% in women consists of RBCs.

If hemoglobin falls below the normal level, as it does in anemia, an unhealthy chain reaction begins: less hemoglobin, less oxygen transported to cells, slower breakdown and use of nutrients by cells, less energy produced by cells, decreased cellular function. If one understands the relationship between hemoglobin and energy, one can understand that an anemic person's complaint will probably be of feeling "tired all the time."

White Blood Cells

Unlike erythrocytes, **leukocytes** (white blood cells [WBCs]) have nuclei, are colorless, and live from a few days to several years. They are primarily involved in body defenses, such as destruction of bacteria and viruses. They number 5000 to 10,000 per mm^3 of blood. Some WBCs can actually leave the bloodstream and move through tissue spaces to fight foreign invaders, such as bacteria. There are two broad categories of white cells: granulocytes and nongranulocytes. The three types of granulocytes are neutrophils, eosinophils, and basophils. The nongranulocytes include lymphocytes and monocytes. A **differential white blood cell count** is an examination in which the different kinds of WBCs are counted and reported as percentages of the total examined. They also may be reported as absolute (actual number) (see Figure 7-1).

Because leukocytes respond predictably to symptoms of infection and recovery, they are a reliable gauge of the state of the body's defenses. That is why the differential WBC is such a common blood test. Although the differential WBC cannot, by itself, be used to diagnose a disease or to discriminate between a bacterial and viral infection, it does reveal activity that points to occult (hidden) infection or that signals the intensity of chemotherapy.

The granulocytes develop from the red bone marrow and contain granules in their cytoplasm. The granules are demonstrated when the cells are stained with Wright's stain (a chemical solution). **Neutrophils** (granular circulating leukocytes essential for *phagocytosis*—the process by which bacteria, cellular debris, and solid particles are destroyed and removed) ingest bacteria and dispose of dead tissue. Neutrophils are the primary phagocytic cells involved in acute inflammatory response. A mature neutrophil is called a segmental neutrophil or "seg" because the nucleus is segmented into two to five lobes connected by strands. They also release lysozyme, an enzyme that destroys certain bacteria. The normal value of neutrophils is 60% to 70%.

Mature neutrophils have a short life span—approximately 7 hours—after which they die, along with the bacteria and debris they have engulfed. Bone marrow thus needs to manufacture neutrophils constantly; normally it stores approximately a 6-day supply. Because neutrophils respond in proportion to the severity of the infection, an overwhelming infection may deplete marrow reserves. When this happens, the marrow releases immature polymorphonuclear leukocytes ("polys"), called bands, which are immature neutrophils that are in the final stages of development. When the band count exceeds 8% of the total number of polys, the marrow has used up its reserve. The presence of excess bands in the peripheral blood is called a shift to the left (i.e., a shift toward immature cells) and indicates severe infection.

Eosinophils are WBCs that play a role in allergic reactions and are effective against certain parasitic worms. Normal values of eosinophils are 1% to 4%. **Basophils** are WBCs that are essential to the nonspecific immune response to inflammation because of their role in releasing histamine (vasodilator) during tissue damage or invasion. Basophils have cytoplasmic granules that contain heparin, serotonin, and histamine. If a basophil is stimulated by an antigen or by tissue injury, it will respond by releasing substances within the granules. This is part of the response seen in allergic and inflammatory reactions. Normal values of basophils are 0.5% to 1%. **Monocytes** are WBCs that function similarly to neutrophils; they circulate in the bloodstream and move into tissue, where they engulf foreign antigens and cell debris. Monocytes are the second type of WBC to arrive at the scene of an injury. They are useful in removing dead bacteria and cells in the recovery stage of acute bacterial infections. Normal values of monocytes are 2% to 6%. The **lymphocytes** are WBCs that are responsible for antibody formation, a special protein that combats foreign invaders, or antigens. They set up the antigen-antibody process, which protects the body. There are two groups of lymphocytes: B cells and T cells. The function of the B cells is to search out, identify, and bind with specific antigens. T cells, when exposed to an antigen, divide rapidly and produce large numbers of new T cells that are sensitized to that antigen. They work together with the B cells to destroy the foreign antigen. Normal values of lymphocytes are 20% to 40% (Table 7-1).

Table 7-1 *Diagnostic Blood Studies*

BLOOD TEST	NORMAL VALUES	DESCRIPTION	CLINICAL SIGNIFICANCE
CBC WITH DIFFERENTIAL			
RBC	Males: 4.7-6.1 million/mm³ Females: 4.2-5.4 million/mm³	Actual cell count	Increased in dehydration, polycythemia, at high altitudes, and with hypoxia; decreased in anemia, leukemia, and posthemorrhage
Hgb	Males:14-18 g/dL Females:12-16 g/dL		Increased in polycythemia, dehydration, chronic obstructive lung disease; decreased in anemia and after hemorrhage
Hct	Males: 42%-52% Females: 37%-47%		Increased with severe burns, shock, severe dehydration, and polycythemia; decreased with severe blood loss, leukemia, and anemia
WBC WITH DIFFERENTIAL			
WBC	5000-10,000/mm³	Actual cell count	Increased neutrophils with a number of bacterial infections, inflammatory but noninfectious diseases (collagen disorder, rheumatic fever, and pancreatitis); increased with infectious diseases (usually of bacterial origin) and with trauma, or leukemia; decreased by chemotherapy, radiation, aplastic anemia, and agranulocytosis
Neutrophils	60%-70%* 3000-7000†		Increased with burns, crushing injuries, diabetic acidosis, and infections; decreased in bone marrow failure following antineoplastic chemotherapy or radiation therapy or in agranulocytosis, dietary deficiencies, and autoimmune diseases
Eosinophils	1%-4%* 50-400†		Increased eosinophils found with allergic and parasitic disorders
Basophils	0.5%-1%* 25-100†		Increased basophils are uncommon and are found with some forms of acute leukemia
Lymphocytes	20%-40%* 1000-4000†		Increased in infectious mononucleosis, measles, certain viruses, infectious hepatitis, and lymphocytic leukemia; decreased in AIDS, lupus erythematosus, and Hodgkin's disease
Monocytes	2%-6%* 100-600†		Increased in the recovery phase of bacterial infections, chronic inflammatory conditions, and monocytic leukemia
Erythrocyte sedimentation rate (ESR)	Male: 0-15 mm/hr Female: 0-20 mm/hr	Rate at which RBCs settle out of a tube of unclotted blood in 1 hour	Increased in tissue destruction; indicates infection when results are compared with elevation in WBC count; ESR is a fairly reliable indicator of the course of disease and can therefore be used to monitor disease therapy, especially for inflammatory autoimmune diseases

*Relative values: expressed as percentage of total WBC.
†Absolute values: expressed in actual numbers × 10⁹/mm³.

Continued

Table 7-1 *Diagnostic Blood Studies—cont'd*

BLOOD TEST	NORMAL VALUES	DESCRIPTION	CLINICAL SIGNIFICANCE
WBC WITH DIFFERENTIAL—cont'd			
Reticulocyte count	0.5%-2%	Number of reticulocytes in whole blood	Increased in bone marrow hyperactivity and hemorrhage; decreased in hemolytic disease
Platelet count	150,000-400,000/mm³	Actual cell count	Increased in granulocytic leukemia; decreased in thrombocytopenia or aplastic anemia
Prothrombin time (PT)	11-12.5 seconds	Rapidity of blood clotting	Detects plasma clotting defects, screens for coagulation, and monitors warfarin (Coumadin) therapy; possible critical values greater than 20 seconds
International Normalized Ratio (INR)	0.7-1.8	The World Health Organization has recommended the PT results now include the use of the INR value; many hospitals are now reporting PT results in both absolute numbers and INR	Therapeutic INR is usually considered to be 2 to 3.5 possible critical values >3.5
Partial thromboplastin time (PTT)	60-70 seconds	Fibrin clot formation	Detects coagulation defects of the intrinsic system and deficiency of plasma clotting; the appropriate dose of heparin can be monitored by the PTT; possible critical values greater than 100 seconds
Bleeding time	1-9 minutes (Ivy method)	Amount of time for a small stab wound to stop bleeding	Prolonged in hemorrhagic disease or with coagulation factor defect
Clotting time	3-9 minutes	Amount of time for blood in a tube to clot	Prolonged with deficiency in coagulation factors or vitamin K; used to monitor anticoagulant therapy

Thrombocytes (Platelets)

Thrombocytes, or platelets, are the smallest cells in the blood. They are circular cell fragments, which do not contain nuclei. They have a life span of 5 to 9 days and number 150,000 to 400,000 per mm³ of blood (see Figure 7-1). They are produced in the red bone marrow and function in the process of hemostasis (the prevention of blood loss). They assist in clotting formation, which seals off a break in the continuity of the walls of the blood vessels (Figure 7-2).

Hemostasis

Hemostasis is a body process that arrests the flow of blood and prevents hemorrhage. Three actions take place: (1) vessel spasm, (2) platelet plug formation, and (3) clot formation. When a vessel has a tear or rupture, the smooth muscle in the walls of the vessel causes it to contract. Platelets rush to the area and attempt to seal the area, which is effective in small vessel tears. The third process, clot formation, is more detailed and occurs in larger injuries. This process can be summarized as follows (see Figure 7-2):

1. Injury
2. Hemorrhage
3. Grouping platelets
4. Thromboplastin released (reacts along with calcium ions)
5. Converts prothrombin to thrombin
6. Links with fibrinogen
7. Formation of fibrin
8. Traps RBCs and platelets
9. Forms clot

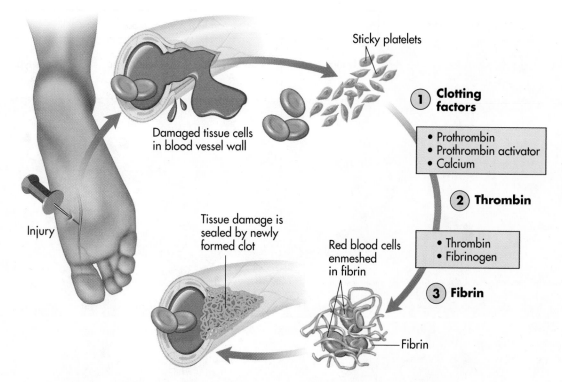

FIGURE **7-2** Blood clotting. The extremely complex clotting mechanism can be distilled into three basic steps: *1,* release of clotting factors from both injured tissue cells and sticky platelets at the injury site; *2,* formation of thrombin; and *3,* formation of fibrin and trapping of red blood cells to form a clot.

Blood Types (Groups)

A person's blood group or type is genetically determined and is inherited from his or her parents. Blood types are determined by the presence or absence of specific antigens on the outer surface of the RBCs. In certain types of blood, the antigens on the RBCs are accompanied by antibodies found in the blood plasma. Every person's blood is one of the following blood types in the ABO system of typing: type **A,** type **B,** type **AB,** or type **O.**

Suppose one has type A blood (as do 41% of Americans). The letter A stands for a certain type of antigen that is present in the plasma membrane of one's RBCs at birth. Because such a person is born with type A antigen, the body does not form antibodies to react with it. In other words, this person's blood plasma contains no anti-A antibodies; it does, however, contain anti-B antibodies. For some unknown reason, these antibodies are present naturally in type A blood plasma. The body did not form them in response to the presence of B antigen. In summary, then, in type A blood the RBCs contain type A antigen and the plasma contains anti-B antibodies.

Correspondingly, in type B blood, the RBCs contain type B antigen and the plasma contains anti-A antibodies. In type AB, as its name indicates, the RBCs contain both type A and B antigens, and the plasma

contains neither anti-A nor anti-B antibodies. The opposite is true of type O blood: Its RBCs contain neither type A nor type B antigens and the plasma contains both anti-A and anti-B antibodies.

Harmful effects or even death can result from a blood transfusion if the donor's RBCs become agglutinated by antibodies in the recipient's plasma. If the donor's RBCs do not contain any A or B antigen, they of course cannot be clumped by anti-A or anti-B antibodies. For this reason the type of blood that contains neither A nor B antigens—namely, type O blood—can be used in an emergency as donor blood without the danger of anti-A or anti-B antibodies clumping its RBCs. Type O blood has therefore been called **universal donor** blood. Similarly, blood type AB has been called the **universal recipient** blood because it contains neither anti-A nor anti-B antibodies in its plasma. Therefore it does not clump any donor's RBCs containing A or B antigens. In a normal clinical setting, however, all blood intended for transfusion is typed and crossmatched carefully to the blood of the recipient for a variety of factors. Figure 7-3 shows the results of combinations of donor and recipient blood.

Two types of reactions can occur: agglutination and hemolyzation. In agglutination the donor cells clump together because of the antibodies; this occludes arter-

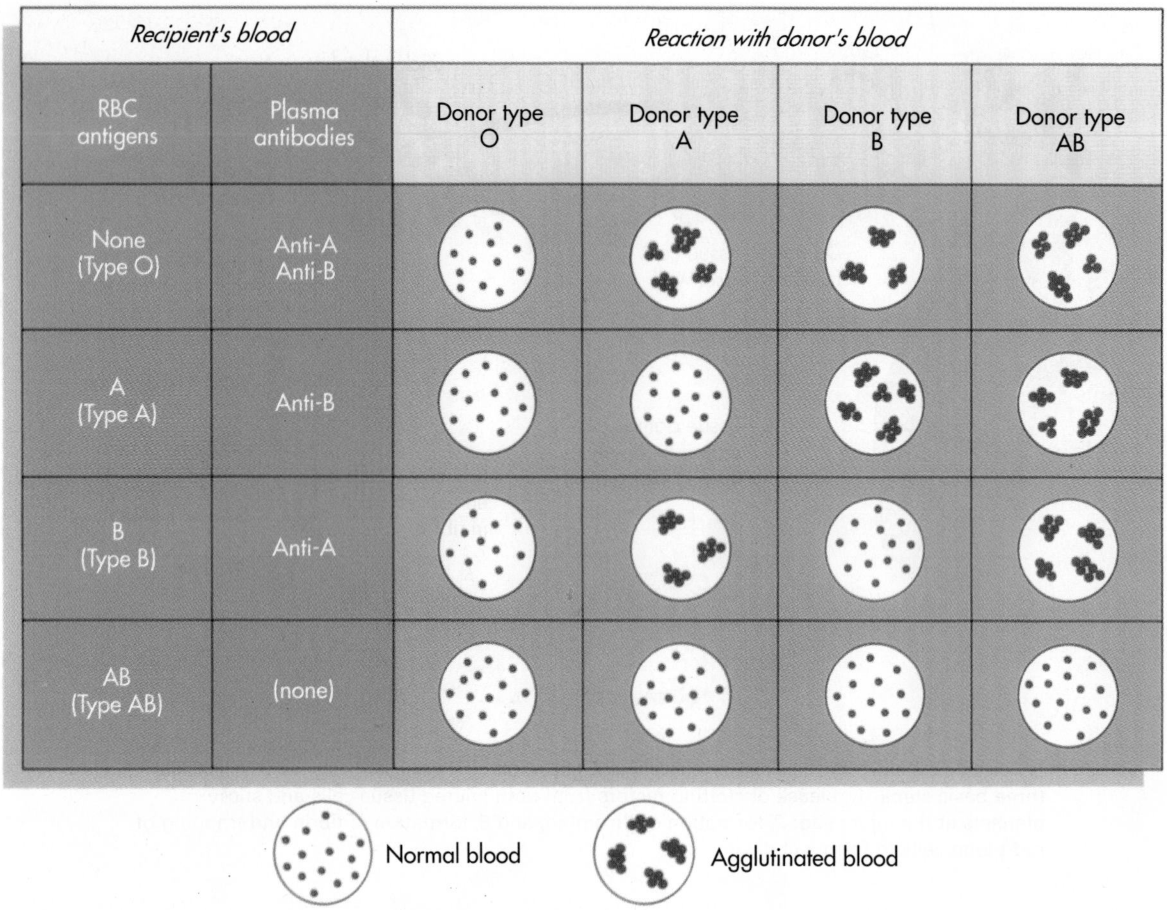

Recipient's blood		Reaction with donor's blood			
RBC antigens	Plasma antibodies	Donor type O	Donor type A	Donor type B	Donor type AB
None (Type O)	Anti-A Anti-B				
A (Type A)	Anti-B				
B (Type B)	Anti-A				
AB (Type AB)	(none)				

Normal blood   Agglutinated blood

FIGURE **7-3** Results of different combinations of donor and recipient blood. The left columns show the recipient's blood characteristics, and the top row shows the donor's blood type.

ies and can result in death. In the second process, hemolyzation, the antibodies cause the RBCs of the recipient to rupture and release their cell contents; this can also lead to death.

Rh Factor

People who have **Rh factor,** which is located on the surface of the RBCs, are said to be Rh positive; people who do not have Rh factor are said to be Rh negative. Eighty-five percent of humans have Rh factor; 15% do not. Normally, human plasma does not contain Rh antibodies; these develop in response to an individual's receiving the wrong type of blood. This occurs if an Rh-negative person receives Rh-positive blood. Within approximately 2 weeks, Rh antibodies are produced and remain in the blood. If the Rh-negative person then receives more Rh-positive blood, a severe reaction occurs because the Rh-positive antibodies react with the donor blood. It hemolyzes the red blood cells, causing them to rupture and lose their contents.

Rh incompatibility is seen most commonly in pregnancy. Fortunately, there is a means for preventing this incompatibility. The mother's blood is tested for antibodies, and if they are present, she can receive an intramuscular dose of RhoGAM—a desensitization drug. This enables her to carry the next infant without the potential complications associated with Rh incompatibility.

LYMPHATIC SYSTEM

The lymphatic system is a subdivision of the cardiovascular system. It consists of lymphatic vessels, the lymph fluid, and the lymph tissue. The system has three basic functions: (1) maintenance of fluid balance, (2) production of lymphocytes, and (3) absorption and transportation of lipids from the intestine to the blood stream.

Lymph and Lymph Vessels

Maintaining the constancy of the fluid around each body cell is possible only if numerous homeostatic mechanisms function effectively together in a controlled and integrated response to changing conditions. The circulatory system provides a key role in bringing many needed substances to cells and then removing the waste products that accumulate as a result of metabolism. This exchange of substances between blood and tissue fluid occurs in capillary beds. Many additional substances that cannot enter or return through the capillary walls, including excess fluid and protein molecules, are returned to the blood as lymph. Lymph is a specialized fluid formed in the tissue spaces and transported by way of specialized lymphatic vessels to eventually reenter the circulatory system. In addition to lymph and the lymphatic vessels, the lymphatic system includes lymph nodes and specialized lymphatic organs such as the thymus and spleen (Figure 7-4).

Lymphatic Tissue

Lymph nodes. Lymph nodes (glands) have two functions: (1) to filter impurities from the lymph (much like an oil filter in a car) and (2) to produce lymphocytes (WBCs). The body contains 500 to 600 lymph nodes. They are small bean-shaped structures, usually appearing in groups. They range from 0.04 to 1 inch (1 to 25 mm) in length. These groups are most numerous in the axilla, groin, abdomen, thorax, and cervical regions (see Figure 7-4). The structure of the lymph node makes it possible for them to perform two functions: defense and WBC production (lymphocytes).

Tonsils. The tonsils are masses of lymphoid tissue embedded in the mucous membrane of the oral cavity and the pharynx. The tonsils protect the body against invasion of foreign substances by producing lymphocytes and antibodies. They also trap bacteria and may become enlarged. The tonsils are larger in children and begin to atrophy (shrink) at about age 7.

Spleen. The spleen is a soft, roughly ovoid, highly vascularized organ located in the upper left quadrant of the abdominal cavity, just below the diaphragm (see Figure 7-4). The spleen is 5 to 6 inches (12.5 to 16 cm) long and 2 to 3 inches (5 to 7.5 cm) wide. It contains lymphatic nodules.

The spleen stores 1 pint of blood, which can be released during emergencies, such as hemorrhage, in less than 60 seconds. This large accumulation of blood gives the spleen its deep purple color. The main functions of the spleen are (1) to serve as a reservoir for blood; (2) to form lymphocytes, monocytes, and plasma cells; (3) to destroy worn-out RBCs; (4) to remove bacteria by phagocytosis (engulfing and digest-

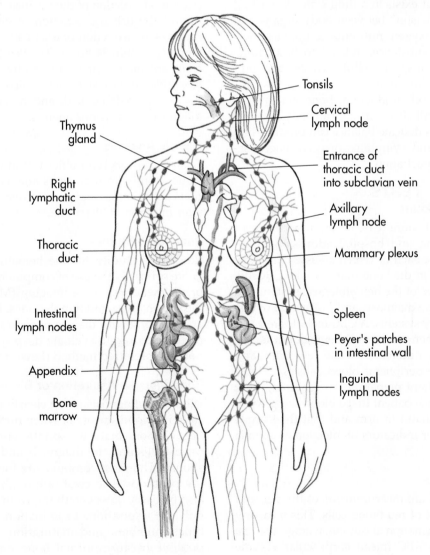

FIGURE **7-4** Principal organs of the lymphatic system.

ing); and (5) to produce RBCs before birth (the spleen is believed to produce red blood cells after birth only in cases of extreme hemolytic anemia).

Thymus. The thymus is located in the upper thorax posterior to the sternum and between the lungs in the mediastinum (see Figure 7-4). The thymus gland functions in utero (before birth) and a few months after birth to develop the immune system. The thymus is responsible for the development of the T lymphocytes of the cell-mediated immune response before they migrate to the lymph nodes and the spleen. At puberty the thymus gland atrophies and is eventually replaced with fat and connective tissue.

DISORDERS OF THE HEMATOLOGICAL AND LYMPHATIC SYSTEMS

The hematological and lymphatic systems include the blood and the organs of blood production—the bone marrow and lymphatic tissue. The blood is the only organ in the body that exists in a fluid state. As such, it functions as the "liaison" between body organs and systems, carrying oxygen, nutrients, antibodies, hormones, and other substances related to body functions. Blood also transports cellular wastes and protects the body from infection.

Disorders of blood production, bone marrow, or lymphatic tissues will affect virtually all body systems. Disturbances in this delicate balance can produce life-threatening signs and symptoms or occurrences, severe pain, and incapacitation.

DIAGNOSTIC TESTS
Complete Blood Count

The complete blood count (CBC) is an important part of routine screening and hospital admission. It involves several tests, each of which assesses the three major cells formed in the bone marrow. The CBC detects many disorders of the hematological system and provides data for the diagnosis and evaluation of disorders in other body systems. A CBC includes red and white cell counts, hematocrit and hemoglobin levels, erythrocyte indices, differential white cell count, and examination of the peripheral blood cells (see Table 7-1). No special patient preparation is required, other than explaining to the patient that a blood sample will be taken from the hand or arm and that the sample will be evaluated for indicators of infection or anemia in the body.

Erythrocyte Indices

Erythrocyte indices are measurements of the size and hemoglobin content of red blood cells. This measurement provides information about the average volume or size of a single RBC (mean corpuscular volume [MCV]). Mean corpuscular hemoglobin (MCH) is a measure of the average amount (weight) of hemoglo-

bin within an RBC. Mean corpuscular hemoglobin concentration (MCHC) is a measure of the average concentration or the percentage of hemoglobin within an RBC.

Peripheral Smear

A peripheral smear often accompanies the differential WBC count and permits examination of the size, shape, and structure of individual RBCs and platelets. This information is useful in differentiating various forms of anemias and blood dyscrasias. All three hematological cell lines (RBCs, WBCs, platelets) can be examined. When adequately prepared and examined microscopically by an experienced technologist, a smear of peripheral blood is the most informative of all hematological tests.

Schilling Test and Megaloblastic Anemia Profile

The Schilling test is a laboratory blood test for diagnosing pernicious anemia. The test measures the absorption of radioactive vitamin B_{12}, before and after parenteral injection of the intrinsic factor, by examination of the urinary excretion of vitamin B_{12}. Normal findings are excretion of 8% to 40% of radioactive vitamin B_{12} within 24 hours. The Schilling test for pernicious anemia is being replaced by a serum test called *megaloblastic anemia profile*, which measures vitamin B_{12}, methylmalonic acid, and homocystine levels for diagnosing pernicious anemia.

Gastric Analysis

Gastric analysis is an older test in determining pernicious anemia. In pernicious anemia the gastric secretions are minimal and the pH remains elevated, even after injection of histamine.

Radiologic Studies

Radiologic studies for the hematological system involve primarily the use of computed tomography (CT) or magnetic resonance imaging (MRI) for evaluating the spleen, liver, and lymph nodes. In the past, lymphangiography with the use of contrast dye was a common procedure to evaluate deep lymph nodes. CT is now the preferred method (Lewis et al, 2004).

Bone Marrow Aspiration or Biopsy

When the diagnosis is not clearly established by peripheral blood smears or when further information is needed, bone marrow aspiration or biopsy is specific for establishing the diagnosis and for treatment response. The most common site for this procedure is the posterior iliac crest, although the sternum can also be used; however, the sternum is generally used only for aspiration. Examination is made of cells: types, numbers, and maturation. The procedure is possible because normal bone marrow is soft and semifluid and can therefore be removed by aspiration through a needle. Bone marrow aspiration is most commonly performed in people with marked anemia, neutropenia (decreased number of WBCs), acute leukemia, and thrombocytopenia (decreased number of platelets). Although complications of bone marrow aspiration are minimal, there is a possibility of penetrating the bone and underlying structures. This hazard is greatest in aspiration procedure involving the sternum.

Lymphangiography

Lymphangiography is a radiologic examination used to detect metastatic involvement of the lymph nodes. Contrast medium is injected into a lymphatic vessel of the foot or hand, followed by radiological visualization of the lymphatic system. This examination is being replaced by CT scanning.

DISORDERS ASSOCIATED WITH ERYTHROCYTES

ANEMIA

Anemia is a disorder characterized by RBC and hemoglobin and hematocrit levels below normal range; anemias also exhibit increased RBC destruction (hemolytic anemia). Anemia causes delivery of insufficient amounts of oxygen to tissues and cells. Erythrocytes are classified according to size, shape, and color. Hemoglobin content is expressed as normochromic or hypochromic anemia, whereas RBC size is usually expressed as macrocytic, microcytic, or normocytic.

Etiology/Pathophysiology

Anemia can be caused by many factors. Anemias may be divided into those that are the result of blood loss (hemorrhage), impaired production of RBCs (bone marrow depression), increased destruction of RBCs (hemolysis), or nutritional deficiencies (long-term iron deficiency). Hemorrhage or blood loss accounts for temporary anemia, whereas nutritional deficit can be the cause of long-term iron-deficiency anemia. Marrow failure is linked to a disease process, toxic exposure, tumor, or unknown causes. A decrease in RBC production or destruction results in a lower number of circulating red blood cells. Bone marrow hematopoietic function manifests the inability to produce the needed quantity.

Loss of the oxygen-carrying element in the blood results in a supply/demand imbalance in vital organs. Peripheral circulation compensates by shunting blood to vital organs, thus causing a hypoxic status in other areas of the body. Rapid hematopoietic effort causes blood cell irregularities (immature RBCs) and inability to produce RBCs, with a resultant decrease of RBC count.

Clinical Manifestations

Most adults do not experience symptoms until the Hgb level is less than 8 g/dL. The older adult, however, may show symptoms with an Hgb concentration less than 10 g/dL. Although each type of anemia has specific signs and symptoms, some are typical of all anemias. These signs and symptoms arise from decreased oxygen-carrying capacity. The following are typical:

Anorexia
Cardiac dilation
Disorientation
Dizziness
Dyspepsia
Dyspnea
Exertional dyspnea
Fatigue
Headache
Insomnia
Pallor (mucous membranes and skin)
Palpitation
Shortness of breath
Systolic murmur
Tachycardia
Vertigo

In older adult patients with impaired cardiopulmonary reserves, be alert to complaints of chest pain, dyspnea on exertion, palpitations, and dizziness.

Assessment

Collection of **subjective data** commonly includes expressions of weakness, dyspnea, fatigue, and vertigo. Anorexia and dyspepsia may accompany headache and insomnia, but the patient generally does not link these complaints to the condition unless questioning leads to this conclusion.

Collection of **objective data** includes observing signs of bleeding or shock (hypovolemic anemia). Laboratory values will show a low RBC count and hematocrit and hemoglobin levels. Pallor of skin and mucous membranes is present, and cardiac symptoms are noted and related to anemia. If the anemia has been a long-term condition, the patient may have ulcerations of the extremities.

Diagnostic Tests

Blood studies will show RBC count and hemoglobin and hematocrit levels to be below normal. Serum iron, total iron-binding capacity, and serum ferritin levels will be below normal. Reticulocyte count is increased because of immaturity of RBCs. A bone marrow study will show a deviation from normal findings. Peripheral blood smears enable identification of abnormalities of shape and color of cells. A megaloblastic anemia profile will reveal decreased levels of vitamin B_{12}.

Medical Management

Intervention depends on the cause. Correction of the disease process may correct or lessen the anemic condition. Transfusion is appropriate for blood loss, as is replacement of iron and vitamin B_{12} if these are deficient. Treatment is often specific to the particular anemia. (See Cultural and Ethnic Considerations for concerns related to blood transfusions.)

Nursing Interventions and Patient Teaching

Nursing diagnoses and interventions for the patient with anemia include but are not limited to the following:

NURSING DIAGNOSES	NURSING INTERVENTIONS
Ineffective tissue perfusion (cardiovascular), related to reduction of cellular components necessary for delivery of oxygen to the cells	Monitor changes in vital signs and in mental alertness. Monitor cardiac rhythms. Monitor Hgb, hematocrit (Hct), and RBCs. Assess baseline arterial blood gases (ABGs) and electrolytes. Note presence/degree of dyspnea, cyanosis, hemoptysis.
Impaired gas exchange, related to RBC, hemoglobin, and hematocrit deficit	Evaluate ability to manage activities of daily living (ADLs), related to O₂ decrease. Assess activity response, dyspnea, and heart rate. Observe for cyanosis, hypoxia, and hypercapnia. Maintain bed rest as necessary and provide range-of-motion (ROM) exercise. Monitor oxygen saturations frequently per pulse oximetry. Administer oxygen as ordered. Explain activity-oxygen deficit relationship.
Activity intolerance, related to O₂ deficit; secondary to decreased hemoglobin and hematocrit	Plan care to provide optimum rest. Assist in identifying factors causing intolerance. Assess ability to perform ADLs, ambulation, and exercise. Assess potential for injury caused by mobility impairment. Teach performing at own rate of ability, to reduce energy expenditure. Monitor hemoglobin and hematocrit levels.

Considerations for education will be tailored to the individual conditions and needs.

Hypovolemic Anemia (Blood Loss Anemia)

Etiology/pathophysiology. RBC and other component deficiencies caused by an abnormally low circulating blood volume from hemorrhage is classified as secondary anemia. Blood loss of 1000 mL or more in an adult can be severe. Such a loss is usually related to internal or external

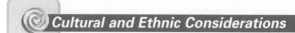

Cultural and Ethnic Considerations

Jehovah's Witness Opposition to Blood Transfusion

There are so many implications for the nurse who provides culturally appropriate nursing interventions to a Jehovah's Witness.

The paramount concern for the nurse is that Jehovah's Witnesses are opposed to homologous blood transfusion (blood obtained from a blood bank or through donations). Jehovah's Witnesses believe that if they receive blood products, there are eternal consequences.

However, many, but not all, Jehovah's Witnesses will submit to certain types of autologous blood transfusions (autotransfusion).

One type of autologous transfusion that might be acceptable is blood retrieved through induced hemodilution at the start of surgery (blood that is directed to storage bags outside the patient's body).

In addition, some Jehovah's Witnesses will permit the use of certain blood volume expanders. Many Jehovah's Witnesses carry a card with the types of blood volume expanders permitted. The nurse should ask the patient for this card, or if the patient is unconscious, examine the patient's personal belongings to find this extremely important card.

The consensus of the Supreme Court of the United States has been that a person of adult majority age has the right to refuse treatment but not to withhold treatment from a minor child.

hemorrhage caused by a surgical procedure, GI bleeding, menorrhagia, trauma, or severe burns.

Loss of blood decreases the amount of circulating fluid and hemoglobin and decreases the amount of oxygen carried to the tissues of the body. The tissues must have oxygen to survive. The average adult has an approximate total blood volume of 6000 mL (6 liters; 12 pints) and can tolerate a loss of up to 500 mL. If the loss approaches 1000 mL, acute complications, such as hypovolemic shock, may occur. The rapidity of blood loss is related to the severity and number of signs and symptoms. The sudden reduction in the total blood volume can lead to hypovolemic shock. RBC count and the hematocrit level drop to half the normal range.

Clinical manifestations. Signs and symptoms include those associated with hypovolemia and hypoxemia: weakness; stupor; irritability; and pale, cool, moist skin. Vital signs demonstrate hypotension, tachycardia, and hypothermia. It is essential to understand that the clinical signs and symptoms the patient is experiencing are more important than the laboratory values. The nurse should be alert to the patient's expression of pain. Internal hemorrhage may cause pain because of tissue distention, organ displacement, and nerve compression. Pain may be localized or referred. Decreased RBC, hemoglobin, and hematocrit levels may not be evident until several days after severe blood loss has occurred. The severity of the patient's signs and symptoms correlates with the severity of the blood loss.

Assessment. Collection of **subjective data** commonly includes complaints of thirst, weakness, irritability, and restlessness.

Collection of **objective data** includes decreased blood pressure; rapid, weak, thready pulse; and rapid respirations. Cold, clammy skin with pallor is noted. Oliguria is often evident. Mental disorientation as well as physical collapse with prostration can occur.

Diagnostic tests. When blood volume loss is sudden, plasma volume has not yet had a chance to increase, the loss of RBCs is not reflected in laboratory data, and values may seem normal or high for 2 to 3 days. However, once the plasma is replaced, the RBC mass is less concentrated. At this time, RBC, hemoglobin, and hematocrit levels are severely decreased, often to half the normal values.

Medical management. In the case of massive hemorrhage, measures are taken to control the bleeding, treat for shock, and replace the volume of circulating fluid with blood transfusion (packed RBCs), plasma, dextran (volume expander), or other IV therapy. Oxygen therapy is ordered to restore decreased available oxygen caused by decreased hemoglobin in the blood. The patient may also need supplemental iron because the availability of iron affects the marrow production of erythrocytes. Oral or parenteral iron preparations are often administered.

Nursing interventions and patient teaching. The nurse will monitor blood and fluid restoration and identify blood loss sites to control the bleeding. Patients should be kept flat and warm. Vital signs should be taken at frequent intervals. Care should be taken to prevent injury to a restless or disoriented patient. Intake and output (I&O) are measured, with careful monitoring of urine output for oliguria caused by decreased renal perfusion.

If the cause of the hemorrhage is a chronic problem, the patient should be taught to monitor bleeding amounts, occasion, and associated factors and to report to the physician immediately for treatment.

Prognosis. Without treatment, death will result. With aggressive treatment, the prognosis is favorable.

Pernicious Anemia

Etiology/pathophysiology. A pernicious disease is one that is capable of causing great injury, destruction, or death. Without treatment, pernicious anemia would be fatal. This type of anemia is the result of a metabolic defect: the absence of a glycoprotein intrinsic factor secreted by the gastric mucosa. Intrinsic secretion fails because of gastric mucosal atrophy. Pernicious anemia is an autoimmune disease; the gastric atrophy of pernicious anemia probably results from destruction of the parietal cells. It is a progressive, megaloblastic, macrocytic anemia primarily affecting older adults. The intrinsic factor is essential for absorption of vitamin B_{12} (cyanocobalamin).

Because the intrinsic factor is not available to combine with vitamin B_{12}, transport of this necessary vitamin to the ileum is prevented (vitamin B_{12} is normally absorbed in the distal ileum). Deficiency of the vitamin affects growth and maturity of all body cells. There is deficiency in the maturation of RBCs in the marrow. The erythrocyte membrane becomes fragile and ruptures easily. This vitamin is related to nerve myelination and, if it is absent, progressive demyelination and degeneration of nerves and white matter occur.

Clinical manifestations. Extreme weakness is noted with dyspnea, fever, and hypoxia. As the condition progresses, weight loss is apparent, as is slight icterus (jaundice) with pallor. The skin color may appear a pale lemon-yellow because of the excessive destruction of the RBCs, which causes the bile pigments to increase in the blood serum. Edema of the legs occurs, as do intermittent constipation and diarrhea.

Assessment. Collection of **subjective data** includes noting the patient's complaints of palpitations, nausea, flatulence, and indigestion. There is soreness and burning of the tongue. Weakness and difficulty swallowing (dysphagia) may occur. Neurological symptoms may develop, including tingling of the hands and feet and loss of the sense of body position (impaired proprioception).

Collection of **objective data** includes observation of a smooth and erythematous tongue, with infection about the teeth and gums. Cerebral signs include mental disorientation, personality changes, and behavior problems. Severe neurological impairments can result, including partial or total paralysis that results from destruction of the nerve fibers of the spinal cord.

Diagnostic tests. The Schilling test shows malabsorption of vitamin B_{12}. This test is being replaced by the serum megaloblastic anemia profile, which will reveal decreased serum levels of vitamin B_{12}. Bone marrow aspiration reveals abnormal RBC development.

The erythrocytes appear large (macrocytic) and have abnormal shapes; serum cyanocobalamin (B_{12}) levels will be reduced. A gastric analysis may be done to determine the cause of the vitamin B_{12} deficiency. Pernicious anemia is caused by an absence of intrinsic factor, from either gastric mucosal atrophy or autoimmune destruction of parietal cells of the stomach. This results in a decrease of hydrochloric acid secretion by the stomach. An acidic environment in the stomach is required for the secretion of intrinsic factor.

Medical management. Cyanocobalamin (vitamin B_{12}) injections, folic acid supplement, and iron replacement are ordered. If the anemia is severe, the patient may be transfused with packed red blood cells. The standard treatment includes initiating vitamin B_{12} replacement therapy; without it, these individuals will die in 1 to 3 years. Treatment is 1000 units of vitamin B_{12} administered intramuscularly daily for 2 weeks, then weekly for 1 month, and finally monthly for life. An intranasal form of cyanocobalamin (Nascobal) is now available. It is a nasal gel that is self-administered once weekly. The patient's blood values should return to normal within 2 months of B_{12} therapy. A CBC will be necessary every 3 to 6 months to monitor the long-term success of treatment.

Nursing interventions and patient teaching. The nursing interventions will depend to some extent on the stage of the disease. A symptomatic approach is appropriate. When the patient is confined to the hospital, vital signs should be checked every 4 hours. Special mouth care should be performed several times daily. The diet should be high in protein, vitamins, and minerals.

Anemic patients are especially sensitive to cold, so additional lightweight, warm blankets may be needed. Interventions should conserve energy and prevent injury.

Nursing diagnoses and interventions for the patient with pernicious anemia include but are not limited to the following:

NURSING DIAGNOSES	NURSING INTERVENTIONS
Risk for injury, related to sensory and motor losses, alteration in mental status	Use bed rest, with side rails up as needed, to prevent patient fatigue and falls caused by weakness. Assist with ambulation to avoid falls. Use bed cradle or footboard to prevent pressure on lower extremities. Apply heat with extreme caution to avoid burning the skin. If heat therapy is required, the patient's skin must be evaluated at frequent intervals to detect erythema. Support patient with patience and reassurance to reduce irritability and depression.
Imbalanced nutrition: less than body requirements, related to sore mouth and tongue, diarrhea, and constipation	Administer vitamin B_{12} and other medications prescribed to promote production of erythrocytes. Encourage diet high in vitamins, iron, and protein to promote production of healthy erythrocytes. Provide meticulous and frequent oral hygiene to promote improved appetite and prevent infection. Offer small, frequent feedings to prevent digestive overload. Observe for diarrhea or constipation and treat as prescribed to avoid fluid and electrolyte imbalance and discomfort.

Patient knowledge in regard to the disease process and the importance of following lifetime therapy of vitamin B_{12} is essential if the disease is to be controlled. Discuss the importance of a diet high in vitamin B_{12}. Activity adjustment when signs and symptoms are present may lessen the patient's stress. The need for assistance with ADLs and for frequent rest periods should be impressed on the patient and significant people involved in the care.

Prognosis. This condition, if untreated, can be considered terminal in 1 to 3 years. With treatment the patient may be asymptomatic. Because the potential for gastric carcinoma is increased in pernicious anemia, the patient should have frequent and careful evaluation for this problem.

Aplastic Anemia

Etiology/pathophysiology. Aplastic anemia or aplasia (a hematological term for a failure of the normal process of cell generation and development) has two etiologic classifications: **congenital** and **acquired.** Congenital origin is caused by chromosomal alterations. Approximately 30% of aplastic anemias that appear in childhood are inherited. Acquired aplastic anemia is directly related to exposure to viral invasion, medications, chemicals (e.g., benzene, insecticides, arsenic, alcohol), radiation, or chemotherapy, in which the hematopoietic tissue is replaced by fatty marrow, causing a defect in RBC production. The causes of 70% of acquired cases of aplastic anemia are idiopathic (cause unknown). It is believed that aplastic anemia is probably an immune-mediated disease.

Depression of erythrocyte production results in lowered hemoglobin and RBCs. Leukopenia and thrombocytopenia may develop. People with aplastic anemia are usually pancytopenic; that is, all three major blood elements (red cells, white cells, and platelets) from the bone marrow are reduced or absent. The incidence of aplastic anemia is low, affecting approximately 4 of every 1 million people.

Clinical manifestations. Repeated infections with high fevers may occur, along with fatigue, weakness, general malaise, dyspnea, and palpitations. Mortality is high from complications of infection and hemorrhage. Bleeding tendencies are reported: petechiae, ecchymoses, bleeding gums, and epistaxis, as well as GI and genitourinary system bleeding.

Assessment. Collection of **subjective data** includes a history of exposure to chemicals such as insecticides and drugs in addition to a family history of aplastic anemia. The patient is questioned about the ability to carry out ADLs without fatigue.

Collection of **objective data** includes monitoring the patient for pallor, signs of infection, and bleeding tendencies. Also, dyspnea and tachycardia may be noted.

Diagnostic tests. A bone marrow study (aspiration biopsy) shows hypoplastic or aplastic fatty deposits, a decrease in cellular elements, and depressed hematopoietic activity. The diagnostic findings are especially important in aplastic anemia because the marrow is hypocellular, with increased yellow marrow (fat content), a finding termed "dry tap." Peripheral blood smears show that blood cells may be normocytic and normochromic.

Medical management. The cause of aplastic anemia must be identified promptly and removed or discontinued. Bone marrow suppression is expected with certain antineoplastic medications or radiation therapy, and laboratory values should be monitored frequently to maintain control.

Blood transfusions are avoided if possible, to prevent iron overloading and the development of antibodies to tissue antigens. Platelet transfusions that are human lymphocyte antigen (HLA) matched are used to treat serious bleeding in a thrombocytopenic patient. Cautious use of blood transfusion is necessary to minimize the risk of rejection for a bone marrow transplant candidate.

A splenectomy may be required in patients with hypersplenism when that is the cause of destruction of normal platelets. Steroids and androgens are sometimes used to stimulate the bone marrow. Immunosuppressive therapy with antithymocyte globulin and cyclosporine has become an important therapy for patients who are not candidates for bone marrow transplantation. Bone marrow transplantation is the treatment of choice in patients younger than the age of 50 who have a compatible donor. Granulocyte-macrophage colony-stimulating factor (GM-CSF) is used as biologic response modifier treatment for aplastic anemia.

Bone marrow transplant. A bone marrow transplant is indicated in certain conditions and diseases such as immunodeficient states, cancer, leukemia, and recurrent aplastic anemia. A matched donor and recipient are essential to avoid rejection or complications. Specimens from twins, siblings, or self (autologous) while in remission are preferred.

After emotional and physical preparation of the patient, blood studies are performed to set baselines and assess the patient's status. A pathogen-free environment is established, with the immunocompromised patient placed on reverse isolation (neutropenic precautions), with monitoring for fever or infection. The medication therapy used in this preparation may include immunosuppressants, antibiotics, and antianxiety agents.

Bone marrow transplants are used increasingly in hematological malignancies following large doses of chemotherapy or radiation therapy. The amount of chemotherapy or radiation that can ordinarily be administered is limited because of its toxicity to the bone marrow. By transplanting bone marrow after these therapeutic modes, much larger therapeutic doses can be administered.

Bone marrow is obtained by multiple marrow aspirations under general or spinal anesthesia, usually yielding 500 to 800 mL of marrow. The marrow is cryopreserved (frozen) until it is used. Shortly after chemotherapy (with or without radiation therapy) is completed, the patient receives the donated marrow through an intravenous catheter. This infusion of marrow is called the **rescue process.** The marrow travels through the bloodstream to the bone marrow, where it begins to manufacture new leukocytes, erythrocytes, and thrombocytes. The infused marrow repopulates the marrow of the patient after several weeks. There is great risk of toxicity to the patient, including infections, marrow rejection, and graft-versus-host disease. Medications supporting graft acceptance include cyclosporine (immunosuppressant) and chemotherapy (to prevent graft-versus-host complications).

Splenectomy. Surgical excision of the spleen may be performed to treat blood dyscrasias with incidence of splenomegaly, to treat trauma to the spleen, or to remove a diseased spleen. Preoperative assessment includes cardiovascular observation, respiratory function determination, and GI evaluation. Postoperatively, these observations are compared with the patient's baseline evaluations, and the patient is observed for any infection or inflammation. Potential complications include infection, hemorrhage, shock, and paralytic ileus. Parenteral therapy is maintained. Nasogastric (NG) suction is used if a paralytic ileus develops. Management of the patient's postoperative pain is addressed. Movement and positioning to prevent infection or postoperative pneumonia are also maintained.

Nursing interventions and patient teaching. Proper observation and care after bone marrow study are essential. Patients with aplastic anemia are highly susceptible to infection, and thus nursing interventions should be directed toward prevention. Strict aseptic techniques must be adhered to for dressing changes and IV site care. Meticulous care to prevent impaired skin and mucous membrane integrity includes avoiding intramuscular injections and avoiding administration of rectal medications or rectal temperatures. Use of protective devices, such as an eggcrate mattress, is indicated. In the presence of thrombocytopenia, the nurse should observe carefully for any signs of bleeding and prevent even the slightest trauma. The patient's urine and stool should also be monitored for occult or gross blood.

Nursing diagnoses and interventions for the patient with aplastic anemia include but are not limited to the following.

NURSING DIAGNOSES	NURSING INTERVENTIONS
Activity intolerance, related to inadequate tissue oxygenation	For hypoxia: Place the patient in a sitting position; observe respiration rate, pulse, and dyspnea; observe skin color and temperature; assist with care; plan rest periods; administer oxygen as needed; monitor laboratory values to improve gas exchange. Monitor pulse oximetry levels carefully. Assist with ADLs as necessary. Encourage patient to engage in activities on a progressive basis as fatigue decreases in response to therapy. Help patient explore feelings associated with fatigue.
Risk for infection, related to increased susceptibility	Maintain reverse isolation to avoid exposure to pathogen. Observe for increase in temperature, pulse, and respirations as signs of infection. Observe the patient for "sniffles," sore throat, anorexia, and pain on urination. Administer antibiotics as ordered to combat specific pathogens. Encourage mobility, turning, coughing, deep breathing, and increased fluids to reduce susceptibility to infection.

 Safety Considerations

Aplastic Anemia

- Prevent infection.
  - a. Use good handwashing technique.
  - b. Avoid contact with those who have infection.
  - c. Avoid sharing eating utensils and bath linens.
  - d. Take a bath or shower every day (or every other day if skin is dry); keep perineal area clean.
  - e. Use good oral hygiene.
  - f. Eliminate intake of raw meats, fruits, or vegetables.
  - g. Report signs of infection immediately to physician.
- Prevent hemorrhage.
  - a. Observe for signs such as blood in urine, stool, and petechiae, and report these to physician.
  - b. Use a soft toothbrush or swab for mouth care.
  - c. Keep mouth clean and free of debris.
  - d. Avoid enemas or other rectal insertions.
  - e. Avoid picking or blowing the nose forcefully.
  - f. Avoid trauma, falls, bumps, and cuts; avoid contact sports.
  - g. Avoid use of aspirin or aspirin preparations (anticoagulant effect).
  - h. Use an electric razor.
  - i. Use adequate lubrication and gentleness during sexual intercourse.
  - j. Avoid intramuscular injections.
- Prevent fatigue.
  - a. Take frequent rest periods between ADLs and activity.
  - b. Avoid excessive workload or heavy lifting, and ask for assistance with strenuous activity.
  - c. Increase time necessary for routine care.
  - d. Decrease activity if shortness of breath, dizziness, or sensation of heaviness in extremities occurs.
  - e. Report signs of increased fatigue.

Everyone with aplastic anemia needs to know how to protect themselves from excessive bleeding. Help the patient maintain a balance between rest and activity. Discuss with the patient how to avoid infection, especially of the respiratory or urinary tract. (Safety Considerations box.)

Prognosis. The prognosis of untreated aplastic anemia is poor (approximately 75% fatal). However, advances in medical management have improved outcomes significantly in aggressively treated patients. The object of care is to produce remission and prolong survival.

Iron Deficiency Anemia

Etiology/pathophysiology. Iron deficiency anemia is a condition in which the RBCs contain decreased levels of hemoglobin.

The most common cause of iron deficiency anemia is excessive iron loss. In adults the most common source is chronic intestinal or uterine bleeding; how-

ever, iron deficiency anemia can also be caused by bleeding from gastric or duodenal ulcers, esophageal varices, hiatal hernias, colonic diverticula, and tumors. The major sources of chronic blood loss are from the GI and genitourinary (GU) systems (Box 7-1).

GI bleeding is often not apparent and therefore may exist for a considerable time before the problem is identified. Loss of 50 to 75 mL of blood from the upper GI tract is required for stools to appear as black or melenic. The color results from the iron in the RBCs. Menstrual blood losses and blood losses related to pregnancy are common causes of iron deficiency anemia in young adult women. Rarely, excessive losses occur through microhemorrhages into lung tissue or from intestinal parasites. Even without excessive blood loss, iron deficiency anemia can also result when the body's demand for iron exceeds its absorption, which commonly occurs in infants, young adolescents, and pregnant women. Less commonly, iron deficiency anemia results from malabsorption of iron caused by diseases such as

Box 7-1 *Causes of Iron Deficiency Anemia*

- Iron deficiency may develop from inadequate dietary intake, malabsorption, blood loss, or hemolysis (breakdown of red blood cells).
- Daily iron intake from food and dietary supplements is adequate to meet the needs of men and older women, but, it may be inadequate for those individuals who have higher iron needs (e.g., menstruating or pregnant women).
- Malabsorption of iron may occur after certain types of gastrointestinal (GI) surgery and in malabsorption syndromes. Iron absorption occurs in the duodenum. Malabsorption of iron may involve disease of the duodenum in which absorption surface is altered or destroyed.
- Blood loss is a major cause of iron deficiency in adults. The major sources of chronic blood loss are from the GI and genitourinary (GU) systems. Common causes of GI blood loss are peptic ulcers, gastritis, esophagitis, diverticulitis, hemorrhoids, and neoplasms. The average monthly menstrual blood loss is about 45 mL and causes the loss of 22 mg of iron.

celiac disease and sprue. Subtotal gastrectomy may lead to iron deficiency caused by **achlorhydria** (loss of hydrochloric acid), occult bleeding, and decreased iron in postgastrectomy diets. Deficiency caused by poor dietary intake is rare in middle-age adults.

Approximately 1 mg of every 10 to 20 mg of iron ingested is absorbed in the duodenum; 5% to 10% of ingested iron is absorbed. This amount of dietary iron is adequate to meet the needs of men and older women, but it may be inadequate for those individuals who have higher iron needs (e.g., children, pregnant and lactating women).

Clinical manifestations. The chief symptoms of iron deficiency anemia are pallor, which is the most common finding, and glossitis (inflammation of the tongue), the second most common. Fatigue, weakness, and shortness of breath also often occur. Signs and symptoms typical of angina and heart failure may also occur.

Assessment. Collection of **subjective data** includes noting that peculiar to iron deficiency anemia are such GI symptoms as glossitis (manifested by inflammation and soreness of the tongue) and **pagophagia** (the desire to eat ice, clays, or starches). The patient may complain of headache, paresthesia, and a burning sensation of the tongue, all of which are caused by lack of iron in the tissues.

Collection of **objective data** includes noting the signs, including pallor and tachycardia. Fingernails may be fragile and may assume the shape of the head of a spoon with a central depression and raised borders. Mucous membranes of the mouth may be inflamed (stomatitis), and lips may be erythemic with cracking at the angles.

Diagnostic tests. The peripheral blood counts show that RBC and hemoglobin levels and the hematocrit are decreased; serum iron levels are low.

Medical management. Iron salts such as ferrous sulfate are administered. The hematocrit level should rise 5% to 15% in 3 weeks and the hemoglobin level to 2 to 5 g/dL. For the body to incorporate 100 mg of iron per day, 900 mg should be administered daily. Iron is administered orally or by injection. Ascorbic acid has been shown to enhance iron absorption. Food sources of iron include meat, fish, poultry, eggs, green leafy vegetables, whole grains, and dried beans. See Box 7-2 for food sources of these nutrients.

Box 7-2 *Food Sources of Iron, Folic Acid, Vitamin B₁₂, Amino Acids, Vitamin C (Nutrients Needed for Erythropoiesis)*

IRON

Organ meats: liver, kidney, heart, and tongue
Muscle meats, especially dark meat from poultry
Eggs
Shellfish
Whole-grain breads and cereals
Iron-enriched or iron-fortified breads and cereal
Dark green vegetables: spinach, Swiss chard, kale, greens (dandelion, beet, and turnip)
Dried fruits: apricots, dates, figs, prunes, and raisins
Legumes and nuts

FOLIC ACID

Green leafy vegetables
Asparagus, broccoli
Organ meats: liver
Meat
Whole-grain breads and cereals
Enriched and fortified breads and cereals
Fish
Legumes

VITAMIN B₁₂

Organ meats: liver and kidney
Muscle meats
Milk and cheese
Eggs

AMINO ACIDS

Eggs
Meat
Milk and milk products (cheese, ice cream)
Poultry
Fish
Legumes
Nuts

VITAMIN C

Citrus fruits
Leafy green vegetables
Strawberries
Cantaloupe

When the patient cannot tolerate oral preparations of iron, parenteral iron therapy is used. The Z-track method of giving iron dextran (DexFerrum) intramuscularly is preferable, to prevent skin staining. Iron sucrose (Venofer) is an intravenous drug used for treatment of iron-deficiency anemia.

Nursing interventions and patient teaching. Because the treatment course is directed toward diagnosis and alleviating the cause, the patient interview is important. Medication therapy for iron replacement is initiated as ordered. Assist to plan for rest periods when fatigue is present.

Education about nutritional needs relative to the condition may prevent this anemia. Foods high in iron include organ meats, white beans, leafy vegetables, raisins, molasses, dried fruit, and egg yolk (see Box 7-2).

Explanation of the side effects of iron therapy is essential to alleviate distress and to extend the therapy for the necessary time (Health Promotion Considerations box). Reporting signs and symptoms to the physician requires knowledge of those that are significant. Diarrhea or nausea is significant, but black, tarry stools are not (these are to be expected with iron therapy).

Prognosis. The prognosis is usually good with correction of the underlying cause and compliance with the medical treatment.

Sickle Cell Anemia

Etiology/pathophysiology. Sickle cell anemia is the most common genetic disorder in the United States. Sickle cell anemia occurs predominantly in the African-American population. A sickle cell is an abnormal, crescent-shaped RBC containing hemoglobin S (Hg-S)—a defective hemoglobin molecule. This anemia is a severe, chronic, incurable condition that occurs in people **homozygous** (having two identical genes inherited from each parent for a given hereditary characteristic) for Hg-S. Sickle cell crisis is an episode of acute "sickling" of erythrocytes, which causes occlusion and ischemia in distal blood vessels. Sickling indicates a clumping or aggregation of these misshapen RBCs, which lodge in small vessels. Sickle cell trait is the **heterozygous** (having two different genes) form of sickle cell anemia whereby the individual has both Hg-S and hemoglobin A (Hg-A) in the RBCs. Signs and symptoms do not occur with this trait. However, the genetic implication is notable. Approximately 1 of every 10 African-Americans has sickle cell trait, and approximately 1 of every 500 has sickle cell anemia. Tissue hypoxia and ischemia occur, causing pain and edema as a result of inflammation. Destruction of fragile RBCs thus inhibits the oxygen-carrying function.

Clinical manifestations. Usually the patient is asymptomatic for the first 10 to 12 weeks of age, at which time most of the fetal hemoglobin (Hbf) has been replaced by Hbs. However, periods of crisis then occur, accelerating the signs and symptoms. Many

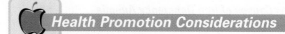

Health Promotion Considerations

Iron Administration

- Iron preparations supplement iron stores.
- Dosages are determined by the elemental iron content of the preparation. Iron supplements may be contraindicated in peptic ulcer disease.
- Side effects include GI upset (nausea, vomiting), constipation or diarrhea, and green to black stools. Elixir may stain teeth.
- Iron is absorbed best from the duodenum and proximal jejunum. Therefore enteric-coated or sustained-release capsules, which release iron farther down in the GI tract, are counterproductive and expensive.
- If side effects develop, the dose and type of iron supplement may be adjusted. Some individuals cannot tolerate ferrous sulfate because of the effects of the sulfate base. However, ferrous gluconate may be an acceptable substitute.
- Iron is best absorbed in an acidic environment. For this reason, to avoid binding the iron with food, iron should be taken about an hour before meals, when the duodenal mucosa is most acidic. Taking iron with vitamin C (ascorbic acid) or orange juice, which contains ascorbic acid, also enhances iron absorption. Gastric side effects, however, may necessitate ingesting iron with meals.
- Do not administer with antacids.
- If a dose is missed, continue with schedule; do not double a dose.
- Iron may interfere with absorption of oral tetracycline antibiotics. Do not take within 2 hours of each other.
- Dilute liquid iron preparations in juice or water, and administer with a straw to avoid staining teeth.
- Check for constipation or diarrhea. Record color (iron turns stools green to black) and amount of stool.
- Iron is toxic, and caution must be taken to store iron preparations out of a child's reach.

people with sickle cell anemia are in reasonably good health the majority of the time. The typical patient is anemic but asymptomatic except during painful episodes. There are definite physical and probable emotional factors (stress) that precipitate a painful episode. Physical factors include events that cause dehydration or change the oxygen tension in the body, such as infection, overexertion, weather changes (cold), ingestion of alcohol, and smoking. Loss of appetite and irritability with weakness follow minor infections. Abdominal enlargement with pooling of blood in the liver, spleen, and other organs may accompany jaundice. Joint and back pain are noted, as is edema of the extremities. Complications include multisystem failure, infarctions, hemorrhage, and retinal damage leading to blindness.

Assessment. Collection of **subjective data** begins with assessing the patient's knowledge and feelings about the disease and factors that appear to precipitate crisis or exacerbate signs and symptoms. Fatigue may be reported when anemia is severe. The primary symptom associated with sickling is pain. During the sickle cell crisis, the pain is severe due to tissue ischemia. Aching of joints, especially those of the hands and feet, is a common complaint. The pain associated with these attacks is often described as deep, gnawing, and throbbing.

Collection of **objective data** includes observing for abdominal enlargement and jaundice, as well as for edema of the extremities and signs of hemorrhage. As a result of the accelerated RBC breakdown, the patient has a characteristic clinical finding of hemolysis (jaundice, elevated serum bilirubin levels).

Diagnostic tests. Electrophoresis of hemoglobin in a patient with sickle cell anemia is specific for detecting sickle cell crisis or anemia. In a patient with sickle cell anemia, more than 80% of hemoglobin as shown by electrophoresis is Hg-S and not Hg-A. A stained blood smear detects anemia only. Hematocrit and hemoglobin levels are below normal values. WBCs are increased with infection. Skeletal roentgenograms will demonstrate bone and joint deformities and flattening. MRI may be used to diagnose a stroke caused by occluded cerebral vessels from sickled cells.

Medical management. Therapeutic care for a patient with sickle cell anemia is essentially supportive. There is no specific treatment for the disease. Therapy is usually directed toward alleviating the symptoms that result from complications of the disease. For example, chronic leg ulcers may be treated with bed rest, antibiotics, warm saline soaks, mechanical or enzyme debridement, and dressings. Pneumovax, *Haemophilus influenzae,* and hepatitis immunizations should be administered.

Sickle cell crisis may require hospitalization. O_2 may be administered to alter hypoxia and control sickling. Rest is encouraged, and fluids and electrolytes are administered to reduce blood viscosity and maintain renal function. Analgesics are used to treat pain. Research has shown that sickle cell crisis pain is often undertreated. To comprehend what sickle cell crisis pain is like, the nurse needs to have a clear understanding of the disease process and of current approaches to pain management (Day, 2001). According to pain experts, parenteral morphine and hydromorphone are the preferred opioid analgesics for acute sickle cell crisis pain. Large doses of continuous (rather than as needed [prn] opioid analgesics are the mainstay of pain management during the acute phase. Patient-controlled analgesia (PCA) may be used during an acute crisis. After discharge, patients often continue on oral opioid analgesics. Health care personnel must overcome their fears of opioid addiction to treat pain optimally and to avoid prolonging the duration of pain. Blood transfusions should be used cautiously to treat a crisis; blood products generally are packed RBCs. Because these patients have an increased need for folic acid, it is important for them to obtain daily supplements.

Hydroxyurea therapy significantly increases HbF levels, reduces hemolysis, increases hemoglobin concentration, and decreases sickled cells.

Results in a multicenter, international trial show that sickle cell disease, until now incurable, can sometimes be cured by a bone marrow transplant. In the investigation trial, 22 people with symptomatic sickle cell disease received bone marrow grafts from human leukocyte antigen (HLA)–identical siblings. In the trial of 22 patients younger than age 16, after 2 years, 2 of the patients died; 16 out of 20 who were alive had no symptoms of sickle cell disease. The four remaining patients rejected the bone marrow graft and their symptoms returned. Recent advances in gene therapy technology provide promise for the future treatment of sickle cell disease (Day, 2001).

Nursing interventions and patient teaching. Supportive treatment follows sign and symptom presentation: hydration and analgesia during crises and dilution of blood with increased fluid intake to reverse sickling. Monitoring the transfusion therapy for evidence of transfusion reaction is vital. Attention to fever and infection is important. Genetic counseling is indicated.

Nursing diagnoses and interventions for the patient with sickle cell anemia include but are not limited to the following:

NURSING DIAGNOSES	NURSING INTERVENTIONS
Pain, related to thrombotic crisis	Place patient in proper anatomic alignment, and protect joints.
	Position patient by slow, gentle handling.
	Apply warmth with soaks or compresses to relieve discomfort.
	Give analgesics as ordered.
Impaired skin integrity, related to altered circulation to tissues, resulting in hypoxia and inadequate nutrition	Remove constrictive clothing to enhance circulation.
	Maintain room and body warmth to avoid discomfort or chilling.
	Initiate ROM exercises; support joints at rest and with movement to stimulate circulation.
	Inspect extremities for adequate circulation.
	Palpate for arterial pulses to assess patency of arterial circulation.
	Monitor blood studies for gas exchange and hematology as indicators of adequate tissue perfusion.

NURSING DIAGNOSES	NURSING INTERVENTIONS
	Place patient on bed rest to decrease resistance to peripheral circulation.
	Elevate affected parts to enhance venous return.
	Implement cleaning procedure (use hydrogen peroxide or normal saline solution) to remove drainage and necrotic tissue.
	Apply sterile dressing or expose affected area to air to promote healing.
	Apply heat with lamp or cradle as ordered to enhance circulation and healing.
	Observe response to evaluate effectiveness of therapy.
	Cut patient's nails and discourage scratching to avoid injury.

Patient teaching should include the following:

- Alert the patient to the need for family testing to determine the presence of Hg-S; genetic counseling is available for carriers.
- Explain how to avoid sickle cell crises: avoid high altitudes, flying in unpressurized planes, dehydration, cold temperatures, iced liquids, and vigorous exercise; use stress-reduction methods.
- Explain to the patient that young pregnant women have a high risk for developing pulmonary and/or renal complications.
- Practice ROM exercises with the patient and encourage regular physical activity to prevent bone demineralization. Explain the need for a balance between rest (physical and mental) and activity, such as ROM and isometric exercises.
- Discuss the principles of good nutrition, such as the importance of protein, calcium, vitamins, and adequate fluids.
- Alert the patient to the signs and symptoms of increased intracranial pressure, to the need to blow the nose gently, to avoid coughing, and to avoid straining on elimination.
- Demonstrate to the patient how to monitor oral intake, urinary output, and urine protein.
- Advise the patient to avoid trauma and extremes in temperature; patients should not smoke and should protect extremities from injury because of impaired circulation.

Prognosis. The prognosis is guarded. In addition to hemolytic anemia, painful crises with multiple infarctions of most organ systems occur. With repeated episodes of sickling, there is gradual involvement of all body systems, especially the spleen, lungs, kidneys, and brain. Bone marrow grafts from HLA-identical siblings are adding hope to sickle cell patients.

Polycythemia (Erythrocytosis)

Etiology/pathophysiology. Two types of polycythemia are **primary polycythemia (polycythemia vera) and secondary polycythemia.** Their etiologies and pathophysiology differ, although their complications and clinical manifestations are similar. Polycythemia vera is a myeloproliferative (characterized by excessive bone marrow production) disorder with hyperplasia of bone marrow; it manifests with an increase in circulating erythrocytes, granulocytes, and platelets. The condition is a stem cell abnormality of unknown cause. Polycythemia vera is characterized by erythrocytosis (an abnormal increase in the number of circulating red blood cells) and increased production of granulocytes and platelets. In polycythemia vera, there is also an elevated WBC with basophilia. Secondary polycythemia is caused by hypoxia rather than by a defect in the evolution of the RBC. Hypoxia stimulates erythropoietin in the kidneys, which in turn stimulates erythrocyte production. The need for oxygen may result from high altitude, pulmonary disease, cardiovascular disease, or tissue hypoxia. Secondary polycythemia is a physiologic response in which the body tries to compensate for a hypoxic problem rather than a pathologic response. In polycythemia vera the pathologic response is a malignancy of the blood cells.

Multiorgan system disease is affected by hyperplastic bone marrow elements. Because of the increased erythrocyte mass, hypervolemic and hyperviscous (sticky) occurrence is two to three times that of normal. The sluggish circulatory process predisposes to infarctions of vital organs.

Clinical manifestations. This disorder's onset is gradual and has a progressive course of some length. It mainly affects men in middle age. Venous distention and platelet dysfunction cause esophageal varices, epistaxis, GI bleeding, and petechiae. Hepatomegaly and splenomegaly from organ engorgement may contribute to patient complaints of satiety and fullness.

Assessment. Collection of **subjective data** includes noting patient complaints of sensitivity to hot and cold. Generalized pruritus may be a striking symptom and is related to histamine release from an increased number of basophils. Headaches, vertigo, tinnitus, and blurred vision are often present.

Collection of **objective data** includes noting eczema and dermatologic changes. The skin may develop an erythemic appearance (plethora). Elevated blood pressure accompanies left ventricular hypertrophy and angina.

Diagnostic tests. Plasma and red blood cell volume are increased. Hemoglobin and hematocrit levels and reticulocyte and erythrocyte counts, as well as platelets (thrombocytes) are elevated, as is WBC count with basophilia. Alkaline phosphatase, uric acid, and histamine levels are noted. Bone marrow examination in polycythemia vera shows hypercellularity of RBCs,

WBCs, and platelets. The basal metabolic rate (BMR) is increased without thyroid function alteration. Splenomegaly is found in 90% of patients with primary polycythemia but does not accompany secondary polycythemia.

Medical management. Repeated phlebotomy decreases blood viscosity: removal of 500 to 2000 mL of blood until the hematocrit level is maintained at 45% to 48%; the procedure is repeated if hematocrit rises to more than 50%. Once the diagnosis of polycythemia vera is made, treatment is directed toward reducing blood volume and viscosity and bone marrow activity. Myelosuppressive agents such as busulfan (Myleran), hydroxyurea (Hydrea), and radioactive phosphorus are often given to inhibit bone marrow activity. Allopurinol may reduce the number of acute gouty attacks.

Nursing interventions and patient teaching. Primary polycythemia vera is not preventable. However, because secondary polycythemia is generated by any source of hypoxia, problems may be prevented by maintaining adequate oxygenation. Therefore controlling chronic pulmonary disease and avoiding high altitudes may be important.

When acute exacerbations of polycythemia vera develop, the nurse has several responsibilities. Fluid intake and output must be judiciously evaluated during hydration therapy to avoid fluid overload (which further complicates the circulatory congestion) and dehydration (which can cause the blood to become even more viscous). If myelosuppressive agents are used, the nurse must administer the drugs as ordered, observe the patient, and teach the patient about medication side effects.

Assessing the patient's nutritional status with the dietitian may be necessary to offset the inadequate food intake that can result from GI symptoms of fullness, pain, and dyspepsia. Activities must be instituted to decrease thrombus formation. The relative immobility normally imposed by hospitalization puts the patient at risk for thrombus formation. Active or passive leg exercises, and ambulation when possible, should be initiated.

Because of its chronic nature, polycythemia vera requires ongoing evaluation. Phlebotomy may need to be performed every 2 to 3 months, reducing the blood volume by about 500 mL each time. The nurse must evaluate the patient for the development of complications.

Nursing diagnoses and interventions for the patient with polycythemia vera include but are not limited to the following:

NURSING DIAGNOSES	NURSING INTERVENTIONS
Ineffective tissue perfusion, cardiopulmonary, cerebral, GI, and peripheral, related to hyperviscosity of fluid and potential bleeding	Have patient maintain comfortable position. When patient is on bed rest, do not raise knee gatch. Provide active or passive ROM exercises q 2-4 hr.
Activity intolerance, related to ischemia	Check peripheral pulses and color and temperature of extremities q 4-6 hr. Report early signs or symptoms of thrombosis or bleeding to physician. If patient has bleeding tendency, avoid invasive procedures when possible. Avoid trauma; provide soft-bristled toothbrush. Encourage avoidance of sodium-rich foods to reduce fluid retention. Encourage adequate exercise and mobility to prevent stasis. Explain disease course and signs and symptoms expected.

The nurse should alleviate deficient knowledge of this condition if it exists. The nurse should emphasize the importance of compliance with the medical and nutritional regimen. Dietary teaching should emphasize avoiding foods that contain iron while increasing the intake of calories and protein (because of BMR increase).

Signs and symptoms that require medical supervision include those associated with thrombosis (pain, edema, or erythema); this must be stressed to the patient. Because this is a chronic illness, emotional support is imperative.

Prognosis. Polycythemia vera is a chronic, life-shortening disorder. Although the incidence is small, leukemia and lymphomas develop in some patients with polycythemia vera. This may occur as a result of the chemotherapeutic drugs used to treat the disease or may be secondary to a disorder in the stem cells that progresses to leukemia. The major cause of morbidity and mortality from polycythemia vera is thrombosis. Permanent cure cannot be achieved today, but remission of many years can be produced.

DISORDERS ASSOCIATED WITH LEUKOCYTES
AGRANULOCYTOSIS
Etiology/Pathophysiology

This potentially fatal condition of the blood is characterized by a severe reduction in the number of granulocytes (basophils, eosinophils, and neutrophils). The white blood count is extremely low (leukopenia) as is the differential neutrophil count—less than 200/mm^3 (neutropenia). Normal neutrophil value is 3000 to 7000/mm^3.

Adverse medication reaction or toxicity is the primary cause of agranulocytosis. However, neoplastic disease, chemotherapy, and radiation therapy are often cited as causative. Viral and bacterial infections are possible causes of the condition. Heredity is also considered.

A suppression of the bone marrow by the causative agent reduces the number and production of white blood cells. Leukocytes, formed in the bone marrow, provide body protection against microorganisms. This protection is ineffective when bone marrow suppression has occurred.

Clinical Manifestations

Fever, chills, headache, and fatigue are symptoms associated with infection and the inflammatory process. Ulcerations of mucous membranes—the mouth, nose, pharynx, vagina, and rectum—are also found. Bronchial pneumonia and urinary tract infections are complications that occur in the later stages.

Assessment

Collection of **subjective data** includes noting the common complaints of fever, extreme fatigue, and prostration. All medications taken, whether prescription or over-the-counter, are considered as possible causes of the condition.

Collection of **objective data** includes observing fever over 100.6° F (38.1° C). Erythema and pain from ulcerations may occur. Ulcerations are cultured for microorganisms. Lung and bronchial auscultation reveals crackles and rhonchi because of trapped exudates.

Possible causative chemical agents are as follows:
Analgesics (Butazolidin)
Antibiotics (chloramphenicol, penicillin derivatives, cephalosporins)
Antiepileptics (phenytoin)
Antihistamines
Antineoplastic drugs (Vincristine)
Antithyroid drugs (propylthiouracil)
Diuretics
Phenothiazides (Thorazine, Prolixin, Sparine, Compazine)
Sulfonamides and derivatives

Diagnostic Tests

Leukocytes with neutrophils differential will be below normal. A bone marrow study will show depression of activity.

Medical Management

The main objective of treatment is to alleviate the factors responsible for bone marrow depression and prevent or treat infection. Blood cultures may be performed when fever is elevated, and cultures may be ordered if ulceration occurs. Transfusions of packed red blood cells (PRBCs) are often ordered. G-CSF (filgrastim [Neupogen]) given subcutaneously can be used to treat a neutropenic patient. Immunocompromised (neutropenic) precautions may also be instituted.

Nursing Interventions and Patient Teaching

A patient with a compromised WBC system is highly susceptible to life-threatening infections. Nursing interventions are directed toward protecting the patient from potential sources of infection, and it is essential to monitor the patient conscientiously to detect the earliest signs of infection so that therapy may be initiated promptly. Meticulous handwashing by medical and nursing personnel and strict asepsis are mandatory.

Nursing diagnosis and interventions for the patient with agranulocytosis include but are not limited to the following:

NURSING DIAGNOSES	NURSING INTERVENTIONS
Risk for infection, related to depressed WBC (leukocytes) production	Maintain scrupulously clean patient environment. Be certain no person with any type of infection is allowed in contact with the patient. Observe for signs and symptoms of infection, such as elevated temperature and chills. Wash hands meticulously and use strict asepsis for procedures. Enforce protective isolation to protect patient from pathogens. Provide high-protein, high-vitamin, high-calorie diet to maintain nutritional status. Encourage patient to take fluids to promote hydration. Monitor heart rate, respirations, blood pressure, and temperature to assess for signs of infection. Observe the patient for extreme fatigue, sore throat or mouth, and fever as signs of infection. Monitor WBC count. Use cooling measures (cooling blanket and tepid baths) to reduce fever if present. Administer antibiotics as ordered to combat specific pathogens. Provide perineal care to maintain hygiene and prevent infection.

Patient teaching should include the following:
- Discuss with the patient the use of frequent, thorough oral hygiene to treat or prevent mouth and pharyngeal infection.
- Explain the need for a soft, bland diet high in protein, vitamins, and calories.

- Encourage a balance between rest and activity to prevent fatigue and generalized weakness.
- Explain the need to avoid crowds, people with infectious diseases, and cold or hot environments; also teach signs and symptoms of infection and appropriate interventions.

Prognosis

Agranulocytosis is a potentially fatal condition because of the possibility of a life-threatening bacterial infection.

LEUKEMIA

Etiology/Pathophysiology

Leukemia is a malignant disorder of the hematopoietic system in which an excess of leukocytes accumulates in the bone marrow and lymph nodes. The cause, while unknown, is attributed to genetic origin, a virus, people previously treated with radiation, or chemotherapeutic agents that are toxic to bone marrow.

Bone marrow is replaced by rapidly developing white cells with abnormal numbers and forms of immature cells found in the circulation and infiltrated into the lymph nodes, spleen, and liver.

The increased numbers of WBCs can lead to infiltration and damage to the bone marrow, lymph nodes, spleen, and organs, including those of the central nervous system (CNS). Leukemic infiltration leads to problems such as hepatomegaly, splenomegaly, lymphadenopathy, bone pain, meningeal irritation, and oral lesions. Hematopoietic function is disturbed by incompetent bone marrow. Increased susceptibility to infection results.

Classification

Leukemia can be classified according to the type of proliferating WBC, or acute versus chronic form. Leukemias can be classified by identifying the type of leukocyte involved, whether it is of myelogenous or lymphocytic origin. By combining the acute and chronic categories with the cell type involved, specific types of leukemia can be identified. Four major types of leukemia are acute lymphocytic leukemia (ALL), acute myelogenous leukemia (AML), chronic myelogenous (granulocytic) leukemia (CML), and chronic lymphocytic leukemia (CLL).

Clinical Manifestations

The clinical manifestations of leukemia are varied. Essentially they relate to problems caused by bone marrow failure and the formation of leukemic infiltrates. Bone marrow failure results from (1) bone marrow overcrowding by abnormal cells and (2) inadequate production of normal marrow elements. The patient is predisposed to anemia and thrombocytopenia.

As leukemia progresses, fewer normal blood cells are produced. The abnormal WBCs continue to accumulate. The leukemic cells infiltrate the patient's organs, leading to problems such as splenomegaly, hepatomegaly, lymphadenopathy, bone pain, meningeal irritation, and oral lesions. Enlarged lymph nodes and painless splenomegaly may be the first sign of the disease in some people.

Diagnostic Tests

The WBC is low, elevated, or excessively elevated. Anemia and thrombocytopenia are noted. Bone marrow biopsy shows immature leukocytes. Chest radiographic examination may show mediastinal node and lung involvement and bone changes. Lymph node biopsy reveals excessive blasts (immature cells). Peripheral blood evaluation and bone marrow examination are the primary methods of diagnosing and classifying the type of leukemia. Further studies such as lumbar puncture and CT scan can be performed to determine the presence of leukemic cells outside of the blood and bone marrow.

Assessment

Collection of **subjective data** includes noting patient complaints regarding symptoms that may seem unrelated at first. Pain in bones or joints is often noticed. Fatigue, malaise, decreased activity tolerance, and irritability are usually present.

Collection of **objective data** includes noting those signs listed in clinical manifestations. Infections are common. Occult blood is detected in laboratory specimens of urine and stool. Abnormalities of skin (petechiae, ecchymoses) and mucous membranes (bleeding) may be present.

Medical Management

The goal of treatment is to achieve remission or to control the symptoms. Treatment is aimed at eradicating the leukemia with chemotherapy or bone marrow transplant. Combination chemotherapy is the mainstay for treating leukemia. The three purposes for using multiple drugs are to (1) decrease drug resistance, (2) minimize the drug toxicity to the patient by using multiple drugs with varying toxicities, and (3) interrupt cell growth at multiple points in the cell cycle. Observation for drug toxicity is imperative (Medications table, Chapter 17).

Tremendous progress in the treatment of leukemia has been made during the past decade, with the use of a complex combination of chemotherapeutic drugs and radiation therapy. Bone marrow and stem cell transplantation may be selected as the treatment of choice in patients with suitable donors if the initial remission of the acute leukemia has been induced (see Chapter 17). Before the transplant, the patient's bone marrow cells and leukemic cells must be killed by massive chemotherapy and total body irradiation. The patient may succumb to infection, hemorrhage, or graft-versus-host disease.

In chronic leukemia, which occurs almost exclusively in adults and develops slowly, the desired objectives of treatment depend on the kind of cells involved. Medications commonly used include chlorambucil (Leukeran), hydroxyurea, corticosteroids, and cyclophosphamide (Cytoxan). Irradiation of lymph nodes is often used, and blood transfusion may be given if anemia is severe. Although medications are not curative in chronic leukemia, they help to prolong life (Medications table).

Nursing Interventions and Patient Teaching

Prevention of infection by immunocompromised (neutropenic) precautions and teaching the avoidance of infectious agents are of utmost importance. Leukopenia (an abnormal decrease in the number of white blood cells to less than 5000 cells/mm³) can be fatal. The usual inflammatory process to control infection is decreased, thus frequent observation for signs and symptoms of infection is necessary. Thrombocytopenia-induced hemorrhage may be life threatening; therefore prevention of this condition through safe, gentle care is a primary consideration. Pain may be controlled through analgesia as ordered and by comfort measures. Coping mechanisms may be strained because of pain, complexities of treatment, side effects and toxicities, change of body image, or fear of death; support of patient and family can be promoted through a positive nurse-patient-family relationship and referral to community support groups.

Nurses have contact with a patient 24 hours a day and can help reverse feelings of abandonment and loneliness by balancing the demanding technical needs with a humanistic, caring approach. Therefore a nurse faces a special challenge in learning how to meet the intense psychosocial needs of a patient with leukemia while continuing to offer the complex physical care that is usually required. Consulting with other health professionals (e.g., psychiatric clinical specialists, oncology clinical specialists, social workers) may help the nurse to develop the skills required to meet the many needs of a patient with leukemia.

From a physical care perspective, the nurse is challenged to make astute assessments and plan care to help the patient survive the severe side effects of chemotherapy. The life-threatening results of bone marrow suppression (anemia, thrombocytopenia, neutropenia) require aggressive nursing interventions. Additional complications of chemotherapy may affect the patient's GI tract, nutritional status, skin and mucosa, cardiopulmonary status, liver, kidneys, and neurological system.

The nurse must be knowledgeable about all drugs being administered. This includes the mechanism of action, purpose, routes of administration, usual doses, potential side effects, safe handling considerations, and toxic effects of the drugs. In addition, the nurse must know how to assess laboratory data reflecting the effects of the drugs. Patient survival and comfort during aggressive chemotherapy are significantly affected by the quality of nursing intervention.

Procedures, meaning of treatments, and care plans should be discussed by the nurse and the patient. The nature of the disease and previous information the patient has received should be discussed. Community resources for support and information are invaluable for education of the patient and family. Expectations of physical abilities, remission, and future plans should be examined. Continuation of medical regimen is encouraged, as is avoidance of situations in which infection can be transmitted. Medication and diet information is important.

Prognosis

Perhaps more dramatically than in any other malignant disorder, chemotherapy has improved the prognosis of children with ALL. Untreated patients have a median survival time of 4 to 6 months. With current therapy of vincristine and prednisone, and an anthracycline drug (daunorubicin or doxorubicin), the median survival rate is about 5 years, and approximately 50% of children with ALL can now be cured. In AML, remission can be achieved in up to 75% of cases; however, relapse will eventually occur in most cases. Only about 20% to 25% of adults with AML experience a 5-year remission.

Overall survival for chronic lymphocytic leukemia is variable. In early stages, median survival rate ranges from 10 to 12½ years; in advanced stages, survival is approximately 18 months (Nursing Care Plan box).

COAGULATION DISORDERS
Etiology/Pathophysiology

Release of blood from the vascular system results from trauma or vessel damage, vessel inadequacy, disturbance of function of platelets or clotting factors, or liver disease (impaired clotting mechanisms).

The clotting mechanism is a hemostatic chain reaction. Vasoconstriction inhibits capillary leakage; hematoma compression provides pressure. Body reaction occurs: arterial blood pressure lowers. Any manifestation that alters this process predisposes the body to hemorrhage. The affected mechanism may be vascular, platelet dysfunction, or plasma coagulation factor alteration. The disorder may be congenital or acquired, possibly secondary to other disease or to medication toxicity.

Clinical Manifestations

Skin and mucous membrane manifestations include petechiae and ecchymoses. Epistaxis and gingival bleeding are common. Circulatory hypovolemia is noted through hypotension; pallor; cool, clammy skin; and tachycardia. GI tract bleeding is common, with abdominal flank pain caused by internal

MEDICATIONS | *Blood and Lymphatic Disorders*

MEDICATION	TRADE NAME	ACTION	SIDE EFFECTS	NURSING IMPLICATIONS
Cyanocobalamin (vitamin B$_{12}$)	Cobex, Vitamin B$_{12}$	Needed for adequate nerve functioning, protein and carbohydrate metabolism, normal growth, RBC development, and cell reproduction	Flushing, diarrhea, itching, rash, hypokalemia	Assess GI functions and potassium levels at beginning of treatment; stress need for patients with pernicious anemia to return for monthly injections; give intramuscularly only
Folic acid (B complex vitamin)	Folvite	Needed for erythropoiesis; increases RBC, WBC, and platelet formation in megaloblastic anemias	Pruritus, rash, general malaise, bronchospasm, slight flushing	Know that drug may be administered by deep intramuscular, subcutaneous, or intravenous routes; do not mix with other medications in same syringe for intramuscular injections
Ferrous sulfate	Feosol, Fer-In-Sol	Replaces iron stores needed for RBC development	Nausea, constipation, epigastric pain, black and red tarry stools, vomiting, diarrhea, discolored urine, staining of teeth	Know that between-meal dosing is preferable but can be given with some foods, although absorption may be decreased; give tablets with orange juice to promote iron absorption; to avoid staining teeth, give elixir iron preparations through straw; know that oral iron may turn stools black
Iron dextran	DexFerrum	Released into the plasma and carried by transferring to the bone marrow, where it is incorporated into hemoglobin	Stained skin at site of injection, fever, chills, headache, sweating, discolored urine, diarrhea	Administer 0.5-mL test dose by preferred route before therapy; wait at least 1 hour before giving remaining portion
Desmopressin acetate	DDAVP, Concentraid	Promotes reabsorption of water by kidneys and increase in plasma factor VIII levels, which increases platelet aggregation, resulting in vasopressor effect	Nasal irritation, congestion, drowsiness, headache, flushing, nausea, abdominal cramps, heartburn, vulval pain, hypertension	Avoid overhydration; assess pulse and blood pressure when giving drug subcutaneously; monitor factor VIII antigen levels and APTT
Filgrastim (G-CSF)	Neupogen	Stimulates proliferation and differentiation of neutrophils	Fever, alopecia, skeletal pain, nausea, vomiting, diarrhea, mucositis, anorexia	Monitor CBC and platelet count before treatment and twice weekly; refrigerate but do not freeze, avoid shaking; store at room temperature for at least 6 hours; discard any vial that has been at room temperature for more than 6 hours

NURSING CARE PLAN

The Patient with Leukemia

Ms. M. is a 26-year-old patient diagnosed with acute lymphatic leukemia. She is married and the mother of a 3-year-old daughter. Ms. M. has been receiving chemotherapy and is immunocompromised, with a differential WBC revealing a neutrophil count of 22%. Her hemoglobin is 8.8 g/dL, and her platelets are 55,000/mm³. Her mouth appears edematous, and she complains of oral tenderness.

NURSING DIAGNOSIS *Risk for infection, related to leukopenia*

Patient Goals/Expected Outcomes	Nursing Intervention	Evaluation
Patient will remain free of infection. Patient or caregiver will identify measures to prevent or control infection. Patient or caregiver will verbalize and report signs and symptoms of infection.	Inspect all body sites for infection at least daily; note and report fever, sore throat, purulent exudate, chills, cough, burning with urination, erythema, edema, tenderness, and pain. Monitor vital signs. Obtain cultures as ordered. Monitor WBC counts and culture reports. Administer antibiotics on time as ordered. Promote and maintain hygiene integrity of skin and mucous membranes. Use aseptic technique in treatments. Teach the patient and family: Necessity of avoiding crowds/people with infections while WBC count less than 1000/mm³. Personal hygiene measures. Signs and symptoms of infection.	Patient demonstrates no signs or symptoms of infection; temperature and WBC are within normal range.

NURSING DIAGNOSIS *Ineffective coping, related to diagnosis and disease process*

Patient Goals/Expected Outcomes	Nursing Intervention	Evaluation
Patient and family will demonstrate measures to effectively cope by verbalizing role of family, significant others, and support groups in therapeutic coping.	Assess coping capabilities of patient and significant others. Discuss disease process and expectations. Alleviate knowledge deficit. Encourage questions and self-expression: listen actively, demonstrate compassion, reassure with touch and personal contact. Assess fear of threat of death: allow time for personal expression and provide one-on-one discussion opportunity.	Patient and family express factors that are causing anxiety and powerlessness.

?CRITICAL THINKING QUESTIONS

1. What would you do if you noticed a visitor who had an obvious upper respiratory infection approaching Ms. M.'s room?
2. What nursing intervention would be most appropriate in providing therapeutic oral hygiene for Ms. M.?
3. State your choice of a bath and ADLs that would be most beneficial for Ms. M.

---

bleeding. CNS involvement ranges from altered response and malaise to loss of consciousness or affected speech.

Assessment

Collection of **subjective data** includes noting a history of bleeding after surgical or dental procedures. Exposure to toxic or hazardous agents or to radiation may

be revealed. Complaint of headache, extremity pain, and numbness is noted. Medications taken (e.g., aspirin) may lead to suspicion of toxicity.

Collection of **objective data** involves observation of pain on pressure to the abdomen, revealing liver and spleen tenderness and perhaps enlargement. Examination of skin and mucous membranes may reveal petechiae, ecchymoses, and occasionally hematoma.

Examination of emesis and stool may show signs of bleeding. Joint examination exhibits motion pain.

Diagnostic Tests

The platelet count will be low. The RBC count will be low with a decreased Hgb level. Coagulation time is altered. Bone marrow studies show abnormal cells.

Medical Management

The underlying cause is assessed and corrected, and replacement transfusions may be ordered. Heparin therapy or medication toxicity is considered as a possible cause. Infections and complications are treated or prevented.

Nursing Interventions

Many times, medical intervention depends on accurate reporting of signs and symptoms and nursing observations. In disorders of coagulation, the nurse should monitor vital signs to note any signs of hypovolemic shock. The patient must be moved gently to prevent trauma to the tissues. The nurse will monitor IV infusions and transfusions as ordered.

PLATELET DISORDERS
THROMBOCYTOPENIA
Etiology/Pathophysiology

A deficiency of the number of circulating platelets or change in the function of platelets alters the process of coagulation. Thrombocytopenia is an abnormal hematological condition in which the number of platelets is reduced to fewer than $150,000/mm^3$. Decreased production occurs in aplastic anemia, leukemia, tumors, and chemotherapy. Decreased platelet survival occurs in the presence of antibody destruction, infection, or viral invasion. Increased platelet destruction is caused by disseminated intravascular coagulation (DIC). Splenomegaly results from entrapment of blood in the spleen.

The most common cause of increased destruction of platelets is **thrombocytopenic purpura,** which may be drug induced or immune thrombocytopenic purpura. This most common acquired thrombocytopenia is a syndrome of abnormal destruction of circulating platelets termed *immune thrombocytopenic purpura* (ITP). It was originally termed idiopathic (cause unknown) thrombocytopenic purpura. However, it is now known that ITP is an autoimmune disease. In ITP, platelets are coated with antibodies. Although these platelets function normally, when they reach the spleen the antibody-coated platelets are recognized as foreign and are destroyed by macrophages in the spleen. If thrombocytopenia is medication induced (Box 7-3), the patient's platelet counts usually return to normal 1 to 2 weeks after the medication is withdrawn. The acute form of ITP is found mostly in children, whereas the chronic form is found among patients of all ages but is more common among women between 20 and 40 years

of age. It is an autoimmune process caused by the production of an autoantibody (immunoglobulin G [IgG]) directed against a platelet antigen.

Clinical Manifestations

The major signs of thrombocytopenia that are observable by physical examination are petechiae and ecchymoses on the skin. Petechiae occur only in platelet disorders. The severity of signs and symptoms correlates with the platelet count. As the level drops to less than $100,000/mm^3$, the risk for bleeding from mucous membranes and in cutaneous sites and internal organs increases. Significant risk for serious bleeding occurs once the count is less than $20,000/mm^3$. When the platelet count is less than $5000/mm^3$, spontaneous, potentially fatal central nervous system or gastrointestinal hemorrhage can occur.

Assessment

Collection of **subjective data** includes questioning the patient about recent viral infections (which may produce a transient thrombocytopenia), medications in current use, and the extent of alcohol ingestion.

Collection of **objective data** includes observing the patient for petechiae and ecchymoses throughout the skin. Epistaxis and gingival bleeding may be noted. Signs of increased intracranial pressure caused by cerebral hemorrhage will be assessed.

Diagnostic Tests

The tests include complete laboratory studies to ascertain the characteristics of all blood cells, which include platelet count, peripheral blood smear, and bleeding time. In addition, a bone marrow aspiration is performed to determine the presence of immature platelets. Examination also reveals the presence or absence of primary bone marrow abnormalities, such as neoplastic invasion or aplastic anemia.

Medical Management

The primary treatments are corticosteroid therapy (because of their ability to suppress the phagocytic response of splenic macrophages) and splenectomy.

| Box 7-3 | *Medications with Thrombocytopenic Effects* |

Aspirin
Digitalis derivatives
Furosemide
Nonsteroidal antiinflammatory agents (azathioprine, D-penicillamine, phenylbutazone, ibuprofen, indomethacin)
Oral hypoglycemics
Penicillins
Quinidine
Rifampicin
Sulfonamides
Thiazides

Other treatments may include intravenous immunoglobulin (IV Ig) or immunosuppressive drugs. Transfusions with platelet concentrates may be used in people with thrombocytopenic bleeding. Platelet transfusions are generally not recommended until the count is below 20,000/mm³ unless the patient is actively bleeding. Plasmapheresis is used to treat ITP by removing antibodies produced by the autoimmune process.

Nursing Interventions and Patient Teaching

The nurse will support the medical treatment regimen, using specific interventions for specific disease causes. If medication toxicity is the cause, the medication is discontinued. Infections are prevented by meticulous asepsis and gentle handling of the patient. Plasma and platelet infusion and whole-blood transfusions are monitored closely for reaction and effects on patients' conditions.

Nursing diagnoses and interventions for the patient with thrombocytopenia include but are not limited to the following:

NURSING DIAGNOSES	NURSING INTERVENTIONS
Ineffective tissue perfusion (cerebral, cardiopulmonary, renal, GI, peripheral), related to bleeding	Monitor vital signs and neurological status. Monitor platelet count. Assess for bleeding and fluid imbalance. Check patient's urine, stool, and emesis for blood. Monitor invasive diagnostic procedure sites for bleeding. Maintain comfort measures and bed rest. Avoid trauma and infection. Monitor patient receiving parenteral fluids and blood components carefully for untoward signs. Monitor potential sites of hemorrhage.
Pain, related to hemorrhage	Assess discomfort and pain level. Assess patient's ability to cope and response to pain. Administer analgesia as ordered and note patient response. Provide education.

An understanding of the disease process and causative agents is necessary in forming a knowledge base for self-care and prevention of trauma or infection. Instructions on signs and symptoms, as well as preventive measures, must be given: avoid trauma, use stool softeners, maintain a high-fiber diet to prevent constipation, check for presence of blood, use a soft toothbrush, and blow nose gently. The nurse should stress the importance of notifying the physician of signs and symptoms of bleeding.

Prognosis

The prognosis is variable, depending on the underlying cause. In ITP, treatment may need to be administered for 3 to 4 weeks before a complete response is seen. In chronic ITP, transient remissions occur. Approximately 80% of patients benefit from splenectomy, resulting in a complete or partial remission.

CLOTTING FACTOR DEFECTS

HEMOPHILIA
Etiology/Pathophysiology

Hemophilia, a hereditary coagulation disorder, is characterized by a disturbance of the clotting factors. In hemophilia A, the more common type, which represents 85% of the total incidence, antihemophilic factor VIII is absent; this factor is essential for conversion of prothrombin to thrombin through thromboplastin component. Hemophilia B (Christmas disease) exhibits a deficiency of factor IX with an absence of plasma thromboplastin component (a plasma protein), resulting in nonformation of thromboplastin.

Hemophilia is an X-linked hereditary trait that affects mainly males; females are carriers. A decrease in the formation of prothrombin activators occurs as a result of the decrease in clotting factors.

The patient with hemophilia was, in the past, at high risk for becoming human immunodeficiency virus (HIV) positive and later developing AIDS because of the need for cryoprecipitate concentrates and the potential for contamination with HIV virus. A number of people with hemophilia A have developed AIDS from transfusions of factor VIII concentrate. Presently, about 90% of older adults severely affected with hemophilia are seropositive for HIV, which was transmitted via replacement therapy. This problem should be eliminated since the inception of testing of all blood donors for evidence of HIV virus and, more recently, with the knowledge that heat treatment of factor VIII concentrates destroys the HIV virus. The use of recombinant replacement factors also is improving long-term survival rates.

Clinical Manifestations

Internal or external hemorrhage occurs with large ecchymoses into tissue—especially muscles, which may show deformity, and joints that become ankylosed. Hemarthrosis, or bleeding into a joint space, is a hallmark of severe disease and usually occurs in the knees, ankles, and elbow. Pain, edema, erythema, and fever accompany hemarthrosis. Small cuts can prove fatal; blood loss from simple dental procedures may be significant. Pain from the hemorrhage damage is significant.

Assessment

Collection of **subjective data** includes noting reports by patient and family of incidents of ecchymoses and hemorrhage from even the slightest trauma. Pain is associated with joint motion.

Collection of **objective data** includes noting the presence of blood in subcutaneous tissues, urine, or stool and noting edematous or immobile joints.

Diagnostic Tests

Factors VIII and IX are absent or deficient. Coagulation profiles reveal a normal platelet count, bleeding time, prothrombin time (PT), and the International Normalized Ratio (INR). The partial thromboplastin time (PTT) is prolonged. Laboratory personnel must be notified of the patient's disorder to alleviate further incidents of trauma as a result of diagnostic procedures (e.g., venipuncture).

Medical Management

Preventing and treating bleeding and relieving pain are the main focuses of care. Transfusions and administration of factor VIII or IX concentrate may be prophylactic or used to stop the hemorrhage. Two different clotting factor concentrates made from human plasma can be used. One, cryoprecipitate, is a clotting factor concentrate rich in factor VIII. Its use is waning because of the associated risk, although small, of viral disease transmission. Additionally, home administration of cryoprecipitate is difficult because it must be stored at low temperatures. The second human-derived product, factor VIII concentrate, is most typically used. A wide variety of products of this type are available, and are all freeze-dried concentrates of factor VIII prepared from pooled plasma from thousands of donors. These products are specially treated to inactivate any viral contamination (such as HIV or hepatitis viruses). Factor IX concentrates are also available and prepared in a similar fashion.

Because human plasma products still carry a very slight risk of infection transmission and require human donors, scientists have used genetic engineering to manufacture factor VIII. This product, recombinant factor VIII, is advantageous because of viral safety, unlimited supply, and lower cost. Recombinant factor VIII is now commercially available for widespread use.

Nursing Interventions and Patient Teaching

The nurse will control hemorrhages in emergency situations by applying pressure and cold to the site. Support and reassurance are imperative. Education of the patient and the entire family is significant because many people may be involved in the patient care. The nurse will monitor transfusions of factor VIII concentrate. The supportive care measures include pain management and genetic counseling. Hemophilia patients should not be given aspirin because it can further complicate the bleeding tendency.

Nursing diagnoses and interventions for the patient with hemophilia include but are not limited to the following:

NURSING DIAGNOSES	NURSING INTERVENTIONS
Ineffective tissue perfusion, related to blood loss from coagulation deficit	Assess for extent of hemorrhage.
	Prevent further hemorrhage or extension.
	Monitor vital signs and laboratory reports.
	Apply cold compresses to bleeding areas.
	Assess for anxiety, shock, disorientation, and decreased urinary output.
	Teach safety precautions to prevent trauma.
	Administer analgesia as ordered.
	Move patient gently and slowly, supporting joints.
	Prevent deformity through support, splints, and physical therapy.
Ineffective coping, related to long-term illness	Discuss disease process, altered lifestyle, and acceptance.
	Suggest genetic counseling.
	Encourage independence.
	Encourage compliance with medical regimen.
	Assess parental knowledge or guilt feelings.
	Be an active listener.
Deficient fluid volume, related to bleeding	Monitor vital signs and level of consciousness for evidence of acute hemorrhage.
	Monitor blood component therapy as ordered to control bleeding.
	Monitor I&O.
	Apply ice pack to affected joint or traumatized area to control bleeding.
	Administer analgesics to relieve joint pain.
	Assess amount, consistency, and frequency of bleeding: • Nose • Joints • Skin • Stool and urine • Pad counts
	Monitor laboratory tests to monitor degree of blood loss.
	Avoid trauma, such as falls, bumps, or injections.

The nurse and patient should discuss avoiding injury and controlling bleeding. Physical activity within limits and avoiding trauma should also be discussed. Wearing a medical alert identification tag is encouraged. Supervision of young patients—as well as informing playmates, teachers, and others—is important. Emergency care teaching includes immobilizing the affected part, applying ice, and notifying the physician. The nurse should discuss diet to prevent obesity, which puts excess pressure on joints. Regular dental care and preventive dental and medical measures are important aspects. Overprotection can sometimes be a factor to discuss. No aspirin or any other medication should be taken except with the physician's knowledge (Home Health Considerations box).

Prognosis

Before the appearance of the HIV virus, the average life span for a person with hemophilia was near normal. Although estimates vary widely of the prevalence of HIV in the hemophiliac population, the majority of severe hemophiliacs who received clotting factor concentrates before 1984 became seropositive for HIV. Now, with the development of methods to

---

Home Health Considerations

Hemophilia

- Home management is a primary consideration for a patient with hemophilia because the disease follows a chronic, progressive course.
- The quantity and length of life may be significantly affected by the patient's knowledge of the illness and understanding of how to live with it.
- The patient and family can be referred to the local chapter of the National Hemophilia Society to encourage association with other individuals who are dealing with the problems associated with hemophilia.
- The patient with hemophilia must be taught to recognize disease-related problems and to learn which problems can be resolved at home and which require hospitalization.
- Immediate medical attention is required for severe pain or edema of a muscle or joint that restricts movement or inhibits sleep and for a head injury, edema in the neck or mouth, abdominal pain, hematuria, melena, and skin wounds in need of suturing.
- Daily oral hygiene must be performed without trauma.
- Aspirin should not be taken because it decreases platelet aggregation.
- Understanding how to prevent injuries is an important consideration. The patient can learn to participate in noncontact sports (e.g., golf) and wear gloves when doing household chores to prevent cuts or abrasions from knives, hammers, and other tools.
- The patient should wear a medical alert tag to ensure that health care providers know about the hemophilia in case of an accident.
- A person with hemophilia who is mature enough or a family member can be taught to administer some of the factor replacement therapies at home.

heat-inactivate the virus, the risk of contracting HIV from clotting factor concentrates is almost nil. With the methods to control HIV transmission and the use of recombinant replacement factors, the average life span for a person with hemophilia is once again near normal.

VON WILLEBRAND'S DISEASE
Etiology/Pathophysiology

von Willebrand's disease is an inherited bleeding disorder characterized by abnormally slow coagulation of blood and spontaneous episodes of GI bleeding, epistaxis, and gingival bleeding caused by a mild deficiency of factor VIII. It is common during postpartum periods, as menorrhagia, and after surgery or trauma. Although similar to hemophilia, its incidence is not limited to males.

Treatment includes administration of cryoprecipitate containing factor VIII, fibrinogen, or fresh plasma. Desmopressin (DDAVP) is becoming the treatment of choice for patients who have a mild form of hemophilia. This drug is a synthetic of the human antidiuretic hormone, vasopressin. It causes an increase in factor VIII release from storage sites in the body. Desmopressin is often administered prophylactically to patients with mild hemophilia who require surgery or dental extractions. Observation and nursing interventions for hemophilia A and B can easily be adapted to von Willebrand's disease.

Prognosis
The prognosis is usually good.

DISSEMINATED INTRAVASCULAR COAGULATION
Etiology/Pathophysiology

Disseminated intravascular coagulation (DIC) is a grave coagulopathy resulting from the overstimulation of clotting and anticlotting processes in response to disease or injury, including septicemia, obstetric complication, malignancies, tissue trauma, transfusion reaction, burns, shock, and snake bites (Box 7-4).

Plasma clotting factors are depleted during widespread clotting within small vessels. This in turn leads to a bleeding disorder and thrombosis. The primary disorder initiates generalized intravascular clotting, which in turn overstimulates fibrinolytic mechanisms. As a result, the initial hypercoagulability is followed by a deficiency in clotting factors with subsequent hypocoagulability and hemorrhaging.

Clinical Manifestations
Bleeding is noted in mucous membranes, venipuncture or surgical sites, GI and urinary tracts, and generally from all orifices, and ranges from occult to profuse. Dyspnea; hemoptysis (blood-tinged spu-

Box 7-4 *Precipitating Causes of DIC*

OBSTETRIC
Abruptio placentae
Acute fatty liver of pregnancy
Amniotic fluid embolism
Hydatidiform mole (intrauterine mass of grapelike
   chorionic villi)
Retained dead fetus
Retained placenta
Toxemia

NEOPLASTIC
Acute leukemias
Adenocarcinomas
Carcinomas
Pheochromocytoma (a vascular tumor of the adrenal
   medulla)
Polycythemia vera
Sarcomas

HEMATOLOGICAL
Blood transfusion reaction
Sickle cell crisis
Thalassemia major (genetic hemolytic anemia;
   occurs in people of Mediterranean origin)

TRAUMA
Aspirin poisoning
Burns
Fat emboli
Heatstroke
Multiple injury
Snake bite
Surgery, particularly if extracorporeal (heart-lung
   machine used) circulation was used
Transplant rejection

OTHER
Acute infectious process/sepsis
Anaphylaxis
Cirrhosis
Glomerulonephritis
Hepatitis
Necrotizing enterocolitis
Purpura
Shock
Systemic lupus erythematosus

From Young, L.M. DIC: the insidious killer. *Crit Care Nurs*, 10(9):27, 1990.
Reprinted with permission of *Critical Care Nurse*.

tum); and diaphoresis with cold, mottled digits are
observed.

Assessment

Collection of **subjective data** includes noting patient
complaints of bone and joint pain. Changes in vision
occur.

Collection of **objective data** includes observing for
occult or obvious bleeding. Purpura on the chest and
abdomen, reflecting fibrin deposits in capillaries, is a
common first sign of DIC. Skin and mucosa color and
the presence of petechiae are noted. Abdominal tenderness may be present. GI bleeding, hematuria, pulmonary edema, pulmonary embolism, hypotension,
tachycardia, absence of peripheral pulses, decreased
blood pressure, restlessness, confusion, seizures, or
coma may be present.

Diagnostic Tests

The coagulation profile shows prolonged clotting. The
platelet count shows marked thrombocytopenia.
Other tests show hypofibrinogenemia and deficits of
factors V, VII, VIII, X, XII.

D-dimer test results are elevated. D-dimer reveals
the breakdown of fibrin and is a specific marker for the
degree of fibrinolysis in the serum.

Medical Management

In keeping with the medical therapeutic approach,
the underlying cause is addressed and corrected and
transfusion replacement and cryoprecipitate are ordered. Heparin therapy will block the subsequent
formation of microemboli by inhibiting thrombin activity. It has no effect, however, on existing clots. The
goal underlying the administration of heparin is to
stop the rapid overproduction of microemboli and
thus allow for reperfusion of vital organs and re-
plenishment of clotting factor supplies. However,
the use of heparin in treating DIC remains controversial. Fibrinolytic inhibitors should be given to
adults. This may be dangerous if the thrombotic
process has not been previously treated with heparin. Packed RBC transfusion should be initiated to
reestablish normal hemostatic potential if the thrombosis is blocked by heparin. Fresh frozen plasma
(FFP) is administered to replace other coagulation
factors.

Nursing Interventions and Patient Teaching

Protection from bleeding and trauma and pressure
to sites of hemorrhage are essential nursing measures. Support and reassurance of the patient may
aid in relieving high stress levels. The patient is
monitored in a quiet, nonstressful environment. The
side rails are padded, and foam or cotton swabs are
used for mouth care. Monitoring vital signs and administering heparin, blood and FFP transfusions,
and cryoprecipitate are necessary. The blood pressure cuff is used infrequently to avoid subcutaneous
bleeding.

Nursing diagnosis and interventions for the
patient with DIC include but are not limited to the
following.

NURSING DIAGNOSES	NURSING INTERVENTIONS
Risk for injury, bleeding, and fluid deficit, related to depleted coagulation factors, adverse effect of heparin (excess heparin, insufficient heparin)	Monitor Hct and Hgb. Examine skin surface for signs of bleeding; note petechiae, purpura, hematomas, oozing of blood from IV sites, drains, and wounds, and bleeding from mucous membranes. Observe for signs of bleeding from GI and genitourinary tracts. Note any hemoptysis or blood obtained during suctioning. Observe for changes in mental status; institute neurological checklist (mental status changes may occur with the decreased fluid volume or with decreasing Hgb). Monitor vital signs. Observe for signs of orthostatic hypotension (drop of greater than 15 mm Hg when changing from supine to sitting position indicates reduced circulating fluids). Avoid IM injections; any needlestick is a potential bleeding site. Apply pressure to oozing site. Prevent trauma to catheter and tubes by proper taping, minimum pulling.

The nurse discusses with the patient and family the signs and symptoms of DIC, which should be reported immediately to the nurse or physician. The patient is taught to self-administer heparin therapy subcutaneously if prescribed. Assist the patient and family to avoid mechanical trauma, such as from a hard toothbrush, blade razor, rough nose blowing, or contact sports.

Prognosis

Mortality rates from DIC vary, depending on degree of severity. Death is usually a result of either uncontrolled hemorrhage or irreversible end organ damage or both.

PLASMA CELL DISORDER
MULTIPLE MYELOMA
Etiology/Pathophysiology

Multiple myeloma, or plasma cell myeloma, is a malignant neoplastic immunodeficiency disease of the bone marrow. Neoplastic plasma cells infiltrate the bone marrow. The tumor, composed of plasma cells, destroys osseous tissue, especially in flat bones, causing pain, fractures, and skeletal deformities.

The specific immunoglobulin produced by the myeloma cells is present in the blood and/or urine and is referred to as the monoclonal protein. This protein is a helpful marker to monitor the extent of the disease as well as the patient's response to treatment. It is measured by serum or urine protein electrophoresis.

It is important to be alert to an older adult patient whose chief complaint is back pain and who has an elevated total serum protein. These patients should be evaluated for possible multiple myeloma. It most frequently occurs in patients older than age 40, with a peak incidence around 55 years of age, and affects twice as many men as women. Onset is gradual and insidious; the disease often goes unrecognized for years while the individual experiences frequent, recurrent bacterial infections. This increased susceptibility to infection follows disturbances of antibody formation by abnormal plasma cells. Suppression of normal antibody levels is seen in this plasma cell tumor disease. The incidence of multiple myeloma has increased and now approaches that of Hodgkin's disease.

Clinical Manifestations

The disease process will show a proliferation of malignant plasma cells and development of single or multiple bone marrow tumors. This is followed by bone destruction with dissemination into lymph nodes, liver, spleen, and kidneys.

The skeletal system symptoms typically involve the ribs, spine, and pelvis. Osteolytic lesions are seen in the skull, vertebrae, and ribs. Vertebral destruction can lead to collapse of vertebrae with ensuing compression of the spinal cord. Individuals complain of bone pain that increases with movement. Some develop pathologic fractures accompanied by severe pain.

In an individual with multiple myeloma, disruption of production of erythrocytes, platelets, and leukocytes occurs because of crowding of the marrow by the abnormal proliferation of plasma cells. This leads to increased infection, anemia, and increased potential for bleeding. Calcium and phosphorus drain from bones, leading to hypercalcemia and renal problems. In addition, cell destruction contributes to the development of hyperuricemia, which, along with the high protein levels caused by the presence of the myeloma protein, can cause renal failure.

Assessment

Collection of **subjective data** includes assessment of the patient's complaints of pain, including location, intensity, and duration. The patient's understanding of the disease, verbalization of discouragement, hopelessness, and desires for emotional and spiritual support should be addressed.

Collection of **objective data** includes assessing the patient's facial expression for signs of increased pain with movement, the ability to perform activities of daily living (ADLs), increased body temperature, increased potential for bleeding, changes in urine characteristics, and effectiveness of medication administration.

Diagnostic Tests

Diagnosis of multiple myeloma is made with radiographic skeletal studies, bone marrow biopsy, and laboratory examination of blood and urine. High serum and urine protein may be present as evidenced in serum or urine electrophoresis. Bony degeneration also causes calcium to be lost in the bones, eventually causing hypercalcemia. Pancytopenia, hypercalcemia, hyperuricemia, and elevated creatinine may be found. In addition, an abnormal globulin known as Bence Jones protein is found in the urine of a patient with multiple myeloma and can result in renal failure.

Radiographic skeletal examinations reveal widespread demineralization, lytic lesions, and osteoporosis. Lytic lesions may be seen on bone roentgenograms but are not well visualized on bone scans. Bone marrow studies reveal large numbers of immature plasma cells, which normally account for only 5% of marrow population.

Medical Management

Treatment is symptomatic, since multiple myeloma is not curable. Radiation and chemotherapy are initiated to reduce tumor size, impede tumor growth, and produce remission. Radiation is used in small doses. The antineoplastic drugs of choice are the alkylating agents, such as melphalan (Alkeran), cyclophosphamide (Cytoxan), chlorambucil (Leukeran), and carmustine (BCNU). Vincristine, doxorubicin (Adriamycin), and dexamethasone can be added for patients who do not respond to alkylating agents. Bone marrow depression occurs as a side effect; therefore the CBC is monitored during treatment.

Hypercalcemia and pain also should be addressed. Analgesics, orthopedic supports, and localized radiation help reduce the skeletal pain. Hospitalization to administer chemotherapy, corticosteroids, and fluids may be required.

Nursing Interventions and Patient Teaching

Care of the patient with multiple myeloma should focus on pain relief, preventing infection and bone injury, administrating chemotherapy and radiation, and maintaining hydration. Ambulation and adequate hydration are used to treat hypercalcemia, dehydration, and potential renal damage. Weight bearing helps the bones reabsorb some calcium, and fluids dilute calcium and prevent protein precipitates from causing renal tubular obstruction.

Because of the potential for pathologic fractures, the nurse must be careful when moving and ambulating the patient. A slight twist or strain in the wrong area (e.g., a weak area in the patient's bones) may be sufficient to cause a fracture. Attention to the psychosocial, emotional, and spiritual needs is also extremely important.

Nursing diagnoses and interventions for the patient with multiple myeloma include but are not limited to the following:

NURSING DIAGNOSES	NURSING INTERVENTIONS
Risk for injury, related to osteoporosis and lytic lesions	Protect from bone injury; use log-roll, turning sheet.
Pain, related to disease process	Administer analgesics as ordered. Provide comfort measures. Assess contributing factors.
Deficient fluid volume, related to impaired renal function	Increase fluid intake to 3000 to 4000 mL/day. Maintain I&O record.

The nurse's responsibilities in patient education include teaching the patient to avoid traumatic bone injury and the importance of avoiding infection. The nurse discusses the importance of adequate hydration and reviews the pain control modalities available. It is also important to identify spiritual resources.

Prognosis

This disease is usually progressive and generally fatal. A patient usually lives for approximately 2 years if untreated. With proper therapeutic treatment, the chronic phase of multiple myeloma may last for more than 10 years. Multiple myeloma is seldom cured, but treatment can relieve symptoms, produce remissions, and prolong life.

LYMPHATIC DISORDERS
LYMPHANGITIS
Etiology/Pathophysiology

Lymphangitis is an inflammation of one or more lymphatic vessels or channels that usually results from an acute streptococcal or staphylococcal infection in an extremity.

Clinical Manifestations

Lymphangitis is characterized by fine red streaks from the affected area in the groin or axilla. The infection is usually not localized, and edema is diffuse. Chills, fever, and local pain accompany headache and myalgia. Septicemia may occur; lymph nodes enlarge.

Medical Management

Administration of penicillin or other antimicrobial drugs controls the infection. Hot, moist heat—soaks or packs—brings comfort.

Nursing Interventions

Aseptic technique promotes healing. Rest and extremity elevation may relieve the pressure.

Prognosis

With treatment, the prognosis is usually good.

LYMPHEDEMA

Etiology/Pathophysiology

Lymphedema is a primary or secondary disorder characterized by the accumulation of lymph in soft tissue and edema. The accumulation of lymph in soft tissue is caused by obstruction, an increase in the amount of lymph, or removal of the lymph channels and nodes. The condition may be hereditary.

If the lymphatic drainage function is disturbed, an inflammatory process may result.

Clinical Manifestations

Massive edema and tightness cause pressure and pain in the affected extremities. It progresses toward the trunk and is aggravated by standing; pressure, as with pregnancy or premenstruation; obesity; and warm, humid environments.

Assessment and Diagnostic Test

Collection of **subjective data** includes the nurse noting the patient's complaints of pain and pressure. Medical history of varicosities, pregnancy, or modified radical mastectomy is important.

Collection of **objective data** includes observation of the extremities for edema and palpation of pedal pulses.

Lymphangiography is used to differentiate lymphedema from venous disorders.

Medical Management

Diuretics and antimicrobials are administered as ordered. Mechanical management includes use of compression pumps and elastic sleeves or stockings on the affected limb. Diet restrictions include limiting sodium and avoiding spicy foods, which would precipitate thirst.

Nursing Interventions and Patient Teaching

The primary goal of care is to increase lymphatic drainage and avoid trauma. Elevation of the extremities while asleep and periodically during the day will facilitate draining the tissues. Massage toward the trunk followed by active exercise (e.g., walking) decreases the edema. Avoidance of constrictive clothing, shoes, or stockings (except elastic stockings) is advisable. Meticulous skin care must be maintained, and every effort must be made to prevent infections.

An important nursing intervention is to provide emotional support for the patient. Body image disturbance related to the appearance of the lymphedematous extremity should be addressed. Emphasizing that lymphedema need not prevent the individual from engaging in routine activity may increase self-esteem.

Nursing diagnosis and interventions for the patient with lymphedema include but are not limited to the following:

NURSING DIAGNOSES	NURSING INTERVENTIONS
Impaired skin integrity, related to impaired lymphatic drainage	Protect engorged tissues. Consider physical therapy or ROM exercises (aids lymphatic flow). Examine skin for impaired skin integrity. Gently handle affected parts. Apply skin-protecting moisturizers or emollients. Teach application of supportive stockings or elastic sleeves.

The patient should be made aware of the progression of the condition and of the cause. If the disorder is long term and ongoing, coping with its effects must be approached. The rationale behind nursing interventions must be explained to enhance the ongoing medical regimen. If unsightly results are permanent, the patient must consider acceptance rather than social isolation.

Prognosis

There is no cure for the disorder, but signs and symptoms can be controlled with compliance to treatment.

HODGKIN'S DISEASE

Etiology/Pathophysiology

Hodgkin's disease is a malignant disorder characterized by painless, progressive enlargement of lymphoid tissue. It affects males twice as frequently as females, and the age incidence curve is bimodal (two separate populations). There is a peak early in life in the second and third decades, and a peak later in life in the sixth and seventh decades. The two peaks in incidence have been suggested as separate diseases. The first incident peak suggests a viral cause. Beginning as an inflammatory or infectious process, it develops into a neoplasm. The exact cause is unknown. Hodgkin's disease is thought to be an immune disorder (T-cell disease).

There are no major risk factors, but the disease occurs more frequently in people who have had mononucleosis (an infection caused by the Epstein-Barr virus [EBV]), have acquired or congenital immune deficiency syndromes, are taking immunosuppressive drugs after organ transplantation, have had a tonsillectomy or appendectomy, or have had diminished or delayed exposure to infections (e.g., someone with few or no siblings) (Thompson & Muscari, 2005).

Lymphoid tissue enlargement is first noticed in the cervical nodes and spleen and is characterized by abnormal or atypical cells. Reed-Sternberg cells are atypical histiocytes consisting of large, abnormal, multinucleated cells in the lymphatic system found in Hodgkin's disease. These cells increase in number, replacing normal cells. The main diagnostic feature of Hodgkin's disease is the presence of Reed-Sternberg cells in lymph node biopsy specimens. The disease is believed to arise in a single location (it originates in lymph nodes in 90% of patients) and then spreads along adjacent lymphatics. It eventually infiltrates other organs, especially the lungs, spleen, and liver. In approximately two thirds of patients, the cervical lymph nodes are the first to be affected. When the disease begins above the diaphragm, it remains confined to lymph nodes for a variable period. Disease originating below the diaphragm frequently spreads to extralymphoid sites such as the liver.

Clinical Manifestations

The initial development is most often enlargement of cervical, axillary, or inguinal lymph nodes. The enlarged lymph nodes are not painful unless they exert pressure on adjacent nerves. Anorexia, weight loss, night sweats, malaise, and extreme pruritus are complaints associated with this condition; they are associated with a poorer prognosis. Low-grade fever may occur. Anemia and leukocytosis follow, with development of complications of respiratory infections.

Assessment

Collection of **subjective data** includes noting the common complaints of malaise and appetite loss. Pruritus is often severe. After the ingestion of even small amounts of alcohol, individuals with Hodgkin's disease may complain of a rapid onset of pain at the site of the disease. The cause for the alcohol-induced pain is unknown. Bone pain occurs later in the disease's course.

Collection of **objective data** includes palpating enlarged cervical and supraclavicular lymph nodes. Splenomegaly, hepatomegaly, and abdominal tenderness are found. Excoriation of skin and evidence of scratching from pruritus are noted. Edema of the face and neck may be noticed. Weight and nutritional status are recorded.

Diagnostic Tests

Peripheral blood studies show anemia (normocytic, normochromic), WBC increase, and an abnormal erythrocyte sedimentation rate. Other blood studies may show hypoferremia caused by excessive iron intake by the liver and spleen, elevated leukocyte alkaline phosphatase from liver and bone involvement, hypercalcemia from bone involvement, hypoalbuminemia from liver involvement. Chest radiographic examination may reveal a mediastinal mass. CT scans can detect retroperitoneal node involvement. Lymph node biopsy that includes laparoscopy for retroperitoneal nodes is performed. Bone marrow biopsy is performed as an important aspect of staging. A CT scan and an ultrasound examination can indicate an enlarged spleen or liver. The presence of Reed-Sternberg cells remains a hallmark of the presence of Hodgkin's disease.

Medical Management

Treatment depends on the staging process (Box 7-5). See Figure 7-5 for nodal involvement, by stage, in Hodgkin's disease.

In general, radiation therapy is used against the localized forms (stages I and II). Combination chemotherapy is used in some early stages in patients believed to have resistant disease or to be at high risk for relapse. Chemotherapy and radiation therapy are used against the generalized forms (stages III and IV). Advances in treatment now enable some stage IIIB and stage IV diseases to be cured with high-dose chemotherapy and bone marrow or peripheral stem cell transplantation. Combination chemotherapy and radiation has been used.

Treatment for Hodgkin's disease involves several drugs, which are usually given in cycles over 6 to 12 months, or for at least 2 months after remission. Until recently, a traditional regimen for Hodgkin's disease had been MOPP. MOPP includes mechlorethamine (Mustargen), vincristine (Oncovin), procarbazine (Matulane), and prednisone. Mechlorethamine is another name for nitrogen mustard. It is one of a group of drugs known as alkylating agents that can cause serious long-term side effects, such as leukemia, particu-

---

Box 7-5 *Clinical Staging System for Hodgkin's Disease*

STAGE I
Abnormal single lymph nodes
Regional or single extranodal site

STAGE II
Two or more abnormal lymph nodes on the same side of the diaphragm
Localized involvement of extranodal site and one or more lymph node regions of the same side of diaphragm

STAGE III
Abnormal lymph node regions on both sides of diaphragm
May be accompanied by spleen involvement
Now subdivided into lymphatic involvement of the upper abdomen in the spleen (splenic, celiac, and portal nodes) (stage III$_1$) and the lower abdominal nodes in the periaortic, mesenteric, and iliac regions (stage III$_2$)

STAGE IV
Diffuse and disseminated involvement of one or more extralymphatic tissues and/or organs— with or without lymph node involvement; the extranodal site is identified as *H*, hepatic; *L*, lung; *P*, pleural; *M*, marrow; *D*, dermal; *O*, osseous

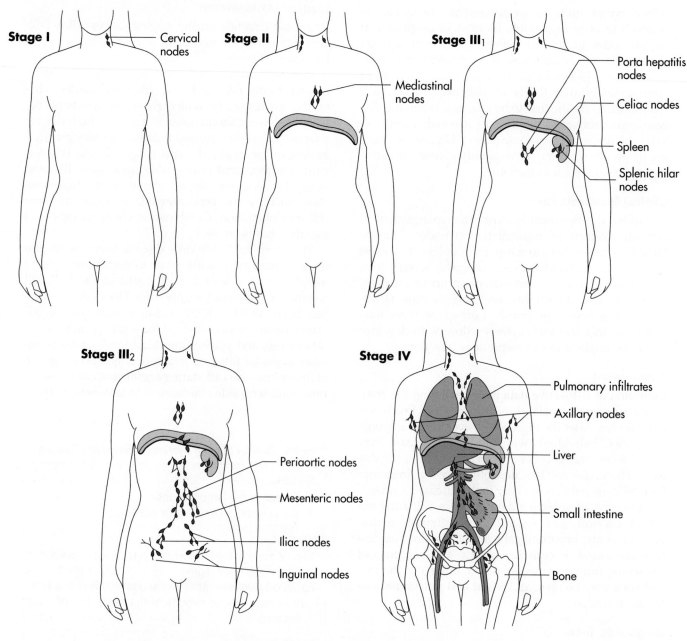

FIGURE **7-5** Nodal involvement by stage in Hodgkin's disease (based on modified Ann Arbor Staging System).

larly when combined with radiation therapy. Oncologists are now choosing a regimen known as ABVD over MOPP, or they're replacing mechlorethamine with cyclophosphamide (Cytoxan) to decrease the likelihood of long-term complications. ABVD includes doxorubicin (Adriamycin), bleomycin (Blenoxane), vinblastine (Velban), and dacarbazine (DTIC-Dome) (Thompson & Muscari, 2005). A biologic response modifier (Neupogen) that stimulates proliferation and differentiation of neutrophils is a treatment option. Neupogen is used to decrease infection in patients receiving antineoplastics that suppress neutrophil production.

Nursing Interventions and Patient Teaching

The nurse will plan care according to the staging level. Awareness of side effects of radiotherapy or chemotherapy is important in preparing the patient to deal effectively with these effects. Comfort measures focus on skin integrity. Soothing baths with an antipruritic medication (as ordered) can be effective. Fever and perspiration may be controlled with medication (with attention to increased fluid intake) plus linen changes as necessary to prevent further skin problems. Extensive tests must be explained to the patient, because there is a tendency toward anxiety and ineffective coping.

Nursing diagnoses and interventions for the patient with Hodgkin's disease include but are not limited to the following:

NURSING DIAGNOSES	NURSING INTERVENTIONS
Impaired skin integrity, related to pruritus and jaundice	Assess condition of skin and level of discomfort. Administer skin care by baths and keep patient clean and dry. Apply calamine lotion, cornstarch, sodium bicarbonate, and medicated powders to relieve pruritus. Maintain adequate humidity and cool room to decrease pruritus. Monitor vital signs for fever; assess for perspiration and change linen, keeping it wrinkle free.
Risk for infection, related to immune system ineffectiveness	Protect the environment and teach the importance of possible reverse isolation. Use meticulous handwashing. Prevent contamination by infectious visitors. Maintain hygiene and cleanliness of area. Monitor vital signs, I&O, respiratory status, and skin integrity.
Anxiety and fear, related to unknown outcome	Instruct patient on symptoms, disease progression, and treatment regimen. Encourage open communication and venting feelings. Encourage questions and problem solving.

Understanding the disease is important to enable personal interaction regarding self-care and retaining independence. Fertility issues may be of particular concern because this disease is frequently seen in adolescents and young adults. In this light the nurse must help ensure that these issues have been addressed soon after diagnosis (Therapeutic Dialogue box). The effect on the patient's life, as well as on significant others, is a prime consideration in patient attitude and adjustment. Realistic approaches to the illness and therapies are imperative. Guidance toward seeking counseling for stress management can be helpful. Special nutritional considerations are discussed concerning excess weight loss or an undernourished condition.

Prognosis

The prognosis is steadily improving. It is dependent on the stage of the disease. The prognosis for untreated patients is about 5 years; those diagnosed and treated in stage I or II have a cure rate greater than 90%, whereas those in stage III or IV have a less favor-

Therapeutic Dialogue

Mr. L. is a 25-year-old with a recent diagnosis of Hodgkin's disease. When the nurse enters Mr. L.'s room, she notes he appears tense and drawn.
NURSE: *You seem tense and preoccupied.*
PATIENT: *Why did this have to happen to me? I just got married and things were going so well. Dr. S. said I would have to have radiation, then chemotherapy. I've heard that can make me sterile.*
NURSE: *The diagnosis of Hodgkin's disease certainly is worrisome for you and your wife.*
PATIENT: *Why do I feel so sad? I just want to cry.*
NURSE: *That is a very natural response; you are grieving because of the loss of a totally healthy body as well as concern over the possibility of being sterile.*
PATIENT: *I don't know what to say to my wife.*
NURSE: *Are you frightened about how she might respond if you would become sterile?*
PATIENT: *Yes, I'm scared; maybe I won't seem as masculine as I am now. I read somewhere about a male being able to store his sperm in a sperm bank before taking radiation and chemotherapy.*
NURSE: *Dr. S. will be stopping in to see you tonight. Would you like to discuss this option with him at that time?*
PATIENT: *I think I'll ask my wife to come up this afternoon and see what she thinks about all of this.*
NURSE: *It is okay for you to let your loved ones know you are afraid.*
PATIENT: *I need to let my wife know my feelings.*
NURSE: *Your desire to have an open communication with your wife is helpful to both of you. I'll stop by and visit with you later.*

able prognosis. A serious consequence of the treatment for Hodgkin's disease is the later development of secondary malignancies. The estimated risk of a secondary cancer is approximately 18% at 15 years after treatment for Hodgkin's disease. The most common secondary malignancies are acute nonlymphoblastic leukemia and non-Hodgkin's lymphoma.

NON-HODGKIN'S LYMPHOMA
Etiology/Pathophysiology

Non-Hodgkin's lymphoma (NHL) is a neoplastic disorder of lymphoid tissue. The condition is starting to be characterized as a neoplasm of the immune system. The cause is unknown, but a viral source is suspected. They are classified according to different cellular and lymph node characteristics. In most cases of NHL, patients who have received immunosuppressive agents have a more than 100 times greater chance of developing NHL. This is probably a result of immunosuppressive agents activating tumor viruses. A herpeslike virus is suspected, but a definite relationship has not been established. It is more common in men older than 60 years of age, whites, and those of Jewish ancestry.

A variety of clinical presentations and courses are recognized from slowly developing to rapidly progressive disease. B-cell lymphomas constitute about 90% of NHL cases. Common names for different types of lymphoma include Burkitt's lymphoma, reticulum cell sarcoma, and lymphosarcoma. There is no hallmark feature in NHL pathology that parallels the Reed-Sternberg cell of Hodgkin's disease. However, all NHLs involve lymphocytes arrested in various stages of development.

Tumors usually start in lymph nodes and spread to lymphoid tissue in the spleen, liver, GI tract, and bone marrow. Involvement of lymphoid tissue also results in malabsorption and bone lesions. NHL is the most commonly occurring hematologic cancer and the fifth leading cause of cancer death. Approximately 54,000 new cases of NHL are diagnosed each year, and approximately 25,000 deaths occur each year. As the population has aged, the incidence of NHL has increased 2% to 3% per year for at least the past 30 years.

Clinical Manifestations

Painless, enlarged lymph nodes are found in the cervical area, and fever, weight loss, night sweats, anemia, pruritus, and susceptibility to infection develop. Pressure symptoms in the involved areas are noted. Pleural effusion, bone fractures, and paralysis are complications. Because the disease is usually disseminated when it is diagnosed, other symptoms will present, depending on where the disease has spread (e.g., hepatomegaly with liver involvement).

Assessment

Collection of **subjective data** includes frequent patient complaints of fatigue, malaise, and anorexia.

Collection of **objective data** includes examination of the abdomen for splenomegaly. Enlarged lymph nodes are also evident. Fever, night sweats, and weight loss are usually present.

Diagnostic Tests

A bone scan may reveal fractures, lesions, and tumor infiltration. Blood studies show hypercalcemia, as well as anemia; leukocytosis; and elevated sedimentation rate, platelet count, and alkaline phosphatase level. A Coombs' test will yield a positive result for antiglobulin. The patient will need a chest roentgenogram; CT scans of the chest, abdomen, and pelvis; a gallium scan; and possibly a lymphangiogram. Biopsies of lymph nodes, liver, and bone marrow are performed to establish the cell type and pattern. Diagnostic studies used for NHL resemble those used for Hodgkin's disease. Staging, as described for Hodgkin's disease, is used to guide therapy.

Medical Management

Once the diagnosis is made, the extent of the disease (staging) will be determined. Accurate staging is crucial to determine the treatment regimen. The therapeutic regimen for NHLs includes chemotherapy and radiation. Some chemotherapy agents used are cyclophosphamide (Cytoxan), vincristine (Oncovin), prednisone, doxorubicin (Adriamycin), bleomycin, and methotrexate. In 1998 the monoclonal antibody rituximab (Rituxan) was approved for the treatment of follicular lymphoma, the most common type of non-Hodgkin's lymphoma. Ibitumomab (Zevalin) is also a monoclonal antibody that can be used in patients who are refractory to Rituxan or in conjunction with it. Other biotherapy agents are being tested in clinical trials, some of which are showing improved survival and remission rates (Gutaj, 2000).

Patients with lymphoma commonly receive radiation to the chest wall, mediastinum, axillae, and neck—the region known as the "mantle field." Some patients will also need radiation to the abdomen; paraaortic area; spleen; and, less commonly, the pelvis.

Chemotherapy is the mainstay of treatment of NHLs that are not localized. High-dose chemotherapy with peripheral blood stem cell or bone marrow transplantation may be indicated. Tumor necrosis factor (TNF) is being used; it has direct cell toxicity and stimulates the immune system. Interferon is being investigated as a treatment option. Older patients have difficulty tolerating the aggressive chemotherapy treatments. This population is increasing in number, and new approaches are being examined.

Nursing Interventions and Patient Teaching

Supportive care of the patient during radiation and chemotherapy is primary in nursing management. Observation for complications follows. Further intervention is similar to that for Hodgkin's disease.

Explanations of the extensive diagnostic workup and its importance for staging the disease for determining the treatment plan are an important focus of patient teaching during the diagnostic period.

Prognosis

The prognosis is influenced by the staging classification. The prognosis for NHL is generally not as good as that for Hodgkin's disease.

NURSING PROCESS *for the Patient with a Blood or Lymphatic Disorder*

The role of the licensed practical nurse/licensed vocational nurse (LPN/LVN) in the nursing process as stated is that the LPN/LVN will:

- Participate in planning care for patients based on patient needs.
- Review patient plan of care and recommend revisions as needed.
- Review and follow defined prioritization for patient care.
- Use clinical pathways/care maps/care plans to guide and review patient care.

Assessment

The nursing data collection is from diverse sources: patient and family observation, physical examination, and diagnostic evaluation results (see Table 7-1).

The **subjective data** collected at the onset of the disease process are generally vague and nonspecific: malaise, fatigue, and weakness. The patient may relate a history of illness, easy bruising, bleeding tendencies with petechiae, and ecchymosis. Integumentary changes—including pruritus, nonhealing cuts and bruises, draining lesions, jaundice, and palpable subcutaneous nodules—may be reported. Edema and tenderness in lymph node regions may be accompanied by pain, sometimes severe. Gastrointestinal (GI) complaints are noted, as well as cardiovascular and respiratory changes. Neurological complaints may include headache, numbness, tingling, paresthesias, and behavioral alteration (Older Adult Considerations box).

Collection of **objective data** uses a system-by-system approach to confirm patient complaints. Manipulation of joints can reveal stiffness and hematoma and may produce pain. Examination of the oral cavity can reveal lesions, ulcers, signs of bleeding, or gingivitis. Cardiovascular and respiratory assessments include breath and heart sound variations and pain or dyspneic positioning. Any patient anxiety is noted, as well as observation for diminished comprehensive ability. Listening and an unhurried interview may reveal many symptoms not previously mentioned.

Nursing Diagnosis

Nursing diagnoses are determined from the assessment, which provides data from which the nurse identifies the patient's problems, strengths, potential complications, and learning needs. Nursing diagnoses for the patient with a blood or lymphatic disorder include but are not limited to the following:

Risk for infection
Injury (trauma) risk for (bleeding, falls)
Fatigue
Deficient knowledge
Acute pain
Chronic pain
Ineffective tissue perfusion
Impaired gas exchange
Activity intolerance
Ineffective coping
Impaired skin integrity

Expected Outcomes/Planning

For most patients the nurse will make more than one nursing diagnosis. Therefore the planning step in the nursing process is to determine the priority for nursing interventions from the list of nursing diagnoses. The nurse can determine the highest priority nursing diagnosis by using Maslow's hierarchy of needs, in

Older Adult Considerations

Blood or Lymphatic Disorder

- The subjective symptoms of hematological disorders (e.g., fatigue, weakness, dizziness, and dyspnea) may be mistaken for normal changes of aging or attributed to other disease processes commonly seen in older adults.
- The most common blood disorders are forms of anemia.
- Decreased production of intrinsic factor in an aging gastric mucosa results in increased incidence of pernicious anemia.
- Many older adults suffer from conditions such as colonic diverticula, hiatal hernia, or ulcerations that can cause occult bleeding. Older adults with these conditions should be observed for iron deficiency anemia.
- Age-related problems such as altered dentition, limited financial resources, difficulty in food preparation, and poor appetite resulting from emotional upset or depression can cause an increased incidence of iron deficiency anemia.
- Severe or persistent anemia can place additional stress on the aging or diseased heart.
- Blood products should be administered with caution because older adults are at increased risk of developing congestive heart failure. Careful assessment of cardiopulmonary function and intake and output is essential.
- Oral administration of iron preparations increases the risk of GI irritation and constipation in older adults.
- Ingestion of large amounts of aspirin and other antiinflammatory medications commonly taken by older adults increases the risk of GI bleeding and can lead to alteration in clotting.
- Chronic lymphocytic leukemia is the most common form seen among older patients. This form of leukemia usually progresses slowly in older adults and is rarely treated.

which the highest priority is generally given to immediate problems that may be life threatening. For example, impaired gas exchange would have a higher priority than ineffective coping.

Planning includes the development of realistic goals and outcomes that stem from the identified nursing diagnosis. Examples of expected patient outcomes for the patient with a blood or lymphatic disorder may include but are not limited to the following:

1. Patient is free of signs and symptoms of an infection.
2. Patient will be free of injury.
3. Patient has no evidence of bleeding (any bleeding is quickly controlled).
4. Patient states that he or she feels rested and able to perform ADLs.
5. Patient states measures needed to prevent infection, hemorrhage, and excessive fatigue.
6. Patient does not complain of shortness of breath with activity.

Implementation

The implementation of the nursing process is the actual initiation of the nursing care plan. Patient outcomes/goals are achieved by performance of the nursing interventions. Nursing interventions for the patient with a blood or lymphatic disorder may include the following:

- Place patient in private room; avoid contact with visitors or staff members who have an infection (in the immunocompromised patient).
- Stress careful handwashing to patient, significant others, and all caregivers.
- Assist in planning daily activities to include rest periods to decrease fatigue and weakness.
- Oxygen is given for dyspnea or excessive fatigue with exertion.
- Patient teaching stresses the disease process and the importance of continued medical follow-up. Of utmost importance in learning is the person's ability to identify the body's signals that blood abnormalities are present. Petechiae, ecchymoses, and gingival bleeding are the warning signs that one should seek medical attention promptly.

Evaluation

To evaluate the effectiveness of nursing interventions, compare patient's behaviors with those stated in the expected patient outcomes. Successful achievement of patient outcomes for the patient with a blood or lymphatic disorder are indicated by the following evaluative measures:

- Patient shows no sign of infection; temperature and WBC are within normal limits.
- Patient has not fallen.
- Patient shows no signs of bleeding (e.g., petechiae, hemorrhage); any bleeding is quickly controlled.
- Patient is able to bathe self in 30 minutes without becoming fatigued.
- Patient is able to correctly explain measures to prevent infection by good handwashing techniques and avoidance of people with infectious conditions.
- Patient is able to explain measures to prevent hemorrhage by avoidance of traumatic injury and avoidance of intramuscular injections.
- Patient states no shortness of breath with activity.

Key Points

- Blood is a thick, red fluid composed of plasma, a light yellow fluid; red blood cells; white blood cells; and platelets, which are suspended in plasma.
- The blood performs several critical functions: It transports oxygen and nutrition to the cells and waste products away from the cells; it regulates acid-base balance (pH) with buffers; and it protects the body against infection and prevents blood loss with special clotting mechanisms.
- Every person's blood is one of the following blood types in the ABO system of typing: type A, type B, type AB, or type O.
- The lymphatic system is a vast, complex network of capillaries, thin vessels, valves, ducts, nodes, and organs that helps to protect and maintain the internal fluid environment of the entire body by producing, filtering, and conveying lymph and by producing various blood cells.
- The tonsils are composed of lymphoid tissue and are responsible for filtering bacteria.
- The thymus gland is composed of lymphoid tissue in utero (before birth) and the early years of life. It aids in the development of the immune system.
- The spleen is also composed of lymphoid tissue and has many functions, such as filtering out old RBCs, storing a pint of blood, producing antibodies, and phagocytosis of bacteria.
- Anemia may be caused by blood loss, impaired RBC production, increased RBC destruction, or nutritional deficiency.
- Weakness and fatigue are major symptoms of anemia. They result from decreased oxygenation from decreased levels of hemoglobin and increased energy needs required by increased RBC production.
- Sickle cell anemia is a hemolytic anemia with a genetic basis; a sickle cell crisis occurs when the RBCs become deoxygenated and sickle shaped, thus causing stasis and obstruction of the microvasculature, leading to organ infarction and necrosis.
- Ingestion of iron compounds or intramuscular Z-track administration of iron dextran (DexFerrum) is part of the therapy for iron deficiency anemia.
- Thrombocytopenia is a decrease in the number of circulating platelets and leads to bleeding; people with thrombocytopenia need to learn how to prevent injury and hemorrhage.
- Hemophilia is a hereditary coagulation disorder; hemophilia A is a lack of coagulation factor VIII, and hemophilia B is a lack of factor IX. Maintenance therapy consists of blood factor replacement therapy and prevention of injury.
- Disseminated intravascular coagulation (DIC) is a coagulation disorder characterized initially by clotting and secondarily by hemorrhage. It results from an alteration in the balance between clotting factors and fibrinolytic factors; the person is usually critically ill.
- People with alterations of WBCs are at high risk of infection because leukocytes are a major factor in the body's defense against invading microorganisms.
- The leukemias are malignant disorders characterized by uncontrolled proliferation of WBCs and their precursors; the cause is unknown, but several theories have been proposed.
- Leukemias may be lymphocytic, monocytic, or myelogenous, and acute or chronic. Acute leukemias have a rapid onset and a short course, if untreated; chronic leukemias have a more insidious onset and longer course. The major therapies for leukemias are chemotherapy and bone marrow transplantation.

- Lymphomas are malignant disorders of the lymphatic system. People with Hodgkin's disease have defective cellular immunity and are therefore at high risk for infection. Non-Hodgkin's lymphoma is a group of lymphoid malignancies. Chemotherapy and radiation are the primary medical treatment for lymphomas.
- Primary polycythemia vera is characterized by excessive bone marrow production that manifests with an increase in circulating erythrocytes, granulocytes, and platelets. Secondary polycythemia is caused by hypoxia rather than a defect in evolution of the RBC.
- Multiple myeloma is a malignant neoplastic immunodeficiency disease of the bone marrow that affects the plasma cells. The specific immunoglobulin produced by the myeloma cells is present in the blood and urine and is referred to as the monoclonal protein.

Go to your free CD-ROM for an Audio Glossary, animations, video clips, and Review Questions for the NCLEX-PN® Examination.

evolve   Be sure to visit the companion Evolve site at http://evolve.elsevier.com/Christensen/adult/ for WebLinks and additional online resources.

CHAPTER CHALLENGE

1. Another name for a red blood cell is:
   1. leukocyte.
   2. monocyte.
   3. erythrocyte.
   4. platelet.

2. The test for a measure of the packed cell volume of red cells expressed as a percentage of the total blood volume is:
   1. hematocrit.
   2. erythrocyte sedimentation rate.
   3. reticulocyte.
   4. differential.

3. The gland that plays a role in the development of the body's immune system is the:
   1. tonsils.
   2. thymus.
   3. spleen.
   4. liver.

4. The compound in the blood that carries oxygen to the cells from the lungs and carbon dioxide away from the cells to the lungs is:
   1. leukocyte.
   2. thrombocyte.
   3. hemoglobin.
   4. erythrocyte.

5. The type of blood that is called the universal donor blood is:
   1. type A.
   2. type B.
   3. type AB.
   4. type O.

6. The spleen is located in which quadrant of the abdominal cavity?
   1. Upper right
   2. Upper left
   3. Lower left
   4. Lower right

7. Ms. W. is immunosuppressed by chemotherapy. She has a WBC count of 1500/mm³, with neutrophils of 20%. Which of the following statements indicates she understands home care instructions relating to her immune system?
   1. Take antibiotics prophylactically
   2. Take large doses of vitamins
   3. Avoid individuals with infections
   4. Use only sterile bed linens

8. Mr. R.'s platelets have dropped to 18,000/mm³. The most appropriate nursing intervention is to:
   1. provide oral hygiene four times per day.
   2. institute bleeding precautions.
   3. order a high-protein diet.
   4. request an order for oxygen per nasal cannula.

9. Mrs. B. tells the nurse that her husband, who has been admitted to the hospital with advanced leukemia, is talking about dying and expressing fears of death. She asks for suggestions for helping with her husband. Which of the following responses by the nurse is best?
   1. "Mr. B. will probably die of another disease before he dies of leukemia."
   2. "Mr. B. is expressing a readiness to be admitted to a hospice."
   3. "Talk of death is natural at this time but will diminish as he feels better."
   4. It's normal to want to talk about death; what we can do is be supportive by listening."

10. Which of the following statements is the most accurate instruction for a patient who is to undergo a bone marrow aspiration?
   1. "There will be no pain, just perhaps a slight discomfort."
   2. "You will be under general anesthesia during the procedure."
   3. "There will be a brief, sharp pain during the aspiration."
   4. "There will be no pain during the procedure but some afterward."

Continued

CHAPTER CHALLENGE—cont'd

11. Ms. D. is a 27-year-old housewife and mother of two children. She is being seen by the nurse at the health maintenance organization for signs of fatigue. She has a history of iron deficiency anemia. Which of the following data from the nursing history indicates that the anemia is not currently managed effectively?

1. Pallor
2. Poor skin turgor
3. Heart rate 68, weak pulse
4. Respirations 18 and regular

12. An important nursing intervention goal to establish for Ms. J., who has iron deficiency anemia, is:

1. use birth control to avoid pregnancy.
2. increase fluids to stimulate erythropoiesis.
3. decrease fluids to prevent sickling of RBCs.
4. alternate periods of rest and activity to balance oxygen supply and demand.

13. The nurse instructs Ms. J. about foods rich in iron. Which of the following foods should be included in the diet?

1. Fresh fruit and milk
2. Cheeses and processed lunch meats
3. Dark green leafy vegetables and organ meats
4. Fruit juices and cornmeal breads

14. Which of the following statements by the patient with pernicious anemia would indicate that she has understood the teaching?

1. "I'll be glad when I can stop the injections and take only oral medicine."
2. "I'll have to take B_{12} shots for the rest of my life."
3. "After a while I'll no longer need to take shots, just the pills."
4. "I was glad to hear that pills are available to treat me."

15. Mr. G. is admitted with polycythemia vera. He has a hemoglobin value of 20 g/dL. A probable treatment that will be ordered is:

1. whole blood transfusion.
2. platelet transfusion.
3. phlebotomy with removal of 800 mL of blood.
4. vitamin B_{12} injection.

16. Which lab finding is a strong indicator of disseminated intravascular coagulation (DIC)?

1. An elevated platelet count
2. An elevated D-dimer test
3. A normal prothrombin time
4. An elevated fibrinogen level

17. In teaching the patient with pernicious anemia about the disease, the nurse explains that it results from a lack of:

1. folic acid.
2. intrinsic factor.
3. extrinsic factor.
4. an RBC enzyme.

18. In addition to the general symptoms of anemia, the patient with pernicious anemia also manifests:

1. neurological symptoms.
2. coagulation deficiencies.
3. cardiovascular disturbances.
4. a decreased immunologic response.

19. A patient with sickle cell anemia asks the nurse why the sickling crisis does not stop when oxygen therapy is started. The nurse explains that:

1. sickling occurs in response to decreased blood viscosity, which is not affected by oxygen therapy.
2. when red cells sickle, they occlude small vessels, which causes more local hypoxia and more sickling.
3. the primary problem during a sickle cell crisis is destruction of the abnormal cells, resulting in fewer RBCs to carry oxygen.
4. oxygen therapy does not alter the shape of the abnormal erythrocytes but only allows for increased oxygen concentration in hemoglobin.

20. A nursing intervention that is indicated for the patient during a sickle cell crisis is:

1. frequent ambulation.
2. application of antiembolism hose.
3. restriction of sodium and oral fluids.
4. administration of large doses of continuous opioid analgesics.

21. Hodgkin's disease occurs more frequently in individuals who have:

1. a history of cancer treated with radiation.
2. been exposed to nuclear explosions.
3. had a tonsillectomy or appendectomy.
4. had an infection of *Helicobacter pylori*.

22. Which statement concerning Hodgkin's disease is correct?

1. The cure rate for stage I or II Hodgkin's disease is greater than 90%.
2. The incidence of Hodgkin's disease has increased over the past 20 years.
3. Hodgkin's disease is considered to be a difficult form of cancer to treat.
4. The occurrence of Hodgkin's disease in the older adult has increased.

23. A patient with hemophilia is hospitalized with acute knee pain and edema. Nursing interventions for the patient include:

1. wrapping the knee with an elastic bandage.
2. placing the patient on bed rest and applying ice to the joint.
3. gently performing ROM exercises to the knee to prevent adhesions.
4. administering nonsteroidal antiinflammatory drugs as needed for pain.

24. During physical assessment of a patient with thrombocytopenia, the nurse would expect to find:
    1. petechiae and purpura.
    2. jaundiced sclera and skin.
    3. tender, enlarged lymph nodes.
    4. splenomegaly.

25. Which of the following nursing interventions are necessary when caring for Ms. L., who has a WBC of 1800/mm³?
    1. Prevent patient contact with people who have respiratory tract infections, influenza.
    2. Wash hands frequently before and after patient contact.
    3. Report temperature elevation.
    4. Monitor hemoglobin.

26. Which of the following are necessary for the maturation of a mature red blood cell?
    1. Vitamin B_{12}
    2. Folic acid
    3. Renal erythropoietic factor
    4. Capric acid
    5. Iron

27. Choose the correct medical management for the patient with DIC:
    1. address and correct underlying cause.
    2. transfusion replacement.
    3. cryoprecipitate.
    4. administer colony-stimulating factor (filgrastim [Neupogen]).
    5. heparin therapy.

28. J., an 8-year-old with hemophilia A, is admitted with uncontrolled bleeding in the left knee joint as a result of a fall from his bicycle. Which of the following are appropriate nursing interventions and medical management?
    1. Applying pressure
    2. Cold applications
    3. Administering cyclophosphamide (Cytoxan)
    4. RBC transfusions
    5. Administering factor VIII concentrate

29. The nurse anticipates that an older adult patient with severe iron deficiency anemia will require which blood product?
    1. Whole blood
    2. Packed red blood cells
    3. Fresh frozen plasma
    4. Frozen red blood cells

8 Care of the Patient with a Cardiovascular or a Peripheral Vascular Disorder

BARBARA LAURITSEN CHRISTENSEN and ELAINE ODEN KOCKROW

Objectives

After reading this chapter, the student should be able to do the following:

Anatomy and Physiology

1. Discuss the location, size, and position of the heart.
2. Identify the chambers of the heart.
3. List the functions of the chambers of the heart.
4. Identify the valves of the heart and their locations.
5. Discuss the electrical conduction system that causes the cardiac muscle fibers to contract.
6. Explain what produces the two main heart sounds.
7. Trace the path of blood through the coronary circulation.

Medical-Surgical

8. Define the key terms as listed.
9. Compare nonmodifiable risk factors in coronary artery disease (CAD) with factors that are modifiable in lifestyle and health management.
10. List diagnostic tests used to evaluate cardiovascular function.
11. Describe five cardiac dysrhythmias.
12. Compare the etiology/pathophysiology, clinical manifestations, assessment, medical management, nursing interventions, diagnostic tests, and prognosis for patients with angina pectoris, myocardial infarction, or heart failure.
13. Specify patient teaching for patients with cardiac dysrhythmias, angina pectoris, myocardial infarction, heart failure, and valvular heart disease.
14. Discuss the etiology/pathophysiology, clinical manifestations, assessment, diagnostic tests, medical management, nursing interventions, and prognosis for the patient with pulmonary edema.
15. Discuss the purposes of cardiac rehabilitation.
16. Compare and contrast the etiology/pathophysiology, clinical manifestations, assessment, diagnostic tests, medical management, nursing interventions, and prognosis for the patient with rheumatic heart disease, pericarditis, or endocarditis.
17. Identify eight conditions that can result in the complication of cardiomyopathy.
18. Discuss the indications and contraindications for cardiac transplant.
19. Identify risk factors associated with peripheral vascular disorders.
20. Describe the effects of aging on the peripheral vascular system.
21. Compare and contrast signs and symptoms associated with arterial and venous disorders.
22. Discuss nursing interventions for arterial and venous disorders.
23. Compare essential (primary) hypertension, secondary hypertension, and malignant hypertension.
24. Discuss the etiology/pathophysiology, clinical manifestations, assessment, diagnostic tests, medical management, and nursing interventions for the patient with hypertension.
25. Discuss the importance of patient education for hypertension.
26. Compare and contrast the etiology/pathophysiology, clinical manifestations, assessment, diagnostic tests, medical management, nursing interventions, and prognosis for patients with arterial aneurysm, Buerger's disease, and Raynaud's disease.
27. Discuss the etiology/pathophysiology, clinical manifestations, assessment, diagnostic tests, medical management, nursing interventions, and prognosis for patients with thrombophlebitis, varicose veins, and stasis ulcer.
28. Discuss appropriate patient education for thrombophlebitis.

Key Terms

Be sure to check out the bonus material on the free CD-ROM, including selected audio pronunciations.

aneurysm (ĂN-ūr-ĭ-zĭm, p. 385)
angina pectoris (ăn-JĬ-nă PĔK-tŏr-ĭs, p. 346)
arteriosclerosis (ăr-tē-rē-ō-sklĕ-RŌ-sĭs, p. 378)
atherosclerosis (ăth-ĕr-ō-sklĕ-RŌ-sĭs, p. 345)
bradycardia (brăd-ē-KĂR-dē-ă, p. 340)
B-type natriuretic peptide (BNP) (p. 337)
cardioversion (kăr-dē-ō-VĔR-zhŭn, p. 336)
coronary artery disease (CAD) (p. 345)
defibrillation (dē-fĭb-rĭ-LĀ-shŭn, p. 342)
dysrhythmia (dĭs-RĬTH-mē-ă, p. 340)
embolus (ĔM-bō-lŭs, p. 351)
endarterectomy (ĕnd-ăr-tĕr-ĔK-tō-mē, p. 384)
heart failure (p. 359)
hypoxemia (hī-pŏk-SĒ-mē-ă, p. 336)
Intermittent claudication (klaw-dē-KĀ-shŭn, p. 376)
ischemia (ĭs-KĒ-mē-ă, p. 346)
myocardial infarction (mī-ō-KĂR-dē-ăl ĭn-FĂRK-shŭn, p. 351)

occlusion (ō-KLŌŌ-zhŭn, p. 351)
orthopnea (ŏr-thŏp-NĒ-ă, p. 361)
peripheral (pĕ-RĬF-ĕr-ăl, p. 375)
pleural effusion (PLŌŌR-ăl ĕ-FŪ-zhŭn, p. 360)
polycythemia (pŏl-ē-sī-THĒ-mē-ă, p. 336)
pulmonary edema (PŬL-mō-nă-rē ĕ-DĒ-mă, p. 366)
tachycardia (tăk-ē-KĂR-dē-ă, p. 340)

OVERVIEW OF ANATOMY AND PHYSIOLOGY

The cardiovascular (circulatory) system is the transportation system of the body. It delivers oxygen and nutrients to the cells to support their individual activities and transports the cells' waste products to the appropriate organs for disposal.

In ancient times the blood was referred to as the "river of life" or "fluid of life." Some even believed it had magical properties. All knew it was necessary to maintain life. This chapter discusses the structure and function of the blood vessels and the heart.

HEART

The heart is a remarkable organ, not much bigger than the fist (Figure 8-1). It is responsible for pumping 1000 gallons of blood every day through the closed circuit of blood vessels. It beats 100,000 times a day and transports the blood 60,000 miles through a network of blood vessels. The heart is a hollow organ composed mainly of muscle tissue with a series of one-way valves.

The heart is located in the chest cavity between the lungs in a region called the **mediastinum** (the mass of organs and tissues separating the lungs; it contains the heart and its greater vessels, the trachea, and the esophagus). Two thirds of the heart lies left of the midline (see Figure 8-1). The wider **base** of the heart lies superior and beneath the second rib. The **apex,** or narrow part, of the heart lies inferiorly, slightly to the left between the fifth and sixth ribs near the diaphragm.

Heart Wall

The heart is composed of three layers: **pericardium, myocardium,** and **endocardium.** The total structure is covered by a two-layered, serous membrane called the **pericardium.** Between the two thin membranes is a serous fluid that allows friction-free movement of the heart as it contracts and relaxes.

The pericardium, a two-layered serous membrane, is the outermost layer of the heart. Between the two thin membranes is a serous fluid that allows friction-free movement of the heart as it contracts and relaxes. The myocardium forms the bulk of the heart wall and is the thickest and strongest layer of the heart. It is composed of cardiac muscle tissue. The contraction of this tissue is responsible for the pumping of the blood. The endocardium (innermost layer) is composed of a thin layer of connective tissue. This structure lines the interior of the heart, the valves, and the larger vessels of the heart.

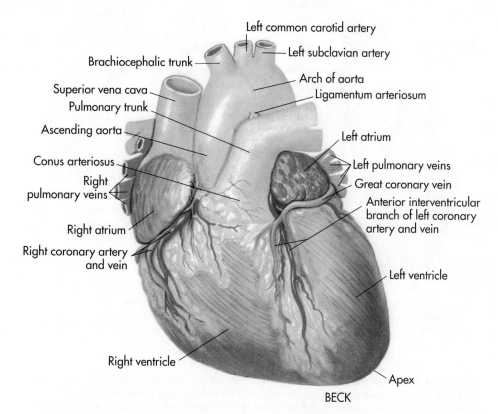

BECK

FIGURE **8-1** Heart and major blood vessels viewed from front (anterior).

Heart Chambers

The heart is divided into a right and left half by a muscular partition called the **septum** (Figure 8-2). The heart has the following four chambers:

1. **Right atrium.** The right atrium is the upper right chamber, and it receives deoxygenated blood from the entire body. The superior vena cava returns blood from the head, neck, arms, and trunk. The inferior vena cava returns blood from the lower body. The coronary sinus returns it from the heart muscle.

2. **Right ventricle.** The right ventricle is the lower right chamber, and it receives blood from the right atrium. Remember that this blood is deoxygenated. The right ventricle pumps blood to the lungs via the **pulmonary artery** to release carbon dioxide and receive oxygen.

3. **Left atrium.** The left atrium is the upper left chamber of the heart. It receives the oxygenated blood from the lungs via the **pulmonary veins.**

4. **Left ventricle.** The left ventricle is the lower left chamber of the heart. It receives the oxygenated blood from the left atrium. It is the thickest, most muscular section of the heart and pumps the oxygenated blood out through the aorta to all parts of the body.

The heart actually functions as two separate pumps—the right side receives deoxygenated blood and pumps it to the lungs; the left side receives the oxygenated blood from the lungs and pumps it throughout the body.

Heart Valves

Located within the heart are four **valves** that keep the blood moving forward and prevent backflow. The heart has two **atrioventricular (AV) valves.** They are located between the atrium and ventricles. The right AV valve is located between the right atrium and right ventricle and is called the **tricuspid** valve because it contains three flaps, or cusps. The left AV valve is composed of two cusps (bicuspid) and is commonly called the **mitral valve.** It is located between the left atrium and left ventricle. Both these valves prevent backflow of blood by rapidly closing. Small cordlike structures, **chordae tendineae,** connect the AV valves to the walls of the heart and work with the **papillary muscles** located in the walls of the ventricles to make a tight seal to prevent backflow when the ventricles contract.

The two remaining valves, the **semilunar valves,** are located at the points where the blood exits the ventricles. The **pulmonary semilunar valve** is located between the right ventricle and the pulmonary artery. Blood is pushed out of the right ventricle and travels

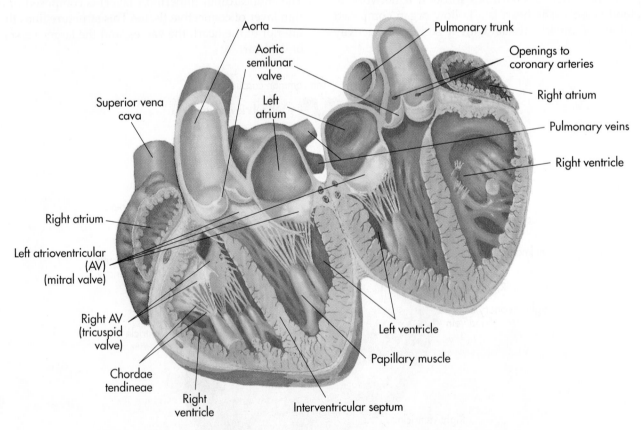

FIGURE **8-2** Interior of the heart. This illustration shows the heart as it would appear if it were cut along a frontal plane and opened like a book. The front portion of the heart lies to the reader's right; the back portion of the heart lies to the reader's left. The four chambers of the heart—two atria and two ventricles—are easily seen.

to the lung via the pulmonary artery. The **aortic semilunar valve** is located between the left ventricle and the aorta. When the left ventricle contracts, the blood is forced into the aorta and the aortic semilunar valve closes. Both of the semilunar valves are composed of three cusps that resemble a half moon, hence the name **semilunar** (see Figure 8-2).

Electrical Conduction System

Heart muscle tissue contains an inherent ability to contract in a rhythmic pattern. This ability is called **automaticity.** If heart muscle cells are removed and placed under a microscope, they continue to beat. In addition, they have the ability to respond to a stimulus in the same way that nerve cells do. This unique property is called **irritability.** Automaticity and irritability are two characteristics that affect the functions of the conduction system. Hormones, ion concentration, and changes in body temperature also affect the following functions:

- Conduction of messages around the heart
- Initiation of heartbeat
- Coordination of beating patterns between the atria and the ventricles

The heartbeat is initiated in the **sinoatrial (SA) node,** which is located in the upper part of the right atrium, just beneath the opening of the superior vena cava (Figure 8-3). Because it regulates the beat of the heart, it is known as the **pacemaker.** Impulses are passed to the AV node, which is located in the base of the right atrium. The impulses are slowed by the AV node to allow the atrium to complete contraction and to allow the ventricles to fill. The impulse then passes to a group of conduction fibers called the **bundle of His (AV) bundle** and divides into right and left branches to travel to smaller branches called the **Purkinje fibers,** which surround the ventricles. The message travels rapidly through the ventricles and causes contraction. This causes emptying of the ventricles.

IMPULSE PATTERN: SA node → AV node → bundle of His → right and left bundle branches → Purkinje fibers

Cardiac Cycle

The cardiac cycle refers to a complete heartbeat. The two atria contract while the two ventricles relax. When the ventricles contract, the two atria relax. The phase

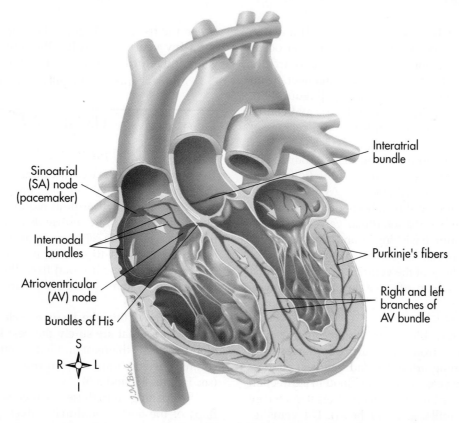

FIGURE **8-3** Conduction system of the heart. Specialized cardiac muscle cells in the wall of the heart rapidly initiate or conduct an electrical impulse throughout the myocardium. The signal is initiated by the SA node (pacemaker) and spreads to the rest of the right atrial myocardium directly, to the left atrial myocardium by way of the bundle of interatrial conducting fibers, and to the AV node by way of the three internodal bundles. The AV node then initiates a signal that is conducted through conduction fibers called the bundle of His and breaks into the right and left branches to travel to smaller branches called the Purkinje fibers, which surround the ventricles.

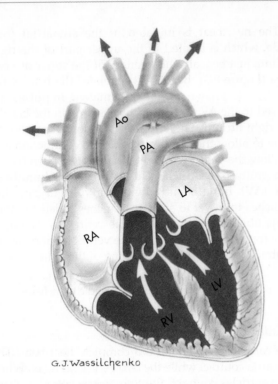

FIGURE **8-4** Blood flow during systole.

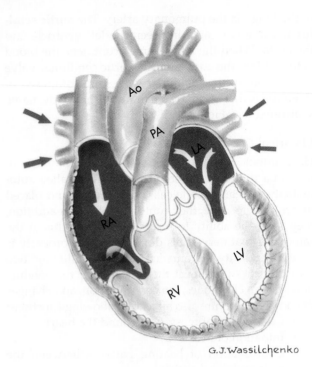

FIGURE **8-5** Blood flow during diastole.

of contraction is called **systole** (Figure 8-4) and the phase of relaxation is called **diastole** (the period of time between contraction of the atria or the ventricles during which blood enters the relaxed chambers from the systemic circulation and the lungs [Figure 8-5]). Complete diastole and systole of both atria and ventricles constitute a cardiac cycle; this takes an average of 0.8 second.

The heart sounds (**lubb** and **dubb**) are produced by closure of the valves. The first sound, **lubb** (long duration and low pitch), is heard when the AV valves close. The second sound, **dubb** (short duration, sharp sound), is heard when the semilunar valves close. Occasionally a murmur (swishing sound) can be heard. This can be a normal functional phenomenon produced by rapid filling of the ventricles or an abnormal condition produced by ineffective closure of the valves.

BLOOD VESSELS

Three main types of blood vessels are organized to carry blood to and from the heart. **Capillaries** (tiny blood vessels joining arterioles and venules) connect the **arteries** (large vessels carrying blood in a direction away from the heart) to the **veins** (vessels that convey blood from the capillaries to the heart). The veins return the blood to the heart. The heart delivers the blood to the arteries, which branch into tiny arteries called **arterioles** (blood vessels of the smallest branch of the arterial circulation), which deliver the blood to the tissues. Within the tissues, microscopic vessels (capillaries) form an extensive (50,000 miles) network that allows exchanges of products and by-products be-

tween the tissues and blood. The capillaries then join with tiny veins, or **venules,** that link with the larger veins and return to the heart. The pattern is as follows:

Artery → arteriole → capillary → venule → vein

CIRCULATION

CORONARY BLOOD SUPPLY

To sustain life, the heart must pump blood throughout the body on a regular, ongoing basis. As a result, the heart muscle or myocardium requires a constant supply of blood containing nutrients and oxygen to function effectively. The delivery of oxygen and nutrient-rich arterial blood to cardiac muscle tissue and the return of oxygen-poor blood from this active tissue to the venous system is called the **coronary circulation** (Figure 8-6).

Blood flows into the heart muscle by way of two small vessels that are surely the best known of all the blood vessels—the right and left coronary arteries. The coronary arteries form a crown around the myocardium (see Figures 8-1 and 8-6).

The openings into these small vessels lie behind the flaps of the aortic semilunar valves (see Figure 8-6). The coronary arteries bring oxygen and nutrition to the myocardium. Once the circulation is completed and the carbon dioxide and waste products have been collected, the blood flows into a large coronary vein and finally into the coronary sinus, which empties into the right atrium. These two main arteries have many tiny branches that serve the heart muscle. If an artery

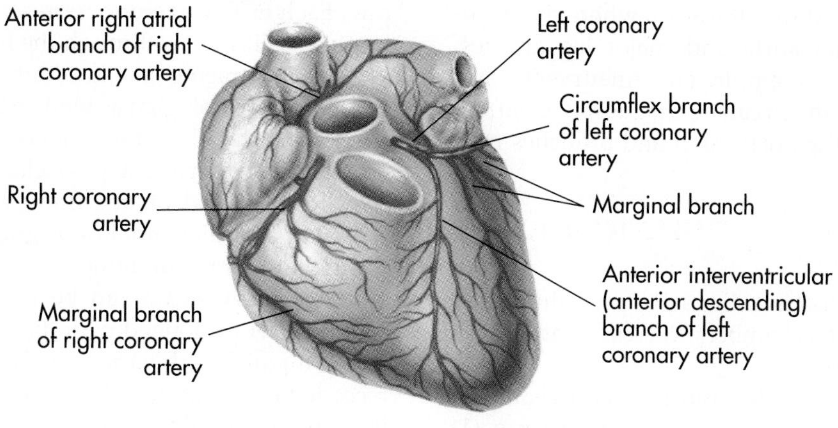

FIGURE **8-6** Arterial coronary circulation (anterior).

becomes occluded, these branches provide collateral circulation (alternate routes) to nourish the heart muscle. If the occlusion is severe, surgery and other procedures may be needed. These treatments are discussed later in this chapter.

SYSTEMIC CIRCULATION

Systemic circulation occurs when blood is pumped from the left ventricle of the heart through all parts of the body and returns to the right atrium. When the oxygenated blood leaves the left ventricle, it enters the largest artery (1 inch [2.5 cm] in diameter) of the body, the **aorta** (the main trunk of the systemic arterial circulation, composed of four parts: the ascending aorta, the arch, the thoracic portion of the descending aorta, and the abdominal portion of the descending aorta). As the blood flows through the artery branches, the branches become smaller in diameter (arterioles). The blood continues to flow into the capillaries. The capillaries surround the cells, and the exchange of oxygen, nutrients, and carbon dioxide and other waste products occurs. The blood proceeds to the tiny venules, then to the larger veins, and finally returns to the right atrium via the largest vein, the **vena cava** (one of two large veins returning blood from the peripheral circulation to the right atrium of the heart).

The blood is now deoxygenated and needs to be replenished with oxygen. It is important to note that the upper portion of the vena cava (superior vena cava) returns deoxygenated blood from the head, neck, chest, and upper extremities. The inferior vena cava returns deoxygenated blood from parts of the body below the diaphragm.

PULMONARY CIRCULATION

The deoxygenated blood will now pass through the pulmonary circulation to pick up the needed oxygen. Blood is pumped from the right atrium to the right ventricle, where it leaves the heart to travel via the pulmonary artery to the lungs. Once the blood reaches the lungs, it travels through arterioles to the capillaries.

The microscopic capillaries surround the **alveoli** (air sacs), where oxygen diffuses into the bloodstream. The capillaries then connect with the venules and finally with the four pulmonary veins, which return the oxygenated blood to the left atrium of the heart. It is then pumped to the left ventricle and to the aorta, and systemic circulation is then repeated. The blood circulation pattern is as follows:

Superior vena cava/inferior vena cava → right atrium → tricuspid valve → right ventricle → pulmonary semilunar valve → pulmonary artery → capillaries in the lungs → pulmonary veins → left atrium → bicuspid valve → left ventricle → aortic semilunar valve → aorta

LABORATORY AND DIAGNOSTIC EXAMINATIONS

Descriptions follow of diagnostic tests to evaluate cardiovascular function.

The nursing responsibilities are to physically prepare the patient for diagnostic procedures and to explain the examination to the patient. Cardiovascular function is evaluated through diagnostic examinations.

DIAGNOSTIC IMAGING

Radiographic examination of the chest provides a film record of heart size, shape, and position and outline of shadows. Lung congestion is also shown, indicating heart failure, perhaps in the earliest stages. Pleural effusion may be noted in left-sided heart failure (HF).

Fluoroscopy, the action-picture radiograph, allows observation of movement. It is invaluable in pacemaker or intracardial catheter placement.

An **angiogram** is a series of radiographs taken after injection of radiopaque dye into an artery. The circulatory process aids in diagnosis of vessel occlusion, pooling in various heart chambers, and congenital anomalies.

An **aortogram** visualizes the abdominal aorta and the major leg arteries by use of dye injected through the femoral artery and into the aorta where dye visualizes the abdominal aorta and major leg arteries. X-ray visualization is employed. Aneurysms and many other abnormalities can be diagnosed. Contrast media to visualize the aortic arch and branches may also be used.

CARDIAC CATHETERIZATION AND ANGIOGRAPHY

Cardiac catheterization is an invasive procedure used to visualize the heart's chambers, valves, great vessels, and coronary arteries.

The passage of a catheter into the heart chambers through a peripheral vessel is used to measure (1) pressure within the heart, and (2) blood-volume relationship to cardiac competence. Valvular defects, arterial occlusion, and congenital anomalies are determined. Blood samples are obtained. Contrast dye may be injected to allow better heart and vessel visualization (angiography). Because iodine is in the contrast medium, sensitivity to iodine is determined before injection to avoid allergic reaction, which could be a dangerous complication of this procedure. Cardiac catheterization is performed under sterile surgical conditions; its invasive nature requires a prior signed consent. The patient lies supine for a designated period with a sandbag over the pressure dressing at the insertion site to prevent hemorrhage. This procedure aids in diagnosis, in prevention of progression of cardiac conditions, and in accuracy in evaluation and treatment of the critically ill patient.

ELECTROCARDIOGRAPHY

The electrocardiogram (ECG) is a graphic study of the electrical activities of the myocardium to determine transmission of cardiac impulses through the muscles/conduction tissue. Each electrocardiogram has three distinct waves, or deflections: the **P wave,** the QRS complex, and the **T wave.** When the heart contracts, the electrical activity is called **depolarization. Repolarization** is the relaxation phase. The P wave represents the depolarization of the atria. The QRS complex represents the depolarization of the ventricles. The T wave represents the repolarization of the ventricles. Atrial repolarization is not represented but does occur; it is covered by the large QRS complex and cannot be seen on the ECG tracing.

A standard ECG has 10 electrodes; 6 are placed on the chest in different positions and 4 on the limbs. A conductive gel is used to enhance the contact and transmission. The patient is in a supine position. However, ambulatory ECGs and exercise/stress test ECGs require position variation. The machine, an electrocardiograph or galvanometer, records the energy wave of each heartbeat through a vibrating needle on graph paper, which feeds through the machine at a standard rate. Each ECG waveform represents a single electrical impulse as it travels through the heart (Figure 8-7).

The ECG tracing is read or interpreted by a cardiac specialist (cardiologist) as well as by internal medicine specialists, family practitioners, pediatricians, and emergency department physicians. The reading can also be displayed on the fluorescent screen (oscilloscope) of a cardiac monitor. A graphic tracing may be printed out by the monitor.

Ambulatory ECGs can be used to monitor heart rhythm over prolonged periods—12, 24, or 48 hours—and compared with various activities or symptoms as recorded in a diary kept by the patient. A Holter monitor (small portable recorder) is attached to the patient by one to four leads, with a 2-pound tape recorder carried on a belt or shoulder strap. The monitor operates continuously to record the patterns and rhythms of the patient's heartbeat. In conjunction with the diary of activities and symptoms kept by the patient, the physician can note various events, times, and medication peaks that affect or precipitate dysrhythmias. An ambulatory ECG is particularly useful for patients whose clinical symptoms indicate heart disorders but may have normal ECG tracings on a resting test.

CARDIAC MONITORS

It is common practice to continually assess the cardiac electrical activity of patients who are known or suspected to have dysrhythmias or who are prone to develop dysrhythmias or to have acute cardiovascular symptoms. This assessment is performed with a cardiac monitor, which displays information transferred via the conductive electrodes, which transfer electrical activity of the heart and relay it to a video display screen. The electrodes are placed on the chest.

Most monitors provide a visual display of cardiac electrical activity and the correct heart rate. Preset alarms warn of heart rates that exceed or drop below limits considered acceptable for each patient and also warn of dysrhythmias.

Ambulatory patients are increasingly monitored by battery-powered ECG transmitters that do not require direct connection of the patient to the oscilloscope. This monitoring is called **telemetry,** which is the electronic transmission of data to a distant location. The electrodes placed on the patient's chest are attached to a transmitter carried by the patient in a pocket or pouch. The transmitter sends a radio signal to a receiver, usually located at the nurse's station.

Patients need telemetry monitoring for various reasons, including a history of cardiac disease, angina pectoris, suspected dysrhythmias, a change in medications, surgery, an electrolyte abnormality, or unexplained syncope. Many of these patients are monitored in a centralized area such as an intermediate care or step-down unit (with monitors at the nurse's station).

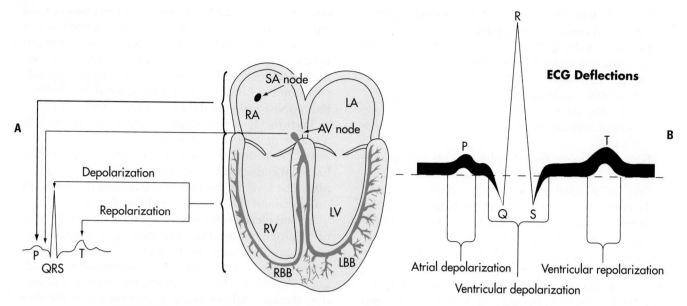

FIGURE **8-7** Normal ECG deflections. **A,** P wave. **B,** Relationship of ECG to cardiac muscle activity. *LBB,* Left bundle block; *RBB,* right bundle block.

But remote telemetry means the patient is on a medical/surgical unit and is being monitored at a separate location, called the **home unit,** which is usually on a critical care unit. Remote telemetry patients are usually stable. But even a stable patient's condition can change rapidly, and telemetry allows continuous heart monitoring to detect abnormalities.

Attachment to a cardiac monitor does not significantly alter a patient's need for nursing interventions. Placement of the monitoring electrodes on the anterior thorax (chest) rather than the extremities leaves the patient relatively free to carry on usual activities. Special attention should be paid to the electrode site to ensure a constant tight seal between the electrode and the skin and to note the development of any skin impairment. The conduction gel dries out, even if the pad is sealed; changing electrodes regularly is recommended. The nurse should also check the telemetry pack for integrity of the lead wires and test the monitoring device's battery with a battery tester. The nurse must also inform the monitoring area whenever the patient is moved off the unit for a diagnostic test, because the patient may go outside the monitor's range. Another important safety measure is *never* to remove telemetry and allow the patient to shower unless the physician has written the order to allow a shower. The patient could be subject to severe dysrhythmia, which would not be detected if the telemetry were removed during showering.

Exercise/stress ECG is another form of monitoring the heart's capability. It is accomplished in a laboratory setting during the performance of a prescribed exertion by the patient. Tasks include use of treadmills, stair climbing, aerobic exercise, and other forms of exertion. Monitored carefully, the patient is coaxed to a limit of exertion to evaluate ischemia, dysrhythmia, and the extent of cardiac capability under extreme circumstances, thus setting the limit of exercise tolerance in cardiac disease. If the patient is unable to tolerate activity, a stress test can be done by administering dipyridamole (Persantine) or adenosine, which mimics the patient's heart under stress/activity.

THALLIUM SCANNING

Thallium 201 is an intracellular ion that is actively transported into normal cells. If the cell is ischemic or infarcted, the thallium will not be picked up and a "cold spot" image is produced. Because the thallium concentrates in tissue with normal blood flow, tissue with inadequate perfusion appears as dark areas on scanning. The radioisotope is injected intravenously while the patient exercises on a treadmill. Breast tissue in the female can produce artifact, leading to a false-positive result. Using technetium 99m sestamibi instead of thallium can help minimize artifact and thus improve accuracy. In patients who cannot tolerate physical exercise, dipyridamole (Persantine) is given before the thallium to physiologically simulate exercise-induced stress.

Echocardiography uses high-frequency ultrasound directed at the heart. The echo, or reflected sound, is graphically recorded. Size, shape, and position of cardiac structures are outlined. The focus of this diagnostic effort is to detect pericardial effusion (collection of blood or other fluid in the pericardial sac), ventricular function, cardiac chamber size and contents, ventricular muscle and septal motion and thickness, cardiac output (ejection fraction), cardiac tumors, valvular function, and congenital heart disorder.

Ejection fraction (EF) of ventricles as demonstrated by an echocardiogram is as follows:

Greater than 60%: normal
40% to 60%: moderate HF
20% to 40%: moderate to severe HF
Less than 20%: severe HF (candidate for heart transplant)

Positron emission tomography (PET) is a computerized radiographic technique that uses radioactive substances to examine the metabolic activity of various body structures. In PET studies the patient either inhales or is injected with a biochemical radioactive substance. Specific color-coded images reveal organs' metabolic functions. Used for the last decade to study dementia, stroke, epilepsy, and tumors, PET is proving its merit in the diagnosis and treatment of cardiac disease. PET's ability to distinguish between viable and nonviable myocardial tissue allows physicians to identify the most appropriate candidates for bypass surgery or angioplasty. PET is also able to accurately detect CAD—noninvasively—in an asymptomatic patient, prompting early intervention that can salvage potentially ischemic myocardium when ischemia is present.

LABORATORY TESTS

History and physical examination as well as blood studies aid the physician in diagnosing and monitoring the cardiovascular disease process. The nurse's responsibility is to prepare the patient by explaining the tests and the preparation required for each test.

Blood cultures to detect growth of bacteria in the blood are crucial to the diagnosis of infective endocarditis.

A **complete blood count** (CBC) is a determination of the number of red and white blood cells per cubic millimeter as well as the white blood cell differential, platelets, hemoglobin, and hematocrit. Low hemoglobin indicates decreased ability to carry oxygen to the cells as well as the condition of anemia; an elevated white blood cell (leukocyte) count indicates infection or inflammation; and an elevated red blood cell (erythrocyte) count indicates that the body is compensating for chronic hypoxemia (an abnormal deficiency of oxygen in the arterial blood) by stimulating red blood cell production by the bone marrow, leading to secondary polycythemia (abnormal increase in the number of red blood cells in the blood). Chronic hypoxemia is often noted in heart failure.

Coagulation studies are useful in monitoring the patient receiving anticoagulant drug therapy, which is prescribed for patients with MI. Coagulation studies are also important in patients who have chronic atrial fibrillation or a patient with atrial fibrillation who is to undergo cardioversion (the restoration of the heart's normal sinus rhythm by delivery of a synchronized electric shock through two metal paddles placed on the patient's chest). Coagulation studies are needed if a myocardial infarction is diagnosed to assess the patient's coagulation status in case fibrinolytics are needed to dissolve the thrombus. These studies include prothrombin time (PT) and International Normalized Ratio (INR) and partial thromboplastin time (PTT).

Erythrocyte sedimentation rate (ESR) is used to monitor or rule out inflammatory conditions of the heart. The sedimentation rate is elevated with MI and bacterial endocarditis and decreases when healing begins. The level of the ESR also indicates the extent of inflammation and infection in rheumatic fever.

Serum electrolyte tests focus on the body's balance of sodium, potassium, calcium, and magnesium, which are necessary for myocardial muscle function. Sodium (Na^+) is necessary for maintaining fluid balance. Potassium (K^+) is required for relaxation of cardiac muscle, and calcium (Ca^{++}) is necessary for contraction of cardiac muscle. Magnesium (Mg^{++}) helps maintain the correct level of electrical excitability in the functioning of nerves and muscles, including the myocardium and cardiac conduction system. The physician compares serum electrolyte levels with ECG changes.

Serum lipids are associated with vascular disease, particularly CAD. Cholesterol and triglycerides bound to plasma proteins are found in the blood as lipoproteins. Density levels vary according to the protein-fat ratio. Serum lipids are associated with risk of cardiovascular disease. An elevated high-density lipoprotein (HDL) is desired, but low-density lipoprotein (LDL) or very-low-density lipoprotein (VLDL) increases the risk for cardiovascular disease (Box 8-1).

Arterial blood gases monitor oxygenation (Pao_2, $Paco_2$) and acid-base balance (pH). This test is useful in patients with unstable cardiac conditions to determine the blood oxygenation process and for evaluation of patients in cardiac failure.

Serum cardiac markers are certain proteins that are released into the blood in large quantities from necrotic heart muscle after a myocardial infarction (MI). These markers, specifically cardiac serum enzymes and troponin I, are important screening diagnostic criteria for an acute MI. The cardiac enzyme creatine kinase (CK) and its isoenzyme, creatine phosphokinase (CK-MB), have been the gold standard for years. However, CK-MB is also found in skeletal muscle and can be elevated by surgery, muscle trauma, and muscular diseases, so it is not a specific indicator for MI. CK and CK-MB start to rise within 2 to 3 hours after the beginning of an MI, peak in 24 hours, and return to normal within 24 to 40 hours (Nagle, 2002). When cardiac cells die, their cellular enzymes are released into circulation. The increase in serum enzymes that occurs after cellular death can demonstrate whether cardiac damage is present and the approximate extent of the damage. Other causes of increased serum enzymes may make the differential diagnosis more difficult.

Troponin I is a myocardial muscle protein released into circulation after a myocardial injury. In the heart there are two subtypes: cardiac-specific troponin T and troponin I. Cardiac troponin T and troponin I are sensitive markers that identify very small amounts of myocardial damage. Troponin T appears in the blood 3 to 5 hours after MI and may remain elevated for up to 21 days. Similar to CK-MB, troponin T is affected by skeletal muscle injury and renal disease. Troponin I is a very sensitive and specific cardiac marker, not influenced by skeletal muscle trauma or renal failure. Troponin I rises 3 hours after MI, peaks at 14 to 18 hours, and returns to normal in 5 to 7 days. Troponin I is very useful in diagnosing an MI (Nagle, 2002). The recent ability to measure myocardial contractile proteins (troponins) in serum is a milestone in the diagnosis of acute MI and acute myocardial damage resulting from other etiologies.

Myoglobin is released into circulation within only a few hours after an MI. Although it is one of the first serum cardiac markers that increases after an MI, it lacks cardiac specificity. Myoglobin is also present in skeletal muscle, so an increase can also be associated with noncardiac causes. In addition, it is rapidly excreted in urine so that blood levels return to normal range within 24 hours after an MI.

B-type natriuretic peptide (BNP) is a neurohormone secreted by the heart in response to ventricular expansion. An elevated BNP greater than 100 pg/mL indicates some heart failure. See p. 362 for detailed description of BNP.

Homocysteine is an amino acid produced during protein digestion. Normal values range from 4 to 14 Umol/L. Increasing evidence suggests that elevated blood levels of homocysteine may act as an independent risk factor for ischemic heart disease, cerebrovascular disease, peripheral arterial disease, and venous thrombosis. Homocysteine appears to promote the progression of atherosclerosis by causing endothelial damage, promoting LDL deposits, and promoting vascular smooth muscle growth. Screening for elevated homocysteine levels (levels greater than 15 μmol/L) should be considered in individuals with progressive and unexplained atherosclerosis despite normal lipoproteins and in the absence of other risk factors. It is also recommended in patients with an unusual family history of atherosclerosis, especially at a young age.

Dietary deficiency of vitamins B_6, B_{12}, or folate is the most common cause of elevated homocysteine. Some researchers believe that elevated levels of homocysteine can be treated by administration of vitamins B_6, B_{12}, and folate. Whether this treatment will reduce the incidence of myocardial infarction remains to be seen (Pagana & Pagana, 2003).

DISORDERS OF THE CARDIOVASCULAR SYSTEM

Cardiovascular disorders continue to be a major health care problem in the United States. Public awareness, modifications in lifestyles, and improvements in medical treatment have contributed to a decline in overall deaths in the past 20 years. The nurse's role in caring for patients with cardiovascular disorders includes an awareness of the prevalence of cardiac disease, knowledge of risk factors and the disease process, implementation of nursing interventions, and patient teaching.

NORMAL AGING PATTERNS

By the time an individual reaches the age of 65 years, any number of physiologic changes have reduced the efficiency of the heart as a pump. Yet the heart still is very capable of functioning adequately unless there is underlying cardiac disease (Older Adult Considerations box).

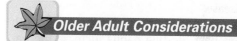

⭐ *Older Adult Considerations*

Cardiac Disease

- Changes in the cardiac musculature lead to reduced efficiency and strength, resulting in decreased cardiac output.
- Disorientation, syncope, and decreased tissue perfusion to organs and other body tissues can occur as a result of decreased cardiac output.
- Aging causes sclerotic changes in blood vessels and leads to decreased elasticity and narrowing of the lumen. Arterial pathology resulting from the aging process causes hypertension because of the increased cardiac effort needed to pump blood through the circulatory system.
- Progressive coronary artery changes can lead to the development of collateral coronary circulation. This can modify the severity of signs and symptoms seen in MI. Angina symptoms may be less pronounced, and dyspnea may replace angina as a key symptom of acute infarction.
- Heart failure can result from rapid intravenous infusion.
- Edema secondary to heart failure may cause tissue impairment in the immobile older adult. Immobility leads to venous stasis, venous ulcer, and poor wound healing. It also increases the risk of venous thrombosis and embolus formation.
- Older adults with cardiac disease often receive several medications, which are often prescribed at lower doses than for younger adults. Even with lower doses of medications, the older adult should be observed closely for signs of toxicity, because the rate of drug metabolism and excretion decreases with age.
- Independent older adults with cardiac conditions should receive adequate teaching regarding medication, diet, and warning signs of complications. They should be encouraged to maintain regular contact with the physician and to seek care at the first sign of problems.

RISK FACTORS

Risk factors have been identified through research methods that indicate predispositions to developing cardiovascular disease. An accumulation of more than one risk factor is indicative of increasing risk for developing cardiovascular disease. Risk factors are classified as those that are nonmodifiable and those that are modifiable.

Nonmodifiable Factors

An important aspect of caring for the patient with a cardiovascular disorder is understanding the risk factors for cardiovascular disease and incorporating them into patient teaching. The nonmodifiable risk factors associated with cardiovascular disorders include the following:

Family history. Familial tendency to develop cardiovascular disease has been documented in the literature. A family member such as a parent or sibling who has a cardiovascular problem before 50 years of age places the patient at greater risk for developing cardiovascular disease.

Age. Normal physiological changes that occur with aging as well as past lifestyle habits increase the patient's risk for developing cardiovascular disease with advancing age. Approximately 50% of all myocardial infarctions (MIs, or heart attacks) occur in people over the age of 65.

Sex. Men are at a greater risk of developing cardiovascular disease than women. Women are affected following menopause because of the decrease in estrogen. The incidence of cardiovascular disease in women 50 years of age and older is increasing. Factors believed to be responsible are increased social and economic pressures on women and changes in lifestyle, including an increased incidence of smoking, use of oral contraceptives, and more women in the workforce. Within the nursing and medical professions, there is a growing awareness of women's increased risk factors.

Cultural and ethnic considerations. African-American males have a higher incidence of hypertension than do whites.

Modifiable Factors

Smoking. Individuals who smoke have a two to three times greater risk of developing cardiovascular disease. This is proportional to the number of cigarettes smoked. Individuals who quit smoking decrease their risk. The nicotine content of cigarettes causes vasoconstriction and the production of carbon monoxide, which place a greater demand on the heart and interfere with oxygen supply.

Hyperlipidemia. Hyperlipidemia is elevated concentrations of any or all lipids in the plasma. The ratio of high-density lipoproteins (HDL) to LDL is the best predictor for the development of cardiovascular disease. Density levels vary according to the protein-fat ratio:

VLDL (very-low-density lipoprotein) contains more fat than protein (primarily triglycerides); triglycerides are the main storage form of lipids and constitute approximately 95% of fatty tissue

LDL (low-density lipoprotein) contains an equal amount of fat and protein (approximately 50%) with moderate amounts of phospholipids cholesterol

Less than 100 mg/dL	Optimal
100 to 129 mg/dL	Near optimal/ above optimal
130 to 159 mg/dL	Borderline high
160 to 189 mg/dL	High
More than 190 mg/dL	Very high

HDL (high-density lipoprotein) contains more protein than fat (serves a protective function, removing cholesterol from tissues). It is suspected that the purpose of HDL is to remove cholesterol from the peripheral tissues and transport it to the liver for excretion. Also, HDL may have a protective effect by preventing cellular uptake of cholesterol and lipids. Low levels (less than 40 mg/dL) are believed to increase a person's risk for CAD, whereas high levels (more than 60 mg/dL) are considered protective (Box 8-1).

A diet high in saturated fat, cholesterol, and calories contributes to hyperlipidemia. Therefore dietary control is an important factor in modifying this risk factor. An overall serum cholesterol level of less than 200 mg/dL is desirable, 200 to 239 mg/dL is borderline high; more than 239 mg/dL is high.

Change in diet is probably the most important method of lowering cholesterol level. Weight reduction, in overweight patients with abnormal lipid profiles, is an essential element of the dietary intervention. In addition to lowering LDL levels, weight reduction leads to a decrease in triglyceride level and blood pressure. A combination of weight reduction and physical exercise has been shown to lend to an improvement in the lipid profile, with a decrease in LDL level, an increase in HDL level, and a decrease in triglyceride levels. Low HDL levels are often familial and only somewhat modifiable.

Cholesterol-lowering drugs are often included in treatment of hyperlipidemia. Cholesterol-lowering drugs are divided into five main groups: bile acid sequestrants, nicotinic acid (niacin), statins such as simvastatin (Zocor), pravastatin (Pravachol), rosuvastatin (Crestor), and fibric acid derivatives such as gemfibrozil (Lopid) and probucol (Lorelco). Pravastatin (Pravachol) reduces the risk of a first MI by about a third in hypercholesterolemic patients with no history of coronary disease. Simvastatin is now allowed by the U.S. Food and Drug Administration (FDA) to add a label statement that states that the drug can reduce deaths by lowering cholesterol.

Hypertension. Hypertension is blood pressure higher than 140/90 mm Hg, which increases an individual's risk of developing cardiovascular dis-

Box 8-1   *Cholesterol Numbers: What Do They Mean?*

YOUR TOTAL CHOLESTEROL NUMBER

A total cholesterol level less than 200 is considered desirable.

HDL CHOLESTEROL NUMBER

The higher the HDL cholesterol level the better, because this means that there are more good lipoproteins to remove adhered cholesterol from the arteries.

LDL CHOLESTEROL NUMBER

The higher the number of bad lipoproteins or LDLs in the blood, the more likely cholesterol is beginning to adhere to the arteries.

TOTAL CHOLESTEROL

Desirable Less than 200
Borderline 200 to 239
High 240 or greater

HDL CHOLESTEROL

Less than 40 low
Greater than 60 high

LDL CHOLESTEROL

Desirable The higher the serum LDL cholesterol level, the more likely cholesterol is beginning to adhere to the arteries. Risk factors must be monitored to assess for probability of development of heart disease. The table below matches risk factors with LDL cholesterol levels.

LDL Cholesterol
Less than 100, optimal
100-129, near optimal/above optimal
130-159, borderline high
160-189, high
Greater than 190, very high

SET LDL CHOLESTEROL GOAL

Once one knows the LDL cholesterol number one can change the diet to help lower the amount of cholesterol in the blood. The table below shows what the target LDL cholesterol goal should be. Reducing the risk factors is important too, so health care providers must make recommendations to assist the patient to maintain acceptable cholesterol levels.

Risk Factors	Start Diet Treatment if LDL Cholesterol:	The LDL Goal is:
No heart disease and fewer than two risk factors other than high LDL cholesterol	**160** or more	Less than **160**
No heart disease but two or more risk factors other than high LDL cholesterol	**130** or more	Less than **130**
Definite heart disease or arterial disease	**100** or more	**100** or less

Modified from the Third Report of National Cholesterol Education Program (NCEP) Expert Panel on Detection, Evaluation and Treatment of High Blood Cholesterol in Adults, 2001.

ease. Adhering to medical therapy for control of elevated blood pressure helps to modify the individual's risk.

Diabetes mellitus. Cardiac disease has been found to be more prevalent in individuals with diabetes mellitus. This is thought to be related to elevated blood glucose levels, which cause damage to the arterial intima and contribute to atherosclerosis. Diabetic patients also have alterations in lipid metabolism and tend to have high cholesterol and triglyceride levels. Adherence to medical therapy for regulating blood glucose levels helps to modify the individual's risk.

Obesity. Excess body weight increases the workload of the heart. It also contributes to the severity of other risk factors. A weight-reduction program and maintenance of an ideal body weight help to modify the individual's risk.

Sedentary lifestyle. Lack of regular exercise has been correlated with increased risk of developing cardiovascular disease. Regular aerobic exercise can improve the heart's efficiency as well as contribute to lowering blood glucose levels, improving the ratio of HDLs to LDLs, reducing weight, lowering the blood pressure, reducing stress, and improving overall feelings of well-being. Some practitioners define regular physical exercise as exercise that occurs at least three to five times a week for at least 30 minutes, causing perspiration and an increase in heart rate (HR) by 30 to 50 beats per minute (BPM). Walking is one of the best forms of exercise.

Stress. The stress response of the body releases catecholamines that increase the heart rate. Catecholamines also affect myocardial cells and may result in cellular damage. The vasoconstriction that thus occurs may be a contributing factor to developing cardiovascular disease. Stress reduction measures may be important in modifying an individual's risk.

Oral contraceptives. The use of oral contraceptives has been linked to the development of cardiovascular disease. The relationship has not been clearly identified. Oral contraceptive use in conjunction with other risk factors is not recommended.

Psychosocial factors. The coronary-prone, or type A, personality has been demonstrated to be more characteristic of people who will develop CAD. The characteristics of type A personality trait include aggressiveness, competitiveness, perfectionism, compulsiveness, and an urgent sense of time. When the type A personality is combined with other risk factors such as age, high lipid levels, and smoking, the risk of heart disease increases.

CARDIAC DYSRHYTHMIAS

A dysrhythmia or arrhythmia refers to any cardiac rhythm that deviates from normal sinus rhythm. Normal sinus rhythm originates in the sinoatrial (SA) node and is characterized by the following:

- Rate: 60 to 100 beats/minute
- P waves: precede each QRS complex—atrial depolarization
- P-R interval: interval between atrial and ventricular repolarization
- QRS complex: ventricular depolarization
- T wave: ventricular repolarization
- Rhythm: regular

A dysrhythmia is the result of an alteration in the formation of impulses through the SA node to the rest of the myocardium. It also results from irritability of myocardial cells that generate impulses, which is independent of the conduction system. Signs and symptoms of dysrhythmia vary, as does treatment, depending on the type and severity of the dysrhythmia. A short overview of each dysrhythmia follows.

Types of Cardiac Dysrhythmias

Sinus tachycardia. Sinus tachycardia is a rapid, regular rhythm originating in the SA. It is characterized by a heartbeat of 100 to 150 or more per minute.

Causes of sinus tachycardia may include exercise, anxiety, fever, shock, medications, hypothermia, heart failure, excessive caffeine, and tobacco use. Tachycardia acts to increase the amount of oxygen delivered to the cells of the body by increasing the amount of blood circulated through the vessels.

Clinical manifestations include occasional palpitations. Many patients are asymptomatic. Other signs and symptoms may include hypotension and angina, if cardiovascular disease is also present.

Medical management is directed at the primary cause. This is a normal rhythm and is not usually caused by a cardiac problem.

Sinus bradycardia. Sinus bradycardia is a slow rhythm originating in the SA node. It is characterized by a pulse rate of fewer than 60 beats per minute. Some sources use a rate of 50 or less as an indication of bradycardia. Causes of sinus bradycardia may include sleep, vomiting, intracranial tumors, MI, drugs (especially patients who are in digitalis toxicity), vagal stimulation, endocrine disturbances, and hypothermia. When found in association with MI, it is a beneficial rhythm because it reduces myocardial oxygen demand. This may be a normal rate and rhythm for an athlete.

Clinical manifestations include fatigue, lightheadedness, and syncope. Some patients are asymptomatic.

Medical management is directed toward the primary cause of the problem and maintaining cardiac output. Atropine may be prescribed to increase the heart rate. A temporary or permanent implantable pacemaker is sometimes necessary (Figures 8-8 and 8-9).

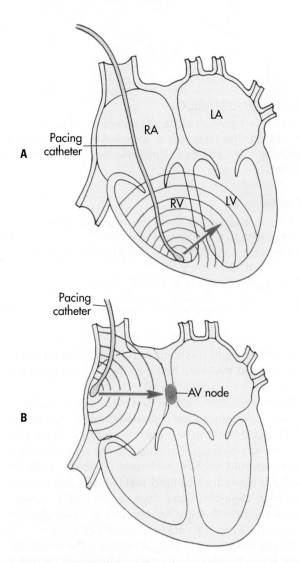

FIGURE **8-8 A,** Ventricular pacing. Impulses are initiated in ventricle. **B,** Atrial pacing. Impulses are initiated in atrium and travel to ventricles by normal conduction system through the AV node.

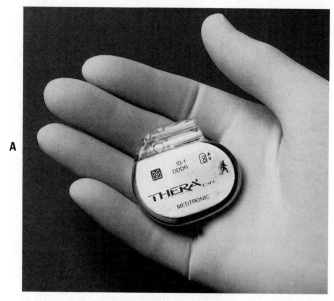

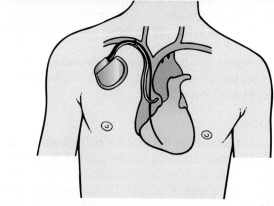

FIGURE 8-9 **A,** A dual-chamber, rate-responsive pacemaker (shown here actual size) from Medtronic, Inc., is designed to detect body movement and automatically increase or decrease paced heart rates based on the level of physical activity. **B,** Cardiac leads, in both the atrium and ventricle, enable a dual-chamber pacemaker to sense and pace in both heart chambers.

Supraventricular tachycardia. Supraventricular tachycardia (SVT) is the sudden onset of a rapid heartbeat. It originates in the atria. It is characterized by a pulse rate of 150 to 250 beats per minute.

Causes of premature atrial tachycardia include drugs, alcohol, mitral valve prolapse, emotional stress, smoking, and hormone imbalance. The cause is typically not associated with heart disease.

Clinical manifestations include palpitations, light-headedness, dyspnea, and anginal pain.

Medical management first looks at how well the patient tolerates the dysrhythmia and at the overall clinical picture. Then the focus is aimed at decreasing the heart rate and eliminating the underlying cause. Specific treatments may include carotid sinus pressure, adenosine (Adenocard), digitalis, calcium channel blockers, propranolol, beta-adrenergic blockers, amniodarone (Cordarone), quinidine, and cardioversion. Persistent,

recurring SVT may ultimately be treated with radiofrequency catheter ablation of the accessory pathway.

Atrial fibrillation. In atrial fibrillation, electrical activity in the atria is disorganized, causing the atria to fibrillate or quiver rather than contract as a unit. Atrial fibrillation is a very rapid production of atrial impulses. The atria beat chaotically and are not contracting properly. It is characterized by an atrial rate of 350 to 600 beats per minute. If untreated, the ventricular response rate may be 100 to 180 beats per minute.

Causes of atrial fibrillation include cardiac surgery, long-standing hypertension, pulmonary embolism, atherosclerosis, mitral valve disease, HF, cardiomyopathy, congenital abnormalities, chronic obstructive pulmonary disease (COPD), and thyrotoxicosis. Clinical manifestations include pulse deficit, palpitations, dyspnea, angina, lightheadedness, syncope, fatigue, change in level of consciousness, and pulmonary edema. Because of ventricular rhythm irregularity and atrial contractions, decreased cardiac output is noted. Thrombi may form in the atria as a result of ineffective atrial contraction and cause embolisms, thus affecting the lungs or periphery (away from the center of the body). An embolized clot may pass to the brain, causing a stroke. Risk of stroke increases fivefold with atrial fibrillation. Risk of stroke is even higher in patients with structural heart disease, with hypertension, and whose age is over 65 years.

Medical management is focused on treating the irritability of the atria, slowing the ventricular response to atrial stimulation, and correcting the primary cause. The goal of therapy is to prevent atrial thrombi from becoming embolisms in the body, such as in the lungs or periphery. Specific treatments for pharmacologic cardioversion may include digitalis, calcium channel blockers such as IV diltiazem (Cardizem), verapamil (Calan, Isoptin), antidysrhythmics such as procainamide (Procan SR, Pronestyl), amiodarone (Cordarone), quinidine, and anticoagulants such as heparin or warfarin (Coumadin). If pharmacologic cardioversion fails, the patient may need electric cardioversion. The Joint Commission on Accreditation of Healthcare Organizations (JCAHO) recommends that patients with atrial fibrillation be prescribed warfarin at discharge. Cardiac output may be impaired, resulting in heart failure, angina, and shock.

Atrioventricular block. Atrioventricular block occurs when a defect in the AV junction slows or impairs conduction of impulses from the SA node to the ventricles. Three types of blocks are seen: first degree, second degree, and third degree. The third-degree block indicates a worsening of the impairment in the AV junction and a complete heart block.

Common causes of AV block include atherosclerotic heart disease, MI, and CHF. Other causes may be digitalis toxicity, congenital abnormality, drugs, and hypokalemia.

Clinical manifestations include no symptoms for first-degree block; vertigo, weakness, and irregular pulse for second-degree block; and hypotension, angina, bradycardia, heart rate often in the 30s, and heart failure for third-degree block.

Medical management evaluates the patient's response and determines the cause of the dysrhythmia. Atropine and isoproterenol may be prescribed. A pacemaker frequently is needed with third-degree block (see Figure 8-8).

Premature ventricular contractions. Premature ventricular contractions (PVCs) are abnormal heart beats that arise from the right or left ventricle. PVCs are early ventricular beats that occur in conjunction with the underlying rhythm. The characteristics of the underlying rhythm remain the same except for the PVC itself and the regularity of the rhythm.

PVCs may originate from more than one location in the ventricles and be caused by irritability of the ventricular musculature, exercise, stress, electrolyte imbalance, digitalis toxicity, hypoxia, and MI.

Clinical manifestations depend on the frequency of PVCs and their effect on the ability of the heart to pump blood effectively. Some patients are asymptomatic; others may experience palpitations, weakness, and lightheadedness. Other symptoms are associated with decreased cardiac output.

Medical management focuses on treating the underlying heart condition. Symptomatic premature ventricular contractions can be treated with β-adrenergic blockers, procainamide (Pronestyl), amiodarone (Cordarone), or lidocaine.

PVC may be a single event or may occur several times in a minute or in pairs or strings. PVCs that last long enough to cause ventricular tachycardia may lead to a patient's death.

Ventricular tachycardia. Ventricular tachycardia (VT) occurs when three or more successive PVCs occur. The ventricular rate is greater than 100/minute and usually is 140 to 240. The rhythm is regular or slightly irregular. Conditions that favor its occurrence include hypoxemia, drug toxicity such as digitalis, quinidine, electrolyte imbalance (e.g., potassium magnesium), and bradycardia. Repeated and more prolonged episodes of ventricular tachycardia in the second week after MI may be a forewarning of ventricular fibrillation and require aggressive evaluation and treatment.

Medical management is focused on intravenously administered procainamide (Pronestyl) or amiodarone (Cordarone), because these drugs depress excitability of cardiac muscle to electrical stimulation and slow conduction in the atria, bundle of His, and ventricles. Lidocaine (Xylocaine) is used only if acute myocardial ischemia or MI is considered to be the cause of VT. If pharmacological measures are unsuccessful, the alternative is cardioversion. Catheter ablation can be helpful. Ongoing VT suppression is obtained with oral beta-adrenergic blockers or calcium channel blockers.

Ventricular fibrillation. Ventricular fibrillation occurs when the ventricular musculature of the heart is quivering. This medical emergency is characterized by rapid and disorganized ventricle pulsation.

The cause is usually myocardial ischemia or infarction. Other causes are untreated ventricular tachycardia, electrolyte imbalances, digitalis or quinidine toxicity, and hypothermia. It may also occur with coronary reperfusion after thrombolytic therapy.

Clinical manifestations are the result of no cardiac output and include loss of consciousness, lack of a pulse, loss of blood pressure and respirations, possible seizures, and sudden death if untreated.

Medical management is focused on providing emergency treatment, including CPR, defibrillation (the termination of ventricular fibrillation by delivering a direct electrical countershock to the patient's precordium), and medications such as lidocaine or procainamide. Defibrillation is the most effective method of terminating ventricular fibrillation and should ideally be performed within 15 to 20 seconds of the onset of the dysrhythmia.

If ventricular fibrillation is not terminated rapidly with defibrillation, brain damage will occur because of the lack of blood flow.

Assessment

Collection of **subjective data** for the patient with a cardiac dysrhythmia includes observing for symptoms associated with the specific dysrhythmia. Symptoms may include palpitations, skipped beats, nausea, lightheadedness, vertigo, anxiety, dyspnea, fatigue, and chest discomfort.

Collection of **objective data** includes immediate visual observation of the patient when ECG monitoring indicates a dysrhythmia. Signs may include syncope, irregular pulse, tachycardia, and tachypnea. Noting the patient's response to the dysrhythmia is important to plan and implement appropriate nursing interventions. Vital signs and observation for signs of decreased cardiac output should be noted.

Diagnostic Tests

ECG monitoring, telemetry, and Holter monitoring are commonly used to confirm the diagnosis of cardiac dysrhythmias.

Medical Management

Treatment varies according to the type of cardiac dysrhythmia. See the Medications table for cardiac dysrhythmias.

Nursing Interventions and Patient Teaching

Nursing interventions focus on symptomatic relief, promotion of comfort, relief of anxiety, emergency action as needed, and patient teaching.

Assess the apical (*not* radial) pulse to obtain an accurate pulse rate when dysrhythmias are present. Be-

MEDICATIONS | *Cardiac Dysrhythmias*

CLASSIFICATION	AGENT	ACTION	NURSING INTERVENTIONS
Cardioglycoside	Digoxin (Lanoxin)	Used to control rapid ventricular rate in atrial fibrillation and to convert paroxysmal supraventricular tachycardia to normal sinus rhythm Increases cardiac force and efficiency, slows heart rate, increases cardiac output	Monitor apical pulse to ensure rate above 60 (call physician if digoxin held) Monitor for digitalis toxicity (nausea, vomiting, anorexia, dysrhythmias, bradycardia, tachycardia, headache, fatigue, visual disturbance)
Antidysrhythmic	Procainamide (Pronestyl) Lidocaine (IV)	IV solutions are given for severe ventricular dysrhythmias Management by suppressing the impulse that triggers dysrhythmias	Observe for new dysrhythmias, dry mouth, blurred vision, hypotension, nausea, dizziness, visual disturbances Monitor heart rate and BP closely
	Disopyramide (Norpace CR) Procainamide (Pronestyl, Procan SR)	For long-term treatment of premature ventricular contractions and ventricular tachycardia as well as atrial fibrillation	Monitor BP and apical pulse Watch for hypotension, bradycardia, tremors, dizziness, nausea, anorexia
	Quinidine sulfate (Quinidex Extentabs) Adenosine (Adenocard)	Conversion of paroxysmal supraventricular tachycardia (PSVT) to normal sinus rhythm by slowing conduction in AV node and restoring sinus rhythm	Monitor BP and pulse rate Assess patient for headache, dizziness, gastrointestinal complaints, new dysrhythmias. Do not give caffeine within 4 to 6 hours of receiving adenosine, because caffeine inhibits the effect of the drug
	Mexiletine HCl (Mexitil) Propafenone HCl (Rythmol) Tocainide HCl (Tonocard)	Decreases excitability of cardiac muscle	Monitor pulse, BP Monitor for diarrhea, visual disturbances, respiratory distress
Beta-adrenergic blockers	Propranolol (Inderal) Sotalol HCl (Betapace) Acebutolol HCl (Sectral) Esmolol HCl (Brevibloc) Metoprolol (Lopressor) Carvedilol (Coreg)	Used to treat supraventricular and ventricular dysrhythmias, persistent sinus tachycardia Decreases myocardial O$_2$ demand, decreases workload of the heart, decreases heart rate	Monitor heart rate and BP carefully. Use caution with patient with bronchospastic disease Monitor for bradycardia, hypotension, new dysrhythmias, dizziness, headache, nausea, diarrhea, sleep disturbances
Calcium channel blockers	Verapamil (Calan, Isoptin) Diltiazem HCl (Cardizem)	Treat supraventricular tachycardia and control rapid rates in atrial tachycardia Produces relaxation of coronary vascular smooth muscle, dilate coronary arteries	Use caution in patients with CHF Monitor apical pulse and BP Watch for fatigue, headache, dizziness, peripheral edema, nausea, tachycardia Both verapamil and diltiazem increase the toxicity of digoxin
Inotropic agent	Dobutamine (Dobutrex) (IV) Dopamine (Intropin) (IV)	Used in severe CHF with pulmonary edema Increases myocardial contractility Increases cardiac output, increases blood pressure, and improves renal blood flow	Monitor blood pressure, heart rate, urinary output continuously during the administration Palpate peripheral pulses, notify physician if extremities become cold or mottled
Anticoagulant	Warfarin (Coumadin)	Used in treatment of atrial fibrillation with embolization to prevent complication of stroke	Assess patient for signs of bleeding and hemorrhage Monitor prothrombin time (PT) frequently during therapy Review foods high in vitamin K. Patient should have consistently limited intake of these foods because these foods will cause levels to fluctuate

cause the rhythm is irregular, take the apical pulse for 1 minute. Assess level of patient's anxiety and degree of understanding, noting both verbal and nonverbal expressions regarding diagnosis, procedures, and treatments.

Provide explanation for the diagnostic and monitoring devices in use. Nursing interventions include monitoring heart rate and rhythm. Administer antidysrhythmic agents as ordered and monitor response. Maintain quiet environment; administer sedation or analgesic medication as ordered. Administer oxygen per protocol.

Nursing diagnoses and interventions for the patient with cardiac dysrhythmias include but are not limited to the following:

NURSING DIAGNOSES	NURSING INTERVENTIONS
Pain, related to ischemia	Administer medications as ordered.
	Teach relaxation techniques.
	Institute position change and support.
	Administer prescribed oxygen.
Decreased cardiac output, related to cardiac insufficiency	Monitor heart rate and rhythm.
	Reduce cardiac workload by encouraging bed rest.
	Elevate head of bed 30 to 45 degrees for comfort.
	Restrict activities as ordered; plan care to avoid fatigue.
	Administer antidysrhythmic agents as ordered.
	Monitor for signs of drug toxicity.
Ineffective coping, related to fear of and uncertainty about disease process	Assist patient with identifying strengths and coping skills.
	Supply emotional support.
	Teach relaxation techniques.
	Assess level of coping ability and family support level.
	Explain purpose of care as related to specific dysrhythmia.

Explain importance of avoiding or stopping smoking or use of nicotine products. Teach the patient about medication therapy and its purposes, desired effects, and dosage and the side effects to report to the physician. Explain the reason for and method of taking pulse rate and rhythm. Explain the need to exercise to tolerance, to avoid strenuous and/or isometric activity, and to check with the physician regarding limitations and allowances. Instruct the patient regarding energy conservation for activities of daily living (ADLs): regular rest periods between activities and for 1 hour after meals; when possible, sit rather than stand when performing a task; stop activity or task if symptoms such as fatigue, dyspnea, or palpitations begin. Stress management is very important to promote healing and prevent further cardiac events.

CARDIAC ARREST

The sudden cessation of cardiac output and circulatory process is termed **cardiac arrest.** Conditions leading to cardiac arrest are severe ventricular tachycardia, ventricular fibrillation, and ventricular asystole. Because of the manifestation of anaerobic tissue cell metabolism and respiratory and metabolic acidosis caused by the absence of O_2–CO_2 exchange, immediate initiation of cardiopulmonary resuscitation (CPR) is indicated to prevent major organ damage. Signs and symptoms of cardiac arrest include abrupt loss of consciousness with no response to stimuli, gasping respirations followed by apnea, absence of pulse (radial, carotid, femoral, and apical), absence of blood pressure, pupil dilation, and development of pallor and cyanosis.

Initiation of CPR is done by the first person to discover the condition. The aim is to reestablish circulation and ventilation. Prevention of severe damage to the brain, heart, liver, and kidneys as a result of anoxia is of primary concern. The *ABCs* of CPR should be remembered: **A**—open *Airway*; **B**—restore *Breathing*; and **C**—restore *Circulation*. Resuscitation measures are divided into two components: basic cardiac life support (BCLs) in the form of CPR and advanced cardiac life support (ACLS).

Advanced cardiac life support involves a systematic approach to treatment of cardiac emergencies with knowledge and skills necessary to provide early treatment. ACLS includes (1) basic life support; (2) the use of adjunctive equipment and special techniques for establishing and maintaining effective ventilation and circulation; (3) ECG monitoring and dysrhythmia recognition; (4) establishment therapies for emergency treatment of patient with cardiac or respiratory arrest; and (5) treatment of patient with suspected acute MI.

Artificial Cardiac Pacemakers

Pacemakers are battery-operated generators that initiate and control the heart rate by delivering an electrical impulse via an electrode to the myocardium. These catheter-like electrodes are placed within the area to be paced: right atrium, right ventricle, or both (see Figures 8-8 and 8-9). External pacemakers deliver impulses to the myocardium through electrode pads placed on the chest wall, which deliver small electrical shocks at an adjustable rate.

A pacemaker maintains a regular cardiac rhythm by electrically stimulating the heart muscle. It is used when patients experience adverse symptoms because of dysrhythmias that cannot be managed by medications alone. These include second- and third-degree AV block, **bradydysrhythmias** (slow and/or irregular heartbeat) and **tachydysrhythmias** (rapid heartbeat that can be regular or irregular).

An external pacemaker is used in emergency situations on a short-term basis, because the shock can be quite uncomfortable. Temporary pacemakers are used for cardiac support following some MIs or open-heart surgery. A permanent pacemaker is placed when other measures have failed to convert the dysrhythmia or conduction problem. The batteries used in permanent pacemakers today are very small, weighing less than an ounce, and can last 15 years or more.

Nursing Interventions and Patient Teaching

After placement of a pacemaker, the nurse closely monitors heart rate and rhythm by apical pulse and by ECG patterns. Vital signs and level of consciousness are checked frequently until stable. The insertion site is observed for erythema, edema, and tenderness, which could indicate the presence of infection. The patient may be on bed rest with the arm on the pacemaker side immobilized for the first few hours, advised to refrain from raising arm above the head for several days, and then allowed to resume normal activity.

The patient should be informed of the necessity to continue medical management, and the nurse should advise that medic-alert identification as well as pacemaker information should be carried. The nurse should emphasize the importance of reporting signs and symptoms of pacemaker failure: weakness, vertigo, chest pain, and pulse changes.

The patient should be taught potentially hazardous situations to avoid. Each pacemaker manufacturer can provide a list of devices that should be avoided by patients with pacemakers. The patient should be told to avoid holding electrical equipment (such as hair dryers or battery-operated toothbrushes) next to the pacemaker. Avoid proximity to high-output electrical generators or to large magnets such as an MRI scanner. This may cause interference, placing the pacemaker in a fixed mode and interfering with its functioning. The patient should be taught to move away from any device that may cause untoward symptoms such as vertigo.

The heart rate of the pulse generator for the pacemaker is set according to the clinical condition of the patient and the desired therapeutic goal. With rare exceptions, the rate is set between 70 and 80 beats per minute. If the heart rate falls below the preset level, notify the physician.

The nurse teaches the patient how and when to take a radial pulse. The pulse should be taken at the same time each day as well as when symptoms of vertigo or weakness occur. The following are important to remember when teaching the patient with a pacemaker:
- List symptoms to expect and to report to physician.
- Promote understanding of medication administration.
- Explain treatment outcomes.
- Explain importance of maintaining prescribed diet and fluid amounts.
- Explain importance of not smoking.

Prognosis

The patient can expect to lead a reasonably normal life with full resumption of most activities as prescribed by the physician.

DISORDERS OF THE HEART

CORONARY ATHEROSCLEROTIC HEART DISEASE

The coronary arteries arise from the base of the aorta just below the semilunar valves (see Figure 8-6). These arteries curve and angle in an attempt to adequately supply the heart muscle with oxygen and nutrients. The shapes, contours, and arrangements of the vessels allow for easy entrapment of substances that interfere with blood flow.

Coronary artery disease (CAD) is the term used to describe a variety of conditions that obstruct blood flow in the coronary arteries. Atherosclerosis (a common arterial disorder characterized by yellowish plaques of cholesterol, lipids, and cellular debris in the inner layers of the walls of large and medium-size arteries) is the primary cause of atherosclerotic heart disease (ASHD). The **lumen** (a cavity or channel within any organ of the body) of the vessel narrows as the disease progresses. Blood flow to the heart is obstructed when this process occurs in the coronary arteries.

Atherosclerosis, the basic underlying disease affecting coronary lumen size, is characterized by changes in the intimal (the innermost layer of a structure, such as the lining membrane of an artery) lining of the arteries. The severity of the disease is measured by the degree of obstruction within each artery and by the number of vessels involved. Obstructions exceeding 75% of the lumen of one or more of the three coronary arteries increase the risk of death.

The basic physiologic changes of the atherosclerotic process result in problems with myocardial oxygen supply and demand. When the myocardial oxygen demand exceeds the supply delivered by the coronary arteries, ischemia results (Figure 8-10). The artery walls also become less elastic and less responsive to blood flow (Cultural and Ethnic Considerations box).

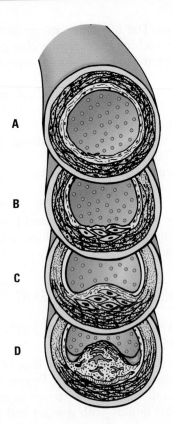

FIGURE **8-10** Progressive development of coronary atherosclerosis. **A,** Injury to intimal wall. **B,** Lipoprotein invasion of smooth muscle cells. **C,** Development of fatty streak and fibrous plaque. **D,** Development of complicated lesion.

ANGINA PECTORIS
Etiology/Pathophysiology

Angina means a spasmodic, cramplike, choking feeling. Pectoris refers to the breast or chest area. Angina pectoris is used to denote the paroxysmal (marked, usually episodic, increase in symptoms) thoracic pain and choking feeling caused by decreased oxygen or anoxia (lack of oxygen) of the myocardium.

Angina pectoris occurs when the cardiac muscle is deprived of oxygen. Atherosclerosis of the coronary arteries is the most common cause. The narrowed lumina of the coronary arteries are unable to deliver enough oxygen-rich blood to the myocardium. When the myocardial oxygen demand exceeds the supply, ischemia (decreased blood supply to a body organ or part, often marked by pain and organ dysfunction) of the heart muscle occurs, resulting in chest pain or angina. Typically angina occurs with an increased cardiac workload brought on by exposure to intense cold, exercise, unusually heavy meals, emotional stress, or any other strenuous activity.

CAD is the nation's number one killer. Many people who die from the disease, however, experience several episodes of unstable angina first. If unstable angina were accurately diagnosed and promptly managed,

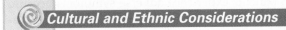

Cardiovascular Disorder

- White, middle-aged men have the highest incidence of coronary artery disease.
- African-Americans, Puerto Ricans, Cubans, and Mexican-Americans have a higher incidence of hypertension than white Americans.
- African-Americans have an early age of onset of CAD.
- African-American women have a higher incidence of CAD than white women.
- American Indians younger than 35 years of age have a heart disease mortality rate twice as high as other Americans.
- Hispanics have a lower death rate from heart disease than non-Hispanics.
- Major modifiable cardiovascular risk factors for American Indians are obesity and diabetes mellitus.

many deaths and much of the disability associated with CAD could be avoided.

Unstable angina is defined as an unpredictable and transient episode of severe and prolonged discomfort that appears at rest, has never been experienced before, or is considerably worse than previous episodes. It mimics an MI in that the discomfort it causes is often described as tightness or a crushing sensation in the chest, arms, back, neck, or jaw. For some patients, unstable angina is a red flag that an MI will occur.

Clinical Manifestations

Pain is the outstanding characteristic of angina pectoris (Figure 8-11). The patient usually describes the pain as a heaviness or tightness of the chest. At times it is thought to be indigestion. The pain is often substernal (below the sternum) or retrosternal (behind the sternum). Pain may radiate to other sites, or it may occur in only one site. The pain often radiates down the left inner arm to the little finger and also upward to the shoulder and jaw. It may also be described as a pressure or a squeezing sensation, but it is not usually described as a sharp pain. Sometimes a patient will experience posterior thoracic or jaw pain only. Other signs and symptoms may accompany the episode of chest pain, such as dyspnea, anxiety, apprehension, diaphoresis, and nausea. The signs and symptoms of angina are often very similar to those of MI. Anginal pain is believed to be a temporary lack of oxygen and blood supply to the heart. It is often relieved by rest or medication such as nitroglycerin, which dilates the coronary arteries and increases the flow of oxygenated blood to the myocardium. Nitroglycerin administered sublingually usually relieves angina symptoms but does not relieve the pain from an MI. This is often used as a preliminary diagnostic tool to quickly differentiate angina from an MI.

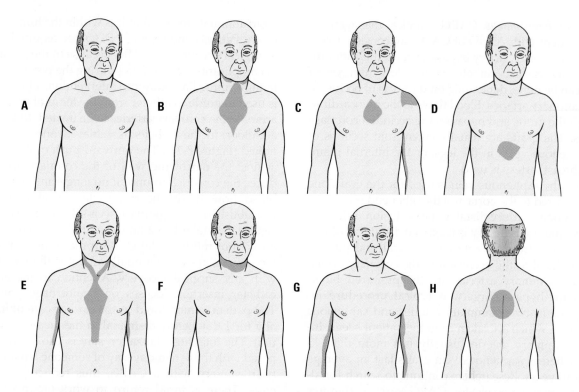

FIGURE **8-11** Sites to which ischemic myocardial pain may be referred. **A,** Upper chest. **B,** Beneath sternum radiating to neck and jaw. **C,** Beneath sternum radiating down left arm. **D,** Epigastric. **E,** Epigastric radiating to neck, jaw, and arms. **F,** Neck and jaw. **G,** Left shoulder and inner aspect of both arms. **H,** Intrascapular.

Assessment

Collection of **subjective data** includes noting the patient's statements regarding the location, intensity, radiation, and duration of pain. The patient may express a feeling of impending death. Precipitating factors that resulted in the development of symptoms should be assessed. Determine what relief measures have been used. Identify whether there have been any changes in the frequency or severity of symptoms that might indicate a progressive worsening of the ischemia.

Collection of **objective data** includes noting the patient's behavior, such as rubbing the left arm or pressing a fist against the sternum. Monitor vital signs and note changes or abnormalities. Increases in pulse rate, blood pressure, and respiratory rate may be noted. Identify the presence of diaphoresis or anxiety.

Diagnostic Tests

The diagnosis of angina pectoris is frequently made on the basis of the patient's history.

The electrocardiogram may reveal findings of ischemia and rhythm changes. Holter monitoring is used to correlate activity with precipitating factors. The exercise stress test is used to determine ischemic changes in a controlled environment. Thallium 201 scanning and PET are used to diagnose ischemic heart disease. Electrocardiogram changes are monitored while the patient exercises on a treadmill. Coronary angiography may be done to determine the extent of CAD.

Medical Management

The focus of medical management is to control symptoms by reducing cardiac ischemia. Cardiovascular risk factors are identified and corrected if possible. Precipitating factors—such as exposure to intense cold, strenuous exercise, smoking, heavy meals, and emotional stress—are identified and avoided. Antiplatelet aggregation therapy is a first-line treatment of angina. Aspirin is the drug of choice. Recent studies indicate that up to a 50% reduction in unstable angina progression to MI occurs with the use of aspirin. Aspirin, even in low doses (81 mg), is effective in inhibiting platelet aggregation. For patients unable to tolerate aspirin, ticlopidine (Ticlid) or clopidogrel (Plavix) may be given (Lewis et al, 2004). Medication therapy to dilate coronary arteries and decrease the workload of the heart consists of vasodilators (nitrates, especially nitroglycerin), beta-adrenergic blocking agents such as propranolol (Inderal), metoprolol (Lopressor), nadolol (Corgard), atenolol (Tenormin), and timolol (Blocadren), and calcium channel blockers such as nifedipine (Procardia), verapamil (Calan, Isoptin), diltiazem (Cardizem), and nicardipine (Cardene). If angina is present, give nitroglycerin sublingually. Repeat dose in 5 minutes if pain does not subside. Repeat two or three times at 5-minute intervals. Call physician if pain has not subsided after third nitroglycerin tablet. High-risk, unstable angina patients should be given supplemental oxygen.

Surgical interventions. **CABG.** Surgical management of the patient with ASHD of CAD may consist of performing a coronary artery bypass graft (CABG) after diagnosis by cardiac catheterization. Any number of grafts can be done, depending on the areas of occlusion in the coronary arteries. Blood flows to the myocardium through the grafts and bypasses the occluded coronary arteries. The grafts are usually taken from sections of the saphenous veins in the legs, or the internal mammary (breast) artery is used.

When the saphenous vein is used for the graft, one end is sutured to the aorta and the other end is sutured to the coronary artery distal to the occlusion. When an internal mammary artery is used, the distal end of this vessel is freed from the anterior chest wall and sutured in place distal to the occlusion in the coronary artery. Internal mammary arteries are the preferred blood vessels for bypass surgery. A typical procedure involves one or two mammary arteries and saphenous vein grafts, which are taken from the patient's legs. Internal mammary arteries usually last more than 15 years, whereas saphenous vein grafts last an average of 5 to 10 years. Researchers continue to search for alternative blood vessels for CABG surgery (Figures 8-12 and 8-13).

PTCA. Another surgical procedure for management of the patient with CAHD is percutaneous transluminal coronary angioplasty (PTCA). PTCA is an invasive procedure performed in the cardiac catheterization laboratory. The technique widens the narrowing in a coronary artery without open heart surgery. "Percutaneous" denotes that the procedure is performed through the skin;

"transluminal" means that it is within the lumen of the artery. Patients undergoing a PTCA are required to sign a surgical permit for a CABG because of the possibility of complications developing during the procedure that require immediate surgical intervention. Fluoroscopy is used to guide a catheter from the femoral or brachial artery to the coronary arteries to be treated. Inflation of a balloon in the catheter is achieved once it is positioned (Figure 8-14). The outward push of the balloon against the narrowing wall of the coronary artery reduces the constriction until it no longer interferes with blood flow to the heart muscle. Vessel patency is reestablished by angioplasty (vessel repair). This procedure may take 1 to 2 hours, with the patient usually awake but mildly sedated. Postprocedure nursing interventions are to continually monitor the patient, as with any surgical recovery. Attention to the area of catheter insertion focuses on hemorrhage potential. The patient is monitored in the cardiac care unit, usually for 1 day before dismissal to the medical-surgical unit. The total hospitalization stay is 1 to 3 days compared with the 4- to 6-day stay of someone having open heart surgery with a CABG, thus reducing hospital costs. There is rapid return to work (approximately 5 to 7 days after PTCA) instead of a 2- to 8-week convalescence after CABG.

Stent placement. Stents are used to treat abrupt or threatened vessel closure following PTCA. Stents are expandable, meshlike structures designed to maintain vessel patency by compressing the arterial walls and resisting vasoconstriction (Figure 8-15). Stents are carefully placed over the angioplasty site to hold the

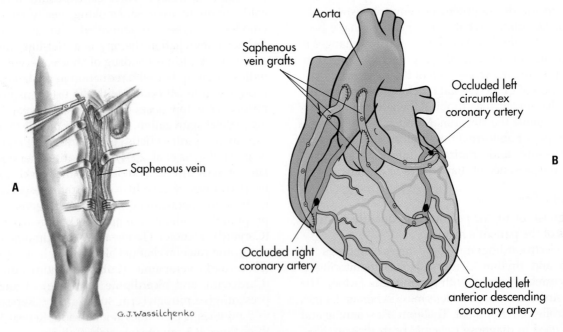

FIGURE **8-12 A,** Saphenous vein. **B,** Saphenous aortocoronary artery bypass or revascularization involves taking a piece of saphenous vein from the leg and creating a conduit for blood from the aorta to the area below the blockage in the coronary artery. A triple bypass is illustrated.

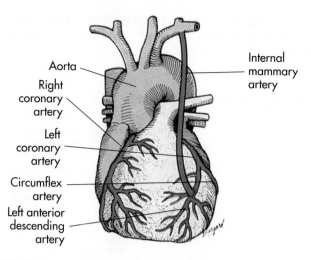

FIGURE **8-13** Coronary artery bypass graft. Internal mammary artery is used; the distal end of this vessel is freed from the anterior chest wall and sutured in place distal to the occlusion in the coronary artery.

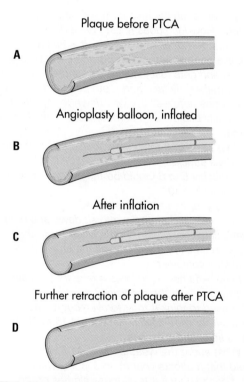

FIGURE **8-14** Percutaneous transluminal coronary angioplasty (PTCA). **A,** Plaque before PTCA. **B,** Inflation of angioplasty balloon. **C,** Plaque after PTCA. **D,** Plaque has retracted even further 6 months after PTCA.

vessel open. Because stents are thrombogenic, the patient must be kept on anticoagulants for at least 3 months. The primary complications from stent placement are hemorrhage and vascular injury. Less common complications are stent thrombosis, acute MI, emergency CABG, and coronary spasms. The possibility of dysrhythmias is always present.

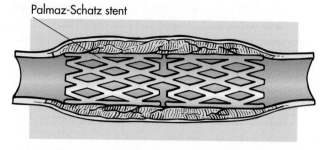

FIGURE **8-15** Palmar-Schatz stent, an articulated stainless steel mesh deployed by balloon inflation.

Nursing Interventions and Patient Teaching

Nursing interventions are based on the individual needs of the patient. They focus on achievement of five major patient outcomes.

1. **Promoting comfort.** Reduce or remove any known factors that are contributing to increased pain. Assess for causes of decreased pain tolerance, such as anxiety, fatigue, or lack of knowledge. Fatigue from increased oxygen demands with a decreased oxygen supply increases pain perception. Promote measures to reduce fatigue, such as providing rest periods. Provide a calm environment to decrease stress and anxiety. Administer sublingual vasodilators, such as nitroglycerin, as ordered. O_2 is administered for high-risk unstable angina patients, as well as those with cyanosis or respiratory distress.

2. **Promoting tissue perfusion.** Instruct patient to avoid becoming overly fatigued and to stop activity immediately in the presence of chest pain, dyspnea, syncope, or vertigo, which indicate low tissue perfusion.

3. **Promoting activity and rest.** Augment (boost or embellish) the patient's activity tolerance by encouraging slower activity or shorter periods of activity with more rest periods. Most people with angina pectoris are able to tolerate mild exercise such as walking or playing golf, but exertion such as running or climbing stairs rapidly causes pain. Anginal pain occurs more easily in cold weather. The key is to avoid overexertion.

4. **Promoting relief of anxiety and feeling of well-being.** Assist the patient to reduce the level of anxiety. The patient should minimize emotional outbursts, worry, and tension. People with angina may need continuing help in accepting situations as they find them. Supportive family members, a spiritual adviser, business associates, and friends can sometimes be of assistance. Relaxation techniques and music therapy may be beneficial to the person with angina pectoris. Support peer groups and behavioral change programs are available. An optimistic outlook helps to relieve the work of the heart. Many people

who learn to live within their limitations live out their expected life span despite the disease.

5. **Teaching patient and family.** Delay teaching until the patient is ready (Therapeutic Dialogue box). The patient needs to be relatively free of pain and excessive anxiety to learn. Promote a positive attitude and active participation of patient and family to encourage compliance. The teaching plan should include information concerning medications, approaches to minimize the events that trigger angina pectoris, effects of exercise on reduction of myocardial oxygen needs, the necessity to stop smoking because of the vasoconstriction of nicotine, and the need for regular medical follow-up (Patient Teaching: Angina Pectoris box).

Nursing diagnoses and interventions for the patient with angina pectoris include but are not limited to the following:

NURSING DIAGNOSES	NURSING INTERVENTIONS
Pain, related to myocardial ischemia	Administer O$_2$ as ordered. Administer prescribed nitroglycerin. Repeat every 5 minutes, three times. If pain is unrelieved, notify physician. Monitor blood pressure and pulse before and after administration of nitroglycerin. Promote rest.

 Therapeutic Dialogue

Mrs. M., a patient with angina, has been admitted for further care, diagnosis, and treatment. After the initial nursing assessment, Nurse G. interviews the patient about the course of her anginal episodes. With the data she gathers, Nurse G. will be able to participate in the development of a program to educate Mrs. M. to minimize or control the attacks.

NURSE: *I would like to ask you some questions, Mrs. M., about the anginal pain you are experiencing.*

PATIENT: *I already told Dr. T. all about those attacks when I visited his office. His nurse, Miss N., has all those records.*

NURSE: *Yes, I know. Your physician has asked us to help you plan a program for preventing or minimizing these attacks. With the information we gather, we can set goals for your care. We can also identify how angina relates to some of your activities.*

PATIENT: *OK, Mrs. G., I would like to understand it better. Perhaps I would be less frightened when it happens. My friend J. told me about her aunt who had angina—she died. That really worries me.*

NURSE: *We hope to decrease some of your fears, Mrs. M., by helping you understand. First, when do your attacks usually occur?*

PATIENT: *Oh, mostly after a real busy day, you know—shopping, or after gardening or housecleaning. But a few times, I had problems after my sister-in-law visited. She and my husband always seem to get into upsetting discussions. They never got along well. She upsets us both—she criticizes everything!*

NURSE: *Have you noticed if a big meal is related to the pain?*

PATIENT: *No, not really . . . well, only when my sister-in-law is there. We hardly ever eat big meals anymore, except when she comes. She expects to be fed well. My husband and I have cut down a lot. Big meals upset our systems—and then her—that harping on old problems and how she thinks we should run our lives! She upsets me so!*

NURSE: *Mrs. M., I think we must talk more on how to handle stressful situations like your sister-in-law. But first,*

could you describe the pain for me: Does it come on suddenly? How long does it last? What does it feel like?

PATIENT: *Oh, no—not all of a sudden. It is just dull at times, like an upset stomach. But then, it travels up in my chest and gets really heavy—like a pressure. Sometimes, it makes my face and teeth hurt; and my arm, too—this one (left)—all the way down to my little finger. If it's a really bad attack, I sometimes feel like I am going to vomit.*

NURSE: *On a scale of 0 to 10, how would you rate most of your angina attacks?*

PATIENT: *Probably 5 to 6 would be the average, but sometimes it's a 10.*

NURSE: *Does your heart beat faster?*

PATIENT: *Oh, yes, and I just have to sit down and be quiet or I can't catch my breath. That's when I take the nitroglycerin. I carry it with me all the time now—in this special little container.*

NURSE: *I see. And how long does it take for the pain to stop after you take the medicine?*

PATIENT: *I used to think it took forever, but my husband—he times it for me—says it lasts about 15 to 20 minutes. I relax a little, and it passes.*

NURSE: *What about the weather, Mrs. M.? Have you noticed that it affects your attacks in any way?*

PATIENT: *I don't know if it is all those clothes or the weather, but I get more pains if I get out in the cold.*

NURSE: *Do you or your husband smoke?*

PATIENT: *Not anymore. I gave up cigarettes when this angina started on me. I noticed the difference, too. Now, I can't even stay in a room if people are smoking. I also cut down on coffee when I retired. Dr. T. said that excessive caffeine isn't good for the angina. All the good things, they have to go when you get old!*

NURSE: *Maybe with some understanding of how certain activities and influences affect your condition, you can find new "good things" for you to enjoy just as much. Soon we will talk again. There are some effective coping methods to decrease your stress when your sister-in-law visits that we can explore.*

NURSING DIAGNOSES	NURSING INTERVENTIONS
	Maintain diet as ordered; if chest pain occurs during eating or immediately after, advise small feedings rather than two or three large meals.
	Balance rest with activity.
	Instruct patient to stop activity at the first sign of chest pain or other symptoms of cardiac ischemia.
Ineffective tissue perfusion, cardiovascular, related to narrowing of coronary arteries	Administer prescribed oxygen.
	Instruct patient that nitroglycerin may need to be taken before exercise and sexual activity to prevent cardiac ischemia.
	Encourage less strenuous or shorter periods of activity interspersed with rest.
	Avoid exercise in cold weather.
	Take prescribed nitroglycerin before activities that will increase the workload of the heart.

Prognosis

The prognosis for the patient with angina pectoris may be grave. Attacks may be intermittent. With early and aggressive management of angina, mortality rate can be reduced and effective management can occur.

MYOCARDIAL INFARCTION
Etiology/Pathophysiology

Myocardial infarction is an occlusion of a major coronary artery or one of its branches with subsequent necrosis of myocardium caused by atherosclerosis or an embolus (a foreign object, a quantity of air or gas, a bit of tissue, or a piece of a thrombus that circulates in the bloodstream until it becomes lodged in a vessel). An obstruction by atherosclerotic process or an embolus may interrupt the blood supply. Coronary occlusion (an obstruction or closing off in a canal, vessel, or passage of the body) is the general term for occlusion of a coronary artery. The occlusion may also be caused by the formation of a thrombus. This is generally referred to as a coronary thrombosis. The occlusion leads to tissue ischemia. Ischemia to the myocardium lasting more than 35 to 45 minutes produces cellular damage and necrosis (Figure 8-16). The ability of the cardiac muscle to contract and pump blood is impaired. The final extent of damage to the surrounding tissues is dependent on the ability to develop collateral circulation. Collateral circulation is the development of new vessels within the heart to compensate for the loss of circulation from the occluded artery. The location of the occlusion and the extent of the tissue damage affect the patient's response to the injury.

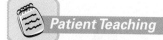 *Patient Teaching*

Angina Pectoris

USE OF NITRATE MEDICATIONS

- Use nitroglycerin prophylactically to avoid pain known to occur with certain activities.
- Burning sensation on tongue indicates nitroglycerin is activated.
- Throbbing sensation in head and flushing may occur.
- Sit and stand slowly after taking nitroglycerin.
- Place nitroglycerin tablets under the tongue at the onset of anginal pain; second tablet can be taken after 5 minutes and third tablet after another 5 minutes if pain is unrelieved.
- Call physician if pain does not subside after third nitroglycerin tablet; go to nearest emergency department; do not drive yourself.
- Always carry nitroglycerin on your person.
- Store nitroglycerin in a dark bottle and keep in a dry place.
- Replenish nitroglycerin supply every 6 months or before expiration date.
- Remove all old nitrate ointment before application of new cream.
- Nitroglycerin patches are placed on patient's skin in the morning and removed at bedtime. This prevents development of tolerance and maintains effectiveness.

WAYS TO MINIMIZE PRECIPITATING EVENTS

- Avoid overexertion.
- Try to reduce stress and anxiety, which cause blood vessels to constrict.
- Avoid overeating, because it places an increased workload on the heart.
- Avoid cold weather (constricts coronary vessels to conserve body heat; hence anginal pain can develop more easily).
- Dress warmly in cold weather.
- Avoid hot, humid conditions (increases workload of the heart).
- Walk downhill and with wind, because walking uphill and against wind increases workload of heart.
- If smoking, cessation is a necessity because of vasoconstriction of arteries from nicotine.

EFFECTS OF EXERCISE PROGRAM IN REDUCTION OF MYOCARDIAL OXYGEN NEEDS

- Engage in a regular exercise program.
- Exercise conditions heart muscle and can decrease oxygen demand during exertion.
- Space exercise period with rest periods.
- Take nitroglycerin before exertion.

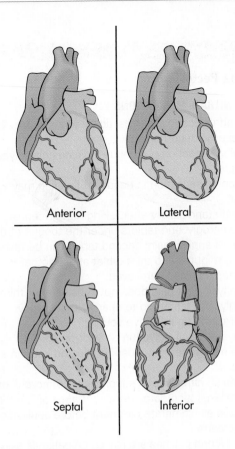

Anterior

Lateral

Septal

Inferior

FIGURE **8-16** Four common locations where myocardial infarctions occur.

The body's response to cell death is the inflammatory process. Within 24 hours, leukocytes infiltrate the area. Enzymes are released from the dead cardiac cells and are important diagnostic indicators. (See the discussion on serum cardiac markers on p. 336.) Phagocytes (neutrophils and monocytes) clear the necrotic debris from the injured area, and by 6 weeks after an MI, scar tissue has replaced necrotic tissue.

Clinical Manifestations

An asymptomatic MI may occur. This is referred to as a silent MI. Many of the symptoms of MI are associated with irreversible ischemia, but they are similar to the signs and symptoms of angina pectoris. The symptoms of an MI are more severe and last longer than those of an angina attack. Pain is the foremost symptom of MI (Box 8-2).

The pain location and radiation to other sites are depicted in Figure 8-11. It is often described as crushing or viselike, an oppressive sensation as though a heavy object is sitting on the chest. The pain is retrosternal (behind the sternum) and in the heart region. It often radiates down the left arm and to the neck, jaws, teeth, and epigastric area. It may occur suddenly, or it may build up over a few minutes. It may occur in conjunction with intense emotion, during exertion, or at rest. The pain is prolonged and more intense than angina pain. It lasts longer than 30 minutes and can last sev-

---

Box 8-2 | *Signs and Symptoms of Myocardial Infarction*

Subjective Data (Symptoms)	Objective Data (Signs)
Heavy pressure or squeezing in center of chest behind sternum	Pallor
	Erratic behavior
	Hypotension, shock
Pain is retrosternal and in heart region, often radiating down the left arm and to the neck, jaw, and teeth	Cardiac rhythm changes
	Vomiting
	Fever
	Diaphoresis
Anxiety	
Dyspnea	
Weakness, faintness	
Nausea	

eral hours. It is not relieved by changes in body position, nitroglycerin, or rest. Physicians often tell patients who call complaining of chest pain to take an aspirin (chewable if they have it) and report to the emergency room. Other signs and symptoms may occur in conjunction with the pain. These include nausea, shortness of breath, dizziness, weakness, diaphoresis, pallor, ashen color, and a sense of impending doom. See Table 8-1 for comparison of signs and symptoms and the medical management of angina pectoris and MI.

Assessment

Collection of **subjective data** includes the onset, location, quality, duration, and radiation of pain. Shortness of breath, dizziness, weakness, and anxiety or fear may be expressed. Identify precipitating factors. Inquire about measures the patient may have tried to relieve the pain.

Collection of **objective data** includes observation of the patient's behavior to determine apprehension and anxiety. Typical vital signs reveal hypotension, pulse abnormalities such as tachycardia, a barely perceptible pulse, and early temperature elevation. Note the presence of diaphoresis; vomiting; ashen color; cool, clammy skin; "labored respirations"; and cardiac dysrhythmias. If possible, ascertain the presence of risk factors. A respiratory assessment should also be made.

Diagnostic Tests

Diagnostic tests are used to confirm the diagnosis of MI. Serum tests are initially obtained. Serum cardiac markers (e.g., CK-MB, myoglobin, troponin I) are released into the vascular system when infarcted myocardial muscle cells die. A sensitive cardiac marker present in serum called **troponin I** has proven useful in detecting ischemic myocardial injury. Troponin I is cardiac specific and therefore a highly specific indicator of an MI. See the discussion of serum cardiac markers on pp. 336 to 337. An elevated white blood cell (WBC)

Table 8-1	*Coronary Artery Disorders*
SIGNS AND SYMPTOMS	**MEDICAL MANAGEMENT**
ANGINA PECTORIS	
Chest pain (substernal, retrosternal), may radiate to neck, jaw, left arm, and shoulder; great anxiety, fear of approaching death; face pale, ashen; pulse variable, usually tense and quick; blood pressure elevated during an attack; usually brought on by exertion, emotional upsets; relieved by rest, nitroglycerin	Avoidance of precipitating factors Reduction of modifiable risk factors Medications: nitrates, beta blockers, calcium channel blockers Oxygen therapy ECG monitoring Aspirin for unstable angina
MYOCARDIAL INFARCTION	
Severe, crushing chest pain; prolonged heavy pressure or squeezing pain in center of chest; may spread to shoulder, neck, arm, fourth and fifth fingers on left hand, teeth, and jaw; may radiate as with angina; not relieved with rest or nitroglycerin; may be associated with dyspnea diaphoresis, apprehension, nausea, and vomiting; signs and symptoms of cardiogenic shock may develop; the pain is prolonged and more intense than angina pain	Relief of pain (O_2), morphine, and other analgesics ECG monitoring Thrombolytic therapy to dissolve clot Reduction of O_2 demand (rest) Prevention of complications (through use of stool softeners, anticoagulants) Treatment of complications (dysrhythmias, HF) Anticoagulants to prevent further clotting

count of 12,000 to 15,000/mm^3 is associated with severe infarcts. The increase begins a few hours after the onset of pain and lasts for 3 to 7 days. The erythrocyte sedimentation rate (ESR) rises during the first week and may remain elevated for several weeks.

Twelve-lead ECG findings that indicate MI include ST segment elevation and the development of Q waves. In time the ST segment returns to normal and the T wave inverts. These ECG changes are important in confirming the diagnosis of MI. A chest radiograph is done to note size and configuration of the heart. More complex tests are occasionally done, including cardiac fluoroscopy, myocardial imaging (thallium scan), echocardiogram, PET, and multigated angiogram (MUGA) scanning (multiple-gated cardiac blood pool imaging). These tests may be done in conjunction with other tests to diagnose MI and determine the severity of CAD.

Medical Management

The focus of medical management is to prevent further tissue injury and limit the size of the infarction. It is extremely important that a patient with a suspected MI is rapidly diagnosed and treated to preserve cardiac muscle. Intervention is designed to facilitate cardiac tissue perfusion and reduce the workload of the heart. Promoting tissue oxygenation, relieving pain, preventing complications, improving tissue perfusion, and preventing further tissue damage are all important medical considerations (Clinical Pathway for Uncomplicated Myocardial Infarction box).

Medications such as morphine and Valium are used to alleviate pain and anxiety. A continuous IV infusion of amiodarone (Cordarone) may be given to the patient who has frequent PVCs, which may precede ventricular fibrillation. The use of prophylactic lidocaine is not recommended by the American College of Cardiology practice guidelines for the treatment of acute MI. However, lidocaine may be a treatment option for the patient who has sustained ventricular tachycardia or ventricular fibrillation (Furry et al, 2000). The use of beta-adrenergic blockers such as atenolol (Tenormin) or metoprolol (Lopressor) early in the acute phase of an MI and during a 1-year follow-up regimen can decrease morbidity. Angiotensin-converting enzyme (ACE) inhibitors may be used following MIs. Their use can help to prevent or slow the progression of heart failure (Medications table for the patient with MI). Oxygen is prescribed to facilitate cardiac tissue perfusion. Attention is given to respiratory difficulties, fluid overload, and cardiac dysrhythmias.

Medical therapy is also directed toward limiting the size and extent of injury by attempting to reperfuse (the reinstitution of blood flow to an area that was ischemic) the occluded coronary artery. Fibrinolytic agents such as streptokinase (Streptase), anistreplase, and tissue plasminogen activator (TPA) such as alteplase are currently used to attempt reperfusion. Thrombolytic therapy is the standard practice in the treatment of acute MI. Thrombolytics salvage heart muscle by minimizing infarct size and maximizing heart function. They lyse (decompose or dissolve) the clot in the occluded coronary artery, reopening the vessel and allowing perfusion (the passage of fluid through a specific organ) of the heart muscle. Remember the adage, "Time is muscle." Fast action to restore myocardial blood flow limits infarct size, preserves heart tissue, and improves the patient's chance of survival and recovery. To be effective, reperfusion must be attained within 3 to 5 hours following the onset of symptoms. Myocardial cells do not die instantly. In most patients, it takes approximately 4 to 6 hours for the entire thickness of the muscle to become necrosed. Reperfusion is most effective in the first 30 minutes to 1 hour. Mortality and infarction size can be significantly reduced if thrombolytic therapy starts within 30 to 60 minutes of symptom onset. Before a

CLINICAL PATHWAY | *Uncomplicated Myocardial Infarction*

Diagnostic Related Group 122   Length of Stay 6.8 Days

Admit Date:_____   Discharge Date:_____

PATHWAY	DAY 1		DAY 2	DAYS 3-4	DAYS 5-6
Clinical Path Implemented (initial):					
Diagnostic Studies	• Chem 7, 12 CBC • Mg • Chest x-ray • PT/PTT q___h • Stool occult blood	• Serum cardiac markers q8h × 2 after initial labs • Pulse oximetry now • Consider ABGs • ECG	• Echocardiogram • Consider serum cardiac markers 24 hr after initial series	Consider: • Serum cardiac markers • Holter monitor	• Consider modified exercise treadmill testing and discharge if negative • If positive, consider cardiac catheterization • Consider signal average ECG (if low EF or significant ventricular ectopy on Holter)
Treatments	• Consider thrombolytic therapy, complete questionnaire, identify eligibility • Oxygen _____ L/min • Cardiac monitoring • Pulse oximetry prn • If chest pain: ECG, SL NTG, call physician				
IV/Meds	• IV heplock • IV fluids____@____ • NTG drip_____ • Heparin • Morphine IVP • Antidysrhythmics • Beta blockers IV/po	• SL NTG _____ • ASA _____ • Implement thrombolytic protocol • Stool softener	• See med sheet	• Consider weaning IV NTG	• Consider discontinuing heparin
Consults	• Cardiology		• Consider cardiac rehab evaluation		
Nursing	• ECG strips every shift prn (rhythm, ST segment analysis) • Monitor chest pain for site, duration, quality, radiation, relief using 0-10 pain scale, notify MD if increasing chest pain or ST elevations or changes in cardiac rhythm • Physical assessment q4h prn × 24 hr, then every shift • Monitor lab values • I&O, admission weight • No IM injections • VS q4h prn • Provide emotional support and assistance to reduce patient/family anxiety				
Diet	• Clear liquids until stable, then 2 g Na, low cholesterol				
Activity and Safety	• Active and passive ROM • BR with bedside commode • Institute cardiac step levels • Routine safety measures		• Cardiac step level _____ • Rest periods after meals	• Cardiac step level _____	• Cardiac step level _____
Teaching Patient and Family	• Orient to unit • Explain diet, meds, activity • Call nurse with chest pain, rate on 0-10 scale • Explain all tests and procedures • Explain relationship among disease process, resulting symptoms, and therapy prescribed		• Explain cardiac step levels • Teach taking of own pulse • Cardiac teaching • Films		
Discharge Planning	• Initial assessment		• Facilitate physician/RN/family conference • Assess need for follow-up care • Review advance directives by date of discharge • To consider: elective cardiac catheterization as outpatient		

ADLs, Activities of daily living; *ASA,* acetylsalicylic acid; *BP,* blood pressure; *bpm,* beats per minute; *BR,* bed rest; *CBC,* complete blood count; *CO,* cardiac output; *ECG,* electrocardiogram; *EF,* ejection fraction; *EMS,* emergency medical system; *HR,* heart rate; *IM,* intramuscular; *I&O,* intake and output; *IV,* intravenous; *IVP,* intravenous pyelogram; *MI,* myocardial infarction; *NTG,* nitroglycerin; *OP,* outpatient; *po,* oral; *prn,* as needed; *PT,* prothrombin time; *PTT,* partial thromboplastin time; *ROM,* range of motion; *RR,* respiratory rate; *SL,* sublingual; *UO,* urinary output; *VS,* vital signs.

Diagnostic Related Group 122   Length of Stay 6.8 Days

Admit Date:_____   Discharge Date:_____

EXPECTED OUTCOMES: UNCOMPLICATED MI

PROBLEM LIST	DAY 1	DAY 2	DAYS 3-4	DAYS 5-6
Meets Expected Outcome (initial)				
Chest pain: Acute MI; validation of chest pain, discomfort, dyspnea	• Verbalizes pain or discomfort on a 0-10 pt scale, with 10, worst pain imaginable; and 0, pain free • Verbalizes dyspnea	• Pain managed • Nonverbal indicators such as grimacing will be absent	• Pain free • Dyspnea resolving	• Pain free at discharge • Denies dyspnea at rest or with activities
Activity intolerance: Imbalance of O_2 supply and demand 2° to decreased CO, dyspnea on exertion	• Identifies activities that precipitate chest pain • Modifies activity as tolerated	• Tolerates bedside commode/chair without chest pain • Participates in ADLs without chest pain • Progressive ROM prn	• Tolerates level of activity • Maintains: RR <24/min, NSR or HR <110 or within 20 bpm of resting HR	• Discharged at anticipated activity tolerance: BP change of <20 mm Hg and pain free • Identifies risks of immobility
Knowledge deficiency: MI and implications for lifestyle changes; states concerns re: chest pain and disease process	• States why admitted to hospital • States importance of notifying RN of chest pain	• Demonstrates readiness to learn • Asks questions, reads MI packet, etc.	• Demonstrates understanding of what an MI and angina are • Lists risk factors • Verbalizes understanding of diet • Selects appropriate items on menu • Takes own pulse	• Verbalizes activity restrictions and rationale • Verbalizes understanding of discharge instructions. Will have completed MI teaching • Has plan to reaccess the EMS • Has discussed potential for OP cardiac catheterization with physician
Anxiety: Real or perceived threat of death, change in health status and unfamiliar environ. Verbalizes fear, is restless; hyperventilates; is withdrawn, angry	• Verbalizes fears and concerns re: hospitalization • Asks questions	• Shows appropriate coping mechanisms • Identifies support systems	• Is coping • Exercises control by making decisions about care	• Verbalizes resources and support systems available to assist on discharge
Decrease in cardiac output: BP <90 mm Hg systolic HR >1200 bpm RR >20 min UO <30 mL/hr	• BP stabilizing • UO >30 mL/hr	• VS stable, hemodynamic parameters stabilized with or without intervention • UO >30 mL/hr • Lungs clear	• BP maintained without IV fluid or vasoactive therapy	• BP stabilized
Potential for bleeding: Risk of hemorrhage 2° to thrombolytics and heparin; bruising	• Verbalizes understanding of reason to notify RN of any bleeding or bruising	• No increased incidence of bruising, bleeding, or hematomas	• No increased incidence of bruising, bleeding, or hematomas	• States risk factors of anticoagulant therapy and when to notify physician

Other parts of this Clinical Pathway include Patient Pathways, Patient Education Documentation Record, and Physician's Orders. Developed by Nanticoke Memorial Hospital, Seaford, DE. Authorized by Molly Metzler, RN, BSN, for Nanticoke Health Services and licensed by the Center for Case Management, Inc., South Natick, MA. This represents an example of a clinical tool for illustrative purposes; clinical pathways at Nanticoke Memorial Hospital are continually being revised or updated.

MEDICATIONS | *Myocardial Infarction*

CLASSIFICATION	AGENT	ACTION
Vasopressors	Dopamine (Intropin)	Raise systemic arterial pressure and cardiac output
Anticoagulants	Heparin	Reduce incidence of clotting
	Warfarin (Coumadin)	
Antiplatelets	Ticlopidine (Ticlid)	Decrease platelet release of thromboxane, so that vasoconstriction and platelet aggregation is decreased
	Aspirin (ASA)	Decrease platelet aggregation
Analgesics	Morphine	Control pain; reduce myocardial oxygen demand
Tranquilizers	Diazepam (Valium)	Decrease anxiety and restlessness
Thrombolytic agents	Streptokinase (Streptase)	Use of thrombolytic (pertaining to dissolution of blood clots) agents when acute MI symptoms are less than 6 hours, preferably 30 minutes to 1 hour duration; these agents restore blood flow and therefore limit infarct size in certain patients
Tissue plasminogen activator (TPA)	Alteplase, recombinant Activase	
Nitrates	Nitroglycerin	Dilate blood vessels by reducing coronary artery spasm, increase coronary artery blood supply, and decrease oxygen demands
	Isosorbide	
	Atenolol (Tenormin)	
Beta-adrenergic blockers	Propranolol (Inderal)	Block Beta-adrenergic stimulation and decrease myocardial oxygen demands, thus decreasing myocardial damage. Decreases incidence of mortality
	Nadolol (Corgard)	
	Metoprolol (Lopressor)	
	Carvedilol (Coreg)	
Calcium channel blockers	Nifedipine (Procardia)	Dilate blood vessels, increase coronary artery blood supply, and decrease myocardial oxygen demands
	Diltiazem (Cardizem)	
	Verapamil (Calan, Isoptin)	
Salicylates	Aspirin	Decrease platelet adhesion and thus decrease thrombosis formation
Antidysrhythmics	Lidocaine (Xylocaine) IV	Treat ventricular dysrhythmias (rarely used except for ventricular tachycardia)
Stool softeners	Surfak	Reduce straining at stool; prevent constipation produced by decreased mobility and use of constipating narcotics
	Colace	
Diuretics	Furosemide (Lasix)	Control edema
Electrolyte replacement	Slow-K	May be necessary when diuretics are used
Inotropic agents	Digoxin (Lanoxin)	Increase the heart's pumping action (contractility)
	Amrinone (Inocor) IV	Indicated when left ventricle failure is present
	Dobutamine (Dobutrex)	

thrombolytic is administered, a thorough history must be obtained. Certain conditions exclude the use of thrombolytics: active internal bleeding, suspected aortic dissecting aneurysm, recent head trauma, history of hemorrhagic stroke within the past year, or surgery within the past 10 days.

Percutaneous transluminal coronary angioplasty may be used instead of thrombolytic therapy as a primary treatment in some cases. This involves advancing a balloon-tipped catheter into the lumen of the obstructed coronary artery. The balloon is inflated intermittently to dilate the artery and improve blood flow (see Figure 8-14). Along with balloon compression, stents may be used to prevent acute closure and restenosis (see Figure 8-15).

Coronary artery bypass graft surgery may be considered for patients with multiple vessel disease and when less invasive interventions, such as thrombolysis and PTCA, have failed (see Figures 8-12, *A* and *B*, and 8-13).

Complications commonly associated with MI include ventricular fibrillation, cardiogenic shock (Table 8-2), heart failure, and dysrhythmias. Other complications may occur, such as ventricular aneurysm, pericarditis, and embolism.

Nursing Interventions and Patient Teaching

Administer oxygen per protocol for 24 to 48 hours and longer if pain, hypotension, dyspnea, or dysrhythmias persist.

Administer medications as prescribed:
- IV morphine sulfate for relief of pain and apprehension and to produce vasodilation. Morphine also decreases myocardial oxygen demands, reduces contractility, and slows the heart rate. Provisions for comfort and rest are essential to reduce stress and increase myocardial oxygen perfusion.
- Heparin therapy or unfractionated or low-molecular-weight heparin such as enoxaparin (Lovenox)

Table 8-2 *Cardiogenic Shock*

Cardiogenic shock, often referred to as pump failure, is an acute and serious complication of MI and heart failure. It is characterized by low cardiac output and peripheral vascular system collapse. Left ventricular function is severely decreased, resulting in an inadequate blood supply to the vital organs. Immediate detection and treatment are necessary to prevent irreversible shock and death. Cardiogenic shock proves fatal in 50% to 80% of cases.

CLINICAL MANIFESTATIONS	SIGNS AND SYMPTOMS	MEDICAL MANAGEMENT	NURSING INTERVENTIONS
Decreased cardiac output	Dysrhythmias, chest pain	Recognition and control of life-threatening signs and symptoms	Monitor vital signs every 5 minutes during acute stage and every 1 hour when stabilized.
Myocardial ischemia	Anxiety, agitation, restlessness, disorientation	Oxygenation promotes tissue perfusion	Administer O$_2$ as ordered.
Cerebral hypoxia	Urinary output diminished or absent	Parenteral fluid acts as a volume expander	Maintain bed rest to reduce myocardial workload and increase oxygenation.
Impaired tissue perfusion	Lactic acid accumulation in blood	Drug therapy:	Monitor acid-base balance.
Renal circulation decreased	Tachycardia, thready pulse, tachypnea	• Vasopressors: raise arterial blood pressure	Monitor urine output hourly to determine adequate kidney perfusion.
Anaerobic metabolism with lactic acidosis	Decreased blood pressure	• Inotropic (digoxin [Lanoxin]): Glycoside: Increases cardiac contraction and strengthen and correct dysrhythmias	Allow nothing by mouth.
Peripheral vascular system collapse	Narrowed pulse pressure	• Adrenergic drugs: dopamine (Intropin) at therapeutic levels increases cardiac output and blood pressure	Initiate bed rest to minimize energy expenditure.
Shock	Cyanosis; cold, moist, pale, clammy	• Sodium bicarbonate: combats lactic acidosis (given sparingly because of the fluid retention it causes)	Administer medications as ordered.
	Decreased peripheral pulses		Provide comfort measures.
	Capillary refill time decreased		
	Hypoactive bowel sounds		

or dalteparin (Fragmin) will inhibit further clotting and prevent coronary artery reocclusion after the thrombolytic therapy opens the vessel.

- Antiplatelet agents such as aspirin (ASA) and ticlopidine (Ticlid) decrease platelet release of thromboxane, which causes vasoconstriction and platelet aggregation. Ticlopidine, an antiplatelet drug, can be ordered for patients allergic to aspirin and should be administered immediately. Nitroglycerin may help patients with left-ventricular infarctions when given intravenously. It reduces cardiac oxygen demand by relaxing vascular smooth muscle and dilating peripheral vessels; it also dilates coronary vessels, improving blood flow to the heart. Administer beta-adrenergic blockers to inhibit cardiotoxicity of catecholamines. Administer lipid-lowering agents such as simvastatin (Zocor), atorvastatin (Lipitor), or rosuvastatin (Crestor) to prevent elevated cholesterol levels.
- Stool softener as prescribed prevents rectal straining. Valsalva's maneuver may cause severe changes in blood pressure and heart rate, which may trigger ischemia, dysrhythmias, or cardiac arrest.

To help the post-MI patient minimize straining, offer the use of a bedside commode or nearby bathroom

whenever possible. Teach mouth breathing to help decrease the severity of straining.

Instruct the patient to avoid excessive fatigue and to stop activity immediately in the presence of chest pain, dyspnea, or faintness. Plan nursing interventions to promote rest and minimize unnecessary disturbances. Monitor vital signs; document rate and rhythm of pulse.

The patient is usually placed on bed rest with commode privileges for 24 to 48 hours. Assist with ADLs. During this period, sedation with Valium or an equivalent may be prescribed to relieve anxiety and restlessness and to promote sleep. After the first 24 to 48 hours, patients are usually encouraged to increase their activity gradually, depending on the size of the infarction. During this period the patient is continually monitored for signs of dysrhythmias, cardiac pain, and changes in vital signs.

Diet is usually withheld until the patient is stabilized. This is important because of the possible need for cardiac catheterization or PTCA/CABG procedure. Liquid diet is progressed as tolerated to regular diet with modifications. A low-fat, low-sodium, easily digested diet is desirable.

Prevention of complications is a primary objective. Antiembolic stockings are used. Ongoing assessment of cardiac status, dyspneic condition, and pulse change (rate, rhythm, and volume) is made and reported.

During hospitalization, many patients experience denial, depression, and anxiety. Anxiety varies in intensity, depending on the severity of the threat as perceived by the patient and on the patient's success in coping.

Nursing diagnoses and interventions for the patient with an MI include but are not limited to the following:

NURSING DIAGNOSES	NURSING INTERVENTIONS
Acute chest pain, related to myocardial ischemia	Assess original pain, assess location, duration, radiation, and onset of new symptoms.
	Administer prescribed analgesics (usually morphine sulfate, which relieves pain, reduces anxiety, causes vasodilation of vascular smooth muscle, and reduces myocardial workload).
	Maintain bed rest and reduced patient activity.
	Administer O_2 as prescribed.
	Record patient's response to pain-relief measures.
	Employ alternative methods of pain relief.
	Provide calm, restful environment for the patient.
Anxiety, related to change in health status and fear of death	Assess for signs and verbal expressions of anxiety and coping mechanisms used.
	Promote restful sleep patterns.
	Reassure through patient education enlisting family support, and allowing positive and negative expression of feelings.
	Remain with patient during periods of highest anxiety; offer reassurance; use calm, but concerned voice.
	Administer antianxiety agents as needed, per physician's order.
	Initiate relaxation techniques (deep breathing, visual imagery, soft rhythmic music).
	Encourage participation in cardiac rehabilitation program.
Decreased cardiac output, related to conduction defects (dysrhythmias) and decreased myocardial pumping action	Assess and monitor vital signs every 4 hours.
	Maintain bed rest with head of bed elevated 30 degrees for first 24 to 48 hours to reduce myocardial oxygen demand.
	Monitor intravenous feedings; infuse according to physician's order.

NURSING DIAGNOSES	NURSING INTERVENTIONS
	Administer prescribed medications such as antidysrhythmics, nitrates, and beta blockers.
	Auscultate breath sounds and heart rate every 4 hours; increase activity level as prescribed by physician's orders.
	Palpate for pedal pulses, assess capillary refill, auscultate bowel sounds, assess for pedal or dependent edema every 4 hours, and strictly monitor I&O.

Patients and their family members need teaching to reassure them of recovery. More than 85% of all patients with an uncomplicated MI return to work. Education should include information covering the resumption of sexual activities. Once patients with an uncomplicated MI are able to climb two flights of stairs without difficulty, they are usually able to resume sexual activities. Approximately 80% of all postcoronary patients will be able to resume sexual activity without serious risks. The other 20% need not abstain totally, but their sexual activity should be limited according to their cardiac capacity.

Cardiac rehabilitation. Participation in a cardiac rehabilitation program should be discussed before discharge from the hospital. A monitored exercise program and continuing education are provided with outpatient cardiac rehabilitation. The physician may prescribe cardiac rehabilitation during the inpatient and outpatient phase of recovery following an MI.

Cardiac rehabilitation services are designated to help patients with heart disease recover faster and return to full and productive lives. Cardiac rehabilitation has two major parts:

1. Exercise training to help the patient learn how to exercise safely, strengthen muscles, and improve stamina. The exercise plan is based on the individual's ability, needs, and interests.
2. Education, counseling, and training to help the patient understand his or her heart condition and find ways to reduce the risk of future heart problems. The cardiac rehabilitation team assists the patient in learning how to cope with the stress of adjusting to a new lifestyle and to deal with fears about the future. Cardiac rehabilitation may last 6 weeks, 6 months, or even longer. Cardiac rehabilitation has lifelong favorable effects (Health Promotion Considerations box and Home Health Considerations box).

Prognosis

It is imperative that medical care be instituted without delay. Many MI patients not treated prior to reaching the hospital die. Delaying specific therapy may cause

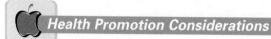

Health Promotion Considerations

Myocardial Infarction

- Teach the effects of MI, the healing process, and treatment regimen.
- Teach the effect of medications in the treatment of MI.
- Teach the association between risk factors and CAD.
- Teach to identify nonmodifiable risk factors.
- Teach to identify modifiable risk factors (especially cigarette smoking and stress). Stop smoking and encourage family and significant others to stop.
- Teach the effect of dietary restrictions on atherosclerotic heart disease (ASHD) or coronary artery disease (CAD): 2 g sodium, 1500 calories, low cholesterol, fluid restrictions.
- Limit total fat intake to 25% to 35% of total calories each day. Limit intake of saturated fats to less than 7% of total fat intake. Teach the patient saturated fats such as shortening, lard, or butter are solid at room temperature; better sources of fat include vegetable, olive, and fish oils.
- Teach the patient to avoid foods high in sodium, saturated fats, and triglycerides. Review alternative ways of seasoning foods to avoid cooking with salt. Explain need to limit intake of eggs, cream, butter, and foods high in animal fat.
- Teach patient to eat 20 to 30 g of soluble fiber every day. Foods such as bran, beans, and peas help lower bad cholesterol (LDL).
- Teach the effect of activity on the heart and the need to participate in a progressive activity plan.
- Refer the patient to social support groups as indicated.
- Teach importance of participating in cardiac rehabilitation services.
- Teach resumption of sexual activity (if appropriate).
- Explain cardiac warning symptoms. Patients and their partners are often unsure which symptoms must be reported. If the patient has a prescription for nitroglycerin, advise to take it when experiencing chest pain and to notify the physician if pain is not relieved within 15 minutes. Other signs to report include shortness of breath, rapid heart rate, dizziness, insomnia, a persistent increase in heart rate or blood pressure, and extreme fatigue following sexual activity.
- Explain what is safe and within what time frame. The joint guidelines of the American College of Cardiology and the American Heart Association recommend that after an "uncomplicated MI" (meaning that the patient was stable and experienced no complications), sexual intercourse can be resumed in a week to 10 days. However, previous studies have found that patients tend to resume sexual activity more gradually than this. A "complicated MI" means that the patient required CPR or had hypotension, serious dysrhythmia, or heart failure while hospitalized. Patients with complicated MIs must resume sexual activity more gradually, depending on their tolerance to exercise and activity. Encourage patients to also talk to their physicians about resuming sexual activity; the type and extent of damage from the MI might influence recommendations. Most patients have concerns about resuming sexual activity after an MI but may not express them to their nurses. Therefore initiating the conversation is the nurse's responsibility.
- Warn against anal sex. Ask patients whether they practice anal sex. If they answer in the affirmative, inform them that anal sex stimulates the vagus nerve, may cause chest pain, and slows down the heart rate and rhythm, impulse conduction, and coronary blood flow. (Steinke, 2000).
- Teach the importance of taking prescribed medications such as beta blockers. The patient who uses beta-adrenergic blockers in the treatment of an acute MI for 1 year following the infarction has a decreased chance of reinfarction and increased survival. Continue with taking lipid-lowering agents such as Zocar, Lipitor, Mevacor, Pravachol or Crestor.

loss of life. The prognosis also depends on the area and extent of the damage and the presence or absence of complications.

HEART FAILURE
Etiology/Pathophysiology

When the heart is no longer able to pump enough blood to sustain the body's metabolic needs, it is referred to as heart failure or cardiac insufficiency. **Heart failure** (HF) is a syndrome characterized by circulatory congestion as a result of the heart's inability to act as an effective pump. This is the traditional definition of heart failure. Because many patients suffer pulmonary or systemic congestion with HF, the syndrome was once called **congestive heart failure.** However, this term has lost favor because it excludes patients who don't experience congestion (McKinney, 1999). The most recent definition is that heart failure should be viewed as a neurohormonal problem in which heart failure progresses as a result of chronic release in the body of substances such as catecholamines (epinephrine and norepinephrine). These substances are capable of exerting toxic effects on the heart and circulatory system (Mann, 1999). Epinephrine and norepinephrine are hormones of the sympathetic nervous system and produce negative effects on the failing heart.

Circulatory congestion and compensatory mechanisms may occur. HF may develop after an MI, in response to prolonged hypertension or diabetes mellitus, or in relation to valvular heart disease or inflammatory heart disease. Other factors associated with HF include infection, stress, hyperthyroidism, anemia, and fluid

Home Health Considerations

Exercise Program after Myocardial Infarction

- During posthospitalization convalescent period, many patients are encouraged to begin a 2- to 12-week walking program.
- This is a structured program designed to have the patient walk 2 miles in less than 60 minutes by the end of the 12 weeks.
- People are encouraged to work through this program at their own rate until they have achieved a pace below a slow jog and their heart rate is below the prescribed rate set by the cardiologist.
- Unfortunately, not all postinfarction patients are physiologically capable of participating in a rigorous exercise program.
- Eventually, most patients are encouraged to participate in a maintenance (lifetime), unsupervised, home-based exercise program designed specifically for them.
- Almost everyone can benefit from some type of cardiac rehabilitation.

---

replacement therapy. HF is the most common diagnosis for the hospitalized patient older than 65 years of age. HF affects about 4.9 million Americans and accounts for 200,000 deaths annually. The increasing prevalence and incidence of heart failure result from both the longer lives of older people and the greater survival of patients with cardiovascular disease.

Because the left ventricle is most often affected by coronary atherosclerosis and hypertension, heart failure usually begins there. If untreated, the condition progresses to right-sided failure. Right ventricular failure can occur separately from left ventricular failure, but its appearance is more often a consequence of left-sided failure. The signs and symptoms of heart failure are the result of decreased cardiac output from impaired cardiac pumping power and congestion that involves the pulmonary system, the venous system, or both (Box 8-3).

Left ventricular failure. When the left ventricle is unable to pump enough blood to meet the demands of the body, major consequences occur. The first is the signs and symptoms of decreased cardiac output. The second is pulmonary congestion. Increased pressure in the left side of the heart backs up into the pulmonary system and the lungs become congested with fluid. Fluid leaks through the engorged capillaries and permeates air spaces in the lungs. If during each heartbeat the right ventricle pumps out just one more drop of blood than the left, then within only 3 hours the pulmonary blood volume will have expanded by 500 mL. Pulmonary edema and pleural effusion (an abnormal accumulation of fluid in the thoracic cavity between the visceral and parietal pleurae) occur. Signs and symptoms of this condition include dyspnea, orthopnea, pulmonary crackles, hemoptysis, and cough.

Box 8-3 | *Classifying Heart Failure*

The New York Heart Association (NYHA) classification is a universal gauge of heart failure severity based on physical limitations.

Class I: Minimal
- No limitations.
- Ordinary physical activity doesn't cause undue fatigue, dyspnea, palpitations, or angina.

Class II: Mild
- Slightly limited physical activity.
- Comfortable at rest.
- Ordinary physical activity results in fatigue, palpitations, dyspnea, or angina.

Class III: Moderate
- Markedly limited physical activity.
- Comfortable at rest.
- Less than ordinary activity causes fatigue, palpitation, dyspnea, or anginal pain.

Class IV: Severe
- Patient unable to perform any physical activity without discomfort.
- Angina or symptoms of cardiac inefficiency may develop at rest. Physical activity increases discomfort.

American College of Cardiology and American Heart Association (ACC/AHA). New guidelines are a complement to NYHA classification.

Stage Definition

A Patient is at high risk for developing heart failure but has no structural disorder of the heart. The patient has a primary condition that is strongly associated with heart failure (such as diabetes, mellitus, hypertension, substance abuse, or history of rheumatic fever) but no signs or symptoms of heart failure.

B Patient has a structural disorder of the heart, such as left ventricular hypertrophy, valvular heart disease, or previous myocardial infarction, but has never developed symptoms of heart failure.

C Patient has past or current symptoms of heart failure associated with underlying structural disease. The patient may display signs of dyspnea or fatigue, but is responding to therapy.

D Patient has end-stage disease and requires specialized treatment strategies that may include mechanical circulatory support, continuous inotropic infusions, heart transplant, or hospice care. These patients are frequently hospitalized and can't be discharged without symptom recurrence.

Right ventricular failure. Right ventricular failure occurs when the right ventricle is unable to pump effectively against increased pressure in the pulmonary circulation. Most often the increased pressure is the result of blood backing up from a failing left ventricle, but right

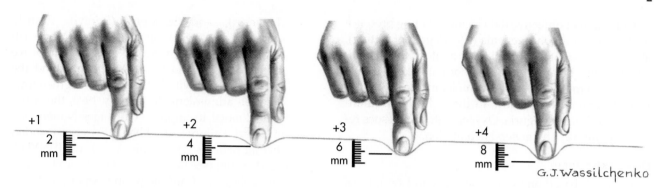

FIGURE **8-17** Scale for pitting edema depth.

Table 8-3 | *Pitting Edema Scale*

SCALE	DEGREE	RESPONSE
1 + Trace	Slight	Rapid
2 + Mild	4 mm (0-¼ in)	10-15 seconds
3 + Moderate	6 mm (¼-½ in)	1-2 minutes
4 + Severe	8 mm (½-1 in)	2-5 minutes

Box 8-4 | *Signs and Symptoms of Heart Failure*

DECREASED CARDIAC OUTPUT
Fatigue
Angina pain
Anxiety
Oliguria
Decreased gastrointestinal motility
Pale, cool skin
Weight gain
Restlessness

LEFT VENTRICULAR FAILURE
Dyspnea
Paroxysmal nocturnal dyspnea (PND)
Cough
Frothy, blood-tinged sputum
Orthopnea
Pulmonary crackles (moist popping and cracking
    sounds heard most often at the end of inspiration)
Evidence of pulmonary vascular congestion with
    pleural effusion, as seen on chest radiograph

RIGHT VENTRICULAR FAILURE
Distended jugular veins
Anorexia, nausea, and abdominal distention
Liver enlargement with right upper quadrant pain
Ascites
Edema in feet, ankles, sacrum; may progress up the
    legs into thighs, external genitalia, and lower
    trunk

ventricular failure can also be a result of chronic pulmonary disease and pulmonary hypertension. Inability of the right ventricle to pump blood forward into the lungs results in peripheral congestion. The right ventricle of the heart is unable to adequately empty its blood volume and thus cannot accommodate all the venous blood that is normally returned to the right side of the heart. Venous blood is reflected backward into the systemic circulation. Increased venous volume and pressure force fluid out of the vasculature into interstitial tissue (peripheral edema). Edema is a sign of increased interstitial fluid and appears in dependent areas of the body such as the sacrum when supine and the feet and ankles while in an upright position. The edema may progress to pitting edema. As right ventricular failure continues, edema may progress up the legs into the thighs, external genitalia, and lower trunk. To check for edema, press down on the tissue for several seconds and lift the finger. If the depression does not fill almost immediately, pitting edema is present (Figure 8-17; Table 8-3).

One liter of fluid equals 1 kg (2.2 pounds); a weight gain of 2.2 pounds will signify a gain of 1 L of body fluid. The liver may become congested, and fluid can accumulate in the abdomen (ascites). Distended neck veins may be observed when the patient is in a sitting position.

Clinical Manifestations

Manifestations of HF are those associated with decreased cardiac output, left ventricular failure, and right ventricular failure (Box 8-4).

Assessment

Collection of **subjective data** includes complaints of dyspnea, orthopnea (an abnormal condition in which a person must sit or stand in order to breathe deeply or comfortably), or paroxysmal nocturnal dyspnea (PND) (sudden awakening from sleep because of shortness of breath), cough, and the precipitating factors and methods for relief. Also listen to the patient's statements that relate to fatigue, anxiety, weight gain from fluid retention, and edema. Physical symptoms and impaired physical function cause psychosocial stress. Patients with New York Heart Association (NYHA) class III or IV heart failure are at very high risk for major depression (Artinian, 2003). Document any pain, anginal or abdominal, and the patient's stated ability to perform ADLs.

Collection of **objective data** includes noting presence of dyspnea, orthopnea, edema (site, degree of pitting), abdominal distention secondary to ascites, weight gain, adventitious breath sounds, abnormal heart sounds (gallop and murmurs), activity intolerance, and jugular vein distention. Blood flow to the kidneys is diminished, resulting in oliguria. Oxygen deficit in tissues results in cyanosis and general debilitation.

Diagnostic Tests

Diagnosis is based on presenting signs and symptoms of congestive heart failure and is confirmed by various diagnostic tests. A chest radiograph reveals pulmonary vascular congestion, pleural effusion, and cardiomegaly (cardiac enlargement). ECG reveals cardiac dysrhythmias. Echocardiography is done to determine valvular heart disease, presence of pericardial fluid, and HF. Echocardiogram is used to determine ejection fraction, and pulmonary artery catheterization is done to assess right and left ventricular function.

Exercise stress testing is done to determine activity tolerance and severity of underlying ischemic cardiovascular disease. **Cardiac catheterization** may be performed to detect cardiac abnormalities and underlying cardiovascular disease. **Multiple gated acquisition scanning** is ordered to evaluate cardiac function, determine ejection fraction, and detect wall motion abnormalities.

Laboratory tests include sodium, calcium, magnesium, and potassium levels. Blood chemistry will reveal elevated blood urea nitrogen (BUN) and creatinine resulting from decreased glomerular filtration; liver function values (alanine aminotransferase [ALT], aspartate transaminase [AST], gamma glutamyltransferase [GT], alkaline phosphatase) will be mildly elevated. **B-type natriuretic peptide (BNP)** is a neurohormone secreted by the heart in response to expansion of ventricular volume and pressure overload. A normal BNP level is less than 100 pg/mL and the patient probably does not have heart failure, whereas a level greater than 100 pg/mL probably is suggestive of heart failure. Levels greater than 700 pg/mL indicate decompensated heart failure (Hobbs, 2003). The higher level of BNP correlates with an increase in the patient's signs and symptoms of heart failure. A BNP is useful in monitoring chronic heart failure (Shatzer, 2004). Arterial blood gases may reveal hypoxemia and acid-base imbalance.

Medical Management

The objectives of medical management include the following:

- Increasing cardiac efficiency with digitalis and vasodilators (nitroglycerin, isosorbide) for expanded output. Angiotensin-converting enzyme (ACE) inhibitors such as captopril (Capoten), enalapril (Vasotec), ramipril (Altace), benazepril (Lotensin), and lisinopril (Prinivil, Zestril); quinapril (Accupril); and fosinopril (Monopril) decrease peripheral vascular resistance, improve cardiac output, and have proven to extend the lives of patients with HF as well as lengthen time between admissions. In January 1999, the Advisory Council to Improve Outcomes Nationwide in Heart Failure (ACTION HF) recommended that all patients with stable class II or III NYHA heart failure (see Box 8-3), or stage C or D American College of Cardiology and American Heart Association (ACC/AHA) heart failure due to left ventricular dysfunction receive a beta blocker to prevent cardiac remodeling. (This occurs when the left ventricle dilates, hypertrophies, and develops a more spherical shape. The shape change stresses the ventricle walls, increases the magnitude of regurgitation through the mitral valve, and depresses mechanical performance.) The only beta blocker that has been approved by the FDA to treat HF is carvedilol (Coreg), an alpha, nonselective beta blocker (McKinney, 1999). It directly blocks the sympathetic nervous system's negative effects on the failing heart. Angiotensin II receptor blockers such as irbesartan (Avapro), losartan (Cozaar), and valsartan (Diovan) selectively and competitively block the vasoconstrictive and aldosterone-secreting effects of angiotensin, leading to vasodilation. Research for their use in HF is in progress. Angiotensin II receptor blockers are not a substitute for ACE inhibitors unless an ACE inhibitor is clearly not tolerated. In 2001, the FDA approved nesiritide (Natrecor) for the intravenous treatment of patients with acutely decompensated congestive heart failure who have shortness of breath (i.e., dyspnea) at rest or with minimal activity. Natrecor is the first of a new drug class, called human B-type natriuretic peptides. It reduces pulmonary capillary pressure, helps improve breathing, and causes vasodilation with increase in stroke volume and cardiac output (Riggs, 2004).
- Lowering oxygen requirements of the body systems with head of bed elevated to 45 degrees to reduce myocardial oxygen demand and decrease circulating volume returning to heart.
- Providing oxygen to the tissues through oxygen therapy if patient is hypoxic.
- Treating edema and pulmonary congestion with diuretics, a sodium-restricted diet, and restriction of fluid intake.
- Weighing patient daily to monitor fluid retention.

Once the workload of the heart is decreased and diuresis of engorged tissues and organs is achieved, the activity ability of the patient will increase. These objectives are achieved by medication therapy and activity per a physician's orders. Medication therapy with digoxin, ACE inhibitors, thiazide, and loop diuretics is a common initial treatment (Medications table for HF).

In acute HF, administration of oxygen and medication should be of first concern. Decreasing oxygen requirements through rest will slow the heart rate and increase cardiac and respiratory reserves. Anxiety produced from the effects of signs and symptoms and the fear of a life-threatening situation can be allayed by reassurance and explanation. Accurate interventions, observation, and reporting reduce the threat of such complications as embolus, thrombophlebitis, MI, and pulmonary edema.

Nursing Interventions

Nursing interventions include measures to prevent disease progression and complications. Vital signs are monitored for changes. Signs of respiratory distress will be noted. The nurse will observe for signs of pulmonary edema. Signs and symptoms of left-sided versus right-sided heart failure are carefully monitored. Urinary output is typically low, and edema is soft and pitting; legs are elevated to decrease edema.

 MEDICATIONS | *Heart Failure*

AGENT	ACTION	NURSING INTERVENTIONS
CARDIAC GLYCOSIDES		
Digitalis preparations, such as digoxin (Lanoxin)	Strengthen cardiac force and efficiency Slow heart rate Increase circulation, effecting diuresis	Monitor apical pulse to ensure rate greater than 60; monitor for toxicity (nausea, vomiting, anorexia, dysrhythmia, bradycardia, tachycardia, headache, fatigue, and blurred or colored vision).
DIURETICS		
Thiazides, such as chlorothiazide (Diuril), hydrochlorothiazide (Esidrix, Hydrodiuril)	Increase renal secretion of sodium Are safe for long-term use Block sodium and water reabsorption in kidney tubules	Monitor electrolyte depletion; weigh daily to ascertain fluid loss.
Sulfonamides (loop diuretic), such as furosemide (Lasix), bumetanide (Bumex)	Act rapidly for less responsive edema	Administer in AM, to prevent nocturia. Monitor for electrolyte depletion. Consider sulfa allergy (furosemide).
Aldosterone antagonist (potassium-sparing), such as spironolactone (Aldactone)	Relieves edema and ascites that do not respond to usual diuretics Blocks sodium-retaining and potassium-excreting properties of aldosterone	Monitor for gastrointestinal irritation and hyperkalemia.
POTASSIUM SUPPLEMENTS		
Potassium (K-Lyte)	Restores electrolyte loss	Monitor blood potassium levels.
SEDATIVES AND ANALGESICS		
Temazepam (Restoril)	Promotes rest and comfort	Monitor rest and sleep benefits.
Morphine	Relieves chest and abdominal pain, reduces anxiety, and decreases myocardial oxygen demands Lessens dyspnea	
NITRATES		
Nitroglycerin (Cardabid)	Dilates arteries, improves blood flow Reduces blood pressure	Monitor blood pressure for hypotension. Monitor for headache and flushing.
ACE INHIBITORS		
Captopril (Capoten) Enalapril (Vasotec) Vamipril (Altace) Benazepril (Lotensin) Lisinopril (Prinivil; Zestril) Univasc (Moexipril) Quinapril (Accupril) Fosinopril (Monopril)	Act as antihypertensives and reduce peripheral arterial resistance and improve cardiac output	Observe patient closely for a precipitous drop in blood pressure within 3 hours of initial dose; monitor blood pressure closely. Monitor blood potassium levels.

Continued

MEDICATIONS | *Heart Failure—cont'd*

AGENT	ACTION	NURSING INTERVENTIONS
β-ADRENERGIC BLOCKERS		
Carvedilol (Coreg)	Directly blocks the sympathetic nervous system's negative effects on the failing heart.	Start gradually, increasing the dosage slowly every 2 weeks as tolerated by the patient.
INOTROPIC AGENTS		
Dobutamine (Dobutrex) (IV) Dopamine HCl (Dopamine HCl, Intropin) (IV)	Low-dose dobutamine (Dobutrex) and low-dose dopamine are relatively safe on med-surg units. In low doses the drugs dilate renal blood vessels, stimulating renal blood flow and glomerular filtration rate, which in turn promotes sodium excretion, often helping CHF patients improve.	Make certain patient not taking monoamine oxidase (MAO) inhibitors, tricyclic depressants, phenytoin (Dilantin), and haloperidol (Haldol). Accurate I&O; assess for dizziness, nausea, vomiting, headache. Assess vital signs carefully q15min for first 2 hours, then q2h for following 4 hours, and finally once a shift Observe carefully for extravasation, tachycardia, bradycardia, angina, palpitations, hypotension, hypertension, azotemia, and anxiety.
Human natriuretic peptides nesiritide (Natrecor)	New class of heart failure drug known as synthetic human B-type Natriuretic Peptides (hBNPs) Nesiritide causes arterial and venous dilation, thereby decreasing systemic vascular resistance and pulmonary arterial pressures. It decreases blood pressure and promotes better left ventricle ejection and increases cardiac output. Nesiritide may also promote diuresis. It is an intravenous treatment of patients with acutely compensated congestive heart failure.	Observe carefully for hypotension. Natrecor should not be used for patients with cardiogenic shock or with a systolic blood pressure <90 mm Hg.

The nurse should also note increase in abdominal girth and total body weight as indicators of fluid retention common in heart failure. The nurse will auscultate lung fields to determine the presence of crackles and wheezes, coughing, and complaints of dyspnea. Restful sleep may be possible only in the sitting position or with the aid of extra pillows. Activity intolerance accompanied by extreme fatigue and anxiety is usually noted. Patients should be assessed for depression. It is important that patients with HF and depression understand that the depression is readily treatable and that there are several approaches to treatment that can be used separately or in combination, including pharmacologic therapy, psychosocial and psychotherapeutic interventions, and cardiac rehabilitation.

The new guidelines also advocate the discussion of end-of-life decisions with the patient and family. Patients should talk with their health care providers about treatment preferences, advance directives, living wills, power of attorney for health care, and life-support issues. Because heart failure is a progressive disease, patients should make these decisions while they are capable of expressing choices. Hospice services, originally developed to assist cancer patients, are now considered to be appropriate for the patient with end-stage heart failure (Bosen, 2002) (Nursing Care Plan box; Box 8-5; Patient Teaching: Heart Failure).

Prognosis

Approximately 10% of patients diagnosed with HF die in the first year, and 50% within 5 years (McKinney, 1999). HF is a chronic condition. With treatment advances, many people now survive for years with damaged hearts. With the advent of ACE inhibitors and new research on the benefits of prescribed exercise, improvement in the quality of life for HF patients is being seen.

NURSING CARE PLAN

The Patient with Heart Failure

Mr. D. is a 61-year-old clinical administrator. He was admitted to the hospital with the diagnosis of heart failure. He has a history of hypertension and coronary artery disease. Six months ago he had a myocardial infarction. He has felt tired for the past 3 weeks and has been experiencing increased dyspnea. He has noticed some edema in his ankles and is concerned about gaining 5 pounds in the past week as well as increasing intolerance to exertion. The nursing admission history revealed:

- Mr. D. has not been taking his antihypertensive medication regularly. He didn't like the side effects and stopped taking the medication, but he was too embarrassed to call his doctor.
- Vital signs revealed an elevated blood pressure.
- Shortness of breath during activities and when lying down
- Pitting edema of both ankles
- Crackles bilaterally in the lungs

NURSING DIAGNOSIS *Decreased cardiac output, related to cardiac insufficiency*

Patient Goals/Expected Outcomes	Nursing Intervention	Evaluation
Patient will have decreased dyspnea with activities and when lying in bed within 24 hours. Patient will have decreased adventitious lung sounds. Patient will have oxygen saturations at 91% with prescribed oxygen within 24 hours. Patient will have vital signs within acceptable levels within 72 hours. Patient will have decreased edema and weight loss of 5 pounds within 72 hours.	Maintain initial bed rest with stress-free environment. Maintain semi-Fowler's to high Fowler's position. Explain and encourage gradual increases in activity to prevent a sudden increase in cardiac workload. Monitor respirations, lung sounds, heart sounds, and vital signs every 4 hours. Palpate pedal pulses, and assess capillary refill every 8 hours. Administer digitalis, diuretics, ACE inhibitors, vasodilators, beta blockers, and antihypertensive medication as prescribed. Monitor I&O and weigh daily. Monitor oxygen saturation with pulse oximetry every 4 hours. Administer prescribed oxygen.	Patient has decreased presence of crackles in lung fields within 24 hours of admission. Patient has an oximetry reading of 91% oxygen saturation with O₂ prescribed within 24 hours of admission. Patient has a heart rate of 80, respiratory rate of 22, and blood pressure of 148/86 within 72 hours of admission. Patient has a weight loss of 5 pounds within 72 hours of admission. Patient has pedal pitting edema decreased to 1+ within 2 days of admission.

NURSING DIAGNOSIS *Anxiety, related to change in health status, lifestyle changes, fear of death, or threats to self-concept.*

Patient Goals/Expected Outcomes	Nursing Intervention	Evaluation
Patient will be able to verbalize anxieties within 48 hours of admission. Patient will be able to demonstrate reduction of anxiety by enjoying periods of rest and sleep undisturbed for 6 hours within 48 hours of admission.	Identify coping techniques. Provide information to decrease fears. Identify support systems. Provide calm, relaxing environment. Administer antianxiety medications per physician's orders as needed. Help patient cope with lifestyle changes. He or she may feel anxious due to changes in body image, family and social roles, and finances. Focus on progress patient is making in managing his or her condition. Encourage patient to participate in health care decisions, and allow him or her to release anger and frustration. Allow patient to sleep undisturbed for 6 hours when vital signs are stable.	Patient is verbalizing anger and frustration over current medical conditions within 48 hours of admission. Patient is sleeping 5 to 6 hours per night within 48 hours of admission.

Continued

NURSING CARE PLAN
The Patient with Heart Failure—cont'd

❓ CRITICAL THINKING QUESTIONS

1. Mr. D. is experiencing severe dyspnea, with the presence of crackles bilaterally in all lung fields. His pulse is 108, and respirations are 33. His nurse enters the room to perform his morning ADLs. The nursing interventions that would be most beneficial would include:

2. On assessing Mr. D.'s skin, the nurse notes 4+ pitting edema in his lower extremities. She also notes a weight gain of 6 pounds in the past 24 hours. For therapeutic diuresis to occur, the medical management would include:

3. Mr. D. puts his light on to request assistance to ambulate. The nurse notes subclavicular retractions and cyanosis of his nailbeds. What would the most appropriate nursing action by the nurse be?

Box 8-5 *Guidelines for Nursing Interventions for the Patient with Heart Failure*

Provide oxygenation.
Administer oxygen by nasal cannula per protocol as prescribed for dyspnea.
Patient should be well supported in semi-Fowler's or high Fowler's position.
Reinforce importance of conservation of energy and planning for activities that avoid fatigue.
Encourage activity within prescribed restrictions; monitor for intolerance to activity (dyspnea, fatigue, increased pulse rate that does not stabilize).
Assist with ADLs as necessary; encourage independence within patient's limitations.
Provide diversionary activity that will assist in conservation of energy.
Monitor for signs of fluid and potassium imbalance; record daily weights, I&O.
Provide skin care, particularly over edematous areas; use prophylactic measures to prevent skin impairment.
Assist in maintaining an adequate nutritional intake while observing prescribed dietary modifications (sodium restrictions).
Monitor for constipation; give prescribed stool softeners.
Give prescribed medications:
  Digitalis (take apical pulse before administration)
  Diuretics (assess for hypokalemia)
  Vasodilators, ACE inhibitors, beta blockers
  Medications to reduce anxiety and promote sleep
Provide patient/family opportunities to discuss their concerns.
Teach patient about the disorder and self-care.

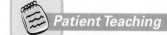 **Patient Teaching**

Heart Failure

- Monitor for signs and symptoms of recurring heart failure and report these signs and symptoms to the physician or clinic:
    Report weight gain of 2 to 3 lb (1 to 1.5 kg) over a short period (about 2 days)
    Shortness of breath
    Orthopnea
    Swelling of ankles, feet, or abdomen
    Persistent cough
    Frequent nighttime urination
- Avoid fatigue and plan activity to allow for rest periods.
- Plan and eat meals within prescribed sodium restrictions.
- Avoid salty foods.
- Avoid drugs with high sodium content (e.g., some laxatives and antacids, Alka-Seltzer); read the labels. Ideally, limit sodium intake to 2 g/day.
- Maintain low-fat diet, with fat intake less than 30% of total calories.
- Eat several small meals rather than three large meals per day.
- Take prescribed medications.
- If several medications are prescribed, develop a method to facilitate accurate administration.
- Digitalis: check own pulse rate daily; report a rate of less than 60/min to physician.
- Take diuretics.
- Weigh self daily at same time of day.
- Eat foods high in potassium and low in sodium (such as oranges and bananas).
- Take vasodilators.
- Report signs of hypotension (lightheadedness, rapid pulse, syncope) to physician.
- Avoid alcohol when taking vasodilators.
- Reinforce the importance of regular exercise once HF is stabilized. Thorough treatment regimen may allow the patient to increase activity level over time. The physician may ultimately recommend 30 to 45 minutes of aerobic exercise three or four times a week to improve patient's well-being (*RN,* June 2000).
- Report to physician for follow-up as directed.

Box 8-6 *Signs and Symptoms of Pulmonary Edema*

Restlessness
Vague uneasiness
Agitation
Disorientation
Diaphoresis
Severe dyspnea
Tachypnea
Tachycardia
Pallor or cyanosis
Cough production of large quantities of blood-
   tinged, frothy sputum
Audible wheezing, crackles
Cold extremities

PULMONARY EDEMA
Etiology/Pathophysiology

Pulmonary edema (the accumulation of extravascular fluid in lung tissues and alveoli, caused mostly by HF) is an acute and extensive, life-threatening complication of heart failure caused by severe left ventricular dysfunction. Fluid from the left side of the heart backs up into the pulmonary vasculature and results in extravascular fluid accumulation in the interstitial space and alveoli. This causes the patient to "drown" in the secretions.

Clinical Manifestations

The patient exhibits signs of severe respiratory distress when pulmonary edema occurs. Frothy sputum is produced from air mixing with the fluid in the alveoli; the sputum is blood-tinged from blood cells that have exuded into the alveoli.

Assessment

See Box 8-6 for signs and symptoms of pulmonary edema.

Diagnostic Tests

Diagnosis is made through signs and symptoms and is supported by chest radiograph and arterial blood gas studies. PaO_2 and $PaCO_2$ may reveal respiratory alkalosis or acidosis.

Medical Management

Medical management involves simultaneous interventions to promote oxygenation, improve cardiac output, and reduce pulmonary congestion. Without emergency treatment, respiratory failure may occur (Table 8-4).

Nursing Interventions

Interventions include administering oxygen. Place patient in an upright position with legs in a dependent position to decrease venous return to the heart, relieving pulmonary congestion and dyspnea. Monitor arterial blood gases and administer drugs as ordered. Aus-

Table 8-4 *Medical Management for Acute Pulmonary Edema*

INTERVENTION	RATIONALE
Patient in high Fowler's position or over side of bed with arms supported on bedside table	Promotes expansion of lungs, legs in dependent position causes venous pooling and reduction in venous return (preload)
Morphine sulfate, 10-15 mg intravenously; titrated	Decreases patient anxiety; relieves pain; slows respirations; reduces venous return; decreases oxygen demand; dilates the pulmonary and systemic blood vessels
Oxygen at 40%-100%; nonrebreather face mask; intubation as needed	Promotes oxygenation; increased tidal volume also promotes removal of secretions from alveoli
Administer sublingual nitroglycerin	Increases myocardial blood flow
Diuretics: furosemide (Lasix), bumetanide (Bumex)	Reduce pulmonary edema by decreasing the fluid in the lungs and increasing excretion through the kidneys
Inotropic agents: dobutamine (Dobutrex), amrinone (Inocor)	Increase myocardial contractility without increasing oxygen consumption; Increase peripheral vasodilation; Increase cardiac output
Nitroprusside (Nitropress)	A potent vasodilator; improves myocardial contraction and reduces pulmonary congestion

cultate lung sounds often. Provide emotional support; remain with patient. Explain all procedures. Monitor vital signs, fluid intake and output (I&O), and serum electrolytes.

Nursing diagnoses and interventions for the patient with pulmonary edema include but are not limited to the following:

NURSING DIAGNOSES	NURSING INTERVENTIONS
Excess fluid volume, related to fluid accumulation in pulmonary vessels	Administer medications as ordered. Carefully monitor I&O. Weigh patient at same time each day. Assess for edema.
Impaired gas exchange, related to fluid in lungs	Assess for signs of hypoxia, such as restlessness, disorientation, and irritability.

NURSING DIAGNOSES	NURSING INTERVENTIONS
Impaired gas exchange, related to fluid in lungs—cont'd	Monitor arterial blood gases per physician's order. Administer oxygen per physician's order. Position patient in high Fowler's position with legs in dependent position or sitting and leaning forward on overbed table to facilitate breathing.
Anxiety, related to fear of suffocation and death	Promote optimal air exchange to decrease anxiety. Assess level of anxiety and coping mechanisms. Deliver nursing interventions in a supportive, kind, and proficient manner. Assess support systems available to patient and mobilize resources.

Prognosis

Pulmonary edema is a grave, life-threatening condition that is usually responsive to aggressive interventions.

VALVULAR HEART DISEASE

Etiology/Pathophysiology

Normal heart valves function to maintain the direction of blood flow through the right atrium, right ventricle, lungs, left atrium, and left ventricle, and to the rest of the body. Heart valves operate by passively opening and closing in response to pressure changes in the heart. The tricuspid valve is located between the right atrium and right ventricle. The pulmonary semilunar valve allows blood to flow through the pulmonary artery into the lungs. The mitral (bicuspid) valve is located between the left atrium and the left ventricle. The aortic semilunar valve allows blood to flow from the left ventricle into the aorta. Valvular disease occurs when the valves are compromised and do not open and close properly. Two problems occur when valves are compromised: **stenosis,** which is a thickening of the valve tissue, causing the valve to become narrow, and **insufficiency,** which occurs when the valve is unable to close completely. Valvular disorders occur in children and adolescents primarily from congenital conditions.

Another prominent factor in the development of valvular disease is a history of rheumatic fever. Clinical symptoms of valvular heart disease tend to occur 10 to 40 years after an episode of rheumatic fever. Because the blood volume and workload of the heart are greater on the left than on the right, the valves affected more frequently are the mitral and aortic. Valvular heart disorders include mitral stenosis, mitral insuffi-

ciency, aortic insufficiency, aortic stenosis, tricuspid insufficiency, tricuspid stenosis, and pulmonary insufficiency and pulmonary stenosis.

Clinical Manifestations

Signs and symptoms seen in valvular disorders are related to decreased cardiac output.

Assessment

Collection of **subjective data** includes noting patient's statement of a history of rheumatic fever and of an inability to perform activities and ADLs without fatigue or weakness. Assessment includes the patient's statement of chest pain, its quality, duration, and onset, as well as precipitating factors and measures that provided relief. The patient may complain of having had heart palpitations. The patient may verbalize feelings of lightheadedness, dizziness, or fainting. The history may include a patient statement of weight gain. Dyspnea, exertional dyspnea, and nocturnal (nighttime) dyspnea as well as orthopnea are often reported, depending on the degree of heart failure.

Collection of **objective data** includes observing for a heart murmur and noting the character and the presence of any adventitious breath sounds (crackles, wheezes) as well as any edema, pitting or nonpitting.

Diagnostic Tests

The diagnostic tests used to confirm a diagnosis of valvular heart disease are chest radiograph, ECG, echocardiogram, and cardiac catheterization.

Medical Management

Medical management includes activity limitations, sodium-restricted diet, diuretics, digoxin, and antidysrhythmics.

Surgical intervention is usually indicated for a patient whose lifestyle is severely affected by valvular heart disease. There are two basic surgical procedures: repair of the valve pathology or replacement of the valve.

When medical therapy no longer alleviates clinical symptoms or when diagnostic evidence exists of progressive myocardial failure, surgery is often performed. The surgery may include the following:

- **Open mitral commissurotomy:** A surgical splitting of the fused mitral valve leaflet for treating stenosis of the mitral valve.
- **Valve replacement:** Replacement of the stenosed or incompetent valve with a bioprosthetic or mechanical valve; commonly used valves include tilting disks, porcine (pig) heterografts (tissue taken from one species and grafted onto another), homografts (a graft of tissue obtained from a member of the same species as the individual receiving it), and ball-in-cage valves.

Nursing Interventions and Patient Teaching

Nursing interventions are focused on assisting with ability to perform ADLs, relieving specific symptoms associated with decreased cardiac output, and promoting comfort.

The nursing interventions include administering the prescribed medications (diuretics, digoxin, and antidysrhythmics). Also included in nursing interventions are recording I&O, daily weight, respiratory rate and rhythm, as well as auscultation of breath sounds, heart sounds, and blood pressure. Assessment also includes a check for capillary perfusion, pedal pulses, and presence of edema. A sodium-restricted diet for control of edema is maintained.

Maintain therapeutic oxygen therapy as prescribed. Discuss with the patient a plan for rest periods, and identify those ADLs that produce fatigue and require assistance for the patient.

Nursing diagnoses and interventions for the patient with valvular heart disease include but are not limited to the following:

NURSING DIAGNOSES	NURSING INTERVENTIONS
Activity intolerance, related to weakness, fatigue, and dyspnea	Balance activities with rest periods. Identify fatiguing activities and obtain assistance as needed. Use oxygen as prescribed by physician.
Excess fluid volume, related to decreased cardiac output	Administer prescribed oxygen, digoxin, diuretics, and antidysrhythmics. Monitor I&O. Weigh patient daily. Perform respiratory assessment. Perform cardiovascular assessment. Inspect for presence of edema. Obtain vital signs routinely. Maintain sodium-restricted diet.

Patient teaching focuses on medications, dietary management, activity limitations, diagnostic tests, surgical interventions, and postoperative care as appropriate for each individual patient. Discuss with the patient the disease process and associated symptoms to report to the physician. Explain to the patient antibiotic prophylaxis to prevent infectious endocarditis. Explain the importance of notifying the dentist, urologist, and gynecologist of valvular heart disease. Patient must remain on higher dosages of warfarin after valve replacement surgery. Prothrombin time is carefully monitored. Discuss with the patient the need to maintain good oral hygiene and regular visits to the dentist.

Prognosis

The prognosis of valvular heart disease is variable, depending on the specific pathology. The prognosis after surgery is fair to good with amelioration (improvement) of signs and symptoms but often without resolution of all abnormalities.

INFLAMMATORY HEART DISORDERS

All cardiac tissues are susceptible to inflammation, and heart failure can be a serious and rapid result of the inflammatory process.

RHEUMATIC HEART DISEASE
Etiology/Pathophysiology

Rheumatic heart disease, a result of rheumatic fever, is an inflammatory disease that predominantly results from a delayed childhood reaction to inadequately treated childhood pharyngeal or upper respiratory tract infection (group A β-hemolytic streptococci). By the 1980s rheumatic fever had almost disappeared in developed countries such as the United States. However, it remained common and severe in most developing countries. Antibiotics, especially penicillin, are responsible for the decline in rheumatic fever. A great deal of interest has been generated by a number of "mini-epidemics"—10 to 75 cases—of acute rheumatic fever during a circumscribed time in a single region. In searching for the cause of the reappearance, researchers have focused on isolating strains of group A streptococci. Researchers have isolated highly virulent strains of the same types that were prevalent in epidemic rheumatic fever more than 30 years ago (Lewis et al., 2004).

Ineffective treatment of infection results in delayed reaction and inflammation of the cardiac tissues as well as the central nervous system, joints, skin, and subcutaneous tissues. Of the individuals affected with rheumatic fever, 90% are between 5 and 15 years of age. The onset of rheumatic fever is usually sudden, often occurring in from 1 to 5 symptom-free weeks after recovery from pharyngitis (sore throat) or from scarlet fever. However, rheumatic fever may progress with symptoms and go undiagnosed and untreated. Years later the patient may develop clinical manifestations of valvular heart disease.

Rheumatic heart disease can affect the pericardium, myocardium, or endocardium. The affected tissue develops small areas of necrosis, which heal, leaving scar tissue. The heart valves are typically the most affected by Aschoff's nodules (vegetative growth) and become fibrous and incompetent. With healing, the valves become thickened and deformed. These changes result in valvular stenosis and insufficiency, varying in extent and severity. Valvular heart disease may be the result.

Clinical Manifestations

Fever, increased pulse, epistaxis, anemia, joint involvement, and nodules on joints and subcutaneous tissue may be noted. Carditis can develop. When valvular involvement occurs, signs and symptoms are specific to each condition.

Assessment

Collection of **subjective data** may reveal joint pain (polyarthritis), as well as abdominal pain. Lethargy and fatigue are also present.

Collection of **objective data** includes skin manifestations of small erythematous circles and wavy lines on the trunk and abdomen that appear and disappear rapidly (erythema marginatum). The nurse may observe involuntary, purposeless movement of the muscles if Sydenham's chorea (St. Vitus' dance), a disorder of the central nervous system, is present. Heart murmur may be auscultated if carditis with valve involvement is present. Rheumatic heart disease is characterized by heart murmurs resulting from stenosis or insufficiency of the valves.

Diagnostic Tests

Diagnosis is made through signs and symptoms and supported by laboratory study results. An echocardiogram is done to determine the extent of damage to the valves and myocardium. An ECG shows cardiac dysrhythmia. Cardiac murmurs or friction rub can be heard. No specific diagnostic test exists for rheumatic fever. Sedimentation rate and leukocyte count will be elevated. The development of serum antibodies against the streptococci (measured by antistreptolysin-O [ASO] titer) may be present. C-reactive protein, elevated in a specimen of blood, is abnormally high.

Medical Management

Intervention is more effective when approach is by preventive measures. Rapid treatment for pharyngeal infection, usually with prolonged antibiotic therapy, is desired. Penicillin is the antibiotic most commonly preferred. Prolonged periods of bed rest have previously been recommended, but now the patient without carditis may be ambulatory as soon as acute symptoms have subsided and may return to normal when the antiinflammatory therapy has been discontinued. When carditis is present, ambulation is postponed until heart failure is controlled. Symptomatic treatment and care are given. Nonsteroidal antiinflammatory drugs (NSAIDs) for joint pain and inflammation is accompanied by application of gentle heat. A well-balanced diet, following the personalized daily food choices and number of servings recommended by the U.S. Department of Agriculture's MyPyramid food planning tool, is supplemented by vitamins B and C and high-volume fluid intake. In some patients, surgical commissurotomy or valve replacement is necessary.

Nursing Interventions and Patient Teaching

Signs and symptoms largely determine the type of nursing interventions. Bed rest during the initial attack is recommended when carditis is present. If polyarthritis is present, the nurse helps minimize joint pain by proper positioning of the patient. After the acute stage, the child or young adult is treated at home. A schedule of daily events is reviewed with the patient and the parents.

Nursing interventions are carried out quickly and skillfully to minimize discomfort and prevent tiring the child. Throughout the course of the disease, the patient and family benefit from emotional support and appropriate diversions.

The focus of teaching is to facilitate an understanding of the disease process, signs, and symptoms, gradually increasing activity levels and medications, including prophylactic use of antibiotics to prevent recurrence. The importance of a nutritional diet should be emphasized as well as when to notify the physician if signs and symptoms develop. Patients with a history of rheumatic fever or evidence of rheumatic heart disease should receive daily prophylactic penicillin by mouth or monthly intramuscular injections of penicillin to prevent streptococcal infection, at least during childhood and adolescence. Patients with evidence of deformed heart valves should be given prophylactic antibiotics before surgery and all dental procedures.

Prognosis

Prognosis depends upon involvement of the heart; carditis can result in a serious heart disease. Valvular heart disease may result.

PERICARDITIS
Etiology/Pathophysiology

Pericarditis is the inflammation of the membranous sac surrounding the heart. It may be manifested as an acute or a chronic condition. Bacterial, viral, or fungal infection is associated with acute pericarditis. It may occur as a complication of noninfectious conditions such as azotemia, acute MI, neoplasms such as lung cancer, breast cancer, leukemia, Hodgkin's disease, lymphoma, scleroderma, trauma after thoracic surgery, systemic lupus erythematosus, radiation, and drug reactions (e.g., from procainamide [Procan SR], and hydralazine [Apresoline]). Fibrosis of the pericardial sac develops in the chronic form.

Fibrous constriction and thickening of the pericardium occur gradually, causing compression severe enough to prevent normal filling during diastole. Surgical removal of the pericardium may be necessary to restore normal cardiac output.

Clinical Manifestations

Pericarditis differs clinically from other inflammatory conditions of the heart in that the presentation of debilitating pain—much like that of MI—is common.

The pain is aggravated by lying supine, deep breathing, coughing, swallowing, and moving the trunk and is alleviated by sitting up and leaning forward. Dyspnea, fever, chills, diaphoresis, and leukocytosis are observed. The hallmark finding in acute pericarditis is pericardial friction rub, grating, scratching, and leathery sounds are detected, as is dysrhythmia.

Decreased heart function to the level of cardiac failure can occur when the heart is compressed by excess fluid in the pericardial sac. Normally only a few drops of fluid are found in the pericardial sac, yet 150 to 200 mL or more may develop with incidence of pericarditis. When pericardial effusion restricts heart movement **(cardiac tamponade)**, a pericardial tap **(pericardiocentesis)** may be performed to remove excess fluid and restore normal heart function.

Assessment

Collection of **subjective data** includes the patient's description of muscle aches, fatigue, and dyspnea. Excruciating chest pain is said to originate precordially and radiate to the neck and shoulders with severe and sudden onset.

Collection of **objective data** includes noting expressed substernal chest pain that radiates to the shoulder and neck, obvious by orthopneic positioning and facial grimace on inspiration. Elevated temperature accompanies chills and may be followed by diaphoresis. A nonproductive cough is often present. Verbalizing anxiety, anticipation of danger, or uneasiness is common. Vital sign changes include a rapid and forcible pulse and rapid, shallow breathing. Pericardial friction rub heart sounds become muffled, and dysrhythmia may be noted by the physician's assessment.

Diagnostic Tests

ECG changes (dysrhythmia) will be noted. Echocardiography will show the presence of pericardial effusion or cardiac tamponade. Laboratory studies will show leukocytosis (10,000 to 20,000/mm^3 will be present), and the sedimentation rate will be elevated. Chest radiographic findings are generally normal or nonspecific in acute pericarditis unless the patient has a large pericardial effusion.

Medical Management

Analgesia for comfort and relief of pain reassures the anxious patient. Oxygen and parenteral fluids are usually given. Antibiotics should be used to treat bacterial pericarditis. The physician prescribes salicylates for increased temperature and antiinflammatory agents (e.g., indomethacin) and corticosteroids for a persistent inflammatory process. These medicines require nursing knowledge of untoward effects and nursing implications in the control of this condition. Surgical intervention—pericardial fenestration (pericardial window) or pericardiocentesis (pericardial tap)—may be per-

formed to provide continuous drainage of pericardial fluid. Complications may include atelectasis and introduction of infectious agents.

Nursing Interventions

Vital signs are carefully evaluated, and lung and heart sounds are auscultated.

The nurse will provide supportive measures and observe for complications in the patient with pericarditis. Bed rest is maintained to promote healing and decrease the cardiac workload. The head of the bed is elevated 45 degrees to decrease dyspnea. Hypothermia treatment may be necessary to reduce elevated temperature. The nurse may remain with the patient if anxiety is present. Explain all procedures thoroughly.

Nursing diagnoses and interventions for the patient with inflammatory heart conditions include but are not limited to the following:

Nursing Diagnoses	Nursing Interventions
Decreased cardiac output, related to inflammatory process	Maintain bed rest with head of bed elevated 45 degrees. Assess vital signs every 2 to 4 hours as indicated by patient's condition. Administer medications as ordered. Monitor I&O. Provide planned rest periods.
Pain, related to inflammatory process	Assess and record pain type and quality. Administer analgesics according to need, as ordered. (Pain is what the patient says it is.) Maintain the patient on bed rest with the head of the bed elevated to 45 degrees and provide a padded overbed table for the patient. Use comfort measures to provide physical and emotional support.
Excess fluid volume, related to ineffective myocardial pumping action	Restrict sodium in diet as prescribed; monitor I&O. Weigh daily; compare values. Administer diuretic therapy as ordered; monitor electrolyte values. Observe respiration and pulse quality. Assess for dyspnea and peripheral edema.

Prognosis

The prognosis is fair in early stages but extremely grave if purulent and fibrinous stages develop.

ENDOCARDITIS

Etiology/Pathophysiology

Endocarditis is an infection or inflammation of the inner membranous lining of the heart, particularly the heart valves. Classified on the basis of cause, it may result from invasion of an organism (**infective endocarditis,** previously known as bacterial endocarditis) or may be the result of injury to the lining. Endocarditis may develop after cardiac surgery, which in itself is traumatic.

People at risk include patients with rheumatic heart disease, congestive heart disease, or degenerative heart disease. With the increasing use of valve replacement, the incidence of prosthetic valve endocarditis has continued to rise. In some cases endocarditis is preceded by intrusive procedures such as dental procedures, minor surgery, gynecological examinations, or insertion of indwelling urinary catheters. Other people at high risk include those who "mainline" street drugs, because of the possibility of bacteremia from contaminated needles and syringes.

The term **bacterial endocarditis** has been replaced by **infective endocarditis** because causative organisms include fungi, chlamydiae, rickettsiae, viruses, and bacteria. The causative organisms—most commonly *Streptococcus viridans, Streptococcus pyogenes, Staphylococcus aureus, Staphylococcus epidermidis,* and enterococci—are deposited on the heart lining or valves. As the organism embeds into the tissue, a vegetative growth perforates the chambers or valve leaflets. Fibrin and calciferous growths of the vegetation may ulcerate and scar the valves or may break away, causing emboli, infection or abscess in organs where they may lodge. The loss of portions of vegetative lesions into the circulation results in embolization. Systemic embolization occurs from left-sided heart vegetation, progressing to organ (particularly the brain, kidneys, and spleen) and limb infarction. Right-sided heart lesions embolize to the lungs. Conditions predisposing to infective endocarditis have changed because of decreasing incidence of rheumatic heart disease, increased recognition and treatment of mitral valve prolapse, the aging population with degenerative heart disease, and IV drug abuse (Lewis et al, 2004). The kidneys and spleen are often affected.

Clinical Manifestations

Occurring in acute or subacute form, signs and symptoms progress either rapidly; in dangerous sequence during the acute phase; or gradually, with damage occurring over a long period.

Assessment

Collection of **subjective data** includes noting patient complaints of influenza-like symptoms with recurrent fever, undue fatigue, chest pain, headaches, joint pain, and chills.

Collection of **objective data** may reveal the significant signs of petechiae in the conjunctiva, oral mucosa, neck, anterior chest, abdomen, and legs and as anemia. Splinter hemorrhages (black longitudinal streaks) may occur in the nailbeds. Weight loss may occur. Pulse is rapid. The onset of a new murmur is frequently noted with infective endocarditis, with the aortic and mitral valves most commonly affected.

Diagnostic Tests

ECG changes and chest radiographic examination denote evidence of HF and heart enlargement. Transesophageal echocardiography and digital imaging using two-dimensional transthoracic echograms can detect vegetation and abscesses on valves. Laboratory findings indicate leukocytosis, increased erythrocyte sedimentation rate (ESR), anemia, and hyperglobulinemia. Blood cultures determine the causative organism, and sensitivity tests indicate the effective antibiotic needed for medical management.

Medical Management

Management relies on rest to decrease the heart's workload. Complete bed rest is usually not indicated unless the temperature remains elevated and there are signs of heart failure. After the blood cultures, massive doses of antibiotics are administered—usually parenterally—to combat the organism. Antibiotic therapy is often as long as a month, or in the case of some organisms, as long as 2 months. Traditionally this has required a prolonged hospitalization for most patients with infective endocarditis. Currently, with the use of newer, more versatile antibiotics (and in light of economic concerns), treatment of patients with infective endocarditis on an outpatient basis is becoming more common.

Priorities include supporting cardiac function and preventing complications, such as emboli and heart failure.

Prophylactic antibiotic treatment is recommended for individuals who are considered at high risk for developing infective endocarditis. Previous valve surgery, preexisting valvular heart disease, or congenital abnormalities may require patients to take infective endocarditis precautions. This involves antibiotic therapy as prescribed by the physician before any invasive procedure such as dental work or minor surgery.

Surgical repair of diseased valves or prosthetic valvular replacement may be necessary if the patient's condition is severe. Valve replacement has become an important adjunct procedure in the management of endocarditis. It is used in more than 25% of cases.

Nursing Interventions and Patient Teaching

The nursing interventions are based primarily on the signs and symptoms. Observation for petechiae, location of pain, vomiting, and fever is a nursing responsibility. If these signs and symptoms are observed, they should be reported at once.

During the acute phase it is essential to maintain the patient on decreased activity and provide a calm, quiet environment. Vital signs should be taken every 4 hours, including apical pulse. When increased activity or ambulation begins, assess pulse before and after to determine the effects on the heart muscle.

Ensuring adequate nutrition is important. Frequently patients have a decreased appetite in conjunction with the disease process. The nurse should provide attractive meals with supplemental between-meal nourishment. Promoting rest and comfort and preventing further inflammation and infection are the focus of nursing interventions while the patient is hospitalized.

Patient teaching focuses on identifying causes, infective endocarditis precautions, and dietary requirements and gradually increasing activity levels as well as teaching the need for prophylactic antibiotics before any invasive procedure if the patient has preexisting valvular heart disease. The patient should be instructed about signs and symptoms that may indicate recurrent infections such as fever, fatigue, malaise, and chills. If any of these signs and symptoms occur, the patient should be aware of the importance of notifying the physician.

Prognosis

Before the advent of antibiotics, patients with infective endocarditis could be expected to live approximately 1 year; prompt treatment with intensive antibiotic therapy will now cure about 90% of patients with this condition.

MYOCARDITIS

Inflammation of the myocardium may originate from rheumatic heart disease; viral, bacterial, or fungal infection; or endocarditis or pericarditis. The cause may be unknown.

Signs and symptoms vary according to the site of manifestation. The patient may have upper respiratory symptoms such as fever, chills, and sore throat. Other possible signs and symptoms include abdominal pain and nausea, vomiting, diarrhea, and myalgia. These generally occur up to 6 weeks before the patient has signs and symptoms of myocarditis, such as chest pain and overt heart failure with dyspnea (Holcomb, 2004). Cardiac enlargement, murmur, gallop, and tachycardia are typically seen in myocarditis. Cardiomyopathy may develop as a complication. Involvement and enlargement of the myocardium may result in dysrhythmias.

Therapy is symptomatic and primarily follows the same approach as that of endocarditis: bed rest, oxygen, antibiotics, antiinflammatory agents, careful assessments, and correction of dysrhythmias.

Recovery may occur; however, cardiomyopathy may develop. As a result, the disease may have a long, benign course, or it may result in sudden death during exercise.

CARDIOMYOPATHY
Etiology/Pathophysiology

Cardiomyopathy is a term used to describe a group of heart muscle diseases that primarily affects the structural or functional ability of the myocardium. This primary dysfunction is not associated with CAD, hypertension, vascular disease, or pulmonary disease.

When cardiomyopathies are classified by cause, two forms are recognized: primary and secondary. Primary cardiomyopathy consists of heart muscle disease of unknown cause and is classified as dilated, hypertrophic, or restrictive. **Dilated cardiomyopathy,** characterized by ventricular dilation, is the most common type of primary cardiomyopathy. **Hypertrophic cardiomyopathy** results in increased size and mass of the heart because of increased muscle thickness (especially of the septal wall) and decreased ventricular size. In **restrictive cardiomyopathy** the ventricular walls are rigid, thus limiting the ventricles' ability to expand and resulting in impaired diastolic filling (Chojnowski, 2004). Secondary cardiomyopathy consists of myocardial disease of known cause as listed below:

A. Infective
1. Viral myocarditis
2. Bacterial myocarditis
3. Fungal myocarditis
4. Protozoal myocarditis
B. Metabolic
C. Nutritional: severe nutritional deprivation
D. Alcohol: individuals who consume large quantities of alcohol over many years may develop dilated cardiomyopathy
E. Peripartum: unexplained cause; may develop in last month of pregnancy or within first few months after delivery
F. Drugs: doxorubicin (Adriamycin), and a variety of medications may lead to cardiomyopathy
G. Radiation therapy
H. Systemic lupus erythematosus
I. Rheumatoid arthritis
J. "Crack" heart: Cardiomyopathy caused by cocaine abuse is seen more frequently now than ever before. Cocaine causes intense vasoconstriction of the coronary arteries and peripheral vasoconstriction, resulting in hypertension. This can result in increased myocardial oxygen needs and decreased oxygen supply to the myocardium and can cause ischemia and infarction. This may lead to an acute MI or ischemic cardiomyopathy. Cocaine also causes high circulating levels of catecholamines. This may lead to further injury to myocardial cells and cause cell

damage leading to ischemic or dilated cardiomyopathy. The cardiomyopathy produced is difficult to treat. Interventions deal mainly with the HF that ensues (Lewis et al, 2004). The patient has a poor prognosis.

Clinical Manifestations

Angina, syncope, fatigue, and dyspnea on exertion are common signs and symptoms. The most common symptom is that of severe exercise intolerance.

Signs and symptoms include those similar to HF. The patient may have signs of both left-sided and right-sided heart failure, including dyspnea, peripheral edema, ascites, and hepatic dysfunction.

Diagnostic Tests

Diagnosis of cardiomyopathy is made by the patient's clinical manifestations and noninvasive and invasive cardiac procedures to rule out other causes of dysfunction. Diagnostic studies include ECG, chest radiograph, echocardiogram, CT scan, nuclear imaging studies, multiple-gated radionuclide angiocardiography (MUGA), cardiac catheterization, and endomyocardial biopsy.

Medical Management

Medical management consists of treatment of underlying cause; heart failure management to slow the progression of the disease and symptoms is initiated. Medications may include diuretics, ACE inhibitors, antidysrhythmics, and beta-adrenergic blockers. Implantation of an automatic internal defibrillator is occasionally done. In patients with advanced disease refractory to medical treatment, cardiac transplantation should be considered. Educate the patient about avoiding strenuous exercise because of the risk of sudden death.

Cardiac transplantation. The first heart transplant was performed in 1967. Since that time, heart transplantation has become the treatment of choice for patients with end-stage heart disease who are unlikely to survive the next 6 to 12 months. Patients with cardiomyopathy account for more than 50% of the cardiac transplant recipients. Dilated cardiomyopathy is the most common type of cardiomyopathy requiring transplantation. Inoperable CAD is the second most common indication for transplantation, accounting for 40% of candidates (Box 8-7).

Once an individual meets the criteria for cardiac transplantation, the goal of the evaluation process is to identify patients who would most benefit from a new heart. In addition to the physical examination, psychological assessment of candidates is valuable. A complete history of coping abilities, family support system, and motivation to follow through with the transplant and the rigorous transplantation regimen is essential. The complexity of the transplant process

---

Box 8-7 | *Indications and Contraindications for Cardiac Transplantation*

INDICATIONS

Suitable physiologic/chronologic age
End-stage heart disease refractory to medical therapy
Dilated cardiomyopathy
Inoperable CAD
Vigorous and healthy individual (except for end-stage cardiac disease) who would benefit from procedure
Compliance with medical regimens
Demonstrated emotional stability and social support system
Financial resources available

CONTRAINDICATIONS

Systemic disease with poor prognosis
Active infection
Active or recent malignancy
Diabetes mellitus, type 1, with end-organ damage
Recent or unresolved pulmonary infarction
Severe pulmonary hypertension unrelieved with medication
Severe cerebrovascular or peripheral vascular disease
Irreversible renal or hepatic dysfunction
Active peptic ulcer disease
Severe osteoporosis
Severe obesity
History of drug or alcohol abuse or mental illness

---

may be overwhelming to a patient with inadequate support systems and a poor understanding of the lifestyle changes required after transplant.

Once potential recipients are placed on the transplant list, they may wait at home and receive ongoing medical care if their medical condition is stable. If their condition is not stable, they may require hospitalization for more intensive therapy. Unfortunately, the overall waiting period for a transplant is long, and many patients die while waiting for a transplant.

Donor and recipient matching is based on body and heart size and ABO type. Tissue crossmatching between donor and recipient is generally not done because of difficulty in obtaining good matches and lack of correlation between match and outcome.

Most donor hearts are obtained at sites distant from the institution performing the transplant. The maximum acceptable ischemic time for cardiac transplant is 4 to 6 hours.

The recipient is prepared for surgery, and cardiopulmonary bypass is used. The usual surgical procedure involves removing the recipient's heart, except for the posterior right and left atrial walls and their venous connections. The recipient's heart is then replaced with the donor heart, which has been trimmed to match. Care is taken to preserve the integrity of the donor sinoatrial (SA) node so that a sinus rhythm may be achieved postoperatively.

Immunosuppressive therapy usually begins while the recipient is in the operating room. Regimens vary but usually include azathioprine (Imuran), corticosteroids, and cyclosporine. Cyclosporine was first used in heart transplantation in 1980. Currently it is used with corticosteroids for maintenance immunosuppression. Its use has resulted not only in reduced rejection, but also in slowing the rejection process so that early treatment can be instituted.

The postoperative care is similar to that of other open heart surgeries. Endomyocardial biopsies via the right internal jugular vein are performed at repeated intervals to detect rejection. In addition, peripheral blood T-lymphocyte monitoring is done to assess the recipient's immune status.

Because the patient is immunosuppressed, nursing interventions should involve prevention of infection, which is the leading cause of death in this population. Many deaths from infection occur during augmented immunosuppressive therapy for acute rejection episodes. Nursing intervention involves a great deal of emotional support and teaching of both the patient and the family, because transplantation is a last resort. In addition, the patient is often a long distance from home and significant others.

Advances in surgical technique and postoperative care have improved early survival rates after cardiac transplantation. Attention is directed toward improvements in immunosuppression and management of long-term complications. Nursing management continues to focus on promoting patient adaptation to the transplant process, monitoring, managing lifestyle changes, and ongoing education of the patient and family. Ongoing data collection and research continues in regard to quality of life, functional level and rehabilitation of the cardiac transplant recipient (Lewis et al., 2004).

Nursing Interventions and Patient Teaching

Nursing interventions focus on relieving symptoms, observing for and preventing complications, and providing emotional and psychological support. Nursing interventions should also focus on monitoring the response to medications and monitoring for dysrhythmias.

Education should focus on teaching patients to adjust their lifestyle to avoid strenuous activity and dehydration. Strenuous exertion is dangerous for this group of patients and should be avoided. The patient should be taught to space activities and allow for rest periods.

Prognosis

Most patients have a severe, progressively deteriorating course, and the majority (particularly those older than 55 years of age) die within 2 years of the onset of signs and symptoms. However, improvement or stabilization occurs in a minority of patients. Death is due to either heart failure or ventricular dysrhythmia. Sudden death resulting from dysrhythmia is a constant threat.

DISORDERS OF THE PERIPHERAL VASCULAR SYSTEM

Peripheral vascular disease is any abnormal condition that affects the blood vessels outside the heart and the lymphatic vessels. The word peripheral means pertaining to the outside, surface, or surrounding area.

The peripheral vascular system consists of arteries, capillaries, and veins. This system supplies oxygen-rich blood to the upper and lower extremities of the body, and returns blood and carbon dioxide from those areas to the heart and lungs. Disorders of the peripheral vascular system occur when circulation to the upper and lower body extremities is compromised.

NORMAL AGING PATTERNS

Degenerative changes occur in the vascular system as part of the normal aging process. These changes affect the walls of the blood vessels and predispose people to problems in the transport of blood and nutrients to the tissues. The inner walls of the blood vessels (tunica interna) become thick and less compliant. A decrease in the elasticity of the middle walls of the blood vessels (tunica media) causes less flexibility. These changes markedly decrease the elasticity and flexibility of the vessels and therefore increase peripheral vascular resistance, causing a rise in blood pressure. This may ultimately lead to an elevation in overall blood pressure. These changes may increase a person's susceptibility to peripheral vascular disease (see Older Adult Considerations box).

RISK FACTORS

Risk factors for peripheral vascular disorders are similar to those for cardiovascular disorders.

An important aspect of caring for the patient with a peripheral vascular disorder is understanding the risk factors and incorporating them into patient teaching.

Nonmodifiable Factors

Age. As a person ages, arteriosclerotic changes occur in the peripheral vascular system, which leads to increased peripheral vascular resistance and decreased blood flow to the tissues.

Gender. Men are more susceptible to arteriosclerotic changes. This gender difference decreases after menopause when the effects of estrogen are no longer present.

Family history. A family history of atherosclerosis increases an individual's risk.

Modifiable Factors

Smoking. Smoking is one of the major contributing factors in the development of peripheral vascular problems. The nicotine in cigarettes causes vasoconstriction and spasms of the arteries, contributes to an elevation in blood pressure, and reduces circulation to the extremities. The carbon monoxide inhaled in cigarette smoke reduces oxygen transport to the tissues.

Hypertension. Increased blood pressure causes wear and damage to the inner arterial walls of the blood vessels, resulting in a buildup of fibrous tissue. This in turn leads to further narrowing of the vessel and increased resistance to blood flow.

Hyperlipidemia. An elevation in serum cholesterol and triglycerides contributes to the buildup of plaque inside the blood vessels.

Obesity. Excessive body weight and body fat contribute to the severity of other risk factors. Extra weight in relation to bone structure and height places an increased workload on the heart and blood vessels and may contribute to congestion in the venous system.

Lack of exercise. Decreased activity may compromise the peripheral vascular system because of a lack of muscle tone. The contraction and relaxation of muscles facilitates the return of blood in the veins to the heart and lungs. Benefits that result from regular physical activity, such as weight and stress reduction and improved vascular tone, are not realized in the sedentary individual.

Emotional stress. Stress contributes to increased blood pressure, increased production of cholesterol, and increased vasoconstriction of the blood vessels.

Diabetes mellitus. Uncontrolled elevated serum glucose levels contribute to the atherosclerotic process, although the exact mechanism by which diabetes mellitus contributes to the development of peripheral vascular disorders is unknown. Elevated serum glucose levels result in circulatory disorders.

Family history. A family history of atherosclerosis increases an individual's risk.

ASSESSMENT

Arterial Assessment

The first symptom of decreased arterial circulation is pain. The pain that initially occurs is from arterial insufficiency and ischemia. Arterial insufficiency occurs when not enough blood is available or able to flow through the arteries to body tissues. Ischemia occurs when the tissue does not receive enough oxygen-rich blood to function normally. Ischemic pain in the lower extremities is usually characterized by a dull ache in the calf muscles. It is often accompanied by leg fatigue and cramping. The pain is brought on by exercise and relieved by rest. It is referred to as intermittent claudication (a weakness of the legs accompanied by cramplike pains in the calves caused by poor circulation of

the arterial blood to the leg muscles). Pain may also be felt in the thighs and buttocks. As arterial disease progresses and becomes chronic, pain occurs even at rest. Burning, tingling, and numbness of the legs may occur at night while the patient is lying down.

Other assessments the nurse makes include palpating and comparing pulses in the extremities. Pulses may be weak, thready, or absent in the affected extremity because of decreased blood flow. Several scales are used to measure pulses. To ensure that the patient's pulses are graded the same way each time, all the nurses should use the same scale, such as the following:

0 Absent
+1 Barely palpable, intermittent
+2 Weak, possibly thready, but constantly palpable and with consistent quality
+3 Normal strength and quality
+4 Bounding, easily palpable, may be visible

The nurse may need to use a Doppler ultrasound device to check the patient's pulses if pulmonary vascular disease (PVD), low blood pressure (BP), edema, or large amounts of subcutaneous tissue impede the assessment. If a Doppler device is used, record pulsation as **present** or **absent** rather than using the numeric scale. For future reference, use a skin marker to indicate where the pulse is present (Willis, 2001). The nurse checks the affected extremity and compares it with the unaffected extremity for color, temperature, skin characteristics, and capillary refill time (Box 8-8).

For a uniform assessment and documentation technique for **veins** and **arteries,** the following mnemonic device, called PATCHES, is helpful:

P for **pulses.** Assess the patient's affected extremity first. Then assess the apical pulse and bilateral temporal, carotid, brachial, radial, femoral, popliteal, posterior tibial, and dorsalis pedis pulses.

Absence of pulses is generally a medical emergency that requires immediate treatment. But in some cases it may be normal, so compare the findings with previous ones or correlate them with the patient's signs and symptoms.

A for **appearance.** Note whether the extremity is pale, mottled, cyanotic, or discolored red, black, or brown. Document areas of necrosis or bleeding and the size, depth, and location of ulcers. As one assesses ulcers, note whether the edges are jagged or smooth and whether the area is painful to touch.

Shiny skin often marks the presence of edema; a dull appearance may signal inadequate arterial blood supply. Look for superficial veins, erythema, or inflammation anywhere on the affected extremity. Standing allows the saphenous veins to fill, so varicosities in the saphenous system are best evaluated with the patient standing. If a line of color change is present, mark it with a skin marker and monitor for changes in location.

Box 8-8 | *Capillary Refill Time*

1. Apply pressure to a toenail or fingernail for several seconds until it blanches (the area loses its color).
2. Relieve the pressure.
3. Note the amount of time it takes for the color to return.
   - The color should return almost instantly—in less than 2 seconds.
   - With an arterial disorder, the time it takes for the color to return will be greater than 2 seconds.

T for **temperature.** If the patient has an arterial problem, his affected extremity will feel cool; if his problem is venous, it will feel normal or abnormally warm. However, problems in arteries and veins are not the only reasons for temperature changes in an extremity; aortoiliac disease, heart failure, hypovolemia, pulmonary embolism, and other conditions can also affect skin temperature by interfering with peripheral blood flow.

C for **capillary refill.** Capillary refill is normally less than 2 seconds, but it may be extended when the patient has PVD. Press on a nail until the nailbed blanches, then release and count how many seconds it takes for normal color to return. Other sites to check capillary refill are the pads of the toes and fingers, the heel, and the thenar eminence on the palm of the hand proximal to the thumb. Although abnormal capillary refill is not diagnostic in itself, it adds valuable data to the assessment (see Box 8-8).

H for **hardness.** Palpate the extremity to determine if the tissues are supple or hard and inelastic. Hardness may indicate long-standing PVD, chronic venous insufficiency, lymphedema, or chronic edema. Hardened subcutaneous skin also increases the risk of stasis ulcers.

E for **edema.** Pitting edema frequently indicates an acute process, and nonpitting edema may be seen with chronic conditions, such as venous insufficiency. Assess both extremities for edema and compare and document the findings.

To assess for pitting edema, gently press the skin on the affected extremity for at least 5 seconds. Release and grade pitting as follows: +1, 2-mm indentation; +2, 4-mm indentation; +3, 6-mm indentation; and +4, 8-mm indentation (see Figure 8-17). The most accurate way to determine the degree of nonpitting edema is to measure the circumference of the extremity and compare measurements versus the other extremity and subsequent measurements. Measure at the point of edema, and then mark the point with a skin marker so everyone will assess the same area. Accuracy is greatest if the measurements are taken at the same time every day, preferably in the morning before the patient ambulates.

S for **sensation.** Vascular discomfort can originate in arteries, veins, or in the microcirculation if the patient has diabetes mellitus. Besides asking the patient about pain, ask if he has other abnormal sensations, such as numbness or tingling. Tingling or tenderness can result from peripheral tissue ischemia, and the patient may tell the nurse his extremity feels abnormally hot or cold (Willis, 2001).

Venous Assessment

Decreased venous circulation leads to edema. When the venous system is not sufficiently returning blood from the tissues to the heart and lungs (venous insufficiency), excess fluid is left in the tissues of the affected extremity (edema). The nurse will assess for edema in the affected extremity and compare it with the unaffected extremity. Venous insufficiency may lead to changes in the pigmentation of the skin.

The nurse assesses the skin for darker pigmentation, dryness, and scaling in the affected extremity. Chronic edema and stasis of blood from venous insufficiency may lead to ulceration of the tissues. These ulcers are referred to as stasis ulcers. Peripheral pulses are usually present with venous insufficiency. Pain, aching, and cramping associated with venous disorders are usually relieved by activity and/or elevating the extremity. Refer to Table 8-5 for a comparison of signs and symptoms associated with arterial and venous disorders.

Diagnostic Tests

Diagnostic tests for peripheral vascular disorders include noninvasive procedures and invasive procedures.

Noninvasive procedures include the following:

- **Treadmill test:** This is an exercise test used to determine blood flow in the extremities after exercising. It is used to identify pain associated with exercise such as claudication.
- **Plethysmography:** Changes in blood volume are assessed in the veins of the calf or other body extremities by using a plethysmograph.
- **Digital subtraction angiography** (DSA): Initially an intravenous contrast solution visible to radiography is administered. This allows blood vessels in the extremities to be visualized by radiography using an image intensifier video system and a television monitor.
- **Doppler ultrasound:** A Doppler ultrasound flowmeter is used to measure blood flow in arteries or veins. This is helpful in assessing intermittent claudication, obstruction of deep veins, and other disorders of peripheral veins and arteries.

Table **8-5** *Comparisons of Signs and Symptoms Associated with Arterial and Venous Disorders*

SIGNS AND SYMPTOMS	ARTERIAL DISORDER	VENOUS DISORDER
Pain	Aching to sharp cramping brought on by exercise; relieved by rest	Aching to cramping pain; relieved by activity or elevating extremity
Pulses	Diminished or absent	Usually present
Edema	Usually absent	Usually present; increases at the end of the day and when extremity is in a dependent position
Skin changes	Cool or cold Dry, shiny Hairless Pallor develops with elevation; becomes erythematous with dangling	Warm, thick, and toughened Darkened pigmentation Stasis ulcers

Invasive procedures include the following:

- **Phlebography or venography,** a radiographic visualization of veins. A contrast medium is administered through a catheter placed in a foot vein. Films are taken to detect filling defects. Venography is used to assess the condition of the deep leg veins and to diagnose deep vein thrombosis.
- **^{125}I-fibrinogen uptake test:** This test is used for looking at acute calf vein thrombosis. When thrombus formation occurs, large amounts of fibrinogen are present at the site of clot formation. When fibrinogen is tagged with iodine 125 (^{125}I) and given intravenously, it can be detected in the bloodstream by a gamma ray detector. This test is costly and time consuming, but accurate.
- **Angiography:** This is done by injection of a contrast medium intravascularly and then visualizing the arteries using radiography.
- **D-dimer:** A serum test. D-dimer is a product of fibrin degradation (change to a less complex form). When a thrombus is present, plasma D-dimer concentrations are usually greater than 1591 ng/mL. The normal range for D-dimer is 68 to 494 ng/mL.
- **Duplex scanning:** This is a combination of ultrasound imaging techniques and Doppler capabilities to determine location and extent of thrombus within veins (most widely used test to diagnose deep vein thrombosis).

ARTERIAL DISORDERS

ARTERIOSCLEROSIS AND ATHEROSCLEROSIS

Arteriosclerosis (a common arterial disorder characterized by thickening, loss of elasticity, and calcification of arterial walls, resulting in a decreased blood supply) is the underlying problem associated with peripheral vascular disorders. **Arteriosclerosis** and **atherosclerosis** are frequently used interchangeably.

Atherosclerosis is characterized by yellowish plaques of cholesterol, lipids, and cellular debris in the inner layers of the walls of large and medium-sized arteries. The result of atherosclerosis is narrowing of the artery. Nutrients and oxygen to the tissue can be reduced, resulting in ischemia to the tissue cells. Because this is a form of arteriosclerosis, the arterial wall also loses its elasticity and becomes less responsive to change in blood volume and pressure. Plaque, once formed in the arteries, is thought to be irreversible. Lesions in the arteries formed from plaque may completely occlude an artery. Atherosclerosis can progress to obstruction, thrombosis, aneurysm development, and rupture.

When the need for oxygen in the tissues exceeds the supply, ischemia occurs and may result in cell death and tissue necrosis. The degree of reduction in blood flow and oxygen determines the amount of ischemia and necrosis that may occur in the tissues. Specific peripheral vascular disorders that stem from arteriosclerosis and atherosclerosis are discussed individually in this chapter.

HYPERTENSION

Hypertension will be considered with peripheral vascular disorders. Hypertension is a risk factor in atherosclerosis, which leads to peripheral vascular disease.

Etiology/Pathophysiology

Normal blood pressure is systolic blood pressure of less than 120 mm Hg and diastolic blood pressure less than 80 mm Hg. Hypertension or high blood pressure occurs when a sustained elevated systolic blood pressure is greater than 140 mm Hg and/or a sustained elevated diastolic blood pressure is greater than 90 mm Hg. A diagnosis is not based on a one-time elevated blood pressure reading, but after averaging two or more elevated blood pressure readings taken on separate occasions. The guidelines adapted from the Seventh Report of the Joint National Committee on Prevention, Detection, Evaluation, and Treatment of High Blood Pressure, National Institutes of Health, National Heart, Lung, and Blood Institute, May 2003, identify people with a blood pressure of 120 to 139 mm Hg systolic or 80 to 89 mm Hg diastolic as being prehypertensive. People whose blood pressure is in the prehypertensive range are at twice the risk for developing hypertension as people with normal values. Although there is no way of predicting in whom high blood pressure will develop, hypertension can be detected easily.

Approximately 60 million Americans have hypertension and an additional 25 million have borderline hypertension. It has been estimated that up to 30% of the adult population in the United States have undiagnosed hypertension. It is difficult to determine exact numbers because most individuals are symptom free.

Arterial blood pressure is the pressure exerted by the blood on the walls of blood vessels. Systolic blood pressure is the greatest force caused by the contraction of the left ventricle of the heart. Diastolic blood pressure occurs during the relaxation phase between heartbeats. Blood flow is determined by the amount of blood the heart pumps with each contraction and how fast the heart beats. Peripheral vascular resistance is affected by the diameter of the blood vessel and the viscosity of the blood. Blood flow and peripheral vascular resistance play an important role in regulating blood pressure. Increased peripheral vascular resistance resulting from vasoconstriction or narrowing of peripheral blood vessels is a common factor in hypertension.

Vasoconstriction and vasodilation are controlled by the sympathetic nervous system and the renin-angiotensin system of the kidney. Stimulation of the sympathetic nervous system and the release of epinephrine and/or norepinephrine cause blood vessel constriction and increased peripheral vascular resistance. The activation of the renin-angiotensin system occurs with decreased blood flow to the kidney. Renin leads to the formation of angiotensin, which is a potent vasoconstrictor. Angiotensin stimulates the secretion of aldosterone, leading to the retention of sodium and water. The result is an increased blood pressure via these physical mechanisms.

Two main types of hypertension exist: **essential (primary)** hypertension and **secondary** hypertension. The occurrence of hypertension increases with age and other risk factors.

Essential (Primary) Hypertension

Essential (primary) hypertension makes up 90% to 95% of all diagnosed cases. Although no generally accepted cause of essential hypertension exists, several theories attempt to explain the mechanisms involved, including arteriolar changes, sympathetic nervous system activation, hormonal influence (renin-angiotensin-aldosterone system stimulation), genetic factors, greater-than-ideal body weight, sedentary lifestyle, increased sodium intake, and excessive alcohol intake. For a long time many experts believed that an increase in systolic blood pressure was a normal part of aging. In fact, some adhered to the theory that "100 mm Hg plus the patient's age" was a tolerable systolic blood pressure in the older adult. Treatment for hypertension was based primarily on the diastolic

reading, and isolated systolic hypertension (ISH) was often not treated.

The Systolic Hypertension in the Elderly Program (SHEP) study results, published in 1991, reported that ISH is now believed to raise the risk of cardiovascular disease and strokes in both middle-aged and older people. It is actually a better overall predictor of cardiovascular morbidity and mortality than diastolic pressure in these two age groups. (Diastolic pressure remains the better predictor of CAD in people younger than 45 years.) ISH is defined as an elevated systolic blood pressure of 140 mm Hg or more with a diastolic blood pressure below 90 mm Hg. The value of treating ISH in older patients has only recently been established, but now those findings are being widely circulated.

Prognosis. With prolonged untreated essential hypertension, the elastic tissue in the arterioles is replaced by fibrous tissue. This process leads to decreased tissue perfusion, especially in the target organs—the heart, kidney, and brain—resulting in deterioration of major organs. CAD and cerebrovascular accident (stroke), the great causes of death and disability, are much more frequent in those who have elevated blood pressure than in those who are normotensive. With treatment, the prognosis is usually good. Risk factors that contribute to the development of essential hypertension are listed in Box 8-9.

Box 8-9 *Risk Factors that Contribute to Development of Essential Hypertension*

NONMODIFIABLE RISK FACTORS
- **Age:** Risk increases as age advances past 30 years old
- **Gender:** Men are more at risk than women
- **Race:** Risk twice as high in African-Americans as in whites
- **Family history:** Risk increases with a family history of hypertension

MODIFIABLE RISK FACTORS
- **Smoking:** Nicotine constricts blood vessels
- **Obesity:** Associated with increased blood volume
- **High-sodium diet:** Increases water retention, which increases blood volume
- **Elevated serum cholesterol:** Leads to atherosclerosis and narrowing of blood vessels
- **Oral contraceptives/estrogen therapy:** May contribute to elevated blood pressure
- **Alcohol:** Increases plasma catecholamines (biologically active amines, epinephrine, and norepinephrine), which leads to blood vessel constriction
- **Emotional stress:** Stimulates the sympathetic nervous system, which leads to blood vessel constriction
- **Sedentary lifestyle:** Regular exercise contributes to lower blood pressure over time

Secondary Hypertension

Secondary hypertension is attributed to an identifiable medical diagnosis. Conditions associated with secondary hypertension are given in Table 8-6.

Prognosis. In most instances, secondary hypertension will subside when the primary disease process is treated or corrected.

Malignant Hypertension

Malignant hypertension is a severe, rapidly progressive elevation in blood pressure (diastolic pressure greater than 120 mm Hg) that causes damage to the small arterioles in major organs (heart, kidneys, brain, eyes). A primary distinguishing finding is inflammation of arterioles (arteriolitis) in the eyes. This type of hypertension is most common in black males under 40 years of age.

Prognosis. Unless medical treatment is successful, the course is rapidly fatal. The most common causes of death are MI, heart failure, stroke, and renal failure.

Clinical Manifestations

Hypertension is essentially a disease without symptoms until vascular changes occur in the heart, brain, eyes, or kidneys. Long-standing, untreated hypertension can cause target organ damage. Advanced target organ damage may account for left ventricular hypertrophy, angina pectoris, myocardial infarction, heart failure, stroke or transient ischemic attack, nephropathy, peripheral arterial disease, or retinopathy. Signs and symptoms usually occur as a result of advanced hypertension. These signs and symptoms may include awakening with a headache, blurred vision, and spontaneous epistaxis (nosebleed).

Assessment

Collection of **subjective data** regarding symptoms, history of hypertension, and knowledge level data may include the following:
- Assess for morning headache in the occipital area, blurred vision.
- Assess for presence of risk factors (see Box 8-9).

- Assess for knowledge level of hypertension: definition, meaning of systolic and diastolic readings, complications of hypertension, possible concerns regarding treatment.
- Collection of **objective data** would include the following:
- Measure the blood pressure in both arms in supine and sitting positions. Previous blood pressure results would be used to compare reading. Two or more blood pressure measurements are taken on two separate occasions.
- Measure height and weight and record.
- Assess and record heart sounds.
- Palpate and record peripheral pulses.

Diagnostic Tests

Diagnostic tests associated with hypertension are those that evaluate the functions of the brain, heart, and kidneys. The results indicate the effects of hypertension on these organs and provide baseline information for future reference. These tests include the following:
- Complete blood count
- Serum levels of sodium, potassium, calcium, hemoglobin, hematocrit
- Lipid profile; fasting blood glucose level
- Creatinine, BUN, urinalysis, intravenous pyelography (effect on kidneys)
- Chest radiograph, ECG, and possible echocardiography (effect on heart)

Medical Management

Medical management is directed at controlling hypertension and preventing complications. The goal in older adults is to keep the blood pressure at less than 140/90 mm Hg. The general goal for younger adults with mild hypertension is to achieve blood pressure less than 131/85. Treatment is based on the severity of the hypertension, associated risk factors, and damage to major organs. Antihypertensive medications along with nonpharmacologic measures are used to lower blood pressure.

Table 8-6 | *Causes of Secondary Hypertension*

CONDITION/DISORDER	MECHANISM
Renal vascular disease	Kidney disease (glomerulonephritis, renal failure, physiologic changes related to type of disease) affects renin and sodium and results in hypertension.
Diseases of the adrenal cortex	Atherosclerotic changes in renal arteries cause increase in peripheral vascular resistance.
Primary aldosteronism	Increase in aldosterone causes sodium and water retention and increases blood volume.
Cushing syndrome	Increase in blood volume.
Pheochromocytoma	Excess secretion of catecholamines increases peripheral vascular resistance.
Coarctation of the aorta	Causes marked elevated blood pressure in upper extremities with decreased perfusion in lower extremities.
Head trauma or cranial tumor	Increased intracranial; pressure reduces cerebral blood flow and stimulates medulla oblongata to raise blood pressure.
Pregnancy-induced hypertension	Cause unknown; generalized vasospasm may be a contributing factor.

Drug therapy. For uncomplicated hypertension, drug treatments include the following (Woods, 1999):

- Diuretics (thiazides, loop diuretics, potassium sparing)
- Beta-adrenergic blockers such as metoprolol (Lopressor), nadolol (Corgard), propranolol (Inderal)
- Angiotensin-converting enzyme (ACE) inhibitors such as captopril (Captopen), enalapril (Vasotec), lisinopril (Prinivil, Zestril)
- Angiotensin II receptor blockers such as valsartan (Diovan), losartan (Cozaar), irbesartan (Avapro)
- Calcium channel blockers such as diltiazem (Cardizem), amlodipine (Norvasc), nifedipine (Procardia)
- Alpha-agonists such as clonidine

Special considerations are as follows:

- Diabetes mellitus: ACE inhibitors
- Heart failure: ACE inhibitors, diuretics
- Myocardial infarction: beta blockers, ACE inhibitors
- African-Americans: calcium channel blockers, diuretics
- Isolated systolic hypertension in older patients: diuretics preferred, long-acting calcium channel blockers

Nonpharmacologic therapy. Measures of nonpharmacologic therapy include the following (Woods, 1999):

- **Lose excess weight.** Being overweight is associated with increased BP, abnormally high blood lipid levels, diabetes mellitus, and coronary artery disease. Limiting calorie intake and increasing physical exercise are the keys to losing weight.
- **Reduce saturated fat.** A patient with high blood lipid levels may require dietary modification or drug therapy to normalize them. A cardinal rule is to limit fat intake to less than 30% of total calories. According to the Dietary Approaches to Stop Hypertension (DASH) study, a low-fat diet rich in fruits and vegetables is recommended.
- **Limit alcohol intake.** Excessive alcohol consumption may contribute to hypertension. A man of normal weight should not drink more than 1 ounce of ethanol per day, the equivalent of 24 ounces of beer, 10 ounces of wine, or 2 ounces of 100-proof whiskey. Women and lightweight men should restrict their intake to half this amount.
- **Exercise regularly.** Thirty to 45 minutes of aerobic exercise three or four times a week helps decrease the risk of hypertension and cardiovascular disease.
- **Reduce sodium intake.** A high sodium intake can increase BP, especially in African-Americans, older adult patients with existing hypertension, and patients with diabetes mellitus. It is recommended limiting sodium intake to 2.4 g/day. Encourage your patient to eat unsalted, unprocessed foods and to read labels when shopping.

- **Consume enough potassium, calcium, and magnesium.** Plenty of potassium in the diet helps decrease BP, so eating potassium-rich fruits and vegetables may improve BP control. Administering potassium supplements to a patient who is hypokalemic as a result of diuretic therapy also combats hypertension. A word of caution: Anyone receiving ACE inhibitors or potassium-sparing diuretics should receive potassium supplements only with extreme caution and close monitoring for hyperkalemia. Low dietary calcium and magnesium may contribute to hypertension; the National Heart and Lung Institute (NHLI) suggests consuming adequate amounts of calcium and magnesium but does not recommend supplementation to combat hypertension.
- **Stop smoking.** Cigarette smoking is one of the leading risk factors of hypertension and heart disease. Smoking also inhibits the effect of antihypertensive medication, so techniques for stopping must be an integral part of patient education. Counseling, support groups, and aids to stop smoking are very effective. Because many people who stop smoking gain weight, make sure a weight management and exercise program is part of the plan.
- **Relaxation techniques/stress management.** Stress management and relaxation techniques have also been shown to offset hypertension and its symptoms.

Nursing Interventions and Patient Teaching

The main focus of nursing interventions is to maintain blood pressure management through patient teaching about hypertension, risk factors, and drug therapy.

Patient compliance is improved with education about side effects of medications, dietary instruction, exercise, and stress-reduction techniques (Box 8-10).

Nursing diagnosis and interventions for the patient with hypertension include but are not limited to the following:

NURSING DIAGNOSES	NURSING INTERVENTIONS
Knowledge, deficient, related to disease process and therapeutic management	Assess level of understanding. Implement teaching plan for hypertension: • Disease process, risk factors • Prescribed medications and side effects; proper dosage and administration; necessity of taking medication, even when blood pressure readings are normal • Dietary restrictions • Exercise program • Relaxation techniques

Box 8-10 *Measures to Increase Compliance with Antihypertensive Therapy*

1. Be sure that patient understands that absence of symptoms does not indicate control of blood pressure; remind patient that symptoms do not occur until advanced stages of the disease.
2. Advise patient against abrupt withdrawal of medication; rebound hypertension can occur.
3. Encourage patient to discuss unpleasant side effects of medication with a health care professional.
4. If remembering to take medications is a problem, discuss alternate ways to remember, such as taking them with certain meals or placing medication in separate containers labeled with times of day.
5. Suggest patient participate in an exercise program with a friend or pay for the program (more likely to participate "to get money's worth").
6. Include family and significant others in the teaching process to provide support and promote adherence to regimen.
7. Explain reason for regular health care follow-up (high blood pressure is a chronic disorder).
8. Contact patients who consistently cancel follow-up appointments.

NURSING DIAGNOSES	NURSING INTERVENTIONS
Knowledge, deficient, related to disease process and therapeutic management—cont'd	• Sexual dysfunction as a potential side effect of adrenergic inhibitors • Compliance with therapy and follow-up appointments Encourage the patient to promptly report any problems to health care professionals for counseling.

ARTERIOSCLEROSIS OBLITERANS
Etiology/Pathophysiology

Arteriosclerosis obliterans is a disorder accompanied by a narrowing or an occlusion of the intima and media of the blood vessel walls. Plaque formation, as a result of the arteriosclerotic process, forms on the internal wall of the blood vessel, causing partial or complete occlusion of the blood vessel. The result is little or no blood flow to the affected extremity. The artery is unable to supply blood and oxygen to the tissues whether the patient is exercising or at rest. Thus, signs and symptoms associated with tissue ischemia appear.

Clinical Manifestations

Pain is the first symptom that occurs from tissue ischemia. The pain generally occurs in the affected extremity in conjunction with sustained activity (see Table 8-5). This is due to the demand of the tissue exceeding the available blood supply. The process of activity → ischemia → pain in an affected extremity is referred to as **claudication.** The pain of claudication subsides with rest; therefore it is frequently referred to as intermittent claudication (a weakness of the legs accompanied by cramping pains in the calves caused by poor circulation of the blood to the muscles). A burning pain at rest or at night is manifested when the disease process is severe. Symptoms of coldness, numbness, and tingling may be associated with the pain. The signs and symptoms to watch for include the classic five P's of arterial occlusion, which are **pain, pulselessness, pallor, paresthesia,** and **paralysis.**

Assessment

Collection of **subjective data** focuses on pain associated with intermittent claudication. Does the pain occur with activity, and is it relieved by rest? Is pain occurring at rest?

Collection of **objective data** includes assessment of pulses in the affected extremity, which may be weak or absent, and comparison with pulses in the unaffected extremity. Other assessment factors may include pallor and hairless, shiny skin that is dry and cool to touch. Chronic arterial occlusion may show assessment findings of rubor (discoloration or erythema [redness] caused by inflammation) or cyanosis, arterial ulcers, cellulitis, or gangrenous changes in the affected extremity.

Diagnostic Tests

A variety of tests are useful to diagnose arteriosclerosis obliterans. Treadmill testing, digital subtraction angiography, Doppler ultrasound, MRI, and angiography may be likely choices.

Medical Management

Medical management is focused on preventing complete arterial occlusion. The most frequently used medications to treat obstructive arterial disorders include anticoagulants, fibrinolytics, and vasodilators. The use of vasodilators is controversial; most studies indicate that these drugs are not effective. Anticoagulants are used to prolong clotting time, thus preventing extension of a clot and inhibiting further clot formation. Heparin and warfarin are the most commonly administered anticoagulants. Fibrinolytics or thrombolytics are useful in dissolving existing thrombi. Urokinase is used in most patients with peripheral arterial occlusive disease. Unlike lytic therapy in MI or pulmonary embolism, in peripheral arterial occlusion the drug is administered directly into the thrombus through a central line that contains proximal and distal infusion wires (see also Complementary & Alternative Therapies box). Surgical intervention for advanced disease includes embolectomy (removal of

![Complementary & Alternative Therapies logo] **Complementary & Alternative Therapies**

Cardiovascular and Peripheral Vascular Disorders

- Vitamin E has been found to be useful in the treatment of intermittent claudication; however, recent studies indicate doses above 400 mg/day increase the risk of intracranial bleeding, especially if used with aspirin.
- A number of herbs have been studied for their circulatory effects. Ginkgo biloba has been found minimally effective for intermittent claudication, as well as for decreased cerebral circulation leading to reduced function. Manifestations of decreased cerebral circulation can include decreased memory, vertigo, tinnitus, and mood swings with anxiety.
- In the treatment of chronic venous insufficiency, horse chestnut seed extract (HCSE, *Aesculus hippocastanum*) may be equivalent to compression stocking therapy. German health authorities have approved HCSE for the treatment of chronic venous insufficiency, as well as for pain and heaviness in the legs and varicose veins. Gastrointestinal side effects may occur but are uncommon.
- Garlic has been studied for its effects on arteriosclerosis and lipids with varying results. The amount of fresh garlic a person would need to eat for a therapeutic dosage is quite high and likely to cause gastric upset. Garlic preparations vary widely in terms of their active constituents.
- Caution must be exercised and patients taking anticoagulants should be advised regarding the use of certain vitamins and herbs, including garlic, ginkgo, and vitamin E. Although natural, these substances can obviously have potent therapeutic activity. This may in part be due to anticoagulant effects, which may potentiate the action of blood-thinning drugs. Health practitioners should be aware of the use of such substances so that any interactions can be monitored safely. Not enough controlled research is available to make definite predictions.
- Herbal remedies used to self-treat peripheral vascular disorders include those for hypertension, varicose veins, atherosclerosis, and vascular spasm. Herbs with antihypertensive action include garlic (*Allium sativum*), hawthorn (*Crataegus oxyacantha*), kudzu (*Pueraria lobata*), nettle (*Urtica dioica*), onion (*Allium cepa*), purslane (*Portulaca oleracea*), reishi mushroom (*Ganoderma lucidum*), and valerian (*Valeriana officinalis*). Ginkgo biloba has also been used for varicose veins and obliterative arterial disease of the lower extremities. Horse chestnut (*A. hippocastanum*) is used for varicose veins and phleblitis, and valerian is used as an antispasmodic. Antihypertensive spices include basil, black pepper, fennel, and tarragon.

Data from Black, J.M. & Hawks, H.J. (2005) *Medical-surgical nursing,* Philadelphia: Saunders.

embolism) or endarterectomy (surgical removal of the lining of an artery, usually performed on any diseased or occluded major artery, such as the carotid, femoral, or popliteal), arterial bypass (Figure 8-18), percutaneous transluminal angioplasty (PTA), or amputation.

Nursing Interventions and Patient Teaching

Nursing interventions will be based on assessment findings and nursing diagnoses. Nursing diagnoses and nursing interventions for the patient with arteriosclerosis obliterans include but are not limited to the following:

NURSING DIAGNOSES	NURSING INTERVENTIONS
Activity intolerance, related to ischemic pain or immobility	Prevent hazards of immobility by turning, positioning, and deep breathing; isometric and range-of-motion exercises.
	Encourage program of balanced exercise and rest to promote circulation.
	Instruct the patient to use pain or intermittent claudication as a guide to limiting activity during exercise
Ineffective tissue perfusion, peripheral, related to decreased arterial blood flow	Place patient's legs in a dependent position relative to the heart to improve peripheral blood flow.
	Avoid raising feet above heart.
	Promote vasodilation by providing warmth to extremities and keeping room warm.
	Teach the patient to avoid vasoconstriction from nicotine, caffeine, stress, or chilling.
	Teach the patient to avoid constrictive clothing such as garters, tight stockings, or belts.
	Administer prescribed medications.
	Teach the patient to avoid crossing the legs.

Prognosis

In advanced disease, ischemia may lead to necrosis, ulceration, and gangrene (particularly of the toes and distal foot) because of the decreased circulation.

ARTERIAL EMBOLISM
Etiology/Pathophysiology

Arterial emboli are blood clots in the arterial bloodstream. They may originate in the heart from an atrial dysrhythmia, MI, valvular heart disease, or congestive heart failure. Other foreign substances such as a de-

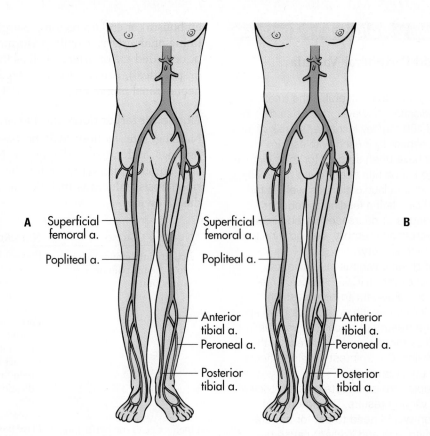

FIGURE **8-18 A,** Femoral-popliteal bypass graft around an occluded superficial femoral artery. **B,** Femoral posterior tibial bypass graft around occluded superficial femoral, popliteal, and proximal tibial arteries.

tached arteriosclerotic plaque or tissue may result in arterial emboli. An embolus becomes dangerous when it lodges within and occludes a blood vessel. Blood flow to the area distal to the lodged embolus is impaired and ischemia occurs. Signs and symptoms depend on the size of the embolus and the amount of circulation that is compromised.

Clinical Manifestations

Sudden loss of blood flow to tissues causes severe pain. Distal pulses are absent and the affected extremity may become pale, cool, and numb. Necrotic changes may occur. Shock may result if the embolus occludes a large artery.

Assessment

Collection of **subjective data** includes determining the onset of pain and numbness and the location, quality, and occurrence of these symptoms.

Collection of **objective data** includes assessing pulses in the affected extremity. Comparison of both extremities to determine skin temperature and color as well as comparison of pulse volumes is of great importance.

Diagnostic Tests

Doppler ultrasonography and angiography are indicated to obtain a diagnosis.

Medical Management

Medications used to treat obstructed arteries include anticoagulants and fibrinolytics or thrombolytics. Anticoagulants are utilized to prevent further clot formation and inhibit extension of a clot. Thrombolytics or fibrinolytics are used to dissolve an existing clot. See the Medications table for Myocardial Infarction on p. 356 for more information on anticoagulants and fibrinolytics.

Endarterectomy (the surgical removal of the intimal lining of an artery) may be selected as the treatment of choice. This involves stripping arteriosclerotic plaques from the intima or inner media of arteries affected by atherosclerosis. Balloon catheters and other instruments are used to accomplish this. Removal of plaques and thrombi increases blood flow and lessens the danger of complications from further emboli or occlusion of an artery.

Embolectomy is another treatment utilized when larger arteries are obstructed. It is the surgical removal of a blood clot. Surgery must be done within 6 to 10 hours of the event to prevent necrosis and loss of the extremity. Endarterectomy and embolectomy may be done together to deal with the existing emboli and prevent recurrence.

Nursing Interventions and Patient Teaching

Nursing interventions are similar to those for arteriosclerosis obliterans in terms of preventing further arterial problems. During the acute phase the patient must be monitored for changes in skin color and temperature of the extremity distal to the embolus. Increasing pallor, cyanosis, and coolness of the skin indicate worsening or occlusion of arterial circulation to the extremity. Keep the extremity warm, but do not apply direct heat.

Nursing diagnoses and nursing interventions for the patient requiring an embolectomy and/or endarterectomy include but are not limited to the following postoperative nursing interventions:

NURSING DIAGNOSES	NURSING INTERVENTIONS
Ineffective tissue perfusion, peripheral, related to decreased arterial blood flow	Monitor skin color and temperature distal to the graft site every hour. Assess sensation and movement in the distal extremity. Assess peripheral pulses and capillary refill in the involved extremity: • Sudden absence of pulse may indicate thrombosis. • Mark location of peripheral pulse with a pen to facilitate frequent assessment. • Use Doppler to monitor if pulses of involved extremity are nonpalpable and compare with pulses of noninvolved extremity. Monitor extremity for edema. Check incision for erythema, edema, and exudate. Monitor and immediately report signs of complications, such as increasing pain, fever, changes in drainage, absent or weakening pulse, change in skin color, limitation of movement, or paresthesia. Promote circulation: • Reposition patient every 2 hours. • Tell patient not to cross legs. • Use a footboard and overbed cradle to keep linens off extremity.

NURSING DIAGNOSES	NURSING INTERVENTIONS
	• Encourage progressive activity when permitted. Avoid sharp flexion in area of graft. Monitor for signs of bleeding secondary to anticoagulation therapy.
Deficient knowledge, related to anticoagulant therapy	Teach patient general action and side effects of prescribed drug; avoid taking medications with aspirin, which also has anticoagulant effect. Instruct patient to take anticoagulant at same time every day; do not stop taking it until advised by physician. Have patient check for signs of bleeding (gum bleeding, epistaxis [nosebleed], ecchymosis [bruising], cuts that do not stop bleeding with direct pressure, blood in urine or stool); report promptly to health care professional. Encourage patient to wear a medic-alert bracelet or carry an identification card containing the drug name, drug dosage, and physician's name in case of emergency. Have patient report for prescribed blood tests (PTT, PT, NR) used to adjust drug dosage. Tell patient not to add dark green and yellow vegetables to diet (contain vitamin K, which counteracts the anticoagulant drug effect). Instruct patient to restrict alcohol intake (increases anticoagulant effect).

Patient teaching is the same as for arteriosclerosis obliterans, with an emphasis on anticoagulant therapy.

Prognosis

Prognosis depends upon the size of the embolus, the presence of collateral circulation, and the proximity to a major organ.

ARTERIAL ANEURYSM
Etiology/Pathophysiology

An aneurysm is an enlarged, dilated portion of an artery. Aneurysms may be the result of arteriosclerosis, trauma, or a congenital defect. Aneurysms of the lower extremities commonly affect the popliteal artery. Other areas predominantly affected are the thoracic and abdominal aorta as well as coronary and cerebral arteries. The aorta is especially prone to aneurysm and rupture because it is continuously exposed to high pressures. Dissections and ruptures are more likely in the thoracic portion of the aorta than in the abdominal portion (Nienaber & Eagle, 2003). An aneurysm starts with a weakened arterial wall that becomes dilated from blood flow and pressure in the area. The pathological effect of this condition is differentiated according to shape and site of presentation (Figure 8-19).

Clinical Manifestations

A large pulsating mass may be the only identifiable factor. Clinical signs and symptoms of a thoracic aortic aneurysm depend on its location. If it compresses adjacent structures, it can cause chest pain, shortness of breath, cough, hoarseness, or dysphagia. If it compresses the superior vena cava, the patient may have edema of the face, neck and arms. An abdominal aneurysm is less common and less complex. In the early stages it is unlikely to cause symptoms. As it expands, however, it may cause pain in the chest, lower back, or scrotum. A pulsatile, nontender upper abdominal mass may be palpated (Nienaber & Eagle, 2003).

Assessment

Collection of **subjective data** by the nurse may reveal a patient whose condition has no subjective symptoms unless the aneurysm is large and impinges on other structures, which can result in pain and inequality of pulses. A thoracic aortic aneurysm can result in chest pain, shortness of breath, or dysphagia.

Collection of **objective data** includes palpation of a large, nontender pulsating mass at the site of the aneurysm.

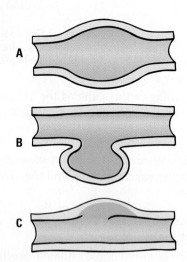

FIGURE **8-19** Types of aneurysms. **A,** Fusiform. **B,** Saccular. **C,** Dissecting.

Diagnostic Tests

Fluoroscopy, chest radiographic studies, CT scan, ultrasound, and arteriography are utilized to diagnose the presence of an aneurysm.

Medical Management

Aneurysms are monitored for complications such as dissection, rupture, formation of thrombi, and ischemia. Control of hypertension is the first priority of care. Surgical intervention may be utilized. The blood vessel may be ligated or grafts may be used to replace the section of the artery that contains the aneurysm or to bypass the aneurysm.

A fusiform or circumferential aneurysm (in which all the walls of the blood vessel dilate more or less equally, creating a tubular swelling) can be removed and repair made with a graft of synthetic fiber, such as Dacron or Teflon, or with another vessel taken from another region of the patient's body. Saccular aneurysms (a yielding of a weak area on one side of the vessel and not involving the entire circumference that causes an outpouching of the vessel wall usually resulting from trauma; it is attached to the artery by a narrow neck) can be removed and the vessel then sutured, or a patch graft can be used to replace the deformity (Figures 8-20 and 8-21).

In repair of a popliteal aneurysm, popliteal blood flow is more enhanced when a homograft/allograft (the transfer of tissue between two genetically dissimilar individuals of the same species, such as a tissue transplant between two humans who are not identical twins) is used.

Nursing Interventions and Patient Teaching

Initial nursing interventions include monitoring the status of an existing aneurysm. The patient should be monitored for signs of rupture of the aneurysm, such as paleness, weakness, tachycardia, hypotension, abdominal pain, back pain, or groin pain.

Postoperative nursing diagnoses and interventions for the patient with arterial aneurysm include but are not limited to the following:

Nursing Diagnoses	Nursing Interventions
Ineffective tissue perfusion, peripheral, related to decreased arterial blood flow	Assess circulation (especially in extremities) by pedal pulse checks and capillary refill assessments. Be alert for complications.
Anxiety, related to feelings of impending death	Examine coping ability. Provide active listening and genuine interest. Maintain therapeutic environment. Administer antianxiety medications as ordered.

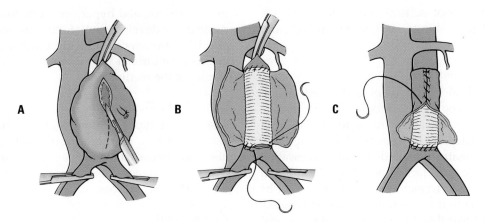

FIGURE **8-20** Surgical repair of an abdominal aortic aneurysm. **A,** Incising the aneurysmal sac. **B,** Insertion of synthetic graft. **C,** Suturing native aortic wall over synthetic graft.

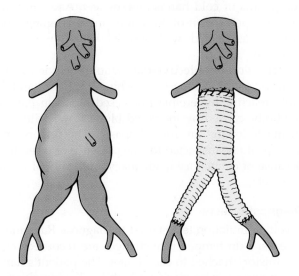

FIGURE **8-21** Replacement of aortoiliac aneurysm with a bifurcated synthetic graft.

Because aneurysm formation is most commonly associated with atherosclerosis, patient teaching is focused on risk factor management, including control of hypertension as well as promotion of tissue perfusion, maintenance of skin integrity, and prevention of infection and injury.

Prognosis

An aneurysm may rupture and cause hemorrhage, resulting in death without emergency surgical intervention. With surgical intervention, the prognosis is often good.

THROMBOANGIITIS OBLITERANS (BUERGER'S DISEASE)
Etiology/Pathophysiology

Thromboangiitis obliterans (Buerger's disease) is an occlusive vascular condition in which the small and medium-sized arteries become inflamed and throm-botic. The cause is not fully understood, but men between the ages of 25 and 40 years who smoke are usually those affected with the disorder. Men are affected 75 times more often than women. The disorder develops in the small arteries and veins of the feet and hands. The wrists and lower legs may also be involved. Occlusion of the arteries leads to ischemia; pain; and in later stages, infection and ulceration. There is a very strong relationship between Buerger's disease and tobacco use. It is thought that the disease occurs only in smokers, and when smoking is stopped, the disease improves.

Clinical Manifestations

The main characteristic is inflammation of vessel walls. The most common symptom is pain with exercise affecting the arch of the foot, also called **instep claudication.** When the hands are involved, the pain is usually bilaterally symmetrical (equal). Pain may occur at rest and be frequent and persistent, particularly when it occurs in the patient who also has atherosclerosis. The skin in the affected extremity may be cold and pale, and ulcers and gangrene may be present. Sensitivity to cold is an outstanding clinical manifestation. An early sign of Buerger's disease may be superficial thrombophlebitis.

Assessment

Collection of **subjective data** includes information about pain, claudication, and sensitivity to cold in affected extremities and risk factor assessment.

Collection of **objective data** includes presence of pulses, skin color, and temperature in the affected extremities.

Diagnostic Tests

There are no diagnostic tests specific to Buerger's disease. Diagnosis is made based on age of onset, history of tobacco use, clinical symptoms, involvement of distal vessels, presence of ischemic ulcerations, and exclusion of diabetes mellitus, autoimmune disease, and proximal source of emboli.

Medical Management

The goal of medical management is directed at preventing disease progression. Modifying risk factors and smoking cessation are a major focus. Smoking causes vasoconstriction and decreases blood supply to the extremities. Treatment includes complete cessation of tobacco use in any form (including secondhand smoke). Nicotine-replacement products should not be used, and trauma to the extremities must be avoided. Patients are told that they have a choice between cigarettes and their affected limbs; they cannot have both. Exercise to develop collateral circulation is encouraged. Surgical intervention, such as amputation of gangrenous fingers and toes, may be indicated. A sympathectomy (a surgical interruption of part of the sympathetic nerve pathways) to alleviate pain and vasospasm may also be performed.

Nursing Interventions and Patient Teaching

Nursing interventions are focused on managing risk factors, promoting tissue perfusion, providing comfort measures, and patient teaching. Care of the extremities to prevent necrosis and gangrene includes hydration and cleanliness. Well-fitting shoes and socks alleviate pressure.

The hazards of cigarette smoking and its relationship to Buerger's disease are the primary focus of patient teaching. The goal is to have the patient quit smoking. None of the palliative treatments are effective if the patient does not stop smoking. Nowhere are the cause and effect of smoking so dramatically presented as with Buerger's disease.

Prognosis

Buerger's disease is a chronic condition. Amputation may be necessary if the condition progresses to gangrene with chronic infection and extensive tissue destruction.

RAYNAUD'S DISEASE
Etiology/Pathophysiology

Raynaud's disease is caused by intermittent arterial spasms. There are intermittent attacks of ischemia of the body—especially the fingers, toes, ears, and nose—caused by exposure to cold or by emotional stimuli.

The attacks may occur secondary to such other conditions as scleroderma (a relatively rare autoimmune disease affecting blood vessels and connective tissue), rheumatoid arthritis, systemic lupus erythematosus, drug intoxication, and occupational trauma. It commonly affects women between 20 and 40 years of age and is more prevalent during the winter months. The exact cause is unknown. It is thought that emotional stress, alterations in the nervous system and immuno-

logical system, and hypersensitivity to cold may play a role in the development of signs and symptoms. Few arterial changes occur initially, but as the disease progresses, the intimal wall thickens and there is hypertrophy of the medial wall.

Clinical Manifestations

The patient typically complains of chronically cold hands and feet. During arterial spasms, pallor, coldness, numbness, cutaneous cyanosis, and pain occur. Chronic Raynaud's disease may result in ulcerations on the fingers and toes.

Assessment

Collection of **subjective data** includes determining underlying disease processes, risk factor evaluation, and complaints of cold hands and/or feet. Assessing the patient's perception of pain, numbness, tingling, and burning associated with arterial spasm would be included.

Collection of **objective data** would include assessment of pallor, coldness, blanching, cyanosis, and finally reactive hyperemia (increased blood in part of the body, caused by increased blood flow) with erythema following an arterial spasm. The fingers and toes would be inspected for the presence of ulceration because of circulatory inadequacy and residual waste products.

Diagnostic Tests

A cold stimulation test is used to diagnose Raynaud's disease. Skin temperature changes are recorded by a thermistor attached to each finger. The patient's hand is submerged in an ice water bath for 20 seconds, and ongoing temperatures are recorded. A comparison is made for baseline data.

Medical Management

Medical therapy is aimed at prevention. Drug therapy may be prescribed to reduce pain and promote circulation. Currently calcium channel blockers are the first-line drug therapy. Calcium channel blockers such as nifedipine (Procardia) and diltiazem (Cardizem) relax smooth muscles of the arterioles. Nifedipine is preferred over diltiazem because it has a stronger vasodilating effect and less effect on the calcium channels in the conduction system in the heart (Lewis et al, 2004). Biofeedback techniques have been used to increase skin temperature and thereby prevent spasms. Relaxation training and stress management are effective for some patients. Temperature extremes should be avoided. The patient should stop using all tobacco products and avoid caffeine and other drugs with vasoconstrictive effects such as amphetamines and cocaine. Surgical interventions may include sympathectomy for symptomatic relief. If the disease is advanced, with ulcerations and gangrene, the involved area may have to be amputated.

Nursing Interventions and Patient Teaching

Nursing interventions are similar to those for other arterial disorders: promoting tissue perfusion, maintaining comfort, and preventing injury and infection. Risk factor management includes stress-reduction techniques and smoking cessation.

Nursing diagnoses and interventions stress patient teaching for the patient with Raynaud's disease, including but not limited to the following:

NURSING DIAGNOSES	NURSING INTERVENTIONS
Deficient knowledge, related to effects of cigarette smoking, stress reduction, and avoiding exposure to cold	Develop teaching plan to include the following: • Effects of smoking on vasoconstriction and arterial blood flow. • Techniques for smoking cessation: stop smoking programs, biofeedback, hypnosis. • Techniques for stress reduction: massage, imagery, music, exercise, lifestyle changes. • Ways of avoiding exposure to cold: layer clothing, wear mittens and warm socks during winter months, use caution when cleaning the refrigerator and freezer, wear gloves when handling frozen food, and avoid occupations that require constant exposure to cold.

Prognosis

Raynaud's disease may be controlled by protecting the body and extremities from the cold and using mild sedatives and vasodilators. Attacks persist but can be controlled. No serious disability develops, but this condition is sometimes associated with the development of rheumatoid arthritis or scleroderma.

VENOUS DISORDERS

Venous disorders occur when the blood flow is interrupted in returning from the tissues to the heart. Changes in smooth muscle and connective tissue make the veins less distensible. The valves in the veins may malfunction, causing backflow of blood. The major venous disorders are thrombophlebitis and varicose veins (Table 8-7).

THROMBOPHLEBITIS
Etiology/Pathophysiology

Thrombophlebitis is inflammation of a vein in conjunction with the formation of a thrombus. It occurs more frequently in women and affects people of all races. The incidence increases with aging. Other factors associated with the development of thrombophlebitis include venous stasis, hypercoagulability (excessive clotting) of the blood, and trauma to the blood vessel wall. Immobilized patients who have had surgical procedures involving pelvic blood vessel manipulation, such as total hip replacement or pelvic surgery, or patients with MI are prone to thrombophlebitis. Thrombophlebitis develops in deep veins (deep vein thrombosis) as well as superficial veins (superficial thrombosis) (Figure 8-22). Thrombophlebitis usually occurs in an extremity, most frequently a leg. Superficial thrombophlebitis is often of minor significance and is treated with elevation, antiinflammatory agents, and warm compresses. Deep vein thrombosis (DVT) is of greater significance and can become dislodged and carried to the lungs in the bloodstream and cause a pulmonary embolus. Pulmonary embolism is a life-threatening complication.

Clinical Manifestations

Pain and edema occur when the vein is obstructed. The size of the calf or thigh may increase in circumference. Active dorsiflexion of the foot may result in calf pain. This is referred to as a positive Homans' sign and may be indicative of thrombophlebitis. Homans' sign is a classic but unreliable sign because it is not specific for deep vein thrombosis. A positive Homans' sign appears in only 10% of DVT patients. Thrombophlebitis of the superficial veins may show signs of inflammation such as erythema, warmth, and tenderness along the course of the vein.

Assessment

Collection of **subjective data** includes characteristics of pain in the affected extremity, noting onset and duration and any history of venous disorders.

Collection of **objective data** includes inspecting the extremity and determining color and temperature (pale and cold if vein is occluded; erythematous and warm if superficial vein is inflamed). Both legs are measured for circumference and comparison and to detect edema.

Diagnostic Tests

Diagnostic tests for deep vein thrombosis include venous Doppler, duplex scanning (the most widely used test), and venogram (phlebogram). A serum D-dimer test will be elevated in DVT. D-dimer is a fibrin degradation fragment that is made from fibrolysis. When a thrombus is undergoing lysis (destruction), it results in increased D-dimer fragments.

Medical Management

Superficial thrombophlebitis is usually treated with bed rest, moist heat, and elevation of the legs. Some physicians believe that complete immobilization is necessary to prevent emboli formation; others believe that clots are sufficiently adhered to vein walls and that mobility improves general circulation and pre-

Table 8-7 *Venous Disorders*

SIGNS AND SYMPTOMS	MEDICAL MANAGEMENT/NURSING INTERVENTIONS
THROMBOPHLEBITIS	
Entire extremity may be pale, cold, and edematous.	Maintain bed rest during acute phase.
Area along vein may be erythematous and feel warm to touch.	Apply warm, moist heat to reduce discomfort and pain per physicians orders.
Homans' sign: pain in calf on dorsiflexion	Elevate extremity, but pillows are not used under the knees, and knees are never bent.
Superficial veins feel indurated (hard) and thready or cordlike and are sensitive to pressure.	Assess circulation of the affected extremity, and skin condition and pulses in all extremities.
Difference in circumference of extremities	Measure calf circumference daily and record.
	Use antiembolism stocking on unaffected extremity.
	Administer heparin or enoxaparin (Lovenox) and warfarin (Coumadin) per physician's orders.
	Administer fibrinolytics (streptokinase) to resolve the thrombus per physician's orders.
	Begin exercise program after acute phase per physician's orders.
VARICOSE VEINS	
Veins appear as darkened, tortuous, raised blood vessels; more pronounced on prolonged standing	Conservative treatment:
Feeling of heaviness in legs	• Elevate legs 10 to15 minutes at least every 2 to 3 hours.
Fatigue	• Wear elastic stockings
Pain and muscle cramps	• Unna's paste boot recommended for older or debilitated person with cutaneous ulcers (see Figure 8-23)
Edema	• Avoid standing for long periods
Ulcers on skin	• Avoid anything that impedes venous flow, such as garters, tight girdles, crossing the legs, and prolonged sitting.
	• Weight reduction if obese
	• Injection of sclerosing solutions for small varicosities
	Surgery:
	• Venous ligation and stripping

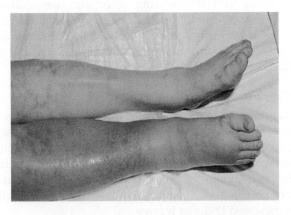

FIGURE **8-22** Deep vein thrombophlebitis.

vents further venous stasis. Drug therapy may include NSAIDs. Deep vein thrombophlebitis requires hospital treatment. The patient is placed on bed rest during the acute phase to prevent embolus. Anticoagulants such as unfractionated heparin administered intra-venously and oral warfarin (Coumadin) are routinely given (Safety Considerations box for the Patient on Anticoagulant Therapy). Fibrinolytics and vasodilators may be prescribed.

Low-molecular-weight heparin (LMWH) is effective for the prevention of venous thrombosis, as well as prevention of extension or recurrence. Enoxaparin (Lovenox), dalteparin (Fragmin) and ardeparin (Normiflo) are three types of low-molecular-weight heparin. LMWH is administered subcutaneously in fixed doses, once or twice daily. LMWH has the practical advantage that it does not require anticoagulant monitoring and dose adjustment. LMWH has a greater bioavailability, more predictable dose response, and longer half-life than heparin with less risk of bleeding complications.

The affected extremity is elevated periodically above heart level to prevent venous stasis and to reduce edema. Specific orders depend on the physician's preference. When the patient begins to ambulate, elastic stockings (antiembolism stockings) are used to

Patient on Anticoagulant Therapy

1. Teach patient on oral warfarin (Coumadin) requirements for frequent follow-up with blood tests (Pt, INR) to assess blood clotting and whether change in drug dosage is required.
2. Teach patient side effects and adverse effects of anticoagulant therapy requiring medical attention.
   - Any bleeding that does not stop after a reasonable amount of time (usually 10 to 15 minutes)
   - Blood in urine or stool or black, tarry stools
   - Unusual bleeding from gums, throat, skin, or nose, or heavy menstrual bleeding
   - Severe headaches or stomach pains
   - Weakness, dizziness, mental status changes
   - Vomiting blood
   - Cold, blue, or painful feet
3. Avoid any trauma or injury that might cause bleeding (e.g., vigorous brushing of teeth, contact sports, inline rollerskating.)
4. Do not take aspirin-containing drugs or nonsteroidal antiinflammatory drugs.
5. Limit alcohol intake to small amounts.
6. Wear a medic-alert bracelet or necklace indicating what anticoagulant is being taken.
7. Avoid marked changes in eating habits, such as dramatically increasing foods high in vitamin K (e.g., broccoli, spinach, kale, greens). Do not take supplemental vitamin K.
8. Inform all health care providers, including dentist, of anticoagulant therapy.
9. Correct dosing is essential and supervision may be required (e.g., patients experiencing confusion.)
10. Do not use herbal products that may alter coagulation (Complementary & Alternative Therapies box).

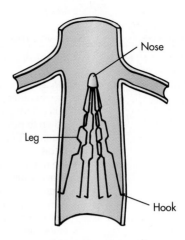

FIGURE **8-23** Inferior vena caval interruption technique using Greenfield stainless steel filter to prevent pulmonary embolism.

compress the superficial veins, increase blood flow through the deep veins, and prevent venous stasis.

Surgery is indicated only when conservative measures have been unsuccessful. A thrombectomy or the **transvenous placement of a grid** or umbrella in the vena cava may be done to prevent the flow of emboli into the lungs. This inferior vena caval interruption device is called a Greenfield filter, which can be inserted percutaneously through superficial femoral or internal jugular veins. When the filter device is opened, the spokes penetrate the vessel walls. The device creates a "sieve-type" obstruction, permitting filtration of clots without interruption of blood flow (Figure 8-23).

Nursing Interventions and Patient Teaching

Early mobilization is the easiest and most cost-effective method to decrease the risk of DVT. Patients on bed rest need to be instructed to change position, dorsiflex their feet, and rotate ankles every 2 to 4 hours. Ambulatory patients should ambulate at least three times per day. Elastic compression stockings (e.g., thromboembolic disease [TED] hose) or an intermittent compression device (ICD) are used for hospitalized patients at risk for DVT. The major emphasis for the patient with thrombophlebitis is preventing complications, promoting comfort, and patient teaching about the disease and prevention of recurrence.

Nursing diagnoses and interventions for the patient with thrombophlebitis include but are not limited to the following:

NURSING DIAGNOSES	NURSING INTERVENTIONS
Ineffective tissue perfusion, peripheral, related to decreased venous blood flow	Confine patient to bed in acute phase. Elevate affected extremity according to physician's orders. Check circulation frequently (monitor pedal pulses, capillary refill). Administer prescribed NSAIDs, anticoagulants, and fibrinolytics. Measure calf or thigh circumference daily. Assess site for signs of inflammation and edema. Have patient wear elastic stockings when ambulatory. Implement graded exercise program as ordered.
Deficient knowledge, related to disease process and risk factors	Develop a teaching plan to prevent venous stasis, including the following: • Avoid prolonged sitting or standing; begin weight reduction if obese. • Avoid crossing the legs at the knee, tight stockings, or garters.

Nursing Diagnoses	Nursing Interventions
Deficient knowledge, related to disease process and risk factors—cont'd	• Elevate legs when sitting. • Do flexion-extension exercises of feet and legs when sitting or lying down to promote circulation and venous return. • Do not massage extremities because of danger of embolization of clots (thrombus breaking off and becoming an embolus). • Take prescribed medication.

Prognosis

A major risk during the acute phase of deep vein thrombophlebitis is dislodgment of the thrombus, which can migrate to the lungs, causing a pulmonary embolus.

VARICOSE VEINS
Etiology/Pathophysiology

A varicose vein is a tortuous, dilated vein with incompetent valves.

The highest incidence of varicose veins occurs in women ages 40 to 60 years. Approximately 15% of the adult population is affected. Causes of varicose veins include congenitally defective valves, an absent valve, or a valve that becomes incompetent. External pressure on the legs from pregnancy or obesity can place a strain on the vessels, and they become elongated and dilated. Poor posture, prolonged standing, and constrictive clothing may also contribute to this problem. The great and small saphenous veins of the legs are most often affected. The vessel wall weakens and dilates, stretching the valves and resulting in an inability of the vessel to support a column of blood. Pooling of blood in the veins or varicosities is the result. Chronic blood pooling in the veins is referred to as **venous stasis.** Hemorrhage can occur if there is trauma to a varicose vein.

Clinical Manifestations

Varicose veins may be primary or secondary. Primary varicosities have a gradual onset and affect superficial veins. Secondary varicosities affect the deep veins and result from chronic venous insufficiency or venous thrombosis. Often no symptoms exist except the appearance of darkened veins on the patient's legs. Symptoms include fatigue, dull aches, cramping of muscles, and a feeling of heaviness or pressure arising from decreased blood flow to the tissues. Signs and symptoms such as edema, pain, changes in skin color, and ulceration may occur from venous stasis.

Assessment

Collection of **subjective data** includes gathering information about predisposing factors: a family history of varicose veins, pregnancy, or other conditions that could cause pressure on the veins. Also to be included are symptoms the patient is experiencing such as aches, fatigue, cramping, heaviness, and pain.

Collection of **objective data** includes inspecting the legs for varicosities, edema, color, and temperature of the skin and observing for ulceration.

Diagnostic Tests

Trendelenburg's test is done to diagnose the ability of the venous valves to support a column of blood by measuring venous filling time. The patient lies down with the affected leg raised to allow for venous emptying. A tourniquet is applied above the knee, and the patient stands. The direction and filling time of the veins are recorded both before and after the tourniquet is removed. When the veins fill rapidly from a backward blood flow, the veins are determined to be incompetent.

Medical Management

Mild signs and symptoms may be controlled with elastic stockings, rest periods, and leg elevation. Sclerotherapy consists of injection of a sclerosing solution at the sites of the varicosities. It is done as an outpatient procedure and produces permanent obliteration (complete occlusion of a part) of collapsed veins and good cosmetic results. Elastic bandages are applied for continuous pressure for 1 to 2 weeks. Surgical intervention is indicated for pain, progression of varicosities, edema, stasis ulcers, and cosmetic reasons. Surgery consists of vein ligation and stripping. The great saphenous vein is ligated (tied) close to the femoral junction. The great and small saphenous veins are stripped out through small incisions made in the inguinal area, above and below the knee and the ankle. The incisions are covered with sterile dressings, and an elastic bandage is applied and is to be worn for at least 1 week.

Nursing Interventions and Patient Teaching

Nursing interventions focus on care of the patient following a surgical procedure, including maintaining comfort, maintaining peripheral circulation and venous return, and patient teaching regarding varicosity prevention and maintenance.

Nursing diagnoses and interventions for the patient with varicose veins include but are not limited to the following:

Nursing Diagnoses	Nursing Interventions
Ineffective tissue perfusion, peripheral, related to impaired venous blood return	Monitor for signs and symptoms of bleeding postoperatively. If bleeding occurs, apply pressure to the wound, elevate the leg, and notify the physician.

NURSING DIAGNOSES	NURSING INTERVENTIONS
	Keep elastic bandage snug and wrinkle free; do not remove bandage for daily dressing change.
	Encourage deep breathing exercises and early ambulation to facilitate venous return.
	Encourage dorsiflexion exercises while in bed or sitting to facilitate venous return.
Deficient knowledge, related to disease process, measures to avoid venous stasis and promote venous return	Develop teaching plan to include: • Avoid anything that can increase pressure above the knees (crossing the legs, sitting in chairs that are too high, wearing garters and knee-high stockings). • Begin regular exercise to promote venous return by contraction of leg muscles. • Avoid prolonged sitting or standing. • Elevate legs when sitting. • Maintain ideal weight. • Wear elastic stockings for support for activities that require prolonged standing or when pregnant.

Prognosis

Varicosities are chronic conditions; the affected person must know how to prevent venous stasis and encourage venous return.

VENOUS STASIS ULCERS
Etiology/Pathophysiology

Venous stasis ulcers or leg ulcers occur from chronic deep vein insufficiency and stasis of blood in the venous system of the legs. Other causes include severe varicose veins, burns, trauma, sickle cell anemia, diabetes mellitus, neurogenic disorders, and hereditary factors. A leg ulcer is an open, necrotic lesion that results when an inadequate supply of oxygen-rich blood and nutrients reaches the tissue (Figure 8-24). The result is cell death, tissue sloughing, and skin impairment. Decreased circulation to the area contributes to the development of infection and prolonged healing.

Clinical Manifestations

Varying degrees of pain may be reported, ranging from mild discomfort to a dull, aching pain relieved by elevation of the extremity. The skin is visibly ulcerated and has a dark pigmentation. Edema may be present. Ulcerations often occur around the medial aspect of the ankle. Pedal pulses are present.

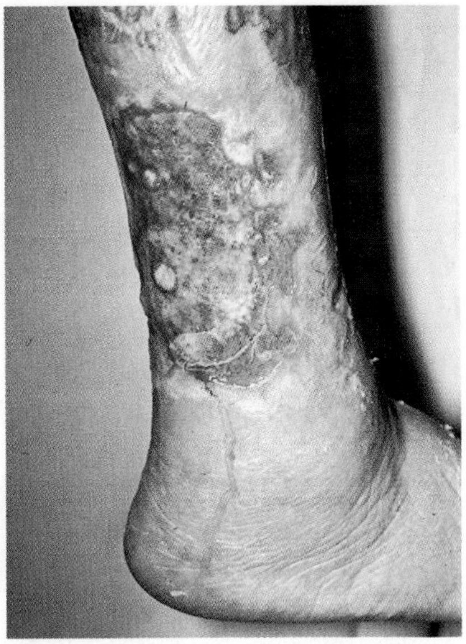

FIGURE **8-24** Venous leg ulcer.

Assessment

Collection of **subjective data** includes onset and duration of pain and successful relief measures. Predisposing factors such as thrombophlebitis, venous insufficiency, and/or diabetes mellitus are noted.

Collection of **objective data** would include inspection of ulcerated areas: size, location, and condition of skin; color; and temperature. Palpate pedal pulses, and observe for presence of edema.

Diagnostic Tests

Diagnostic tests utilized to confirm venous insufficiency and stasis are venography and Doppler ultrasonography.

Medical Management

Management is focused on promoting wound healing and preventing infection. Diet is very important to ensure adequate protein intake, because large amounts of protein in the form of albumin are lost through the ulcers. Also vitamin A and C and the mineral zinc are administered to promote tissue healing. Debridement of necrotic tissue, antibiotic therapy, and protection of the ulcerated area are usual treatments. Debridement may be mechanical, such as applying wet-to-dry dressing to the wound. The dressing is applied damp; when dry, it is removed, pulling off the debris that has adhered to the dressing. Debridement can be chemical, which is the use of enzyme ointments such as fibrinolysin deoxyribonuclease (Elase) placed over the ulcer to break down necrotic tissue. Surgical debridement using a scalpel is done when other measures are not successful. Protection of ulcerated areas may be accomplished with the use of an Unna's paste boot (Figure 8-25). This boot protects the ulcer and provides constant and even support to the area. A moist, impregnated gauze is wrapped around the patient's foot

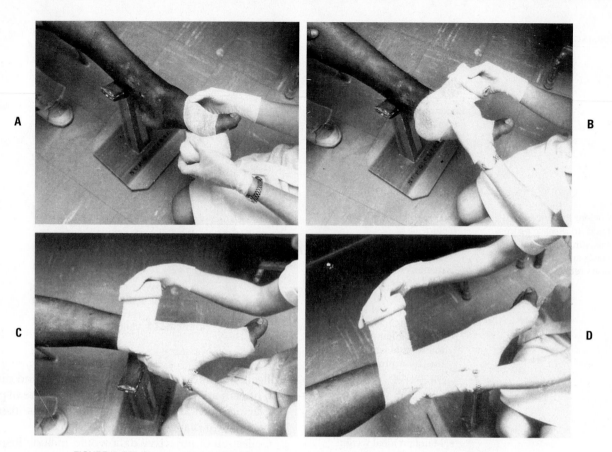

FIGURE **8-25** Nurse applying Unna's paste boot using specially impregnated gauze. Most ulcers are on inferior aspect of patient's foot.

and leg. It hardens into a "boot" that may be left on for 1 to 2 weeks, although it may be changed more often if there is copious drainage.

Nursing Interventions and Patient Teaching

Nursing interventions focus on promoting wound healing, promoting comfort, maintaining peripheral tissue perfusion, preventing infection, and patient teaching.

Nursing diagnoses and interventions for the patient with venous stasis ulcers include but are not limited to the following:

NURSING DIAGNOSES	NURSING INTERVENTIONS
Impaired skin integrity, related to open ulceration	Perform dressing changes perphysician's order, using wet-to-dry technique, topical drug treatments, and Unna's boot therapy. Assess wound for signs and symptoms of infection. Provide antibiotic therapy as prescribed. Encourage nutritional intake to promote wound healing.

NURSING DIAGNOSES	NURSING INTERVENTIONS
Ineffective tissue perfusion, peripheral, related to insufficent venous circulation	Elevate extremities when sitting or lying to promote venous return and decrease incidence of edema and venous stasis. Use overbed cradle to protect extremities from pressure of bed linens. Use cotton between toes to prevent pressure on a toe ulcer. Assess level of discomfort.

Patient teaching focuses on preventing infection, maintaining peripheral tissue circulation, avoiding venous stasis, and proper wound care and dressing changes. See previous nursing diagnoses and interventions.

Prognosis

Venous stasis ulcers are a chronic condition caused by chronic venous insufficiency and delayed healing. Most venous ulcers heal with therapy.

NURSING PROCESS *for the Patient with a Cardiovascular Disorder*

The role of the licensed practical nurse/licensed vocational nurse (LPN/LVN) in the nursing process as stated is that the LPN/LVN will:

- Participate in planning care for patients based on patient needs
- Review patient's plan of care and recommend revisions as needed
- Review and follow defined prioritzation for patient care
- Use clinical pathways/care maps/care plans to guide and review patient care

Systemic cardiac assessment provides the nurse with baseline data useful for identifying the physiologic and psychosocial needs of the patient.

Assessment

The nurse begins assessment of the patient with a cardiovascular disorder by performing a physical assessment and by obtaining a complete health history. The physical assessment includes level of consciousness, vital signs, lung sounds (crackles, wheezes), bowel sounds, apical heart sounds (strength, regularity of rhythm) and pedal pulses, capillary refill, skin color (pallor, cyanosis), turgor, temperature and moisture, and presence of edema. The history includes a description of symptoms, when they occurred, their course and duration, location, precipitating factors, and relief measures. Specific signs and symptoms the nurse should be aware of include the following:

- **Pain.** The character, quality, radiation, and associated symptoms must be noted. Ask patient to rate pain on a scale of 1 to 10. Determine what, if anything, relieved the pain, such as rest or medication such as nitroglycerin sublingually. Chest pain is the primary complaint when patients have symptoms of heart disease. Some patients with ischemia have pain in the jaw and left shoulder. The patient may use the following terms to describe the pain: dull, sharp, pressure, squeezing, crushing, viselike, grinding, or radiating. Precipitating onset is noted. Pain originating from cardiac muscle ischemia (decreased blood supply to a body organ or part) is anxiety producing. It may lead to other signs and symptoms such as nausea, vertigo, or diaphoresis. Chest pain is significant in indicating cardiac ischemia or damage.
- **Palpitations.** Characterized by rapid, irregular, or pounding heartbeat, palpitations may be associated with cardiac dysrhythmias (any disturbance or abnormality in a normal rhythmic pattern) or cardiac ischemia. Patients may begin to notice the heartbeat and describe it as "pounding" or "racing." This can be frightening for the patient.

- **Cyanosis.** A bluish discoloration of the skin and mucous membranes caused by an excess of deoxygenated hemoglobin in the blood, cyanosis results from decreased cardiac output and poor peripheral perfusion.
- **Dyspnea.** Dyspnea is characterized by difficulty breathing or shortness of breath. Dyspnea with activity should also be noted. This symptom is referred to as **exertional dyspnea** and is commonly associated with decreased cardiac function.
- **Orthopnea.** Orthopnea is an abnormal condition in which a person must sit or stand to breathe deeply or comfortably.
- **Cough.** The cough may be dry or productive and results from a fluid accumulation in the lungs. The patient may describe it as irritating or spasmodic. Dyspnea may be associated with it. The production of sputum should be observed for frothiness or hemoptysis (see discussion of pulmonary edema).
- **Fatigue.** Fatigue is a feeling of exhaustion and activity intolerance associated with decreased cardiac output. The patient may be unable to perform ADLs. Depression may accompany this or be a result of it.
- **Syncope.** Syncope or fainting is a brief lapse of consciousness caused by transient cerebral hypoxia. It is usually preceded by a sensation of lightheadedness. It can result from a sudden decrease in cardiac output to the brain as a result of dysrhythmia (bradycardia or tachycardia) or decreased pumping action of the heart.
- **Diaphoresis.** This is the secretion of sweat, especially profuse secretion; it is associated with clamminess. Diaphoresis is a result of decreased cardiac output and poor peripheral perfusion.
- **Edema.** Weight gain of more than 3 pounds in 24 hours may be indicative of heart failure. The mechanism leading to edema in heart failure is the inability of the heart to pump efficiently or accept venous return, causing retrograde blood flow and an excessive amount of circulating blood volume. This increased blood volume results in increased hydrostatic pressure and an increase of fluid to the interstitial spaces.

Nursing Diagnosis

The nurse assesses the patient's cardiovascular system and identifies characteristics that reveal a nursing diagnosis. Nursing diagnoses for cardiovascular problems may include the following:

- Activity intolerance
- Anxiety
- Decreased cardiac output
- Ineffective coronary tissue perfusion

- Excess fluid volume
- Impaired gas exchange
- Deficient knowledge (specify)
- Pain

Expected Outcomes/Planning

The nurse plans appropriate interventions to meet the needs of patients with cardiovascular problems. The nurse is in the unique position of ongoing patient monitoring and is able to participate in the development of nursing diagnoses, assist in the selection of appropriate interventions, and document the plan of care. Teaching throughout the hospital stay and when preparing for discharge is important. Reinforcement of good health habits improves the likelihood for compliance with the plan of care.

Implementation

Nursing interventions for the patient with a cardiovascular disorder include enhancing cardiac output, promoting tissue perfusion, promoting adequate gas exchange, improving activity tolerance, and promoting comfort. Patient teaching emphasizes adherence to diet and exercise and medication protocols and strategies for balancing activity, getting rest, and reducing stress.

Evaluation

The nurse evaluates the expected outcomes as the final step of the nursing process and determines their effectiveness. The nurse may participate in the revision of the plan and nursing interventions when necessary.

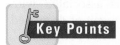 **Key Points**

- The cardiovascular system is composed of the heart, blood vessels, and lymphatic structures.
- The functions of the cardiovascular system are to deliver oxygen and nutrients to the cells and to remove carbon dioxide and waste products from the cells.
- The heart is a large pump (the size of a human fist) that propels blood through the circulatory system.
- The heart is composed of four chambers: two atria and two ventricles.
- There are two coronary arteries; they supply the heart with nutrition and oxygen.
- The electrical pattern of impulse starts with the sinoatrial (SA) node, which is the pacemaker of the heart; it initiates the heartbeat. This impulse travels to the atrioventricular (AV) node. From here the impulse travels to a bundle of fibers called the bundle of His and divides into right and left bundle branches and finally to the Purkinje fibers.
- There are three kinds of blood vessels organized for carrying blood to and from the heart: the arteries, veins, and capillaries.

- Risk factors for developing coronary artery disease (CAD) are classified as nonmodifiable and modifiable.
- Nonmodifiable risk factors for CAD include advancing age, being of the male gender or African-American race, and a positive family history of CAD.
- Major modifiable risk factors for CAD include cigarette smoking, hyperlipidemia, stress, obesity, sedentary lifestyle, and hypertension. A diet high in cholesterol and saturated fats contributes to risk factors.
- An important aspect of caring for the patient with a cardiovascular disorder is understanding the risk factors and incorporating them into patient teaching.
- Major diagnostic tests to evaluate cardiovascular function may include chest radiograph, arteriography, cardiac catheterization, electrocardiography (ECG), echocardiogram, telemetry, stress test, positron emission tomography (PET), and thallium scanning.
- Common laboratory examinations to evaluate cardiovascular function are blood cultures, complete blood count (CBC), prothrombin time (PT), International Normalized Ratio (INR); partial thromboplastin time (PTT), erythrocyte sedimentation rate (ESR), serum electrolytes, lipids (VLDL, LDL, HDL), triglycerides, arterial blood gases (ABGs), B-type natriuretic peptide (BNP), and serum cardiac markers. Troponin I is a myocardial muscle protein released into circulation after myocardial injury and is useful in diagnosing a myocardial infarction.
- Coronary artery disease (CAD) is the term used to describe a variety of conditions that obstruct blood flow in the coronary arteries.
- When the myocardial oxygen demand exceeds the myocardial oxygen supply, ischemia of the heart muscle occurs, resulting in chest pain or angina.
- Patient teaching to minimize the pain of angina pectoris will include nitroglycerin before exertion, small feedings rather than two or three larger meals, exercise periods with rest periods, stopping activity at first sign of chest pain, avoiding exposure to extreme weather conditions, ceasing to smoke, and seeking a calm environment.
- The subjective data of a patient with MI may include heavy pressure or squeezing pressure in the chest, retrosternal pain radiating to left arm and jaw, anxiety, nausea and dyspnea.
- Major objective data for the patient with MI include pallor, hypertension, cardiac rhythm changes, vomiting, fever, and diaphoresis.
- Possible nursing diagnoses for the patient with MI may include pain (acute), tissue perfusion (ineffective), activity intolerance, decreased cardiac output, anxiety, and constipation.
- Cardiac rehabilitation services are designed to help patients with heart disease recover faster and return to full and productive lives. Cardiac rehabilitation improves patient compliance.
- Heart failure (HF) leads to the congested state of the heart, lungs, and systemic circulation as a result of the heart's inability to act as an effective pump. The most recent definition is that heart failure should be viewed as a neurohormonal problem in which heart failure progresses as a result of chronic release in the body of substances such as catecholamines (epinephrine and

norepinephrine). These substances are capable of toxic effects on the heart.

- It is important for the nurse to realize that 1 L of fluid equals 1 kg (2.2 pounds); a weight gain of 2.2 pounds will signify a gain of 1 L of body fluid.
- Signs and symptoms of HF with left ventricular failure include dyspnea; cough; frothy, blood-tinged sputum; pulmonary crackles; and evidence of pulmonary vascular congestion with pleural effusion.
- Signs and symptoms of HF with right ventricular failure include edema in feet, ankles, and sacrum, which may progress into the thigh and external genitals; liver congestion; ascites; and distended jugular veins.
- Medical management of HF includes increasing cardiac efficiency with digitalis, vasodilators, and ACE inhibitors; beta blocker (Coreg) for mild to moderate HF; lowering oxygen requirements through bed rest; providing oxygen to the tissues through oxygen therapy if the patient is hypoxic; treating edema and pulmonary congestion with a diuretic and a sodium-restricted diet; and weighing daily to monitor fluid retention.
- Nursing interventions for the patient with valvular heart disease include administering the prescribed medications (diuretics, digoxin, and antidysrhythmics); monitoring I&O and daily weight; auscultating breath sounds and heart sounds; taking blood pressure; and assessing capillary perfusion, pedal pulses, and presence of edema.
- Patient teaching for the patient with valvular heart disease includes dietary management, activity limitations, and the importance of antibiotic prophylaxis before invasive procedure.
- Most patients with cardiomyopathy have a severe, progressively deteriorating course, and the majority older than age 55 years die within 2 years of the onset of signs and symptoms.
- Peripheral vascular disease is any abnormal condition that affects the blood vessels outside the heart and the lymphatic vessels.

- Arteriosclerosis is the underlying problem associated with peripheral vascular disorders.
- Hypertension occurs when there is a sustained elevated systolic blood pressure greater than 140 mm Hg and/or sustained elevated diastolic blood pressure of less than 90 mm Hg on two or more such readings.
- The main focus of nursing interventions for the patient with hypertension is to maintain blood pressure management through patient teaching, risk factor recognition, and drug therapy as well as dietary management, exercise, and stress-reduction techniques.
- An aneurysm is an enlarged, dilated portion of an artery and may be the result of arteriosclerosis, trauma, or a congenital defect.
- The hazards of cigarette smoking and its relationship to thromboangiitis obliterans (Buerger's disease) are the primary focuses of patient teaching.
- The two major venous disorders are thrombophlebitis and varicose veins.
- Thrombophlebitis results in calf pain upon dorsiflexion of the foot, which is referred to as a positive Homans' sign.
- Patient teaching to avoid thrombophlebitis includes the following: avoid prolonged sitting or standing, reduce weight if obese, do dorsiflexion-extension exercises of feet and legs, do not cross legs at the knees, and elevate legs when sitting.

Go to your free CD-ROM for an Audio Glossary, animations, video clips, and Review Questions for the NCLEX-PN® Examination.

evolve   Be sure to visit the companion Evolve site at http://evolve.elsevier.com/Christensen/adult/ for WebLinks and additional online resources.

CHAPTER CHALLENGE

1. The blood that is pumped out of the left ventricle contains:

   1. a full supply of oxygen.
   2. impurities that must be removed by the liver.
   3. a high percentage of carbon dioxide.
   4. all the wastes to be delivered to the organs of excretion.

2. The heart contracts in the following patterns:

   1. right atrium, left atrium, then the ventricles.
   2. both atria, then both ventricles.
   3. right atrium, right ventricles, then the left atrium, left ventricles.
   4. ventricles, then atria.

3. The interior lining of the heart, the valves, and the large vessels of the heart are together called the:

   1. endocardium.
   2. myocardium.
   3. pericardium.
   4. epicardium.

4. Valve flaps prevent the backflow of blood from the pulmonary artery into the:

   1. lung.
   2. right atrium.
   3. right ventricle.
   4. left atrium.

Continued

CHAPTER CHALLENGE—cont'd

5. The normal period in the heart cycle during which the muscle fibers lengthen, the heart dilates, and the cavities fill with blood, roughly the period of relaxation, is called:
   1. systole.
   2. pulse pressure.
   3. diastose.
   4. diastole.

6. The right atrium receives blood from the:
   1. superior and inferior venae cavae.
   2. pulmonary veins, pulmonary arteries.
   3. superior and inferior venae cavae and coronary sinus.
   4. membranous septum, coronary sinus.

7. When Mr. J. is receiving heparin therapy, the nurse should:
   1. observe him for cyanosis.
   2. remember that a sedimentation rate is ordered for monitoring blood coagulation.
   3. give the injection intramuscularly.
   4. observe emesis, urine, and stools for blood.

8. Mr. S., 72 years of age, is admitted to the medical floor with a diagnosis of HF. In HF an increase in abdominal girth, increase in total body weight, and pitting edema are indications of:
   1. fluid retention.
   2. electrolyte imbalance.
   3. disorganized ventricle pulsation.
   4. AV node dysfunction.

9. T. C., 10 years of age, is diagnosed with rheumatic fever. Of all the manifestations that may be seen in rheumatic fever, the one that may lead to permanent complications is:
   1. Sydenham's chorea.
   2. erythema marginatum.
   3. subcutaneous nodules.
   4. carditis.

10. Ms. L., 67 years of age, has a diagnosis of hypertension. She is being dismissed from the hospital. Her teaching should include:
   1. instruction in consuming a bland diet.
   2. encouragement to take medicines until blood pressure is controlled.
   3. encouragement to begin a vigorous exercise program.
   4. education on continuing to take antihypertensive medications as prescribed.

11. Mr. M. is an 86-year-old patient who is receiving D 5½ NS per IV at 83 mL/hour on the electronic infusion pump. It is vitally important that the IVs of older adult patients be monitored carefully because:
   1. these patients do not get dehydrated very easily.
   2. they may get a fluid overload of the circulatory system.
   3. of the increased risk of infection in the veins.
   4. of the danger of thrombophlebitis developing in the peripheral system.

12. Mr. A. is a 34-year-old patient with a history of IV drug use. He is diagnosed with acute infective endocarditis. Nursing interventions for this patient would include:
   1. early ambulation and activity progression.
   2. restricted activity for several weeks.
   3. low-calorie diet.
   4. dilution of blood by increased fluid intake.

13. Mr. K. is a 62-year-old patient with a history of angina pectoris. To decrease the pain from angina pectoris, Mr. K. should:
   1. take a cardiac glycoside at first symptom of cardiac pain.
   2. be careful to avoid taking more than three or four nitroglycerin pills daily.
   3. take nitroglycerin sublingually qid.
   4. take nitroglycerin sublingually at the first sign of chest discomfort.

14. Ms. J. has an arterial occlusive disorder. Patient teaching for arterial occlusive disorders would include:
   1. encouraging the patient to ambulate frequently.
   2. the importance of avoiding exposure to cold and chilling.
   3. teaching self-massage of the legs with lotion.
   4. maintaining a reduced-calorie diet.

15. Ms. R., 75 years of age, is diagnosed with heart failure. The nursing diagnosis of activity intolerance, related to dyspnea and fatigue, would be appropriate. Choose the appropriate nursing intervention in keeping with this diagnosis.
   1. Plan frequent rest periods.
   2. Allow patient to shower.
   3. Encourage patient to perform all ADLs.
   4. Encourage fluid intake of 3000 L/day.

16. A postmyocardial patient being prepared for discharge should be instructed to:
   1. remain inactive until healing is complete.
   2. remain at home and avoid exposure to cold temperatures.
   3. begin a cardiac rehabilitation program.
   4. perform isometric exercises in a relaxed environment.

17. Dependent edema of the extremities, enlargement of the liver, oliguria, jugular vein, and abdominal distention are signs and symptoms of:
    1. right-sided heart failure.
    2. left-sided heart failure.
    3. cardiac dysrhythmias.
    4. valvular heart disease.

18. The primary function of patient teaching following a myocardial infarction is:
    1. focusing education on an understanding of the disease process.
    2. to assist the patient to develop a healthy lifestyle.
    3. focusing on precipitating causes and onset of pain.
    4. to educate the patient on causative factors that initiate cardiac vasoconstriction.

19. An important nursing intervention when caring for a patient with remote telemetry is to:
    1. allow patient independence by permitting patient to shower.
    2. never remove telemetry and allow patient to shower unless physician has written the order to allow a shower.
    3. encourage use of stair climbing, aerobic exercise, and other forms of exertion to promote collateral circulation.
    4. be cognizant that special microphones, attached to the patient's chest, pick up cardiac sounds produced by pressure changes in the heart.

20. Signs and symptoms of cardiogenic shock could include:
    1. warm, dry skin.
    2. decreasing blood pressure and weak, rapid pulse.
    3. flushed face, restlessness.
    4. polyuria and dysuria.

21. Modifiable risk factors for coronary artery disease (CAD) include which of the following?
    1. Diabetes, family history
    2. Family history, smoking
    3. Smoking, heredity
    4. High cholesterol, obesity

22. The name of the neurohormone released from the left ventricle in response to volume expansion and pressure overload that has emerged as the blood marker for the identification of individuals with CHF:
    1. A-type natriuretic peptide (ANP).
    2. Troponin I.
    3. B-type natriuretic peptide (BNP).
    4. CPK peptide.

23. The normal range for the above blood marker is:
    1. 0 to 100 pg/mL.
    2. 500 to 900 pg/mL.
    3. 0.003 to 1 pg/mL.
    4. 400 to 500 pg/mL.

24. _____ is a myocardial muscle protein released into circulation after myocardial injury and is useful in diagnosing a myocardial infarction.

Care of the Patient with a Respiratory Disorder

BARBARA LAURITSEN CHRISTENSEN and ELAINE ODEN KOCKROW

Key Terms

Be sure to check out the bonus material on the free CD-ROM, including selected audio pronunciations.

adventitious (ăd-věnt-TĬ-shŭs, p. 406)
atelectasis (ă-tě-LĔK-tă-sĭs, p. 440)
bronchoscopy (brŏng-KŎS-kō-pē, p. 409)
cor pumonale (kŏr pŭl-mō-NĂ-lē, p. 451)
coryza (kō-RĪ-ză, p. 419)
crackles (KRĂK-ŭlz, p. 406)
cyanosis (sī-ă-NŌ-sĭs, p. 416)
dyspnea (DĬSP-nē-ă, p. 406)
embolism (ĔM-bō-lĭz-ŭm, p. 446)
empyema (ĕm-pī-Ē-mă, p. 437)
epistaxis (ĕp-ĭ-STĂK-sĭs, p. 412)
exacerbation (ĕg-zăs-ĕr-BĀ-shŭn, p. 455)
extrinsic (ĕk-STRĬN-zĭk, p. 457)
hypercapnia (hī-pĕr-KĂP-nē-ă, p. 455)
hypoventilation (hī-pō-věn-tĭ-LĀ-shŭn, p. 440)
hypoxia (hī-PŎK-sē-ă, p. 407)
intrinsic (ĭn-TRĬN-zĭk, p. 457)
orthopnea (ŏr-thŏp-NĒ-ă, p. 406)
pleural friction rub (PLOO-răl FRĬK-shŭn rŭb, p. 406)
pneumothorax (nū-mō-THŌ-răks, p. 441)
sibilant wheeze (SĬB-ĭ-lănt wēz, p. 406)
sonorous wheeze (sŏ-NŌR-ŭs wēz, p. 406)
stertorous (STĔR-tĕr-ŭs, p. 413)
tachypnea (tăk-ĭp-NĒ-ă, p. 440)
thoracentesis (thō-ră-sĕn-TĒ-sĭs, p. 404)
virulent (VĬR-ū-lĕnt, p. 427)

OVERVIEW OF ANATOMY AND PHYSIOLOGY

Experiencing choking or struggling to breathe causes a sensation of panic, serving as a reminder that one cannot live without air. For the millions of cells throughout the body to carry out their specialized activities, they must have a continuous supply of oxygen. External respiration, or breathing, is the exchange of oxygen and carbon dioxide between the lung and the environment. As air is inhaled, it is warmed, moistened, and filtered to prepare it for use by the body. The respiratory system works with the cardiovascular system to deliver the oxygen to the cells, where it provides the cells with energy to carry out metabolism. Internal respiration is the exchange of oxygen and carbon dioxide at the cellular level. Oxygen enters the cells while carbon dioxide leaves them. The gases diffuse across the cell membrane into the bloodstream, which plays the role of transporter. Failure of the respiratory system or cardiovascular system has the same result: rapid cell death from oxygen starvation. Figure 9-1 shows the structure of the respiratory organs.

UPPER RESPIRATORY TRACT
Nose

Air enters the respiratory tract through the nose. The air is filtered, moistened, and warmed as it enters the two nasal openings (nares) and travels to the nasal cavity. The nasal septum separates the nares. This entire area is lined with mucous membrane, which is vascular. This provides the warmth and moisture necessary. Normally a liter of moisture is secreted by this membrane every day.

Lateral to the nasal cavities are three scroll-like bones called **turbinates** or **conchae** (Figure 9-2), which cause the air to move over a larger surface area. This increase in surface area allows the air more time for warming and moisturizing. Lining the nasal cavities are tiny hairs, which trap dust and other foreign particles and prevent them from entering the lower respiratory tract.

Communicating with the nasal structures are paranasal sinuses (Figure 9-3). They are called the **frontal, maxillary, sphenoid,** and **ethmoid cavities.** They are hollow areas that make the skull lighter. It is believed they give resonance to the voice. They are lined with mucous membranes continuous with the nasal cavity. Because of this, nasal infections can cause sinusitis, which is uncomfortable and difficult to treat.

The receptors for the sense of smell are located in the mucosa of the nasal cavities. They are the nerve endings of the olfactory nerve, the first cranial nerve. The nasolacrimal ducts, or tear ducts, communicate with the upper nasal chamber. Hence, when an individual cries, there are copious nasal secretions.

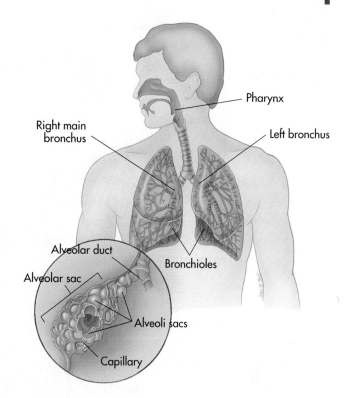

FIGURE **9-1** Structural plan of the respiratory organs showing the pharynx, trachea, bronchi, and lungs. Inset shows the grapelike alveolar sacs where the interchange of oxygen and carbon dioxide takes place through the thin walls of the alveoli. Capillaries surround the alveoli.

Pharynx

The **pharynx** (a tubular structure about 5 inches [13 cm] long extending from the base of the skull to the esophagus and situated just in front of the vertebrae), or throat, is the passageway for both air and food. At the distal end of the pharynx are three subdivisions: (1) **nasopharynx** (most superior portion), (2) **oropharynx** (posterior to mouth), and (3) **laryngopharynx** (directly superior to larynx) (see Figure 9-2).

The eustachian tubes enter either side of the nasopharynx, connecting it to the middle ear. Because the inner lining of the pharynx and the eustachian tube are continuous, an infection of the pharynx can spread easily to the ear. This is very common in children. The adenoids (pharyngeal tonsils) are in the nasopharynx, whereas the palatine tonsils are in the oropharynx.

Larynx

The **larynx** (Figure 9-4, *A*) or organ of voice, is supported by nine areas of cartilage and connects the pharynx with the trachea. The largest area of cartilage is composed of two fused plates and is called the **thyroid cartilage,** or **Adam's apple.** It is the same size in women and men until puberty. At puberty, it produces a large projection in the neck of the man due to its enlargement. The **epiglottis,** a large leaf-shaped area of cartilage, pro-

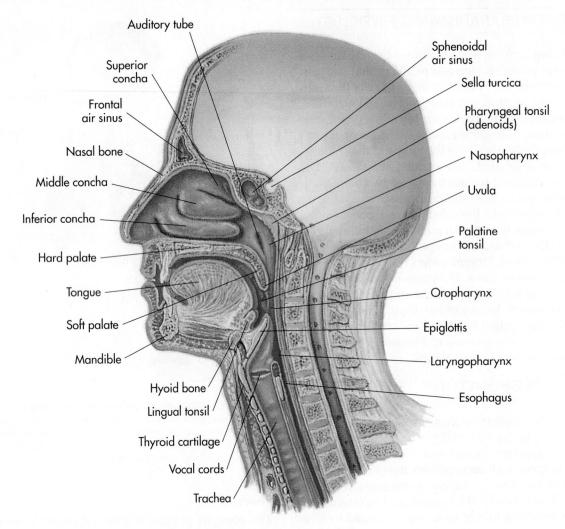

Auditory tube

Superior concha

Frontal air sinus

Nasal bone

Middle concha

Inferior concha

Hard palate

Tongue

Soft palate

Mandible

Hyoid bone

Lingual tonsil

Thyroid cartilage

Vocal cords

Trachea

Sphenoidal air sinus

Sella turcica

Pharyngeal tonsil (adenoids)

Nasopharynx

Uvula

Palatine tonsil

Oropharynx

Epiglottis

Laryngopharynx

Esophagus

FIGURE **9-2** Sagittal section through the face and neck.

tects the larynx when swallowing. It covers the larynx tightly to prevent food from entering the trachea and directs the food to the esophagus (Figure 9-4, *B*).

The larynx contains the vocal cords. During expiration, air rushes over the vocal cords, which causes them to vibrate. This enables speech to occur. The opening between the vocal cords is the glottis.

Trachea

The **trachea** (Figure 9-5), or windpipe, is a tubelike structure that extends approximately 5 inches (11 cm) to the midchest, where it divides into the right and left bronchi. It lies anterior to the esophagus and connects the larynx with the bronchi. The ventral (anterior) surface of the tube is covered in the neck by the isthmus (narrow connection) of the thyroid gland. It contains C-shaped cartilaginous rings that keep it from collapsing. The open part of the C-shaped rings lies posterior to the column anterior to the esophagus, which allows for expansion of the esophagus during swallowing while still maintaining patency of the trachea. This is necessary for uninterrupted breathing. The entire

structure is lined with mucous membranes and tiny **cilia** (small, hairlike processes on the outer surfaces of small cells, aiding metabolism by producing motion or current in a fluid) that sweep dust or debris upward toward the nasal cavity. Any large particles initiate the cough reflex, which is a protective mechanism that aids in the evacuation of foreign material. Sometimes, because of an airway obstruction, it becomes necessary to perform a tracheostomy (a surgical opening into the trachea through which an indwelling tube may be inserted). Once this procedure is completed, the individual breathes through the tracheal opening rather than the nose. The opening is below the larynx, so air cannot pass over the vocal cords. The vocal cords cannot vibrate, and speech becomes physiologically impossible.

LOWER RESPIRATORY TRACT
Bronchial Tree

As the trachea enters the lungs, it divides into the right and left bronchi. The right bronchus enters into the right lung. It is larger in diameter and more vertical in descent. The left bronchus enters the left lung. It is

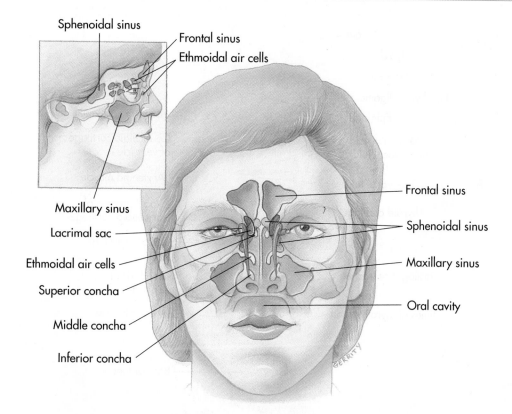

FIGURE **9-3** Projections of paranasal sinuses and oral nasal cavities on the skull and face. Note the connection between the sinuses and nasal cavity.

smaller in diameter and slightly horizontal in position. Because of this design, foreign objects that are aspirated generally enter the right bronchus.

The large bronchi continue to divide into smaller structures called **bronchioles.** These structures continue to divide into smaller, tubelike structures called **terminal bronchioles** or **alveolar ducts.** All these structures are lined with ciliated mucous membrane, as is the trachea. The end structures of the bronchial tree are called **alveoli.** These saclike structures resemble a bunch of grapes. A single grapelike structure is called an alveolus (Figures 9-1 and 9-6). It is in this terminal structure of the bronchial tree that gas exchange takes place. Each alveolus is surrounded by a blood capillary, where diffusion of carbon dioxide and oxygen occurs. Alveoli are very effective in gas exchange, mainly because they are extremely thin walled; each alveolus lies in contact with a blood capillary. In addition, each alveolus is coated with a thin covering of surfactant. Surfactant reduces the surface tension of the alveolus and prevents it from collapsing after each breath (see Figure 9-6).

The lungs contain millions of alveoli; they give shape and form to the lungs. They are filled with air, and lung tissue would float if it was put in water. This tiny, grapelike structure is the most important feature of the respiratory system. It is here that the oxygen diffuses into the cardiovascular system.

MECHANICS OF BREATHING
Thoracic Cavity

The lungs occupy almost all the thoracic cavity except the centermost area—the mediastinum—which contains the heart and great vessels. This cavity, the interpleural space, is enclosed by the sternum, ribs, and thoracic vertebrae.

Lungs. The lungs are large, paired, spongy cone-shaped organs (see Figure 9-5). The right lung weighs approximately 625 g; the left lung weighs approximately 570 g. The right lung contains three lobes; the left lung contains only two lobes. Located approximately 1 inch (2.5 cm) above the first rib is the narrow part—the apex—of each lung. The broad, inferior part—the base of the lungs—lies in the diaphragm.

The lungs receive their blood supply, which comes directly from the heart, through the pulmonary arteries. By the time the blood reaches the lung capillaries, it is "low" in oxygen content. Because alveolar air is rich in oxygen, diffusion will cause movement of oxygen from the area of high concentration. Diffusion of carbon dioxide also occurs between blood and lung capillaries and alveolar air. Blood flowing through the lung capillaries is high in carbon dioxide. After carbon dioxide is diffused into the alveoli and oxygen is diffused into the blood, carbon dioxide leaves the body by expiration of air from the lungs.

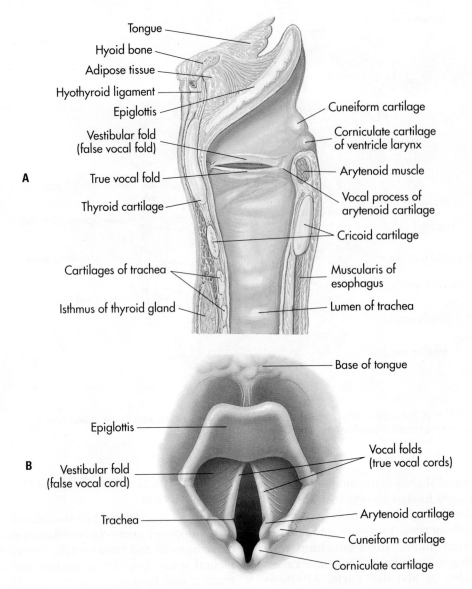

Tongue

Hyoid bone

Adipose tissue

Hyothyroid ligament

Epiglottis

Cuneiform cartilage

Corniculate cartilage
of ventricle larynx

Vestibular fold
(false vocal fold)

True vocal fold

Arytenoid muscle

Vocal process of
arytenoid cartilage

Thyroid cartilage

Cricoid cartilage

Muscularis of
esophagus

Cartilages of trachea

Isthmus of thyroid gland

Lumen of trachea

A

Base of tongue

Epiglottis

Vocal folds
(true vocal cords)

B

Vestibular fold
(false vocal cord)

Trachea

Arytenoid cartilage

Cuneiform cartilage

Corniculate cartilage

FIGURE **9-4 A,** Sagittal section through the larynx. **B,** Larynx and vocal cords as viewed from above through a laryngeal mirror.

The blood, now rich in oxygen, is returned to the heart for circulation to the body via the pulmonary veins to the left atrium.

The surface of each lung is covered with a thin, moist, serous membrane called the **visceral pleura.** The walls of the thoracic cavity are also covered with the same type of membrane called the **parietal pleura.** The pleural cavity around the lungs is an airtight vacuum that contains negative pressure. The air in the lungs is atmospheric pressure and is higher than the pleural cavity. The negative pressure assists in keeping the lungs inflated. The visceral and parietal pleura produce a serous secretion, which allows the lung to slide over the walls of the thorax while breathing. Usually the body produces the exact amount of serous secretion needed. If too much serous secretion is produced, it results in an accumulation of fluid in the pleural space, which is called **pleural effusion.** This causes the pleural space to become distended and puts pressure on the lungs, making it difficult to breathe. The physician may decide to remove the fluid. In this case a thoracentesis will be performed. A needlelike instrument is inserted into the pleural space and the fluid is removed.

Respiratory Movements and Ranges

The rhythmic movements of the chest walls, ribs, and associated muscles when air is inhaled and exhaled make up the respiratory movements. The combination of one inspiration and one expiration makes one respiration. At rest the normal inspiration lasts about 2 seconds and expiration about 3 seconds.

Room air, when inhaled, contains about 21% oxygen; exhaled air contains 16% oxygen and 3.5% carbon dioxide. This represents the actual amount of oxygen used from a single breath.

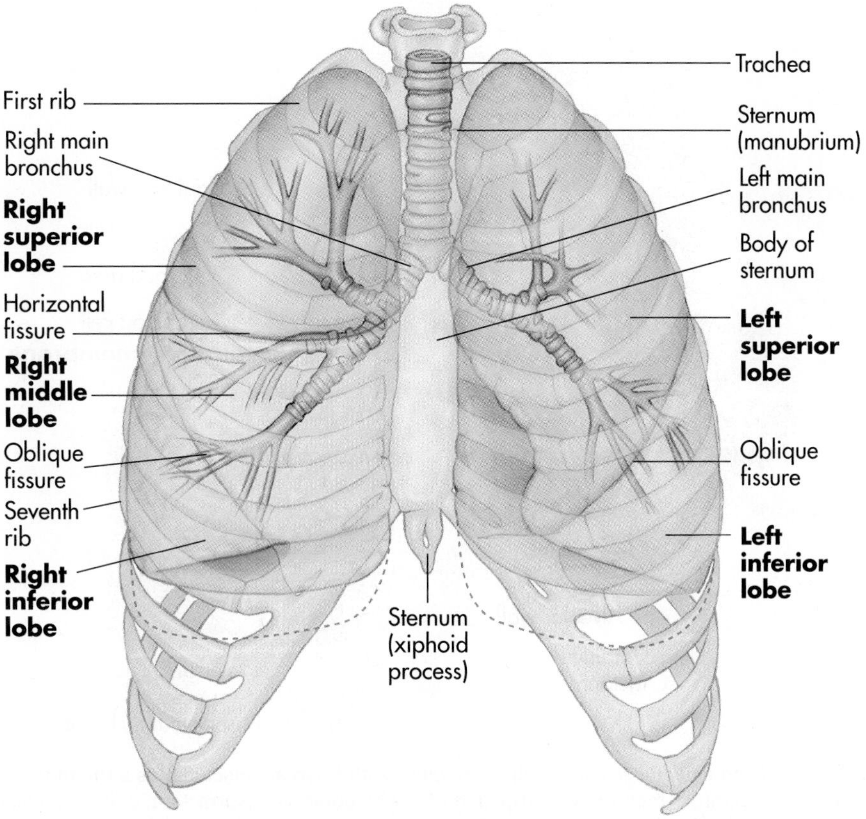

FIGURE **9-5** Projection of the lungs and trachea in relation to ribcage and clavicles. Dotted line shows location of dome-shaped diaphragm at the end of expiration and before inspiration. Note that apex of each lung projects above the clavicle. Ribs 11 and 12 are not visible in this view.

The normal range of respiration for an adult at rest is 14 to 20 breaths per minute. This rate can be affected by many variables: age, sex, activity, disease, and body temperature. For example, the respiratory rate for a newborn is 40 to 60 breaths per minute; early school-age, 22 to 24 breaths; teenagers, 20 to 22 breaths. The normal range for women is usually higher than that for men.

Members of the health care team should assess all factors influencing the patient's respirations and should count the respirations without the patient's awareness to prevent alterations in the breathing pattern.

REGULATION OF RESPIRATION
Nervous Control

The medulla oblongata and pons of the brain are responsible for the basic rhythm and depth of respiration. The rhythm can be modified according to the demands of the body. Other parts of the nervous system help to coordinate the transfer from inspiration to expiration.

Chemoreceptors located in the carotid and aortic bodies are specialized receptors that are sensitive to blood carbon dioxide level, blood oxygen levels, and blood acid levels. When stimulated by increasing levels of blood carbon dioxide, decreasing levels of blood oxygen, or increasing blood acidity, these receptors send nerve impulses to the respiratory centers, which in turn modify respiratory rates.

Carbon dioxide, which is present in the blood as carbonic acid, is considered the chemical stimulant for regulation of respiration. Therefore the more carbon dioxide in the blood, the more acidic the blood becomes. After exhalation the blood becomes more alkaline. The normal pH of the blood is 7.35 to 7.45—a narrow range. Deviation from this range causes the patient to develop either acidosis or alkalosis.

ASSESSMENT OF THE RESPIRATORY SYSTEM

The function of the respiratory system is gas exchange (oxygen and carbon dioxide) at the alveolar/capillary level. This function depends on the lungs' capability for contraction and expansion, which in turn is influenced by musculoskeletal and neurological functions.

The respiratory system is always included in a physical assessment of the patient's general health. Certain types of patients require more extensive assessments: those with acute or chronic respiratory or cardiac conditions, those with a history of respiratory impairment related to trauma or allergic reactions, or those who have recently undergone surgery or anesthesia. Be-

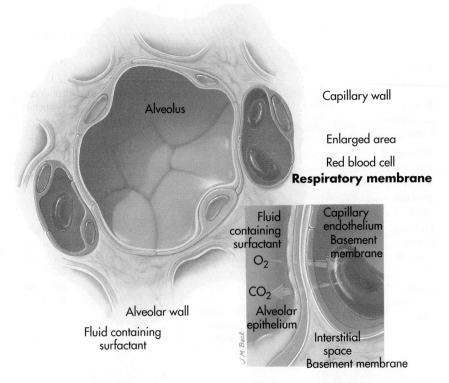

FIGURE **9-6** Each alveolus is continually ventilated with fresh air. Inset shows a magnified view of the respiratory membrane composed of the alveolar wall (surfactant, epithelial cells, and basement membrane), interstitial fluid, and the wall of a pulmonary capillary (basement membrane and endothelial cells). Carbon dioxide and oxygen diffuse across the respiratory membrane.

cause physical and emotional responses are often correlated, the nurse should also inquire about any accompanying anxiety or stress. This information should be obtained in an unhurried, matter-of-fact manner.

The respiratory assessment will include collection of **subjective data.** During the interview the patient should be encouraged to describe any symptoms, such as shortness of breath, dyspnea on exertion, or cough. Dyspnea, or difficulty breathing, is a subjective experience that only the patient can accurately describe. Data should include onset; duration; precipitating factors; and relief measures, such as position and use of over-the-counter or prescribed medications. If the patient has reported a cough, the nurse will ask for a description of the cough—productive or nonproductive; harsh, dry, or hacking; and color and amount of mucus expectorated. This information should be recorded as direct quotes from the patient when possible.

The nurse will then gather **objective data.** Assessment begins with observation. The patient's expression, chest movement, and respirations all provide valuable visual clues. There may be times when the patient cannot verbalize distress, but the wide-eyed, anxious look on the patient's face reflects the fear of suffocating. Flaring nostrils indicate that the patient is struggling to breathe, which is usually a late sign of respiratory distress. Initial observation by the nurse

will yield information on the patient's skin color and turgor. The nurse will note any obvious respiratory distress, wheezes, or orthopnea (an abnormal condition in which a person must sit or stand in order to breathe deeply or comfortably).

To continue this assessment, the nurse will auscultate all lung fields, anteriorly and posteriorly, noting the presence of adventitious sounds (abnormal sounds superimposed on breath sounds, including sibilant wheezes [formerly called simply **wheezes**], sonorous wheezes [formerly called simply **rhonchi**], crackles [formerly called **rales**], and pleural friction rubs). Sibilant wheezes are musical, high-pitched, squeaking or whistling sounds, caused by the rapid movement of air through narrowed bronchioles. Sonorous wheezes are low-pitched, loud, coarse, snoring sounds. They are often heard on expiration.

Crackles are short, discrete, interrupted crackling or bubbling sounds that are most commonly heard during inspiration. The sound of crackles is similar to that produced by hairs being rolled between the fingers while close to the ear. They are thought to occur when air is forced through respiratory passages narrowed by fluid, mucus, or pus. They are associated with inflammation or infection of the small bronchi, bronchioles, and alveoli. Pleural friction rubs are low-pitched, grating or creaking lung sounds that occur when inflamed pleural

Table 9-1 *Adventitious Breath Sounds*

TYPE	CHARACTERISTICS	COMMENTS
Crackles (rales)	Brief, not continuous; more common in inspiration; interrupted crackling or bubbling sounds, similar to those produced by hairs being rolled between the fingers close to the ear	Caused by fluid, mucus, or pus in the small airways and alveoli
Fine crackles	As described above; high-pitched, sibilant crackling at end of inspiration	Found in diseases affecting bronchioles and alveoli
Medium crackles	As described above; medium pitch, more sonorous, moisture sound during midinspiration	Associated with diseases of small bronchi
Coarse crackles	As described above; loud, bubbly sound in early inspiration	Associated with diseases of small bronchi
Sonorous wheezes (rhonchi)	Deep, running sound that may be continuous; loud, low, coarse sound (like a snore) heard at any point of inspiration or expiration	Caused by air moving through narrowed tracheobronchial passages (caused by secretions, tumor, spasm); cough may alter sound if caused by mucus in trachea or large bronchi
Sibilant wheezes (wheezes)	High-pitched, musical, whistlelike sound during inspiration or expiration; sound may consist of several notes or one, and may vary from one minute to the next	Caused by narrowed bronchioles; bilateral wheeze often result of bronchospasm; unilateral, sharply localized wheeze may result from foreign matter or tumor compression
Pleural friction rub	Dry, creaking, grating, low-pitched sound with a machinelike quality during both inspiration and expiration; loudest over anterior chest	Sound originates outside respiratory tree, usually caused by inflammation; over the lung fields it suggests pleurisy; over the pericardium it suggests pericarditis with a pericardial friction rub. To distinguish the two, ask the patient to hold the breath briefly. If the rubbing sound persists, it is a pericardial friction rub because the inflamed pericardial layers continue rubbing together with each heartbeat; a pleural rub would stop when breathing stops

Box 9-1 *Signs and Symptoms of Hypoxia*

- Apprehension, anxiety, restlessness
- Decreased ability to concentrate
- Disorientation
- Decreased level of consciousness
- Increased fatigue
- Vertigo
- Behavioral changes
- Increased pulse rate; as hypoxia advances, bradycardia results
- Increased rate and depth of respiration; as hypoxia progresses, shallow, slow respirations develop
- Elevated blood pressure; if O_2 deficiency is not corrected, blood pressure will decrease
- Cardiac dysrhythmias
- Pallor
- Cyanosis (may not be present until hypoxia is severe)
- Clubbing
- Dyspnea

surfaces rub together during respiration (Table 9-1). The nurse can also assess chest movement. He or she should note if the chest expands equally on both sides; chest expansion on one side only may indicate serious pulmonary complications. The nurse should note retraction of the chest wall between the ribs and under the clavicle during inspiration. This can signal late-stage respiratory distress. Another important aspect in collecting objective data is to be alert for signs and symptoms of hypoxia (an oxygen deficiency) (Box 9-1).

LABORATORY AND DIAGNOSTIC EXAMINATIONS

A variety of tests are used to evaluate respiratory status and identify respiratory conditions. Other tests include diagnostic imaging, laboratory work, and more invasive measures. Nurses should be familiar with these tests so they can adequately prepare the patient.

CHEST ROENTGENOGRAM

Usually referred to as chest radiographs, chest roentgenograms are an essential diagnostic tool for evaluating disorders of the chest. A chest radiograph provides visualization of the lungs, ribs, clavicles, humeri, scapulae, vertebrae, heart, and major thoracic vessels. This test gives information on alterations in size and location of the pulmonary structures and blood flow, as well as identifies the presence of lesions, infiltrates, foreign bodies, or fluid. A chest radiograph also identifies whether a disorder involves the lung parenchyma (the tissue of an organ as distinguished from supporting or connective tissue) or the interstitial spaces. Chest radiographs can also confirm pneumothorax, pneumonia, pleural effusion, and pulmonary edema. The chest radiographic examination can be performed at different angles for greater clarification. The nurse should have the patient wear a hospital gown tied in back. Pins must not be used. Any article of clothing containing metal (e.g., a bra with metal hooks) or jewelry must be removed, since the metal will produce a shadow on the film.

COMPUTED TOMOGRAPHY
Chest CT Scan

Computed tomography (CT) **scans** of the lungs take pictures of small layers of pulmonary tissue, usually to identify a pulmonary lesion. These views can be diagonal or cross-sectional, with a scanner rotating at various angles. Although this test is painless and noninvasive and results in little radiation exposure, patient teaching is necessary before the procedure to offer explanations and allay anxiety.

Helical/spiral CT chest scan. **Helical** (also called spiral or volume-averaging) **CT scanning** represents a marked improvement over standard CT scanning. The helical CT scan continuously obtains images. This produces faster and more accurate images. Because the helical CT can image the abdomen and chest in less than 30 seconds, the entire study can be performed with one breath-hold. Furthermore, when contrast material is used, the entire region can be imaged in just a few seconds after the contrast injection, thereby further improving contrast imaging (Pagana & Pagana, 2003).

Pulmonary angiography (pulmonary arteriography). **Pulmonary angiography (pulmonary arteriography)** uses a radiographic contrast material injected into the pulmonary arteries; pulmonary angiography permits visualization of the pulmonary vasculature. Angiography is used to detect pulmonary embolism and a variety of congenital and acquired lesions of the pulmonary vessels.

When pulmonary embolism is suspected, lung scanning should be performed first. If the lung scan is normal, pulmonary embolism is ruled out. If the scan is equivocal, however, the diagnosis of pulmonary embolism is questionable because pathologic processes (e.g., emphysema, pneumonia) also may cause abnor-

malities on the lung scan. Definitive diagnosis for pulmonary embolism may require pulmonary angiography (Pagana & Pagana, 2003).

Ventilation-perfusion scan (V/Q scan). **Ventilation-perfusion (V/Q) scanning** is used primarily to check for the presence of a pulmonary embolism. An intravenous (IV) radioisotope is given for the perfusion portion of the test, and the pulmonary vasculature is outlined and photographed. For the ventilation portion of the test, the patient inhales a radioactive gas that outlines the alveoli, and another photograph is taken. Normal scans show homogeneous radioactivity. Diminished or absent radioactivity suggests lack of perfusion or airflow (Lewis et al, 2004).

PULMONARY FUNCTION TESTING (PFT)

Pulmonary function tests are performed to assess the presence and severity of disease in the large and small airways. PFT is composed of various procedures to obtain information on lung volume, ventilation, pulmonary spirometry, and gas exchange. Lung volume tests refer to the volume of air that can be completely and slowly exhaled after a maximum inhalation (**vital capacity** [VC]). **Inspiratory capacity** (IC) is the largest amount of air that can be inhaled in one breath from the resting expiratory level. **Total lung capacity** (TLC) is calculated to determine the volume of air in the lung after a maximal inhalation. Ventilation tests evaluate the volume of air inhaled or exhaled in each respiratory cycle. Pulmonary spirometry tests evaluate the amount of air that can be forcefully exhaled after maximum inhalation. These tests require the use of a spirometer.

One of the most important tools for diagnosing respiratory diseases is gas exchange, which identifies the capacity for carbon dioxide to be diffused. This component of PFT determines the degree of function in the pulmonary capillary beds in contact with functioning alveoli.

MEDIASTINOSCOPY

A mediastinoscopy is a surgical endoscopic procedure in which an incision is created in the suprasternal notch, allowing the endoscope to be passed into the upper mediastinum. This is performed to gather a sample of lymph nodes for biopsy for tumor diagnosis. Because these lymph nodes receive lymphatic drainage from the lungs, they are of diagnostic value for malignant tumors. This procedure is performed in the operating room, and the patient usually receives a general anesthetic agent.

LARYNGOSCOPY

Laryngoscopy can be performed for either direct or indirect visualization of the larynx. Indirect laryngoscopy is probably the most common procedure for assessment of respiratory difficulties; this entails the use of a laryngeal mirror in the awake patient's mouth for visualization. This procedure can be used for biopsy or polyp excision.

Direct laryngoscopy requires local or general anesthesia and exposes the vocal chords with a laryngoscope passed down over the tongue.

BRONCHOSCOPY

A **bronchoscopy** is performed by passing a bronchoscope into the trachea and bronchi. By use of either a rigid bronchoscope or a flexible fiberoptic bronchoscope (the instrument of choice in most cases), the larynx, trachea, and bronchi can be visualized (Figure 9-7). Diagnostic bronchoscopic examination includes observation of the tracheobronchial tree for (1) abnormalities, (2) tissue biopsy, and (3) secretions collected for cytological (cell) or bacteriological examination. A local anesthetic agent may be used, but an intravenous general anesthetic agent is usually given. The patient is treated as a surgical patient. Nursing interventions for patients after bronchoscopy are as follows:

1. Patient is on NPO status until gag reflex returns, usually about 2 hours after the procedure.
2. Patient is in semi-Fowler's position and turns on either side to facilitate removal of secretions, unless the physician specifies another position.

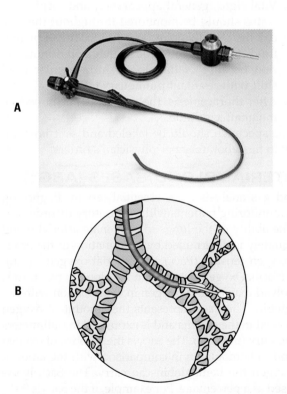

FIGURE 9-7 Fiberoptic bronchoscope. **A,** The transbronchoscopic balloon-tipped catheter and the flexible fiberoptic bronchoscope. **B,** The catheter is introduced into a small airway and the balloon inflated with 1.5 to 2 mL of air to occlude the airway. Bronchial alveolar lavage is performed by injecting and withdrawing 30-mL aliquots of sterile saline solution, gently aspirating after each instillation. Specimens are sent to the laboratory for analysis.

3. Patient is monitored for signs of laryngeal edema or laryngospasms, such as stridor or increasing dyspnea.
4. If lung tissue biopsy is taken, sputum is monitored for signs of hemorrhage; blood-streaked sputum can be expected for a few days after biopsy.

SPUTUM SPECIMEN

Sputum samples frequently are obtained for microscopic evaluation, such as Gram stain and culture and sensitivity (Box 9-2). For the range of sputum characteristics, see Box 9-3.

CYTOLOGIC STUDIES

Cytologic tests can be performed on any body secretion, such as sputum or pleural fluid, to detect the presence of abnormal or malignant cells.

LUNG BIOPSY

Lung biopsy may be done transbronchially or as an open-lung biopsy. The purpose is to obtain tissue, cells, or secretions for evaluation. Transbronchial lung

---

Box 9-2 | *Guidelines for Sputum Specimen Collection*

1. Explain to the patient that the sputum must be brought up from the lungs. Patients who have difficulty producing sputum or who have very tenacious sputum may be dehydrated. Encourage fluid intake.
2. Collection of sputum specimen should occur before prescribed antibiotics are started.
3. Collect specimens before meals to avoid possible emesis from coughing.
4. Instruct patient to inhale and exhale deeply three times, then inhale swiftly, cough forcefully, and expectorate into the sterile sputum container. Usually early morning samples are collected on 3 consecutive days.
5. If your patient cannot raise sputum spontaneously, a hypertonic saline aerosol mist may help to produce a good specimen. Instruct the patient to take several normal breaths of the mist, inhale deeply, cough, and expectorate.
6. Instruct patient to rinse mouth with water before expectorating into sterile specimen bottle to decrease sputum contamination.
7. Notify staff as soon as a specimen is collected so it can be properly labeled and sent to the laboratory without delay.
8. Sputum samples can also be obtained indirectly, such as with nasotracheal suctioning with a catheter or transtracheal aspiration. Care must be taken to ensure that the suction catheters remain sterile. A physician's order must be obtained for endotracheal suctioning.

Box 9-3 **Range of Sputum Characteristics**

COLOR	CONSISTENCY
Clear	Frothy
White	Watery
Yellow	Tenacious
Green	
Brown	**BLOOD**
Red	All the time
Pink-tinged	Occasionally
Streaked with blood	Early morning
ODOR	
None	
Malodorous	

biopsy involves passing a forceps or needle through the bronchoscope for a specimen. Specimens can be cultured or examined for malignant cells. Nursing interventions are the same as for fiberoptic bronchoscopy. Open-lung biopsy is used when pulmonary disease cannot be diagnosed by other procedures. The patient is anesthetized, the chest is opened with a thoracotomy incision, and a biopsy specimen is obtained.

THORACENTESIS

Thoracentesis is the surgical perforation of the chest wall and pleural space with a needle for the aspiration of fluid for diagnostic or therapeutic purposes or for the removal of a specimen for biopsy (Figure 9-8). Indications for a thoracentesis include the following:
- Removal of fluid for diagnostic purposes
  —The pleural fluid can be examined for specific gravity, white blood cell count, red blood cell count, protein, and glucose.
  —The fluid can be cultured for pathogens and checked for the presence of abnormal or malignant cells.
  —The gross appearance of the fluid, the quantity obtained, and the location of the site of the thoracentesis should be recorded.
- Biopsy of the pleura
- Removal of fluid when it is a threat to patient safety or comfort
- Instillation of medication into the pleural space

Nursing interventions for the patient undergoing thoracentesis include the following:
1. Explain the procedure; obtain a written consent; every means should be used to relieve the patient's anxiety.
2. The procedure is usually carried out in the patient's room. The patient sits on the edge of the bed with the head and arms resting on a pillow placed on an overbed table. Patients who cannot sit up should be turned to the unaffected side with the head of the bed elevated 30 degrees.

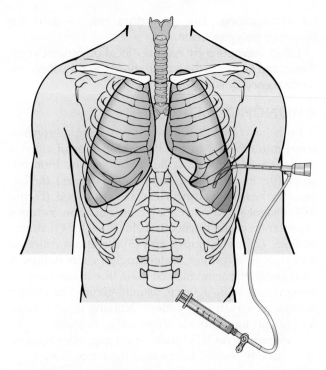

FIGURE **9-8** Thoracentesis. The needle has penetrated the fluid-filled pleural space to remove fluid.

3. Vital signs, general appearance, and respiratory status should be monitored throughout the procedure. Usually no more than 1300 mL of pleural fluid should be removed within a 30-minute period because of the risk of intravascular fluid shift with resultant pulmonary edema.
4. After thoracentesis, the patient is positioned on the unaffected side.

The specimen should be labeled and sent immediately to the laboratory per physician's orders.

ARTERIAL BLOOD GASES (ABGs)

Blood gas analysis is an essential test in diagnosing and monitoring patients with respiratory disorders.

The ability of the lungs to oxygenate arterial blood adequately is determined by examination of the arterial oxygen tension (PaO_2) and arterial oxygen saturation (SaO_2). Oxygen is carried in the blood in two forms: dissolved oxygen and oxygen in combination with hemoglobin. The PaO_2 represents the amount of oxygen dissolved in the plasma and is expressed in millimeters of mercury (mm Hg). The SaO_2 is the amount of oxygen bound to hemoglobin in comparison with the amount of oxygen the hemoglobin can carry. The SaO_2 is expressed as a percentage. For example, if the SaO_2 is 90%, then 90% of the hemoglobin attachments for oxygen have oxygen bound to them (Box 9-4).

The PCO_2 is a measure of the partial pressure of CO_2 in the blood. PCO_2 is referred to as the respiratory component in acid-base determination, because this value is primarily controlled by the lungs. As the CO_2 level

Box 9-4 | *Guidelines for Interpreting ABGs*

1. Examine each value by itself.
   Normal ABGs
   pH   7.35-7.45
   $Paco_2$ 35-45 mm Hg
   Pao_2 80-100 mm Hg
   HCO_3^- 21-28 mEq/L
   Sao_2 95%
2. Determine whether the pH reflects acidity or alkalinity.
   pH of 7.35 and lower = acidity
   pH of 7.45 and higher = alkalinity
3. Which other value corresponds with that condition?
   NOTE: $Paco_2$ reflects respiratory factors; HCO_3^- reflects metabolic factors.
   CO_2 is a potential acid, so CO_2 of greater than 45 = more acidity.
   HCO_3^- is a basic (alkaline) substance, so HCO_3^- greater than 45 = more alkalinity.
   EXAMPLE: A patient with acute exacerbation of COPD has the following ABGs:
   pH   7.42
   $Paco_2$ 49 mm Hg
   Pao_2 50 mm Hg
   HCO_3^- 31 mEq/L
   Sao_2 84%
   Because the pH is within a normal range, this is a compensated respiratory problem. The kidneys have increased the amount of bicarbonate they put into the blood to bring the pH to a normal level.

Table 9-2 | *Acid-Base Disturbances and Compensatory Mechanisms*

ACID-BASE DISTURBANCE	MODE OF COMPENSATION
Respiratory acidosis	Kidneys will retain increased amounts of HCO_3^- to increase pH.
Respiratory alkalosis	Kidneys will excrete increased amounts of HCO_3^- to lower pH.
Metabolic acidosis	Lungs "blow off" CO_2 to raise pH.
Metabolic alkalosis	Lungs retain CO_2 to lower pH.

This test yields definitive information on the patient's respiratory status and metabolic balance. The procedure is performed at the bedside. A heparinized syringe and needle are used to withdraw 3 to 5 mL of arterial blood, usually from the radial artery. Other possible sites include femoral or brachial arteries. After the sample is obtained, the nurse must place direct pressure on the puncture site for a minimum of 5 minutes to prevent hematoma formation and blood loss. If the patient is on anticoagulants, maintain pressure for 20 minutes or longer until bleeding stops. Place the capped syringe in a basin of crushed ice and water to preserve the gas and pH levels of the specimen. Send the properly labeled specimen to the laboratory immediately.

The blood gas values (see Box 9-4) assess the patient's metabolic (acid-base) status by measuring the pH. Carbon dioxide tension is measured by $Paco_2$ and will assess the patient's ventilation. Oxygen saturation (Pao_2 and Sao_2) is also measured.

PULSE OXIMETRY

Pulse oximetry is a noninvasive method of providing continuous monitoring of Sao_2 (saturation of oxygen) for assessment of gas exchange. The system consists of a probe that looks like a large clothespin and is applied to a finger, toe, earlobe, or the bridge of the nose. The probe has a light-emitting sensor that shoots narrow beams of red and infrared light through the tissue and a light-receiving sensor that measures the amount of light being absorbed by oxygenated and deoxygenated hemoglobin in pulsating arterial blood. The probe is connected to a computer with a monitor that displays hemoglobin oxygen saturation and pulse rates (Figure 9-9). A pulse oximeter will beep if the patient's Sao_2 registers outside of the limits set in response to the physician's order.

For decades, physicians have relied on arterial blood gas (ABG) analysis to evaluate gas exchange and oxygen transport. As valuable as this test is, ABG results reflect a patient's oxygenation status at only one mo-

increases, the pH decreases. Therefore, the CO_2 level and the pH are inversely proportional. The Pco_2 level is elevated in primary respiratory acidosis and decreased in primary respiratory alkalosis. Because the lungs compensate for primary metabolic acid-based derangements, Pco_2 levels are affected by metabolic disturbances as well. In metabolic acidosis the lungs attempt to compensate by "blowing off" CO_2 to raise pH. In metabolic alkalosis the lungs attempt to compensate by retaining CO_2 to lower pH.

The bicarbonate ion (HCO_3^-) is a measure of the metabolic (renal) component of the acid-base equilibrium. This ion can be measured directly by the bicarbonate value or indirectly by the CO_2 content. As the HCO_3^- level increases, the pH also increases; therefore the relationship of bicarbonate to pH is directly proportional. HCO_3^- is elevated in metabolic alkalosis and decreased in metabolic acidosis. The kidneys also are used to compensate for primary respiratory acid-base derangements. For example, in respiratory acidosis, the kidneys attempt to compensate by reabsorbing increased amounts of HCO_3^-. In respiratory alkalosis the kidneys excrete HCO_3^- in increased amounts in an attempt to lower pH through compensation (Table 9-2).

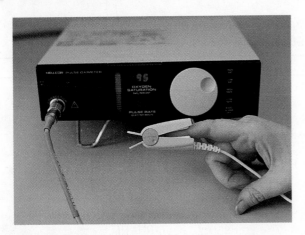

FIGURE **9-9** Portable pulse oximeter with spring-tension digit probe displays oxygen saturation and pulse rate.

ment in time. Today, pulse oximetry permits continuous, noninvasive monitoring of SaO_2. Oximetry technology allows the nurse to assess minute-to-minute changes in arterial saturations, intervene before hypoxemia produces obvious and serious signs and symptoms, and evaluate the patient's response to treatment.

An SaO_2 of 90% to 100% is needed to adequately replenish O_2 in plasma. The ability of hemoglobin to feed oxygen to the plasma weakens significantly when the SaO_2 drops below 85%. An SaO_2 less than 70% is considered life threatening.

Arterial oxygen saturation can be quickly and noninvasively determined through pulse oximetry. Severe circulatory problems may diminish the accuracy of the reading. If oximetry results seem questionable, the physician will usually order ABG tests. A pulse oximeter can detect a change within 6 seconds. To get optimal results, remember these points:

- Do not attach the transducer to an extremity that has a blood pressure cuff or arterial catheter in place; these devices reduce blood flow.
- Place the probe over a pulsating vascular bed.
- While the probe is on your patient, protect it from strong light (such as direct sunlight), which can affect the reading.
- Avoid excess patient movement to ensure accuracy.
- Remember that hypothermia, hypotension, and vasoconstriction can affect readings.

DISORDERS OF THE UPPER AIRWAY

EPISTAXIS
Etiology/Pathophysiology
The underlying cause of epistaxis (a bleeding from the nose) is congestion of the nasal membranes, leading to capillary rupture. This condition is frequently caused by injury and occurs more frequently in men.

Epistaxis can be either a primary disorder or secondary to other conditions. It can be related to menstrual flow in women, as well as hypertension. Other causes include local irritation of nasal mucosa, such as dryness, chronic infection, or trauma (e.g., injury, vigorous nose blowing, or nose picking). A prime consideration of epistaxis is the many capillaries in the nasal passages.

Clinical Manifestations
The primary observation is the presence of bright red blood draining from one or both nostrils. With a severe nasal hemorrhage, adults can lose as much as 1 L of blood per hour, but this loss is not prolonged. Exsanguination (loss of blood to the point at which life can no longer be sustained) from the usual epistaxis is rare.

Assessment
Collection of **subjective data** includes interviewing the patient and asking the patient to relate the duration and severity of bleeding and identification of precipitating factors, if possible.

Collection of **objective data** involves assessing the presence of bleeding from one or both nostrils. The nurse will also need to determine whether the bleeding is occurring in the anterior or posterior portion of the nasal passageway. The nurse will assess the patient's blood pressure; temperature, pulse, and respirations (TPR); and any evidence of hypovolemic shock. Severe bleeding results in a drop in blood pressure, which may cause the bleeding to stop.

Diagnostic Tests
A hemoglobin and hematocrit determination will aid in establishing an estimate of the blood loss. Prothrombin time (PT), international normalized ratio (INR), and partial thromboplastin time (PTT) will assist in identifying contributing factors, such as a bleeding tendency and clotting abnormalities. A rhinoscopy may be performed to locate the bleeding site as well as possible causes and treatment. This procedure involves inserting a lighted nasal speculum into the nasal cavity.

Medical Management
There are many possible treatments for epistaxis, including nasal packing with cotton saturated with 1:1000 epinephrine to promote local vasoconstriction. Cautery can be either electrical (in which the bleeding vessel is burned [cauterized]) or chemical (in which a silver nitrate stick is applied to the site of the bleeding). Posterior packing of the nasal cavity may be needed, or use of a balloon tamponade may be required. This is done by inserting a Foley-like catheter into the nose and inflating the balloon after it is placed posteriorly. Traction is then placed on the catheter so

the vessel in the area is compressed. Also, some physicians will prescribe antibiotics (penicillin) after the bleeding is controlled to minimize risk of infection.

Nursing Interventions and Patient Teaching

Nursing interventions include the following:

1. Keep the patient quiet.
2. Place the patient in a sitting position, leaning forward, or if that is not possible, in a reclining position with head and shoulders elevated.
3. Apply direct pressure by pinching the entire soft lower portion of the nose for 10 to 15 minutes.
4. Apply ice compresses to the nose and have the patient suck on ice.
5. Partially insert a small gauze pad into the bleeding nostril, and apply digital pressure if bleeding continues.
6. Monitor for signs and symptoms of hypovolemic shock.

Nursing diagnoses and interventions for the patient with epistaxis include but are not limited to the following:

NURSING DIAGNOSES	NURSING INTERVENTIONS
Ineffective tissue perfusion, cerebral and/or cardiopulmonary, related to blood loss	Assess vital signs and level of consciousness every 15 minutes and report any changes. Document estimated blood loss.
Risk for aspiration, related to bleeding	Elevate head of bed; place patient in Fowler's position with the head forward; patient should be encouraged to let the blood drain from the nose. Pinch nostrils; have the patient breathe through the mouth; apply ice compresses over the nose (however, the primary benefit of the application of ice is that it requires the patient to remain still); assist patient to clear secretions. Maintain airway patency. Instruct patient to expectorate any blood or clots rather than swallow them, which could cause nausea and vomiting.

The patient (and the family; if possible) should be instructed not to pick, scratch, or otherwise irritate the nares. To prevent recurrent hemorrhage, the patient is warned not to blow the nose vigorously and to avoid dryness of the nose. The patient and family should be instructed regarding the risks of foreign objects inserted in the nose (this is especially important in pediatric patients). The use of vaporizer to keep nasal mucous membranes moist should be encouraged as well as the use of saline or nasal lubricants.

Prognosis

With treatment, prognosis is good.

DEVIATED SEPTUM AND NASAL POLYPS
Etiology/Pathophysiology

Common conditions that cause nasal obstruction include nasal polyps or deviated septum caused by congenital abnormality or, more likely, injury.

The septum deviates from the midline and can cause a partial obstruction of the nasal passageway. Nasal polyps are tissue growths on the nasal tissues that are frequently caused by prolonged sinus inflammation; allergies are often the underlying cause.

Clinical Manifestations

The major manifestations of nasal septal deviations and polyps are stertorous (pertaining to a respiratory effort that is strenuous and struggling, provoking a snoring sound) respirations, dyspnea, and sometimes postnasal drip.

Assessment

Collection of **subjective data** includes establishing the presence of previous injuries or infections, allergies, and sinus congestion. The patient will offer complaints of dyspnea.

Collection of **objective data** involves the nurse attempting to identify the condition and its location. The rate and character of the patient's respirations must be noted.

Diagnostic Tests

Sinus radiographic studies will depict the presence of shadowy sinuses when nasal polyps are present, and a shift of the nasal septum will be evident with a septal defect. A deviated septum may also be present on visual examination.

Medical Management

These conditions frequently require surgical correction. Nasoseptoplasty may be done to reconstruct, align, and straighten the nasal septum; this is the operation of choice for deviated nasal septum. Another alternative is nasal polypectomy to remove the polyps. Actions include nasal packing to control bleeding, for 24 hours, and then maintaining nasal mucosa hydration with nasal irrigation of saline or application of a light layer of petroleum to the external nares to prevent drying. Medications include (1) corticosteroids (prednisone), which will cause polyps to decrease or disappear; and (2) antihistamines for allergy signs and symptoms, to decrease congestion in both septal deviations and polyps. Antibiotic agents (penicillin) may be used in both conditions to prevent infection. Analgesics (acetaminophen [Tylenol]) may be given to relieve the headache that occurs with septal deviation.

Nursing Interventions and Patient Teaching

Nursing interventions are generally aimed at maintaining airway patency and preventing infection. Postoperative intervention for nasal surgery will include monitoring closely for infection or hemorrhage and maintaining patient comfort.

Nursing diagnoses and interventions for the patient with deviated septum and nasal polyps include but are not limited to the following:

NURSING DIAGNOSES	NURSING INTERVENTIONS
Ineffective airway clearance, related to nasal exudate	Document patient's ability to clear secretions, and note respiratory status. Elevate head of bed, and apply ice compresses to the nose to decrease edema, discoloration, discomfort, and bleeding. Change nasal drip pad as needed, documenting color, consistency, and amount of exudate.
Risk for injury, related to trauma to bleeding site associated with vigorous nose blowing	Assess and report exudate (as stated above). Instruct patient against blowing nose in immediate postoperative period, because this could increase bleeding, edema, and ecchymosis.

The patient should be instructed to contact the physician if bleeding or infection develops. The patient should be instructed to use nasal sprays and drops judiciously because of the possible rebound effect on nasal mucous membranes. The patient should be reminded to avoid nose blowing, vigorous coughing, or Valsalva's maneuver (technique in which the patient holds the breath and bears down as if straining during a bowel movement) for 2 days postoperatively. The nurse should remind the patient that facial ecchymosis and edema may persist for several days after surgery.

Prognosis

With surgical correction, the prognosis is excellent.

ANTIGEN-ANTIBODY ALLERGIC RHINITIS AND ALLERGIC CONJUNCTIVITIS (HAY FEVER)
Etiology/Pathophysiology

These atopic allergic conditions are a result of antigen-antibody reactions occurring in the nasal membranes, nasopharynx, and conjunctiva from inhaled or contact allergens. Many infants, children, and adults have these seasonal or perennial conditions, which often result in absences from school and work.

Rhinitis and conjunctivitis occur as the result of antigen-antibody reaction. Ciliary action slows; mucosal gland secretion increases; leukocyte (eosinophil) infiltration occurs; and because of increased capillary permeability and vasodilation, local tissue edema results.

Common allergens causing allergic rhinitis and conjunctivitis (hay fever) are tree, grass, and weed pollens; mold spores; fungi; house dusts; mites; and animal dander. Other allergens include some foods, drugs, and insect stings.

Clinical Manifestations

Acute ocular manifestations include edema, photophobia, excessive tearing, blurring of vision, and pruritus.

Individuals with rhinitis complain of excessive secretions or inability to breathe through the nose because of congestion and/or edema.

Serious otitis media symptoms can occur if the eustachian tubes are occluded. These symptoms occur more in childhood, with the individual complaining of ear fullness, ear popping, or decreased hearing.

Assessment

The initial complaints of seasonal rhinitis and conjunctivitis include severe sneezing, congestion, pruritus, and lacrimation (watery eyes). Cough, epistaxis, and headache may also occur. More chronic signs and symptoms include headache, severe nasal congestion, postnasal drip, and cough. If these are not treated, chronic sufferers eventually develop secondary infections, such as otitis media, bronchitis, sinusitis, and pneumonia.

Diagnostic Tests

In allergic rhinitis, on physical examination the mucosa of the turbines is usually pale because of venous engorgement, which is in contrast to the erythema of viral rhinitis. When symptoms are extremely bothersome, a search for offending allergens may be helpful. This can be done by skin testing or serum radioallergosorbent test (RAST).

Medical Management

Treatment goals are to relieve signs and symptoms and prevent infections and other complaints, such as malaise, extreme fatigue, and severe headaches. Avoiding the allergen is effective. Perennial use of antihistamines is recommended. Changing from one antihistamine to another seasonally may help to impede tolerance to any one medication.

Decongestants may be added and used intermittently for 3 to 5 days if congestion occurs. Common over-the-counter decongestants—such as phenylephrine, pseudoephedrine, chlorpheniramine, and phenylpropanolamine—are contained in familiar products such as Actifed, Triaminic, and Robitussin.

Lodoxamide (Alomide) four times a day is the recommended treatment for mild to moderately severe allergic conjunctivitis.

Long-term, consistent use of topical or nasal corticosteroids is highly recommended. Included are beclomethasone (Vancenase, Beconase), dexamethasone (Decadron, Turbinaire), flunisolide (Nasalide), fluticasone (Flonase), and budesonide (Rhinocort). Corticosteroids require a prescription.

Pressure headaches may require opioid analgesics until signs and symptoms are relieved. Hot packs over facial sinuses offer relief if headache is related to sinus congestion.

Nursing Interventions and Patient Teaching

These illnesses are self-limiting, so the nurse focuses on health promotion and maintenance teaching to provide for self-care management.

The nurse's responsibilities in patient education are as follows:
- Teach patient ways to avoid allergen.
- Teach patient self-care management through symptom control.
- Teach medication action and usage; assess for medication effectiveness.

OBSTRUCTIVE SLEEP APNEA
Etiology/Pathophysiology

Obstructive sleep apnea (OSA) is a condition characterized by partial or complete upper airway obstruction during sleep, causing apnea and hypopnea. **Apnea** is the cessation of spontaneous respirations; **hypopnea** is abnormally shallow and slow respirations. Airflow obstruction occurs when the tongue and the soft palate fall backward and partially or completely obstruct the pharynx. The obstruction may last from 15 to 90 seconds. During the apneic period, the patient experiences severe hypoxemia (decreased PaO_2) and hypercapnia (increased $PaCO_2$). These changes are ventilatory stimulants and cause the patient to partially awaken. The patient has a generalized startle response, snorts, and gasps, which causes the tongue and soft palate to move forward and the airway to open. Apnea and arousal cycles occur repeatedly, as many as 200 to 400 times during 6 to 8 hours of sleep.

Sleep apnea occurs in 2% to 10% of the population.

Clinical Manifestations/Assessment

Clinical manifestations of sleep apnea include frequent awakening at night, insomnia, excessive daytime sleepiness, and witnessed apneic episodes. The patient's bed partner may complain about the patient's loud snoring. More than a nuisance, snoring is a hallmark of OSA. The snoring may be so loud that both people cannot sleep in the same room. Other symptoms include morning headaches (from hypercapnia, which causes vasodilation of cerebral blood vessels), personality changes, and irritability. Systemic hypertension, cardiac dysrhythmias, and stroke are serious complications that may occur.

Symptoms of sleep apnea alter many aspects of a patient's lifestyle. Chronic sleep loss predisposes to diminished ability to concentrate, impaired memory, failure to accomplish daily tasks, and interpersonal difficulties. The male patient may experience impotence. Driving accidents are more common in habitually sleepy people. Family life and the patient's ability to maintain employment are also often compromised. As a result, the patient may experience severe depression. Risk factors for OSA include the following:
- Male gender: About twice as many men as women have OSA.
- Older age: Although younger patients can develop OSA, the incidence increases with age, probably due to weight gain and loss of pharyngeal muscle strength.
- **Obesity:** An obese person's pharynx may be infiltrated with fat, and the tongue and soft palate may be enlarged, crowding the air passages. An obese individual may also have a short, thick neck, which increases the susceptibility to obstruction.
- Nasal allergies, polyps, or septal deviation decrease the diameter of the pharynx.
- Receding chin: A person with a receding chin may not have enough room in the pharynx for the tongue, thus contributing to obstructions.
- Pharyngeal structural abnormalities: A person with OSA may have enlarged tonsils, an elongated uvula, and especially long tongue, or a soft palate that rests on the base of the tongue. Any of these structural abnormalities can impinge on the airway (Tate & Tasota, 2002).

Appropriate referral should be made if problems are identified. Cessation of breathing reported by the bed partner is usually a source of great anxiety because of the fear that breathing may not resume.

Diagnostic Tests

Diagnosis of sleep apnea is made during sleep with the use of polysomnography. The patient's chest and abdominal movement, oral airflow, nasal airflow, SpO_2, ocular movement, and heart rate and rhythm are monitored, and time in each sleep stage is determined. A diagnosis of sleep apnea requires documentation of multiple episodes of apnea (no airflow with respiratory effort) or hypopnea (airflow diminished 30% to 50% with respiratory effort). Polysomnography may be carried out in a sleep laboratory, or the patient may be taught to attach monitoring leads for a home sleep study.

Medical Management/Nursing Interventions

Mild sleep apnea may respond to simple measures. The patient should be instructed to avoid sedatives and alcoholic beverages for 3 to 4 hours before sleep. Referral to a weight loss program may help, because excessive weight exacerbates symptoms. Symptoms resolve in half of the patients with OSA who use an oral appliance during sleep to prevent airflow obstruction. Oral appliances bring the mandible and tongue forward to enlarge the airway space, thereby preventing airway occlusion. Some individuals find a support group beneficial in which concerns and feelings can be expressed and strategies discussed for resolving problems.

In patients with more severe symptoms, nasal continuous positive airway pressure (nCPAP) may be used. With nCPAP the patient applies a nasal mask that is attached to a high-flow blower (Figure 9-10). The blower is adjusted to maintain sufficient positive pressure (5 to 15 cm H$_2$O) in the airway during inspiration and expiration to prevent airway collapse. Some patients cannot adjust to exhaling against the high pressure. A technologically more sophisticated therapy, bilevel positive airway pressure (BiPAP), capable of delivering a higher pressure during inspiration (which the airway is most likely to be occluded) and a lower pressure during expiration (when the airway is least likely to be occluded), may be helpful and is better tolerated. Although nCPAP is highly effective, compliance is poor even if symptoms of sleep apnea are relieved.

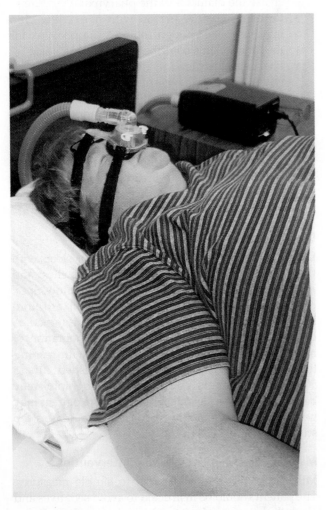

FIGURE **9-10** Nasal continuous positive airway pressure (nCPAP). The patient applies a nasal mask attached to a blower to maintain positive pressure.

If other measures fail, sleep apnea may be managed surgically. The two most common procedures are uvulopalatoplasty, pharyngoplasty (UPP, UPPP, or UP³) and genioglossal advancement and hyoid myotomy (GAHM). UPPP involves excision of the tonsillar pillars, uvula, and posterior soft palate with the goal of removing the obstructing tissue. GAHM involves advancing the attachment of the muscular part of the tongue on the mandible. When GAHM is performed, UPPP is generally done as well. Symptoms are relieved in up to 60% of patients. Laser-assisted uvulopalatoplasty (LAUP) is a new surgical procedure that has been used to treat OSA (Lewis et al, 2004).

UPPER AIRWAY OBSTRUCTION
Etiology/Pathophysiology

Upper airway obstruction is precipitated by a recent respiratory event, such as traumatic injury to the airway or surrounding tissues. Common airway obstructions include dentures; aspiration of vomitus or secretions; and, the most common airway obstruction in an unconscious person, the tongue.

Altered physiology includes any condition that could produce airway obstruction, such as laryngeal spasm caused by tetany resulting from hypocalcemia. Another cause may be laryngeal edema caused by injury.

Clinical Manifestations

The main signs are stertorous respirations, altered respiratory rate and character, and apneic periods.

Assessment

Collection of **subjective data** is limited because a patient is unable to talk when the airway is obstructed. The nurse therefore must make a prompt and accurate assessment of objective data.

Collection of **objective data** includes prompt assessment for signs of hypoxia (an inadequate, reduced tension of cellular oxygen; see Box 9-1), cyanosis (slightly bluish, grayish, slatelike, or dark purple discoloration of the skin resulting from the presence of abnormal amounts of reduced hemoglobin in the blood), stertorous respirations, and wheezing or stridor (harsh, high-pitched sounds during respiration, caused by obstruction). As hypoxia progresses, the respiratory centers in the brain (medulla oblongata and pons) are depressed, resulting in bradycardia and shallow, slow respirations.

Diagnostic Tests

Because this is a medical emergency, no diagnostic tests are needed. This condition is diagnosed by a prompt and accurate assessment.

Medical Management

The patient may require an emergency tracheostomy to remove the obstruction. Depending on the cause of the obstruction, an artificial airway may need to be inserted to maintain patency. Examples of artificial airways include pharyngeal, endotracheal, and tracheal.

Nursing Interventions and Patient Teaching

The most immediate nursing intervention will be that of opening the airway and restoring patency. This may be accomplished by properly repositioning the patient's head and neck, or it may require further maneuvers. The head-tilt/chin-lift technique is recommended by the American Heart Association because it minimizes further damage in the presence of a suspected cervical neck fracture. With a foreign body airway obstruction, the Heimlich maneuver is used.

Nursing diagnoses and interventions for the patient with an airway obstruction include but are not limited to the following:

Nursing Diagnoses	Nursing Interventions
Ineffective airway clearance, related to obstruction in airway	Reestablish and maintain secure airway. Administer oxygen as ordered. Suction as needed, and assess patient's ability to mobilize secretions. Monitor vital signs and breath sounds closely.
Risk for aspiration, related to partial airway obstruction	Monitor respiratory rate, rhythm, and effort. Assess patient's ability to swallow secretions by elevating the head of the bed. Assess and document breath sounds. Facilitate optimal airway and functional swallowing by elevating head of bed. Note amount, color, and characteristics of secretions. Suction as needed.

The best goal of education is prevention. The patient and family should be taught how to assess for airway patency. Appropriate use of the Heimlich maneuver should be provided. Rationale for all treatments and procedures should be explained.

Prognosis

With immediate medical and nursing intervention, the prognosis is good; without emergency intervention, the condition is life threatening.

CANCER OF THE LARYNX
Etiology/Pathophysiology

Squamous cell carcinoma of the larynx is increasing in frequency. Laryngeal cancers occur most often in people older than age 60; 90% of laryngeal cancers occur in men. This fact appears to be correlated to prolonged tobacco use (cigarettes, pipes, cigars, chewing tobacco, smokeless tobacco) and heavy alcohol use, chronic laryngitis, vocal abuse, and family history. Because of the increase in the number of women who are heavy smokers, their incidence of carcinoma of the larynx is increasing.

Laryngeal cancer limited to the true vocal cords is slow growing because of decreased lymphatic supply; however, elsewhere in the larynx there is an abundance of lymph tissue, and cancer in these tissues spreads rapidly and metastasizes early to the deep lymph nodes of the neck.

Clinical Manifestations

Progressive or persistent hoarseness is an early sign. Any person who is hoarse longer than 2 weeks should seek medical treatment. Signs of metastasis to other areas include pain in the larynx radiating to the ear, difficulty swallowing (dysphagia), a feeling of a lump in the throat, and enlarged cervical lymph nodes.

Assessment

Collection of **subjective data** includes assessing the onset and duration of symptoms. A complaint of referred pain to the ear (otalgia), as well as difficulty breathing (dyspnea) or swallowing, should be noted.

Collection of **objective data** includes examining sputum for the presence of blood **hemoptysis** (expectorating blood from the respiratory tract).

Diagnostic Tests

Visual examination of the larynx with direct laryngoscopy is done to determine the presence of laryngeal cancer. A computed tomography (CT) scan or magnetic resonance imaging (MRI) may be performed to detect local and regional spread. A health history will be helpful in making the diagnosis, and a biopsy and microscopic study of the lesion will be definitive.

Medical Management

Treatment will be determined by the extent of tumor growth. Radiation therapy or surgery is often performed. If the tumor is limited to the true cord without limitation of cord movement, then radiation therapy is the best course of treatment. Surgical intervention is considered when extension of the tumor becomes affixed to one of the cords or extends upward or downward from the larynx, and it may include either a total or partial laryngectomy or a radical neck dissection. A partial laryngectomy is done to remove the diseased vocal cord and possibly a portion of thyroid cartilage, requiring the placement of a temporary tracheostomy, which will be closed when the edema has decreased. A total laryngectomy is performed when the cancer of the larynx is advanced and requires the placement of a permanent tracheostomy. Because the patient can no longer breathe through the nose, the sense of smell is absent. The voice is also absent, because the larynx is removed. There is no connection between the patient's mouth and trachea.

A radical neck dissection to remove cervical lymph nodes is often done in conjunction with a total laryngectomy in those patients who have a high risk of metastasis to the neck from carcinoma of the larynx. This surgery entails removal of the submandibular salivary gland, sternocleidomastoid muscle, spinal accessory nerve, and the internal jugular vein, which results in one-sided shoulder droop.

Nursing Interventions and Patient Teaching

Airway maintenance through proper suctioning techniques is important. Skin integrity surrounding the tracheal opening should be assessed; the nurse should be alert for signs of infection.

The nurse should monitor intake and output (I&O) balance and assist with tube feedings as ordered. The nurse should explain to the patient that the tube feedings are temporary and that normal eating may begin again when healing occurs in a few weeks. The nurse should weigh the patient daily and assess hydration status for the need for additional fluids; note skin turgor and observe for diarrhea.

Because of neck and facial disfigurement and loss of voice, a thorough psychosocial assessment and resultant interventions will be beneficial. The nurse should encourage communication through writing and facial and hand gestures. Often no one else can give a patient reassurance that speech can be regained as well as a fellow patient who has undergone the same surgical intervention. Many cities have a Lost Chord Club or a New Voice Club, and the members are willing to visit hospitalized patients. Several options are available to restore speech. A speech therapist should meet with the patient following a total laryngectomy to discuss voice restoration options. These options include use of a voice prosthesis, esophageal speech, and an electrolarynx.

Nursing diagnoses and interventions for the patient with a tracheostomy include but are not limited to the following:

NURSING DIAGNOSES	NURSING INTERVENTIONS
Ineffective airway clearance, related to secretions or obstruction	Suction secretions as needed. Provide tracheostomy care according to protocol; ensure the availability of emergency equipment (oxygen and tracheostomy tray). Offer small, frequent feedings, and give liquid or pureed food as tolerated to prevent choking. Teach patient stoma protection. Assess respiratory rate and characteristics every 1 to 2 hours.

NURSING DIAGNOSES	NURSING INTERVENTIONS
	Auscultate lung sounds, monitor SaO$_2$ every 4 hours. Maintain head of bed elevation of 30 degrees or higher. Turn, cough, and encourage deep breathing every 2 to 4 hours. Auscultate lung sounds. Provide constant humidity. Suction laryngectomy tube as needed (prn), using aseptic technique; instruct patient to inhale as catheter is advanced. Clean inner cannula of laryngectomy tube every 2 to 4 hours and prn, using a solution of normal saline and hydrogen peroxide. Suction trachea prn.
Impaired communication, verbal, related to removal of larynx	Provide patient with implements for communication, including pencil, paper, Magic Slate; picture books, or electronic voice device. Keep call light or bell by patient's hand at all times. If possible, ask patient questions that require only a yes or no response to avoid fatigue and frustration. Refer patient to local support groups and the local chapter of the American Cancer Society. Assist with speech rehabilitation. Review instructions about esophageal and electro-esophageal speech. Reinforce need for regular follow-up with speech pathologist and surgeon after discharge.

Techniques of airway maintenance—such as oxygen usage, deep breathing, and coughing—should be explained. The importance of dietary management in relationship to airway maintenance should be discussed. Optimal communication should be encouraged through speech rehabilitation and community support groups.

Prognosis

If tumor is limited to the true cord, the cure rate is 80% to 90%. The prognosis in primary supraglottic and subglottic cancer is poor.

RESPIRATORY INFECTIONS
ACUTE RHINITIS
Etiology/Pathophysiology

Acute rhinitis (or acute coryza), known as the **common cold,** is an inflammatory condition of the mucous membranes of the nose and accessory sinuses. It is characterized most typically by edema of the nasal mucous membrane. The common cold is usually caused by one or more viruses; however, it may become complicated by a bacterial infection. Signs and symptoms usually are evident within 24 to 48 hours after exposure. Sinus congestion causes increased sinus drainage, leading to postnasal drip. The postnasal drip causes throat irritation, headache, and earache. Most people with colds contaminate their hands when coughing or sneezing, thus contaminating everything they touch. Others become infected when touching the telephone, computer, or anything else that has been touched by the person with a cold. Also, many colds are believed to be spread through shaking hands with a person who has a cold.

Clinical Manifestations

An increased amount of thin, serous nasal exudate and a productive cough are two of the most common signs. Sore throat and fever are often present. If the infection remains uncomplicated, it generally subsides in a week.

Assessment

Collection of **subjective data** includes the patient's complaints of sore throat, dyspnea, and congestion of varying duration.

Collection of **objective data** includes noting the color and consistency of the nasal exudate. A visual examination of the throat may reveal erythema, edema, and local irritation. The nurse will also document the presence and duration of fever.

Diagnostic Tests

Throat and sputum cultures will indicate the presence and nature of microorganisms.

Medical Management

Medical management is aimed at accurate diagnosis and prevention of complications. No specific treatment is available for the common cold. Among the medications used are (1) aspirin or acetaminophen for analgesia and reduction of temperature (aspirin is not used in infants, children, and adolescents because of the danger of developing Reye syndrome); and either (2) a cough suppressant for a dry, nonproductive cough; or (3) an expectorant for a productive cough. If the presence of a secondary bacterial infection is confirmed, an antibiotic agent (e.g., erythromycin) is prescribed (Complementary & Alternative Therapies box).

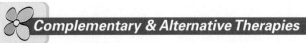
Complementary & Alternative Therapies

Respiratory Disorders

- Herbal medicines for respiratory problems include remedies for nasal discharge and congestion, cough, sore throat, fever and headache, and immunostimulant effects. Ephedra *(Ephedra sinica, Ephedra vulgaris)* is a stimulant and is illegal in some areas. Expectorants include anise *(Pimpinella anisum)*, coltsfoot *(Tussilago farfara)*, and horehound *(Marrubium vulgare)*. Coltsfoot and horehound are also believed to have antitussive action.
- Sore throat remedies include mint *(Mentha piperita* [peppermint], *Mentha spicata,* [spearmint]) and slippery elm *(Ulmus rubra)*. Remedies for the fever and headache that may accompany colds and influenza include boneset *(Eupatorium perfoliatum)*, feverfew *(Tanacetum parthenium)*, and white willow *(Salix purpurea, S. fragilis, S. daphnoides)*.
- Stimulants of the immune system, believed to help ward off colds and flu, include echinacea *(Echinacea angustifolia, E. pallida, E. purpurea)* and goldenseal *(Hydrastis canadensis)*.
- Some interventions that nurses can initiate that contribute to comfort in patients experiencing dyspnea include the following:
  Breathing exercises
  Relaxation therapy
  Massage
  Acupuncture
  Hypnosis
  Visualization
- Some believe that reflexology helps relieve congestion.
- Facial massage with diluted aromatic oils is believed by some to open occluded sinuses and relieve congestion. These essential oils include lavender, eucalyptus, peppermint, or tea tree oil.

Nursing Interventions and Patient Teaching

Nursing interventions are aimed at promoting comfort. Such measures include encouraging fluids and applying warm, moist packs to sinuses.

Nursing diagnoses and interventions for the patient with acute rhinitis include but are not limited to the following:

NURSING DIAGNOSES	NURSING INTERVENTIONS
Ineffective airway clearance, related to nasal exudate	Encourage fluids to liquefy secretions and aid in their expectoration. Use vaporizer to moisten mucous membranes and prevent further irritation.

Continued

Nursing Diagnoses	Nursing Interventions
Health-seeking behaviors: illness prevention, related to preventing exacerbation or spread of infection	Remind patient and family of health maintenance behaviors to decrease risk of illness, such as adequate fluid and nutritional management and sufficient rest. Teach importance of hygiene measures to decrease spread of infection.

The patient should be taught correct handwashing technique and proper disposal of tissues used for nasal secretions. The nurse should instruct the patient to limit exposure to others during the first 48 hours and to check the temperature every 4 hours.

Prognosis

Signs and symptoms are resolved in 2 to 10 days. Even though the common cold does not cause death, its economic importance is vast because it is the greatest cause of absenteeism in industry and schools.

ACUTE FOLLICULAR TONSILLITIS
Etiology/Pathophysiology

Acute follicular tonsillitis can be an acute inflammation of the tonsils. It is the result of an air- or foodborne bacterial infection, often *Streptococcus*. It can also be viral, but this occurs less often. If it is caused by group A β-hemolytic streptococci, sequelae such as rheumatic fever, carditis, and nephritis must be considered. It appears to be most common in school-age children. Signs and symptoms of tonsillitis include sore throat, fever, chills, and anorexia. The tonsils become enlarged and often contain purulent exudate.

Clinical Manifestations

Acute follicular tonsillitis manifests itself clinically with enlarged, tender, cervical lymph nodes. Fever may be present with chills, general muscle aching, and malaise. Laboratory data reveal an elevated white blood cell count.

Assessment

Collection of **subjective data** includes monitoring the severity of throat pain and the possibility of referred pain to the ears. Headache or joint pain should be noted.

Collection of **objective data** includes a visual examination that shows increased throat secretions and enlarged, erythematous tonsils.

Diagnostic Tests

Throat cultures will identify the causative microorganism, most commonly β-hemolytic streptococci. A complete blood count will be done to determine if the white blood count is elevated. It is not uncommon for the white blood count to be 10,000 to 20,000/mm³.

Medical Management

If antibiotics to which the offending organism is sensitive are administered early, infection subsides. When an elective tonsillectomy and adenoidectomy (T&A) is performed, the tonsils and adenoids are surgically excised. This procedure occurs in people who have recurrent attacks of tonsillitis. The procedure is usually performed from 4 to 6 weeks after an acute attack has subsided. Either general or local anesthesia is used. When a T&A is performed, hemostasis is of utmost importance, because the patient can lose a large amount of blood through hemorrhage without demonstrating any outward signs of bleeding. The physician may be able to control minor postoperative bleeding by applying a sponge soaked in a solution of epinephrine to the site. The patient who is bleeding excessively often is returned to the operating room for surgical treatment to stop the hemorrhage.

Medications used in tonsillitis include analgesics and antipyretics (e.g., acetaminophen) and antibiotic agents (e.g., penicillin). Warm saline gargles are also beneficial.

Nursing Interventions and Patient Teaching

One of the primary nursing goals for acute tonsillitis is to provide meticulous oral care, which will promote comfort and assist in combating infection. An important postoperative nursing intervention is to observe and report if the patient exhibits frequent swallowing, because this is often a subtle but reliable indication of excessive bleeding.

Postoperative care for tonsillectomy includes maintaining intravenous fluids until the nausea subsides, at which time the patient may begin drinking ice cold liquids. The diet will be advanced to custard and ice cream and then to a normal diet as soon as possible. An ice collar should be applied to the neck for comfort and to reduce bleeding by vasoconstriction. Vital signs must be monitored to assess for hemorrhage, postoperative fever, or other complications. Comfort measures are important, and emotional support is essential.

Nursing diagnoses and interventions for the patient with acute follicular tonsillitis include but are not limited to the following:

Nursing Diagnoses	Nursing Interventions
Pain, related to inflammation/irritation of pharynx	Assess degree of pain and need for analgesics. Document effectiveness of medication, and offer analgesic as ordered. Maintain bed rest, and promote rest. Offer warm saline gargles, ice chips, and ice collar as needed.

Nursing Diagnoses	Nursing Interventions
Risk for deficient fluid volume, related to inability to maintain usual oral intake because of painful swallowing	Assess hydration status by noting mucous membranes, skin turgor, and urine output. Encourage Popsicles, ice chips, and increased oral intake: cold liquids, sherbet, and ice cream will be best tolerated; carbonated drinks may be taken if patient tolerates; avoid offering citrus juices, because they may burn the throat.
Risk for aspiration, related to postoperative bleeding	Maintain patent airway; keep patient lying on side as much as possible to prevent aspiration. Observe for vomiting of dark brown fluid; patient may have "swallowed" blood during surgery. Watch for frequent swallowing, which may indicate bleeding; check frequently with flashlight to see if blood is trickling down posterior pharynx.

The patient or family should be instructed that the patient should complete the entire course of the prescribed antibiotic. If patient has had surgery (T&A), dietary instruction should be offered regarding appropriate foods and liquids. The nurse should teach the patient to avoid attempting to clear the throat immediately after surgery (may initiate bleeding) and to avoid coughing, sneezing, or vigorous nose blowing for 1 to 2 weeks. Most surgeons no longer prescribe aspirin for pain after tonsillectomy, since it increases the tendency to bleed; acetaminophen or other aspirin substitute is usually ordered. The nurse should remind the patient to avoid overexertion and should ascertain that the patient and family know how to reach the physician in case of increased pain, fever, or bleeding.

Prognosis

Tonsillitis is usually self-limited, but serious complications—such as sinusitis, otitis media, mastoiditis, rheumatic fever, nephritis, or peritonsillar abscess—may occur.

LARYNGITIS
Etiology/Pathophysiology

Laryngitis often occurs secondary to other respiratory infections. Laryngeal inflammation is a common disorder that can be either chronic or acute. Acute laryngitis may cause severe respiratory distress in children younger than 5 years of age because the relatively small larynx of the young child is subject to spasm when irritated or infected and readily becomes partially or totally obstructed.

Acute laryngitis often accompanies viral or bacterial infections. Other causes include excessive use of the voice or inhalation of irritating fumes. Chronic laryngitis is usually associated with inflammation of laryngeal mucosa or edematous vocal cords.

Clinical Manifestations

Clinical manifestation includes hoarseness of varying degrees or even complete voice loss. The throat will feel scratchy and irritated, and the patient may have a persistent cough.

Assessment

Collection of **subjective data** includes the patient reporting progressive hoarseness and a cough that may be productive or may be dry and nonproductive. The nurse should attempt to identify any precipitating factors such as excessive voice use or increased exposure to inhaled irritants.

Collections of **objective data** includes the nurse evaluating the patient's voice quality as well as the characteristics (color, consistency, and amount) of sputum produced.

Diagnostic Tests

Laryngoscopy will reveal abnormalities (edema, drainage) of vocal cords and erythematous laryngeal mucosa.

Medical Management

If the laryngitis is due to a virus, there is no specific therapy; if it is bacterial, medications include antibiotics (such as erythromycin). Analgesics/antipyretics for comfort, antitussives to relieve cough (such as Phenergan with codeine), and throat lozenges to promote comfort and decrease irritation are useful.

Nursing Interventions and Patient Teaching

General interventions include use of warm or cool mist inhalation via vaporizer. The patient should be encouraged to rest the voice by limiting verbal communication.

Nursing diagnoses and interventions for the patient with laryngitis include but are not limited to the following:

Nursing Diagnoses	Nursing Interventions
Pain, related to pharyngeal irritation	Assess level of pain, and offer medications to promote comfort. Use steam inhalation as ordered.
Impaired communication, verbal, related to edematous vocal cord	Instruct patient on the importance of resting the voice. Provide other means for communication (written word, gestures). Anticipate patient's needs whenever possible.

If the patient receives antibiotic agents, the nurse should instruct him to finish the entire prescribed course. The patient should be reminded of the need to limit use of the voice. Patients who smoke should be encouraged to quit and also to limit exposure to irritating fumes.

Prognosis

Prognosis is good in adults. In the infant and young child, respiratory edema can result in respiratory distress.

PHARYNGITIS
Etiology/Pathophysiology

Pharyngitis may be either chronic or acute. It is the most common throat inflammation and frequently accompanies the common cold. Pharyngitis is usually viral in origin but can be caused by hemolytic streptococci, staphylococci, or other bacteria. There is increased evidence of gonococcal pharyngitis caused by the gram-negative diplococcus *Neisseria gonorrhoeae*. A severe form of acute pharyngitis often is referred to as **strep throat** because the streptococcus organism is commonly the cause. This disorder is contagious for 2 or 3 days after the onset of signs and symptoms.

Clinical Manifestations

Pharyngitis manifests itself clinically by a dry cough, tender tonsils, and enlarged cervical lymph glands. The throat appears erythematous, and soreness may range from slight scratchiness to severe pain with difficulty swallowing.

Assessment

Collection of **subjective data** includes any reported pharyngeal discomfort, presence of fever, or any difficulty swallowing.

Collection of **objective data** includes palpating for enlarged, edematous glands and associated tenderness and noting elevated temperature.

Diagnostic Tests

Throat cultures will be done to document presence or absence of a bacterial infection.

Medical Management

Commonly ordered medications include antibiotics, such as penicillin or erythromycin, to (1) treat severe infections; or (2) prevent superimposed infections, particularly in people who have a history of rheumatic fever or bacterial endocarditis. Analgesics/antipyretics, such as acetaminophen, are used to promote comfort.

Nursing Interventions and Patient Teaching

The nurse should offer throat rinses/gargles and encourage oral intake. The importance of adequate rest and use of a vaporizer to increase humidity should be emphasized.

Nursing diagnoses and interventions for the patient with pharyngitis include but are not limited to the following:

NURSING DIAGNOSES	NURSING INTERVENTIONS
Impaired oral mucous membrane, related to edema	Provide warm saline gargles to promote comfort. Assess level of pain and offer medications as ordered. Encourage oral intake of fluids. Offer frequent oral care.
Deficient fluid volume, risk for, related to decreased oral intake as a result of painful swallowing	Observe and record patient's hydration status. Monitor I&O and patient's temperature. Maintain IV therapy if indicated.

The nurse should perform and document medication teaching, including the importance of completing the entire prescribed course of antibiotics and any side effects of medications. The patient should be instructed to avoid exposure to inhaled irritants and to use preventive measures, such as using a vaporizer and maintaining adequate fluid intake.

Prognosis

Signs and symptoms will usually resolve in 4 to 6 days unless secondary complications develop.

SINUSITIS
Etiology/Pathophysiology

Sinusitis can be chronic or acute, involving any sinus area, such as maxillary or frontal. This infection can be either viral or bacterial in origin and often is a complication of pneumonia or nasal polyps.

The underlying pathophysiology begins with an upper respiratory infection that leads to a sinus infection.

Clinical Manifestations

The patient with sinusitis often complains of a constant, severe headache with pain and tenderness in the particular sinus region. Frequently there is a purulent exudate.

Assessment

Collection of **subjective data** includes the patient reporting a decreased appetite or nausea. The patient may also complain of generalized malaise, headache, and pain in the sinus region.

Collection of **objective data** involves the nurse assessing vital signs, particularly temperature, and also assessing the character and amount of drainage.

Diagnostic Tests

Sinus radiographic studies are frequently done to depict cloudy or fluid-filled sinus cavities. A simple way to diagnose sinusitis is with transillumination. This procedure involves shining a light in the mouth with the lips closed around it; infected sinuses will look dark, and normal sinuses will transilluminate.

Medical Management

Nasal windows or other surgical incisions can be created to allow better drainage and removal of diseased mucosal tissue. One of the most common surgical procedures to relieve chronic maxillary sinusitis is the Caldwell-Luc operation, which is a radical antrum operation involving the creation of an incision under the lip to remove diseased mucosal and bone tissue.

Medications used to treat sinusitis include antibiotic agents (penicillin), analgesics to relieve headache (acetaminophen [Tylenol], possibly with codeine), antihistamines (azatadine [Optimine]) to reduce congestion and secretions, and vasoconstrictors in the form of nasal sprays (Afrin) to reduce local vascular congestion.

Nursing Interventions and Patient Teaching

Steam inhalation and warm, moist packs will facilitate drainage and promote comfort.

Nursing diagnoses and interventions for the patient with sinusitis include but are not limited to the following:

Nursing Diagnoses	Nursing Interventions
Ineffective breathing pattern, related to nasal congestion	Assess respiratory status frequently, noting any changes; mouth breathing may be necessary because of nasal airway/sinus discomfort.
Pain, related to sinus congestion	Document comfort level. Assess need for analgesics, and document patient response. Elevate head of bed to promote drainage of secretions. Apply warm moist packs four times a day to promote secretion drainage and provide relief.

The aim of patient education is to prevent recurrence or complications of sinus infection. The patient should be instructed to be alert to signs and symptoms of sinusitis so early treatment can be obtained.

Prognosis

Prognosis for uncomplicated sinusitis is good; complications include cavernous sinus thrombosis and spread of infection to bone, brain, or meninges, which can result in meningitis, osteomyelitis, or septicemia.

DISORDERS OF THE LOWER AIRWAY

ACUTE BRONCHITIS
Etiology/Pathophysiology

Usually acute bronchitis is secondary to an upper respiratory infection, but it can be related to exposure to inhaled irritants. Inflammation of the trachea and bronchial tree causes congestion of the mucous membranes, which results in retention of tenacious secretions. These secretions can become a culture medium for bacterial growth.

Clinical Manifestations

Acute bronchitis manifests itself by a productive cough, diffuse rhonchi/wheezes, dyspnea, chest pain, and low-grade temperature. Generalized malaise and headache are also common symptoms.

Assessment

Collection of **subjective data** includes the patient's complaints of feeling poorly and experiencing headache and aching tightness in the chest.

Collection of **objective data** involves a nursing assessment that includes monitoring vital signs frequently, checking breath sounds, and noting the presence of wheezes or basilar crackles.

Diagnostic Tests

The usual diagnostic aids include a chest radiographic examination to ensure clear lung fields and a sputum specimen to determine the presence of associated bacterial infections.

Medical Management

A quick recovery is promoted by preventing further infectious complications. The physician may order sputum cultures periodically to ascertain that there is no secondary infection.

Medications that are frequently prescribed are cough suppressants (codeine), antitussives (dextromethorphan [Pertussin]), antipyretics (Tylenol), and bronchodilators (terbutaline [Brethine]). Antibiotics, such as ampicillin, may be ordered to combat an infectious process or to prevent its occurrence.

Nursing Interventions and Patient Teaching

The goal of nursing interventions is to facilitate recovery and prevent secondary infections. Such actions include placing the patient on bed rest to conserve energy, using a vaporizer to add humidity to inhaled air, and increasing fluid intake.

Nursing diagnoses and interventions for the patient with acute bronchitis include but are not limited to the following.

NURSING DIAGNOSES	NURSING INTERVENTIONS
Risk for infection, related to retained pulmonary secretions	Assess for signs and symptoms of infection: fever, dyspnea, color and characteristics of sputum production. Administer antipyretics and antibiotics as ordered.
Ineffective airway clearance, related to tenacious pulmonary secretions	Assess patient's ability to move secretions; also note any increase in retained pulmonary secretions. Facilitate airway clearance by elevating head of bed and liquefying secretions by use of humidifier and adequate fluid intake (3000 to 4000 mL/day). Suction as needed. When offering fluids, avoid dairy products, which tend to produce more tenacious secretions.

The patient should be instructed on measures that will prevent exacerbation or recurrence of infection. Such measures include stressing the importance of increasing oral fluid intake, incorporating rest periods between activities, and teaching the patient the signs that may indicate worsening infection (purulent sputum and increased dyspnea). Medication teaching would involve emphasizing the importance of adhering to prescribed medication regimen and using analgesics and antipyretics to reduce fever and malaise. The nurse should teach the patient to limit exposure to others, who may spread infection, and to avoid smoking or other irritating fumes.

Prognosis

Prognosis for acute bronchitis is good.

LEGIONNAIRES' DISEASE
Etiology/Pathophysiology

The causative microorganism of this disease is *Legionella pneumophila*, first identified in 1976 when it caused a pneumonia outbreak at a convention of the American Legion in Philadelphia, Pennsylvania. *L. pneumophila* is a gram-negative bacillus not previously recognized as an agent of human disease. This organism thrives in water reservoirs, such as in air conditioners and humidifiers, and is transmitted through airborne routes. The *Legionella* microbe can progress in two different forms: influenza or Legionnaires' disease. The latter characteristically results in life-threatening pneumonia. This pneumonia causes lung consolidation and alveolar necrosis. The disease progresses rapidly (less than 1 week) and can result in respiratory failure, renal failure, bacteremic shock, and ultimately death.

Clinical Manifestations

Clinical manifestations include significantly elevated temperature, headache, nonproductive cough, diarrhea, and general malaise.

Assessment

Collection of **subjective data** includes noting the patient's complaints of dyspnea, headache, and chest pain on inspiration.

Collection of **objective data** includes many significant signs associated with this infectious process. A significantly elevated temperature (102° to 105° F [38.8° to 40.5° C]) bears close watching and may require immediate interventions. Another sign the patient will exhibit is a nonproductive cough with difficult and rapid breathing. Auscultation of lungs will reveal crackles or wheezes. Because of the high fever and extreme respiratory effort, tachycardia and signs of shock may be present. Hematuria may develop, indicative of resulting renal impairment.

Diagnostic Tests

Diagnostic tests to confirm *L. pneumophila* infection are cultures of blood, sputum, and pulmonary tissue or fluid. Chest radiographic studies will show patchy infiltrates and small pleural effusions.

Medical Management

The physician may need to place the patient on assisted ventilation, which requires intubating the patient through an oral or nasal airway or directly via the trachea. Close observation for disease progression is required. The patient may also require temporary renal dialysis because of acute kidney failure.

To control and compensate for impaired/ineffective respiratory function, the patient will require oxygen therapy, possibly even mechanical ventilation. The patient will need adequate IV fluid therapy to maintain hydration and electrolyte status.

Antibiotic agents (erythromycin) will be given intravenously early in the course of the disease and then orally for a prolonged period to treat the infection. Rifampin is also beneficial. Antipyretics will be administered to reduce the patient's temperature. The patient may also require vasopressors (dopamine or dobutamine) and analgesics to treat shock signs and promote comfort.

Nursing Interventions and Patient Teaching

The patient will be maintained on bed rest, and I&O will be monitored.

Nursing diagnoses and interventions for the patient with Legionnaires' disease include but are not limited to the following:

NURSING DIAGNOSES	NURSING INTERVENTIONS
Ineffective tissue perfusion, cardiopulmonary or renal, related to lack of oxygen	Monitor and report signs and symptoms of impending shock (decreased blood pressure and increased pulse). Administer vasopressor drugs as ordered. Maintain hydration status and urinary output. Assess changes in level of consciousness. Assist with acute hemodialysis if indicated.
Ineffective breathing pattern, related to respiratory failure	Assess signs and symptoms of respiratory failure. Note respiratory rate, rhythm, and effort. Be alert for cyanosis and dyspnea. Assist with oxygen therapy or mechanical ventilation as ordered. Facilitate optimal ventilation—patient in semi-Fowler's position if condition tolerates; suction as needed. Have patient cough and deep breathe every 2 hours if able. Identify associated factors, such as ineffective airway clearance, pain, and altered level of consciousness.

Because of the many alarming actions necessary to treat this disease and its complications, patient and family education is important. The nurse should instruct the patient and family on the purpose of respiratory support—oxygen therapy or ventilator assistance—and how to use these procedures for the greatest benefit. Explanations should be provided of all procedures before their implementation. The purpose of hemodialysis and why it is required should be explained. The nurse should stress the importance of controlling the patient's temperature and fluid and electrolyte status. Emotional support should be offered to the patient and family as needed.

Prognosis

Legionnaires' disease is a severe, often fatal disease. The mortality has been 15% to 20% in a few localized epidemics.

SEVERE ACUTE RESPIRATORY SYNDROME (SARS)
Etiology/Pathophysiology

Severe acute respiratory syndrome (SARS) is a serious acute respiratory infection caused by a coronavirus. The virus spreads by close contact between people. SARS is most likely spread via droplets in the air. It is possible that SARS may also be spread from touching objects that have become contaminated.

Clinical Manifestations

In general, SARS begins with a fever greater than 100.4° F (38° C). Other manifestations may include headache, an overall feeling of discomfort, and muscle aches. Some people also experience mild respiratory symptoms. After 2 to 7 days, SARS patients may develop a dry cough and shortness of breath, difficulty breathing, or hypoxia. About 20% of patients with SARS need intubation and mechanical ventilation (Lewis et al, 2004).

Diagnostic Tests

A chest radiograph will be ordered. In the early stages of SARS, the chest radiograph may be normal. In some patients a chest radiograph may later reveal some interstitial infiltrates that progress to a patchy appearance.

A SARS diagnosis can later be made from detection of serum antibodies or positive tissue cultures. Blood specimen for lab tests, nasopharyngeal and oropharyngeal swabs, and nasopharyngeal aspirate will be obtained. Bronchoalveolar lavage may be used to obtain secretions from the lower respiratory tract. Reverse transcription polymerase chain reaction tests may be done on serum, stool, and nasal secretions.

Initially, the patient's white blood cell count will be normal or low. In about 50% of cases, platelet counts are 50,000 to 150,000/mm³ (normal range, 150,000 to 400,000/mm³). Early in the respiratory phase, creatine phosphokinase levels (CPK) may be as high as 3000 units/L (normal, 5 to 200 units/L) (Parini, 2003).

Additional criteria to establish a diagnosis of SARS include travel within 10 days of symptom onset to an area with current community transmission of SARS—recently including mainland China (particularly Beijing), Hong Kong, Vietnam, Singapore, Taiwan, and Toronto—or close contact within 10 days of symptom onset with a person suspected of having SARS (Katz & Hirsch, 2003).

Medical Management

Because the disease is severe, treatment needs to be started based on the symptoms and before the cause of the illness is confirmed. First, people who are suspected of having SARS should be placed in respiratory isolation, including use of an appropriate disposable particulate respirator mask to protect other patients and health care workers. Although there is no definitive treatment, antiviral medications (such as ribavirin), antibiotics, and corticosteroids may be used, although antibiotics will not help with SARS (because it is believed to be caused by a *virus*), they may be used in cases in which the person also has a bacterial infection.

Nursing Interventions/Patient Teaching

The infection control nurse must notify the local public health department. Respiratory isolation with meticulous hand hygiene is carried out to prevent the spread of SARS. When the patient's respiratory status returns to baseline, the patient will be discharged home. The patient can go out in public and return to work 10 days after the fever has resolved and respiratory symptoms are improving or absent (Parini, 2003).

Prognosis

About 80% to 90% of infected people start to recover after 6 to 7 days. However, 10% to 20% go on to develop severe breathing problems and may need mechanical ventilation to breathe. The risk of death is higher for this group and appears to be linked to the person's preexisting health conditions. People older than age 40 are more likely to develop severe breathing problems (Lewis et al, 2004).

ANTHRAX
Etiology/Pathophysiology

Anthrax infection is caused by the spore-forming bacterium *Bacillus anthracis.* Found in nature, anthrax most commonly infects wild and domestic hoofed animals. It is spread through direct contact with the bacteria and its spores—dormant, encapsulated bacteria that become active when they enter a living host.

In humans, anthrax gains a foothold when spores enter the body via the skin, intestines, or lungs. It is not contagious by person-to-person contact, so treating family members and others in contact with an infected person is not recommended unless they were exposed to the same source of infection.

Three types of anthrax. Anthrax symptoms depend on the initial site of infection. The three types of anthrax are:

1. **Cutaneous anthrax,** the most common type, occurs after bacteria or spores enter the skin through a cut or abrasion. Within several days of exposure, a pruritic reddened macule or papule develops, followed by vesicle formation. The lesion resembles an insect bite at first, until black eschar appears at the center of the lesion and the site becomes edematous. Although a patient may develop bacteremia if the organism enters his or her bloodstream, cutaneous anthrax is rarely fatal if it is treated with antibiotics.

2. **Gastrointestinal (GI) anthrax,** the least common type, occurs after ingestion of the organism in contaminated, undercooked food. Spores can germinate in the mouth, esophagus, stomach, or small and large intestines, causing ulcers. Inflammation of the GI tract can cause nausea, vomiting, fever, abdominal pain, and diarrhea. Unless treated early, a patient may die from sepsis.

3. **Inhalational anthrax,** the most deadly type, develops when spores are inhaled deeply into the lungs. Immune cells sent to fight the lung infection carry some bacteria back to the lymph system, allowing the infection to spread to other organs.

Initial symptoms of inhalational anthrax resemble those of the common cold or influenza, except that the patient usually will not develop an increased amount of thin, clear nasal exudate. Subsequent breathing problems may be mistaken for pneumonia, delaying diagnosis. Other severe symptoms, including hemorrhage, tissue necrosis, and lymph edema, are caused by bacterial toxins. Death usually results from blood loss and shock.

Diagnostic Tests

A chest x-ray helps differentiate inhalational anthrax from pneumonia. A widening mediastinum from lymphadenopathy is characteristic of inhalational anthrax infection; infiltrates characterize pneumonia.

No single reliable screening test for anthrax is currently available, although the Mayo Clinic recently announced development of a rapid DNA test to identify anthrax in people and the environment. Using standard precautions, obtain specimens for a blood smear and culture and a chest x-ray for anyone with symptoms of inhalational anthrax. A nasal swab is not recommended to diagnose anthrax infection. For a patient suspected of cutaneous anthrax, obtain a culture specimen from the lesion's vesicular fluid. Obtain a specimen for stool culture if intestinal anthrax is suspected.

Medical Management

Antibiotic treatment is indicated for anyone diagnosed with anthrax or exposed to anthrax spores. For both children and adults, ciprofloxacin (Cipro) has been considered the treatment of choice for all three forms of anthrax because of concerns that genetically engineered anthrax strains might resist older antibiotics. However, most anthrax strains are susceptible to many other antibiotics, including penicillin and doxycycline (Vibramycin).

The Centers for Disease Control and Prevention (CDC) recommend a 60-day course of therapy to ensure eradication of inactive spores, as well as bacteria. An alternative treatment for postexposure prophylaxis is 30 days of antibiotics and three doses of the anthrax vaccine if it is available. (The anthrax vaccine is not currently recommended for the general public in the absence of anthrax exposure.) Consult the U.S. Food and Drug Administration (FDA) and CDC websites for the prescribing information for children and other treatment updates.

In October 2001, the FDA issued new labeling for several older antibiotics effective against anthrax. Concerned about drug resistance, the FDA has urged health care providers to avoid prescribing antibiotics indiscriminately (*Nursing*, 2002).

TUBERCULOSIS
Etiology/Pathophysiology

In 1882, Robert Koch identified the tubercle bacillus (*Mycobacterium tuberculosis*) as the causative agent for tuberculosis (TB). TB is a chronic pulmonary and extrapulmonary (outside of the lung) infectious disease acquired by inhalation of a dried droplet nucleus containing a tubercle bacillus into the alveolar structure of the lung. It is characterized by stages of early infection (frequently asymptomatic), latency, and a potential for recurrent postprimary disease. It most commonly affects the respiratory system, but other parts of the body such as gastrointestinal and genitourinary tracts, bones, joints, nervous system, lymph nodes, and skin may become infected (Cultural and Ethnic Considerations box).

Tuberculosis infection is different from tuberculosis disease. It is important to differentiate **infection** with TB from **active disease.** Although infection always precedes the development of active disease, only about 10% of infections progress to active disease. Tuberculosis infection is characterized by the presence of mycobacteria in the tissue of a host who is free of clinical signs and symptoms and who demonstrates the presence of antibodies against the mycobacteria. Tuberculosis disease is manifest as pathological and functional signs and symptoms indicating destructive activity of mycobacteria in host tissue. Transmission is primarily by inhalation of minute dried-droplet nuclei (each containing a single tubercle bacillus), coughed or sneezed into the air by a person whose sputum contains virulent (capable of producing disease) tubercle bacilli.

A common misconception about TB is that it is easily transmitted. In fact, most people exposed to TB do not become infected. The body's first line of defense, the upper airway, prevents most inhaled TB organisms from ever reaching the lungs. If the inhaled particles are small enough, the organisms can survive in the upper respiratory tract, reach the alveoli, and establish infection. Less commonly, transmission may occur by ingestion or by invasion of the skin or mucous membranes.

TB had been epidemic in the Western world. With the introduction of pharmacological management in the late 1940s and early 1950s, there was a dramatic decrease in the prevalence of TB. TB had been responsible for one third of the deaths of young adults in Europe. Following Koch's discovery, improvement in living conditions, sanitation, and the development of effective drug therapy and treatment brought about a steady decline in mortality attributable to TB. Shortly after the centennial of Koch's work, eradication of the disease in the United States by the year 2010 was considered a realistic goal.

Two decades later, there is less reason for optimism. Approximately 15 million Americans are infected with the TB bacillus, and TB case rates in the United States rose by 18% from 1985 to 1991. Now, because of renewed efforts at prevention and detection, the number of TB cases has declined below the 1985 rate of 9.3 cases per 100,000 people to its lowest rate ever of 5.8 cases per 100,000 people in 2000.

TB still presents a serious health problem. Although the number of U.S.-born people with active TB has decreased, the number of foreign-born U.S. residents with the disease has increased more than 65% since 1986. More than two thirds of reported cases occur in racial and ethnic minorities, particularly among Hispanics and African-Americans (Boutotte, 1999). Most alarming, a growing percentage of new cases of TB are resistant to the drugs that are traditionally used to fight the disease.

TB has been particularly prevalent among people infected with the human immunodeficiency virus (HIV). The status of the host's immune system is the major determinant for the development of active TB. The disease occurs most often in individuals with incompetent immune systems, such as HIV-infected people, older adults, people receiving immunosuppressive therapy, and the malnourished.

Hospitals are a high-risk setting for TB transmission, and health care workers are at high occupational risk for TB infection. Until recently the vulnerability of hospital workers to TB infection had not been empha-

---

🌀 Cultural and Ethnic Considerations

Tuberculosis

- Tuberculosis in the United States tends to be a disease of the older population, urban poor, minority groups, and patients with acquired immunodeficiency syndrome (AIDS).
- At all ages the incidence of tuberculosis among nonwhites is at least twice that of whites.
- Ethnic groups that have a high incidence of tuberculosis include foreign-born people from Asia, Africa, and Latin America.
- Southeastern Asian, Haitian, and Hispanic immigrants have incidence rates of tuberculosis similar to those of the countries from which they came.

sized. This complacency is changing with the wide publicity accompanying the increase of TB (Box 9-5).

In the lung, pulmonary macrophages ingest TB bacteria. Macrophages engulf the organisms, but do not kill them. Instead they surround them and wall them off in tiny, hard capsules called **tubercles.** Macrophages activate lymphocytes, and within 2 to 10 weeks, activated lymphocytes usually control the initial infection in the lung and nonpulmonary sites. Nonmultiplying tubercle bacilli can survive, often more than 50 years in human tissue.

Most people who become infected with the TB organism do not progress to the active disease stage. They remain asymptomatic and noninfectious. They will have a positive tuberculin skin test, and chest radiographs will be negative. These people still retain a lifelong risk of developing reactivation TB if the immune system is compromised.

Clinical Manifestations

The clinical manifestations are insidious. Generally there is fever, weight loss, weakness, and a productive cough. Later in the disease, daily recurring fever with chills, night sweats, and hemoptysis is seen.

Assessment

Collection of **subjective data** includes the patient reporting loss of muscle strength and weight loss.

Collection of **objective data** includes evaluating and recording the amount, color, and characteristics of sputum produced.

Box 9-5 *High-Risk Groups to Screen for TB*

- HIV-infected people
- Close contacts (especially children and adolescents) of people with active infectious TB
- People with conditions that increase the risk of active TB after infection, such as silicosis, diabetes, chronic renal failure, history of gastrectomy, weight 10% below ideal body weight, prolonged corticosteroid or other immunosuppressive therapy, some hematologic disorders (leukemia and lymphomas, for example), and other malignancies
- People born in countries with a high prevalence of TB
- Substance abusers, such as alcoholics, IV drug users, and cocaine or crack users
- Residents of long-term care facilities, nursing homes, prisons, mental institutions, homeless shelters, and other congregate housing settings
- Medically underserved low-income populations, including racial and ethnic minorities, homeless people, and migrant workers
- Health care workers and others who provide service to any high-risk group

---

Diagnostic Tests

Diagnostic evaluation for pulmonary TB includes a Mantoux tuberculin skin test. The tuberculin skin test is used to identify people infected with the TB organism. A positive reaction can detect infection 2 to 10 weeks after exposure to the tubercle bacillus. To read the test 48 to 72 hours later, measure and record the subsequent induration (an area of hardened tissue); do not measure the erythema (redness). A negative reaction is less than 5 mm. If the patient is infected with tuberculosis (whether active or dormant), lymphocytes will recognize the purified protein derivative antigen in the skin test and cause a local indurated reaction. Generally, the larger the reaction is, the greater the likelihood that the person is infected with the TB organism. However, a negative reaction doesn't rule out infection. An infected person whose immune system has been weakened by disease, drugs, or old age may have a limited or negative reaction. If the test is negative and the physician strongly suspects tuberculosis, a "second-strength" tuberculin test can be used. If this test is then negative, the patient does not have tuberculosis. Other diagnostic tests that are used to confirm the diagnosis of pulmonary tuberculosis are chest radiograph and evaluation of sputum specimens for mycobacterial organisms. Sputum specimens can be rapidly smeared, stained, and screened for the presence of acid-fast organisms. Mycobacteria are one of the few organisms that are characteristically acid-fast. Three positive acid-fast smears constitute a presumptive diagnosis of TB and indicate the need for treatment. The diagnosis of tuberculosis is confirmed if TB bacilli grow in culture, a process that may take 6 to 8 weeks. A new test, nucleic acid amplification (NAA), is a rapid diagnostic test for TB. Test results are available in a few hours. This does not replace routine sputum smears and cultures but it offers a health care provider increased confidence in the diagnosis. All patients with tuberculosis must be reported to the appropriate public health authority for case follow-up and investigation of contacts.

Medical Management

Drug therapy is the mainstay of tuberculosis treatment. Infectiousness declines rapidly once drug therapy is initiated, even before sputum smears become negative. Cough frequently also declines with drug therapy.

Tuberculosis isolation (acid-fast bacillus, or AFB) is isolation for patients with pulmonary TB who have a positive sputum smear or a chest radiograph that strongly suggests current (active) TB. Laryngeal TB is also included in this isolation category. In general, infants and young children with pulmonary TB do not require isolation precautions because they rarely cough and their bronchial secretions contain few AFB, compared with adults with pulmonary TB. If there is question of infectiousness in the adult TB patient, hospitalized patients usually remain in respiratory isolation during their hospital stay.

Compared with most other infectious diseases, treatment for TB is lengthy, typically 6 to 9 months, and sometimes longer for extrapulmonary disease. If treatment is not continued for a long period of time, some of the TB organisms will survive and the patient will be at risk for a relapse.

Treatment therapy now involves multiple drugs to which the organisms are susceptible. If only one drug is given, the patient may become resistant to it. Treatment of TB usually consists of a combination of at least four drugs, each of which helps prevent the emergence of organisms resistant to the other, thus increasing the therapeutic effectiveness of treatment. The drugs that are used to treat tuberculosis are categorized as first-line drugs and second-line drugs. First-line drugs are isoniazid (INH); rifampin (rifampicin); rifampin and isoniazid (Rifamate), with a fixed combination of 300 mg rifampin and 150 mg isoniazid per capsule; pyrazinamide; ethambutol; and streptomycin. In 1998 the U.S. Food and Drug Administration (FDA) approved rifapentine (Priftin), the first new TB drug to become available in the United States in 10 years. Although it is similar to rifampin, rifapentine has a longer half-life and can be taken less frequently. Second-line drugs are ethionamide, para-aminosalicylate sodium (PAS), cycloserine, capreomycin, kanamycin, amikacin, levofloxacin, ofloxacin, and ciprofloxacin (Medications table).

The monitoring of patients with TB is critically important; the failure to complete prescribed medication treatment accounts for most treatment failures. To ensure compliance and to help prevent the development of drug-resistant strains of the tubercle bacillus, there may be circumstances when it may be necessary for the health care worker to watch the patient take the medications, which is referred to as directly observed therapy (DOT).

Nursing Interventions and Patient Teaching

If TB is suspected, permission to place the patient in acid-fast bacilli (AFB) isolation precautions should be requested immediately. These precautions would include the use of isolation rooms with a negative air pressure so that air flows into, rather than out of, the room. Doors and windows must be kept closed to maintain airflow control. Room air should be exhausted directly to the outside and not recirculated to other rooms. Also included in AFB isolation precautions is the use of particulate respiration masks (because AFB particles pass through standard masks). Although TB is not easily transmitted, it is more easily transmitted in closed spaces and in areas with poor ventilation and no environmental controls.

Perhaps the simplest, most effective technique for stopping TB at the source is kindly insisting that patients cover their noses and mouths when coughing or sneezing.

In order to assist the patient's compliance to the prescribed medication regimen, the nurse must develop a supportive relationship with the patient.

Nursing interventions are focused on preventing complications and illness transmission.

Nursing diagnoses and interventions for the patient with tuberculosis include but are not limited to the following:

NURSING DIAGNOSES	NURSING INTERVENTIONS
Ineffective breathing pattern, related to pulmonary infection process	Monitor breathing for evidence of dyspnea or signs and symptoms of pneumothorax. Evaluate degree of respiratory effort and assist as needed. Assess expectorated sputum for hemoptysis. Assist immobile patient to turn, cough, and deep breathe every 2 to 4 hours to prevent pooling of secretions.
Risk for infection, (patient contacts), related to viable *Mycobacterium tuberculosis* in respiratory secretions	Obtain specimen for culture (incorrect collection and handling may destroy or contaminate specimen, thus interfering with diagnostic results). Employ AFB isolation until antimicrobial therapy is successfully initiated for sputum-positive patients to prevent transmission of organisms. Employ drainage and secretion precautions until wounds from patient with extrapulmonary tuberculosis stop draining to prevent transmission of organism. Instruct the patient to cough and sneeze into tissue and properly dispose of to prevent organism transmission.

The nurse should teach the patient techniques of proper disposal and handwashing related to coughing and sneezing. These measures will decrease the spread of infection. The nurse should explain the vital importance of adhering to the medication regimen as ordered and the need for prolonged treatment. The patient should be instructed on medication, dosage, frequency, and possible side effects. The nurse should emphasize the need to report hemoptysis, dyspnea, vertigo, or chest pain. The patient should be reminded to maintain adequate fluid and nutritional requirements.

Text continued on p. 433

MEDICATIONS | *Respiratory Disorders*

MEDICATION	TRADE NAME	ACTION	SIDE EFFECTS	NURSING IMPLICATIONS
Acetylcysteine	Mucomyst	Mucolytic agent; also used as antidote in acetaminophen overdose	Nausea, vomiting, rhinorrhea, mucorrhea, bronchospasm	Store product in refrigerator; bad taste may be masked by mixing with soft drink when using as antidote
Aminophylline	Many	See theophylline	See theophylline	See theophylline
Azatadine	Optimine, also available in numerous combination allergy and cold preparations	Antihistamine; blocks allergic response through histamine receptor blockade	Drowsiness, confusion, dry mouth, constipation, urinary retention, blurred vision, increased viscosity of respiratory secretions	Avoid use with alcohol or other CNS depressants; avoid driving and other hazardous activities
Short-acting beta$_2$-receptor agonists (albuterol, others)	Proventil, Ventolin	Beta$_2$-receptor agonists; cause bronchodilation cardiac, palpitations, angina or chest pain, cardiac dysrhythmias	Anxiety, headache, insomnia, dizziness, restlessness, tachy-metered dose inhaler is crucial to achieve therapeutic response; instruct patients carefully	Use with caution in cardiac disease Teach patient that paradoxic bronchospasm may occur and to stop drug immediately and call physician Teach proper use of inhaler
Long-acting beta$_2$-receptor agonists (salmeterol)	Serevent	Causes bronchodilation Uses—prevention of exercise-induced asthma	Tremors, anxiety, insomnia, headache, stimulation, tachycardia, dry mouth, bronchospasm	Avoid use of OTC medications; extra stimulation may occur Use with caution in cardiac disorders, hyperthyroidism, hypertension, and narrow-angle glaucoma
Corticosteroids (prednisone, methylprednisolone, hydrocortisone, others)	Deltasone, others (prednisone); Medrol, others (methylprednisolone); Cortef, others (hydrocortisone)	Antiinflammatory agent	Short-term—sodium and water retention, hypokalemia, hyperglycemia, euphoria Long-term—osteoporosis, increased susceptibility to infection, poor wound healing, bruising, thinning of skin, Cushingoid weight distribution, cataracts, glaucoma, peptic ulcer disease, myopathy, muscle weakness, suppression of endogenous glucocorticoid production	Do not discontinue medication abruptly; dosage must be slowly tapered down; patient should carry identification on person signaling steroid use; take with food or milk to minimize upset
Fluticasone (inhaled corticosteroid)	Flovent			
Epinephrine	Adrenalin, many others	Beta$_1$- and beta$_2$-receptor agonist, causes	Tachycardia, palpitations, angina, chest pain, myocardial	Use with extreme caution in cardiac disease; do not use

MEDICATIONS | *Respiratory Disorders—cont'd*

MEDICATION	TRADE NAME	ACTION	SIDE EFFECTS	NURSING IMPLICATIONS
Epinephrine—cont'd		bronchodilation and cardiac stimulation, alpha$_1$ agonist activity may cause vasoconstriction	infarction, cardiac dysrhythmias, hypertension, restlessness, agitation, anxiety	OTC cough or cold preparations; do not use discolored preparations
Ethambutol	Myambutol	Antitubercular agent	Optic neuritis, blurred vision or decreased visual acuity, hyperuricemia, exacerbation of gout, drowsiness, confusion, GI effects, hepatoxicity, thrombocytopenia	Patient should have baseline visual examination at start of therapy; emphasize that long-term therapy is required for cure
Isoniazid (INH)	Nydrazid, others	Antitubercular agent	Peripheral neuopathy, hepatotoxicity, SLE-like syndrome, hyperglycemia, bone marrow suppression	Monitor liver function, emphasize that long-term therapy is required; instruct patient to report numbness or tingling of extremities
Leukotriene modifiers; leukotriene receptor antagonists (zafirlukast, montelukast); leukotriene synthesis inhibitors (zileuton)	Accolate, Singulair, Zyflo	Interferes with the synthesis or blocks the action of leukotrienes, causing both bronchodilator and antiinflammatory effects; for long-term treatment of asthma	Accolate—hepatic dysfunction, systemic eosinophilia, headache, infection, nausea, asthenia, abdominal pain; Singulair—tiredness, fever, abdominal pain, dizziness; Zyflo—headache, abdominal pain, asthenia, dyspepsia	Monitor for eosinophilia, worsening pumonary symptoms, cardiac complications, and/or neuropathy Administer after meals for GI symptoms
Oxymetazoline	Afrin, others	Vasoconstrictor, used for nasal congestion	Local nasal irritation, dryness, rebound congestion	Do not use for more than 4 consecutive days to minimize rebound congestion
Para-aminosalicylate sodium (PAS)	Many	Antitubercular agent	Nausea, vomiting, diarrhea, abdominal pain, hypersensitivity reactions, hepatotoxicity, leukopenia, thrombocytopenia	Take with food; discard if discolored; use with caution in peptic ulcer disease or congestive heart failure; emphasize that long-term therapy is required
Potassium iodide	Many; also available in numerous combination preparations	Expectorant, mucokinetic agent	Hypersensitivity, rash, metallic taste, burning in mouth or throat, GI irritation, headache, parotitis, hyperkalemia	Do not use in pregnant women; mix with fruit juice to mask taste

Continued

MEDICATIONS | *Respiratory Disorders—cont'd*

MEDICATION	TRADE NAME	ACTION	SIDE EFFECTS	NURSING IMPLICATIONS
Pyrazinamide	Many	Antitubercular agent	Hyperuricemia, exacerbation of gout, hepatotoxicity	Monitor liver function tests and serum uric acid levels; instruct patient not to use alcohol; emphasize that long-term therapy is required
Rifampin	Rifadin, Rimactane	Antitubercular agent	Flulike syndrome, hematopoietic reactions, hepatotoxicity, rash, red-orange coloration of bodily fluids, shortness of breath, heartburn, sore mouth and tongue, dizziness, confusion	Give on empty stomach; emphasize that long-term therapy is required; may accelerate metabolism of other drugs, including theophylline, oral contraceptives, and warfarin; instruct patient that body fluids may be discolored; may cause permanent staining of soft contact lenses
Rifapentine	Priftin	Antitubercular agent	Hepatotoxicity, hyperuricemia, neutropenia, pyuria, proteinuria, rash, anemia, leukopenia, arthralgias, nausea, vomiting, dyspepsia, pseudomembranous colitis	Monitor liver function tests, and serum uric acid. Monitor WBC count. Tell the patient that rifapentine may produce red-orange discoloration of body tissues and/or fluids (e.g., skin, teeth, tongue, urine, feces, saliva, sputum, tears, cerebrospinal fluid). Emphasize importance of not missing any doses
Theophylline (aminophylline is a salt of theophylline)	Many	Bronchodilator	Anxiety, restlessness, insomnia, headache, seizures, tachycardia, cardiac dysrhythmias, nausea, epigastric pain, hematemesis, gastroesophageal reflux, tachypnea	Do not crush sustained-release preparations; contents of pellet-containing capsules may be sprinkled over food; avoid caffeine; use with caution in peptic ulcer disease or cardiac dysrhythmias; metabolism affected by other medications (erythromycin, ciprofloxacin, cimetidine, rifampin); monitor serum concentrations

Prognosis

Active TB requires a long course of drug ingestion—6 to 9 months minimum, and often longer—to result in an arrest of the disease. As many as 50% of patients fail to complete therapy as prescribed. Numerous drug-resistant tuberculosis cases have been reported in HIV-infected people with TB. These infections were characterized by rapid disease progression, with 4 to 16 weeks from diagnosis to death and mortality rates of 72% to 89%.

Nonmultiplying tubercle bacilli can survive more than 50 years in human tissue and can become reactivated when the patient has a compromised immune system.

PNEUMONIA
Etiology/Pathophysiology

Pneumonia is an inflammatory process of the respiratory bronchioles and the alveolar spaces that is caused by an infection. It can also be caused by oversedation, inadequate ventilation, or aspiration.

Pneumonia can occur in any season but is most common during winter and early spring. People of all ages are susceptible, but pneumonia is more common among infants and older adults. Pneumonia is often caused by aspiration of infected materials into the distal bronchioles and alveoli. Certain individuals are especially susceptible, including people whose normal respiratory defense mechanisms are damaged or altered (those with chronic obstructive pulmonary disease, influenza, or tracheostomy and those who have recently had anesthesia); people who have a disease affecting antibody response; people with alcoholism, in whom there is increased danger of aspiration; and people with delayed white blood cell response to infection. Increasingly, nosocomial pneumonia (acquired in the hospital) is a cause of morbidity and mortality (Health Promotion Considerations box).

Pneumonia is a communicable disease; the mode of transmission is dependent on the infecting organism. Pneumonia is classified according to the offending organism rather than the anatomical location (lobar or bronchial) as was the practice in the past.

Pneumonia can be caused by bacteria, viruses, mycoplasma, fungi, and chemicals. Currently, about half of pneumonia cases are caused by bacteria and half by virus. Up to 96% of bacterial pneumonia is caused by four organisms: *Streptococcus pneumoniae* (pneumococcal), hemolytic streptococcus type A, *Staphylococcus aureus*, and *Haemophilus influenzae* (type B). Nonbacterial or atypical pneumonia is caused by *Mycoplasma pneumoniae*, *L. pneumophila* (Legionnaires' disease), and *Pneumocystis jiroveci* (formerly *carinii*) pneumonia.

Aspiration pneumonia is frequently called necrotizing pneumonia because of the pathological changes in the lungs. Aspiration pneumonia occurs most commonly as a result of aspiration of vomitus when the patient is in an altered state of consciousness due to a

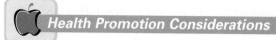

Health Promotion Considerations

Pneumonia

- There are many nursing interventions to help prevent the occurrence of, as well as the morbidity associated with, pneumonia.
- Teach the individual to practice good health habits, such as proper diet and hygiene, adequate rest, and regular exercise, to maintain the natural resistance to infecting organisms.
- The individual at risk for pneumonia (e.g., the chronically ill, older adult) should be encouraged to obtain both influenza and pneumococcal vaccines.
- In the hospital, the nursing role involves identifying the patient at risk and taking measures to prevent the development of pneumonia.
- The patient with altered consciousness should be placed in positions (e.g., side lying, upright) that will prevent or minimize the risk of aspiration. The patient should be turned and repositioned at least every 2 hours to facilitate adequate lung expansion and to discourage pooling of secretions.
- The patient who has difficulty swallowing (e.g., stroke patient) needs assistance in eating, drinking, and taking medication to prevent aspiration.
- The patient who has recently had surgery and others who are immobile need assistance with turning and deep breathing measures at frequent intervals and use of incentive spirometer.
- The nurse must be careful to avoid overmedication with opioids or sedatives, which can cause a depressed cough reflex and accumulation of fluid in the lungs.
- The gag reflex should be present in the individual who has had local anesthesia to the throat before the administration of fluids or food.
- Strict medical asepsis and adherence to infection control guidelines should be practiced by the nurse to reduce the incidence of nosocomial infections. Health care providers should wash their hands each time before they provide care to a patient. Comply with current CDC hand hygiene guidelines.

seizure, drugs, alcohol, anesthesia, acute infection, or shock. Aspiration pneumonia may be acquired through foreign body aspiration or may follow aspiration of toxic materials, such as gasoline or kerosene.

The causative agents of bacterial aspiration pneumonia include *S. aureus*, *Escherichia coli*, *Klebsiella pneumoniae*, *Pseudomonas aeruginosa*, and *Proteus* species.

The pathophysiology of pneumonia depends on the causative agent. Bacterial pneumonia is marked by an alveolar suppurative (process of pus formation) exudate with consolidation of infection. Mycoplasmal and viral pneumonia produce interstitial inflammation with no consolidation or exudate. Fungal and mycobacterial pneumonias are marked by patchy distribution that may undergo necrosis with the development of cavities. Aspiration pneumonia presents with various physiological responses depending upon the pH of the aspirated substance.

An overview of the pathophysiology is as follows: (1) pulmonary cilia cannot remove accumulating secretions from the respiratory tract; (2) these retained secretions then become infected; (3) inflammation of some part of the respiratory tract develops, leading to a localized edema; (4) this causes decreased oxygen–carbon dioxide exchange. This process can begin in the bronchi or in the lobe of one lung, and it can become more extensive.

Clinical Manifestations

There are many significant signs and symptoms seen in pneumonia. A productive cough is very common; color and consistency of sputum will vary depending on the type of pneumonia present. Severe chills, ele-vated temperature, and increased heart and respiratory rates may accompany the painful, productive cough (Older Adult Considerations box).

Clinical manifestations are dependent on the type of pneumonia:

- **Streptococcal, pneumococcal:** Sudden onset; chest pain; chills; fever; headache; cough; rust-colored sputum; crackles and possibly friction rub; hypoxemia as blood is shunted away from area of consolidation; cyanosis; area of consolidation visible on chest radiograph; sputum culture needed to determine causative agent
- **Staphylococcal:** Many of same signs as strepto-coccal; sputum copious and salmon colored
- **Klebsiella:** Many of the same signs and symptoms as streptococcal; onset more gradual; more bronchopneumonia (inflammation of the termi-

---

Older Adult Considerations

Respiratory Disorder

- Signs and symptoms of pneumonia are often atypical in older adults. Fever, cough, and purulent sputum may be absent. Generalized signs and symptoms such as lethargy, disorientation, dyspnea, tachypnea, chills, chest pain, and vomiting, as well as an unexpected exacerbation of coexisting conditions, should be viewed with suspicion because they may indicate pneumonia in the older adult.
- Adequate hydration is very important for the older person with pneumonia. It helps liquefy secretions and promotes expectoration.
- Many older adults have difficulty expectorating. This slows resolution of congestions and increases the difficulty of obtaining sputum specimens. Because deep breathing and coughing are difficult, the older person may require suctioning to remove respiratory secretions. This should be done with discretion because too-frequent suctioning can stimulate increased production of secretions.
- Older adults, particularly those living in an institution, should have routine skin tests for tuberculosis. Many older adults were exposed to tuberculosis during their childhood and have positive results on skin tests. These individuals should receive routine chest radiographic studies. Older adults who have histories of inactive tuberculosis should be watched for recurrence of active tuberculosis. Signs and symptoms are often vague and include loss of appetite and weight loss.
- Older immigrants and immunosuppressed older adults should be watched closely for drug-resistant strains of tuberculosis.
- Provided that there is no serious disease of the respiratory tract, the older person is generally able to maintain adequate ventilation and oxygenation.

- However, changes of aging do have an effect on respiratory function:
  —Drier mucous membranes and decreased number of cilia affect the older individual's ability to humidify inhaled air and trap debris. These, in turn, increase the risk for inflammation and irritation of the upper respiratory tract.
  —Kyphosis and calcification of costal cartilage are common changes. These restrict expansion of the thoracic cavity and lead to a barrel-chested appearance.
  —Intercostal muscles and the diaphragm lose elasticity, resulting in a decreased ability to breathe deeply and cough.
  —The elasticity of airways and alveoli decreases, alveoli thicken, and pulmonary blood flow decreases, resulting in an increased risk for impaired gas exchange.
- Years of exposure to air pollution, smoke, and mechanical irritants increase the risk for respiratory disease in older adults, particularly those who have emphysema and chronic bronchitis.
- Inactivity and immobility increase the risk of stasis pooling of respiratory secretions. This increases the risk of pneumonia.
- Neurological damage as a result of strokes, Parkinson's disease, and other conditions are increasingly common in the older adult. Any neurological disorder that decreases the gag or swallow reflexes increases the risk of aspiration of fluids and food, with resultant trauma to the respiratory tract.
- Cor pulmonale with right-sided heart failure, as well as left-sided heart failure with pulmonary congestion, are common complications of chronic obstructive pulmonary disease in the older adult.

nal bronchioles and alveoli) visible on chest radiograph; if treatment delayed beyond second day after onset, patient will become critically ill; mortality will be high

- **Haemophilus:** Commonly follows upper respiratory infection; low-grade fever; croupy cough; malaise; arthralgias; yellow or green sputum
- **Mycoplasmal:** Gradual onset; headache; fever; malaise; chills; cough severe and nonproductive; decreased breath sounds and crackles; chest radiograph clear; white blood cell count normal
- **Viral:** Signs and symptoms generally mild; cold symptoms; headache; anorexia; myalgia (tenderness or pain in muscles); irritating cough that produces mucopurulent or bloody sputum; bronchopneumonic type of infiltration on chest radiograph; white blood cell count usually normal; rise in antibody titers

Assessment

Collection of **subjective data** includes obtaining the patient's description of the history, onset, and duration of cough. The patient may complain of fever and night sweats.

Collection of **objective data** involves nursing assessment measures, including checking the level of consciousness and vital signs, especially temperature and respirations, every 2 hours or as ordered. The color, consistency, and amount of sputum produced should be noted. The nurse should inspect the thorax to determine the patient's use of accessory muscles in respiratory effort and note any cyanosis or dyspnea. The nurse will observe and document if the patient needs to use abdominal muscles or intercostal muscles to adequately breathe. On auscultation, the nurse will hear crackles on inspiration and possibly a pleural effusion.

Diagnostic Tests

Blood and sputum cultures will help in identification of organisms. Sputum for culture and sensitivity should be collected before initiation of antibiotic therapy, to identify the causative agent. Chest radiographic studies will reveal changes in density, primarily in the lower lobes. White blood cell count will be normal or even low in viral or mycoplasmal pneumonia, whereas it will be elevated in bacterial pneumonia. Leukocytosis is found in the majority of patients with bacterial pneumonia, usually with a white blood cell (WBC) count greater than $15,000/mm^3$ with a shift to the left. Pulmonary function tests may be done to determine whether lung volume is decreased, and ABG values will be determined to identify altered gas exchange. Pulse oximetry will be ordered to monitor oxygen saturation of arterial blood levels. Oximetry is invaluable for rapid and continuous assessment of oxygen needs.

Medical Management

If an accumulation of pus in the pleural space (empyema) occurs, the physician will insert a chest tube for drainage. The physician will also prescribe oxygen therapy and physiotherapy—chest percussion and postural drainage. Patients should be encouraged to cough and deep breathe to maximize ventilatory capabilities.

Commonly prescribed medications include antibiotics—penicillin, erythromycin, cephalosporin, and tetracycline—depending upon causative organism and sensitivity. Currently there is no definitive treatment for viral pneumonia. Analgesics and antipyretics (acetaminophen [Tylenol] or aspirin), expectorants, and bronchodilators are often prescribed. Humidification with humidifier or nebulizer if secretions are tenacious and copious is useful. Oxygenation is prescribed if the patient has oxygen saturation of less than 91%. Venturi mask or nasal cannula is commonly used.

A vaccine is now available for the most common and important bacterial pneumonia, streptococcal (also called pneumococcal) pneumonia. Pneumococcal vaccine is indicated primarily for the individual considered at risk who (1) has chronic illnesses such as lung and heart disease and diabetes mellitus, (2) is recovering from a severe illness, (3) is 65 years of age or older, or (4) is in a nursing home or other long-term care facility. This is particularly important because the rate of drug-resistant streptococcus pneumonia is increasing. The current recommendation is that pneumococcal vaccine is good for the person's lifetime. However, in the immunosuppressed individual at risk for development of fatal pneumococcal infection, it is recommended that revaccination should be considered every 5 years.

Nursing Interventions and Patient Teaching

Nursing strategies are aimed at assisting the patient to conserve energy. The nurse should allow rest periods and should facilitate optimal air exchange by placing the patient in high Fowler's position. Place the patient on the side with the "good lung down." The "good lung down" position benefits those with unilateral pulmonary pathology, including unilateral pneumonia. In pneumonia and many other pulmonary problems, PaO_2 rises when the healthy lung is dependent or "good lung down." When the unimpaired lung is down, this better ventilated lung also is vastly better perfused. Studies have revealed that hypoxia worsened when patients were placed on their back or side with the affected (sick) lung down.

Nursing interventions also include assessing the patient to identify inability to move secretions. If inability is identified, assist with appropriate measures (such as coughing, positioning, suctioning, and liquefying secretions). Promptly administer bronchodilators, mucolytics, and expectorants per protocol as prescribed to dilate bronchioles and remove secretions. Carefully and frequently auscultate chest for quality of breath sounds and adventitious sounds. Note cough and sputum characteristics and document. Provide hydration to liquefy secretions and replace fluids. Fluid intake of at least 3 L per day is important in the supportive treatment of pneumonia. If oral intake cannot be maintained, IV administration of fluids and electrolytes may be necessary for the acutely ill patient. If the patient has heart failure, fluid intake must be individualized.

An intake of at least 1500 calories per day should be maintained to provide energy for the increased metabolic processes in the patient. Small, frequent meals are better tolerated by the dyspneic patient.

Nursing diagnoses and interventions for the patient with pneumonia include but are not limited to the following:

NURSING DIAGNOSES	NURSING INTERVENTIONS
Ineffective breathing pattern, related to inflammatory process and pleuritic pain	Assess ventilation, including evaluation of breathing rate, rhythm, and depth; chest expansion; presence of respiratory distress such as dyspnea, shortness of breath, nasal flaring, pursed-lip breathing, or prolonged expiratory phase; and use of accessory muscles.
	Auscultate lungs for crackles, wheezes, and pleural friction rub.
	Identify contributing factors such as airway clearance or obstruction problem or weakness.
	Encourage increased fluid intake to 3 L/day, unless contraindicated, to liquefy secretions for easier expectoration.
	Maintain patient in position that facilitates ventilation (head of bed in semi-Fowler's position or patient sitting and leaning forward on overbed table).
Impaired gas exchange, related to alveolar-capillary membrane changes secondary to inflammation	Assess patient to identify signs—such as restlessness, disorientation, and irritability—that may indicate body's response to altered blood gas states (hypoxia).
	If necessary and with physician consultation, administer oxygen by nasal cannula or Venturi mask to maintain oxygen saturations above 90%.
	Carefully monitor body temperature, which may fluctuate due to alterations in metabolism or infection.

The nurse should teach the patient and family the following:

- Deep breathing and coughing techniques
- The importance of handwashing to prevent the spread of the disease
- Facts about and the importance of prescribed medications such as antibiotics, including the action, dosage, frequency of administration, and side effects
- Information regarding the specific type of pneumonia the patient has, treatment, anticipated response, possible complications, and probable disease duration
- That a change in health status must be reported to the patient's health care providers (indicators or change may include a change in sputum characteristics or color, decreased activity tolerance, fever despite the antibiotics, increasing chest pain, or a feeling that things are not getting better)
- The importance of consuming large quantities of fluid
- Adaptive exercise and rest techniques
- The availability of streptococcal pneumonia (pneumococcal) vaccine

Prognosis

The disease usually resolves within 2 to 3 weeks with proper treatment. However, pneumonia is the most common cause of death from infectious disease in North America. It is also considered to be the major cause of disease and death in critically ill patients. Despite the use of antibiotics, pneumonia still accounts for 27.7 of every 100,000 deaths.

Bacterial aspiration pneumonia has a poor prognosis even with antibiotic therapy. It may cause extensive lung damage, resulting in lung abscess or empyema. Mortality is 70% with *P. aeruginosa*, 45% with *E. coli*, 35% to 50% with *K. pneumoniae*, and 15% to 50% with *S. aureus*.

PLEURISY
Etiology/Pathophysiology

Pleurisy is an inflammation of the visceral and parietal pleura. Pleurisy can be caused by either a bacterial or viral infection. The underlying physiological change is an inflammation of any portion of the pleura. It may occur spontaneously but more frequently results as a complication of pneumonia, pulmonary infarctions, viral infections of the intercostal muscles, pleural trauma, or early stages of tuberculosis or lung tumor.

Clinical Manifestations

One of the first symptoms of pleurisy may be a sharp inspiratory pain, often radiating to the shoulder or abdomen of the affected side. The pain felt in pleurisy is caused by stretching of the inflamed pleura. If pleural effusion develops, pain subsides and fever and dry cough occur. Other signs and symptoms include dyspnea, cough, and elevated temperature.

Assessment

Collection of **subjective data** is awareness of a patient's complaint of chest pain on inspiration. The patient may also report an elevated temperature.

Collection of **objective data** includes the nurse's assessment of the nature of inspiratory pain, noting its radiation points. The nurse should monitor vital signs, especially temperature, every 2 or 4 hours. Respiratory rate and rhythm should be monitored and documented, noting dyspnea. On auscultation of the lungs, the nurse will hear a pleural friction rub.

Diagnostic Tests

The presence of a pleural friction rub may be considered to be diagnostic. Chest radiographic examination is of limited value in diagnosing pleurisy unless there is the presence of a pleural effusion if fluid accumulates.

Medical Management

The physician may inject an anesthetic block around the vertebra to block the intercostal nerves, thus relieving pain. Prescribed medications may include antibiotics (penicillin) to combat the infection and analgesics (meperidine [Demerol] or morphine) to decrease pain when the patient takes deep breaths and coughs. Antipyretics (Tylenol) are used for fever. Oxygen may be administered.

Nursing Interventions and Patient Teaching

The patient should be positioned comfortably on the affected side to splint the chest, and heat may be applied to the area.

Nursing diagnoses and interventions for the patient with pleurisy include, but are not limited to, the following:

Nursing Diagnoses	Nursing Interventions
Pain, related to stretching of the pulmonary pleura as a result of fluid accumulation	Assess patient's pain level and need for analgesics; administer as needed, documenting effectiveness. Assist with splinting affected side when patient coughs and deep breathes.
Impaired gas exchange, related to pain on inspiration and expiration	Assess patient's level of consciousness, noting any increase in restlessness or disorientation, which may indicate ineffective breathing. Auscultate lungs for wheezes, crackles, and pleural friction rub.

Nursing Diagnoses	Nursing Interventions
	Reposition patient every 2 hours to prevent pooling of secretions and to promote optimal lung expansion. Elevate head of bed to facilitate optimal ventilation.

The patient should be instructed to be alert to signs and symptoms of exacerbation—purulent sputum production, further increase in temperature, and increased pain. The nurse should teach the patient to effectively cough every 2 hours and to splint the affected side.

Prognosis

Prognosis is usually excellent. Complications of atelectasis or secondary infection such as pneumonia may develop.

PLEURAL EFFUSION/EMPYEMA
Etiology/Pathophysiology

Once the pleural lining is inflamed (as in pleurisy), fluid can accumulate in the pleural space. This accumulation of fluid is known as **pleural effusion.** Pleural effusion is rarely a disease by itself but occurs as a secondary problem when the physiological pressure in the lungs and pleurae is disturbed. If the fluid becomes infected, it is called empyema.

The pathophysiology of pleural effusion lies in the alteration of pressure gradients or surface characteristics of capillaries. Empyema may be acute or can become chronic. In acute empyema there is inflammation of the affected area with a thin layer of fluid. If this goes untreated, the fluid thickens and the pleura becomes scarred and fibrosed, losing its elasticity.

Clinical Manifestations

Pleural effusion is generally associated with other disease processes, such as pancreatitis, cirrhosis of the liver, pulmonary edema, congestive heart failure, kidney disease, or carcinoma involving altered capillary permeability. Empyema is usually seen as a result of bacterial infection, as in pneumonia, tuberculosis, or blunt chest trauma. The patient may have a persistent fever in spite of receiving antibiotics.

Assessment

Collection of **subjective data** includes the patient verbalizing complaints of dyspnea and air hunger. The patient may also disclose feelings of fear and anxiety related to decreased levels of oxygen.

Collection of **objective data** in both pleural effusion and empyema includes the nurse's assessment of signs and symptoms of respiratory distress, such as nasal flaring, tachypnea, dyspnea, and decreased breath sounds. Breath sounds and vital signs, especially temperature, should be assessed frequently.

Diagnostic Tests

Effusions or pleural fluid will be evident on chest radiographic examination. Often a thoracentesis (needle inserted into pleural space to aspirate excess fluid) will be done not only to obtain a specimen for culture to identify the causative agent, but to relieve the dyspnea and discomfort.

Medical Management

Usually this condition requires a thoracentesis to remove fluid from the pleural space. A possible danger resulting from this procedure is removing fluid too rapidly; less than 1300 to 1500 mL at one time is recommended.

A chest tube may be inserted for continuous drainage and medication instillation. This tube will be sutured into place and covered with a sterile dressing.

The patient may have a thoracic drainage system in use. To prevent the lung from collapsing, a closed system is used, which maintains the lung cavity's normal negative pressure.

Under normal conditions, intrapleural pressure is below atmospheric pressure (approximately 4 to 5 cm H_2O below atmospheric pressure during expiration and approximately 8 to 10 cm H_2O below atmospheric pressure during inspiration). If intrapleural pressure becomes equal to atmospheric pressure, the lungs will collapse. Chest tubes with attached drainage systems are placed in the pleural cavity to drain fluid, blood, or air from the pleural cavity and to reestablish a negative pressure that will facilitate expansion of the lung, restoring normal intrapleural pressure.

With this procedure one or, more commonly, two thoracotomy tubes are inserted into the pleural space and are attached to a closed-system, water-seal drainage. One catheter is inserted through a stab wound in the anterior chest wall; this is referred to as the **anterior tube.** It is used to remove air from the pleural space. The second tube is inserted through a stab wound in the posterior chest and is referred to as the **posterior tube.** It is primarily for the drainage of serosanguineous fluid or purulent exudate. The posterior (lower) tube may be larger in diameter than the anterior (upper) tube to prevent it from becoming occluded with exudate or clots (Figure 9-11).

When chest tube drainage is initiated, a 2-L clear glass bottle may be used, although other commercial devices (Figure 9-12) are now usually used. Approximately 300 mL of sterile water, or enough to fill the bottle 1 to 2 cm from the bottom, is added so the end of the glass rod is under water to maintain water-seal drainage and prevent air from entering the pleural cavity (Figure 9-13).

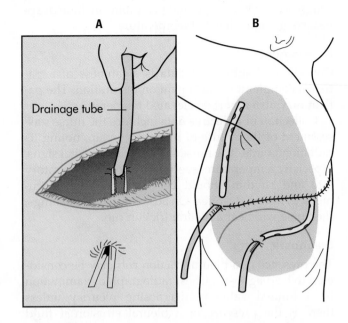

FIGURE 9-11 A, Drainage tube inserted into pleural space. **B,** Note that anterior and posterior tubes are placed well into pleural space.

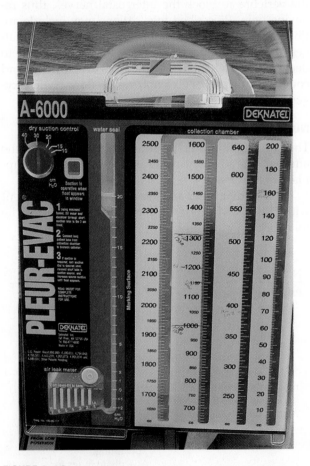

FIGURE 9-12 Pleur-Evac, a disposable, commercial chest drainage system.

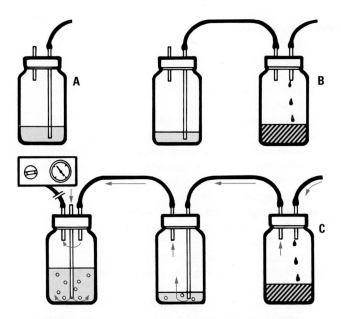

FIGURE **9-13** Water-sealed, closed-chest drainage system. **A,** One-bottle system. **B,** Two-bottle system. **C,** Three-bottle system with suction.

Nursing Interventions and Patient Teaching

General nursing measures include placing the patient on bed rest. The patient may be receiving oxygen therapy; if so, frequent oral care will help prevent drying of mucous membranes. Also, the nurse should encourage effective coughing and deep breathing techniques and respiratory treatments. If the patient has had a thoracentesis, a large sterile dressing will be applied, and the nurse will assess the dressing for drainage, noting the color and amount.

The nurse must ensure that patency of the chest tube system is maintained so that it can drain fluid adequately. Areas of concern for maintaining chest tubes and closed chest drainage bottles are the following:

- **Proper system function:** ensuring that the water in the water-seal chamber fluctuates when suction is applied; there should not be any bubbling in the water seal, because this indicates an air leak.
- **Potential atelectasis resulting from hypoventilation:** assessing for increased dyspnea; checking chest radiographic studies frequently to compare degree of lung consolidation.
- **Increased air in the pleural space:** noting any air leaks in the system; ensuring tubing is secure and remains patent.
- **Complication of infection:** noting an increase in white blood cells, elevated temperature, and presence of purulent drainage.

While the chest tube is in place, the nurse will usually position the patient on the unaffected side to keep the tube from becoming kinked; however, the patient may assume any position of comfort in bed. There is no contraindication to ambulation with a chest tube in

place, as long as the water-seal bottle remains below the level of the chest. Never elevate the drainage system to the level of the patient's chest, because this will cause fluid to drain back into the pleural cavity. The nurse must facilitate coughing and deep-breathing procedures at least every 2 hours and auscultate breath sounds frequently. The nurse will document the amount and characteristics of pleural fluid drainage by marking and documenting the drainage level on the container at the end of each shift. Write date and hour on container so that amount of drainage can easily be determined (Box 9-6). The nurse can usually prevent a chest tube from being accidentally removed by careful attention to securing connections and positioning drainage tubes. The nurse must be diligent to keep tubing as straight as possible and coiled loosely. Do not let the patient lie on it. Tubing should never be placed over the side rails.

The patient will receive antibiotic agents and the nurse should administer them as ordered.

Nursing diagnoses and interventions for the patient with pleural effusion/empyema include but are not limited to the following:

NURSING DIAGNOSES	NURSING INTERVENTIONS
Impaired gas exchange, related to ineffective breathing pattern	Assess for changes in level of consciousness, such as disorientation, restlessness, or irritability, because these may indicate increasing hypoxia as a result of ineffective breathing.
	Monitor ABGs and pulse oximetry.
	Encourage coughing and deep breathing to rid secretions and facilitate lung expansion.
	Reposition patient every 2 hours to prevent pooling of secretions.
	Assess for atelectasis.
Self-care deficit, related to mobility restriction	Assess patient's ability to care for self, and assist when needed.
	Encourage increasing activity level when fever is reduced.

The nurse should explain all procedures before their implementation. The patient should be prepared emotionally for chest tube insertion. The patient and family should be taught about his condition and the healing process. The nurse should instruct the patient on effective coughing and deep-breathing techniques.

Prognosis

The prognosis is variable, depending on the patient's overall health status.

Box 9-6 *Guidelines for Care of Patient with Chest Tubes and Water-Seal Drainage*

1. Keep all tubing as straight as possible and coiled loosely below chest level. Do not let patient lie on it.
2. Keep all connections between chest tubes, drainage tubing, and the drainage collector tight, and tape at connections.
3. Keep the water-seal and suction control chamber at the appropriate water levels by adding sterile water as needed because water loss by evaporation may occur.
4. Mark the time measurement and the fluid level on the drainage chamber according to the prescribed orders. Marking intervals may range from once per hour to every 8 hours. Any change in the quantity or characteristics of drainage (e.g., clear yellow to serosanguineous) should be reported to the physician and recorded. Record output on chart.
5. Observe for air bubbling in the water-seal chamber and fluctuations (tidaling). If no tidaling is observed (rising with inspiration and falling with expiration in the spontaneously breathing patient; the opposite occurs during positive-pressure mechanical ventilation), the drainage system is occluded or the lungs are reexpanded. If bubbling increases, there may be an air leak.
6. Bubbling in the water seal may occur intermittently. When bubbling is continuous and constant, the source of the air leak may be determined by momentarily clamping the tubing at successively distal points away from the patient until the bubbling ceases. Retaping tubing connections or replacing the drainage apparatus may be necessary to correct the air leak.
7. Monitor the patient's clinical status. Vital signs should be taken frequently, lungs auscultated, and the chest wall observed for any abnormal chest movements.
8. Never elevate the drainage system to the level of the patient's chest because this will cause fluid to drain back into the lungs. Secure the drainage system to the metal drainage stand or racks. The drainage chamber should not be emptied unless it is in danger of overflowing.
9. Encourage the patient to breathe deeply periodically to facilitate lung expansion, and encourage range-of-motion exercises to the shoulder on the affected side.
10. Check the position of the chest drainage system. If it is overturned and the water seal is disrupted, return the system to an upright position and encourage the patient to take a few deep breaths, followed by forced exhalations and cough maneuvers.
11. Do not strip or milk chest tubes routinely because this increases pleural pressures.
12. If the drainage system breaks, place the distal end of the chest tubing connection in a sterile water container at a 2-cm level as an emergency water seal.
13. Chest tubes are not clamped routinely. Clamps with rubber protection are kept at the bedside for special procedures such as changing the chest drainage system and assessment before removal of chest tubes.

ATELECTASIS
Etiology/Pathophysiology

Atelectasis (an abnormal condition characterized by the collapse of lung tissue, preventing the respiratory exchange of carbon dioxide and oxygen) occurs from occlusion of air (blockage) to a portion of the lung. Atelectasis is a common postoperative complication resulting from shallow breathing. All or part of the lung collapses, usually as a result of hypoventilation (an abnormal condition of the respiratory system that occurs when the volume of air that enters the alveoli and takes part in gas exchange is not adequate for the metabolic needs of the body), which then leads to bronchial obstruction caused by mucous accumulation. Accumulation of secretions, a foreign body, or a tenacious plug of mucus may completely occlude a bronchus, closing off all air to a portion of the patient's lung. Atelectasis can also be the result of compression of lung tissue caused by emphysema, pneumothorax, or tumor.

The altered physiology depends on the site and degree of occlusion. If the mainstem bronchus is obstructed, there will be severe ventilatory compromise. When a small bronchiole becomes obstructed, as with secretion accumulation, there are fewer signs and symptoms because the respiratory system will try to compensate. However, in either case, atelectasis can lead to stasis pneumonia (because the retained secretions are rich in nutrients for the growth of bacteria) as well as lung damage.

Clinical Manifestations

The patient will display dyspnea, tachypnea (an abnormally rapid rate of breathing), pleural friction rub, restlessness, hypertension, and elevated temperature.

Assessment

Collection of **subjective data** includes the patient complaining of severe shortness of breath (dyspnea) requiring much effort, which results in fatigue. The patient may also verbalize a feeling of air hunger and resulting anxiety.

Collection of **objective data** includes noting decreased breath sounds and crackles on auscultation. The nurse should assess vital signs frequently because hypertension will be present at first, followed by hypotension. Respiration rate and amount of effort required for breathing should be noted. The patient may exhibit altered levels of consciousness caused by hypoxia.

Diagnostic Tests

Serial chest radiographic studies (repeated radiographic examinations of same area done for comparison) will demonstrate atelectatic changes. ABGs will reveal a PaO_2 of less than 80 mm Hg initially; this generally improves within the first 24 hours. Pulse oximetry will reveal oxygen saturation levels below 90%. $PaCO_2$ will be normal or low, because of hypoventilation. A bronchoscopy may reveal a bronchial obstruction.

Medical Management

Ventilation maintenance with intubation is often required. Incentive spirometry 10 times every hour while awake helps provide visual feedback of respiratory effort. Respiratory therapy with oxygen will be ordered. Chest physiotherapy with postural drainage will be administered. The patient may require suctioning. Prescribed medications may include bronchodilators (Proventil) to dilate bronchioles and facilitate secretion removal, antibiotics to prevent infection, and mucolytic agents (acetylcysteine) to reduce viscosity of secretions.

Nursing Interventions and Patient Teaching

Postoperatively, patients should be reminded to cough, deep breathe, and change positions every 1 to 2 hours. Effective coughing is essential in mobilizing secretions. If secretions are present in the respiratory passages, deep breathing often will move them up to stimulate the cough reflex and then they can be expectorated. Administer analgesia to relieve pain and facilitate ventilatory effort. Provide emotional support. Early ambulation is encouraged. Nursing diagnoses and interventions for the patient with atelectasis include but are not limited to the following:

NURSING DIAGNOSES	NURSING INTERVENTIONS
Ineffective airway clearance, related to inability to clear secretions	Assess patient's ability to move secretions, and assist if needed. Encourage use of incentive spirometer 10 times every hour while awake Encourage adequate hydration to liquefy secretions. Auscultate breath sounds frequently, documenting and reporting any changes. Assess color, consistency, and amount of secretions removed via either coughing or suction.
Ineffective coping, related to invasive medical regimen	Assess the patient's ability to comply with the prescribed regimen and to cooperate with caregivers. Identify patient's emotional support systems.

The nurse should instruct the patient on proper techniques for effective coughing and deep breathing, as well as other measures to facilitate optimal air exchange, such as increasing movement and changing position. Medication teaching should address the rationale for prescribed medications, as well as side effects.

Prognosis

Prognosis is dependent upon age and preexisting illness of the patient.

PNEUMOTHORAX
Etiology/Pathophysiology

Pneumothorax is a collection of air or gas in the pleural space, causing the lung to collapse. It can be secondary to a ruptured bleb on the lung surface (as in emphysema) or a severe coughing episode. It can be caused by a penetrating chest injury in which the pleural lining is punctured, fractured ribs, or injury to the pleura from insertion of a subclavian catheter, or a spontaneous pneumothorax can occur suddenly without an apparent cause (Figure 9-14).

When the pleural space is penetrated, air enters, thus interrupting the normal negative pressure. Consequently the lung cannot remain fully inflated.

Clinical Manifestations

The patient may present with a recent chest injury. There will be decreased breath sounds on the affected side and a sudden, sharp, pleuritic chest pain with dyspnea. The patient may be diaphoretic and exhibit an increased heart rate, tachypnea, and dyspnea. There will be a cessation of normal chest movements on the affected side. With a pneumothorax resulting from penetrating injury, there will be a sucking sound heard on inspiration.

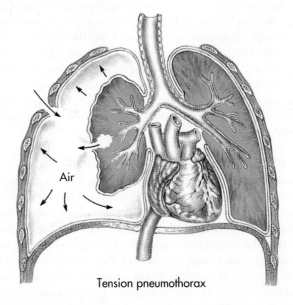

Air

Tension pneumothorax

FIGURE 9-14 Pneumothorax (complete collapse of the right lung).

As intrathoracic pressure increases in the pleural space, the lung collapses. Because lung tissue no longer expands, the mediastinum may shift to the unaffected side (mediastinal shift), which is subsequently compressed. As the intrathoracic pressure increases, cardiac output is altered because there is decreased venous return and compression of the great vessels.

Assessment

Collection of **subjective data** may include reporting a recent penetrating chest injury or severe coughing episode. The patient may also complain of shortness of breath of sudden onset and may indicate feelings of anxiety associated with air hunger.

Collection of **objective data** involves a nursing assessment that includes frequent vital signs, noting any change in respiratory and cardiac rate and rhythm. On auscultation the nurse will note bilaterally unequal breath sounds, diminished on the affected side. Color, characteristics, and amount of sputum should be noted.

Diagnostic Tests

Important findings to aid in diagnosis will come from the patient's history. For example, the patient may report a recent chest injury or a precipitating respiratory condition, such as COPD. Chest radiographic examination shows the presence of pneumothorax. ABGs will show a decrease in pH and PaO_2, with an increased $PaCO_2$.

Medical Management

Surgery may be done to insert a chest tube (thoracotomy). The chest tube is inserted in the fifth and sixth intercostal spaces at the midaxillary line. The chest tube is attached to a water-seal drainage system. Intermittent positive pressure may be administered.

Another approach to correcting a pneumothorax is the use of a Heimlich valve, which is typically used as a stopgap measure until chest tube therapy can be started. The valve attaches to a chest tube and is inserted into the chest. As the patient exhales, air and fluid drain through the valve into a plastic bag. When the patient inhales, however, the flexible tubing in the valve collapses, preventing secretions and air from reentering the pleura.

Nursing Interventions and Patient Teaching

General measures include maintaining airway patency and providing adequate oxygenation. The nurse will need to assess and document patency of the chest tube system, keeping it free from kinks. If a chest tube is inserted, the nurse must note the color and amount of drainage and assess integrity of the drainage system. The nurse will monitor blood pressure and place the patient in high Fowler's position to promote airway clearance and lung expansion. Pain may be controlled

by administering appropriate analgesics, but the use of respiratory depressants is avoided.

Nursing diagnoses and interventions for the patient with pneumothorax include but are not limited to the following:

NURSING DIAGNOSES	NURSING INTERVENTIONS
Ineffective breathing pattern, related to nonfunctioning lung	Assess respiratory rate and rhythm, and note any signs of respiratory distress, such as dyspnea, use of accessory muscles, nasal flaring, and anxiety.
	Provide chest tube care, maintaining secure placement.
	Facilitate ventilation by elevating head of bed, and administer oxygen as ordered.
	Suction as needed to remove secretions.
	Encourage adaptive breathing techniques to decrease respiratory effort.
	Encourage rest periods interspersed with activities.
Fear, related to feeling of air hunger	Assess patient's feelings of fear related to health concerns and feeling of air hunger.
	Identify positive coping methods, and support their use.
	Determine support systems available to patient.

The nurse should explain the rationale for treatments—oxygen therapy and chest tube drainage—before their implementation. Effective breathing techniques and the need for ongoing medical care should be reinforced. The nurse should instruct the patient to limit exposure to people who may have infections, such as upper respiratory infection or influenza. The patient is advised not to smoke but to drink fluids copiously, to avoid fatigue and strenuous activity, and to report any signs and symptoms of recurrence (e.g., chest pain, difficulty breathing, or fever) to the physician.

Prognosis

The lung will usually reexpand within several days. The chest tube is removed by the physician when a chest radiograph shows that the lungs are completely expanded.

LUNG CANCER
Etiology/Pathophysiology

The incidence of lung cancer has been steadily increasing during the past 50 years in both men and women. In 1987, cancer of the lung surpassed breast cancer to become the number one cancer killer of women. Thus lung cancer is now the leading cause of death from cancer in both men and women. Lung cancer causes 34% of cancer deaths in men. The American Cancer Society predicts that in 2003 about 171,900 Americans will be diagnosed with lung cancer and 157,200 will die of this devastating disease; 72% of people have regional or distant metastases at diagnosis. Tumors may result from metastasis anywhere in the body or may appear as primary tumors. Metastasis from the colon and kidney is common. Metastasis to the lung may be discovered before the primary lesion is known, and sometimes the location of the primary lesion is not determined during the person's life. It has been linked primarily with cigarette smoking. A history of smoking, especially for 20 years or more, is considered to be a prime risk factor. The more cigarettes someone smokes each day, the higher the risk.

Approximately 80% to 90% of lung tumors are linked to cigarette smoking. "Passive smoking" (breathing in sidestream smoke) is qualitatively similar to mainstream smoking; involuntary (secondhand) smoking poses a risk for the development of lung cancer in nonsmokers. Occupational exposures, such as asbestos, radon, and uranium are also risk factors. It is suspected that air pollutants may increase risk.

The mortality of people with lung cancer depends primarily on the specific type of cancer and the size of the tumor when detected.

Lung cancer is classified by microscopic study of the tumor. Treatment is based on the type and extent of the disease, using two major classifications. Small cell lung cancer (SCLC) is very aggressive and occurs in approximately 20% of patients with lung cancer; non–small cell lung cancer (NSCLC), including adenocarcinoma, accounts for 30% to 32% of lung cancer, squamous cell carcinoma accounts for 30% of lung cancers, and large cell carcinoma occurs in about 9% of cases.

Most people who develop the disease are older than 50 years of age.

Clinical Manifestations

Lung cancer is insidious because it is usually asymptomatic in the early stages. If the lesion is located peripherally, there are few symptoms and it may not be discovered until visualized on a routine chest radiographic examination. If the peripheral lesion perforates the pleural space, a pleural effusion will result and severe pain will occur. Central lesions originate from a larger branch of the bronchial tree. These lesions cause obstruction and erosion of the bronchus. Signs and symptoms are cough, hemoptysis, dyspnea, fever, and chills. Auscultation may reveal wheezing on the affected side as well. Phrenic nerve involvement causes paralysis of the diaphragm.

As the disease progresses, metastasis may occur, along with weight loss, fatigue, decreased stamina, and changes in functional status. Pain is unlikely unless the tumor is pressing on a nerve or the cancer has spread to the bones. Primary lung tumors usually metastasize to the liver or to nearby structures, such as the esophagus, heart pericardium, skeletal bone, and brain.

Assessment

Collection of **subjective data** includes the patient's complaints of a chronic cough and of hoarseness. The patient may also report weight loss and extreme fatigue. The nurse should interview the patient regarding a family history, especially a history of cigarette smoking and of exposure to occupational irritants.

Collection of **objective data** includes assessing the cough, noting color (especially blood streaked) and consistency of sputum, as well as frequency, duration, and precipitating factors. Also the nurse should assess the characteristics of the cough (moist, dry, hacking) and effect of body position and should identify with the patient what, if anything, helps to relieve the cough. The lungs should be auscultated to determine if unilateral wheezing or crackles are present. Invasion of the superior vena cava causes edema of the neck and face and is called **superior vena cava syndrome.**

Diagnostic Tests

Chest radiographic studies and CT scan of the chest are used to identify the location and size of the tumor. MRI may be used along with or instead of CT scans. Positron emission tomography (PET), a newer diagnostic tool, may become the standard imaging study to detect lung cancer once enough data are accumulated to confirm its efficacy. When the lesion is on the lung periphery, the physician can obtain specimens via percutaneous fine needle aspiration guided by fluoroscopy or CT. Bronchoscopy with biopsy or brushings for cytologic findings will indicate the presence of malignant cells. Sputum cytology can identify malignant cells, but results are positive in only 20% to 30% of lung cancer cases. A mediastinoscopy may be done to determine whether spread of the tumor to the lymph nodes has occurred. Scalene lymph node biopsy is also done to determine metastasis. This biopsy is performed in the supraclavicular area.

Medical Management

The treatment of lung cancer depends on the type and stage of lung cancer. Unfortunately, most patients are not diagnosed early enough for curative surgical intervention. It is estimated that one third of the patients are inoperable when first seen, and one third are found to be inoperable on exploratory thoracotomy. Of the third who are operable, the surgical mortality is 10% for pneumonectomy and 2% to 3% for lobectomy. A pneumonectomy is the most common surgical treatment. This consists of removing the entire lung. Because there is no lung left to require reexpansion, drainage tubes are usually not necessary. The fluid remaining in that area will consolidate eventually, which will help prevent a mediastinal shift. A lobectomy is performed when one lobe is involved rather than the entire lung. If only a portion of a lobe of a lung is involved, a segmental resection is done. Both a lobectomy and segmental resection require chest tube insertion with water-seal drainage to facilitate lung reexpansion (see Figures 9-12 and 9-13). Video-assisted thoracoscopic surgery allows surgeons to remove tumors through a small keyhole incision in the chest cavity. Radiation therapy and chemotherapy are often done in conjunction with surgery to enhance recovery for NSCLC. An oral drug called gefitinib (IRESSA) has been approved for NSCLC as a monotherapy in patients with locally advanced or metastatic NSCLC after failure of first-line treatment with both platinum-based and docetaxel chemotherapies (*Nursing*, 2004) (Home Health Considerations box). In SCLC, chemotherapy alone or combined with radiation has largely replaced surgery as a treatment of choice because regardless of staging, SCLC is considered to be metastatic at diagnosis. A large percentage of these patients experience remission; in a few cases the remission has been long lasting. At present about one third of the patients who have surgery experience tumor spread.

Among the promising biologic response modifiers are interferon-α, interleukin-2, interleukin-4, tumor necrosis factor, and monoclonal antibodies. The last are being investigated alone and in combination with radioisotopes, toxins, and standard chemotherapeutic drugs to see if they can identify and destroy cancer cells with specific antigens (Dest, 2000).

Nursing Interventions and Patient Teaching

Whether treatment offers comfort or cure, the patient needs comprehensive nursing interventions. From patient education to symptom management to emotional support, the nursing interventions can improve the quality of life and help the patient and family cope with a frightening diagnosis. Nursing intervention is often directed at postsurgical interventions, including facilitating recovery and preventing complications by promoting effective airway clearance through frequent repositioning, coughing, and deep breathing. Encourage use of incentive spirometry. Explain the importance of changing position (to prevent atelectasis) and exercising the legs and feet (to prevent deep vein thrombosis [DVT]). Administer supplemental oxygen and monitor oxygen saturation levels. If a patient has chest tubes to H_2O, seal drainage, assess for patency, and record the amount, color, and consistency of drainage. Carefully assess lung sounds and record findings. The nurse will assess vital signs frequently. After routine postoperative vital signs check, the patient will be checked every 2 hours to ascertain stability; as progress is made, the patient will be checked every 4 hours.

Prescribed medications are primarily antineoplastic agents to prevent or reduce tumor growth. Medications will be given also for symptomatic relief: opioid analgesics for pain control, antipyretics for fever, and antiemetics for nausea.

Nursing diagnoses and interventions for the patient with lung cancer include but are not limited to the following:

🏠 Home Health Considerations

Lung Cancer

- If the patient with lung cancer smokes, teach her or him that stopping smoking can improve pulmonary function, minimize postoperative complications, decrease the risk of pneumonia, and improve appetite during treatment.
- The patient who has had a surgical resection of the lung with intent to cure should be followed up carefully after discharge for manifestations of metastasis.
- The patient and family should be told to contact the physician if symptoms such as hemoptysis, dysphagia, chest pain, and hoarseness develop.
- For many individuals who have lung cancer, little can be done to significantly prolong their lives.
- Many people with lung cancer require palliative and hospice care. Encourage the patient and her or his family to adjust their expectation and adapt their goals from controlling disease to improving symptom relief.
- Radiation therapy and chemotherapy can be used to provide palliative relief from distressing symptoms.
- Constant pain becomes a major problem. Measures used to relieve pain must be achieved.

NURSING DIAGNOSES	NURSING INTERVENTIONS
Ineffective airway clearance, related to lung surgery	Facilitate optimal breathing by placing patient in a sitting position. Assist with position changes frequently. Promote coughing and deep breathing, providing necessary splinting. Encourage early ambulation to mobilize secretions. Encourage incentive spirometer.
Fear, related to cancer, treatment, and prognosis	Monitor changes in communication patterns with others. Monitor expressions, such as worthlessness, anxiety, powerlessness, abandonment, or exhaustion. Listen and accept expressions of anger without personalizing reaction.

NURSING DIAGNOSES	NURSING INTERVENTIONS
	Encourage patient to identify problem, redefine situation, obtain needed information, generate alternatives, and focus on solutions.

The nurse should teach the patient effective coughing techniques. The patient and family should be instructed regarding nutritional needs and importance of maintaining physical mobility. If the patient smokes, encourage quitting and encourage family members to stop also. Encourage eating a diet high in protein and calories. The nurse should also instruct the patient and family regarding signs and symptoms that could indicate recurrence of metastasis, such as fatigue, weight loss, increased coughing or hemoptysis, central nervous system changes, and arm or shoulder pain. Identify resources in the community, such as the American Cancer Society and the American Lung Association, that can assist the patient and family with information, support groups, and equipment needed.

Prognosis
Only 10% to 15% of lung cancer patients live 5 years or longer after diagnosis. The survival rate is 40% for cases detected in a localized stage; only 20% of lung cancers are discovered that early.

PULMONARY EDEMA
Etiology/Pathophysiology
Pulmonary edema is an accumulation of serous fluid in interstitial lung tissue and alveoli resulting from:
- Severe left ventricular failure resulting from a weakened myocardium due to a myocardial infarction
- Inhalation of irritating gases
- Rapid administration of intravenous fluids (whole blood, plasma, or fluids)
- Barbiturate or opiate overdose

Cardiogenic pulmonary edema usually accompanies underlying cardiac disease in which the failure of the left ventricle causes pooling of fluid to back up into the left atrium and into pulmonary veins and capillaries. The most common cause of pulmonary edema is increased capillary pressure from left ventricular failure.

As the pulmonary capillary pressure exceeds the intravascular pressure, serous fluid is rapidly forced into the alveoli. Fluid rapidly reaches the bronchioles and bronchi, and patients literally begin to drown in their own secretions. As oxygen decreases, the person shows signs of severe respiratory distress.

Pulmonary edema is acute and extensive and may lead to death unless treated rapidly.

Clinical Manifestations
The primary signs and symptoms of pulmonary edema are dyspnea and related breathing disturbances. Labored respirations; tachypnea; tachycardia; cyanosis; and, especially, pink (or blood-tinged), frothy sputum are the most obvious signs. The patient may also exhibit restlessness or agitation because of the altered tissue perfusion and resulting hypoxia and respiratory failure.

Assessment
Collection of **subjective data** includes noting the patient's complaints of severe dyspnea and a feeling of impending death.

Collection of **objective data** involves the nurse assessing for signs of respiratory distress. Such signs include nasal flaring and sternal retractions with inspiration, as well as rapid, stertorous respirations; hypertension; tachycardia; restlessness; and disorientation. On auscultation the nurse will most likely hear wheezing and crackles. On physical examination the nurse will often note a sudden weight gain caused by fluid retention; decreased urinary output as a result of retained fluid in the pulmonary vasculature; and a productive cough of frothy, pink sputum.

Diagnostic Tests
Chest radiographic examination will reveal fluid infiltrates, indicating alveolar edema, increased pleural space fluid (pleural effusion), and enlarged heart (cardiomegaly). ABGs are altered, with varying PaO_2 and $PaCO_2$ levels. There may be respiratory alkalosis or acidosis. Sputum cultures are done periodically to rule out a bronchopulmonary infection.

Medical Management
The physician will order oxygen therapy and may intubate the patient for adequate ventilation support. Medications will include diuretics to reduce alveolar and systemic edema by increasing urinary output (furosemide [Lasix]) and an opioid analgesic, usually morphine sulfate, to decrease respiratory rate, lower the patient's anxiety level, reduce venous return, and dilate both the pulmonary and systemic blood vessels thus improving the exchange of gases. IV nitroprusside (Nipride) is a potent vasodilator that improves myocardial contraction and reduces pulmonary congestion. Because of its potent effects on the vascular system, it is the drug of choice for the patient with pulmonary edema. Medications such as cardiotonic glycosides (digoxin [Lanoxin]), will be used to treat underlying causative conditions.

Nursing Interventions and Patient Teaching
An important nursing measure is accurate assessment and documentation to identify changes in the patient's condition. This includes assessment of respiratory sta-

tus and frequent monitoring of I&O, vital signs, ABGs, pulse oximetry, and electrolyte values. The nurse maintains oxygenation therapy as ordered—commonly delivered by Venturi mask at 40% to 70% concentration. Mechanical ventilation may be required; in this case the intubated patient needs oral care and tracheostomy care according to protocol. Optimal air exchange must be facilitated by maintaining the patient in high Fowler's position. A patent IV line must be maintained, usually at a very slow rate to keep the vein open for medication administration (i.e., 30 mL/hour) per infusion pump. This prevents adding even more fluid to the overloaded patient. The patient requires extremely close monitoring of cardiac status and accurate measuring and recording of I&O.

Nursing diagnoses and interventions for the patient with pulmonary edema include but are not limited to the following:

Nursing Diagnoses	Nursing Interventions
Impaired gas exchange, related to excess fluid in pulmonary vessels interfering with oxygen diffusion	Be alert to any signs indicating altered ventilation, such as restlessness, irritability, disorientation, or apprehension. Monitor ABGs and notify physician of any change. Monitor vital signs frequently, including cardiac rhythm. Administer oxygen therapy as ordered and document patient response. Administer diuretics, bronchodilators, morphine sulfate, cardiotonic glycosides, and other medications as ordered.
Excess fluid volume, related to altered tissue permeability	Assess indicators of patient's fluid volume status, such as breath sounds and skin turgor. Monitor I&O accurately. Monitor electrolyte values closely, and notify physician of alterations. Administer diuretics as ordered, and note patient response. Weigh patient daily on same scale at same time of day with same amount of bed linen and patient clothing. Provide low-sodium diet to prevent excess fluid retention.

The patient should be taught effective breathing techniques. Medication teaching regarding actions, side effects, and dosage of prescribed medications should be given to the patient and family. The patient and family should be instructed on a low-sodium diet and referred to the dietitian for follow-up. The nurse should emphasize to the patient and family the signs and symptoms to observe that would indicate alteration in health, such as productive cough (noting the color and characteristics of sputum), activity intolerance, or the presence of dyspnea.

Prognosis

The prognosis for acute pulmonary edema is guarded and may lead to death unless treated rapidly.

PULMONARY EMBOLUS
Etiology/Pathophysiology

The most common pulmonary perfusion abnormality, pulmonary embolism (PE), is caused by the passage of a foreign substance (blood clot, fat, air, or amniotic fluid) into the pulmonary artery or its branches, with resulting obstruction of the blood supply to lung tissue and subsequent collapse. PE usually occurs in patients identified to be at risk, such as the following:

- Those with prior thrombophlebitis
- Those who have recently had surgery, been pregnant, or given birth
- Women who are taking contraceptives on a long-term basis
- Those with a history of congestive heart failure, obesity, or immobilization from fracture; immobilization appears to be a key consideration

Venous stasis, venous wall injury, and increased coagulability of blood cause the formation of a venous thrombus. The thrombus (usually in the deep veins of the lower extremities) dislodges and travels through the venous circulation; it passes through the right side of the heart and enters the pulmonary artery, where it becomes lodged.

Once an embolus obstructs pulmonary blood flow, a ventilation/perfusion (V/Q) mismatch develops: an area of lung is ventilated but not perfused. The obstruction hinders oxygenation of the blood. Atelectasis develops, and pulmonary vascular resistance increases. As a result of this, arterial hypoxia develops.

Clinical Manifestations

A pulmonary embolus may manifest itself by a sudden, sharp, constant, nonradiating, pleuritic chest pain that worsens with inspiration. Because PE impairs gas exchange, there is acute, unexplained dyspnea. The respiratory rate will be rapid. In small areas of infarction, presenting signs and symptoms are a small amount of hemoptysis, pleuritic chest pain, elevated temperature, and increased white blood cell count. In large areas of infarction, symptoms include hypoxia, hemoptysis, hypotension, diaphoresis, and tachypnea. Regional bronchoconstriction, atelectasis, and pulmonary edema develop, along with decreased surfactant production. Lung sounds will be diminished, and wheezes may be present.

Assessment

Collection of **subjective data** includes noting the patient's report of presence and degree of dyspnea and chest pain. Nursing assessment will also include identifying the presence of associated risk factors.

Collection of **objective data** involves the nurse assessing for pleuritic pain and noting the nature of the patient's cough. Further assessment includes breath sounds, vital signs, and being alert for tachycardia and tachypnea. On auscultation the nurse will note any crackles, decreased breath sounds over the affected area, and the presence of a pleural friction rub. In assessing the psychological response of the patient, the nurse will document the presence and degree of anxiety, which is often correlated to air hunger.

Diagnostic Tests

ABGs will be significantly altered, depicting hypoxia. The pH remains normal unless respiratory alkalosis develops early from hyperventilation as respiratory drive diminishes. Respiratory acidosis with hypoxemia often follows.

Initially, the chest radiograph is normal. After 24 hours the radiograph may reveal small infiltrates secondary to atelectasis. Chest radiographic examination will also show an enlarged main pulmonary artery. In most cases of PE, the chest radiograph is normal and is useful only to rule out pulmonary edema or pneumothorax.

A helical, also called spiral CT, scan of the lung to visualize the pulmonary vasculature will be ordered. This new type of noninvasive scan can be performed in a few seconds and is replacing the V/Q scan, although the V/Q scan is still used in smaller facilities where a spiral CT may not be available. If the V/Q scan result is intermediate or low probability but the physician still suspects a PE based on the patient's signs and symptoms and risk factors, he may order a pulmonary angiogram (Lazzara, 2001).

Pulmonary arteriogram is the "gold standard" for detecting PE because it provides direct anatomical view of the pulmonary vessels to assess perfusion defects. ABG analysis is important. A D-dimer serum test is drawn. D-dimer is a product of fibrin degration (change to a less complex form). When a thrombus or embolus is present, plasma D-dimer concentrations are usually greater than 1591 ng/mL. The normal range for D-dimer is 68 to 494 ng/L. In the event that the D-dimer levels are elevated, a venous Doppler study or duplex scanning is indicated to look for a DVT.

Positive results from venous ultrasound are helpful in diagnosing DVT.

Medical Management

When there are multiple pulmonary emboli present, an umbrella filter may be placed in the inferior vena cava to retain the emboli, preventing their migration to other parts of the body.

The physician will prescribe anticoagulant therapy, for example, oral Coumadin or subcutaneous low-molecular-weight heparin (enoxaparin sodium [Lovenox]) or dalteparin (Fragmin), to prevent clot formation. Initially heparin will be administered intravenously, by way of either continuous infusion on a pump or intermittent boluses.

Heparin doesn't dissolve an existing thrombus; its role is to keep it from enlarging and to prevent more thrombi from forming while the body's natural fibrinolytic mechanism lyses (destruction of red blood cells) the existing clot. The effectiveness of heparin is determined by monitoring PTT values, which should be maintained at $1\frac{1}{2}$ to 2 times the control (or normal) values. In the event of overheparinization resulting in profound bleeding, the treatment is intravenous administration of protamine sulfate. Heparin therapy is gradually tapered (it may take several days). Oral anticoagulation (warfarin [Coumadin]) is initiated. The patient will take warfarin for up to 1 year. Effectiveness of warfarin therapy is determined by monitoring PT and INR values; with the goal being $1\frac{1}{4}$ to $1\frac{1}{5}$ times the control (or normal) values. Vitamin K reverses the effects of warfarin. Fresh frozen plasma may be required in cases of severe bleeding.

A massive PE must be dissolved using thrombolytics such as tissue plasminogen activator (tPA) or streptokinase (Streptase).

Nursing Interventions and Patient Teaching

General nursing interventions include applying thromboembolic disease (TED) stockings and elevating the lower extremities. The nurse should check peripheral pulses and frequently measure bilateral calf circumference to check for occlusion caused by a clot. The head of the bed may be slightly elevated, and oxygen will be administered by mask or nasal cannula to facilitate optimal gas exchange. The patient will promote lung expansion by coughing and deep breathing.

Related nursing interventions will include assessing for signs of bleeding: epistaxis, hemoptysis, bleeding from gums or rectum, and ecchymosis. Other general nursing interventions will include keeping the patient adequately hydrated, placing the patient on bed rest for the first few days, and gradually increasing activity.

Nursing diagnoses and interventions for the patient with pulmonary embolus include but are not limited to the following.

Nursing Diagnoses	Nursing Interventions
Impaired gas exchange, related to alteration in pulmonary vasculature	Assess sensorium and vital signs every 2 hours or as needed, noting any changes indicative of altered oxygenation/ventilation. Elevate head of bed 30 degrees to improve ventilation. Administer oxygen as ordered. Monitor ABGs frequently, reporting any increase or decrease of $PaCO_2$ and PaO_2 of more than 10 mm Hg.
Ineffective protection, related to risk of prolonged bleeding or hemorrhage secondary to anticoagulation therapy	Monitor vital signs for indicators of profuse bleeding or hemorrhage resulting from anticoagulant therapy: hypotension, tachycardia, and tachypnea. At least once a shift, check stool, urine, sputum, and vomitus for occult blood using agency-approved method for testing per protocol. At least once a shift, inspect wounds, oral mucous membranes, any entry site of an invasive procedure, and nares for evidence of bleeding. To prevent hematoma formation, avoid giving IM injection unless it is unavoidable. Teach patient the necessity of using sponge-tipped applicators and mouthwash for oral care to minimize the risk of gum bleeding. Instruct patient to shave with an electric rather than a bladed razor.

Medication teaching is a major nursing concern. Oral anticoagulation often becomes a lifelong regimen that bears close monitoring, so the nurse must assess the patient's present knowledge base and expand on it. Preventive measures are also important, especially in the postoperative period. The nurse should teach the patient techniques to reduce venous pooling (which could precipitate thrombophlebitis), such as position changes and wearing nonrestrictive clothing. The patient must be told to avoid crossing the legs while in a sitting or lying position and also to avoid standing in one place for a prolonged period, because these activities increase venous pooling. The nurse should teach the rationale and application procedure for TED hose. Explain that the patient should put them on in the morning before getting out of bed. The patient and family should be instructed on signs and symptoms of

pulmonary embolism to report to the physician, such as chest pain and dyspnea. Blood-tinged sputum or blood in the urine, which could result from anticoagulant therapy, should also be reported.

Prognosis

Early diagnosis and appropriate treatment reduce mortality to 5%. Untreated PE carries a 30% mortality rate. Although most pulmonary emboli resolve completely and leave no residual deficits, some patients may be left with chronic pulmonary hypertension.

ADULT RESPIRATORY DISTRESS SYNDROME (ARDS)
Etiology/Pathophysiology

ARDS is not a disease but a complication that occurs as a result of other disease processes. There are many causes of ARDS, which results from either a direct or indirect pulmonary injury. Possible causes include viral or bacterial pneumonia, chest trauma, aspiration, inhalation injury, near drowning, fat emboli, sepsis, or any type of shock. Drug overdoses, renal failure, and pancreatitis are also known to be causative factors, as well as COPD, neuromuscular defects with Guillain-Barré syndrome, and myasthenia gravis. Among these, sepsis is the most common precursor of ARDS.

Regardless of the cause of ARDS, there is a certain sequela of events in the body's response that remains the same. The surface of the alveolar capillary membrane becomes altered, causing increased permeability, which then allows fluid to leak into the interstitial spaces and alveoli. This creates pulmonary edema and hypoxia. The alveoli lose their elasticity and collapse, which causes the blood to be shunted through the impaired alveoli, hence interfering with oxygen transport. The damaged capillaries allow plasma and red blood cells to leak out, resulting in hemorrhage. ARDS is characterized by pulmonary artery hypertension, which results from vasoconstriction.

Clinical Manifestations

ARDS manifests itself in 12 to 24 hours after injury, resulting in lung tissue damage or hypovolemic shock; 5 to 10 days after sepsis development, the patient will experience respiratory distress with altered breath sounds. There may be altered sensorium as a result of an elevated $PaCO_2$ and decreased PaO_2. Additional signs will be cardiovascular in nature: tachycardia, hypotension, and decreased urinary output.

Assessment

Collection of **subjective data** involves a nursing assessment that will include background information and a history of the present illness (obtained from family members, because the patient is usually too ill to give details).

Collection of **objective data** involves the nurse being an astute observer of any change in the patient's condition, no matter how small or gradual. The nurse must make an accurate and thorough initial assessment so such changes will be quickly recognized. Initial assessment includes identifying and documenting respiratory rate, rhythm, and effort. Signs of dyspnea should be noted, such as nasal flaring, sternal and subclavicular retractions, or cyanosis. The nurse should auscultate the lungs and document the presence of crackles or wheezing and should maintain close observation of vital signs. Frequent assessment of the level of consciousness, with particular attention to increased restlessness or lethargy, is necessary.

Diagnostic Tests

Pulmonary function tests will be done to determine the ease or difficulty of oxygen in crossing the alveolar capillary membrane. ABGs will show definitive changes: the PaO_2 will be decreased (less than 70 mm Hg), the $PaCO_2$ will be increased (greater than 35 mm Hg), and the bicarbonate ion will be decreased (less than 22 mEq/L). Initially, HCO_3^- increases in an attempt to buffer the elevated $PaCO_2$ level, thereby maintaining pH in the normal range. The pH will be elevated initially but will steadily decrease as the patient's condition deteriorates. A chest radiographic examination will depict thickened bronchial margins and possibly diffuse infiltrates.

Medical Management

The medical plan focuses on supportive treatment by maintaining adequate oxygenation and treating the cause—drug overdose, infections, or inhaled toxins. Medications commonly used to treat associated conditions include corticosteroids and diuretics to treat pulmonary edema, aiding in restoring lung tissues to their normal structure and function. Morphine sulfate is commonly given to sedate restless patients and decrease respiratory rate. When the patient is intubated and ventilator dependent, a neurological blocking agent, such as pancuronium (Pavulon), may be administered to suppress the patient's own respiratory effort, relying on the controlled ventilator assistance.

Other medications may include cardiotonic glycosides (digoxin) to enhance cardiac function and antibiotic agents to prevent the complication of infection.

An experimental treatment is being used in which nitric oxide gas is inhaled, causing local vasodilatation and maximizing perfusion in ventilated areas of the lungs and often significantly improving oxygenation. Nitric oxide is usually administered via a face mask; if the patient is ventilator dependent, however, the ventilator is the mode of delivery.

Nursing Interventions and Patient Teaching

The goal of nursing interventions is to provide adequate oxygenation and ventilation and to treat the multisystem responses caused by ARDS. Nursing intervention includes knowledge of mechanical ventilator settings and effects. Nursing intervention correlated to this is pertinent to intubated patients, such as suctioning, providing oral care, and assessing for signs of inadequate ventilation. ABGs as well as pulse oximetry should be monitored closely and any changes reported.

Current studies are being done that suggest some people with ARDS demonstrate a marked improvement in PaO_2 when turned from the supine to prone position. Not all patients respond to prone positioning. Prone positioning is typically reserved for patients with refractory hypoxemia who do not respond to other strategies to increase PaO_2 (Balas, 2000).

Also, an accurate, ongoing assessment of cardiac function is important. The nurse should be alert for and document any rate or rhythm changes. The RN will notify the physician of any changes.

The nurse should assess vital signs and identify the presence of an elevated temperature so that cultures can be obtained to treat infections.

Nursing diagnoses and interventions for the patient with ARDS include but are not limited to the following:

NURSING DIAGNOSES	NURSING INTERVENTIONS
Impaired gas exchange, related to tachypnea	Monitor ABGs and report any changes.
	Address any factors that would contribute to restlessness and anxiety, because they increase the body's oxygen demand and will exacerbate the patient's already serious condition.
	Administer oxygen per order, assessing and recording patient response.
	Monitor electrocardiogram changes.
	Report any changes in vital signs and any change in patient's level of response, no matter how small or gradual.
Ineffective breathing pattern, related to respiratory distress	Assess respiratory rate, rhythm, and effort, being alert to signs of dyspnea.
	Facilitate optimal ventilation by proper positioning.
	Maintain airway patency by encouraging frequent coughing and deep breathing if able, or suctioning as needed.

The nurse should teach the patient effective breathing techniques, emphasizing the importance of frequent position changes and coughing and deep breathing. If the patient is intubated, the nurse should explain all procedures before their implementation and should explain the importance of working with the ventilator and not trying to breathe independently.

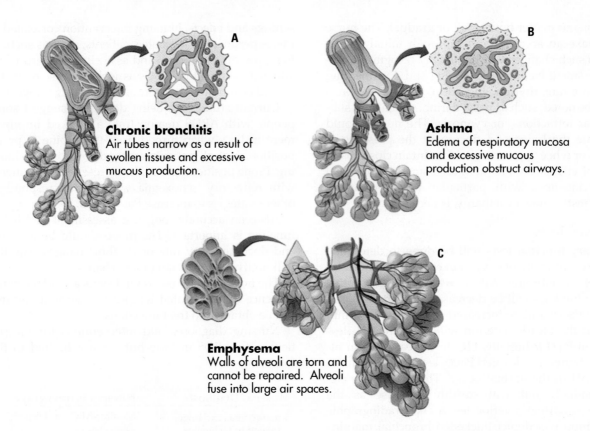

FIGURE **9-15** Disorders of the airways in patients with chronic bronchitis, asthma, and emphysema. **A,** Chronic bronchitis. Excessive amounts of mucus accumulate in the airways, obstructing airflow and impairing ciliary function. **B,** Asthma. Bronchial smooth muscle constricts in response to irritants, resulting in airflow obstruction and wheezing. **C,** Emphysema. Proteolytic enzymes destroy lung tissue, resulting in enlarged air sacs and impaired gas exchange.

The patient should be reassured that the ventilator will breathe for him and that those breaths will be more effective than his own. The nurse should explain to the patient and family the importance of using rest and activity appropriately. Explanations of the purpose and side effects of all medications should be offered.

Prognosis
ARDS affects an estimated 150,000 to 200,000 people each year, with mortality rates of 40% with severe ARDS and 100% when the condition is associated with the failure of two other organs.

CHRONIC OBSTRUCTIVE PULMONARY DISEASE

Chronic obstructive pulmonary disease (COPD) is a progressive and irreversible condition that is characterized by diminished inspiratory and expiratory capacity of the lungs. It is a chronic respiratory condition that obstructs the flow of air to or from the patient's bronchioles (Figure 9-15). COPD includes emphysema, chronic bronchitis, asthma, and bronchiectasis. All diseases included in COPD are characterized by **chronic airflow limitation,** which accurately describes the underlying pathology.

EMPHYSEMA
Etiology/Pathophysiology

Emphysema symptoms usually develop when the patient is in his or her 40s, with disability increasing by age 50 to 60. This condition is characterized by changes in the alveolar walls and capillaries: thus emphysema is primarily an **alveolar disease** (Figure 9-15, C).

Emphysema is an abnormal permanent enlargement of the alveoli distal to the terminal bronchioles, accompanied by destruction of their walls. There is usually an overlap between chronic bronchitis and emphysema. The bronchi, bronchioles, and alveoli become inflamed as a result of chronic irritation. Because of bronchiole lumen narrowing, air becomes trapped in the alveoli during expiration, causing alveolar distention (Figure 9-16). The alveoli then rupture and scar, losing their elasticity. Oxygen in the arterial blood decreases and CO_2 increases. This process is worsened by cigarette smoking and other inhaled irritants. Cigarette smoking is by far the most common cause of emphysema and chronic bronchitis. Risk factors for emphysema are the same as for chronic bronchitis, with one addition: heredity. An inherited form of emphysema is caused by a deficiency of alpha antitrypsin (ATT), a lung protective protein produced by the liver.

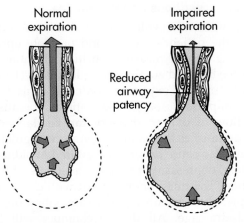

FIGURE **9-16** Mechanisms of air trapping in emphysema. Damaged or destroyed alveolar walls no longer support and hold airways open. Alveoli lose their property of passive elastic recoil. Both of these factors contribute to collapse during expiration.

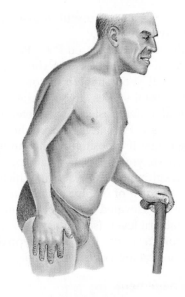

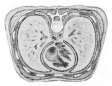

FIGURE **9-17** Barrel chest. Note increase in AP diameter.

ATT deficiency accounts for less than 1% of emphysema in the United States. There is a lag of 30 to 35 years, on average, between taking up smoking and onset of signs and symptoms. The patient is disabled because all available energy must be used for breathing. COPD can lead to cor pulmonale, an abnormal cardiac condition characterized by hypertrophy of the right ventricle of the heart as a result of hypertension of the pulmonary circulation. Cor pulmonale results in the presence of edema in the lower extremities as well as in the sacral and perineal area, distended neck veins, and enlargement of the liver with ascites. Cor pulmonale is a late complication of emphysema.

Clinical Manifestations

The primary symptom of emphysema is dyspnea on exertion, which becomes progressively more severe. Eventually dyspnea occurs at rest. Initially there is little sputum production, but later it becomes copious. The patient will eventually appear barrel chested (an increased anteroposterior diameter caused by overinflation) and begin using accessory muscles for breathing (Figure 9-17). Spontaneous pursed-lip breathing and chronic weight loss with emaciation ensue.

Assessment

Collection of **subjective data** includes a nursing assessment that details a history of onset of symptoms. The nurse should note duration and intensity of dyspnea, cough, and sputum production (documenting color and amount). Also the patient's reported history of smoking and exposure to in-halants, and family history of respiratory disorders should be determined.

Collection of **objective data** includes assessment of presenting signs, such as tachycardia, tachypnea, peripheral cyanosis, and clubbing of fingers. The most outstanding feature of clubbing is a lateral and longitudinal curvature of the nails accompanied by soft tissue enlargement, presenting a bulbous (bulb-shaped), shiny appearance. This occurs late in the disease. Hypoxemia (especially during exercise) may be present, but hypercapnia does not develop until late in the disease. The person is characteristically underweight, but the exact cause for this is not well understood. One possibility is that the patient is in a hypermetabolic state with increased energy requirements that are partly due to the increased work of breathing.

Diagnostic Tests

An important goal of the diagnostic workup is to determine the major disease component of COPD, the severity of the disease, and the impact of the disease on the patient's quality of life. A history and physical examination are extremely important in a diagnostic workup of the patient.

Pulmonary function tests will be done to measure total lung capacity, which will be decreased with COPD. Residual volume is increased, as are compliance and airway resistance. Ventilatory response is decreased. Pulse oximetry is useful in assessing oxygen saturation in arterial blood.

ABGs will reveal a decreased PaO_2. $PaCO_2$ will often be increased late in the disease. A chest radiographic examination will show hyperinflation of the lungs, widened intercostal spaces, and flattened diaphragm with increased anteroposterior diameter (associated with barrel chest). Hematological studies should be done to determine if a positive alpha$_1$-antitrypsin assay exists (an enzyme deficiency causing airway abnormalities resulting in emphysema), which is present in an inherited form of emphysema. Complete blood count will reveal elevated erythrocytes and hemoglobin and hematocrit levels (secondary polycythemia, as a compensatory response to chronic hypoxia). This is also a late manifestation of emphysema.

Medical Management

The medical plan will include long-term management with home oxygen therapy and chest physiotherapy as needed. In an acute exacerbation the patient may require mechanical ventilation.

Prescribed medications will include bronchodilators such as beta-adrenergic agonists (such as short-acting albuterol (Proventil) and long-acting inhaled salmeterol (Serevent) or theophyllines. Anticholinergics such as ipratropium (Atrovent) are also effective bronchodilators. Bronchodilators enlarge the bronchioles for greater oxygenation and ease of secretion clearance, and corticosteroids to decrease pulmonary inflammation and obstruction. Corticosteroids are usually prescribed only during an acute exacerbation because of the many side effects seen in long-term steroid therapy. Antibiotics are frequently ordered to reduce the risk of infection related to retained pulmonary secretions. Diuretics will assist with fluid removal. Pulmonary therapy can help mobilize secretions and improve oxygenation.

Many physicians are prescribing pulmonary rehabilitation therapy to include aerobic exercise such as walking. This increases the body's capacity to take up and use oxygen through the sustained rhythmic contraction of large muscle groups. Prescribed exercise training improves aerobic capacity, endurance, and strength; improves and maintains functional performance in day-to-day life; and reduces breathlessness and fatigue during exertion (Covey & Larson, 2004).

During an acute exacerbation, severe dyspnea can produce considerable anxiety, restlessness, or irritability in the patient. The patient with COPD must be carefully monitored because of the increased risk for respiratory failure from CNS depressants. The patient should be carefully evaluated for hypoxemia before a CNS depressant is prescribed (Clinical Pathway box).

Nursing Interventions and Patient Teaching

Nursing intervention will be directed at attempting to decrease the patient's anxiety and promote optimal air exchange. Such measures include elevating the head of the bed and administering **low-flow** (1 to 2 L by nasal cannula) oxygen as ordered. (This is extremely important for COPD patients, because a higher flow of oxygen delivery can be dangerous, since it diminishes the brain's respiratory [regulatory] center and can cause respiratory failure.) Avoid use of respiratory depressants to ensure adequate alveolar ventilation. The nurse should assist with chest physiotherapy, which includes percussion, vibration, and postural drainage. All three techniques will help loosen secretions to be expectorated; it sometimes takes several hours after chest physiotherapy before the patient can expectorate loosened secretions. Increasing oral intake of fluids will liquefy secretions, thus aiding in their removal. Additionally, the use of a humidifier will enhance this process. Frequent oral care will promote comfort. The nurse should allow sufficient rest periods and should assist the patient in activities of daily living (ADLs) to prevent decrease in oxygen saturation levels.

The nurse can assist the patient in maintaining nutritional intake by advising rest for 30 minutes before eating. This will conserve energy and decrease dyspnea.

The patient with emphysema has a markedly increased need for protein and calories to maintain an adequate nutritional status. A high-protein, high-calorie diet should be divided into five or six small meals a day. Oral fluid intake should be maintained at 2 to 3 L/day unless contraindicated (because of congestive heart failure, for example). Instruct the patient to drink fluids between meals, rather than with meals, to reduce gastric distention and pressure on the diaphragm. Perform frequent oral hygiene to freshen the patient's mouth after coughing exercises and before meals.

Cessation of cigarette smoking in the early stages is probably the most significant factor in slowing the progression of the disease and improving pulmonary function. The use of nicotine replacement therapy and the newer, nonnicotine medication bupropion (Zyban) may be helpful in minimizing the effects of nicotine withdrawal. These adjunctive therapies should be combined with other modalities such as support groups, education materials, and behavior modification programs. Regardless of the method used to stop smoking, the most important factor is that the person is committed to stopping.

The patient with COPD should have a vaccination with influenza virus vaccine yearly; pneumococcal revaccination is recommended every 5 years for the patient with COPD.

CLINICAL PATHWAY | Chronic Obstructive Pulmonary Disease

Northwest Community Healthcare
Coordinated Caremap Summary
Timeframe (minutes, hours, days, weeks visits)
Diagnostic Related Group 88   COPD
National Length of Stay: 6.0 Days

Code status: _____
NWCH: 6.0 days

Physician: _____
Demographics: Older adult (usually older than 65) with chronic illness

AREA OF TREATMENT	TIMEFRAME	CLINICAL FOCUS	EXPECTED OUTCOMES
Emergency Department	2-4 hr	• Open airway (breathing) • Chest discomfort • Fluid intake and balance • Rule out infection • Anxiety	• Improved oxygen levels in blood • Breathing easier • Lung sounds show improved air movement • Anxiety addressed • Underlying infection addressed
Hospital	6 days	• Diet and nutritional needs • Physical condition • Airway • Chest discomfort	• Improvement in oxygen levels in blood • Ease of breathing improved • COPD teaching protocol followed • Chest discomfort reduced • Nutritional needs addressed
Physician's Office	First visit 7-14 days after discharge with regular checkups thereafter	• Chronic airway problems • Recent illness resolved	• Return to previous level of functioning

This plan has been reviewed and discussed with me.

Patient's Name _____   Signature _____

CATEGORIES OF CARE	AREA: ED	TIME: 2-4 HR	AREA: HOSPITAL	TIME: DAY 1
Consults	MESA physician on call/attending Respiratory care tech		Dietitian prn Discharge Planner prn	
Tests/Specimens	Chest x-ray, ABGs/pulse oximetry, CBC, electrolytes, ECG, UA (cultures)			
Treatments/Therapy • Respiratory status	*Respiratory status addressed* Date_____ Initials_____ • Decreasing anxiety • Less dyspnea • Improved ABGs • O₂ • Nebulizer treatments/bronchodilator • Pursed-lip breathing **Assess:** Vital signs q1h and prn Respiratory assessment q1h and prn Level of anxiety	Mental status Sputum	*Improving respiratory status from ED* Date_____ Initials_____ • Decreasing anxiety • Improving pulse oximetry/ABGs • Less dyspnea • O₂ • Nebulizer treatments/bronchodilator **Assess:** Vital signs q4h Respiratory assessment q4h	Sputum Level of anxiety Mental status
Fluid Balance	*Hydration status addressed* Date_____ Initials_____ • IVs per MD order • I&O **Assess:** Breath sounds Presence of peripheral edema Skin turgor Mucous membranes dry/moist		*Stabilizing hydration status balanced I&O* Date_____ Initials_____ • Daily weight • IVs per MD order • I&O **Assess:** Breath sounds Presence of peripheral edema	Skin turgor Mucous membranes dry/moist

Partial critical pathway for COPD. The complete plan is for a 6-day hospitalization. Developed by Northwest Community Hospital, Arlington Heights, IL. Licensed by the Center for Case Management, South Natick, MA.

CBC, Complete blood count; *ER*, emergency room; *NWCH*, Northwest Community Hospital; *SO*, significant other; *SOB*, shortness of breath.

Continued

CLINICAL PATHWAY | *Chronic Obstructive Pulmonary Disease—cont'd*

CATEGORIES OF CARE	AREA: ED	TIME: 2-4 HR	AREA: HOSPITAL	TIME: DAY 1
Diet	As tolerated		*Nutritional needs addressed* Date_____ Initials_____ • O_2 cannula for meals if on face mask • Obtain order for dietitian to see for nutritional assessment if indicated • Good oral hygiene **Assess:** Nutritional status____Albumin____Weight____	
Medications	Medications per MD's order		*Demonstrates proper use of MDI if ordered* Date_____ Initials_____ • Refer to patient teaching protocol	
Activity	*Expresses acceptable breathing comfort level* Date_____ Initials_____ • Head of bed up • Overbed table with pillow to lean on • Keep head in good alignment with patent airway **Assess:** Decreased dyspnea with positioning Able to expectorate secretions		• Out of bed as tolerated • Up in chair tid **Assess:** Current physical condition Ability to complete ADLs Current baseline activity level Patient response to activity • Increased SOB • Increased anxiety	
Miscellaneous	*Patient/SO verbalizes understanding need for admission* Date_____ Initials_____ • Type of unit • Admitting process		*Become familiar with proper breathing techniques during ADLs/activities* Date_____ Initials_____ • Pursed-lip breathing (refer to teaching protocol)	
Discharge Planning			• Refer to discharge plan if indicated **Assess:** Current living arrangements Discharge planning needs Level of independence Use of O_2/home Initials [ ] [ ] [ ] D E N	

Nursing diagnoses and interventions for the patient with emphysema include but are not limited to the following:

NURSING DIAGNOSES	NURSING INTERVENTIONS
Ineffective airway clearance, related to narrowed bronchioles	Assess patient's ability to mobilize secretions, intervening as needed. Encourage coughing and deep breathing, frequent position changes, and increased oral intake (up to 2000 mL/day). Elevate head of bed; suction as needed. Assist with respiratory treatments. Auscultate lungs, reporting any changes in lung sounds.

NURSING DIAGNOSES	NURSING INTERVENTIONS
Activity intolerance, related to imbalance between oxygen supply and demand, secondary to inefficient work of breathing	Organize care so that periods of activity are interspersed with periods of at least 90 minutes of undisturbed rest. Assist patient with active ROM exercises to build stamina and prevent complications of decreased mobility. Monitor patient's respiratory response to activity. Activity intolerance is indicated by excessively increased respiratory rate (e.g., increased more than 10 breaths/minute above patient's baseline) and depth, dyspnea, and use of accessory muscles of respiration.

Home Health Considerations

Chronic Oxygen Therapy at Home

- Improved prognosis has been noted in patients with COPD who receive nocturnal or continuous O_2 to treat hypoxemia.
- The longer that the continuous daily use of O_2 is maintained, the greater the improvement.
- Periodic reevaluations are necessary for the patient who is using chronic supplemental O_2 in the home.
- Home O_2 systems are usually rented from a company that sends a respiratory therapist or pulmonary nurse specialist to the patient's home.
- The therapist teaches the patient how to use the O_2 system, how to care for it, and how to recognize when the supply is running low and needs to be reordered.
- Post "No smoking" warning signs where they can be seen in the home.
- Do not use electric razors, portable radios, open flames, wool blankets, or mineral oils in the area where oxygen is in use.
- Do not allow smoking in the home.

The nurse should instruct the patient and family (1) on the importance of not smoking and of reducing exposure to other inhaled irritants and (2) effective breathing techniques (such as pursed-lip breathing) and relaxation exercises for anxiety control. Teach the patient about the dangers of increased oxygen intake to a patient dependent on hypoxic drive for ventilation. Also, the nurse should teach the patient and family (1) how to prevent infection, and (2) symptoms that should be reported to the physician (Home Health Considerations; Therapeutic Dialogue; Nursing Care Plan boxes).

Prognosis

Emphysema is usually irreversible. COPD is the fourth leading cause of death in the United States. COPD affects about 16 million Americans with about 120,000 deaths each year.

CHRONIC BRONCHITIS
Etiology/Pathophysiology

Chronic bronchitis is characterized by a recurrent or chronic productive cough for a minimum of 3 months a year for at least 2 years. It is caused by physical or chemical irritants and recurrent lung infections. Cigarette smoking is by far the most common cause of chronic bronchitis. Workers exposed to dust, such as coal miners and grain handlers, also are at higher risk. The underlying process is an impairment of cilia, so they can no longer move secretions. Mucous gland hypertrophy causes hypersecretion, altering cilia function (see Figure 9-15, *A*). Excessive mucus is trapped in edematous airways, obstructing airflow. The lining of

Therapeutic Dialogue

Mr. O., a 91-year-old, lives at home with his wife of 38 years. He was admitted to the hospital with acute exacerbation *(an increase in the seriousness of a disease or disorder as marked by greater intensity in the signs or symptoms of the patient) of emphysema. Mr. O. has a 24-year history of emphysema, with progression of signs and symptoms. Signs and symptoms that he manifests are exertional dyspnea, expectoration of copious amounts of tenacious mucus, fatigue, and fear of suffocation.*
PATIENT: *Will it always be like this? I'm so short of air.*
NURSE: *Are you frightened?*
PATIENT: *I'm not afraid of dying, but I worry about having to fight for my air.*
NURSE: *(gently touches Mr. O's arm) Try taking slow, deep breaths, and concentrate on remaining calm.*
PATIENT: *Sometimes I can't even get to the bathroom and do my business—much less help my wife with the dishes or even fill the bird feeder.*
NURSE: *Do you feel you are becoming a burden?*
PATIENT: *I have to be good to my wife. I want to have something left to give her.*
NURSE: *I notice you are breathing more easily. I will be back to check on you, and perhaps we can continue this conversation.*

the bronchial tubes becomes inflamed and eventually scarred. The patient cannot clear tenacious mucus and it becomes a medium for bacteria and infection. This increased airway resistance leads to bronchospasm. There is an altered oxygen–carbon dioxide exchange hypoxia (an inadequate, reduced tension of cellular oxygen) and hypercapnia (greater than normal amounts of carbon dioxide in the blood).

Clinical Manifestations

Primary signs include a productive cough, most pronounced in the mornings (this is often overlooked by cigarette smokers). There is also increased dyspnea and use of accessory muscles.

A complication of chronic bronchitis is cor pulmonale, which is hypertrophy of the right side of the heart resulting from pulmonary hypertension. Cyanosis develops, often accompanied by right ventricular failure. The patient with chronic bronchitis often has a characteristic reddish blue skin (resulting from chronic hypoxia, which stimulates erythropoiesis, thus resulting in polycythemia, cyanosis, and dependent edema).

Assessment

Collection of **subjective data** includes obtaining a detailed history of smoking or exposure to irritants, as well as family history of respiratory disorders. Also, the patient's current medication and treatment regimen should be determined.

NURSING CARE PLAN

The Patient with Emphysema

Mr. O. is a 91-year-old patient admitted with an exacerbation of COPD. His respirations are 32 and labored. He has nasal flaring and his nail beds are cyanotic. He has a barrel chest and digital clubbing. He states he has a productive cough and "can't get my air." It is noted he expectorates tenacious yellow mucus. He appears anxious during the assessment.

NURSING DIAGNOSIS *Ineffective airway clearance, related to tenacious secretions and expiratory airflow obstruction*

Patient Goals/Expected Outcomes	Nursing Intervention	Evaluation
Patient will maintain patent airway as evidenced by decreased rhonchi, wheezes, tachypnea, dyspnea, and ABG values within limits (for this patient).	Assess lung sounds every 2 to 4 hours. Encourage turning, coughing, and deep breathing every 2 to 4 hours. Suction prn. Explain all medications used in inhalation therapy and assist with treatment. Monitor effectiveness. Ensure hydration: oral intake for 2 to 3 L/day to liquefy secretions for easier expectoration.	Patient's respiratory status remains within baseline for this patient. Patient has normal breath sounds upon auscultation. Patient is able to expectorate sputum without difficulty.

NURSING DIAGNOSIS *Ineffective breathing pattern, related to decreased lung expansion secondary to chronic air flow limitations*

Patient Goals/Expected Outcomes	Nursing Intervention	Evaluation
Following treatment intervention, patient's breathing pattern improves as evidenced by patient maintaining respiratory rate within 5 of baseline. Patient will demonstrate relaxed appearance.	Assess for indicators of respiratory distress (agitation, restlessness, decreased level of consciousness, and use of accessory muscles of respiration). Auscultate breath sounds; report a decrease in breath sounds or an increase in adventitious breath sounds. Instruct patient in the use of pursed-lip breathing, which provides internal stability to the airways and may prevent airway collapse during expiration. Administer bronchodilator therapy as prescribed. Monitor patient's response to prescribed O_2 therapy. Be aware that high concentrations of O_2 can depress the respiratory drive in individuals with chronic CO_2 retention. Avoid use of respiratory depressants to ensure adequate alveolar ventilation.	Patient's arterial blood gases are within normal values. Patient has absence of adventitious breath sounds. Patient is sleeping for 5 to 6 hours without respiratory distress.

? CRITICAL THINKING QUESTIONS

1. Mr. O. turns on his light and states that he is "unable to get my air." The nurse notes subclavicular retractions and a respiratory rate of 36. His oxygen is flowing at 1 L per nasal cannula. Nursing interventions that will decrease his dyspnea include:

2. While the nurse is performing an assessment on Mr. O., he states, "I'm so tired of fighting to breathe that I wish I could just go to sleep and never wake up." An appropriate response would be:

3. During vital signs assessment, the nurse notes that Mr. O.'s temperature is 102° F, the pulse rate is 110, and the respiratory rate is 44. The nurse knows that Mr. O.'s COPD places him at a high risk for:

Collection of **objective data** includes assessing the patient's productive cough, noting characteristics and amount of sputum. The nurse should assess the severity of dyspnea and presence of wheezing and should note the patient's level of restlessness. Also, when vital signs are checked, special attention should be paid to tachycardia, tachypnea, and elevated temperature.

Diagnostic Tests

Chest radiographs taken early in the disease may not show abnormalities. Later in the disease the finding will show abnormalities. An electrocardiogram (ECG) may be normal or show signs indicative of right ventricular failure. An echocardiogram can be used to evaluate right-sided ventricular as well as left ventricular function.

A CBC will show increased erythrocytes, hemoglobin, hematocrit, and white blood cell count. Polycythemia develops as a result of increased production of red blood cells secondary to the body's attempt to compensate for chronic hypoxemia. Hemoglobin concentrations may reach 20 g/dL or more. ABG values will reveal respiratory acidosis, hypoxia, and hypercapnia. Pulse oximetry is valuable to assess oxygen saturation levels in arterial blood. There will be an alteration in pulmonary function studies that reveals airflow limitation on expiration, increased airway resistance and residual volume, and often electrolyte abnormalities. Oximetry levels should be monitored on all patients with hypoxia.

Medical Management

The medical plan is aimed at minimizing the disease progression and facilitating optimal air exchange by reducing spasms and secretions.

Three main classes of bronchodilators are typically used to treat COPD. To reverse bronchospasm, the health care provider may order beta-adrenergic agonists such as short-acting albuterol (Proventil) and long-acting salmeterol (Serevent); or the theophyllines, anticholinergics, such as ipratropium, are also effective as bronchodilators. Corticosteroids are helpful in reducing airway inflammation. Long-term use of systemic steroids can lead to many adverse reactions, including osteoporosis. Inhaled steroids have fewer systemic effects and are preferred. Mucolytics such as guaifenesin to break up tenacious mucus may be helpful (Wisniewski, 2004). Antibiotic agents (erythromycin) are commonly ordered.

Nursing Interventions and Patient Teaching

The nurse should provide adequate hydration to liquefy secretions and aid in their removal. The patient must be suctioned as needed and maintained on low-flow oxygen to maintain SaO$_2$ above 90%). The nurse should offer frequent oral hygiene and provide rest periods. The nutritional needs are similar to those of the patient with emphysema.

Nursing diagnoses and interventions for the patient with chronic bronchitis include but are not limited to the following:

NURSING DIAGNOSES	NURSING INTERVENTIONS
Ineffective breathing pattern, related to retained pulmonary secretions	Assess degree of dyspnea, noting nasal flaring, sternal retractions, and pursed-lip breathing. Instruct on effective breathing techniques. Suction as needed.
Fatigue, related to increased respiratory effort	Assess degree of fatigue, and with patient, use problem-solving techniques to explore techniques for decreasing fatigue. Provide treatments in calm, unhurried manner. Identify support systems and refer if needed. Encourage adequate periods of rest.

The nurse should teach the patient effective breathing techniques and instruct the patient and family on avoidance of infection exposure. Instruct the patient to notify the physician at the first sign of a respiratory infection. Usually the best indication of such an infection is a change in the color, consistency, or amount of sputum. Medication teaching should be provided, including action, rationale, and side effects. The nurse should stress the importance of increasing fluid intake, unless contraindicated. The patient and family should be encouraged not to smoke. Encourage a patient who smokes to join a smoking cessation program and teach about prescription and over-the-counter medications to assist with quitting smoking.

Prognosis

Chronic bronchitis is usually irreversible. COPD is the fourth leading cause of death in the United States, after heart disease, cancer, and traumatic injuries.

ASTHMA
Etiology/Pathophysiology

Asthma is a broad clinical syndrome and an airway pathology. It involves episodic increased tracheal/bronchial responsiveness to various stimuli, resulting in widespread narrowing of the airways, which usually improves either spontaneously or with treatment. It is classified as extrinsic or intrinsic. **Extrinsic** is caused by external factors, such as environmental allergens (pollens, dust, feathers, animal dander, foods, etc.); **intrinsic** is from internal causes, not fully understood but often triggered by respiratory infection. Recurrence of attacks is greatly influenced by secondary factors, by mental or physical fatigue, and by emotional factors.

Asthma can result from an altered immune response or increased airway resistance and altered air exchange. An acute asthma attack is caused by an antigen-antibody reaction in which histamine is released. There are three mechanisms involved (see Figure 9-14, *B*):

- Recurrent, reversible obstruction of airflow in the bronchioles and smaller bronchi secondary to bronchospasm. The muscles around the bronchioles tighten and narrow the air passages.
- Increased capillary permeability resulting in edema of mucous membranes with increased narrowing of airways and increased mucus secretion.
- An acute inflammatory response in the mast cells of the lungs, caused by exposure to an asthma trigger. These cells release histamine and other inflammatory agents. Systemic immune system cells release substances that cause circulating inflammatory cells to migrate to the lungs.

Clinical Manifestations

Mild asthma is manifested by dyspnea on exertion and wheezing. Symptoms are usually controlled by medications. An acute asthma attack usually occurs at night and will include tachypnea, tachycardia, diaphoresis, chest tightness, cough, expiratory wheezing, use of accessory muscles, and nasal flaring. The wheezing sound characteristic of asthma is caused by air forcing its way through the narrowed bronchioles and by vibrating mucus. There will also be increased anxiety and diaphoresis. The patient will exhibit a productive cough of copious, thick mucus. Asthma can be triggered by external factors (e.g., dust, mold, or lint) or precipitated intrinsically by a respiratory infection or exercise.

Status asthmaticus is a severe, unrelenting, life-threatening attack that fails to respond to usual treatment. Symptoms of an acute attack are present, and the trapped air leads to exhaustion and respiratory failure. An axion describes status asthmaticus: "The longer it lasts, the worse it gets, and the worse it gets, the longer it lasts" (Lewis et al, 2004).

Assessment

Collection of **subjective data** includes noting that the patient may report asthma-related factors: medications, self-care regimen, precipitating factors, and anxiety.

Collection of **objective data** includes the nurse assessing the presence of cyanosis, the amount of respiratory effort, and vital signs. The patient may assume a "hunched forward" position in an attempt to get more air. The nurse should auscultate the lungs for wheezing.

Diagnostic Tests

To diagnose asthma the physician will order ABGs and pulmonary function tests. The chest radiographic examination will reveal lung hyperinflation related to air trapping, and a flat diaphragm related to increased intrathoracic volume. Pulmonary function tests are performed to assess airway reversibility during and after an asthma attack. Normal values for these tests vary, depending on the patient's age, weight, and sex. In an acute asthma episode the patient will not be able to perform a complete pulmonary function study, but the nurse can check the peak expiratory flow rate.

A sputum culture should be obtained from the patient to rule out any secondary infection. A CBC will reveal an increased eosinophil count in the differential, which is indicative of an allergic response. If the patient has been taking theophylline, a blood sample should be drawn to determine whether the prescribed dose of theophylline is maintained at a therapeutic level; the acceptable therapeutic range is 10 to 20 mcg/mL. This will also reduce the risk of complications as a result of toxicity.

Medical Management

Medication management of asthma can be placed in two categories: maintenance therapy and acute (or rescue) therapy. **Maintenance therapy** is to prevent and minimize symptoms and the medications are to be taken on a regular basis. These include the long acting beta$_2$-agonist salmeterol (Serevent), which is to be used for prophylactic use only; inhaled corticosteroids, such as fluticasone (Flovent); cromolyn; and theophylline.

A recent group of drugs called leukotriene inhibitors is now available for the prophylaxis and chronic treatment of asthma. Leukotrienes are chemicals present in the body that are powerful bronchoconstrictors and vasodilators; some also cause airway edema and inflammation, thus contributing to the symptoms of asthma. Two new groups of drugs called leukotriene receptor antagonists (zafirlukast [Accolate], montelukast [Singulair]) and leukotriene synthesis inhibitors (zileuton [Zyflo]) are being used for the treatment of asthma. These drugs interfere with the synthesis or block the action of leukotrienes. A major advantage of these drugs is that they have both bronchodilator and antiinflammatory effects. It is recommended that these drugs not be used as the only therapy for treatment of persistent asthma. A broad range of patients, from those with mild symptoms to those with more severe asthma, can benefit from leukotriene modifiers. Leukotriene modifiers are not indicated for use in the reversal of bronchospasms in acute asthma attacks. They are indicated for the chronic treatment of asthma (Miracle and Winston, 2000). (See Medications: Respiratory Disorders, p. 430.)

Acute (or **rescue**) **therapy** works to immediately relieve symptoms of an asthma attack. The drugs involved include short-acting inhaled beta₂-agonist albuterol (ventolin, Proventil), by metered dose inhaler (MDI) using spacer devices or nebulizer; oral or IV corticosteroids; and epinephrine. A recent study showed that inhaled corticosteroids, given with short-acting beta₂-agonists, may be better and faster than IV corticosteroids at treating an acute exacerbation (Miracle and Winston, 2000). Short-acting beta₂-agonists (ventolin, Proventil) work to quickly relax the muscles around the airway. See the Medications table. Epinephrine, given subcutaneously or intramuscularly, may be considered in an emergency when symptoms haven't been relieved by the use of a beta₂-agonist. Epinephrine acts as a bronchodilator. Although the value of administering aminophylline in the treatment of acute asthma has been questioned, IV aminophylline may be considered if the asthma is severe or there is minimal or no response to short-acting inhaled beta₂-agonists.

In acute asthma, oxygen (O_2) therapy should be started immediately, and its administration should be monitored by pulse oximetry, and in more severe cases by measurement of ABGs.

Using a peak flowmeter can help the patient manage asthma. This device measures peak expiratory flow rate (PEFR)—the flow of air in a forced exhalation in liters per minute, which is a good indicator of lung function. Peak flow monitoring measures how well air moves out of the lungs when blown out as hard and fast as possible. Peak flow measurement can help the patient detect early signs of asthma episodes before symptoms occur. Normal peak flow is 80% to 100% of the value predicted for the patient based on height, weight, age, and sex. Severe, persistent asthma is characterized by a peak flow less than 60% of the value predicted. A severe, life-threatening exacerbation of asthma is characterized by a peak flow less than 50% of the patient's predicted value.

Once the acute event is over, the medical plan includes identification of precipitating factors and promoting optimal health. Elimination of allergen or countermeasures, such as desensitization or hyposensitization, are desirable.

Nursing Interventions and Patient Teaching

Nursing intervention includes administering prescribed medications, ensuring adequate fluid intake and optimal ventilation. Measures to facilitate these goals include incorporating rest periods into activities and interventions; elevating the head of the bed; teaching effective breathing techniques, such as pursed-lip breathing; correct use of peak flowmeter; and providing oxygen therapy as ordered. The nurse should monitor vital signs and electrolytes. Kind and empathetic emotional support is vital.

Nursing diagnoses and interventions for the patient with asthma include but are not limited to the following:

NURSING DIAGNOSES	NURSING INTERVENTIONS
Ineffective breathing pattern, related to narrowed airway	Assess ventilation, and be alert for signs of increasing dyspnea, such as using accessory muscles, nasal flaring, dyspnea, pursed-lip breathing, or prolonged expiration.
	Maintain position to facilitate ventilation.
	Administer prescribed medications.
	Assist with administration of respiratory treatments.
	Provide care in calm, unhurried manner.
	Attempt to minimize exposure to dust and other irritants by maintaining clean environment and use of humidifier.
	Maintain adequate hydration.
Ineffective health maintenance, related to possible allergens in the home	Implement mutual problem-solving to explore with patient and family what stimulants may be in home environment, such as allergens.
	Facilitate allergy testing if needed.
	Teach the patient and family importance of avoiding exposure to known irritants.

The nurse should educate the patient and family to identify signs and symptoms and recognize asthma "triggers" and avoid them or lessen their effects, to avoid recurrent attacks. The patient should be instructed on relaxation techniques to use to manage anxiety. The importance of health maintenance measures, such as adequate fluid intake and effective breathing techniques, should be stressed.

The patient needs to be taught to take prescribed medications correctly and on time, to monitor the peak flowmeter to recognize the early signs of an asthma attack and begin treatment immediately, and to follow the program treatment steps during an attack. The goal is to provide a good control of symptoms with the least possible medication.

Prognosis

Asthma is the leading cause of chronic illness in childhood. The Centers for Disease Control and Prevention report that after a 15-year decline, the death rate for asthma has increased by 50% over the last 10 years. It is a disheartening statistic, because treatment and education can reduce or eliminate asthma attacks.

If status asthmaticus is not reversed, death will ensue.

BRONCHIECTASIS
Etiology/Pathophysiology

Bronchiectasis is a gradual, irreversible process that involves chronic dilation of bronchi and that eventually destroys bronchial elastic and muscular elements. This pulmonary muscle tone is gradually lost after one or, as is generally the case, repeated pulmonary infections in children and adults.

This condition is usually secondary to failure of normal lung tissue defenses (as caused by cystic fibrosis, foreign body, or tumor). It occurs as a complication of recurrence of an inflammation/infection process that gradually alters the pulmonary structures.

Clinical Manifestations

Signs and symptoms occur after a respiratory infection. The signs and symptoms usually seen are dyspnea, cyanosis, and clubbing of fingers. There are paroxysms of coughing upon arising in the morning and when lying down. This severe coughing produces copious amounts of foul-smelling sputum. Fatigue, weakness, and a loss of appetite are also noted.

Assessment

Collection of **subjective data** includes noting the patient's report of difficulty breathing, weight loss, and fever.

Collection of **objective data** includes the nurse hearing fine crackles and wheezes in the lower lobes on auscultation. The patient will exhibit a prolonged expiratory phase and increased dyspnea. Hemoptysis is seen in 50% of the patients.

Diagnostic Tests

Chest radiographic examination will be essentially normal, but inflammation and mediastinal shift may be the result of overinflation of specific lobes. Sputum cultures can rule out the presence of a bacterial infection. CBC may show the presence of polycythemia, caused by pulmonary insufficiency (hypoxia). Pulmonary function tests will show a decreased forced expiratory volume.

Medical Management

Oxygen will be ordered at low flow volume. The patient may require surgery if there is no response to more conservative measures, such as medications, chest physiotherapy, and adequate hydration. If surgery is needed, the affected area will be removed (lobectomy).

Medications include mucolytic agents (acetylcysteine [Mucomyst]), as well as antibiotics and bronchodilators.

Nursing Interventions and Patient Teaching

General nursing interventions include using a cool mist vaporizer to provide humidity and increasing oral intake of fluids to aid in secretion removal. The nurse should assess vital signs and lung sounds every 2 to 4 hours. The patient should be suctioned as needed and assisted to turn, cough, and deep breathe every 2 hours. The nurse should assist with chest physiotherapy.

Nursing diagnoses and interventions for the patient with bronchiectasis include but are not limited to the following:

Nursing Diagnoses	Nursing Interventions
Ineffective airway clearance, related to retained pulmonary secretions	Assess patient's ability to mobilize secretions, assisting as needed. Encourage postural drainage and coughing; suction if needed. Encourage frequent position changes to facilitate secretion mobility and removal. Maintain adequate hydration. Administer mucolytic agents as ordered, and note patient response.
Impaired physical mobility, related to decreased exercise tolerance	Assess patient's activity tolerance, and promote adaptive techniques, such as incorporating rest periods into activities. Promote a gradual increase of activity, noting patient tolerance. Problem-solve with patient and family to identify methods of energy conservation and ways to implement them into lifestyle.

The nurse should teach the patient and family environmental awareness (avoidance of smoke, fumes, and irritating inhalants). Smoking should be discouraged and appropriate rest/exercise practices should be taught. The nurse should perform medication teaching, including dosage, rationale, and side effects. The patient and family should be instructed on signs and symptoms of a secondary infection. The nurse should ensure that the patient knows how to reach the physician after discharge.

Prognosis

Bronchiectasis is a chronic disease. Surgical removal of a portion of the patient's lung is the only cure.

NURSING PROCESS *for the Patient with a Respiratory Disorder*

The role of the licensed practical nurse/licensed vocational nurse (LPN/LVN) in the nursing process as stated is that the LPN/LVN will:

- Participate in planning care for patients based on patient needs
- Review patient's plan of care and recommend revisions as needed
- Review and follow defined prioritzation for patient care
- Use clinical pathways/care maps/care plans to guide and review patient care

Assessment

As the nurse begins care of the patient admitted with a respiratory disorder, a thorough immediate, and accurate nursing assessment is an essential first step. The assessment should include the patient's level of consciousness, vital signs, lung sounds (crackles, wheezes, pleural friction rub) and oximetry level. The patient should be asked if he has shortness of breath, dyspnea on exertion, or cough. If the patient has a cough, the nurse should ask whether it is productive or nonproductive and regarding the amount as well as the color of the sputum expectorated. The nurse will observe the patient's facial expressions as well as signs of respiratory distress such as flaring nostrils, substernal or clavicular retractions, asymmetrical chest wall expansion, and abdominal breathing.

Nursing Diagnosis

The nurse assists in the development of nursing diagnoses. Nursing diagnoses specific to the patient with a respiratory disorder include but are not limited to the following:

- Ineffective airway clearance
- Ineffective breathing pattern
- Impaired gas exchange
- Anxiety
- Activity intolerance
- Imbalanced nutrition: less than body requirements

Expected Outcomes/Planning

The overall goals are that the patient with a respiratory disorder will have (1) effective breathing patterns, (2) adequate airway clearance, (3) adequate oxygenation of tissues, and (4) a realistic attitude toward compliance to treatment. The care plan may include the following goals:

Goal #1: Patient achieves improved activity tolerance.
Outcome: Patient reports less discomfort with exercise.
Goal #2: Patient maintains a patent airway.
Outcome: Patient clears airway by coughing.

Implementation

Maintaining the patient's optimal level of health is important in reducing respiratory symptoms. Nursing interventions may include improving the patient's activity tolerance. This results in the patient's increased ability to perform activities of daily living while not increasing dyspnea.

Evaluation

The nurse evaluates the expected outcomes and determines their effectiveness. The nurse should notify the physician if the patient's respiratory status does not improve immediately.

Goal #1: Patient achieves improved activity tolerance.
Evaluation: Assess patient's exercise tolerance.
Goal #2: Patient maintains a patent airway.
Evaluation: Auscultate lungs after hearing patient cough.

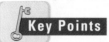

Key Points

- When air is inhaled, it is warmed, moistened, and filtered to prepare it for use by the body.
- The most important structure of the respiratory system is the alveolus; it is here that actual air exchange occurs.
- For breathing to occur, pressure changes must occur within the thoracic cavity.
- The combination of one inspiration plus one expiration equals one respiration, or one respiratory movement.
- The primary function of the respiratory system is to exchange oxygen and carbon dioxide at the alveolar-capillary level.
- The ability of the lungs to expand and contract depends on musculoskeletal and neurological functions, as well as physiologic conditions affecting the respiratory system.
- Activity tolerance is frequently altered as a result of decreased oxygenation/ventilation.
- Anxiety can exacerbate pulmonary disorders, increasing the body's need for oxygen.
- Breathing exercises can improve ventilation.
- Effective breathing techniques include elevating the head and chest to maintain airway patency; deep breathing and coughing exercises to facilitate lung expansion; and pursed-lip breathing to decrease the effort of breathing.
- Adequate fluid intake and humidity help moisten secretions, thus aiding in their clearance.
- A thorough psychosocial assessment and resultant interventions are necessary for the patient with a laryngectomy, because of loss of voice and neck and facial disfigurement.
- Severe acute respiratory syndrome (SARS) is a serious acute respiratory infection caused by a coronavirus.
- People who are suspected of having SARS should be placed in respiratory isolation, including use of an appropriate disposable particulate respirator to protect other patients and health care workers.

- Clinical manifestations of sleep apnea include frequent awakening at night, insomnia, excessive daytime sleepiness, witnessed apneic episodes, morning headaches, personality changes, and irritability.
- Chest drainage serves a twofold purpose: it (1) drains air, blood, or fluid from the pleural space; and (2) restores negative pressure. It requires a water seal to prevent air from reentering the pleural space.
- Techniques used in chest physiotherapy include percussion, vibration, and postural drainage.
- Nursing interventions after thoracic surgery that assist in preventing complications by promoting effective airway clearance are (1) frequent repositioning, (2) coughing, and (3) deep breathing.
- Studies have revealed that hypoxia worsens when patients are placed on their backs or sides with the affected (sick) lung down.
- Low-flow oxygen therapy is required for patients with COPD, because higher oxygen concentrations depress the body's own respiratory regulatory centers.
- Hospitals are a high-risk setting for TB transmission, and health care workers are at high occupational risk for TB infection.

- Because pulmonary embolism (PE) impairs gas exchange, its hallmark is acute, unexplained dyspnea with abrupt, constant, nonradiating pain that worsens with inspiration.
- Patients with respiratory disorders must reduce exposure to infection, because infection will further increase the body's oxygen demands.
- Chronic obstructive pulmonary disease includes emphysema, chronic bronchitis, asthma, and bronchiectasis.
- Transmission of tuberculosis is primarily by inhalation of minute droplet nuclei (each containing a single tubercle bacillus) coughed or sneezed by a person whose sputum contains tubercle bacilli.
- Pulse oximetry is a noninvasive method providing continuing monitoring of SaO_2 (saturation of oxygen).

Go to your free CD-ROM for an Audio Glossary, animations, video clips, and Review Questions for the NCLEX-PN® Examination.

evolve Be sure to visit the companion Evolve site at http://evolve.elsevier.com/Christensen/adult/ for WebLinks and additional online resources.

CHAPTER CHALLENGE

1. Rapid and deeper respirations are stimulated by the respiratory center of the brain when:

   1. oxygen saturation levels are greater than 90%.
   2. carbon dioxide levels increase.
   3. the alveoli contract.
   4. the diaphragm contracts and lowers its dome.

2. The tendency of molecules of a substance (gaseous, liquid, or solid) to move from a region of high concentration to one of lower concentration is the passive process in which the exchange of gases between the blood capillary and alveolar area occurs. This process is called:

   1. osmosis.
   2. filtration.
   3. diffusion.
   4. transport.

3. Each alveolus is coated with a thin lipoprotein covering that prevents it from collapsing after each breath; this covering is:

   1. LDH.
   2. isoenzyme.
   3. surfactant.
   4. sebum.

4. The walls of the thoracic cavity are lined with a serous membrane composed of tough endothelial cells called:

   1. visceral pleura.
   2. apneustic serosa.
   3. pneumotaxic serosa.
   4. parietal pleura.

5. The exchange of oxygen and carbon dioxide in external respiration takes place in the:

   1. lungs.
   2. bronchioles.
   3. capillaries and the body cells.
   4. alveoli and pulmonary capillaries.

6. Mr. K., age 73, is diagnosed with chronic bronchitis. He is very dyspneic and must sit up to breathe. An abnormal condition in which there is discomfort in breathing in any but an erect sitting position is:

   1. orthopnea.
   2. dyspnea.
   3. orthopsia.
   4. Cheyne-Stokes.

7. Ms. C., age 45, is being evaluated to rule out pulmonary tuberculosis. Which finding is most closely associated with TB?

   1. Leg cramps
   2. Night sweats
   3. Skin discoloration
   4. Green-colored sputum

8. The health care workers caring for Ms. C., who is diagnosed with active tuberculosis, are instructed in methods of protecting themselves from contracting tuberculosis. The Centers for Disease Control and Prevention currently recommend that health care workers who care for TB-infected patients:

   1. ask the patient to wear a mask while in isolation.
   2. wear a surgical mask.
   3. wear a small-micron, fitted filtration mask.
   4. receive the BCG vaccine.

9. The physician ordered a blood culture and sputum specimen to be obtained for Mr. G., a patient who has pneumonia. These diagnostic tests should be collected:
   1. after initiation of antibiotic therapy.
   2. the morning following admission.
   3. before initiation of antibiotic therapy.
   4. at the first elevated temperature.

10. Ms. V., age 62, has just returned to her room following a bronchoscopy. No food or fluids should be given after the examination until:
    1. total absence of blood-streaked sputum.
    2. the head nurse gives the order.
    3. her gag reflex returns.
    4. she is up and about and steady on her feet.

11. Mr. M. was in a motor vehicle accident and has a lacerated pleura secondary to fractured ribs. To promote reexpansion of his lung, what type of thoracic drainage system was used?
    1. Open system to promote negative pressure
    2. Closed system to maintain the lungs' normal negative pressure
    3. Closed system to maintain the lungs' positive pressure
    4. Closed system to allow air to enter the pleural cavity for reexpansion

12. Mr. R., 45 years old, is a second-day postoperative patient recovering from thoracic surgery. A very therapeutic nursing intervention would include:
    1. coughing and deep breathing the patient by splinting the anterior and posterior chest.
    2. splinting the anterior chest for coughing.
    3. placing the patient in a supine position.
    4. allowing the patient to sleep uninterrupted for 8 hours.

13. Mr. A., age 71, is admitted with an exacerbation of COPD. He has dependent edema and ascites as well as dyspnea. A complication that may occur in COPD, in which some of the capillaries surrounding the alveoli are destroyed, resulting in pulmonary hypertension, blood returning to the right side of the heart, and signs and symptoms of right-sided HF is:
    1. pulmonary edema.
    2. cor pulmonale.
    3. tetralogy of Fallot.
    4. acyanotic heart disease.

14. Mr. F., age 52, had a laryngectomy due to cancer of the larynx. Discharge instructions are given to Mr. F. and his family. Which response, by written communication from Mr. F. or verbal response by the family, will be a signal to the nurse that the instructions need to be reclarified?
    1. Report swelling, pain, or excessive drainage.
    2. The suctioning at home must be a clean procedure, not sterile.

    3. Cleanse skin around stoma bid, use hydrogen peroxide and rinse with water, pat dry.
    4. It is acceptable to take over-the-counter medications now that condition is stable.

15. Most pulmonary embolisms (PEs) originate from:
    1. deep vein thrombosis (DVT).
    2. ventilation/perfusion (V/Q) mismatch.
    3. increased pulmonary vascular resistance.
    4. right-sided heart failure.

16. Chest pain from pulmonary embolism (PE) typically:
    1. radiates to the neck and jaw.
    2. is unchanged by deep breathing.
    3. is pleuritic and worsens upon inspiration.
    4. radiates to the abdomen and back.

17. In the treatment of asthma, peak-flow monitoring is important to help the patient manage the asthma. Peak-flow monitoring measures:
    1. the inspiratory capacity of the lungs.
    2. the residual volume of the lungs.
    3. the vital capacity of the lungs.
    4. how well air moves out of the lungs during forceful exhalation.

18. The primary goal for the patient with bronchiectasis is that the patient will:
    1. have no recurrence of disease.
    2. have normal pulmonary function.
    3. maintain removal of bronchial secretions.
    4. avoid environmental agents that precipitate inflammation.

19. A patient was seen in clinic for an episode of epistaxis, which was controlled by placement of anterior nasal packing. During discharge teaching, the nurse instructs the patient to:
    1. avoid vigorous nose blowing and strenuous activity.
    2. use aspirin or aspirin-containing compounds for pain relief.
    3. apply ice compresses to the nose every 4 hours for the first 48 hours.
    4. leave the packing in place for 7 to 10 days until it is removed by the physician.

20. TB is spread by:
    1. contact with clothing, bedding, or food.
    2. eating from utensils used by an infected person.
    3. inhaling the TB bacteria after a person coughs, speaks, or sneezes.
    4. talking with an individual with TB.

21. Which type of medication is used as rescue medication in an acute asthma exacerbation?
    1. Methylxanthines
    2. Leukotriene modifiers
    3. Long-acting beta$_2$-agonists
    4. Short-acting beta$_1$-agonists

Continued

CHAPTER CHALLENGE—cont'd

22. Asthma is best characterized as:
    1. an inflammatory disease.
    2. a steady progression of bronchoconstriction.
    3. an obstructive disease with loss of alveolar walls.
    4. a chronic obstructive disorder characterized by mucus production.

23. A patient with COPD asks why the heart is affected by the respiratory disease. The nurse's response to the patient is based on the knowledge that cor pulmonale is characterized by:
    1. pulmonary congestion secondary to left ventricular failure.
    2. excess serous fluid collection in the alveoli caused by retained respiratory secretions.
    3. right ventricular hypertrophy secondary to increased pulmonary vascular resistance.
    4. right ventricular failure secondary to compression of the heart by hyperinflated lungs.

24. A patient with tuberculosis has a nursing diagnosis of noncompliance. The nurse recognizes that the most common etiologic factor for this diagnosis in patients with TB is:
    1. fatigue and lack of energy to manage self-care.
    2. lack of knowledge about how the disease is transmitted.
    3. little or no motivation to adhere to a long-term drug regimen.
    4. feelings of shame and the response to the social stigma associated with TB.

25. Three types of anthrax are:
    1. cutaneous, gastrointestinal, inhalational.
    2. renal, gastrointestinal, CNS.
    3. musculoskeletal, inhalational, adrenal.
    4. cutaneous, endocrine, gastrointestinal.

26. To get optimal results from pulse oximetry, which of the following statements are correct? (More than one answer may be correct.)
    1. Do not attach the transducer to an extremity that has a blood pressure cuff in place.
    2. While the probe is in place, protect it from decreased light, which can affect the reading.
    3. Place the probe over a pulsating vascular bed.
    4. Remember that hypothermia, hypotension, and vasoconstriction can affect readings.

27. Ineffective airway clearance related to tracheobronchial obstruction and/or secretions is a nursing diagnosis for a patient with COPD. Which of the following nursing interventions are correct? (More than one answer may be correct.)
    1. Offer small, frequent, high-calorie, high-protein feedings.
    2. Encourage generous fluid intake.
    3. Restrict fluid intake to decrease congestion.
    4. Have patient turn and cough every 2 hours; teach effective coughing technique.

28. Ineffective breathing pattern related to decreased lung expansion during an acute attack of asthma is an appropriate nursing diagnosis. Which nursing intervention(s) is(are) correct?
    1. Place patient in a supine position.
    2. Administer oxygen therapy as ordered.
    3. Remain with patient during acute attack to decrease fear and anxiety.
    4. Incorporate rest periods into activities and interventions.
    5. Maintain semi-Fowler's position to facilitate ventilation.

29. The patient with respiratory acidosis will demonstrate which of the following? (More than one answer may be correct.)
    1. Disorientation
    2. pH of less than 7.35
    3. pH of more than 7.44
    4. Rapid respirations

30. The appropriate nursing intervention for Mr. K., age 40, diagnosed with active tuberculosis would be:
    1. place the patient in drainage and secretion precautions.
    2. place the patient in acid-fast bacilli (AFB) isolation precautions.
    3. maintain the patient in enteric isolation.
    4. It is inappropriate to place Mr. K. in any isolation precautions.

31. Patient teaching for a patient postoperatively following a tonsillectomy and adenoidectomy would include which of the following: (Select more than one answer.)
    1. Avoid attempting to clear the throat, coughing, and sneezing.
    2. Avoid vigorous nose blowing for 1 to 2 weeks.
    3. Resume foods and fluids as tolerated.
    4. Take aspirin, gr 10 every 4 hours.
    5. Notify the physician in case of increased pain, fever, or bleeding.

32. If the patient has an epistaxis, the correct nursing interventions would include which of the following? (More than one answer may be correct.)
    1. Place the patient in Fowler's position with the head forward.
    2. Place the patient in Fowler's position with the head extended.
    3. Compress the nostrils tightly below the bone and hold for 10 minutes or longer.
    4. Place ice compresses over the nose.

33. In pulmonary edema, the medical management will often include which of the following? (More than one answer may be correct.)
    1. IV infusion at 150 mL/hr
    2. Furosemide (Lasix) IV
    3. Oxygen therapy
    4. Orthopneic position
    5. Morphine sulfate to decrease respiratory rate

The nursing diagnosis for a patient with pulmonary edema, excess fluid volume, related to altered tissue permeability is appropriate. Which of the following nursing interventions for this diagnosis is(are) correct? (More than one answer may be correct.)

1. Assess indicators of patient's fluid volume status, such as breath sounds, skin turgor, and pedal/sacral/periorbital edema.
2. Monitor intake and output accurately.
3. Administer diuretics as ordered.
4. Weigh daily.
5. Provide regular diet with normal sodium intake.

The nurse should educate the patient in the proper techniques to use for the collection of sputum specimen. Which of the following guidelines are correct? (More than one answer may be correct.)

1. Explain to the patient the need to bring the sputum up from the lungs.
2. Encourage fluid intake.
3. Collect specimens after meals when patient feels stronger.
4. Notify staff as soon as specimen is collected so it can be sent to the laboratory without delay.
5. Place sputum specimen in sterile container.

Medical management and nursing interventions of the patient with pulmonary embolism usually include which of the following? (More than one answer may be correct.)

1. Bed rest
2. Administration of intravenous heparin per protocol
3. Semi-Fowler's position
4. Administering vitamin K subcutaneously
5. Oxygen per mask or nasal cannula

10 Care of the Patient with a Urinary Disorder

ALITA K. SELLERS

Objectives

After reading this chapter, the student should be able to do the following:

Anatomy and Physiology

1. Describe the structures of the urinary system, including functions.
2. List the three processes involved in urine formation.
3. Compare the normal components of urine with the abnormal components.
4. Name three hormones and their influence on nephron function.

Medical-Surgical

5. Define the key terms as listed.
6. Describe the alterations in renal function associated with disorders of the urinary tract.
7. Select nursing diagnoses related to alterations in urinary function.
8. Prioritize the special needs of the patient with urinary dysfunction.
9. Appraise the changes in body image created when the patient experiences an alteration in urinary function.
10. Identify the effects of aging on urinary system function.
11. Adapt teaching methods for the patient with urinary disorders.
12. Discuss the effect of renal disease on family function.
13. Incorporate pharmacotherapeutic and nutritional considerations into the nursing care plan of the patient with a urinary disorder.
14. Investigate community resources for support for the patient and significant others as they face lifestyle changes from chronic urinary disorders and treatments.

Key Terms

Be sure to check out the bonus material on the free CD-ROM, including selected audio pronunciations.

anasarca (ăn-ă-SĂR-kă, p. 498)
anuria (ă-NŪ-rē-ă, p. 503)
asthenia (ăs-THĒ-nē-ă, p. 484)
azotemia (ă-zō-TĒ-mē-ă, p. 487)
bacteriuria (băk-tēr-ē-Ū-rē-ŭh, p. 483)
costovertebral angle (kŏs-tō-VĔR-tē-brăl ĂNG-gŭl, p. 487)
cytologic evaluation (sī-tō-LŎJ-ĭk ē-văl-ū-Ā-shŭn, p. 493)
dialysis (dī-ĂL-ĭ-sĭs, p. 506)

dysuria (dĭs-Ū-rē-ă, p. 474)
hematuria (hēm-ă-TŪ-rē-ă, p. 484)
hydronephrosis (hī-drō-nĕ-FRŌ-sĭs, p. 489)
ileal conduit (ĭl-ē-ăl KŎN-dū-ĭt, p. 510)
micturition (mĭk-tū-RĬSH-ŭn, p. 489)
nephrotoxin (nĕf-rō-TŎK-sĭn, p. 511)
nocturia (nŏk-TŪ-rē-ă, p. 484)
oliguria (ōl-ĭ-GŪ-rē-ă, p. 498)
prostatodynia (prŏs-tĕ-tō-DĬN-ē-ă, p. 486)
pyuria (pī-Ū-rē-ă, p. 484)
residual urine (rĕ-ZĬ-dū-ăl Ū-rĭn, p. 481)
retention (rē-TĔN-shŭn, p. 480)
urolithiasis (ū-rō-lĭ-THĪ-ă-sĭs, p. 490)

OVERVIEW OF ANATOMY AND PHYSIOLOGY

Each day, the cells throughout the body metabolize ingested nutrients. This process provides energy for the body and produces waste products. As proteins break down, nitrogenous waste—urea, ammonia, and **creatinine** (a nitrogenous compound produced by metabolic processes in the body)—is produced. Excretion of these waste products is the primary function of the kidneys. The kidneys also assist in regulating the body's water, electrolytes, and acid-base balance. The urinary system is probably the most important system in maintaining homeostasis.

The urinary system is composed of two kidneys, which produce urine by removing waste, excess water, and electrolytes from the blood; two ureters, which transport the urine from the kidneys to the bladder; one bladder, which collects and stores urine; and one urethra, which transports the urine from the bladder to the outside of the body for elimination (Figure 10-1). This chapter will explore the filtering process, the composition of urine, and the pathway of urine removal from the body.

KIDNEYS

The kidneys lie behind the parietal peritoneum (retroperitoneal), just below the diaphragm on each side of the vertebral column. Kidneys are dark red, bean-shaped organs that are 4 to 5 inches (10 to 12 cm) long, 2 to 3 inches (5 to 7.5 cm) wide, and about 1 inch (2.5 cm) thick. Because of the size and shape of the liver, the right kidney lies slightly lower than the left.

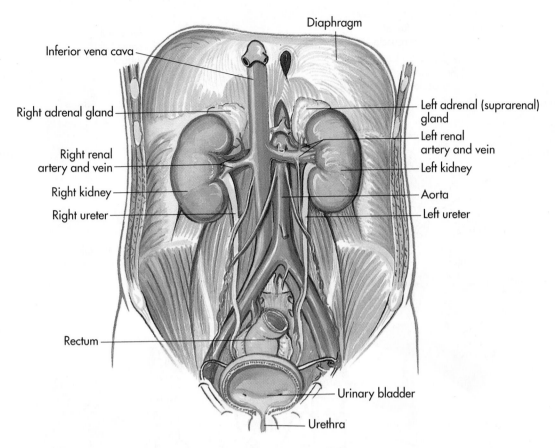

FIGURE **10-1** Locations of urinary system organs.

The kidneys are surrounded by a layer of adipose tissue that anchors them in place. Near the center of the medial border of the kidney is a notch or indentation called the **hilus** where the ureter, blood vessels, and nerves enter and exit the kidney.

Gross Anatomical Structure

The outer covering of the kidney is composed of a strong layer of connective tissue called the **renal capsule.** Directly beneath the renal capsule is the renal **cortex.** It contains 1.25 million renal tubules. These tubules are part of the microscopic filtration system. Immediately beneath the cortex is the **medulla,** which is a darker color. The medulla contains the triangular **pyramids.** Continuing inward, the narrow points of the pyramids **(papillae)** empty urine into the calyces. The *calyces* are cuplike extensions of the renal pelvis that guide urine into the renal pelvis. The **renal pelvis** is an expansion of the upper end of the ureter; the ureter in turn drains the finished product, urine, into the bladder (Figure 10-2).

Microscopic Structure

Nephron. Each kidney contains more than 1 million nephrons. The **nephron** is the functional unit of the kidney, resembling a microscopic funnel with a long stem and two convoluted sections (Figure 10-3). It is responsible for filtering the blood and processing the urine. The nephron has three major functions: (1) con-

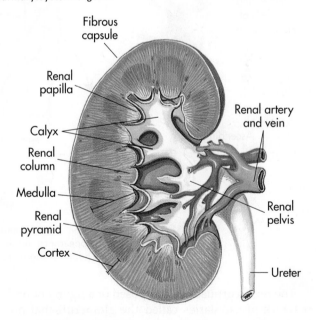

FIGURE **10-2** Coronal section through right kidney.

trolling body fluid levels by selectively removing or retaining water; (2) assisting with the regulation of the pH of the blood; and (3) removing toxic waste from the blood. Approximately 60 times a day, the body's entire volume of blood is filtered through the kidneys. A nephron consists of two main structures: the renal corpuscle and the renal tubule.

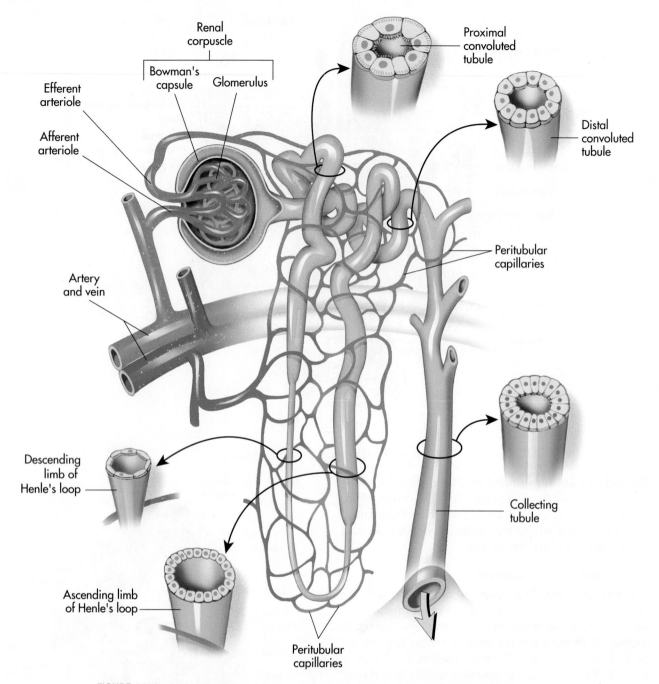

FIGURE **10-3** The nephron unit. Cross sections from the four segments of the renal tubule are shown. The differences in appearance in tubular cells seen in a cross-section reflect the differing functions of each nephron segment.

The renal corpuscle is composed of a tightly bound network of capillaries called the **glomeruli** that are held inside a cuplike structure, **Bowman's capsule.** The renal arteries (right and left) branch off the abdominal aorta and enter the kidney at the hilus. The renal arteries continue branching until blood is delivered to the glomerulus by the afferent arteriole. The blood leaves the glomerulus through the efferent arteriole to the peritubular capillary. Blood finally reaches the renal veins and flows into the inferior vena cava.

The renal tubule becomes tightly coiled (at the proximal convoluted tubule), makes a sudden straight drop, and curves back upward like a hairpin (at the loop of Henle, or nephron loop) and becomes tightly coiled again (at the distal convoluted tubule). The convoluted tubule terminates at the collecting tubule/duct. Several collecting ducts unite in a pyramid and open at the papilla to empty urine into the associated calyx.

The juxtaglomerular apparatus is formed as the distal convoluted tubule makes contact with the afferent and efferent arterioles. This specialized structure plays a role in blood pressure control (Figure 10-4). Blood pressure (hydrostatic pressure) determines the glomerular filtration rate (GFR).

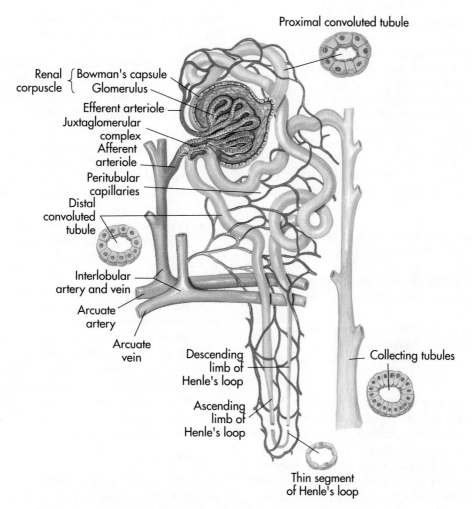

FIGURE **10-4** Cross-section from the four segments of the renal tubule.

Table 10-1 | *Functions of Parts of the Nephron in Urine Formation*

PART OF NEPHRON	PROCESS IN URINE FORMATION	SUBSTANCES MOVED AND DIRECTION OF MOVEMENT
Glomerulus	Filtration	Water and solutes (sodium and other ions, nitrogen wastes, urea, uric acid, creatinine, glucose, and other nutrients) filter through the glomeruli into Bowman's capsule
Proximal convoluted tubule	Reabsorption	Water and solutes
Loop of Henle	Reabsorption	Sodium and chloride ions
Distal convoluted and collecting tubules	Reabsorption	Water, sodium, and other chloride ions
	Secretion	Ammonia, potassium ions, urea, uric acid, creatinine, hydrogen ions, and some drugs

Reabsorption begins as soon as the filtrate reaches the tubule system. The filtrate contains important products needed by the body: water, glucose, and ions may be absorbed. In fact, 99% of the filtrate is returned to the body (see Figure 10-4).

In summary, the three phases of urine formation (Table 10-1) and location of the processes are as follows:

1. **Filtration** of water and blood products occurs in the glomerulus of Bowman's capsule.

2. **Reabsorption** of water, glucose, and necessary ions back into the blood occurs primarily in the proximal convoluted tubules, loop of Henle, and the distal convoluted tubules. This process reclaims important substances needed by the body.

3. **Secretion** of certain ions, nitrogenous waste products, and drugs occurs primarily in the distal convoluted tubule. This process is the reverse of reabsorption; the substances move from the blood to the filtrate.

Box 10-1 *Major Functions of the Kidneys*

Urine formation: Glomerular filtration, tubular reabsorption, and secretion. Each day, the body forms 1000 to 2000 mL of urine

Fluid and electrolyte control: Maintain correct balance of fluid and electrolytes within a normal range by excretion, secretion, and reabsorption

Acid-base balance: Maintain pH of blood (7.35 to 7.45) at normal range by directly excreting H^+ ions and forming bicarbonate for buffering

Excretion of waste products: Direct removal of metabolic waste products contained in the glomerular filtrate

Blood pressure regulation: Regulate blood pressure by controlling the circulating volume and renin secretion

Red blood cell (RBC) production: Erythropoietin secreted by kidneys stimulates bone marrow to produce RBCs

Regulation of calcium-phosphate metabolism: Vitamin D activation regulated by kidneys

Hormonal influence on nephron function. When the body has suffered increased fluid loss through hemorrhage, diaphoresis, vomiting, diarrhea, or other means, the blood pressure drops. These events decrease the amount of filtrate produced by the kidneys. The posterior pituitary gland releases antidiuretic hormone (ADH). ADH causes the cells of the distal convoluted tubules to increase their rate of water reabsorption. This action returns the water to the bloodstream, which increases the blood pressure to a more normal level and causes the urine to become concentrated. See Box 10-1 for major functions of kidneys.

URINE COMPOSITION AND CHARACTERISTICS

The word **urine** comes from one of its components, uric acid. Each day, the body forms 1000 to 2000 mL of urine; this amount is influenced by several factors, such as mental and physical health, oral intake, and blood pressure. Urine is 95% water; the remainder is nitrogenous wastes and salts. It is usually a transparent yellow with a characteristic aromatic odor. Normal urine is yellow because of urochrome, a pigment resulting from the body's destruction of hemoglobin. Urine is slightly acidic, with a pH of 4.6 to 8.0. Healthy urine is sterile, but at room temperature it rapidly decomposes and develops the odor of ammonia as a result of the breakdown of urea.

URINE ABNORMALITIES

A urinalysis, which studies the physical, chemical, and microscopic properties of urine, can give important diagnostic information. If the body's homeostasis has been compromised, certain substances may spill into the urine. Some of the more common substances include:

- **Albumin:** The presence of albumin in the urine (albuminuria) indicates possible kidney disease, increased blood pressure, or toxicity of the kidney cells from heavy metals.
- **Glucose:** The presence of sugar in the urine (glycosuria) most often indicates a high blood glucose level. The blood glucose level rises above the renal threshold (the point at which the kidney tubules can no longer reabsorb), and the glucose spills into the urine.
- **Erythrocytes:** The presence of erythrocytes in the urine (hematuria) may indicate infection, tumors, or kidney disease. Occasionally an individual may have a renal calculus (kidney stone) and irritation produces hematuria.
- **Ketone bodies:** The presence of ketone bodies in the urine, ketoaciduria (also called ketonuria), occurs when excessive quantities of fatty acids are oxidized. This condition may be seen with diabetes mellitus, starvation, or any other metabolic condition in which fats are rapidly catabolized.
- **Leukocytes:** The presence of leukocytes (white blood cells [WBCs]) occurs when there is an infection in the urinary tract.

URETERS

Once the urine has been formed in the nephrons, it passes to the paired ureters. Ureters are actually extensions of the kidney pelvis and extend downward 10 to 12 inches (25 to 30 cm) to the lower part of the urinary bladder. As the ureters leave the kidneys, they are retroperitoneal and pass under the urinary bladder before entering it.

As the ureters enter the bladder (ureterovesical junction), the mucous membrane folds, acting as a valve to prevent backflow of urine.

URINARY BLADDER

The urinary bladder (Figure 10-5) is a temporary storage pouch for urine. It is composed of collapsible muscle and is located anterior to the small intestine and posterior to the symphysis pubis. As the bladder fills with urine, it rises into the abdominal cavity and can be palpated. The bladder can hold 750 to 1000 mL of urine. When the bladder contains approximately 250 mL of urine, the individual has a conscious desire to urinate. This is because the stretch receptors become activated and a message is sent to the spinal cord. A moderately full bladder holds 450 mL (1 pint) of urine.

Two sphincters, the internal and external, control the release of the urine. The internal sphincter located at the bladder neck is composed of involuntary muscle, and as the bladder becomes full, the stretch receptors cause contractions, pushing the urine past the in-

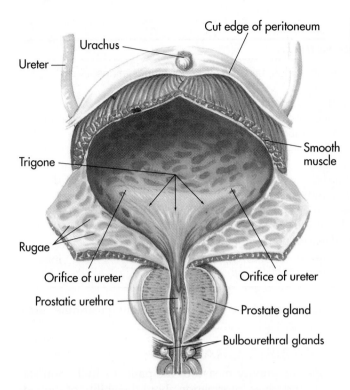

FIGURE **10-5** The male urinary bladder, cut to show the interior. Note how the prostate gland surrounds the urethra as it exits the bladder.

ternal sphincter. The urine then presses on the external sphincter, which is composed of skeletal or voluntary muscle at the terminus of the urethra.

URETHRA

The **urethra** is the terminal portion of the urinary system. It is a small tube that carries urine by peristalsis from the bladder out of its external opening, the **urinary meatus.** In females it is embedded in the anterior wall of the vagina vestibule and exits between the clitoris and the vaginal opening. The female urethra is approximately $\frac{1}{4}$ inch in diameter and $1\frac{1}{2}$ inches long. In males the urethra is approximately 8 inches long, passing through the prostate gland and extending the length of the glans penis. In the male the urethra serves two functions: as a passageway for urine and a passageway for semen.

NORMAL AGING OF THE URINARY SYSTEM

With aging the kidneys lose part of their normal functioning capacity; in fact, by 70 years of age, the filtering mechanism is only 50% as efficient as at 40 years. This occurs because of decreased blood supply and loss of nephrons.

In aging the female bladder loses tone and the perineal muscles may relax; resulting in stress incontinence. In the aging male the prostate gland may become enlarged, leading to constriction of the urethra.

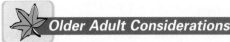

Older Adult Considerations

Urinary Disorder

- Urinary frequency, urgency, nocturia retention, and incontinence are common with aging. These occur because of weakened musculature in the bladder and urethra, diminished neurological sensation combined with decreased bladder capacity, and the effects of medications such as diuretics.
- Urinary incontinence is a leading reason for institutional placement of older adults.
- Urinary incontinence can lead to a loss of self-esteem and result in decreased participation in social activities.
- Older women are at risk for stress incontinence because of hormonal changes and weakened pelvic musculature.
- Older men are at risk for urinary retention because of prostatic hypertrophy.
- Urinary tract infections in older adults are often associated with invasive procedures such as catheterization, diabetes mellitus, and neurological disorders.
- Inadequate fluid intake, immobility, and conditions that lead to urinary stasis increase the risk of infection in the older adult.
- Frequent toileting and meticulous skin care can reduce the risk of skin impairment secondary to urinary incontinence.

Incomplete emptying of the bladder in both males and females increases the possibility of urinary infection (Older Adult Considerations box).

LABORATORY AND DIAGNOSTIC EXAMINATIONS

Diagnostic tests for urinary tract conditions include laboratory tests, diagnostic imaging, and endoscopic procedures. Nursing responsibilities vary according to the studies performed. Nurses need to be aware of specific patient variables that may influence test results: state of hydration, nutritional status, or trauma (Cultural & Ethnic Considerations box). Patient preparation for diagnostic testing includes a brief description of the purpose of the procedure and what the patient can expect to happen during the test.

URINALYSIS

The most common urinary diagnostic study is the urinalysis. Table 10-2 provides a description of normal and abnormal constituents in the urine and possible factors that will influence test results. A urinalysis may be done in relation to conditions of other body systems because of the role of the kidneys in maintaining

Table 10-2 *Urinalysis*

CONSTITUENT	NORMAL RANGE	INFLUENCING FACTORS
Color	Pale yellow to amber	Diabetes insipidus, biliary obstruction, medications, diet
Turbidity	Clear to slightly cloudy	Phosphates, WBCs, bacteria
Odor	Mildly aromatic	Medication, bacteria, diet
pH	4.6 to 8	Stale specimen, food intake, infection, homeostatic imbalance
Specific gravity	1.003 to 1.030	State of hydration, medications
Glucose	Negative	Diabetes mellitus, medications, diet
Protein	Negative	Renal disease, muscle exertion, dehydration
Bilirubin	Negative	Liver disease with obstruction or damage, medications
Hemoglobin	Negative	Trauma, renal disease
Ketones	Negative	Diabetes mellitus, diet, medications
Red blood cells	Up to 2	Renal or bladder disease, trauma, medications
White blood cells	0 to 4 LPF	Renal disease, urinary tract infection
Casts	Rare	Renal disease
Bacteria	Negative	Urinary tract infection

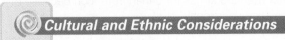

Cultural and Ethnic Considerations

Urinary Disorder

A cultural assessment reflects a dynamic process in which the health care team seeks to understand the patient and gain insights about the meanings of care, health, and well-being. Integral components of a cultural assessment include communication, time orientation, space, pain, religious beliefs, taboos, customs, dietary practices, health practices, family roles, and views of death. Professional discussion of urinary problems requires *ardent* sensitivity because of the association of the urinary system with the reproductive system and the associated cultural taboos surrounding sexuality. Often the patient's self-image and sexual performance are affected by altered urinary function. It is important for the nurse to be sensitive to the patient's feelings, guiding the interview to ensure accurate assessment while maintaining the patient's dignity.

homeostasis. Urinalysis is completed on a clean-catch or catheterized specimen. Urine culture and sensitivity may be done to confirm suspected infections, to identify causative organisms, and to determine appropriate antimicrobial therapy. Cultures are also obtained for periodic screening of urine when the threat of a urinary tract infection (UTI) persists.

There are various reagent strips available to test urine for abnormal substances. The strips are a quick reference that can be used in a clinical setting or at home. Easy-to-follow instructions accompany the specific reagent strips. Because the kidneys excrete substances in varying amounts and rates during a 24-hour period, the nurse may be responsible for collecting a 24-hour urine sample. The first voiding is discarded and the time noted at the beginning of the 24-hour urine collection. For the next 24 hours all urine is collected and placed in a special laboratory container. Common substances measured to monitor kidney

function include total urine protein, creatinine, urea, uric acid levels, and catecholamines.

SPECIFIC GRAVITY

Specific gravity measures the patient's hydration status and gives information about the ability of the kidneys to concentrate urine. Specific gravity is decreased by high fluid intake, reduced renal concentrating ability, diabetes insipidus, and diuretic use; it is increased in dehydration due to fever, diaphoresis, vomiting, diarrhea, and medical conditions such as diabetes mellitus (diabetic ketoacidosis or hyperglycemic hyperosmolar nonketotic coma) and inappropriate secretion of antidiuretic hormone. The value ranges between 1.003 and 1.030, with the lower values suggesting more dilute urine (Pagana & Pagana, 2003).

BLOOD (SERUM) UREA NITROGEN

Blood urea nitrogen (BUN) is a laboratory test used to determine the kidney's ability to rid the blood of the nonprotein nitrogen (NPN) waste and urea, which results from protein breakdown (catabolism). The acceptable serum range for BUN is 10 to 20 mg/dL. For a more accurate test result, the patient should receive nothing by mouth (NPO) for 8 hours before blood sampling. If the BUN is elevated, preventive nursing measures should be instituted to protect the patient from possible disorientation or seizures.

BLOOD (SERUM) CREATININE

This test measures the amount of creatinine in the blood. Creatinine is a catabolic product of creatine, which is used in skeletal muscle contraction. The daily production of creatine, and subsequently creatinine, depends on muscle mass, which fluctuates very little. Creatinine, as with BUN, is excreted entirely by the kidneys and is therefore directly proportional to renal excretory function. Thus, with normal renal excretory function, the serum creatinine level should remain constant and normal. Only renal disorders—such as glomerulonephritis, pyelonephritis, acute tubular necrosis, and urinary obstruction—will cause an abnormal elevation in creatinine.

The serum creatinine test, as with BUN, is used to diagnose impaired renal function. However, unlike BUN, the creatinine level is affected very little by dehydration, malnutrition, or hepatic function. The creatinine level is interpreted in conjunction with the BUN. The acceptable serum creatinine range is 0.5 to 1.1 mg/dL (female), 0.6 to 1.2 mg/dL (male) (Pagana & Pagana, 2003).

CREATININE CLEARANCE

Creatinine, a nonprotein nitrogen (NPN) substance, is present in blood and urine. Creatinine is generated during muscle contraction and then excreted by glomerular filtration. Levels are directly related to muscle mass and are usually measured for a 24-hour period. During the testing period, excessive physical activity should be avoided. A fasting blood sample is drawn at the onset of testing and another at the conclusion. Discard the initial specimen and start the 24-hour timing at that point. All urine in the 24-hour period is collected because any deviation will alter test results. An elevation in serum levels with a decline in urine levels indicates renal disease. Normal ranges follow: **serum,** 0.5 to 1.1 mg/dL (female), 0.6 to 1.2mg/dL (male); **urine,** 87 to 107 mL/min (female), 107 to 139 mL/min (male), (Pagana & Pagana, 2003).

PROSTATE-SPECIFIC ANTIGEN

Prostate-specific antigen (PSA) is an organ-specific glycoprotein produced by normal prostatic tissue. Measurement of PSA has largely replaced prostatic acid phosphatase (PAP) because it is a more accurate test. Test results elevate with tissue manipulation; therefore a blood sample should be obtained before physical examination. Normal range is less than 4 ng (nanogram)/mL. Elevated PSA levels result from prostate cancer, benign prostatic hypertrophy, and prostatitis.

OSMOLALITY

Assessment of urine **osmolality,** which measures the weight of the solute compared with its own weight, may be preferred over specific gravity. Plasma osmolality may be done in conjunction with the urine sampling when pituitary disorders are suspected. Results provide information of the concentration ability of the kidney.

KIDNEY-URETER-BLADDER RADIOGRAPHY

A kidney-ureter-bladder (KUB) radiograph assesses the general status of the abdomen and evaluates the size, structure, and position of the urinary tract structures. No special preparation is necessary. The nurse should explain that the procedure involves changing position on the radiography table, which may be un-comfortably firm. Abnormal findings related to the urinary system may indicate tumors, calculi, glomerulonephritis, cysts, and other conditions.

INTRAVENOUS PYELOGRAM (IVP)/INTRAVENOUS UROGRAPHY (IVU)

IVP/IVU evaluates structures of the urinary tract, filling of the renal pelvis with urine, and transport of urine via the ureters to the bladder. It is vital that the nurse determine whether the patient has an allergy to iodine (or iodine-containing foods such as iodized salt, saltwater fish, seaweed products, vegetables grown in iodine-rich soils) because it is the base of the radiopaque dye that will be injected into a vein for this and other radiologic examinations. If the patient has previously had an allergic reaction, the physician may order a corticosteroid or an antihistamine to be administered before testing or, as an alternative, may order ultrasonography.

Because kidneys and ureters are positioned in the retroperitoneal space, gas and stool in the intestines interfere with radiographic visualization. Preparation usually includes a light supper, a non–gas-forming laxative, and NPO 8 hours before testing. In planning the testing regimen, the nurse should schedule urography before barium-based studies. When the dye is injected, the patient will experience a warm, flushing sensation and a metallic taste. During the procedure, vital signs will be monitored frequently. Radiographs will be taken at various intervals to monitor movement of the dye. Abnormal findings may indicate structural deviations, hydronephrosis, calculi within the urinary tract, polycystic kidney disease, tumors, and other conditions.

RETROGRADE PYELOGRAPHY

Retrograde pyelography involves examination of the lower urinary tract with a cystoscope under aseptic conditions. The urologist injects radiopaque dye directly into the ureters to visualize the upper urinary tract. Urine samples can be obtained directly from the renal pelvis. Additional retrograde studies include the following:

- **Retrograde cystography:** Radiopaque dye is injected through an indwelling catheter into the urinary bladder for visualization of the urinary bladder to evaluate its structure or to determine the cause of recurrent infections.
- **Retrograde urethrography:** A catheter is inserted and dye injected as with the cystography to assess the status of the urethral structure.

VOIDING CYSTOURETHROGRAPHY

Voiding cystourethrography is used in conjunction with other diagnostic studies to detect abnormalities of the urinary bladder and urethra. Preparation includes an enema before testing. An indwelling catheter is inserted into the urinary bladder, and dye is injected to outline the lower urinary tract. Radiographs are taken, and the catheter is then removed. The patient will be asked to void while radiographs are being taken. Some patients may experience embarrassment or anxiety related to the procedure and should be given the opportunity to express their feelings. Structural abnormalities, diverticula, and reflux into the ureter may be detected.

ENDOSCOPIC PROCEDURES

Endoscopic procedures are visual examinations of hollow organs using an instrument with a scope and light source. Because of the invasive nature of the procedure, an informed consent is necessary, and because the procedure is most often performed in the surgical suite, preoperative preparation is indicated (see Chapter 2). The urologist performs the procedure.

Cystoscopy is a visual examination to inspect, treat, or diagnose disorders of the urinary bladder and proximal structures. Patient preparation includes a description of the procedure. Usually the procedure is carried out using a local anesthetic after the patient has been sedated. Patient safety is paramount when the patient is sedated.

The patient will be placed in lithotomy position for the procedure, which may produce embarrassment and anxiety. The thought of a scope being passed while the patient is awake may intensify these feelings. The nurse should provide an opportunity for the patient to verbalize feelings.

The scope is passed under aseptic conditions after a local anesthetic is instilled into the urethra. The patient will experience a feeling of pressure as the scope is passed. Continuous fluid irrigation of the bladder is necessary to facilitate visualization. Care after the procedure includes hydration to dilute the urine. The first voiding after the procedure should be monitored, assessing time, amount, color, and any dysuria (painful or difficult urination). The nurse can expect the first voiding to occasionally be blood tinged due to the trauma of the procedure.

The urologist can perform a brush biopsy via a ureteral catheter during a cystoscopy. A nylon brush is inserted through the catheter to obtain specimens from the renal pelvis or calyces. Nephroscopy (renal endoscopy) is done using the percutaneous (through the skin) route and provides direct visualization of the upper urinary structures. The urologist can obtain biopsy or urine specimens or remove calculi.

RENAL ANGIOGRAPHY

Renal angiography aids in evaluation of blood supply to the kidneys, evaluates masses, and detects possible complications after kidney transplantation. The patient should have oral intake withheld the night before the procedure. The procedure requires the passing of a small radiopaque catheter into an artery (usually the femoral artery) to provide a port for the injection of radiopaque dye. Therefore, when the procedure is completed, the patient will need to lie flat in bed for several hours to minimize the risk of bleeding. The puncture site should be assessed for bleeding or hematoma, and the pressure dressing at the site should be maintained. Circulatory status of the involved extremity will be assessed every 15 minutes for 1 hour, then every 2 hours for 24 hours.

RENAL VENOGRAM

A renal venogram will provide information about the kidney's venous drainage. Access for the radiopaque catheter is the femoral vein. The patient will be monitored afterward for bleeding at the puncture site.

COMPUTED TOMOGRAPHY

A computed tomography (CT) scan differentiates masses of the kidney. Images are obtained by a computer-controlled scanner. A radiopaque dye may be injected to enhance the image. A serum urea and creatinine level are obtained prior to use of radiopaque dye. The dye is not used if inadequate renal function is noted. The nurse informs the patient that the table on which he or she is placed and the machine "taking pictures" will move at intervals and that it is very important to lie still. The CT body-scanning unit will take multiple cross-sectional pictures at several different sites, creating a three-dimensional map of the kidney structure. Visualization of the adrenals, bladder, and prostate may also be done.

MAGNETIC RESONANCE IMAGING (MRI)

MRI uses nuclear magnetic resonance as its source of energy to obtain a visual assessment of body tissues. There is no special preparation of the patient for MRI other than removal of all metal objects that might be attracted by the magnet. Patients with metal prostheses—such as heart valves, orthopedic screws, or cardiac pacemakers—cannot undergo MRI.

It should be emphasized that the examination area will be confining and that a repetitive "pounding" sound will be heard (somewhat like the sound of a muffled jackhammer). MRI can be used for various diagnoses of pathologic conditions of the renal system.

RENAL SCAN

A radionuclide tracer substance that will be taken up by renal tubular cells or excreted by the glomerular filtrate is injected intravenously. A series of computer-generated images will then be made. The scan will provide data related to functional parenchyma (the essential parts of an organ that are concerned with its function). No special preparation is needed. The nurse must check facility policy concerning the disposal of the patient's urine for the first 24 hours. The pregnant nurse should refrain from caring for this patient during this time.

ULTRASONOGRAPHY

Ultrasonography is a diagnostic tool that uses the reflection of sound waves to produce images of deep body structures. The nurse should inform the patient that the procedure requires the application of a conducting jelly on the skin over the area to be studied; this improves the transmission of sound waves. The sound waves are of a very high frequency that is inaudible to the human ear and will be converted into electrical impulses that will be photographed for study.

Ultrasonography of the kidney will visualize size, shape, and position of the kidney and delineate any irregularities in structure. Deviations from normal findings may indicate tumor, congenital anomalies, cysts, or obstructions. No special preparations are necessary.

TRANSRECTAL ULTRASOUND

Transrectal ultrasound instrumentation of the prostate gland provides clear prostatic tumor images that otherwise might go undiagnosed. Transrectal ultrasound–guided biopsy can be performed to provide samples of prostatic tissue from various areas with minimal discomfort to the patient.

RENAL BIOPSY

The kidney can be biopsied by an open procedure similar to other surgical procedures on the kidney or by the less invasive method of needle biopsy, also called a **percutaneous biopsy.** The patient should understand that pain may be experienced during the procedure and that instructions, such as holding the breath, must be followed. Bed rest is instituted for 24 hours after the procedure. Mobility is restricted to bathroom privileges for the next 24 hours, and gradual resumption of activities is allowed after 48 to 72 hours.

URODYNAMIC STUDIES

Urodynamic studies are indicated when neurological disease is suspected of being an underlying cause of incontinence. The studies evaluate detrusor reflex. The patient may experience embarrassment and slight discomfort. During cystometrogram a catheter is inserted into the bladder, then connected to a cystometer, which measures bladder capacity and pressure. The patient will be asked about sensations of heat, cold, and urge to void and will be instructed at times to void and change position.

Cholinergic and anticholinergic medications may be administered during urodynamic studies to determine their effects on bladder function. (A cholinergic drug, such as Urecholine, stimulates the atonic bladder; an anticholinergic drug, such as atropine, brings an overactive bladder to a more normal level or function.)

Associated testing includes rectal electromyography, which involves placement of an electrode and urethral pressure profile, which necessitates the use of a special catheter connected to a transducer to evaluate urethral pressures.

MEDICATION CONSIDERATIONS

The kidneys filter a wide range of water-soluble products from the blood, including medications. The kidney's effectiveness in removing certain medications from the blood may be affected by various conditions, such as renal disease, changes in the pH of urine, and age. Patients with renal disease will be administered reduced doses of medications to minimize further damage or drug toxicity. Alteration in urinary pH affects the absorption rate of certain medications. Older patients may have decreased physiological functioning, diminishing the kidneys' capacity for excretion of drugs. Diminished kidney function interferes with the filtration of water-soluble medications.

The medications included in this discussion are representative of those that act directly to effect the function of the kidney or are used to treat urinary disorders. Miscellaneous medications that affect the urinary system are included in Table 10-3.

DIURETICS TO ENHANCE URINARY OUTPUT

Diuretics are administered to enhance urinary output. This action is achieved by increasing the kidney's filtration of sodium, chloride, and water at different sites in the kidney. Diuretics are used in the management of a variety of disorders, such as heart failure and hypertension. Diuretics are classified by chemical structure, as well as the site and type of action on the kidney.

Thiazide Diuretics

Thiazide diuretics (*prototype,* chlorothiazide) act at the distal convoluted tubule to impair sodium and chloride reabsorption, leading to excretion of electrolytes and water. The thiazide diuretic, chlorothiazide (Diuril), effects electrolytes to cause hypokalemia (extreme potassium depletion in blood), hyponatremia (decreased sodium concentration in blood), and/or hypercalcemia (excessive amounts of calcium in blood). The effect on acid-base balance is hypochloremic alkalosis, which occurs from a deficiency of chloride. The main use is the management of systemic edema and the control of mild to moderate hypertension, although it may take a month to achieve the full antihypertensive effect. Diuril is contraindicated in anuria.

Loop (or High-Ceiling) Diuretics

Loop, or **high-ceiling, diuretics** act primarily in the ascending loop of Henle to inhibit tubular reabsorption of sodium and chloride. This group is the most potent of all diuretics and may lead to significant elec-

Table 10-3 | *Miscellaneous Medications that Affect the Urinary System*

MEDICATION	FUNCTIONAL CLASS	USE	SPECIAL CONSIDERATIONS
Oxybutynin chloride (Ditropan)	Spasmolytic	Reduce bladder spasms (neurogenic bladder)	Assess voiding pattern.
Bethanechol chloride (Urecholine)	Cholinergic stimulant	Urinary bladder stimulant (urinary retention, neurogenic atony)	Assess for hypotension.
Phenazopyridine (Pyridium, Urogesic)	Nonnarcotic analgesic	Anesthetic on mucosa of urinary tract	Assess decrease in urinary symptoms. Urine may turn red-orange. Report yellowing of sclera.
Flavoxate (Urispas)	Spasmolytic	Relieve nocturia, incontinence, dysuria	Assess decrease of urinary symptoms.
Finasteride (Proscar)	Androgen hormone inhibitor	Prevent benign prostatic hyperplasia	Monitor urine output. May cause impotence. Pregnant women should avoid handling crushed pills.
Tevazosin hydrochloride (Hytrin)	Antihpertensive and benign prostate hyperplasia agent	In benign prostatic hyperplasia, causes relaxation of smooth muscle and improves urine flow	Assess for hypotension. Assess voiding pattern.

trolyte depletion. These diuretics are effective to use for patients with impaired renal function.

The loop diuretic prototype, furosemide (Lasix), effects electrolytes to cause hypokalemia, hypochloremia, hyponatremia, hypocalcemia (abnormally low blood calcium), and/or hypomagnesia (decreased magnesium in the blood). The effect on acid-base balance is the development of hypochloremic alkalosis. Lasix is used in nephrotic syndrome, heart failure, and pulmonary edema. Side effects are those associated with rapid fluid loss: vertigo, hypotension, and possible circulatory collapse.

Potassium-Sparing Diuretics

Potassium-sparing diuretics act on the distal convoluted tubule to inhibit sodium reabsorption and potassium secretion. Potassium-sparing diuretics decrease the sodium-potassium exchange. Although the actions of these medications are varied, they all conserve potassium that is usually lost with sodium in diuresis. But, because they are weak, they are usually used in combination with other diuretics. Potassium-sparing diuretics are contraindicated in patients who experience hyperkalemia, because further retention of potassium could cause a fatal cardiac dysrhythmia. There are two types of potassium-sparing diuretics: aldosterone antagonists and nonaldosterone antagonists.

The aldosterone antagonist prototype, spironolactone (Aldactone), acts to block aldosterone in the distal tubule to promote potassium uptake in exchange for sodium secretion. Although it can be used in combination with other diuretics primarily in the treatment of

hypertension and edema, spironolactone is most frequently used for its potassium-sparing quality.

The nonaldosterone antagonist prototype, triamterene (Dyrenium), acts directly to reduce ion transportation in the tubule, though there is little diuretic effect. Triamterene is instead used to help limit the potassium-wasting effect of other diuretics.

Osmotic Diuretics

Osmotic diuretics act at the proximal convoluted tubule to increase plasma osmotic pressure, causing redistribution of fluid toward the circulatory vessels. Osmotic diuretics are used to manage edema, promote systemic diuresis in cerebral edema, decrease intraocular pressure, and improve renal function in acute renal failure. In acute renal failure, osmotics are used to attempt to prevent irreversible failure, but they are contraindicated in advanced states of renal failure.

The osmotic diuretic prototype, mannitol (Osmitrol), acts by increasing osmolarity of glomerular filtrate; decreasing reabsorption of water electrolytes; and increasing urinary output, sodium, and chloride, which actually has minimal effect on acid-base balance. Mannitol is used specifically to prevent/treat the oliguric phase of acute renal failure, promote systemic diuresis in cerebral edema, and decrease intraocular pressure. Careful assessment of the cardiovascular system before the administration of mannitol is essential because of the high risk of inducing heart failure. Avoid extravasation (escape of the medication from the blood vessel into the tissues), which may lead to tissue irritation or necrosis.

Carbonic Anhydrase Inhibitor Diuretics

The **carbonic anhydrase inhibitor diuretic** prototype, acetazolamide (Diamox), interferes with the bonding of water and carbon dioxide by the enzyme carbonic anhydrase (an enzyme present in red blood cells) at the proximal convoluted tubule. Although it has limited usefulness as a diuretic, acetazolamide is used to lower intraocular pressure.

Nursing Interventions

Because patients receiving diuretics often have complicated disease conditions such as heart failure and pulmonary edema, nursing interventions include monitoring for signs and symptoms of fluid overload: changes in pulse rate, respirations, cardiac sounds, and lung fields. Daily morning weights should be recorded for the patient receiving diuretics. Accurate intake and output (I&O) records should be kept, and blood pressure, pulse, and respirations should be documented 4 times a day until the medication is regulated and the vital signs stabilize. BUN, serum electrolytes, and urine are assessed as ordered. Diet instruction to the patient and family should include a warning to avoid overuse of salt in cooking or as a table additive. A number of salt substitutes are currently on the market; however, the long-term effects of those potassium preparations are not known and could further complicate the renal patient's condition. The use of most diuretics, with the exception of the potassium-sparing diuretics, requires adding daily potassium sources (e.g., baked potatoes, raw bananas, apricots, or navel oranges). In some cases it is necessary for the physician to order potassium supplements to be taken in combination with the diuretic.

It is important to note that as a diuretic is effective, there may be a resultant increase in the serum concentration of other medications. Careful monitoring of this potentiating effect is essential for safe nursing management to prevent toxicity from other medications. For example, as diuretics effectively decrease the volume of extracellular fluid, the serum level of digoxin may increase proportionately, resulting in digitoxicity. Special considerations should be used in the selection and management of diuretics in the treatment of children, adolescents, and the older adult.

MEDICATIONS FOR URINARY TRACT INFECTIONS

Certain antimicrobial agents are administered primarily to treat infections within the urinary tract. The appropriate medication is selected according to Gram-stain sensitivity of the organism.

Urinary antiseptics act to inhibit bacteria growth and are used to prevent and treat urethritis and cystitis. Caution should be used to determine if the patient is pregnant, because all of these agents have not been sufficiently tested for use during pregnancy. Urinary antiseptics are divided into four groups: quinolones, nitrofurantoins, methenamines, and fluoroquinolones. Examples of each group follow.

Quinolone. Nalidixic acid (NegGram) is used to treat UTIs caused by gram-negative microbes (e.g., *Escherichia coli* and *Proteus mirabilis*). The common side effects are drowsiness, vertigo, weakness, nausea, and vomiting. The use of nalidixic acid is contraindicated in renal impairment.

Nitrofurantoin. Nitrofuran compound (Macrodantin) is effective against both gram-positive and gram-negative microbes (e.g., *Streptococcus faecalis*, *E. coli*, and *P. mirabilis*) in the urinary tract. Common side effects are loss of appetite, nausea, and vomiting.

Methenamine. Methenamine mandelate (Mandelamine) suppresses fungi and gram-negative and gram-positive organisms (e.g., *E. coli*, staphylococci, and enterococci). Acidification of the urine with an acid-ash diet or other acidifiers to a pH of less than 5.5 is necessary for effective action. Methenamine mandelate is used for patients with chronic, recurrent urinary traction infections as a preventive measure after the use of antibiotics that clear the infection. Although side effects are rare, they may include nausea, vomiting, skin rash, and urticaria (hives).

Fluoroquinolone. Norfloxacin (Noroxin) is a broad-spectrum antibiotic effective against gram-positive and gram-negative organisms (e.g., *E. coli*, *P. mirabilis*, *Pseudomonas*, *Staphylococcus aureus*, *Staphylococcus epidermidis*, and others) used in the treatment of UTIs, gonorrhea, and gonococcal urethritis. Administration should be with a full glass of water 1 hour before or 2 hours after meals or the use of antacids.

Nursing Interventions

Precautions should be taken in the nursing care of patients receiving antibiotics for UTIs. The nurse should do each of the following:

1. Check all medications the patient is using for potential negative drug interactions.
2. Hydrate the patient to produce daily urine output of 2000 mL, unless contraindicated.
3. Instruct the patient to take all the medication, even though the symptoms may subside quickly.
4. Soothe skin irritations with cornstarch or a bath of bicarbonate of soda or dilute vinegar.
5. When indicated, teach the patient to use the acid-ash diet to help maintain a urine pH of 5.5.
6. Observe the patient receiving nalidixic acid (NegGram) for visual disturbances and offer appropriate assistance for ambulation or transfer.
7. Monitor the patient receiving nitrofurantoin (Macrodantin) for signs of allergic response (such as erythema, chills, fever, and dyspnea). If these signs or symptoms develop, medication should be discontinued and the physician notified (trial doses of this medication may be used

Box 10-2 *Acid-Ash and Alkaline-Ash Foods*

ACID-ASH FOODS*

Meat, whole grains, eggs, cheese, cranberries, prunes, and plums

ALKALINE-ASH FOODS

Milk, vegetables, fruits (except cranberries, prunes, and plums)

*Acid-ash diets should be supplemented with vitamins C and A and folic acid.

to detect possible allergic reaction before administering full dosage).

8. Report continuing signs of infection.

NUTRITIONAL CONSIDERATIONS

The nutritional needs of the patient with a urinary tract disorder vary with each disease process. Some general guidelines include provision of food choices and number of servings as recommended by the U.S. Department of Agriculture's MyPyramid nutrition planning tool (www.mypyramid.gov) and daily intake of 2000 mL of water, unless contraindicated. Unique nutritional requirements are discussed with each disorder. An example of unique dietary modifications with urinary lithiasis is noted in Box 10-2. The presence of other systemic diseases, such as diabetes mellitus, will require strict adherence to those restrictions as well.

MAINTAINING ADEQUATE URINARY DRAINAGE

Urine clears the body of waste materials and aids in the balance of electrolytes. Conditions that interfere with urinary drainage may create a health crisis. Therefore it is important to reestablish urine flow as soon as possible to prevent the buildup of toxins in the bloodstream.

Patients at risk for difficulty with urine elimination include patients who have undergone surgical procedures of the bladder, prostate, or vagina; patients with primary urological problems, such as urethral stricture; and those who are critically ill with multisystem problems.

Urinary catheters are used to maintain urine flow, to divert urine flow to facilitate healing postoperatively, to introduce medications by irrigation, and to dilate or prevent narrowing of some portions of the urinary tract. Catheters may be used for intermittent or continuous urinary drainage. Urinary catheters may be introduced into the bladder, ureter, or kidney. The type and size of urinary catheter used are determined by the location and cause of the urinary tract

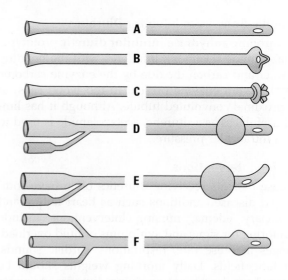

FIGURE **10-6** Different types of commonly used catheters. **A,** Simple urethral catheter. **B,** Mushroom or Pezzer (can be used for suprapubic catheterization). **C,** Winged-tip or malecot. **D,** Indwelling with inflated balloon. **E,** Indwelling with coudé tip. **F,** Three-way indwelling (the third lumen is used for irrigation of the bladder).

problem. Catheters are measured by the French (Fr) system. Urethral catheters range in size from 14 to 24 Fr for adult patients. Ureteral catheters are usually 4 to 6 Fr. The physician always inserts ureteral catheters. The nurse is usually responsible for the insertion of indwelling urethral catheters.

TYPES OF CATHETERS

Different types of catheters are used for different purposes (Figure 10-6). The **coudé catheter** has a tapered tip and is selected for ease of insertion when enlargement of the prostate gland is suspected. The curved stylet is used to assist the physician in the insertion of a urethral catheter in a male patient. The **Foley catheter** is designed with a balloon near its tip so the balloon may be inflated after insertion, holding the catheter in the urinary bladder for continuous drainage. **Malecot** and **Pezzer,** or **mushroom, catheters** are used to drain urine from the renal pelvis of the kidney. The **Robinson catheter** has multiple openings in its tip to facilitate intermittent drainage. **Ureteral catheters** are long and slender to pass into the ureters. The **whistle-tip catheter** has a slanted, larger orifice at its tip to be used if there is blood in the urine. The **cystostomy, vesicostomy,** or **suprapubic catheter** is introduced by the physician through the abdominal wall above the symphysis pubis. This catheter is used to divert urine flow from the urethra as needed to treat injury to the bony pelvis, urinary tract, or surrounding organs; strictures; or obstruction. The catheter is inserted via surgical incision or puncture of the abdominal and bladder walls with a trocar cannula. The catheter is connected to a sterile closed drainage system and secured to avoid accidental removal; the wound is covered with a sterile dressing. When the lower urinary tract has healed, the patient's ability to void is tested by clamping the catheter so the patient can try to void naturally. When the measured residual urine is consistently less than 50 mL, the catheter is usually removed and a sterile dressing is placed over the wound.

An **external (Texas** or **condom)** catheter is not actually a catheter but rather a drainage system connected to the external male genitalia. This noninvasive appliance is used for the incontinent male to minimize skin irritation from urine. The appliance is removed daily for cleansing and inspection of the skin. Use of the external catheter allows for a more normal lifestyle for the patient.

NURSING INTERVENTIONS AND PATIENT TEACHING

Nursing interventions for the patient with a urinary drainage system include employing a number of principles to prevent and detect infection and trauma:

1. Follow aseptic technique to avoid introduction of microorganisms from the environment. Never rest the collecting bag on the floor.
2. Record intake and output (I&O). For precision monitoring, such as hourly urine output, add a urometer to the drainage system. If urine output falls to less than 50 mL/hour, first check the drainage system for proper placement and function before contacting the physician.
3. Adequately hydrate the patient to flush the urinary tract.
4. Do not open the drainage system after it is in place except to irrigate the catheter, and then only with a specific order from the physician. It is important to maintain a closed system to prevent urinary infections.
5. Perform catheter care twice daily and as needed, using standard precautions. Each institution has a specific protocol for catheter care. Cleanse perineum with mild soap and warm water, rinse well, and pat dry. At times an antiseptic solution or ointment may be ordered to use at the catheter incision site.
6. Check the drainage system daily for leaks.
7. Avoid placement of the urinary drainage bag above the level of the catheter insertion, which would cause urine to reenter the drainage system and contaminate the urinary tract.
8. Prevent tension on the system or backflow of urine while transferring the patient.
9. Ambulate the patient if possible to facilitate urine flow. If the patient's activity must be restricted, turn and reposition every 1½ hours.
10. Avoid kinks or compression of the drainage tube that may cause pooling of the urine within the urinary tract. Gently coil excess tubing, secure with a clamp or pin to avoid dislodging the catheter, and release the tubing before transferring or repositioning the patient.
11. Gently inspect the entry site of the catheter for blood or exudate that may indicate trauma or infection. Observe the color and composition of the urine to note any blood or sediment. During drainage of the collection bag, note the presence of malodor.
12. Collect specimens from the catheter by cleansing the drainage port with alcohol, then withdrawing the urine by using a sterile adapter and a sterile 10-mL syringe, using standard precautions. Send the urine specimen immediately to the laboratory.
13. Report and record assessment findings and interventions initiated.

After the urinary catheter is removed, the patient may experience difficulty voiding until bladder tone and sensation return. If the patient complains of urinary retention, the nurse should institute the following measures:

1. If necessary, urination may be stimulated by running water, placing the patient's hands in water, or pouring water over the perineum. If the last method is attempted, the amount of water used should be subtracted in calculating the correct amount voided.
2. If the patient's condition permits, it is preferable for a female to sit on a bathroom stool or commode, and preferable for a male to stand to void.

The patient may experience some dribbling of urine after voiding as a result of dilation of the sphincter from the catheter. The time, amount, and color of the urine output should be recorded.

Nursing diagnoses and interventions for the patient with a urinary catheter include but are not limited to the following:

NURSING DIAGNOSES	NURSING INTERVENTIONS
Risk for trauma, related to insertion and maintenance of the catheter	Maintain sterile technique during insertion. Use smallest size of catheter possible. Lubricate catheter. Secure catheter to leg, as appropriate. Provide adequate fluids. Administer urinary analgesic as ordered. Allow enough slack in tubing for patient to move about freely while in bed. **Evaluation:** Patient reports no discomfort from catheter. Inspect insertion site to determine if area is clean and without signs of possible infection or bleeding.

Continued

NURSING DIAGNOSES	NURSING INTERVENTIONS
Risk for infection, related to invasive use of catheter	Use aseptic technique. Complete meticulous catheter care. Maintain closed urinary drainage system. Avoid placement of drainage bag above level of catheter insertion (meatus). Avoid reflux of urine. Encourage adequate fluid intake. Administer antimicrobials as ordered. **Evaluation:** Temperature remains within normal limits. Patient reports no burning, etc. Color, odor, and clarity of urine normal.

The patient should be instructed about proper transfer from bed, chair, or stretcher and taught the principles of catheter care. Fluid intake should be encouraged to flush the urinary system.

Self-Catheterization

Self-catheterization may be the intervention of choice for the patient who experiences spinal cord injury or other neurological disorders that interfere with urinary elimination. Intermittent self-catheterization promotes independent function for the patient. At home there is less risk of cross-contamination than in the hospital, so the catheterization procedure can be safely modified as a clean technique, although the nurse will instruct the patient using strict surgical asepsis in the hospital because of the risk of infection there. The need for the patient to be alert for signs and symptoms of infection and to have periodic evaluations by the physician should be emphasized. Institutional guidelines for catheter insertion technique should be followed.

Bladder Training

Bladder training involves developing the use of the muscles of the perineum to improve voluntary control over voiding; bladder training may be modified for different problems. In preparation for the removal of a urethral catheter, the physician may order a clamp/unclamp routine to improve bladder tone. For the patient with stress incontinence, the muscles of the perineum are exercised to assist in stopping urine flow. The nurse instructs the patient to perform **Kegel,** or **pubococcygeal, exercises** by tightening the muscles of the perineal floor. The patient can perhaps develop awareness of the appropriate muscle group by trying to stop the flow of urine during voiding. Having identified the correct muscles and the feeling of their con-

traction, the patient can be directed to tighten the muscles of the perineum, holding that tension for 10 seconds, then relaxing for 10 seconds. The exercises should be done initially in groups of 10, building to groups of 20, four times a day. Because muscle control develops gradually, it may take 4 to 6 weeks to develop control of leakage.

For habit training, a voiding schedule is established. The nurse monitors the patient's voiding for a few days to identify patterns, or schedules voiding times to correlate with the patient's activities. Typical voiding times are on arising, before each meal, and at bedtime. The patient is assisted to void as scheduled. After a few days, the scheduled voiding pattern is evaluated by identifying its effectiveness in keeping the patient continent. The schedule is modified until continence is established. Fluid intake and medications may influence voiding patterns (i.e., the patient may need to void 30 minutes after the ingestion of coffee or furosemide in response to the diuretic effect). Reduction of fluid intake during the hours preceding bedtime may aid in keeping the patient dry during sleep.

PROGNOSIS

The outcome of patient treatment and nursing care planning/intervention for the patient with urinary disorders is dependent on multiple variables: age, pre-existing health conditions, general health status, complications, compliance, and available family and community support.

DISORDERS OF THE URINARY SYSTEM

ALTERATIONS IN VOIDING PATTERNS
URINARY RETENTION
Etiology/Pathophysiology

Urinary retention is the inability to void even with an urge to void. It may be acute or chronic. With urinary retention the patient may not be able to empty the bladder, creating urinary stasis and increasing the possibility of infection.

Urinary retention may occur from a variety of causes: secondarily in response to stress; interference with the sphincter muscles during surgery to the perineum; occlusion of the urethra by calculi, infection, or tumor; medication side effects; or perineal trauma secondary to vaginal delivery. With chronic urinary retention the bladder capacity may be exceeded and the urine may overflow the bladder, causing incontinence.

Clinical Manifestations

The signs and symptoms of urinary retention are sometimes vague and easily overlooked. The bladder becomes increasingly distended and may be palpated above the symphysis pubis. Urinary retention may cause the patient considerable discomfort and anxiety.

Assessment

Collection of **subjective data** includes noting patient complains of frequency with or without symptoms of burning, urgency, nocturia, and occasionally acute discomfort. Initial symptoms may not seem to be directly associated with urinary retention.

Collection of **objective data** includes assessing urinary bladder distention: palpable ovoid (egg-shaped) bladder arising suprapubically, voiding frequently, voiding small amounts, and episodes of incontinence. Patients with diminished sensorium, as from spinal cord injury or organic brain disorder, may show signs of restlessness and irritability without direct complaints about difficulty voiding.

Medical Management

Mechanical methods, such as the use of urinary catheters or the surgical release of obstructions, may be necessary for the treatment of urinary retention. Urinary analgesics and antispasmodics are administered as prescribed to enhance patient (relaxation) comfort.

Nursing Interventions

The primary goal of nursing intervention is the reinstitution of normal voiding patterns. Regardless of the pathologic findings and medical intervention, the nurse can greatly aid in the return of adequate voiding by supporting the patient's efforts with a private, relaxed environment. Bladder training approaches may assist the patient to empty the bladder. Warm showers or sitz baths may promote relaxation of the abdominal, gluteal, and sphincter muscles. Warm beverages may help the patient relax. If possible, the patient should be permitted whatever position is preferred for voiding: for the female, sitting on a commode or bathroom stool is best; for the male, standing may be more natural.

When continence is established, the patient may be catheterized intermittently to determine whether the bladder is emptying. The patient should void, and the amount should be measured. The patient should be catheterized immediately after the voiding, and the amount should be measured. The amount retained in the bladder is residual urine and should be less than 50 mL. If the underlying pathologic condition remains unchanged, this patient may still be at risk for again developing retention. It is therefore important to teach the patient and/or primary caretaker to be observant for signs and symptoms of urinary retention and to notify the physician immediately if they return.

Nursing diagnosis and interventions for the patient with urinary retention include but are not limited to the following:

NURSING DIAGNOSES	NURSING INTERVENTIONS
Impaired urinary elimination, related to sensory/motor impairment, neuromuscular impairment, or mechanical trauma	Establish urinary drainage. Develop voiding schedule. Teach Kegel exercises. Assist with skin care. Suggest use of protective clothing. Engage patient in social activities. Teach importance of adequate fluid intake. **Evaluation:** Patient verbalizes understanding of factors that alter urinary pattern. Patient reports return of normal urination pattern.

URINARY INCONTINENCE

Urinary incontinence (UI) may be the most common health problem in women. Although stress incontinence is not the only cause of UI, it is the one most frequently mentioned. Stress incontinence is the involuntary loss of urine during physical exertion or when coughing, sneezing, or laughing. Because of embarrassment, stress UI may be underreported, and thus its sociologic and economic influence is impossible to assess. However, UI is a major reason older adults are admitted to long-term care facilities.

Etiology/Pathophysiology

Urinary incontinence is the involuntary loss of urine from the bladder. The patient may be totally incontinent, have dribbling, or experience leakage while lifting or sneezing (stress incontinence).

Incontinence may arise as a complication of many disorders, such as infection within the urinary tract, loss of sphincter control, or sudden change in the pressure within the abdomen. Incontinence may be permanent, as with spinal cord trauma, or temporary, as with pregnancy. Women with weakened structures of the pelvic floor are prone to stress incontinence. Although incontinence may occur in patients of any age, loss of control of urination is a particular problem for the older adult.

Physical activities that involve exertion such as heavy lifting, jobs that require long periods of standing, and sports that include high-impact activity may increase an individual's risk for UI.

Urinary incontinence may also result from physiologic conditions such as obesity, chronic lung disease, smoking, pelvic floor injury, and surgery.

Lack of estrogen in postmenopausal women contributes to atrophy of the vaginal and urethral walls with subsequent loss of muscle tone that may result in postvoiding urine retention and possible prolapse of the bladder.

Clinical Manifestations

The cardinal sign of urinary incontinence is the involuntary loss of urine, which may or may not be the primary reason the patient seeks treatment.

Assessment

Collection of **subjective data** includes seeking information concerning the patient's inability to control the urine. A woman may complain of urine leaking when she coughs, sneezes, lifts heavy objects, or during intercourse.

Collection of **objective data** includes the nurse being alert for clues that the patient is experiencing difficulty controlling the flow of urine. The assessment guidelines should be followed to clarify the patient's complaints. Although more common in women, UI is a common symptom for men who have benign prostatic hypertrophy, and should be included in the assessment.

Medical Management

The management of incontinence depends on the underlying cause. If the problem arises from a disorder within the neck of the bladder, surgical repair may be necessary. In certain patients, stress incontinence related to sphincter weakness may be treated with collagen implant injections. The patient may require temporary or permanent urinary diversion or management with an indwelling catheter. New appliances and drugs on the market are being used for the control of UI.

The incontinence pessary, which is inserted into the vagina and designed to support the bladder, may help manage episodes of stress incontinence in some women. Close-fitting absorbent pads may be effective in managing mild leakage.

Estrogen replacement for the treatment of UI is controversial and its reported effectiveness is varied. Topical administration of prednisone and estrogen may help to restore loss of turgor and elasticity of the vaginal submucosa.

Transdermal oxybutynin (Oxytrol) is effective in reducing the symptoms of an overactive bladder with few side effects. This medication is being evaluated for use by the U.S. Food and Drug Administration (FDA).

A new self-catheterization system is available for patients who must maintain intermittent self-catheterization. The Self-Cath Closed System is designed for patient convenience and minimization of bacterial contamination.

An artificial urinary sphincter is a surgical option to reestablish continence, though there is controversy over its use.

Nursing Interventions

The incontinent patient may reduce fluid intake to decrease voiding, but without adequate fluids, urine may become more concentrated, irritating the bladder mucosa and increasing the urge to urinate. Bladder training exercises should be taught to improve the tone of the perineal muscles. Establish a 2-hour schedule for the patient to go to the bathroom. Once continence has been achieved, the schedule goal may be raised to 3 hours. Use of protective undergarments may help keep the patient and the patient's clothing dry. For the female patient, Kegel exercises are helpful; 10 repetitions, 5 to 10 times a day is suggested to improve muscle tone.

Incontinence pads of different absorbancy are available in most grocery stores and pharmacies. They can add to the patient's confidence to participate in social activities.

Alcoholic and caffeinated drinks stimulate urgency and urination; advise the patient not to drink too much liquid just before bedtime.

Many patients who are incontinent have low self-esteem. The nurse can be supportive by listening, encouraging the patient to express feelings, and providing kind reassurances. Never scold!

NEUROGENIC BLADDER
Etiology/Pathophysiology

Neurogenic bladder means the loss of voluntary voiding control, resulting in urinary retention or incontinence. Neurogenic bladder is caused by a lesion of the nervous system that interferes with normal nerve conduction to the urinary bladder. The lesion may be caused by a congenital anomaly (e.g., spina bifida), a neurological disease (e.g., multiple sclerosis), or trauma (as in spinal cord injury). The two types of neurogenic bladder are **spastic** and **flaccid.**

Spastic (reflex or automatic) bladder is caused by a lesion above the voiding reflex arc (upper motor neuron) that results in a loss of sensation to void and a loss of motor control. The bladder wall then atrophies, decreasing bladder capacity. Release of the urine occurs on reflex, with little or no conscious control.

A flaccid (atonic, nonreflex) bladder, caused by a lesion of a lower motor neuron, continues to fill and distend, with pooling of urine and incomplete emptying. Because of the accompanying loss of sensation, the patient may not even experience discomfort that would indicate retention.

Clinical Manifestations

Identification of the disease process is the first step in assessing the potential problem of neurogenic bladder. Prevention of complications is a major concern; infection occurs from urinary stasis and repeated catheterization. Retention of urine may lead to backup of urine (reflux) into the upper urinary tract and to the distention of the structures of the urinary tract.

Assessment

Collection of **subjective data** includes noting patient complaints consistent with the pathophysiology of the neurogenic bladder: diaphoresis, flushing and nausea prior to reflex incontinence, or infrequent voiding.

Collection of **objective data** involves investigating the urinary status of the patient at risk for neurogenic bladder; this includes patients with a congenital anomaly, a neurological disease, or a spinal cord injury. The patient with a spastic bladder will experience urinary incontinence, whereas the patient with a flaccid bladder will describe infrequent voiding.

Diagnostic Tests

Diagnostic testing is completed to assess the type and extent of damage to the urinary tract; chemistry studies monitor change in BUN and creatinine levels. Radiographic studies outline structural changes that occur.

Medical Management

Patients identified at risk for neurogenic bladder should be closely monitored. Assessment of urinary function should be started early in the course of treatment and antibiotics given to treat signs of infection. The patient is aided by the use of parasympathomimetic medication (e.g., bethanechol chloride [Urecholine]) to increase the contractility of the bladder. It may be necessary for the patient to use intermittent self-catheterization or a urinary collection system if continence is not achieved.

Sacral nerve modulation (sacral neuromodulation) and stimulation. There are a number of electronic devices to modulate nerve impulses that are being used experimentally and in clinical practice for treating various bladder problems: urinary frequency, urgency, incontinence, chronic pain, and interstitial cystitis.

Sacral nerve stimulation for urinary urge incontinence is the use of a permanently implantable electrical stimulation device to change neuronal activity in the sacral efferent and afferent nerves to reduce urinary urge incontinence.

The Interstim device, marketed by Medtronic Inc., delivers continuous low-level electrical impulses to the bladder and urethral sphincters via the sacral nerve. It corrects urinary incontinence by modulating the neural reflexes, reducing stimulation to an overactive bladder, or boosting stimulation to an underactive one. The action of the impulses is unknown.

Four electrodes are connected to a battery-operated generator. The wire is inserted into the sacral foramen through a 2-cm incision. The end of the wire is tunneled across subcutaneous tissue, exits on the patient's back, and is connected to a temporary generator attached to the outside of the body. The patient tests this temporary implant for 1 to 2 weeks. If the patient achieves 50% continence, a permanent implant is put in place.

Nursing Interventions and Patient Teaching

The goal for management of the patient with neurogenic bladder is to establish urinary elimination and prevent complications. Because of the disturbance of neurological function, it may not be possible to reinstate normal voiding function. The patient with a spastic bladder may be placed on a bladder training program, with self-stimulation used every 2 hours to empty the bladder: the patient tries to initiate voiding using bladder compressions achieved by applying pressure to the abdomen suprapubically or by digital stimulation of the anal sphincter. Residual urine is then measured by catheterization. As the patient becomes more proficient in emptying the bladder, the times between the catheterizations are increased until voiding is achieved independently.

It is important to educate the patient to be alert for signs of the bladder becoming distended.

Management of the patient with a flaccid bladder is similar. The patient may be placed on a 2-hour voiding schedule for bladder training. Issues of self-esteem are crucial for this patient to remain in social settings. The nurse should provide a supportive, sensitive environment for the patient to discuss ways to adapt to an altered self-image.

URINARY TRACT INFECTIONS

A urinary tract infection (UTI) is the presence of microorganisms in any urinary system structure. **Bacteriuria** (presence of bacteria in the urine) is the most common of all nosocomial infections; most are associated with the use of urinary catheters. UTIs are common in older patients, related to bladder obstruction, insufficient bladder emptying, decreased bactericidal secretions of the prostate, and increased perineal soiling in females. Immobility, sensory impairment, and multiple organ impairment may increase the probability of infection in the older adult. Females are more susceptible to UTIs than males because the urethra is short and proximal to the vagina and rectum.

Etiology/Pathophysiology

UTIs are caused by pathogens that enter the urinary tract, with or without the presence of symptoms. Normally the flushing of the urinary tract with urine is sufficient to keep pathogens washed away. However, some conditions interfere with this process; urinary obstruction, neurogenic bladder, ureterovesical or urethrovesical reflux, sexual intercourse, and catheterization may introduce bacteria into the urinary system. Many chronic health states predispose the patient to a UTI: diabetes mellitus, multiple sclerosis, spinal cord injuries, hypertension, and diseases of the kidney.

Changes in urinary tract homeostasis allow the concentration of bacteria and increase the risk of infection. The patient with a compromised immune system does not seem to be predisposed to UTI infections, but once the infection is established, that patient will have difficulty recovering. Infections of the lower urinary tract increase the risk of infection of the upper urinary tract, especially if untreated.

Gram-negative microorganisms (e.g., *E. coli, Klebsiella, Proteus,* or *Pseudomonas*) that commonly infect the urinary tract are usually from the gastrointestinal tract and ascend through the urinary meatus. Normally the body's defenses keep infections in check and clear them from the system before signs and symptoms appear. If there is incomplete emptying of the bladder or reflux of urine, the retained urine supports growth of bacteria.

Clinical Manifestations

The common signs and symptoms associated with UTI are urgency, frequency, burning on urination, and microscopic to gross (visible without aid of microscope) hematuria. UTIs are identified by the location of the infection: urethritis (urethra), cystitis (urinary bladder), pyelonephritis (kidney), and prostatitis (inflammation of the prostate gland). Infections of the bladder are said to be *lower* UTIs, whereas infections of the kidneys are *upper* UTIs.

Assessment

Collection of **subjective data** includes noting patient complaints of pain or burning on urination, urgency, frequency, and nocturia (excessive urination at night). The patient may also have related asthenia (a general feeling of tiredness and listlessness). Abdominal discomfort, perineal pain, or back pain may be present, depending on the extent of the disease process and site of infection.

Collection of **objective data** involves palpation of the lower abdomen, which may produce discomfort over the urinary bladder. Urine may be cloudy or blood tinged.

Diagnostic Tests

Urine culture and bacteriologic tests confirm the diagnosis. For patients with repeated UTIs or systemic disease, more detailed urologic studies, such as an IVP and a voiding cystogram, are completed to assess the extent of involvement and damage to the structures of the urinary tract. Microscopic inspection of the urine often reveals bacteria, hematuria (blood in the urine), and pyuria (pus in the urine). Prostatitis is confirmed by patient history and culture of prostatic fluid or tissue.

Medical Management

The goal of medical management is to eliminate bacteria from the urinary tract, thereby relieving symptoms, preventing damage to renal structures, and preventing spread of infection to other body systems. Antiinfective medications are prescribed in either oral or parenteral single or multiple doses, depending on the severity of the infection, microbial sensitivity, cost, and the medications the patient can tolerate. Urinary antiseptics, such as methenamine mandelate (Mandelamine), may be used prophylactically in recurrent infections. Some of these medications are instilled directly into the bladder. If the infection is complicated by obstruction, that obstruction should be removed. If

the patient experiences neurogenic bladder or other retention, the use of intermittent catheterization permits urinary drainage (see Complementary & Alternative Therapies box).

Nursing Interventions

Nursing intervention should be supportive, with patient education for adequate hydration and hygiene. Because there is a strong tendency for these infections to recur by either reinfection or persistent infection, patient education must include early detection. Comfort measures include a regimen of antiinfective agents, urinary analgesics (e.g., phenazopyridine [Pyridium]), adequate fluid intake, and perineal care. If treatment is effective, the patient should receive relief quickly. Infection may spread from the urinary system to other parts of the body. **Urosepsis** is septic poisoning due to retention and absorption of urinary products in the tissues.

Because of the high incidence of nosocomial urinary tract infections, regular staff in-service review of basic procedures for catheter insertion and maintenance is important. Patient education for those who practice self-catheterization should include return demonstration to evaluate the success of maintaining clean technique.

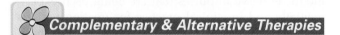
Complementary & Alternative Therapies

Urinary Disorders

- Cranberry (cranberry plus, ultra cranberry) has been used to prevent urinary tract infections (UTIs), particularly in women prone to recurrent infection. It has also been known to treat acute UTI. Patients should be monitored for lack of therapeutic effect.
- Echinacea stimulates the immune system and treats UTI. Patients with HIV infections, including AIDS and patients with tuberculosis, collagen disease, multiple sclerosis, or other autoimmune disease should avoid use. Should not be used in place of antibiotic therapy.
- Sea holly (*Eryngium campestre*) aboveground plant parts have a mild diuretic effect. Roots have antispasmodic effect. Aboveground parts are used in UTI and prostatitis; roots are used to treat kidney and bladder calculi, renal colic, kidney and urinary tract inflammation, and urinary retention.
- Nettle (*Utrica dioica*) is presently being investigated as an irrigation for the urinary tract and also to treat benign prostatic hypertrophy (BPH). Patients with fluid retention caused by reduced cardiac or renal activity should not use this herb.
- Caffeine increases urine production.
- Some believe that acupuncture applied to the abdominal meridian may help relieve cystitis.
- Some advocate that a massage with diluted rosemary, juniper, or lavender may aid in relieving pain associated with cystitis.

URETHRITIS

Etiology/Pathophysiology

Urethritis, inflammation of the urethra, is classified by the presence or absence of gonorrhea. Nongonorrheal urethritis is called **nonspecific urethritis (NSU).** NSU may be caused by monilial or trichomonal infections in women. Bacteria are present normally in the urethra but do not cause problems unless the integrity of the mucous membrane or tissues is interrupted, as when a catheter is in place or trauma has occurred.

Clinical Manifestations

The clinical manifestations include inflammation of the urethra with pus formation in the mucus-forming glands within the lining of the urethra. Gonorrheal urethritis is evidenced by acute infection of the mucous membrane of the urethra that causes a purulent exudate from the meatus; the patient feels discomfort and burning on urination.

Assessment

Collection of **subjective data** should be done with an awareness that the patient may be asymptomatic or may complain of dysuria, urethral pruritus, and urethral discharge. Women may complain of vaginal discharge or vulvar irritation.

Collection of **objective data** includes light palpation of the lower abdomen, which may produce discomfort over the urinary bladder. Inspection of the urethra may reveal purulent exudates or inflammation. Culture and sensitivity may be ordered; follow the procedure for your institution.

Diagnostic Tests

These are usually limited to a Gram stain of the exudate to identify the pathogen.

Medical Management

The first step in medical management is prevention of injury to the urethra during catheterization or sexual intercourse. Comfort measures include a regimen of antibiotics, adequate fluid intake to flush the system, and special care of the perineum using clean technique.

Patients with continuous catheter drainage have used either a bedside bag or a leg bag for urine collection. Studies are under way to test a drainage system designed for the bag to be worn around the waist and can be maintained closed for 24 hours. Other product benefits from this experimental drainage system include improved ambulation, increased activities of daily living (ADLs), and increased social and mental well-being.

Nursing Interventions

These should focus on patient education: avoid sexual activity until the infection clears; take all medications, especially antibiotics, to ensure the infection is resolved; use condoms for protection from reinfection; and instruct sexual partners to be evaluated for urethritis to prevent continuing infections.

CYSTITIS

Etiology/Pathophysiology

Cystitis is an inflammation of the wall of the urinary bladder, usually caused by urethrovesical reflux, introduction of a catheter or similar instrument, or perhaps contamination from feces. Cystitis is most common in women, due to ease of entrance of pathogens through the short urethra, even during voiding.

The most common microorganism causing acute cystitis is *E. coli.* Conflicting data exist about the role of bubble baths, clothing, and hygiene in increasing the risk of cystitis in women. Cystitis in men usually occurs secondary to another infection, such as prostatitis or epididymitis.

Clinical Manifestations

The common signs and symptoms associated with cystitis are dysuria, urinary frequency, and pyuria.

Assessment

Collection of **subjective data** includes assessment of the lower abdomen, which may produce discomfort over the urinary bladder. Patient complaints include burning on urination, dysuria (painful or difficult urination), frequency, urgency, and nocturia.

Collection of **objective data** includes a clean-catch or catheterized urinalysis with culture and sensitivity to aid in confirming the diagnosis and in determining the appropriate treatment.

Diagnostic Tests

Microscopic inspection of the urine often reveals bacteria and hematuria. A voiding cystogram may be used to identify reflux of urine into the bladder. Diagnosis is confirmed by a clean-catch, midstream urinalysis that reveals a bacterial count greater than 100,000 organisms/mL.

Medical Management

For cystitis without the complications of obstruction or other underlying pathologic conditions, medical management consists of short-term therapy with an antiinfective agent. If the treatment is effective, the patient should receive relief quickly. A repeat urinalysis 1 to 3 days after initiation of the medication confirms the effectiveness of the intervention.

Nursing Interventions and Patient Teaching

This should focus on teaching because there is a strong tendency for these infections to recur by either reinfection or persistent infection. The patient should be encouraged to drink 2000 mL of fluid per day. Accurate I&O should be recorded.

Teaching must include early detection. Long-term prophylaxis with low doses of medication may be necessary. Currently available is a simple urine test, Chem Strip LN, which allows the patient to test the urine at the first sign of infection and to call the physician for a prescription (see Safety Considerations).

Prognosis

Successful treatment is contingent upon the patient's ability to maintain adequate flushing of the urinary tract and completion of the antiinfective cycle.

INTERSTITIAL CYSTITIS
Etiology/Pathophysiology

Interstitial cystitis (IC) is a chronic pelvic pain disorder with recurring discomfort or pain in the urinary bladder and surrounding region. It affects predominantly middle-aged white women. The pathophysiology is unknown, but bacteria do not trigger it. Instead, it seems to be caused by a breech in the bladder's protective mucosal lining that allows urine to seep through to the bladder wall, resulting in pain, inflammation, and small vessel bleeding. Because IC cannot be diagnosed with a urine test, other urinary conditions are ruled out. Small bleeding sites may be visualized via endoscopy.

Clinical Manifestations

The common signs and symptoms associated with IC are similar to those of cystitis: dysuria, urinary frequency, microscopic bleeding.

Assessment

Collection of **subjective data** includes complaints of discomfort over the urinary bladder, dysuria, frequency, urgency, and nocturia.

Collection of **objective data** includes assessment of the lower abdomen, which may produce discomfort over the urinary bladder, as well as the lower quad-

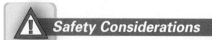

Safety Considerations

Cystitis

- Teach the female to cleanse perineal area anteriorly to posteriorly to prevent contamination of pathogens (especially *Escherichia coli*) from the rectum to the short urethra.
- Encourage drinking 2000 mL of liquids per day unless contraindicated.
- Instruct the patient to take all the prescribed medications even though symptoms may subside quickly.
- Teaching must include early detection. Currently available is a sample urine test, ChemStrip LN, which allows the patient to test the urine at the first sign of infection of the bladder and call the physician for a prescription.
- Teach patients, particularly females, to drink cranberry juice to help prevent urinary infections.

rants of the abdomen. A clean-catch midstream sample for urinalysis is used to rule out infection.

Cystoscopy and tissue biopsy are used to establish a differential diagnosis.

Medical Management

Intersitital cystitis is difficult to treat. Medications are prescribed for pain and inflammation. Current research investigations of the use of low-dose cyclosporine A (Neoral, Sandimmune), doxycycline (Vibramycin), and pentosan polysulfate sodium show favorable results in relieving symptoms.

Surgical interventions include studies of the effect of sacral nerve root stimulation via implantation of electrodes; cystectomy, with the creation of a urostomy; and urinary diversion. It is important to note that some patients continue to experience pain even after surgery.

Nursing Interventions and Patient Teaching

Nursing interventions should focus on pain control and comfort measures. Because all medications have side effects, patients must consult their physician before taking any prescription or over-the-counter medication. Pelvic floor exercise may be helpful in decreasing urgency and nocturia. Although there is no special nutritional regimen, some patients identify foods that seem to aggravate their symptoms. Patients may be asked to keep a daily bladder diary; this information can be used to make treatment decisions. The patient and significant other(s) will need psychosocial support to face an uncertain outcome.

Patient information is available at the National Institute of Diabetes and Digestive and Kidney Diseases (NIDDK) at http://kidney.niddk.nih.gov.

Prognosis

Only about half of the patients with IC recover fully. Until researchers find a cause and an effective treatment, symptoms will continue.

PROSTATITIS
Etiology/Pathophysiology

Prostatitis, defined as inflammation and/or infection of the prostate gland, is actually a group of diseases. Bacterial prostatitis is caused by infectious organisms such as *Pseudomonas* and *Streptococcus faecalis* traveling up the urethra. Nonbacterial prostatitis may result from a variety of reasons related to occlusion of the urethra (e.g., enlargement of the prostate gland).

Prostatodynia (pain in the prostate gland) presents with neither inflammation nor infection but demonstrates the other symptoms typical of prostatitis.

Clinical Manifestations

The patient experiences a burning sensation, discomfort in the perineum, dysuria, frequency, and urgency. Edema of the prostate gland may serve as an obstruction, causing urinary retention as a complication to the prostatitis. Pooling of urine may also foster stone formation. Other complications are epididymitis, pyelonephritis, and bacteremia (the presence of bacteria in the blood). Although the patient may be asymptomatic, the symptoms of acute bacterial prostatitis are often the same as a UTI, with pain in the low back, perineum, or rectum. Because of a potential for relapse, the condition may become chronic.

Diagnostic Tests

Diagnosis is confirmed by patient history and culture of prostatic fluid or tissue. The expressed prostate secretion (EPS) is considered useful in the diagnosis of prostatitis. EPS is obtained using a premassage and postmassage test. The patient is asked to void into a specimen cup just before and just after a vigorous prostate massage. Prostatic massage (for EPS) should be avoided if acute bacterial prostatitis is suspected, because compression is extremely painful and can increase the risk of bacterial spread. Transabdominal ultrasound or MRI may be done to rule out an abscess on the prostate. A urinalysis and urine culture as well as a WBC and blood cultures may also be performed.

Assessment

Collection of **subjective data** includes noting complaints of chills and low back and perineal pain. Chronic bacterial prostatitis causes dysuria; urgency; frequency; nocturia; and pain in the lower abdomen or back, perineum, or genitalia.

Collection of **objective data** involves assessing for elevated temperature and palpation of the prostate gland by the physician by rectal examination, which may reveal the prostate to be firm, edematous, and tender.

Medical Management

If the condition is infectious, management focuses on control of the infection and prevention of the complications of abscess formation or bacteremia. Antibiotics commonly used for acute and chronic bacterial prostatitis include trimethoprim-sulfamethoxazole (Bactrim), ciprofloxin (Cipro), and floxacin (Floxin). Doxycycline (Vibramycin) or tetracycline may be prescribed for those patients with multiple sex partners. Antibiotics are usually given orally for up to 4 weeks for acute bacterial prostatitis. However, if the patient has high fever or other signs of impending sepsis, hospitalization and intravenous antibiotics are prescribed. Patients with chronic bacterial prostatitis are given oral antibiotic therapy for 4 to 16 weeks.

Anti-inflammatory agents are the most common agents used for pain control in prostatitis, but these provide only moderate pain relief. Opioid analgesics can be used, but because this pain can be chronic in nature, the use of opioids should be approached cautiously. The pain resolves as the infection is treated.

Nursing Interventions and Patient Teaching

Regardless of the pathologic basis, comfort measures used are analgesics, sitz baths, and stool softeners to reduce pain, edema, spasm, and straining pressure in the pelvis.

Teaching includes the medication regimen. Sexual arousal and intercourse should be avoided in acute prostatitis so the prostate can rest; however, intercourse may be beneficial in the treatment of chronic prostatitis. Follow-up with the physician is crucial because of the likelihood that the disorder will become chronic.

Prognosis

Prostatitis is difficult to cure and requires long periods of antibiotic treatment. The patient may not see the need of continuing antibiotic therapy after the initial symptoms have subsided. It is imperative that he understand the importance of taking all the antibiotic prescribed.

PYELONEPHRITIS
Etiology/Pathophysiology

Pyelonephritis is an inflammation of the structures of the kidney—the renal pelvis, renal tubules, and interstitial tissue. Pyelonephritis is almost always caused by *E. coli.*

Pyelonephritis is usually seen in association with pregnancy; chronic health problems, such as diabetes mellitus or polycystic or hypertensive kidney disease; insult to the urinary tract from catheterization; or infection, obstruction, or trauma. Careful management of these disorders is important to prevent pyelonephritis.

The kidney becomes edematous and inflamed, and the blood vessels are congested. The urine may be cloudy and contain pus (pyuria), mucus, and blood. Small abscesses may form in the kidney.

Clinical Manifestations

Acute pyelonephritis may be unilateral or bilateral, causing chills, fever, prostration, and flank pain. Repeated episodes of pyelonephritis lead to a chronic disease pattern, with atrophy of the kidney as the nephrons are destroyed. Studies have also shown that chronic pyelonephritis may develop in association with other renal diseases unrelated to infection processes. Azotemia (the retention in the blood of excessive amounts of nitrogenous compounds) develops if enough nephrons are nonfunctional.

Assessment

Collection of **subjective data** includes noting that in acute pyelonephritis the patient will become acutely ill, with malaise and pain in the costovertebral angle (CVA) (one of two angles that outline a space over the kidneys). CVA tenderness to percussion is a common finding in pyelonephritis. In the chronic phase the patient may show unremarkable symptoms, such as nausea and general malaise.

Collection of **objective data** includes assessing the patient for signs of infection: elevated temperature, chills, and pus in the urine. Systemic signs occur as a result of the chronic disease: elevated blood pressure and gastrointestinal irritation such as vomiting and diarrhea.

Diagnostic Tests

Diagnosis is confirmed by bacteria and pus in the urine and leukocytosis. A clean-catch or catheterized urinalysis with culture and sensitivity identifies the pathogen and determines appropriate antimicrobial therapy. An IVP will identify the presence of obstruction or degenerative changes caused by the infectious process. Assessment of BUN and creatinine levels of the blood and urine may be used to monitor kidney function.

Medical Management

The patient with mild signs and symptoms may be treated on an outpatient basis with antibiotics for 14 to 21 days. Parenteral antibiotics are often given initially in the hospital to establish high serum and urinary medication levels. When initial treatment resolves the acute symptoms and the patient is able to tolerate oral fluids and medications, the person may be discharged on a regimen of oral antibiotics for an additional 14 to 21 days. Antibiotics are selected according to results of urinalysis culture and sensitivity and may include broad-spectrum medications such as ampicillin or vancomycin combined with an aminoglycoside (e.g., tobramycin [Nebcin], gentamicin [Garamycin]); other treatment options include trimethoprim-sulfamethoxazole (Bactrim, Septra) and fluoroquinolones such as ciprofloxin (Cipro) and ofloxin (Floxin).

Adequate fluids (at least eight 8-oz glasses per day) are encouraged. Urinary analgesics such as phenazopyridine (Pyridium) is helpful. Follow up urine culture is indicated.

Nursing Interventions and Patient Teaching

Nursing diagnoses and interventions for the patient with pyelonephritis include but are not limited to the following:

NURSING DIAGNOSES	NURSING INTERVENTIONS
Risk for infection, related to bacteria in the urinary tract	Monitor urine character, malodor. Encourage oral fluids. Instruct to void when urge is felt. Encourage perineal hygiene.
Health-seeking behaviors, related to desire for prevention of further renal disease	Assess knowledge level concerning measures to prevent recurrence of symptoms. Discuss personal health habits: diet, exercise. Discuss treatment plan with patient and family.

The patient should be taught to identify the signs and symptoms of infection: elevated temperature, flank pain, chills, fever, nausea and vomiting, urgency, fatigue, and general malaise. The patient should also be taught indications, dose, length of course, and side effects of the medications. The nurse should emphasize the importance of follow-up care with the physician on a routine basis and when signs of infection arise..

Prognosis

Prognosis is dependent upon early detection and successful treatment. Baseline assessment for every patient must include urinary assessment because pyelonephritis may occur as a primary or secondary disorder.

OBSTRUCTIVE DISORDERS OF THE URINARY TRACT
URINARY OBSTRUCTION
Etiology/Pathophysiology

Obstruction at any point within the urinary tract can adversely affect function and alter structure. Causes of obstruction include strictures, kinks, cysts, tumors, calculi, and prostatic hypertrophy. Obstruction may lead to alterations in blood chemistry; infection that thrives as a result of urine stasis; ischemia due to compression; or atrophy of renal tissue.

Clinical Manifestations

The patient may be unaware of any problems initially if the obstruction is partial, allowing urine to drain and kidney function to remain within normal limits. With prostatic hypertrophy the obstructive process may be so gradual that the patient ignores the vague symptom of dull flank pain and seeks medical attention only when urination becomes acutely difficult. Acute pain occurs as the musculature is stretched by increasing pressure from urine accumulation and as muscular contractions increase in an attempt to move urine past the obstruction. This acute pain is called renal colic and is a classic symptom of renal calculi.

Assessment

Collection of **subjective data** includes the patient's cardinal complaint of a sensation of needing to void but only being able to void small amounts. Pain may range from dull flank pain to acute, incapacitating pain. Nausea often accompanies acute pain.

Collection of **objective data** includes noting on physical assessment if the bladder is palpable suprapubically because of urine retention. The affected kidney may also be palpable. Retention with overflow occurs when the patient is unable to completely empty the urinary bladder and it quickly refills, causing the urge to void again. The nurse should assess time and amount of voidings.

Diagnostic Tests

As a quick evaluation the physician may order a kidney, ureter, and bladder (KUB) radiograph. Renal ultrasonography or IVP will provide definitive information about structural changes. Other diagnostic tests may include visual examinations with the aid of endoscopy and a blood chemistry profile.

Medical Management

Initial intervention will be to establish urine drainage and relieve discomfort. Conservative measures include insertion of an indwelling catheter, analgesic (usually opioid), and an anticholinergic agent (Atropine) to decrease smooth muscle motility. It may be necessary to establish urine drainage surgically by inserting a catheter directly into the bladder through the abdominal wall (suprapubic cystostomy), into a ureter (ureterostomy), or into the kidney (nephrostomy).

Surgical correction of an obstruction in the urinary system may be aided by the use of a tube, called a stent. Stent insertion is used for patients who are poor operative risks. A meshlike tube or coil-shaped device is inserted through an endoscope into the ureter. The stent holds the tubular structure open to facilitate drainage. Stents may be permanent or temporary. The patient should be closely monitored for signs of infection, obstruction, and pain.

Nursing Interventions

These procedures require observation for hemorrhage, maintaining aseptic care of the surgical site, restoring optimal urinary function, and providing a safe environment to prevent injury and infection.

Prognosis

The prognosis is variable, depending on the cause of the obstruction. If surgical correction is successful, the prognosis is excellent.

HYDRONEPHROSIS
Etiology/Pathophysiology

Hydronephrosis (the dilation of the renal pelvis and calyces) may be congenital or may develop at any time. It can occur either unilaterally or bilaterally. Hydronephrosis is caused by obstructions in the urinary tract. An obstruction may be located in the lower urinary tract, in the ureters, or in the kidneys. The location of the obstruction will determine whether one or both kidneys are affected.

An obstruction generates pressure from accumulated urine that cannot flow past the obstruction. This pressure may cause functional and anatomical damage to the renal system. The renal pelvis and ureters dilate and hypertrophy. This pressure, if prolonged, causes fibrosis and loss of function in affected nephrons. If the condition is left untreated, the kidney may be destroyed.

Clinical Manifestations

Hydronephrosis can occur without any symptoms as long as kidney function is adequate and urine can drain. The amount of pain is proportional to the rate of stretching of urinary tract structures. Slowly developing hydronephrosis may cause only a dull flank pain, whereas a sudden occlusion of the ureter, such as may occur from a calculus, causes a severe stabbing (colicky) pain in the flank of the abdomen. Nausea and vomiting, which often accompany hydronephrosis, are caused by a reflex reaction to the pain and will usually subside when the pain is controlled.

Assessment

Collection of **subjective data** involves questioning the patient about the presence of pain, including location, intensity, and character, and about the presence of nausea. The patient's voiding pattern should be discussed: frequency, difficulty starting a stream of urine, dribbling at the end of micturition (voiding), nocturia, and burning on urination. Any history of obstructive disorders should be noted.

Collection of **objective data** includes assessing patients suspected of having hydronephrosis for vomiting, hematuria, urinary output, edema, a palpable mass in the abdomen, bladder distention on palpation, and tenderness over the kidneys or bladder.

Diagnostic Tests

A urinalysis and serum renal function studies that include measurement of urea and creatinine are obtained. Cystoscopy may be performed with or without retrograde pyelogram. Radiographic examinations may include IVP/IVU, KUB radiograph, CT scan, and/or ultrasound evaluation. Sometimes a renal biopsy is performed.

Medical Management

Management is usually conservative if the condition is not severe. Surgical intervention is used to relieve the obstruction and preserve renal function. If the kidney is severely damaged, a nephrectomy may be necessary. If infection is present, antiinfective medications are administered: penicillin in combination with a sulfonamide (Gantrisin) or a sulfamethoxazole (Septra, Bactrim). Opioids, such as morphine and meperidine, in combination with antispasmodic drugs, such as propantheline (Pro-Banthīne) and belladonna preparations, are usually necessary to relieve severe, colicky pain.

Nursing Interventions and Patient Teaching

Nursing interventions for the patient with hydronephrosis include administering medications as ordered, monitoring intake (intravenous and oral) and output, observing for signs and symptoms of infection, and monitoring vital signs. The nurse will need to encourage the patient to take fluids and will also assess the patient for pain. Any drainage tubes will need to be kept open and anchored to avoid inadvertent displacement. If a catheter is present, catheter care will be necessary. If surgery has been performed, the dressing must be observed, because drainage of urine may continue for some time. The area should be kept clean and dry to avoid excoriation of the skin. All procedures should be explained to the patient and family.

Patient teaching should include an explanation of the abnormality, along with the signs and symptoms of infection or obstruction. Measures to prevent infection should be explained, such as adequate fluid intake, perineal hygiene daily with mild soap and water (drying thoroughly), and regular emptying of the bladder.

Prognosis

Prognosis is directly proportional to the degree of urinary system destruction and the need for surgical intervention.

UROLITHIASIS

Urolithiasis (formation of urinary calculi) can develop in any area of the urinary tract. Urolithiasis is a general term that encompasses all urinary calculi, but they are also named specifically to indicate where they are located or formed: nephrolithiasis (stones in the kidney), ureterolithiasis (stones in the ureter), and cystolithiasis (stones in the bladder). Other descriptive terms are **lithiasis,** and **calculi** (the formation of stones).

Etiology/Pathophysiology

Urolithiasis develops from minerals that have precipitated out of solution and adhere, forming stones that vary in size and shape. The event that initiates stone formation remains elusive, but some individuals are known to be predisposed: people who are immobile, are hyperparathyroid (calcium leaves the bones and accumulates in the bloodstream), or have recurrent UTIs. Individual history and some foods, nutrients, and medications contribute to development of stones. Thorough assessment and analysis of the composition of the stones guides medical and nursing management.

Clinical Manifestations

Size and degree of mobility of the stone influence symptomatology. The patient with renal colic will seek care immediately, whereas a person with a less mobile stone may not seek assistance until signs of infection or hydronephrosis occur.

Assessment

Collection of **subjective data** may include the patient with mobile calculi complaining of intractable pain (pain that is unrelieved by ordinary medical measures and is usually accompanied by nausea and vomiting). The patient describes the pain as starting in the flank and radiating into the groin, the genitalia, and the inner thigh. The patient with a less mobile stone will have signs and symptoms associated with urinary infection or hydronephrosis.

Collection of **objective data** includes the nurse assessing for the presence of hematuria (gross or microscopic on urinalysis) and vomiting.

Diagnostic Tests

Diagnostic tests include KUB and IVP/IVU radiography, ultrasound, cystoscopy, and urinalysis. Other tests may be ordered to determine stone content, presence of infection, and alterations in blood chemistry that may influence stone formation. Twenty-four-hour urine examination may be done to detect abnormal excretion of calcium oxalate, phosphorus, or uric acid.

Medical Management

Antiinfective agents may be administered in the presence of infection or prophylactically. If stones are not passed, invasive techniques may be indicated. Stones in the lower tract can be removed by cystoscopy with stone manipulation or by surgical incision (Figure 10-7). Terminology describes the location: ureterolithotomy, pyelolithotomy, and nephrolithotomy. Chemolytic agents, either alkylating or acidifying agents, may be instilled to dissolve stones. Extracorporeal shock wave lithotripsy is an alternative to surgery. The patient is submerged in a special tank of water and ultrasonic shock waves are used to pulverize the stone. Urine must still be strained, even if a catheter is in place. Renal colic may still occur as the patient passes the stone fragments. Long-term management may include dietary adjustments to influence the urine pH or to decrease availability of certain substances to discourage stone formation. Moderate reduction of calcium phosphorus and purine-containing foods may be beneficial when stones are caused by metabolic abnormalities. Some foods to be avoided include cheese, greens, whole grains, carbonated beverages, nuts, chocolate, shellfish, and organ meat. Adequate daily fluid intake of 2000 mL will help cleanse the urinary tract (unless clinically contraindicated). Some physicians encourage diets that alter the urine pH, to produce a less favorable environment for stone formation. Drug therapy will be specific to stone composition: in calcium stone formation, sodium cellulose phosphate binds with ingested calcium and prevents its absorption; aluminum hydroxide gel will bind with excess phosphorus, allowing intestinal excretion rather than urinary excretion; allopurinol (Zyloprim) reduces serum urate levels, thereby facilitating reabsorption of urate crystals.

Nursing Interventions and Patient Teaching

Stones are more likely to be passed if the patient remains active and increases fluid intake. If pain is so severe as to require opioid medication, the nurse must exercise discretion in allowing the patient out of bed. If nausea inhibits oral intake, the physician may order

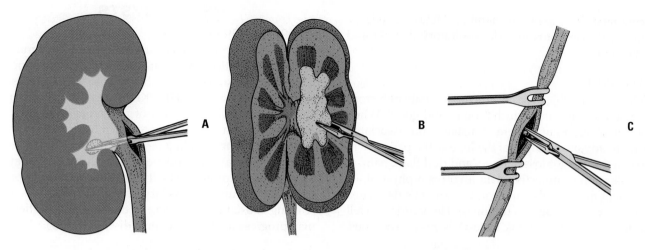

FIGURE **10-7** Location and methods of removing renal calculi from upper urinary tract.
A, Pyelolithotomy, removal of stone through renal pelvis. **B,** Nephrolithotomy, removal of
staghorn calculus from renal parenchyma (kidney split). **C,** Ureterolithotomy, removal of stone
from ureter.

supplemental intravenous fluids. All urine will be
strained. Because stones may be any size, even the
smallest speck must be saved for assessment. The
nurse should encourage fluids and administer analgesics as ordered. Urine is assessed for possible hematuria. BUN and creatinine are monitored for indications of continuing urinary obstruction.

Nursing diagnoses and interventions for the patient
with urolithiasis include but are not limited to the
following:

Nursing Diagnoses	Nursing Interventions
Pain, related to mobility of renal calculus (and/or surgery)	Assess nature, location, intensity, duration of pain. Provide nonpharmacologic comfort measures: reposition, quiet environment, diversional activities. Offer analgesics, noting response.
Urinary retention, related to obstruction	Assess bladder distention. Monitor I & O. Assist with mobility as tolerated. Strain urine, if appropriate. Use measures to facilitate bladder emptying: privacy, running water, sitting/standing position.

Prescribed diet, including fluid intake, should be
discussed, as well as home medications (their purpose,
dose, refills, and side effects). The patient should avoid
inactivity by walking frequently. The need for follow-
up with the physician should be emphasized, including keeping scheduled appointments and reporting
difficulty of urination.

Although opinions vary greatly as to benefits of dietary restrictions, the nurse may be responsible for
clarifying diet instructions. Fluid intake should be en-

couraged to at least 2000 mL of fluid in 24 hours, unless contraindicated. People who are calcium stone
formers may need to curtail their intake of dietary calcium (dairy products, antacids) to within minimum
recommended dietary allowance (RDA) guidelines.
New research on the impact of diet on the development of calcium oxalate kidney stones concludes that
restricting consumption of animal protein and salt in
combination with normal calcium intake reduces the
risk of kidney stones better than the traditional low-
calcium diet (Moyad, 2003).

Prognosis

Prognosis is related to the location of the stone and the
extent of invasive procedures necessary to remove the
stone. A certain population is categorized as "stone
formers" and consequently are at risk for recurrence.

RENAL TUMORS
Etiology/Pathophysiology

More common in men than in women, renal tumors
are primarily adenocarcinomas that develop unilaterally and are often quite large when first detected. Renal cell carcinoma as a primary malignant tumor appears to arise from cells of the proximal convoluted
tubules. Risk factors include smoking; familial incidence; and preexisting renal disorders, such as adult
polycystic kidney disease and renal cystic disease secondary to renal failure. Transitional cell tumors of the
renal pelvis cause hematuria and can be confirmed by
cytologic study.

Clinical Manifestations

The most common signs and symptoms are intermittent, painless hematuria, misleading the patient to defer seeking medical attention. Other signs and symptoms appear after the malignant process has advanced:
weight loss, dull flank pain, a palpable mass in the

flank area, and gross hematuria. Metastatic-related signs and symptoms include respiratory distress and bone pain.

Assessment

Collection of **subjective data** includes a patient history of blood in the urine, which "comes and goes." When the bleeding occurs, there is usually no associated pain. In advanced stages of the illness, the patient will experience weight loss, fatigue, and dull flank pain.

Collection of **objective data** involves a physical assessment that reveals a mass in the patient's flank area in the advanced stages of the illness. Hematuria, as well as signs related to systemic metastasis, may be obvious.

Diagnostic Tests

Urinalysis will reveal hematuria in most patients. IVP will detect a renal mass, and ultrasonography will define composition of the mass in most instances. If indicated, other tests will be used to evaluate the status of other body systems; these include scans, MRI, and renal arteriography.

Medical Management

Patients with localized disease usually respond well to radical nephrectomy. Radiation therapy and chemotherapy provide minimal benefit.

Nursing Interventions and Patient Teaching

Care of the patient with surgery of the urinary tract will be addressed later in this chapter.

Nursing diagnoses and interventions for the patient with renal tumors include but are not limited to the following:

Nursing Diagnoses	Nursing Interventions
Ineffective coping, related to powerlessness	Encourage patient to express feelings. Assist patient to identify personal strengths and coping skills. Actively listen. Support realistic hope: answer questions honestly.
Impaired physical mobility, related to pain/discomfort	Plan activities when pain control is greatest. Encourage active/passive range of motion exercises. Assess need for assistive devices.

The patient should be instructed about community resources, support groups, and home health care. The nurse should emphasize the importance of follow-up care, including following discharge instructions and keeping return appointment.

Prognosis

Prognosis is directly related to the stage of the disease process when diagnosis is made.

RENAL CYSTS

Etiology/Pathophysiology

A single renal cyst may occur without clinical significance, but multiple cysts interfere with kidney function. The most significant problems arise with **polycystic kidney disease (PKD).** PKD is a genetic disorder characterized by the growth of numerous fluid-filled cysts, which can slowly replace much of the kidney. A patient with long-standing renal insufficiency or a dialysis patient may develop polycystic disease. Kidney function is compromised by the pressure of the cysts on kidney structures, secondary infections, and tissue scarring caused by rupturing of the cysts. The patient may progress to end-stage renal disease (ESRD).

Clinical Manifestations

Signs and symptoms are influenced by the degree of kidney structure involvement. The most common site is the collecting ducts, which fill with urine and/or blood. As the disease progresses, fewer nephrons are available to maintain normal kidney function.

Assessment

Collection of **subjective data** includes noting the most common symptoms of abdominal and flank pain, followed by headache, gastrointestinal complaints, voiding disturbances, and a history of recurrent UTIs.

Collection of **objective data** involves an initial assessment that includes observation for systemic changes. The nurse should closely monitor blood pressure, which is usually elevated, and hematuria. Document the degree of patient complaints and response to intervention.

Diagnostic Tests

Diagnosis is established by family history, physical examination, excretory urography, and imaging of cysts on radiographic examination or sonography. Blood chemistry results, such as urea and creatinine levels, are used to monitor the level of kidney function.

Medical Management

There is no specific treatment for PKD. Medical treatment is aimed at relief of pain and symptoms of the disease. Heat and analgesics may relieve some of the discomfort caused by the enlarging kidneys. If the patient bleeds, heat should be discontinued and the patient should be placed on bed rest. Hypertension is treated vigorously with antihypertensive agents, diuretics, and fluid and dietary modifications. Because infections are common, antibiotics are often prescribed. As the disease progresses, dialysis or renal transplantation may be required.

Nursing Interventions

Individual complaints and the severity of the disease process will influence nursing interventions. Patients and family members need to be given information about the availability of genetic counseling. The nurse should emphasize the need to report any changes in health status to the physician.

Prognosis

Prognosis with a single cyst is favorable but guarded with polycystic disease because of the chronic nature of the disease.

TUMORS OF THE URINARY BLADDER
Etiology/Pathophysiology

Tumors of the urinary bladder range from benign papillomas to invasive carcinomas. The bladder is the most common site of cancer in the urinary tract, occurring more often in men than in women. Papillomas have the potential to become cancerous and are removed when detected.

Clinical Manifestations

The patient may delay seeking medical attention because the primary sign of bladder cancer is painless, intermittent hematuria.

Assessment

Collection of **subjective data** may include symptoms such as changes in voiding patterns, signs of urine obstruction, or renal failure, depending on the extent of the disease process.

Collection of **objective data** includes assessing the patient's understanding of current health status, which will aid the nurse in planning teaching interventions. Accurate documentation of the time and amount of voiding, including the urine description, is indicated.

Diagnostic Tests

Diagnostic tests include cystoscopy to obtain tissue samples for cytologic evaluation (study of cells). Kidney function tests will assist in evaluation of overall renal status.

Medical Management

The patient with local disease may be treated by removing the tissue by burning with an electric spark (fulguration), laser, instillation of chemotherapy agents, or radiation therapy. These individuals need to be closely monitored with cytologic studies and cystoscopy, since the recurrence rate is as high as 60%. A partial or total cystectomy may be performed to remove invasive lesions. With complete removal of the urinary bladder, urinary diversion is necessary. (See the discussion of the ileal conduit or sigmoid conduit on pp. 510-511 and in Figure 10-13.)

Nursing Interventions and Patient Teaching

The importance of follow-up care for the patient with papilloma must be emphasized. Care of the patient with bladder cancer will be influenced by the extent of the disease process, medical treatment, coincidental illness, and the patient's response to treatment. Observation of voiding patterns and urine character are necessary to monitor response to these therapies.

Patient teaching is indicated so that the patient can return to optimum performance of activities of daily living. Suggested interventions are addressed under surgical interventions later in this chapter.

Prognosis

There is a direct relationship between the prognosis and the extent of the disease process when diagnosed. The other most important aspect in recovery is the patient's adaptability to any changes in urinary elimination as a result of treatment.

CONDITIONS AFFECTING THE PROSTATE GLAND
BENIGN PROSTATIC HYPERTROPHY
Etiology/Pathophysiology

The prostate gland encircles the male urethra at the base of the urinary bladder. Its function is secretion of an alkaline fluid that helps neutralize seminal fluid and increases sperm motility. Benign prostatic hypertrophy (BPH), enlargement of the prostate gland, is common in men older than 50 years of age. The cause is unclear but may be influenced by hormonal changes. The prostate enlarges, exerting pressure on the urethra and vesicle neck of the urinary bladder, which prevents complete emptying.

Clinical Manifestations

The patient will have symptoms associated with urinary obstruction. Other clinical manifestations include complications of urinary obstruction, such as UTI, hematuria, oliguria, and signs of renal insufficiency.

Assessment

Collection of **subjective data** includes the patient describing the urine stream as difficult to start, slow, and painful, with complaints of frequency and nocturia (awakened by urgency to void two or more times). Collectively these symptoms may be referred to as **prostatism** (any condition of the prostate gland that causes retention of urine in the bladder).

Collection of **objective data** involves the nurse eliciting information about voiding patterns to aid in determining the severity of the obstruction.

Diagnostic Tests

On rectal examination the physician may palpate the enlarged prostate gland, which has an elastic consistency. The hypertrophied prostate is symmetrically enlarged with a uniform, boggy presentation. Severity of the process can be determined through detecting alterations in blood chemistry, by measuring residual urine, or by cystoscopy or IVP. Cytologic evaluation will determine whether the process is benign or malignant.

Medical Management

Treatment is based on the degree of occlusion as well as signs and symptoms. Pharmacologic agents such as avodart (Dusteride) convert testosterone to dihydrotestosterone, a key enzyme in the development and growth rate of prostate hyperplasia. This medication may take 3 to 6 months to shrink the prostate gland, decreasing its size as much as 25%. Terazosin (Hytrin) is an antihypertensive that dilates arteries and veins and decreases contractions in smooth muscle of the prostatic capsule. This decreases symptoms of prostatic hyperplasia (urinary urgency, hesitancy, nocturia).

Nursing Interventions

Initial management is aimed at relieving the obstruction, usually by insertion of a Foley catheter. Care must be taken to avoid rapid decompression of the bladder to prevent rupture of mucosal blood vessels. Usually no more than 1000 mL of urine should be removed from a distended bladder initially. Physician's orders should be followed for the individual patient.

Prostatectomy (removal of the prostate gland) is indicated to relieve and/or prevent further obstruction of the urethra. The physician will choose the surgical approach for the prostatectomy after thorough appraisal of the patient. Preoperatively the physician may order an enema to reduce the possibility of the patient's straining to defecate after surgery, which could cause bleeding. Other preoperative preparations are standard, as noted in Chapter 2. There are four surgical techniques by which a prostatectomy may be done; they are presented in Box 10-3 and Figure 10-8.

With BPH, a transurethral resection of the prostate (TURP) is less invasive and less stressful for the patient, especially the older patient or the patient with coincidental illness. Removal of the tissue is done through the urethra. With this procedure the outer capsule of the prostate gland is left in place, maintaining the continuity between the bladder and the lower urethra (see Figure 10-8, *A*). Care of this patient is centered on observation of urine character and maintaining patency of the Foley catheter.

The patient who has a TURP may have continuous closed bladder irrigation or intermittent irrigation to prevent occlusion of the catheter with blood clots, which would cause bladder spasms. The patient and family need to know that hematuria is expected after prostatic surgery. Vital signs and urine color will be monitored every 2 hours for the first 24 hours to detect early signs of complications. With continuous bladder irrigation (CBI) the urine will be light red to pink, and with intermittent irrigation the urine will be a clear, cherry red. Continuous irrigation is achieved by using a three-way catheter (one lumen for irrigation fluid, one for urine drainage, and one to the retention balloon) or by using two catheters (Foley and suprapubic—one for irrigation fluid and one for urine drainage). The irrigant is an isotonic solution. To determine urine output, the nurse will subtract the amount of irrigation fluid used from the Foley catheter output to calculate urine output. This is reported as "actual urine output." Catheter drainage tubes should be checked frequently for kinks that would occlude urine flow and cause bladder spasms. The patient should be advised not to try to void around the catheter because this will contribute to bladder spasms. Hemorrhage is always a possibility. Belladonna and opium (B&O) rectal suppositories are helpful to relieve bladder spasms but are not used in the retropubic approach because rectal stimulation is contraindicated.

Routine postoperative care is instituted. Prolonged sitting is to be avoided because the resulting increased intraabdominal pressure may cause the operative site to bleed. The catheter is removed when the urine becomes clear. The patient is informed that initially he may experience frequency, voiding small amounts with some dribbling. He should be instructed to void with the first urge to prevent increased bladder pressure against the operative site.

Some physicians may request that samples of the most recent voiding be saved for assessment. When the patient voids, the nurse records the time, amount, and color of each voiding.

Laser ablation of the prostate has become increasingly successful in the treatment of benign prostatic hypertrophy. A transurethral, ultrasound-guided, laser-induced prostatectomy (TULIP) is the usual treatment. Sloughing of the tissue may be delayed, but blood loss is minimal. Dysuria and the need for longer catheterization may be necessary.

A suprapubic or abdominal approach will require dressing observations and changes. When a suprapu-

---

Box 10-3 | *Four Prostatectomy Techniques*

1. **Transurethral prostatectomy** is done by approaching the gland through the penis and bladder using a resectoscope, a surgical instrument with an electric cutting wire for resection and cautery to resect the lobes away from the capsule (Figure 10-8, *A*).
2. **Suprapubic prostatectomy** is accomplished by an incision through the abdomen; the bladder is opened, and the gland is removed from above with the finger (Figure 10-8, *B*).
3. **Radical perineal prostatectomy** requires an incision through the perineum between the scrotum and the rectum (Figure 10-8, *C*).
4. **Retropubic prostatectomy** is the method in which a low abdominal incision is made, but the bladder is not opened. The gland is removed by making an incision into the capsule encasing the gland (Figure 10-8, *D*).

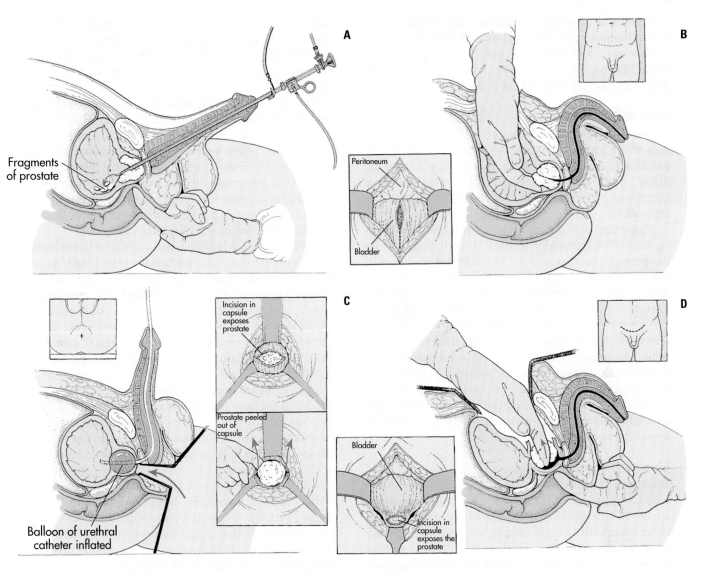

Fragments of prostate

Balloon of urethral catheter inflated

Peritoneum

Bladder

Incision in capsule exposes prostate

Prostate peeled out of capsule

Bladder

Incision in capsule exposes the prostate

FIGURE 10-8 Four types of prostatectomies. **A,** Transurethral resection of prostate gland by means of resectoscope. Note enlarged prostate gland surrounding urethra and tiny pieces of prostatic tissue that have been cut away. **B,** Suprapubic. **C,** Radical perineal. **D,** Retropubic prostatectomy.

bic catheter is present, it will be observed for unobstructed flow and color of the urine and monitored for total output.

Prognosis

Prognosis is favorable without residual effects. Problems with urine dribbling vary depending on the individual patient response.

CANCER OF THE PROSTATE
Etiology/Pathophysiology

Prostatic cancer is common in men older than 50 years of age. This insidious cancer usually starts as a nodule on the posterior portion of the prostate without noticeable symptoms. When the tumor causes urinary symptoms, the cancer is in advanced stages. At this point, metastasis is common; frequent sites are the pelvic lymph nodes and bone. Regular rectal examinations and prostate-specific antigen (PSA) measure-

ment to detect abnormalities of the prostate gland lead to early treatment and an increased survival rate.

Clinical Manifestations

The patient will have signs and symptoms related to urinary obstruction. Other signs and symptoms will be determined by the presence and/or degree of metastasis.

Assessment

Collection of **subjective data** involves understanding that the patient with prostatic cancer may have no symptoms until the disease is advanced. The patient may seek medical intervention for benign prostatic hypertrophy (BPH), which often accompanies prostate cancer, or when he experiences back pain or sciatica that occurs from metastatic changes in the bony pelvis. The patient may complain of dysuria, frequency, and nocturia.

Collection of **objective data** includes noting metastatic changes in the lymph glands of the pelvis and in the bones of the lower spine, pelvis, and hips with associated signs. Hematuria may or may not be present, depending on the stage of the malignancy.

Diagnostic Tests

On rectal examination by the physician, the involved area of the prostate gland will feel firm and fixed with hardened nodules typically in the posterior lobe of the gland. Definitive diagnosis is made by cytologic examination. Prostate cells can be obtained by needle aspiration.

PSA is increasing considerably the odds of early diagnosis. PSA, normally secreted and disposed of by the prostate, increases in the bloodstream in cancer of the prostate as well as in the harmless condition of BPH. The normal PSA is 0 to 4 ng/mL. It is very important to monitor even a slight increase in PSA levels. Elevated PSA levels mean further diagnostic evaluation is needed. In cases when PSA levels are high but a digital exam is normal, the imaging technique of transrectal ultrasound is proving increasingly helpful in detecting cancer tumor of the prostate gland too small to be palpated rectally. Other tests, such as a bone scan and serum alkaline phosphatase, will be performed to assess the degree of metastasis.

Medical Management

Treatment is based on the stage of the cancer—whether it has spread beyond the wall of the prostate, and to what extent—and the age of the patient. In an older man with an estimated remaining life span of 5 to 10 years, controlling the disease with radiation or hormone therapy may be enough. In many cases, particularly in men older than 70 years of age, prostate cancer grows slowly, and hormone therapy can hold the disease at bay for several years.

Localized prostate cancer can be cured by radiation therapy or surgery. Radiation therapy also is used when the cancer has spread to just outside the gland, in an attempt to destroy cancer cells and shrink the prostate.

The operation to remove the prostate is called a radical prostatectomy. Radical prostatectomy by the perineal approach is used in patients with early-stage clinical disease and is considered one of the most effective ways of eradicating the tumor. This procedure involves removing the entire prostate, including the true prostatic capsule, seminal vesicles, and a portion of the bladder neck. The remaining portion of the bladder neck is reanastomosed to the urethra. The retropubic approach often is used first, because it provides access to the pelvic lymph nodes (pelvic lymphadenectomy) and affords more urinary control and less stricture formation.

A nerve-sparing prostatectomy procedure is being used with a retropubic and perineal approach in an attempt to prevent impotence and reduce the likelihood of urinary incontinence. This procedure is not guaranteed because the extent of surgical resection needed to confine the disease is not known before the surgery.

The three goals of a radical prostatectomy are removing all the tumor, preserving urine control, and preserving sexual function. Extent of sexual function may not be known for 6 to 12 months postoperatively. This patient will need emotional support related to the cancer and the possibility of impotence as a result of the surgery. Preoperative teaching should include an opportunity for the patient and his partner to discuss optional treatments and mortality rate.

When the capsule of the prostate gland is removed, as with the perineal approach, there is no longer a connection between the bladder and the lower urethra. The area where these two structures are reconnected is usually supported by placement of a Foley catheter. Extreme care must be taken not to cause tension on the catheter, which would disturb the surgical area. The catheter will remain indwelling for several postoperative days.

In cases of advanced prostatic cancer, hormonal deprivation therapy may be used in an attempt to alter the tumor growth by blocking androgen (testosterone) production. Hormone deprivation therapy includes estrogens, gonadotropin-releasing hormone analogs, and antiandrogens. Luteinizing hormone–releasing hormone (LHRH) drugs act by causing an initial surge in luteinizing hormone (LH) and testosterone, rapidly followed by a decline in testosterone level similar to that achieved by castration. The primary forms of LHRH agonists are leuprolide (Lupon) and goserelin (Zoladex). Alternatives to LHRH agonists include oral nonsteroidal antiandrogens, including bicalutamide (Casodex), flutamide (Eulexin), and nilutamide (Niladron) (Black & Hawks, 2005). Palliative therapy for patients with metastatic disease also may include orchiectomy (removal of the testes). Bilateral orchiectomy may be used to eliminate 95% of testosterone production, a step that is useful in managing metastatic disease. The patient may receive relief from such symptoms as pain or obstruction, but may, however, experience feminization, increased incidence of cardiac disease, thrombophlebitis, pulmonary embolus, and stroke. Additional therapies are instituted to treat these side effects.

Radiation therapy may be used in advanced stages of the illness as primary or palliative treatment. Management of disseminated disease with cytotoxic drugs has been marginally successful.

Because cure for cancer of the prostate is possible only when the tumor is discovered early, it is important to teach all male patients older than the age of 40 to have annual or biannual rectal examinations and yearly PSA serum levels.

Nursing Interventions and Patient Teaching

Postoperative nursing management is similar to that for perineal surgery, with special attention to maintenance of bowel and bladder function while keeping the surgical wound clean and avoiding pressure on the perineum and wound. Adequate fluid intake, modification of dietary selections, and perineal exercises may be used to promote regulation of bowel and bladder function. Extreme care must be taken to prevent trauma to the perineum, which could lead to fistula formation. Rectal temperature-taking, enemas, and use of rectal tubes are therefore forbidden. Extreme care must be taken not to create tension on the Foley catheter, which would disturb the surgical area. The nurse observes the color of the urine for signs of bleeding. The patient will also have a tissue drain inserted during surgery to promote drainage from the wound in the perineum. Initially there may be some small amount of urine from the drain, but this should cease in 1 or 2 days. Surgical asepsis should be followed during dressing changes. Irrigation of the perineum may be ordered to cleanse the wound and soothe the patient. Comfort measures and analgesics should be administered as ordered for pain control in the lower back, pelvis, upper thighs, and operative site.

Nursing diagnoses and interventions for the patient undergoing prostate surgery include but are not limited to the following:

NURSING DIAGNOSES	NURSING INTERVENTIONS
Risk for fluid volume, deficient, related to hemorrhage/decreased fluid intake	Monitor signs/symptoms of fluid deficit: decreasing BP, increasing BP, dyspnea. Observe catheter(s) for urine color and amount. Avoid manipulation of rectum by thermometer/rectal tube.
Ineffective sexuality patterns related to surgical trauma/altered body function	Encourage verbalization of sexual concerns. Provide privacy with significant other to discuss concerns. Inform physician of patient concerns. Explore professional resources: clergy, sexual counselors.

Because urinary incontinence may occur postoperatively, the nurse should teach the patient how to keep himself clean. He may need to discuss feelings of depression about his altered body function. Modifying lifestyle and maintaining confidence are important for his return to preillness function.

- Emphasize the need for adequate fluid intake, exercise, and rest.
- Instruct the patient in pain-relieving measures (e.g., exercise, warmth, and medication).

- Discuss alternate expressions of sexuality, the value of sexual counseling, and the possibility of recovering some or all of sexual function after treatment is completed.

Discuss new pharmacologic agents that act as adjuvants in the treatment of cancer and for pain relief during the postoperative recovery period.

Prognosis

There is a direct correlation between prognosis and the extent of the disease process when diagnosed. Grading of the tumors (well, moderately, or poorly differentiated) correlates with the prognosis; the more poorly differentiated the tumor, the poorer the prognosis is. Pathologists use a system called the **Gleason score** to rank cell differentiation. A low score of 2 through 4 is good; a high score of 7 through 10 is not. The treatment goal for the localized disease process is a cure; palliation is used for the extended disease process.

URETHRAL STRICTURES

Etiology/Pathophysiology

A urethral stricture is a narrowing of the lumen of the urethra that interferes with urine flow. Narrowing may be congenital or acquired. Acquired strictures may be caused by chronic infection, trauma, tumor, or as a complication of radiation treatment of the pelvis.

Clinical Manifestations

Signs and symptoms include dysuria, weak stream, splaying (spreading out) of the urine stream, nocturia, and increasing pain with bladder distention. In the presence of infection, fever and malaise may be apparent.

Assessment

Collection of **subjective data** includes noting a patient complaint of difficulty initiating the urine stream and the stream seeming to spray more than usual or even seeming to "fork."

Collection of **objective data** includes assessing for signs that may indicate an infectious process and gathering information to describe the infectious process to describe the extent of the stricture and possible presence of an obstruction.

Diagnostic Tests

Diagnosis can be confirmed by a voiding cystourethrogram, which demonstrates stricture. Additional diagnostic studies help evaluate damage caused by the obstruction.

Medical Management

Correction of the stricture may be achieved by dilation with metal sounds or surgical release (internal urethrotomy).

Nursing Interventions

Care includes adequate hydration to decrease discomfort when voiding and monitoring urine output. Mild analgesics should be sufficient to relieve discomfort. Sitz baths may encourage voiding. Reconstruction (urethroplasty) of the urethra may require temporary urinary diversion. After the procedure a splinting catheter will support the suture line. Care must be taken not to cause tension on the catheter.

Prognosis

Prognosis after surgical correction or dilation is favorable.

URINARY TRACT TRAUMA

Etiology/Pathophysiology

Any patient with a history of traumatic injury should be assessed for involvement of the urinary tract. Such injuries may include contusions or rupture of the urinary structures. A patient who has undergone abdominal surgery should also be observed for incidental injury sustained during the operation. Traumatic invasion of the urinary tract may be evident in open wounds to the lower abdomen, such as with gunshot or stab wounds. Trauma to the bladder can occur from a fractured pelvis. Contusion or laceration of the urethra may lead to urethral stricture and possible impotence in males secondary to soft tissue, blood vessel, and nerve damage.

Clinical Manifestations

Urine output should be monitored hourly for amount and color. Any evidence of hematuria should be reported. The patient is assessed for abdominal pain and tenderness, which may indicate internal hemorrhage, peritonitis, or seepage of urine into the tissues.

Assessment

Collection of **subjective data** involves understanding that the trauma patient may be unable to relate any symptoms that would aid in the assessment of urinary tract involvement. If the patient is able to respond, any reference to the signs of hematuria is extremely important.

Collection of **objective data** includes a comprehensive assessment of the trauma patient reviewing all body systems. Assessment related to the urinary tract includes hourly measurement of I&O; observation of urine character or difficulty voiding; evaluation of complaints of abdominal, flank, or referred shoulder pain; and evaluation of abdominal distention and girth.

Diagnostic Tests

Diagnosis of traumatic involvement of the urinary tract may be aided by KUB radiograph, IVP, urinalysis, excretory urogram, and cystoscopy.

Medical Management

Surgical intervention will be necessary for correction of tears or rupture of the integrity of the urinary tract, to reinstate urine flow. If damage to the structures is severe, removal of the kidney or bladder may be necessary with the creation of urinary diversion as discussed later in this chapter.

Management of possible hemorrhage and prevention of infection are necessary preoperatively and postoperatively.

Nursing Interventions

Nursing responsibility centers on identifying individuals at risk and detecting variations in assessment findings that indicate trauma to the urinary tract. The nurse should document and report all findings.

Prognosis

Prognosis depends on the extent and location of the trauma.

IMMUNOLOGICAL DISORDERS OF THE KIDNEY

NEPHROTIC SYNDROME

Etiology/Pathophysiology

Nephrotic syndrome (nephrosis) is a group of signs characterized by marked proteinuria, hypoalbuminemia, and edema. Several events may precipitate the signs of nephrotic syndrome; the primary form of nephrosis occurs in the absence of glomerulonephritis or systemic disease, with the inciting event being an upper respiratory infection or allergic reaction.

Physiologic changes in the glomeruli interfere with selective permeability. Blood protein is allowed to pass into the urine (proteinuria), causing a loss of serum protein (hypoalbuminemia). This decreases serum osmotic pressure, thus allowing fluid to seep into interstitial spaces, and edema occurs.

Immune responses, both humoral and cellular, are altered in nephrotic syndrome; as a result, infection is an important cause of morbidity and mortality.

Clinical Manifestations

The patient has severe generalized edema (anasarca), anorexia, fatigue, and altered renal function.

Assessment

Collection of **subjective data** includes noting patient complaints of loss of interest in eating, a constant feeling of being tired, foamy urine from the presence of protein, and decreased urine output (oliguria).

Collection of **objective data** includes the nurse assessing the degree of fluid retention by monitoring daily weight, intake and output, respiratory effort, and level of consciousness. The patient may relate problems with "swelling" of his face, hands, and feet. Skin integrity is assessed to determine special needs.

Diagnostic Tests

Blood chemistry findings include hypoalbuminemia and hyperlipidemia. Renal biopsy provides identification of the type and extent of tissue change. Other diagnostic testing will be performed to identify the specific underlying cause.

Medical Management

Medical management depends on the extent of tissue involvement and may include the use of corticosteroids (Prednisone); antineoplastic agents for immunosuppressive effect; loop diuretics; and a low-sodium, high-protein diet for therapeutic management of edema. Hypoproteinemia may be treated with normal serum albumin and protein-rich nutrition replacement therapy.

Nursing Interventions and Patient Teaching

Nursing intervention includes monitoring of fluid balance (weight, measuring abdominal girth, I&O), bed rest in the presence of extreme edema (recumbent position may initiate diuresis), and assessing for electrolyte imbalance. Skin care is very important, as is a gradual increase in activity as the edema is resolved.

Diet includes protein replacement using foods that provide high biologic value (meat, fish, poultry, cheese, eggs) and restriction of sodium to decrease edema. Blood pressure is often elevated and should be monitored closely for changes.

As the patient begins to convalesce, the teaching plan includes the following:

- Medication regimen: type, dosage, side effects, and need to take all doses prescribed
- Nutrition teaching: high protein, low sodium
- Self-assessment of fluid status: monitor weight, presence of edema
- Signs and symptoms indicating need for medical attention (increase in edema, fatigue, headache, infection)
- Need for follow-up care

Prognosis

In approximately 25% of children and 50% to 75% of adults who develop nephrosis, the disease progresses to renal failure within 5 years. In other individuals (particularly children), there may be remissions or nephrotic syndrome may exist in a chronic form. Other than treating the underlying illness, little can be done to prevent a recurrence of nephrosis.

NEPHRITIS

Nephritis encompasses a number of kidney disorders characterized by inflammation of the kidney—involving the glomeruli, tubules, or interstitial tissue—and abnormal function. Included in this group of disorders are acute and chronic glomerulonephritis.

Acute Glomerulonephritis

Etiology/pathophysiology. The health history commonly reveals that the onset of acute glomerulonephritis was preceded by an infection, such as a sore throat or skin infection (most commonly β-hemolytic streptococci 2 to 3 weeks earlier, or other preexisting multisystem diseases, such as systemic lupus erythematosus. The infectious disease process triggers an immune response that results in inflammation of glomeruli that allows excretion of red blood cells and protein in the urine. This condition is common in children and young adults.

Clinical manifestations. It is not unusual for family members to first note that the individual has "swelling" of the face, especially around the eyes. Some patients may be acutely ill with a multitude of symptoms, whereas others may be diagnosed on routine examination with only vague symptoms.

Assessment. Collection of **subjective data** includes noting that the patient relates symptoms indicative of anorexia, nocturia, malaise, and exertional dyspnea.

Collection of **objective data** includes assessment of skin integrity and general condition of skin; the presence, degree, and nature of edema with associated difficulty in breathing upon exertion, when recumbent, or as evidenced by changes in lung and heart sounds (unusual heart sounds, crackles over lung fields, distention of neck veins); hematuria with changes in urine color from "cola" to frank sanguineous; or changes in voiding, decrease in amount of urine output, or dysuria.

Diagnostic tests. Diagnostic tests will reveal elevation of BUN, serum creatinine, potassium, erythrocyte sedimentation rate (ESR), and antistreptolysin-O titer (ASO titer). Urinalysis will show red blood cells, casts, and/or protein.

Medical management. Medical management includes treatment of primary symptoms while preventing complications to cerebral and cardiac function. Serum electrolyte levels (sodium and potassium) may indicate a need to adjust dietary intake of sodium and potassium. Level of consciousness should be monitored when the BUN is elevated. Bed rest and fluid intake adjustments are guided by urinary output until diuresis is adequate.

A prophylactic antimicrobial agent, such as penicillin, may be administered for several months after the acute phase of the illness to protect against recurrence of infection. Diuretics may be prescribed to control fluid retention and antihypertensives to reduce blood pressure.

Nursing interventions and patient teaching. Nursing intervention will be guided by individual patient needs, focusing on control of symptoms and prevention of complications. Dietary intake will include protein restrictions (to decrease blood urea levels), with carbohydrates providing a source of energy.

Nursing interventions include monitoring I&O and vital signs. Level of activity will be determined by the degree of edema, hypertension, proteinuria, and hematuria, since excessive activity may increase these signs (Health Promotion Considerations: The Patient with Nephritis box).

Because of the long-term nature of glomerulonephritis, patient teaching is important. Proteinuria and hematuria may exist microscopically even when other symptoms subside. Although fatigue may be present, these patients usually feel well; therefore they often must be convinced of the need to continue prescribed treatment and to return for follow-up care. Teaching includes the following:

- Nature of the illness and effect of diet and fluids on fluid balance and sodium retention.
- Diet teaching regarding prescribed sodium and fluid restrictions (provide written information regarding sodium content of foods, as necessary).

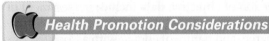

Health Promotion Considerations

The Patient with Nephritis

ACTIVITY

Bed rest until edema and blood pressure are reduced.
Encourage quiet diversional activities.
Ambulate gradually with assistance.
Space activity to lessen fatigue.

FLUID BALANCE MAINTENANCE

Implement dietary restrictions.
Monitor I&O.
Document reactions to medication.

DIET THERAPY

Protein restrictions to decrease nitrogenous wastes.
Sodium restrictions to prevent further fluid retention.
Increase calories for energy source.

DRUG THERAPY

Prophylactic antibiotics.
Antihypertensives.
Diuretics.
Drug interactions, side effects to expect and report.

HEALTH MAINTENANCE

Recovery may be extended.
Urine will be monitored for albumin and RBCs by physician.
Teach early signs of fluid retention.
Signs and symptoms may resolve and then become worse.
Normal activities may be resumed after urine is free of albumin and RBCs for a month, though the patient is not considered cured until the urine is free of albumin and RBCs for 6 months.
Report hematuria, headache, edema.

Include information about protein restrictions and carbohydrate sources.

- Medication regimen (dose, frequency, side effects, need to continue per physician instructions).
- Need to pace activities with rest if fatigue is present.
- Avoidance of trauma and infection (may exacerbate the illness).
- Signs and symptoms indicating need for medical attention (hematuria, headache, edema, hypertension).
- Importance of follow-up health care.

Prognosis. The prognosis of acute poststreptococcal glomerulonephritis is generally good; however, some patients develop chronic glomerulonephritis and end-stage renal disease (ESRD), requiring dialysis or renal transplantation.

Chronic Glomerulonephritis

Etiology/pathophysiology. With chronic glomerulonephritis there is usually no indication of an inciting event. Occasionally the patient with acute glomerulonephritis will progress to a chronic phase. Because other chronic illnesses, (e.g., diabetes mellitus or systemic lupus erythematosus) may mask the symptoms of renal degeneration, many patients will not seek medical attention until renal function is compromised. Chronic glomerulonephritis is characterized by slow, progressive destruction of glomeruli with related loss of function. The kidney will atrophy (actually decrease in size).

Clinical manifestations. Signs and symptoms may include malaise, morning headaches, dyspnea with exertion, visual and digestive disturbances, edema, and fatigue. Physical findings include hypertension, anemia, proteinuria, anasarca, and cardiac and cerebral manifestations.

Assessment. Collection of **subjective data** includes the patient complaints of fatigue and a decreased ability to perform ADLs as a result of dyspnea and decreasing ability to concentrate. Investigate complaints of morning headaches—their location, pattern, and character—and note presence of any visual disturbance.

Collection of **objective data** includes the nurse's clarifying outward manifestations of the headache and respiratory effort that may interfere with daily task performance. Assess mental functioning, irritability, slurred speech, ataxia, or tremors. Careful assessment of the degree of edema will be documented, noting specific location and response to pressure by pressing the fingers into the edematous area and observing for pitting (see Chapter 8, Figure 8-17). Note skin color, ecchymoses (irregularly formed hemorrhagic areas of the skin) or rash, dry skin, and scratching. Observe urine color and amount. Monitor vital signs, including a chest assessment for cardiac and pulmonary signs of fluid retention: unusual heart sounds, crackles over lung fields, distention of neck veins.

Diagnostic tests. Early disease shows albumin and RBCs in the urine, although renal function test results are within normal limits. With advanced destruction of nephrons, the specific gravity becomes fixed and blood levels of nonprotein nitrogen wastes (creatinine and urea) increase. Creatinine clearance may be as low as 5 to 10 mL/minute, compared with the normal range of 107 to 139 mL/minute in men and 87 to 107 mL/minute in women.

Medical management. Medical management includes control of secondary side effects as discussed with acute glomerulonephritis, with the use of renal dialysis and possible kidney transplantation to provide elimination of wastes from the body.

Nursing interventions and patient teaching. Nursing interventions for the patient with chronic glomerulonephritis represent a special challenge. This patient has already suffered major damage to the kidney filtration system. It is crucial that the patient's condition not be further compromised by infection or other complications. Changes in vital signs and diagnostic tests are monitored to aid in choosing proper nursing interventions. Interventions parallel those noted with nephrotic syndrome and acute glomerulonephritis. Chronic glomerulonephritis may progress to ESRD, necessitating related nursing interventions (Health Promotion Considerations: The Patient with Nephritis box).

Nursing diagnoses and interventions for the patient with chronic glomerulonephritis include but are not limited to the following:

NURSING DIAGNOSES	NURSING INTERVENTIONS
Excess fluid volume, related to decreased urine output	Assess understanding of therapeutic interventions. Note I&O every hour (or more often). Monitor signs/symptoms of fluid excess: weight gain, hypertension, edema, dyspnea. Provide ice chips for thirst with prescribed diet. Monitor and report abnormal laboratory results.
Activity intolerance, related to renal dysfunction	Assess level of activity tolerance. Encourage patient to report activities that increase his or her fatigue. Plan activities to minimize fatigue.

The focus for patient teaching must be preventive health maintenance, emphasizing a health-promoting lifestyle, with prevention and early treatment of infections.

Prognosis. Some people with minimal impairment in renal function continue to feel well and show little progression of disease. With other individuals the progression of renal deterioration may be slow but steady and end in renal failure. In still other individuals the progression of disease is rapid.

RENAL FAILURE

Renal failure is characterized by the inability of the kidneys to remove wastes, concentrate urine, and conserve or eliminate electrolytes. Diabetes mellitus is the most common cause of kidney failure, accounting for more than 40% of new cases. Other predisposing concurrent illnesses include burns, trauma, heart failure, volume depletion, and renal disease. Nursing interventions to prevent the development of renal failure include adequate hydration, prevention of infections, monitoring for signs and symptoms of shock, and teaching drug side effects to report immediately.

ACUTE RENAL FAILURE
Etiology/Pathophysiology

Kidney function may be altered by interference with the kidney's ability to be selective in filtering blood or by an actual decrease in blood flow to the kidneys. A number of medical conditions can lead to acute renal failure (ARF), such as hemorrhage, trauma, infection, and decreased cardiac output. The course of ARF is divided into phases. In the **oliguric phase,** BUN and serum creatinine levels rise while urine output decreases. The oliguric phase may last from several days to 4 to 6 weeks.

Some patients may experience the nonoliguric form, usually caused by nephrotoxic antibiotics, with which urinary output may exceed 2 L per day.

In the **diuretic phase,** blood chemistry levels begin to return to normal and urine output increases. Return to normal or near-normal function occurs in the **recovery phase.**

Clinical Manifestations

The patient may experience anorexia, nausea, vomiting, edema, and associated signs and symptoms of diminished renal function.

Assessment

Collection of **subjective data** includes the patient report of experiencing lethargy, loss of appetite, nausea, and headache.

Collection of **objective data** involves physical findings that will depend on the progression of the disease process. The nurse assesses for dry mucous membranes, poor skin turgor, urine output of less than 400 mL/24 hours, vomiting, diarrhea, and anasarca. Assessment findings may include central nervous system manifestations of drowsiness, muscle twitching, and seizures.

Diagnostic Tests

Physical assessment, history, and elevated blood chemistry tests such as BUN and creatinine (azotemia) will confirm diagnosis. After the patient is stabilized, further studies may be done to assess for residual damage.

Medical Management

Measures include administration of fluids and osmotic preparations to prevent decreased renal perfusion, manage fluid volume, and treat electrolyte imbalances. Renal dialysis may be necessary to manage systemic fluid shifts, especially cardiac and respiratory, and may be effective in removing some nephrotoxins.

Diet should be protein sparing, high in carbohydrates, and low in potassium and sodium. Drug therapy may include diuretics to increase urine output (e.g., furosemide [Lasix], hydrochlorothiazide [Hydrodiuril]). Potassium-lowering agents are used to remove potassium through the gastrointestinal tract; sodium polystyrene sulfonate (Kayexalate) is administered orally, per NG tube or as a retention enema. Antibiotics that are not dependent on kidney excretion are used to eradicate or prevent infection. Whatever combination of drug therapy is utilized, dosage and administration times will require adjustment according to the level of kidney function.

Nursing Interventions and Patient Teaching

Accurate documentation of urine output is necessary to identify the level of renal function. Azotemia may be revealed by blood chemistry studies. The patient with azotemia must be observed for changes in level of consciousness. Fluid status, vital signs, and response to therapies must be closely monitored. Frequent skin care with tepid water to remove urea crystals will be comforting. Box 10-4 lists nursing intervention guidelines. Dialysis presents special nursing challenges, discussed later in this chapter.

Teaching includes the following:
- Identifying preventable environmental or health factors contributing to the illness (such as hypertension, nephrotoxic drugs)
- Teaching dietary restrictions and medication regimen
- Reporting signs and symptoms of infection and of returning renal failure to physician
- Instructing patient concerning activity
- Emphasizing need for ongoing follow-up care
- Providing nutritional support with specialized enteral formulas, which may contain essential amino acids and minerals, in addition to replacement of electrolytes (especially sodium to match insensible loss) and provision of caloric needs; nutritional assessment with appropriate modifications is made daily

Prognosis

Recovery from an episode of ARF depends on the underlying illness, condition of patient, and careful supportive management given during the period of kidney shutdown. The leading cause of death is infection, such as that of the urinary tract, lungs, and peritoneum. Mortality from fluid overload and acidosis

---

Box 10-4 *Nursing Intervention Guidelines for the Patient Undergoing Hemodialysis*

PATIENT TEACHING
Reinforce explanation of dialysis procedure
Inform of community resources
Explain dietary restrictions
Self-care, general

MONITORING DURING DIALYSIS
Maintain asepsis and universal precautions
Weigh before and after treatment
Obtain vital signs every 30 to 60 minutes (BP in arm without fistula)
Maintain orientation (thought processes may be altered)
Assess for hemorrhage resulting from heparin use during dialysis
Monitor equipment (interruption of procedure)

ACTIVITY
Diversions (reading, television, sleep)
Comfort (reclining, sitting, lying)
Dietary intake (may be hungry or nauseated)

CARE AFTER DIALYSIS OR BETWEEN TREATMENTS
Schedule fluid intake within restrictions
Monitor signs of fluid and electrolyte imbalance
Assess the access site for signs of infection, adequate circulation
Post signs regarding location of access site; do not take blood pressure or perform a venipuncture on arm with access site
Auscultate arteriovenous fistula for bruit (adventitious sound of venous/arterial origin heard on auscultation); palpate arteriovenous fistula for thrill (abnormal tremor felt on palpation of fistula)
Assess, document, and report changes in general status
Skin care: bathe with tepid water to remove urea deposit

---

has been reduced as a result of dialysis and other forms of therapy. There is potential for recovery of renal function in patients who survive the acute episode of tubular insufficiency. Although kidney tissue may regenerate more completely after toxic injury than ischemia, both forms usually show return to normal or near-normal renal function.

For those in whom ARF has been caused by glomerular disease or severe infection of kidney tissue, the prognosis may not be as favorable. Return of renal function is determined by the extent of scarring and destruction of functional renal tissue that has occurred during the acute episode of kidney failure.

CHRONIC RENAL FAILURE (END-STAGE RENAL DISEASE)

Etiology/Pathophysiology

Chronic renal failure, or end-stage renal disease (ESRD), exists when the kidneys are unable to regain normal function. ESRD develops slowly over an extended period as a result of kidney disease or other disease processes that compromise renal blood perfusion. As much as 80% of nephrons may be severely impaired before loss of renal function is detected. The most common causes of ESRD are pyelonephritis, chronic glomerulonephritis, glomerulosclerosis, chronic urinary obstruction, severe hypertension, diabetes mellitus, gout, and polycystic kidney disease. Whatever the cause, dialysis or kidney transplantation will be needed to maintain life.

ESRD represents a significant health problem worldwide, resulting in the death of thousands and financial crisis for the patients and their families. The government does actively help defray costs through the Medicare program.

Clinical Manifestations

The onset of signs and symptoms may be so gradual and the signs and symptoms so vague that the patient is unable to identify when the problems started. When questioned, the patient may be able to relate occurrences that seemed insignificant at the time. The clinical picture is usually unique to the individual. Common symptoms are headache; lethargy; asthenia (decreased strength or energy); anorexia; pruritus; elimination changes; anuria (urinary output less than 100 mL/day); muscle cramps or twitching; impotence; characteristic dusky yellow-tan, or gray skin color from retained urochrome pigments; and signs and symptoms characteristic of central nervous system involvement, such as disorientation and mental lapses.

Other associated conditions are responsible for many of the symptoms. Azotemia develops as excessive amounts of nitrogenous compounds build in the blood. Anemia occurs when the production of renal erythropoietin is decreased as a result of loss of kidney function. Acidosis, hypertension, and glucose intolerance may be present as a result of the insult to homeostasis.

Assessment

Collection of **subjective data** will include noting patient complaints of joint pain and edema; severe headaches; nausea; anorexia; intermittent chest pain; weakness; and in particular, fatigue, intractable singultus (hiccups), decreased libido, menstrual irregularities, and impaired concentration. The clinical consequences of renal failure are far reaching, affecting nearly every body system.

Collection of **objective data** involves a nursing assessment that may yield unremarkable results, except for signs and symptoms that support the patient complaints.

Uremic encephalopathy affects the central nervous system. Usually the first sign is a reduction in alertness and awareness. Respirations will become Kussmaul (abnormally deep, very rapid sighing respirations) in character, and coma develops. The accumulation of urates results in halitosis with a urine odor and "uremic frost" on the skin in the form of a white powder.

Diagnostic Tests

Diagnosis of ESRD is confirmed by elevated BUN of at least 50 mg/dL and serum creatinine levels greater than 5 mg/dL, electrolyte imbalance (including a decreased number of bicarbonate and magnesium and an increased number of potassium, sodium, and phosphatase ions), and other indicators related to the underlying cause. Renal function studies assess the degree of damage and/or level of renal function.

Medical Management

Medical management is instituted to conserve renal function as long as possible. Renal dialysis is initiated when necessary, and the patient may be prepared for renal transplantation. Drug therapy may include anticonvulsants to control seizure activity (phenytoin [Dilantin], diazepam [Valium]), antianemics, vitamin supplements to counteract nutritional deficiencies, antiemetics (prochlorperazine [Compazine]), antipruritics (cyproheptadine [Periactin]), and biologic response modifiers to stimulate red cell production (epoetin alfa [Epogen]) to treat anemia caused by a reduced production of erythropoietin. Iron deficiency anemia must be treated with ferrous sulfate orally or iron dextran (DexFerrum per Z-track IM method) before Epogen (EPO) will be effective.

Nursing Interventions and Patient Teaching

Nursing interventions focus on restoring homeostasis. Measures to control fluid and electrolyte balance vary greatly, according to unique needs of the individual patient. Nutritional therapy is aimed at preserving protein stores and preventing production of additional protein waste products that the kidney would have to clear. High biologic proteins are used to provide the essential amino acids.

The diet is high in calories from carbohydrates and fats from polyunsaturated sources (to maintain weight and spare protein), at least 2500 to 3000 calories daily. Other dietary restrictions are related to the patient's degree of acidosis. Potassium is retained, so foods high in potassium are restricted. Sodium is controlled at a level sufficient to replace sodium loss without causing fluid retention.

Nursing interventions for ARF are also instituted for ESRD. Emphasis is placed on emotional support for the patient who faces role changes and invasive treatments such as dialysis and/or kidney transplantation. As discussed in the Health Promotion Considerations for the patient with renal failure, fluid balance is of prime importance. The patient may have fluid equal to the amount excreted in the urine plus about 300 to 600 mL to compensate for **insensible** (imperceptible) **fluid loss** (fluid lost through the lungs, perspiration, and feces). Salt substitutes are not advised, because most contain potassium. If seizure activity occurs, safety measures need to be instituted to provide for patient protection (Nursing Care Plan box) (see also Chapter 14).

Patient teaching should emphasize food exchanges and fluid intake within restrictions prescribed for that patient. Patient should be encouraged to increase activity as tolerated, maintain

---

 Health Promotion Considerations

The Patient with Renal Failure

FLUID AND ELECTROLYTE BALANCE

Assess I&O (hourly may be indicated).
Weigh daily (same time, same clothing, same scale).
Assess overt (open to view) signs of hydration status (edema, turgor).
Assess covert (hidden) signs of hydration status (breath sounds, laboratory studies, and so on).

NUTRITION

Provide prescribed diet.
Guide patient food selection.
Plan fluid intake per shift within prescribed limits and according to patient preference.
Reinforce diet instructions as indicated.

COMFORT AND SAFETY

Provide quiet environment (sound and lighting).
Space nursing interventions to conserve patient energy.
Medicate as needed for comfort.

Skin care to alleviate discomfort resulting from pruritus.
Mouth care as needed.
Maintain asepsis during procedures.
Prevent exposure to pathogens.

COPING BEHAVIORS

Listen (patient and significant other).
Refer to pastoral care or religious support group.
Provide private times with significant others.
Offer interview with social services.

DOCUMENTATION AND REPORTING

Document all relevant findings.
Maintain open communications with supervisory staff.
Adjust nursing care plan as indicated to meet changing patient needs.
Dietary restrictions: food exchange, measuring fluids, food diary.
Health promotion/illness prevention measures.

NURSING CARE PLAN

The Patient with End-Stage Renal Disease (ESRD)

Mr. J., a 37-year-old high school basketball coach, visited his family doctor with complaints of weight gain, decreasing strength, increasing inability to concentrate, and morning headaches. Physical examination revealed severe hypertension, yellow-gray skin color, and pale mucous membranes. After diagnostic studies reveal chronic glomerulonephritis with ESRD, Mr. J. is admitted to the hospital to stabilize his condition.

NURSING DIAGNOSIS *Excess fluid volume, related to compromised renal regulatory mechanism, as evidenced by systemic edema*

Patient Goals/Expected Outcomes	Nursing Intervention	Evaluation

The patient will be able to reduce fluid to precrisis level	Record baseline assessment data
	Create chart for patient monitoring of
	  —Daily weight
	  —Intake and output
	  —Edema
		Patient able to complete daily self-monitoring with 1 lb weight loss daily × 3

The patient will modify diet to exclude foods/fluids that foster sodium, potassium, and water retention	Teach nutritional guidelines for dietary and fluid parameters with scheduling Evaluate daily/prn for systemic edema: girth, skin turgor, respiratory rate and quality Monitor for manifestations of electrolyte imbalance Teach patient and significant other about the type, cause, and treatment for fluid and electrolyte imbalance, as appropriate	Patient able to order daily diet and fluids within prescribed parameters

NURSING CARE PLAN

The Patient with End-Stage Renal Disease (ESRD)—cont'd

NURSING DIAGNOSIS *Powerlessness, related to sudden onset of life-altering illness as evidenced by patient statements: "I've always tried to take care of myself—look where it got me. Nowhere! Now I have to face my own death!"*

Patient Goals/Expected Outcomes	Nursing Intervention	Evaluation
The patient will be empowered to assist in planning own care and in goal achievement.	Provide a presence of support for the patient. Explain plans and procedures before scheduled times, according to patient's ability to understand. Negotaiate with patient when changes are necessary. Accept patient's expression of self and values. Include significant other in planning for the patient's maximum role in self-management. Communicate unique patient planning arrangements for continuity with all treatment team members.	Patient voices a sense that the staff is sensitive to his needs. Patient seems to be able to plan modifications in work and home schedules to accommodate health needs.

NURSING DIAGNOSIS *Deficient knowledge, related to health education and home maintenance for ESRD*

Patient Goals/Expected Outcomes	Nursing Intervention	Evaluation

The patient will describe the fundamental characteristics of ESRD and treatment options.	Assess the amount and depth of the patient's information about ESRD.
	Collaborate with physician and treatment team about individualizing established institutional protocol for care of the patient with ESRD:
	1. What happens when kidneys fail?
	2. Treatment options
	   a. Hemodialysis
	   b. Peritoneal dialysis
	   c. Kidney transplantation
	3. Inpatient versus outpatient care
	4. Financing treatment
	5. Teaching aids
	6. Organizations that can help
	Plan time to listen to the patient's and family's concerns and fears.
	Allow time for questions and answers and teaching reinforcement each day.
	Arrange (with patient's permission) opportunity for patient and family to meet with a patient/family who is positively adapting to ESRD.
	Be consistent in scheduling treatments with primary health care providers.
	Participate in end-of-life planning, when and if appropriate.
		
		Patient is able to correctly answer basic questions about treatment options.
		
		Patient is able to correctly answer questions from teaching and is open to pose new questions.

? CRITICAL THINKING QUESTIONS

1. Mr. J. complains of loss of appetite as well as a limited choice of foods to eat. Helpful suggestions to improve his nutritional status would include:

2. Mr. J. establishes a therapeutic nurse-patient relationship with Nurse B. He confides that he is having marital problems partly due to his inability to have a satisfactory sexual relationship with his wife. An appropriate response by the nurse would be:

3. The nurse notes Mr. J.'s disinterest in his therapeutic regimen of diet, medications, and fluid restrictions. He states, "What's the use? I will never be well again." Therapeutic interventions would include:

impeccable skin care, prevent infection and injury, and develop coping behaviors to adapt to lifestyle for patient, family, and caretaker.

CARE OF THE PATIENT REQUIRING DIALYSIS

Dialysis (a medical procedure for the removal of certain elements from the blood by virtue of the difference in their rates of diffusion through an external semipermeable membrane or, in the case of peritoneal dialysis, through the peritoneum) mimics kidney function, helping to restore balance when normal kidney function is interrupted temporarily or permanently. Dialysis involves either diffusion of wastes, drugs, and/or excess electrolytes and/or osmosis of water across a semipermeable membrane into a dialysate fluid that is prescribed specific to individual patient needs. Dialysis is achieved by the process of hemodialysis or peritoneal dialysis.

HEMODIALYSIS

Hemodialysis requires an access to the patient's circulatory system to route blood through the artificial kidney (dialyzer) for removal of wastes, fluids, and electrolytes and then return the blood to the patient's body. Temporary methods include subclavian or femoral catheters or an external shunt placed in the nondominant forearm (Figure 10-9). In ESRD, access can be achieved by constructing a direct or a graft arteriovenous fistula (Figure 10-10). The AV fistula is preferred for permanent access.

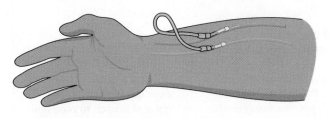

FIGURE **10-9** External arteriovenous shunt.

Hemodialysis is usually scheduled three times a week for 3 to 6 hours. Patients can be maintained on dialysis therapy indefinitely. Other patients may be maintained while waiting for kidney transplantation.

In a comparative study of the use of daily versus traditional hemodialysis on alternative days, researchers found that the more frequent hemodialysis decreased the risk of fatal nonrenal complications of acute renal failure (Schiffl et al, 2002).

Medical Management

Medical management includes continuation of previously instituted therapies. Blood levels of drugs excreted by the kidney must be closely monitored to maintain therapeutic levels and to prevent toxic accumulations. Dose adjustments are affected by glomerular filtration rate, dialysis, vomiting, and doses missed during hospital treatments. Medication may include antihypertensives, cardiac glycosides, antibiotics, and antidysrhythmics. The patient is instructed not to take over-the-counter medications without consulting the physician.

Nursing Interventions

Nursing interventions are dictated by individual patient conditions. The patient receiving renal dialysis may have other acute or chronic problems. Most patients are dialyzed on an outpatient basis. (General nursing intervention guidelines are noted later in Box 10-6 and the ESRD Nursing Care Plan.) Psychosocial aspects of care for patients receiving dialysis are illustrated in the Therapeutic Dialogue.

Nurses have a key responsibility for maintaining access sites and preventing and/or managing infection. Optimally, a structured teaching program will be used, with individualization of patient teaching strategies to accommodate culture and knowledge level.

PERITONEAL DIALYSIS

Peritoneal dialysis can be performed with a minimum of equipment and by the patient who is ambulatory. Unlike hemodialysis, peritoneal dialysis is performed 4

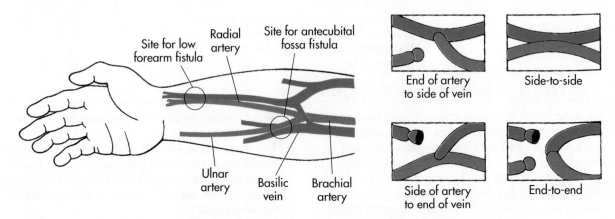

FIGURE **10-10** Internal arteriovenous fistula. Types of fistula construction.

Therapeutic Dialogue

Mr. J., student nurse, enters Mr. K.'s room to complete the initial morning assessment and finds him crying while struggling to get out of bed.

NURSE: *Mr. K, what's wrong? (general lead, allows patient to describe)*

PATIENT: *Oh, nothing!*

NURSE: *(therapeutic silence, remains attentive, gives time)*

PATIENT: *Nothing is going right. I might as well be dead!*

NURSE: *What's wrong? (general lead, patient didn't answer, encourages description)*

PATIENT: *I was trying to get up to take a shower, but I'm so weak I can't get myself out of bed.*

NURSE: *That must be frustrating. (voicing the implied)*

PATIENT: *That's an understatement! Look at me! I'm 37 years old; I should be in my prime but instead I'm gaining weight; can't do my job because I can't concentrate. How am I supposed to feel?*

NURSE: *It must be frightening to experience all these changes. It would be understandable for you to be scared. (validating feelings)*

PATIENT: *I am scared! What if I never get better? I read this article about someone younger than I am who had the same thing and he died when he had to go on dialysis.*

NURSE: *What do you think will happen to you? (general lead, encourages description without prescribing response)*

PATIENT: *Well, I don't know. The doctor keeps avoiding my questions and I see myself being less able to do anything. Maybe I am afraid—afraid of dying.*

NURSE: *(therapeutic silence, allows time for reflection)*

PATIENT: *Well, I never thought I'd say that—being afraid to die. It doesn't seem so frightening to say. I guess I didn't trust myself to be honest with myself or anyone else.*

NURSE: *Being honest with yourself is an important step to understanding. (pause) It seems, too, that you may not have accurate information about your illness. Let's plan to talk with your doctor about what you can reasonably expect—things you will be able to do, limitations, and things that you can do to enhance your physical and emotional health (summarizing and goal setting for individualized patient teaching and discharge planning).*

PATIENT: *That sounds great, Mr. J. I really do want to do whatever I can to improve my chances of a better life. Would you help me get up to shower?*

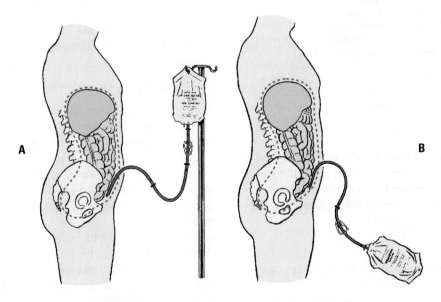

FIGURE **10-11** Peritoneal dialysis. **A,** Inflow. **B,** Outflow.

times a day, 7 days a week. One exchange cycle usually requires 30 to 40 minutes. The principle of osmosis and diffusion through a semipermeable membrane is the same as in hemodialysis, but the peritoneum is used as the semipermeable membrane instead of the artificial kidney. Peritoneal dialysis is contraindicated for those individuals with systemic inflammatory disease, previous abdominal surgery, and chronic back pain, among others.

To facilitate peritoneal dialysis, the physician places a catheter into the peritoneal space under aseptic conditions (Figure 10-11). The dialyzing fluid is then instilled for a predetermined period, then drained. The patient with ESRD may be maintained on peritoneal dialysis, continuous ambulatory peritoneal dialysis (CAPD), or continuous cycle peritoneal dialysis (CCPD). Nocturnal intermittent peritoneal dialysis can be done three to five times per week for 10 to 12 hours.

The patient is taught how to do the dialysis, which allows for more freedom. Although hemodialysis can also be done at home using strict aseptic technique, it is much more expensive and confining than CAPD.

Nursing Interventions

Common complications associated with peritoneal dialysis guide nursing interventions. Hypotension may occur with excessive sodium and fluid removal. Peritonitis may arise from sepsis. Pain and hemorrhage may accompany instillation of the dialysate. Box 10-5 lists nursing intervention guidelines for peritoneal dialysis.

Nursing diagnoses and interventions for the patient undergoing dialysis include but are not limited to the following:

NURSING DIAGNOSES	NURSING INTERVENTIONS
Ineffective role performance, related to chronic illness, treatment side effects	Encourage verbalization of self-concept. Assist in identifying personal strengths. Assist patient and significant others with clarifying expected roles and those that must be relinquished or altered. Support grief work if loss of role has occurred.
Ineffective tissue perfusion, peripheral, related to risk of disconnection/clotting of vascular access	Avoid taking BP and venipuncture in arm with fistula/cannula. Auscultate for bruits. Observe access site for skin color and condition. After dialysis, inspect needle puncture sites for bleeding.

A new bioartificial kidney device, the Renal Assist Device, appears to more completely replace the functions of the failed kidney and is in clinical trials in the treatment of critically ill patients with acute renal failure (Dirkes & Kozlowski, 2003).

Prognosis

The patient with effective medical management can be maintained indefinitely on dialysis.

SURGICAL PROCEDURES FOR URINARY DYSFUNCTION

If damage to the urinary system cannot be corrected by medical management, surgical intervention may be necessary for temporary or permanent resection of the affected organ, such as when kidney function is lost. Dialysis is a viable management alternative, but a kidney transplant is preferable. It may become necessary for the patient to have a live or cadaver kidney replace

---

Box 10-5 *Nursing Intervention Guidelines for the Patient Undergoing Peritoneal Dialysis*

PATIENT TEACHING
Explanation of procedure
Signs of complications
Diet and/or fluid restrictions
Medication (schedule in relation to dialysis time)
Dialysate should be body temperature to lessen discomfort

MONITORING DURING DIALYSIS
Weigh before and after procedure
Hemorrhage (smoky, pink, or red-tinged dialysate)
Type of dialysate (tailored to patient needs)
Amount and timing of dialysate instillation
Vital signs

CARE BETWEEN DIALYSES
Signs of peritonitis (pain, fever, cloudy fluid)
Strict aseptic care of catheter site
Weigh daily

---

the damaged kidney. Common surgical interventions and nursing intervention priorities are listed in Table 10-4. Preoperative and intraoperative management measures are the same as for major abdominal surgery and general anesthesia (see Chapter 2). Suggested nursing diagnoses include those for abdominal surgery.

NEPHRECTOMY

Nephrectomy is the surgical removal of the kidney. Postoperative management for surgical removal of the kidney is based on the prevention and detection of hemorrhage by monitoring vital signs, especially pulse and blood pressure; observation for restlessness and for GI complications of nausea, vomiting, and abdominal distention; and establishment of adequate urinary drainage. I&O are recorded. If the thoracic cavity is opened during surgery, the patient will have chest tubes (see Chapter 9). Pain may compromise respiratory efficiency. Analgesics are administered as ordered to facilitate lung expansion and the patient's activity level. The patient is repositioned every 2 hours and ambulated as ordered. Dressings are changed according to the physician's order, and the amount and color of any drainage is recorded.

Patient Teaching

This includes instructing the patient to avoid heavy lifting, maintain hydration of 2000 mL each day unless contraindicated, monitor output, avoid use of alcohol, and avoid respiratory infections and hazardous activities that may cause assault to the remaining kidney.

Table 10-4 | *Surgical Intervention and Nursing Intervention Priorities*

SURGICAL INTERVENTION	NURSING INTERVENTION PRIORITIES
Nephrostomy: surgical procedure in which an incision is made on the flank of patient, so that a catheter can be inserted into the kidney pelvis for drainage	Meticulous skin care, assessment for hemorrhage, accurate I&O
Nephrectomy: surgical removal of the kidney	Assessment for hemorrhage, promotion of respiratory effort, accurate I&O
Cystectomy: surgical removal of the bladder	Promotion of urinary drainage via ileal conduit, I&O
Ureterosigmoidostomy: surgical procedure in which a ureter is implanted in the sigmoid colon of the intestinal tract	Meticulous skin care, monitoring of electrolyte imbalance, assessment of signs and symptoms of infection
Cutaneous ureterostomy: surgical implantation of the terminal ends of the ureter under the skin	Meticulous skin care, assessment of urinary obstruction, accurate I&O

Prognosis

Complete recovery from nephrectomy is expected in the absence of any complication.

NEPHROSTOMY

Nephrostomy is an incision to drain the pelvis of the kidney. Catheters are used to drain the wound. Care must be given to prevent obstruction of the catheters with blood clots postoperatively. The amount and nature of drainage from the catheters is measured and recorded, and dressings are changed frequently, keeping the skin clean using surgical sepsis. The patient is turned and positioned to the affected side when ordered to facilitate drainage and assist in respiratory ventilation. Never clamp a nephrostomy catheter (tube); acute pyelonephritis may result. If ordered by the physician, irrigation of a nephrostomy catheter is performed using strict aseptic technique. Gentle instillation of no more than 5 mL of sterile saline solution at one time prevents renal damage.

KIDNEY TRANSPLANTATION

There are special considerations for nursing interventions for a kidney transplantation recipient. Preoperative nursing intervention is complicated by the patient's fear and anxiety about transplantation and about possible rejection of the implanted organ. The patient is dialyzed until surgery can be satisfactorily completed. In surgery the nonfunctioning kidney remains in place and the donor kidney is positioned in the iliac fossa anterior to the crest of the ileum. The ureter is anastomosed into either the patient's ureter or bladder (Figure 10-12).

Postoperatively the patient is assessed for signs of rejection and infection: apprehension, generalized edema, fever, increased blood pressure, oliguria, edema, and tenderness over the graft site. An immunosuppressive agent, such as cyclosporine (Sandimmune), is used alone or in conjunction with steroids. Cyclosporine is considered an effective drug in suppressing the im-

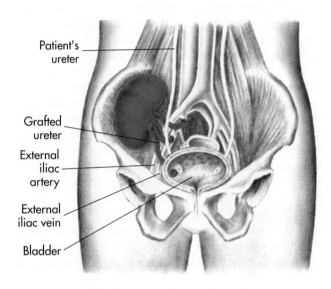

Patient's ureter

Grafted ureter

External iliac artery

External iliac vein

Bladder

FIGURE **10-12** Renal transplantation.

mune system's efforts to reject tissue while leaving the recipient sufficient immune activity to combat infection. Mycophenolate (CellCept) and tacrolimus (Prograf) are drugs now used to prevent rejection of kidney transplants; they are used in combination with corticosteroids. Immunosuppressive therapy increases the risk for infection and possible steroid-induced bleeding.

Patient Teaching

Home follow-up becomes a life pattern for the transplantation patient. Patient education is extensive: diet, fluids, daily weights, strict I&O measurements, prevention of infection, and avoidance of activities that may compromise the integrity of the urinary tract. Community support groups, sponsored by the National Association of Patients on Hemodialysis and Transplantation, Inc., assist the patient and family to adapt to living with dialysis and transplantation. The

National Kidney Foundation has a written protocol for the procurement of organs for donation.

Prognosis

Success of renal transplantation parallels the individual patient's general health status and compliance to the treatment plan. Transplantation offers the only possibility of return to a normal lifestyle for the ESRD patient.

URINARY DIVERSION

Several types of procedures are used to divert the flow of urine when required for treatment of bladder cancer, invasive cancer of the cervix, neurogenic bladder, and congenital anomalies. Often a cystectomy, which is the surgical removal of the bladder, is performed.

The cystectomy patient presents a unique challenge because of the need to create an artificial port for urine elimination. The most common urinary diversion procedure is the ileal conduit (Bricker's procedure or ileal loop). In an ileal conduit procedure the ureters are implanted into a loop of the ileum that is isolated and brought to the surface of the abdominal wall (Figure 10-13). Occasionally a segment of the sigmoid colon is isolated and used instead of the ileum to form a sigmoid conduit. The integrity of bowel function is maintained with the anastomosis of the remaining intestine. A drainage bag (urostomy bag or appliance) is fitted over the stoma to contain the constant drainage of urine. Continual urine drainage prevents increased pressure within the conduit that would cause backflow to the kidneys, compromise the circulatory integrity of the conduit, or rupture the surgical anastomosis. Decreased urine output and low abdominal pain may signal the onset of such problems. Complications of this procedure are wound infection, dehiscence, urinary leakage, ureteral obstruction, small bowel obstruction, stomal gangrene, atrophy of the stoma, pyelonephritis, renal calculi, and/or a compromised respiratory status secondary to incisional pain.

Postoperatively, urine flow is measured hourly. Output less than 30 mL/hour should be reported to the physician immediately. A healthy stoma will appear moist and pink and may even bleed slightly. The skin around the stoma should be inspected daily for signs of bleeding, excoriation, and infection. There will be mucus present in the urine from the intestinal secretions. Large quantities of water should be ingested to flush the ileal conduit. Any odor of urine about the patient may indicate an infection or leak of urine from the drainage bag. Early signs of urinary leakage (indicating a leak in an anastomosis) include increased abdominal girth, fever, and drainage through the incision, tubes, or drains. Ureteral separation from the conduit may cause urine to seep into the peritoneal cavity; observe the patient for signs and symptoms of peritonitis such as fever, abdominal pain and rigidity, and absence of bowel sounds.

Care of the patient with an ileal conduit is a nursing challenge because of the continual drainage of urine through the stoma.

To change the urostomy bag, remove and drain it. Cleanse the skin with water, and apply the new appliance as outlined in the institution's standards of care. When the peristomal skin is healed, the bag is emptied at 2- to 3-hour intervals and at night a straight drainage tube is connected to a drainage bag. A permanent urostomy bag can be left in place 4 to 7 days if it remains sealed. The nurse should recommend that the patient have two bags, so one can be worn while the other is washed. Some patients prefer to use disposable bags. Odor is controlled by using deodorant drops or tablets in the urostomy bag; avoiding odor-producing foods, such as beans, onions, cabbage, asparagus, high-fiber wheat, simple sugars, and milk in the lactose-intolerant patient; and cleansing the urostomy bag with a vinegar and water rinse and thoroughly drying.

The **continent ileal urinary reservoir,** or **Kock pouch,** is created by implantation of the ureters into a segment of the small intestine that has been surgically removed from the rest of the bowel and anastomosed to the abdominal wall. Control of urine flow is achieved by the use of a nipplelike valve that prevents leakage of urine. To drain the urine from the reservoir, the patient inserts a catheter through the valve at regular intervals, thus minimizing the reabsorption of waste materials from the urine and reflux into the ureters (Figure 10-14).

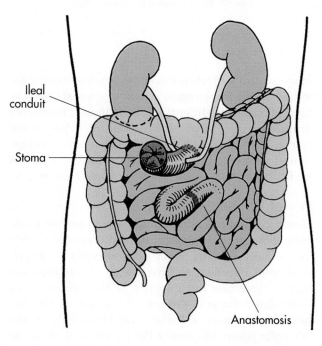

Ileal conduit

Stoma

Anastomosis

FIGURE **10-13** Ileal conduit or ileal loop.

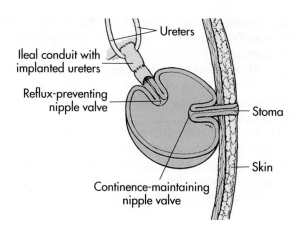

lleal conduit with implanted ureters

Reflux-preventing nipple valve

Ureters

Stoma

Skin

Continence-maintaining nipple valve

FIGURE **10-14** Kock pouch.

Patient Teaching

Patient teaching centers on the task of lifestyle adaptation: care of the stoma, nutrition, fluid intake, maintaining self-esteem in light of altered body image, modifying sexual activities, and early detection of complications. Patient teaching begins with appliance selection, sizing the stoma, and changing the appliances. The home health nurse can assist the patient in modifying care to the home environment and by providing support during this stressful adjustment period (Home Health Considerations box).

Prognosis

Although the patient may fully recover without recurrence, the day-to-day challenges of managing a urinary diversion will be permanent.

NURSING PROCESS *for the Patient with a Urinary Disorder*

The role of the licensed practical nurse/licensed vocational nurse (LPN/LVN) in the nursing process as stated is that the LPN/LVN will:

- Participate in planning care for patients based on patient needs
- Review patient's plan of care and recommend revisions as needed
- Review and follow defined prioritzation for patient care
- Use clinical pathways/care maps/care plans to guide and review patient care

Assessment

Assessment of the urinary tract is included in baseline data for all patients. The assessment includes **subjective data:** the patient's description of urination patterns and associated sensations, such as complaints of burning or pain upon urination or difficulty maintaining the urine stream. The nurse supplements subjective data with **objective data** by assessing for signs of fluid overload or depletion. The skin provides easily assessed clues about the patient's state of hydration.

For example, dryness and pruritus (itching) can occur as a result of electrolyte imbalance or the buildup of waste products.

Careful attention should be given to assessment of high-risk populations. Urinary disorders are associated with a number of systemic malformations and structural anomalies in newborns. Pediatric patients, especially girls, are susceptible to urinary tract infections because of the short urethra. Geriatric patients may experience weakened musculature and sphincter tone, with resultant difficulty in bladder control. In male patients, enlargement of the prostate gland may interfere with initiating and maintaining an adequate urine stream.

Occupational and environmental factors also contribute to the development of renal disease. Nephrotoxins are substances with specific destructive properties for the kidneys. Sources include industrial exposure to heavy metals, such as lead and mercury, and medical treatment with cisplatin, aminoglycoside antibiotics (Gentamicin or Kanamycin), nonsteroidal anti-inflammatory drugs (NSAIDs), or radiopaque contrast media.

Other vulnerable populations include those patients experiencing systemic changes from altered health states, such as pregnancy, diabetes mellitus, or hypertension. Most susceptible are those with conditions that directly compromise renal function: trauma, fluid depletion or retention, and especially those patients with active or suspected renal disease.

Nursing Diagnosis

Assisting in the analysis of assessment data is the next step in nursing care planning. Analysis leads to conclusions about the patient's health status. These data are clustered, and North American Nursing Diagnosis Association (NANDA)–approved nursing diagnoses that describe the patient's problems are selected. Suggested nursing diagnoses are included with the discussion of each urinary tract disorder. These nursing diagnoses serve as the foundation for care planning:

Impaired urinary elimination
Ineffective tissue perfusion: renal
Acute pain; chronic pain
Risk for infection
Risk for deficient fluid volume
Excess fluid volume
Ineffective sexuality patterns
Deficient knowledge

Note that suggested priority nursing diagnoses and interventions appear throughout the text with each disorder.

Expected Outcomes/Planning

Assisting in planning begins with the identification of desired outcomes, stated in terms of patient-centered goals. For the patient with a urinary disorder, the nursing care priority is the short-term goal to reestablish urinary flow and renal function. Long-term planning for the patient and family or significant other focuses on prevention of complications and quick response to recurrence of problems. Goals are individualized to reflect the unique patient experience and are modified to adapt to the patient's changing health status and urinary elimination management.

Goal #1: The patient will achieve control of the elimination of urine.

Outcome: Patient reports effective management of normal patterns of urination.

Goal #2: The patient will use self-modification to prevent and detect symptoms of urinary disorders for early signs and symptoms of recurrent urinary tract infection.

Outcome: Patient reports no signs or symptoms of recurrent urinary difficulty.

Implementation

Implementation of the plan of care is the fourth step of the nursing process. Nursing interventions specific to patient needs help ensure individualized care. Activities may be modified or delayed based on the patient's condition. Written documentation of the nursing action and the patient response is an important part of this phase.

Evaluation

Evaluation of urinary status is determined by success in attaining expected outcomes. Monitoring of urine output and character is continual. Because of the tendency of some urinary disorders to become chronic, the need for patient involvement in the prevention of complications is vitally important. Avoidance of risk factors and early detection of symptoms is essential to limit damage to the urinary tract.

Goal #1: The patient will experience normal patterns of urinary elimination.

Evaluation of outcome: Patient reports return to own normal voiding.

Goal #2: The patient will monitor self for early signs and symptoms of recurrent urinary tract infection.

Evaluation of outcome: Patient is able to correctly answer questions about signs and symptoms and appropriate measures to take for treatment.

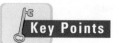
Key Points

- The kidneys lie retroperitoneally, just below the diaphragm.
- The functioning unit of the kidney is the nephron.
- The kidneys rid the body of wastes and excess electrolytes, maintain water and electrolyte balance, and maintain acid-base balance.
- Kidney function is achieved by the processes of filtration, secretion, and reabsorption.
- Assessment of the urinary tract is included in baseline data for all patients.
- The subject of urinary problems is an embarrassing topic for many patients. The nurse must be sensitive to the patient's feelings and be supportive.
- Aging may have a negative influence on urinary function, but many problems can be corrected.
- Hydration status is monitored by daily weights, I&O, laboratory studies, inspection of the skin and mucous membranes, and assessing the level of consciousness.
- A large percentage of nosocomial infections involve the urinary tract.
- Proper care of urinary catheters will decrease the chance of urinary tract infections.
- Surgical intervention may be indicated for urinary dysfunction that cannot be corrected by medical management.
- Dialysis, which mimics kidney function, may be used temporarily or as a long-term therapy.
- Dietary, fluid, and medication modifications may be necessary for the patient with urinary dysfunction.
- Sacral nerve stimulation for urinary urge incontinence is conducted with a permanently implanted electrical stimulation device that changes neuronal activity in the sacral efferent and afferent nerves to reduce urinary urge incontinence.

Go to your free CD-ROM for an Audio Glossary, animations, video clips, and Review Questions for the NCLEX-PN® Examination.

evolve Be sure to visit the companion Evolve site at http://evolve.elsevier.com/Christensen/adult/ for WebLinks and additional online resources.

CHAPTER CHALLENGE

1. When reading the urinalysis report, the nurse recognizes this result as abnormal:
   1. turbidity clear.
   2. pH 6.0.
   3. glucose negative.
   4. red blood cells, 15 to 20.

2. Following a renal angiography, the patient assessment priority is the:
   1. blood pressure.
   2. respiratory effort.
   3. puncture site.
   4. urinary output.

3. The nursing care plan includes teaching the patient Kegel exercises. The nurse will teach the patient to alternately tighten and relax which group of muscles?
   1. Perineal floor
   2. Pubococcygeal
   3. Abdominis rectus
   4. Detrusor

4. The physician has talked to Mr. D. and his wife about the treatment plan for Mr. D.'s bladder cancer. Later, Mr. D. tells the nurse he doesn't understand what the doctor is going to do. The most appropriate response by the nurse would be:
   1. "Okay. I'll explain it to you again."
   2. "Make a list of questions for the doctor."
   3. "Try not to think about the treatment."
   4. "Tell me what you know about the treatment."

5. Which of the following activities would be harmful for the incontinent patient?
   1. Restricting fluid intake
   2. Drinking only water
   3. Fluid intake of 2000 mL per day
   4. Restricting acidic fruit juice intake

6. The nurse recognizes that the most common causative organism in pyelonephritis is:
   1. *Candida albicans.*
   2. *Klebsiella.*
   3. *Escherichia coli.*
   4. *Pseudomonas.*

7. The most important factor to foster patient compliance with the treatment plan is to provide the patient with:
   1. a set time schedule to follow.
   2. data on success rates.
   3. written information of the plan.
   4. an active role in the planning.

8. When scheduling the administration of furosemide (Lasix) it would be in the patient's best interest to schedule the medication to be given at:
   1. 9 AM
   2. 12 PM (noon)
   3. 2100
   4. 12 AM (midnight)

9. In discussion with the ESRD patient about dietary needs, the nurse recognizes that foods highest in potassium include:
   1. apples, applesauce, grapes, and raisins.
   2. bananas, nuts, and chocolate.
   3. grapefruit, tomatoes, oranges, and bananas.
   4. milk, grapefruit, orange juice, and sugar.

10. Which of the following patient reports indicates (phenozopyridine HCl (Pyridium) is being effective?
    1. Decreased bladder spasms
    2. Decrease in burning
    3. Increased urine output
    4. Increased pain tolerance

11. When calculating actual urine output during continuous bladder irrigations the nurse would:
    1. measure and record all fluid output in the drainage bag.
    2. measure the total output and deduct the amount of irrigation solution used.
    3. add the total of all intravenous and irrigation solutions and deduct output.
    4. measure total output and deduct the total intravenous solutions.

12. What statement by the patient indicates the need for further teaching before renal angiography?
    1. "I will miss having breakfast."
    2. "I know the nurse will be checking my pulse after the test."
    3. "I'm glad I don't have to stay in bed after the test."
    4. "I had a test similar to this 3 years ago."

13. The nurse performs a catheterization immediately after the patient voids and obtains 30 mL residual urine. The next step would be to:
    1. document the procedure with outcome data.
    2. continue the catheterization routine after each voiding.
    3. restrict fluid intake after dinner.
    4. immediately notify the physician of the results.

14. Which of these goals would have priority in planning care of the aging patient with urinary incontinence?
    1. Recognizes the urge to void
    2. Mobility necessary for toileting independently
    3. Episodes of incontinency decrease
    4. Drinks a minimum of 2000 mL of fluid per day

Continued

CHAPTER CHALLENGE—cont'd

15. The goal for peritoneal dialysis is to:
    1. remove toxins and metabolic waste.
    2. produce rapid fluid shifts.
    3. increase clearance of dialysate flow.
    4. restore normal kidney function.

16. In postoperative care of the patient with an arteriovenous shunt, the nurse should:
    1. secure the shunt with an elastic bandage.
    2. notify the physician if a bruit or thrill is present.
    3. change the shunt if clotting occurs.
    4. use strict surgical asepsis for dressing changes.

17. The teaching priority for the patient with acute renal failure is:
    1. treatment of hyponatremia.
    2. prevention of infection.
    3. maintenance urine output at 50 mL/hour.
    4. control of caloric intake.

18. The ESRD patient receiving hemodialysis is at risk for:
    1. sepsis.
    2. renal insufficiency.
    3. anemia.
    4. *Klebsiella* infection.

19. The primary function of the kidney is:
    1. regulation of enzymes.
    2. filtration of water and blood products.
    3. collection of urine from the body.
    4. control of the adrenal glands.

20. The priority short-term goal for disorders of the urinary system is:
    1. patient confidentiality.
    2. privacy.
    3. education for patient and family.
    4. normal patterns of urinary elimination.

21. Assessment of the patient with a urinary disorder may be complicated by:
    1. European practices to withhold personal information.
    2. marital status.
    3. coexisting pathology.
    4. social taboos surrounding sexuality.

22. When the nurse makes rounds, she discovers that there is no urine drainage from a postoperative patient's Foley catheter. The first nursing action is to:
    1. ensure patency.
    2. irrigate until clear.
    3. call the physician.
    4. insert larger lumen catheter.

23. Which of the following problems constitutes a medical emergency?
    1. Anuria
    2. Polyuria
    3. Dysuria
    4. Dyspnea

24. The most common cause of renal failure is:
    1. trauma.
    2. diabetes mellitus.
    3. cancer.
    4. heart failure.

25. The clinical findings in the oliguric phase of acute renal failure include:
    1. BUN and creatinine levels rise.
    2. urine output increases.
    3. signs of impending shock.
    4. increased blood flow to the kidneys.

26. During postoperative care of the patient with an ileoconduit, which of these findings represents an emergency?
    1. Abdominal pain
    2. Presence of mucus in the urine
    3. Nausea and vomiting
    4. Absence of bowel sounds

27. Choose all of the correct answers for the patient with cystitis.
    1. Teach the patient to drink cranberry juice to treat and prevent UTIs.
    2. Teach the female patient to cleanse the perineal area from anterior to posterior to prevent rectal *E. coli* contamination of the urethra.
    3. Encourage the patient to drink 2000 mL of fluid per day, unless contraindicated.
    4. Instruct the patient that it is acceptable to stop taking prescribed medications when symptoms subside.

28. Renal calculi may result from which of the following? (Choose all correct answers.)
    1. Stasis of urine caused by obstruction or quadriplegia
    2. Infections of urinary tract
    3. Hyperparathyroidism, which causes increase in calcium metabolism
    4. Diabetes mellitus

29. The collection of subjective and objective data for the patient with acute glomerulonephritis could include which of the following? (Choose all correct answers.)

    1. Periorbital edema
    2. Anorexia
    3. Hypotension
    4. Frankly sanguineous urine

30. In preparing a patient for an IVP, careful preparation is necessary. These nursing interventions would include which of the following? (Choose all correct answers.)

    1. NPO for about 12 hours before examination.
    2. Ascertaining whether patient has allergy to magnesium
    3. Giving prescribed bowel prep
    4. Instructing patient concerning IVP

11 Care of the Patient with an Endocrine Disorder

BARBARA LAURITSEN CHRISTENSEN

Objectives

After reading this chapter, the student should be able to do the following:

Anatomy and Physiology

1. List and describe the endocrine glands and their hormones.
2. Explain the action of the hormones on their target organs.
3. Define the negative feedback system.
4. Describe how the hypothalamus controls the anterior and posterior pituitary glands.

Medical-Surgical

5. Define the key terms as listed.
6. Discuss the etiology/pathophysiology, clinical manifestations, assessment, diagnostic tests, medical management, nursing interventions, patient teaching, and prognosis for patients with acromegaly, gigantism, dwarfism, diabetes insipidus, syndrome of inappropriate antidiuretic hormone (SIADH), hyperthyroidism, hypothyroidism, goiter, thyroid cancer, hyperparathyroidism, hypoparathyroidism, Cushing syndrome, and Addison's disease.
7. List four tests used in the diagnosis of hyperthyroidism.
8. Discuss the medications commonly used to treat hyperthyroidism and hypothyroidism.
9. Explain how to test for Chvostek's sign, Trousseau's sign, and carpopedal spasms.
10. List two significant complications that may occur after thyroidectomy.
11. Differentiate between the clinical manifestations of Cushing syndrome and those of Addison's disease.
12. Describe the etiology/pathophysiology, clinical manifestations, assessment, diagnostic tests, medical management, nursing interventions, patient teaching, and prognosis for the patient with diabetes mellitus.
13. Explain the interrelationship of nutrition, exercise, and medication in the control of diabetes mellitus.
14. Discuss the various insulin types and their characteristics.
15. Describe the proper way to draw up and administer insulin.
16. Discuss the various classes of oral hypoglycemic medications to treat type 2 diabetes mellitus.
17. Differentiate between the signs and symptoms of hyperglycemia and hypoglycemia.
18. Differentiate among the signs and symptoms of diabetic ketoacidosis, hyperglycemic hyperosmolar nonketotic coma, and hypoglycemic reaction.
19. List five nursing interventions that foster self-care in the activities of daily living of the patient with diabetes mellitus.
20. Discuss the acute and long-term complications of diabetes mellitus.

Key Terms

Be sure to check out the bonus material on the free CD-ROM, including selected audio pronunciations.

Chvostek's sign (KHVŎS-tĕks sīn, p. 529)
dysphagia (dĭs-FĀ-jē-ă, p. 529)
endocrinologist (ĕn-dō-krī-NŎL-ŏ-jĭst, p. 523)
glycosuria (glī-kōs-Ū-rē-ă, p. 544)
hirsutism (HĔR-sōōt-ĭszm, p. 538)
hyperglycemia (hī-pĕr-glī-SĒ-mē-ă, p. 543)
hypocalcemia (hī-pō-kăl-SĒ-mē-ă, p. 536)
hypoglycemia (hī-pō-glī-SĒ-mē-ă, p. 550)
hypokalemia (hī-pō-kă-LĒ-mē-ă, p. 538)
idiopathic hyperplasia (ĭd-ē-ō-PĂTH-ĭk hī-pĕr-PLĀ-zhă, p. 521)
ketoacidosis (kē-tō-ă-sĭ-DŌ-sĭs, p. 544)
ketone bodies (KĒ-tōn bŏd-ēz, p. 543)
lipodystrophy (lĭp-ō-DĬS-trō-fē, p. 550)
neuropathy (nōō-RŎP-ē-thē, p. 554)
polydipsia (pŏl-ē-DĬP-sē-ă, p. 544)
polyphagia (pŏl-ē-FĀ-jă, p. 544)
polyuria (pŏl-ē-Ū-rē-ă, p. 544)
Trousseau's sign (trōō-SŌZ sīn, p. 529)
turgor (TŬR-gŏr, p. 524)
type 1 diabetes mellitus (tīp 1 dī-ă-BĒ-tēz MĚL-ĭ-tŭs, p. 542)
type 2 diabetes mellitus (tīp 2 dī-ă-BĒ-tēz MĚL-ĭ-tŭs, p. 542)

OVERVIEW OF ANATOMY AND PHYSIOLOGY

ENDOCRINE GLANDS AND HORMONES

Glands may be divided into two broad categories: exocrine and endocrine. **Exocrine glands** secrete through a series of ducts (sebaceous and sudoriferous glands of the skin). Their secretions are protective and functional. Endocrine glands are ductless; they release their secretions directly into the bloodstream. Their secretions have a regulatory function.

The endocrine system is composed of a series of ductless glands whose work is closely related to the nervous system. Both systems control homeostasis through communication within the systems. The endocrine system communicates more slowly through the use of **hormones,** which are chemical messengers that travel through the bloodstream to their target organ. When the hormone reaches its target, a metabolic change occurs.

The total weight of all the endocrine glands is less than half a pound, yet they exert a very powerful influence. The slightest change in hormonal levels can upset the metabolic balance of the entire body. Hormones can increase or decrease a normal body process by exerting their effects on a target organ. Too much or too little of a given hormone can affect other hormones, and for this reason they are somewhat interrelated. The endocrine glands (Figure 11-1) have a generalized effect on the patient's metabolism, growth, development, reproduction, and many other bodily activities.

The amount of hormonal release is controlled by a **negative feedback** (a decrease in function in response to stimuli) system. Information is constantly being exchanged between the target organ and the pituitary

gland via the bloodstream regarding the effect of the hormone on the target organ.

Pituitary Gland

The pea-sized **pituitary gland** (hypophysis) is one of the most powerful glands in the body. It has been called the "master gland" because through the negative feedback system it exerts its control over the other endocrine glands. It works closely with the hypothalamus of the brain and is located in the cranial cavity in a small saddlelike depression in the sphenoid bone. It is divided into two segments, each with specialized hormones. The first segment is called the **anterior pituitary** (adenohypophysis); the second is called the **posterior pituitary** (neurohypophysis). The hypothalamus actually produces the hormones of the posterior pituitary and releases them for storage in the posterior pituitary gland; they are released from here as a result of nerve impulses received from the hypothalamus.

Anterior pituitary gland. Six major hormones are secreted by the anterior pituitary gland, which constitutes about 75% of the total weight of the pituitary gland. Five hormones are called **tropic** hormones, because they are responsible for the stimulation of other endocrine glands. Prolactin, the remaining hormone, causes the mammary glands to produce milk. These hormones and their functions are shown in Figures 11-2 and 11-3.

Posterior pituitary gland. Two hormones are released by the posterior pituitary when the hypothalamus stimulates their release. They are **oxytocin** and **antidiuretic hormone** (ADH) (see Figure 11-2). Oxytocin promotes the release of milk and stimulates uterine contractions during labor. ADH causes the kidneys to conserve water by decreasing the amount of urine produced. It also causes constriction of the arterioles in the body, which results in increased blood pressure (BP). This hormone is sometimes referred to as **vasopressin,** because of its effect on blood pressure.

Thyroid Gland

The **thyroid gland** is butterfly shaped, with one lobe lying on either side of the trachea (Figure 11-4). It lies just below the larynx. The lobes are connected by the **isthmus.** The gland is very vascular and receives approximately 80 to 120 mL of blood per minute.

The thyroid gland secretes **thyroxine** (T_4) and **triiodothyronine** (T_3). Adequate oral intake of iodine is necessary for the formation of thyroid hormones. These hormones regulate three main functions: (1) growth and development, (2) metabolism, and (3) activity of the nervous system. Their function is controlled by the release of thyroid-stimulating hormone (TSH) from the pituitary gland.

Calcitonin is a hormone also released by the thyroid gland. It decreases blood calcium levels by causing calcium to be stored in the bones.

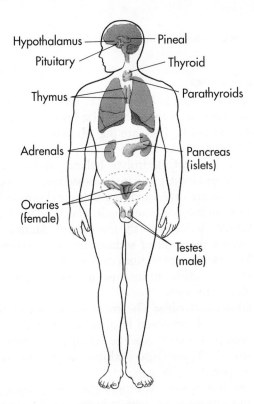

Hypothalamus — **Pineal**
Pituitary — **Thyroid**
Thymus — **Parathyroids**
Adrenals — **Pancreas (islets)**
Ovaries (female) — **Testes (male)**

FIGURE **11-1** Location of the endocrine glands in the female and male bodies. Thymus gland is shown at maximal size at puberty.

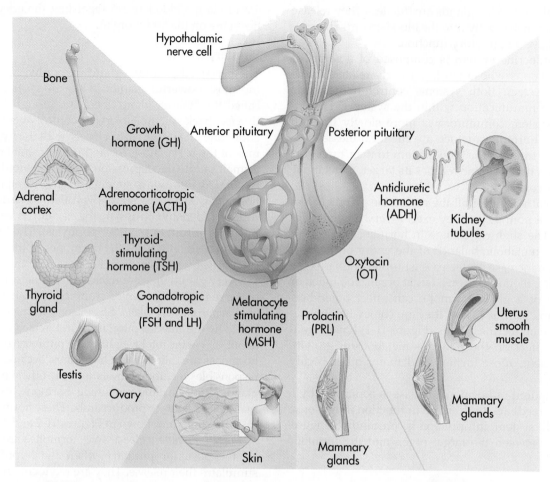

FIGURE **11-2** Pituitary hormones. Principal anterior and posterior pituitary hormones and their target organs.

Parathyroid Glands

The four parathyroid glands are located on the posterior surface of the thyroid gland (see Figure 11-4) and secrete parathyroid hormone (parathormone). As an antagonist to calcitonin from the thyroid, **parathormone** tends to increase the concentration of calcium in the blood. It also regulates the amount of phosphorus in the blood.

The delicate balance of calcium in the blood is extremely important for normal body function. When calcium blood levels are low, the nerve cells become excited and stimulate the muscles with too many impulses, resulting in spasms **(tetany)**. When blood calcium levels are abnormally high, heart function becomes impaired; this can result in death. Under its influence, two changes occur in the kidneys: it increases the reabsorption of calcium and magnesium from the kidney tubules and accelerates the elimination of phosphorus in the urine.

Adrenal Glands

The adrenal glands (suprarenal glands) are small, yellow masses that lie atop the kidneys. Both glands contain an outer section, the adrenal cortex, and a smaller inner section, the adrenal medulla (Figure 11-5).

Adrenal Cortex

The adrenal cortex is divided into three separate layers. Each layer secretes a particular hormone, all three are called **steroids.** They are the following:

- **Mineralocorticoids:** These are primarily involved in water and electrolyte balance and indirectly manage blood pressure. Aldosterone, the principal mineralocorticoid, regulates sodium and potassium levels by exerting its effects on the kidney tubules. It decreases the level of potassium and increases the level of sodium in the bloodstream. The retention of sodium causes retention of water, which leads to an increase in blood volume and blood pressure.

- **Glucocorticoids:** The most important of these is cortisol (involved in glucose metabolism and provides extra reserve energy in times of stress). These also exhibit antiinflammatory properties.

- **Sex hormones:** Androgens are male hormones and estrogens are female hormones. In the adult the release of these hormones from the adrenal glands is relatively small; their impact on the system is insignificant.

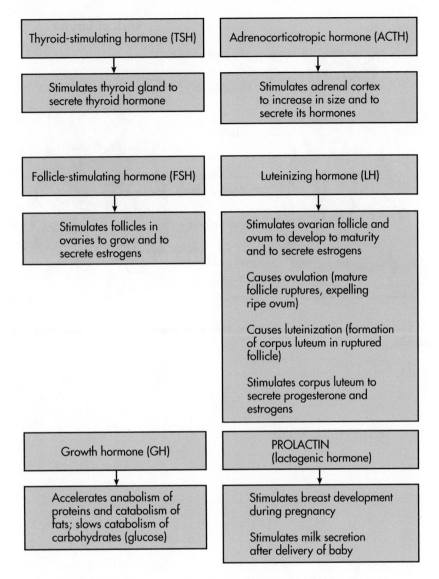

FIGURE **11-3** Names and functions of anterior pituitary hormones.

Adrenal Medulla

The cells composing the adrenal medulla arise from the same type of cells as does the sympathetic nervous system. Two hormones are released during times of stress: (1) epinephrine (adrenaline), and (2) norepinephrine. They can cause the heart rate and blood pressure to increase, the blood vessels to constrict, and the liver to release glucose reserves for immediate energy. This is a systemic preparation of the body for a "fight or flight" response needed in times of crisis.

Pancreas

The pancreas is an elongated gland that lies posterior to the stomach. It is a very active organ, composed of both exocrine and endocrine tissue. The endocrine tissue of the pancreas contains more than a million tiny clusters of cells known collectively as the islets of Langerhans. These cells secrete two major hormones:

(1) **insulin** (a hormone secreted in response to increased levels of glucose in the blood), secreted by the **beta cells;** and (2) **glucagon** (a hormone secreted in response to decreased levels of glucose in the blood), secreted by the **alpha cells.** Insulin and glucagon play a major role in carbohydrate, fat, and protein metabolism.

Female Sex Glands

Deep in the lower abdominal region, lying to the left and right of the uterus, are two almond-shaped **ovaries,** the major sex glands of the woman. The ovaries begin their production of hormones at puberty. Two hormones are released: **estrogen** (responsible for the development of secondary sex characteristics, such as axillary hair, pubic hair, and maturation of the reproductive organs) and **progesterone** (maintains the preparation of the reproductive organs that was initiated by the estrogen). See Chapter 12 for more information.

Back of larynx

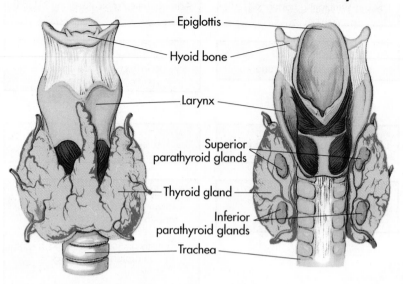

FIGURE **11-4** Thyroid and parathyroid glands. Note their relations to each other and to the larynx and trachea.

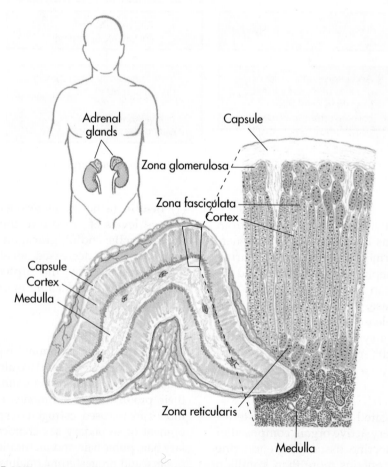

FIGURE **11-5** Structure of the adrenal gland. The zona glomerulosa of the cortex secretes abundant amounts of glucocorticoids, chiefly cortisol. The zona reticularis secretes minute amounts of sex hormones and glucocorticoids. A portion of the medulla is visible at the bottom of the illustration.

The **placenta** is a temporary endocrine gland that forms and functions during pregnancy. During this time the ovaries become inactive and the placenta releases the estrogen and progesterone needed to maintain the pregnancy. For a more in-depth discussion, refer to Chapter 12.

Male Sex Glands

Suspended outside the body in the **scrotum,** a saclike structure, are the two oval sex glands called the **testes.** They release the hormone **testosterone,** which is responsible for the development of the male secondary sex characteristics, including the appearance of axillary, pubic, and facial hair; maturation of the reproductive organs; deepening of the voice; and the development of muscle and bone mass. Testosterone is necessary for sperm formation.

Thymus Gland

The thymus gland lies in the upper thorax, posterior to the sternum (see Figure 11-1). It produces the hormone thymosin, which plays an active role in the immune system. T lymphocytes (a type of white blood cell) are stimulated to carry out immune reactions to certain types of antigens. The thymus gland programs this information into the T lymphocytes in utero and during the first few months of life.

Pineal Gland

The pineal gland is a small, cone-shaped gland located in the roof of the third ventricle of the brain (see Figure 11-1). It secretes the hormone **melatonin,** which seems to inhibit reproductive activities by inhibiting the gonadotropic hormones. This is particularly important in preventing the sexual maturation of the child's body until adulthood. It is thought to induce sleep, may affect mood, and has an impact on menstrual cycles.

DISORDERS OF THE PITUITARY GLAND (HYPOPHYSIS)

ACROMEGALY
Etiology/Pathophysiology

An overproduction of somatotropin (growth hormone, or GH) in the adult causes acromegaly, a condition that affects an estimated 250 people in the United States each year. The cause may be either idiopathic hyperplasia (an increase in number of cells without a known cause) of the anterior lobe of the pituitary gland or tumor growth. Unfortunately, growth changes that occur in acromegaly are irreversible, even with adequate medical or surgical intervention.

Clinical Manifestations

Manifestations of acromegaly begin gradually, usually in the third or fourth decade of life. Typically there is an average of 7 to 9 years between the initial onset of signs and symptoms and final diagnosis. The subsequent overabundance of growth hormone produces many changes throughout the patient's body, including enlargement of the cranium and lower jaw, with separation and malocclusion of the teeth, bulging forehead, bulbous nose, thick lips, enlarged tongue, and generalized coarsening of the facial features. Enlargement of the tongue results in speech difficulties and the voice deepens as a result of hypertrophy of the vocal cords. Figure 11-6 reveals coarse facial features. The hands and feet become enlarged, as do the heart, liver, and spleen; muscle weakness usually develops. Joints may hypertrophy and become painful and stiff. Male patients may become impotent, and female patients may develop a deepened voice, increased facial hair growth, and amenorrhea. If a tumor is present, pressure on the optic nerve may cause partial or complete blindness. Severe headaches commonly occur.

Assessment

Collection of **subjective data** includes determining the presence of headaches or visual disturbances and any precipitating factors. Muscle weakness and its effect on the patient's ability to perform activities should be evaluated. Patients should be encouraged to verbalize emotional responses to sexual problems (such as impotence in males and masculinization in females).

Collection of **objective data** includes ongoing assessment of bone enlargement and joint involvement, evidenced by gait changes and increasing inability to perform other activities. The interval between doses of pain medication should be evaluated. Changes in vital signs that may herald the onset of early heart failure include dyspnea, tachycardia, weak pulse, and hypotension.

Diagnostic Tests

Diagnosis of acromegaly is based on the patient's history and the clinical manifestations, as well as computed tomography (CT) scan, magnetic resonance

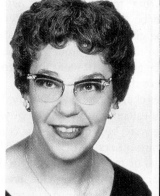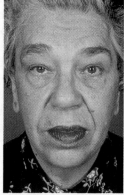

FIGURE **11-6** *Right:* This patient has coarse facial features typical of acromegaly. *Left:* Compare the patient's face several years before she developed the pituitary tumor.

imaging (MRI), and cranial radiographic evaluation. A complete ophthalmologic examination, including visual fields, is usually performed because a very large tumor of the pituitary gland potentially causes pressure on the optic chiasm or optic nerves. Laboratory tests confirm the presence of elevated serum GH and plasma insulin-like growth factor–1 (IGF-1) levels. The definitive test for acromegaly is the oral glucose challenge test. Normally GH concentration falls during an oral glucose challenge test, but in acromegaly, these levels do not fall (Quabbe, 2001). The patient's oral intake is restricted for 8 hours before this test.

Medical Management

Medical treatments include dopamine agonists such as cabergoline (Dostinex) and somatostatin analogs (which inhibit GH), such as octreotide (Sandostatin, Depot) and lanreotide SR (Ipstyl), especially in patients who are not candidates for surgery or radiation therapy. These drugs are used in an attempt to suppress growth hormone secretion. Surgical treatment may include either cryosurgery (the use of subfreezing temperatures to destroy tissue) or transsphenoidal removal of tumor tissue. New irradiation procedures using proton beam therapy have been used to destroy GH-secreting tumors. Proton beam treatment uses very low doses of radiation, and therefore it is much less destructive to adjacent tissues, such as the hypothalamus and temporal lobes, than conventional radiation therapy.

Nursing Interventions and Patient Teaching

Nursing interventions are mainly supportive. The presence of muscle weakness, joint pain, or stiffness warrants assessment of the ability to perform activities of daily living (ADLs). The presence of headache may impair the patient's ability to socialize and may also impede education. Worsening headaches may indicate tumor progression. The diet should be soft and easy to chew, because jaw muscles and the temporomandibular joint may be involved. The patient should be encouraged to chew thoroughly, and the nurse should allow adequate time during meals, assisting when necessary. Fluids should be encouraged often. Nonopioid analgesics may be given for pain relief. Visual impairment may increase the risk of injury for these patients, so care should be taken to prevent them from stumbling into furniture or dropping objects.

As the body undergoes change, the patient may develop problems with self-esteem and may feel physically unattractive. There may be difficulties in communicating with significant others, which can lead to disturbances in individual or family coping methods. Other complications of acromegaly are related to the enlargement of the liver, spleen, and heart. Cardiac dysrhythmias may develop, and the patient may experience heart failure. Abdominal girth may increase as a result of weight gain and inactivity, and respiratory difficulty may occur.

Nursing diagnoses and interventions for the patient with acromegaly include but are not limited to the following:

Nursing Diagnoses	Nursing Interventions
Disturbed body image, related to enlargement of the hands, feet, tongue, jaw, and soft tissue	Convey respect and non-judgmental acceptance of patient as a person. Help the patient set achievable short-term goals.
Activity intolerance, related to physical weakness	Assess patient's current activity level and priorities for activity performance. Discuss with patient alternate ways of performing activities.

The patient should remain under the supervision of a physician so that any complications can be diagnosed promptly and treated adequately. The patient should be taught exercises that can be performed at home, such as active range of motion of joints of the extremities and of the neck, to help prevent muscle atrophy and loss of movement.

Prognosis

Even with adequate medical or surgical treatment, the physical changes are irreversible, and the patient is prone to developing complications.

GIGANTISM
Etiology/Pathophysiology

Gigantism usually results from an oversecretion of GH as a result of hyperplasia of the anterior pituitary; this hyperplastic tissue may develop into a tumor. Another possible cause is a defect in the hypothalamus, which directs the anterior pituitary to release excess amounts of GH.

Clinical Manifestations

When overproduction of GH occurs in a child before closure of the epiphyses, there is an overgrowth of the long bones, which results in the attainment of great height, accompanied by increased muscle and visceral development. There is an increase in weight, but body proportions are usually normal. Despite their size, these patients are usually quite weak. Other kinds of gigantism may be caused by certain genetic disorders or by disturbances in sex hormone production. Once identified, these children should be referred for further medical evaluation and follow-up.

Assessment

Collection of **subjective data** includes assessment of the patient's understanding of the disease process, as well as his or her ability to verbalize emotional responses.

Collection of **objective data** requires frequent measurement of height. The patient's use of adaptive coping measures should be assessed, as well as his or her family interactions.

Diagnostic Tests

The GH-suppression test (also called the **glucose-loading test**) may be done to evaluate GH levels. In the patient with gigantism, baseline levels of GH will be high.

Medical Management

Medical management of children with gigantism may include surgical removal of tumor tissue or irradiation of the anterior pituitary gland, with a subsequent replacement of pituitary hormones as indicated. The physician should then observe the child for the development of related complications, such as hypertension, heart failure, osteoporosis, thickened bones, and delayed sexual development.

Nursing Interventions and Patient Teaching

Nursing interventions primarily include early identification of children who are experiencing increased growth rates compared with other children in their age group. There are potential problems with self-image, especially if the child is a preteen who is a great deal taller than peers. Girls usually suffer more emotional trauma in this situation than boys do. The nurse must be understanding and compassionate and accentuate the positive aspects of being tall.

Nursing diagnoses and interventions for the patient with gigantism include but are not limited to the following:

NURSING DIAGNOSES	NURSING INTERVENTIONS
Chronic low self-esteem, related to irreversible body changes	Be genuinely interested in and concerned about the patient. Help patient to identify problems in relating to others.
Ineffective coping, related to personal vulnerability	Assess patient's coping behaviors, stresses, and adaptive skills. Provide positive feedback.

Early diagnosis of these patients is essential, because proper medical management can retard the height a child will reach. The importance of regular visits to the pediatrician or pediatric endocrinologist (a physician who specializes in endocrinology) should be stressed to the parents.

Prognosis

With new medical and surgical advances, the expected life span of these patients is longer. However, their life expectancy is still shorter than that of the average individual.

DWARFISM
Etiology/Pathophysiology

A condition with a deficiency in growth hormone is called **hypopituitary dwarfism.** Most cases are idiopathic, but a small number can be attributed to an autosomal-recessive trait. In some cases there is also a lack of adrenocorticotropic hormone (ACTH), TSH, and the gonadotropins.

Clinical Manifestations

The most common clinical manifestation of dwarfism is that the child is a great deal shorter than his or her peers. These patients usually appear well proportioned and well nourished but appear younger than their chronologic age. There may be problems with dentition as the permanent teeth erupt, because the jaws are underdeveloped. Sexual development is usually normal but delayed. Many people with hypopituitary dwarfism are able to reproduce normal offspring, unless there is an accompanying deficiency in gonadotropins. Because only a small number of children who experience short stature or delayed growth suffer from dwarfism, it is crucial that the diagnostic workup be thorough.

Assessment

Collection of **subjective data** includes assessment of the patient's understanding of the disease process, as well as emotional responses to it. A family history of dwarfism may reveal previously successful coping strategies. The patient should be encouraged to verbalize feelings. Normal intelligence is displayed by most of these children. The child's growth pattern should be compared with that of siblings and other relatives at comparable age periods. The child's history usually reveals a normal birth weight. It is important to determine when the child's growth retardation was first noted.

Collection of **objective data** includes regular measurement of height and weight to determine responses to GH and other hormones that may be administered. Current height and weight should be compared with standard growth charts.

Diagnostic Tests

Diagnostic tests include radiographic evaluation of the wrist for bone age and a skull series to rule out a pituitary tumor. Definitive diagnosis is based on finding decreased plasma levels of GH. The patient's oral intake should be restricted after midnight for this test.

Medical Management

Medical treatment involves replacement of GH by injection, as well as the addition of other specific hormones as needed to correct deficiencies. If a tumor is the cause of dwarfism, surgery is usually indicated.

Nursing Interventions and Patient Teaching

Particular care should be exercised to identify children with growth problems. The physician will correlate the onset of growth retardation with symptoms of headache, visual disturbances, or behavior changes that might indicate tumor, so the nurse should be alert for these. The nurse should be careful not to make the parents feel guilty about any delay in seeking medical attention for their child.

Nursing diagnoses and interventions for the patient with dwarfism include but are not limited to the following:

NURSING DIAGNOSES	NURSING INTERVENTIONS
Disturbed body image, related to negative self-perception	Encourage patient to verbalize feelings about body. Respect patient's need for privacy while performing personal hygiene.
Deficient knowledge, related to age level and learning ability	Explain diagnostic and therapeutic measures, considering patient's level of understanding. Praise patient's efforts to cooperate with plan of treatment.

The child should be encouraged to wear age-appropriate clothing and engage in activities with peers, because major problems with self-esteem can occur in dwarfism. The child's abilities and strengths should be emphasized instead of his or her physical size.

Prognosis

Most of these patients lead fairly normal lives, and many become parents of normal children. Complications experienced are often of the musculoskeletal and cardiovascular systems.

DIABETES INSIPIDUS
Etiology/Pathophysiology

Diabetes insipidus (*diabetes:* "like a sieve or siphon"; *insipidus:* "tasteless") is a transient or permanent metabolic disorder of the posterior pituitary in which ADH is deficient. The condition may be either primary or secondary to other conditions, such as head injury, intracranial tumor, intracranial aneurysm, or infarct. Infections, such as encephalitis or meningitis, have been known to cause diabetes insipidus.

Diabetes insipidus occurs when either the secretion or action of antidiuretic hormone (ADH) goes awry.

Clinical Manifestations

Diabetes insipidus is characterized by marked polyuria and intense polydipsia. The urine is very dilute, looking much like water, with a low specific gravity (1.001 to 1.005)—the normal being 1.003 to 1.030. Urinary output may exceed 2 to 20 L in a 24-hour period, whereas the average is 1.5 L. Patients typically may lose as much as 200 mL of urine an hour for more than 2 consecutive hours. The patient craves cold or iced water and may drink 4 to 20 L of fluid daily, yet may become severely dehydrated and have increased levels of sodium in the blood (hypernatremia). Even when unconscious after surgery or head trauma, these patients continue to produce copious quantities of urine. If untreated, diabetes insipidus can lead to signs and symptoms associated with hypovolemic shock, including changes in level of consciousness, tachycardia, tachypnea, and hypotension. However, unlike hypovolemic shock, diabetes insipidus causes an increase in urine output rather than a decrease.

Assessment

Collection of **subjective data** includes evaluation of the patient's understanding of the relationship of symptoms (such as thirst and polyuria) to the underlying cause. The patient should be able to verbalize the importance of not restricting oral fluids. The severity of thirst should be assessed. The patient may be very embarrassed about the constant need to drink and then empty the bladder and may voluntarily restrict social contacts and work activities. The patient is weak, tired, and lethargic.

Collection of **objective data** to be assessed includes skin turgor (the normal resiliency of the skin) and color and specific gravity of the urine, and intake and output (I&O) should be carefully monitored. The skin is dry, turgor is poor, and body weight is lost. Constipation may occur. The patient should be weighed daily in the early morning, before breakfast. The nurse should determine the presence of nocturia.

Diagnostic Tests

Diagnosis is based on clinical manifestations, as well as urinary specific gravity and urinary ADH measurement. The urine specific gravity often drops below 1.003, the serum sodium level increases to more than 145 mEq/L (normal serum sodium level is 135 to 145 mEq/L). The serum osmolality may be greater than 300 mOsm/kg (normal is 280 to 300 mOsm/kg). The fluid deprivation (water deprivation) test may be ordered to determine how well the pituitary is producing ADH and to help rule out other causes. A CT scan and radiographic evaluation of the sella turcica (the "Turkish saddle"–shaped depression in the sphenoid bone that houses the pituitary gland) may be done.

Medical Management

Medical treatment involves intravenous, subcutaneous, intranasal, or oral administration of ADH preparations in the form of DDAVP (desmopressin acetate). Several other drugs are available for ADH replacement, including aqueous vasopressin (Pitressin [IM or intranasal]), vasopressin tannate [IM], and lysine vasopressin (Diapid [intranasal]). Coffee, tea, and other beverages containing caffeine are usually eliminated from the diet because of their possible diuretic effect. If the patient cannot match the urinary losses through oral intake, he is at risk for dehydration and severe hypernatremia. IV fluids will be needed.

Nursing Interventions and Patient Teaching

Because of the potential for fluid volume deficiency, the urinary output of pediatric and unconscious patients should be carefully monitored. Skin turgor should be assessed frequently, as should the condition of oral mucous membranes. The patient should be weighed daily and fluid intake and output should be recorded daily. Oral fluids should not be limited in an effort to reduce urinary output.

Conscientious nursing interventions are an essential part of the treatment plan. Nursing diagnoses and interventions for the patient with diabetes insipidus include but are not limited to the following:

Nursing Diagnoses	Nursing Interventions
Deficient fluid volume, risk for, related to excessive urine production	Assess for signs and symptoms of dehydration (dry oral mucous membranes, poor skin turgor, soft eyeballs, lowered BP, rapid pulse). Monitor electrolyte status carefully Measure intake and urinary output. Obtain daily weight.
Impaired skin integrity, risk for, related to altered state of hydration	Inspect skin for erythema, cyanosis, vesicles, and lesions. Prevent pressure on skin and skeletal prominences by turning and ambulating patient, use of sheepskin, eggcrate mattress, or other measures. Increase fluid intake up to 2600 mL/day if possible. Encourage patient to eat food adequate in calories, protein, and vitamin C to promote healthy skin.

The patient should be instructed to wear medic-alert jewelry, such as a necklace or bracelet, stating the diagnosis of diabetes insipidus. It is important that the patient remain under medical supervision for monitoring of the metabolic state, because the condition may worsen with time.

Prognosis

The prognosis depends on the etiology. Those patients who survive will usually be dependent on medication for the rest of their lives. With proper treatment, most patients can expect to live a relatively normal life.

SYNDROME OF INAPPROPRIATE SECRETION OF ANTIDIURETIC HORMONE

Syndrome of inappropriate antidiuretic hormone (SIADH) occurs when the pituitary gland releases too much ADH. In response to ADH, the kidneys reabsorb more water, decreasing urine output and expanding the body's fluid volume. The patient experiences hyponatremia, hemodilution, and fluid overload without peripheral edema.

Etiology/Pathophysiology

ADH regulates the body's water balance. Synthesized in the hypothalamus, ADH is stored in the posterior pituitary gland. When released into the circulation, it acts on the kidney's distal tubules and collecting ducts, increasing their permeability to water. This decreases urine volume, because more water is being reabsorbed and returned to the circulation, which increases blood volume.

When the body's system of checks and balances malfunctions—whether from a tumor, medication, unrelated disease process, or some other cause—ADH may be released continuously, causing SIADH.

ADH is released in response to stress. Be alert to patients who have the following risk factors and who are also in pain or undergoing stressful procedures:

Medications
- General anesthetics
- Opiates
- Barbiturates
- Thiazide diuretics
- Oral hypoglycemics
- Oxytocin

Malignancies
- Small-cell cancer of the lung
- Duodenal cancer
- Pancreatic cancer

Nonmalignant pulmonary diseases
- Tuberculosis
- Lung abscess
- Pneumonia

Nervous system disorders
- Head trauma
- Cerebral vascular thrombosis
- Cerebral atrophy
- Acute encephalitis
- Meningitis
- Guillain-Barré syndrome

Miscellaneous
- Hypothyroidism
- Lupus erythematosus

Clinical Manifestations

Clinically, SIADH is characterized by hyponatremia and water retention that progresses to water intoxication. The severity of the patient's condition depends on how hyponatremic he or she becomes and how rapidly fluid accumulates. Most signs and symptoms appear when serum sodium levels fall below 125 mEq/L.

Assessment

Collection of **subjective data** includes vague complaints. Hyponatremia triggers the earliest symptoms, which being rather nonspecific could indicate other disorders. These symptoms include weakness, muscle cramps, anorexia, nausea, and headache.

Collection of **objective data** includes assessment for hyponatremia. Hyponatremia may trigger diarrhea. The patient may also be disoriented and irritable and may demonstrate a weight gain. Fluid intake will exceed urine output. The patient will not develop peripheral edema, because excess fluid is accumulating in the vascular system and not in the interstitial spaces.

As water intoxication progresses and serum becomes more hypotonic, brain cells expand (become edematous), so later signs of SIADH are neurological. The patient will become progressively lethargic, with marked personality changes. The patient will have seizures, and the deep tendon reflexes will diminish or disappear altogether.

Diagnostic Tests

Laboratory tests will show hyponatremia (sodium less than 135 mEq/L). The blood urea nitrogen and creatinine will be low to normal. Urine specific gravity will be greater than 1.032, and urine sodium will be elevated.

Medical Management

The physician will order fluid restriction. Initially fluids may be restricted to 800 to 1000 mL of fluid per day. However, with severe hyponatremia fluids may be restricted to 500 mL per day.

Daily fluid intake should equal fluid output. If fluid restriction is adequate, a gradual increase in serum sodium along with a decrease in body weight will be shown.

A hypertonic saline solution will be ordered per intravenous route via infusion pump at a very slow rate to avoid too rapid a rise in sodium. This is necessary to correct sodium imbalance and to pull water out of edematous brain cells.

Medications such as demeclocycline (Declomycin), a tetracycline derivative, in a dosage of 300 mg orally four times daily may be ordered. The physician may also prescribe lithium carbonate. Both of these drugs interfere with the antidiuretic action of ADH and cause polyuria. Diuretics such as furosemide (Lasix)—40 to 80 mg orally daily in divided dosages or 20 to 40 mg intravenous (IV) daily—may be prescribed.

Treatment must also be directed at eliminating the underlying problem. Surgical resection, radiation, or chemotherapy may be indicated for malignant neo-

plasms. If the causative factor is a medication, it is discontinued.

The loss of potassium and other electrolytes from diuresis should be monitored closely as well as I&O to prevent hypovolemia.

Nursing Interventions and Patient Teaching

Nursing interventions for SIADH focus on a continual assessment of the patient's condition to determine if his or her condition is improving, not deteriorating. Every 3 to 4 hours a neurological examination is performed, and the patient's hydration status is assessed. The nurse should auscultate lung sounds every 2 to 4 hours to check for crackles that would indicate overhydration, and changes should be reported and documented immediately.

Serum electrolytes, urine sodium, and urine specific gravity are observed carefully because overcorrection can cause hypernatremia.

A daily weight is necessary at the same time and on the same scales. I&O are closely monitored; output is the guide to regulating intake.

The nursing goal is to control the patient's intake and to minimize discomfort. Explain why fluids are being restricted; allow the patient to divide allotted fluids and to choose the fluids, if possible. Fluids should be high in sodium (milk, orange or tomato juice, and beef or chicken broth). Salty foods should be avoided (potato chips or bacon, for example), because they will make the patient more thirsty.

Frequent mouth care is essential to maintain the integrity of oral mucous membranes. Steps must be taken to prevent skin impairment. Keep the patient and family members informed with simple explanations, such as that pain and anxiety can aggravate SIADH. If nausea is present (because of water intoxication), obtain an order for an antiemetic to be administered 30 minutes before meals.

Nursing diagnoses and interventions for the patient with SIADH include but are not limited to the following:

NURSING DIAGNOSES	NURSING INTERVENTIONS
Excess fluid volume, related to decreased urine output	Obtain daily weight, same scales, same time.
	Assess and record I&O.
	Monitor laboratory results.
	Administer medications as ordered.
	Maintain dietary and fluid restrictions (fluids should be high in sodium; avoid salty foods).
	Monitor IV infusions (such as 5% sodium chloride over several hours).

Nursing Diagnoses	Nursing Interventions
Risk for impaired oral mucous membrane, related to fluid restrictions of 100 ml per 24 hours	Provide frequent oral care; avoid alcohol-based mouthwashes and lemon glycerin swabs. Provide water-soluble lubricant for lips. Allow patient to choose fluids and to divide the allotted amount (such as one half in morning, one third in evening, and the remainder during the night). Offer simple explanation for fluid restrictions. If ordered, administer antiemetics 30 minutes before meals.

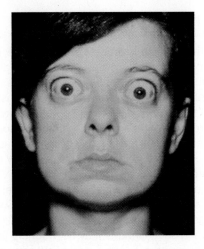

FIGURE **11-7** Exophthalmia of Graves' disease.

Patient teaching should be an ongoing part of nursing care. Be certain the patient understands the treatment plan, the rationale behind it, and the expected outcome. The teaching should include providing information about signs and symptoms of SIADH and telling the patient that the physician should be alerted if any changes are noted. SIADH can recur following discharge.

Prognosis

SIADH is potentially dangerous but treatable. If signs and symptoms are recognized early and intervention is appropriate, the prognosis is good; without treatment, coma and death occur.

DISORDERS OF THE THYROID AND PARATHYROID GLANDS

HYPERTHYROIDISM
Etiology/Pathophysiology

Hyperthyroidism—also called **Graves' disease,** exophthalmic goiter, and thyrotoxicosis—is a condition in which there is increased activity of the thyroid gland, with overproduction of the thyroid hormones thyroxine (T_4) and triiodothyronine (T_3). As a result, all the patient's metabolic processes are exaggerated. Although the exact cause of hyperthyroidism is unknown, it may result from extreme physical or emotional stress. It may occur during pregnancy, in adolescence, and in the presence of infection. There may be a genetic basis or autoimmune factors. The condition affects an estimated 2% of women but is seen much less often in men (only 0.2%). The highest frequency is in the 30- to 50-year age group.

Clinical Manifestations

Clinical manifestations are numerous and varied and are mild to severe. There is usually visible edema of the anterior portion of the neck as a result of enlargement of the thyroid. In severe cases, exophthalmos (bulging of the eyeballs) may occur, usually attributable to periorbital edema (Figure 11-7).

Assessment

Collection of **subjective data** includes assessment of the ability to concentrate and the presence of memory loss. The patient may complain of dysphagia or may be hoarse. There is usually weight loss, even in the presence of a voracious appetite. The patient appears very nervous, jittery, and excitable and may experience insomnia. These patients are emotionally labile and may overreact to stressful situations.

Collection of **objective data** includes assessment of changes in the vital signs. The pulse is usually rapid, blood pressure is elevated, and a bruit may be auscultated over the thyroid. The skin is warm and flushed, and the hair is fine and soft. Female patients may cease to menstruate. Elevated body temperature may be accompanied by intolerance to heat, with profuse diaphoresis. The presence of tremors of the hands should be noted. Behavior changes may include hyperactivity and clumsiness. Daily weighing usually shows weight loss.

Diagnostic Tests

Diagnostic tests usually include those in Box 11-1.

Medical Management

Medical management for hyperthyroidism may include administration of drugs that block the production of thyroid hormones, such as propylthiouracil (PTU) or methimazole (Tapazole) (Table 11-1). This may be followed after the acute stage by ablation therapy using a therapeutic dose of radioactive iodine (^{131}INaI or ^{125}INaI), based on the patient's age, clinical manifestations, and estimated weight of the thyroid. This is done in an effort to destroy some of the hypertrophied thyroid tissue. Ablation therapy using radioactive iodine is

| Box 11-1 | *Diagnostic Tests for Hyperthyroidism*

T_3 **(serum triiodothyronine):** Measures the T_3 level in the blood serum. Normal is 65 to 195 ng/dL. As with the thyroxin (T_4 test), the serum T_3 is an accurate measurement of thyroid function. T_3 is less stable than T_4. An elevated T_3 determination is clinically important in the patient who has a normal T_4 level but has all the signs and symptoms of hyperthyroidism. In this patient the test may identify T_3 thyrotoxicosis.

T_4 **(serum thyroxine):** Measures the T_4 level in the blood serum. Normal is 5 to 12 mcg/dL. Some medications such as oral contraceptives, steroids, estrogens, and sulfonamides may be withheld for several hours before the T_3 and T_4 tests, but food and fluids are not withheld. Elevated levels of these tests usually indicate hyperthyroidism.

Free T_4: Measures active component of total T_4. Normal values are 1 to 3.5 ng/dL. Because level remains constant, this is considered a better indication function than T_4. This is useful in diagnosing hyperthyroidism and hypothyroidism. High free T_4 suggest hyperthyroidism; low free T_4 suggest hypothyroidism.

Thyroid-stimulating hormone (TSH): Measures level of TSH. Normal values are 0.3 to 5.4 mcg/mL, considered the most sensitive method for evaluating thyroid disease. Generally recommended as first diagnostic test for thyroid dysfunction. TSH is suppressed in hyperthyroidism and elevated in hypothyroidism.

Radioactive iodine uptake test (RAIU): Radioactive iodine, ^{131}I, is given by mouth to the fasting patient. After 2, 6, and 24 hours, a scintillator is held over the thyroid to measure how much of the isotope has been removed from the bloodstream. A hyperactive thyroid may remove up to 90% of the drug. This test may be affected by prior ingestion of iodine-containing substances or foods. It is necessary to obtain a signed consent form for this test. Also, any allergy to iodine should be noted on the request form, along with medications currently being taken. No radiation precautions are necessary.

Thyroid scan: [131]I is given to the patient either orally or intravenously. If an IV dose is given, the scan may be done in 30 to 60 minutes. A scintillation camera positioned over the patient's thyroid sends images that are received on an oscilloscope and may be printed out on special paper. A consent form must be signed for this test. No radiation precautions are necessary.

| Table 11-1 | *Medications Commonly Used to Treat Hyperthyroidism and Hypothyroidism*

MEDICATIONS	COMMON SIDE EFFECTS
HYPERTHYROIDISM	
Iodine or iodine products (potassium or sodium iodide with strong iodine solution, potassium iodide, Lugol's solution)	Nausea, vomiting, diarrhea, abdominal pain
Radioactive iodine ([131]INaI or [125]INaI)	Sore throat, edema or pain in neck, temporary loss of taste, nausea, vomiting, painful salivary glands
Methimazole (Tapazole), propylthiouracil (Propyl-Thoracil, PTU)	Rash or pruritus, vertigo, nausea, vomiting, loss of taste, paresthesias, abdominal pain
HYPOTHYROIDISM	
Levothyroxine sodium (Levothroid, Synthroid, Eltroxin)	Nervousness, irritability, tremors, insomnia, tachycardia, hypertension, palpitations, cardiac dysrhythmias, vomiting, diarrhea, nausea, appetite changes, weight loss, menstrual irregularities, leg cramps, fever
Liothyronine sodium (Cytomel, Tertroxin)	
Liotrex (Euthroid, Thyrolar)	
Thyroglobulin (Proloid)	
Thyroid (Armour Thyroid, Thyro-Teric, Westthroid)	

the gold standard for treating hyperthyroidism. The patient usually begins to notice a decrease in symptoms within 6 to 8 weeks after the dose of the drug. An unfortunate sequela of this treatment in most patients is the development of hypothyroidism. For this reason the patient must have adequate follow-up medical supervision. If a patient develops hypothyroidism after treatment, levothyroxine therapy will be needed. [131]I is not a radiation hazard to the nonpregnant patient but is absolutely contraindicated during pregnancy. Pregnant nurses should not care for this patient for several days.

Surgery has fallen out of favor because of possible serious complications, such as hemorrhage, hypoparathyroidism, and vocal cord paralysis. However, surgery may still be indicated for patients who cannot tolerate antithyroid drugs or are not candidates for ablation therapy (Holcomb, 2003).

Surgical treatment for hyperthyroidism is subtotal thyroidectomy, a procedure in which approximately five sixths of the thyroid is removed. Surgery is usually delayed, if possible, until the patient is in a normal thyroid (euthyroid) state, because of the risk of excess bleeding during thyroidectomy, as well as postoperative thyroid crisis. Patients who have only mild hyperthyroidism will rarely be admitted to the acute care hospital. They will be followed by the physician in an office or clinic setting. However, the hospital nurse may come in contact with the patient because of admission for a different condition and will also care for these patients before and after thyroidectomy.

Nursing Interventions and Patient Teaching

The hyperthyroid patient has a need for more nutrients because of increased metabolism, so diet therapy usually consists of food high in calories, vitamins (especially the B vitamins), minerals, and carbohydrates. Between-meal snacks are offered. Food should be soft and easily swallowed if there is dysphagia (difficulty in swallowing). Coffee, tea, and colas should be avoided because of their stimulant effect. Preoperative nursing interventions for the patient who is scheduled for a thyroidectomy should stress keeping the environment as stable as possible to prevent emotional strain. Visitors may have to be limited to ensure adequate time for the patient to rest. The room should be quiet and cool, not above 23° C (74° F). The nurse should encourage food and fluids to help replace electrolytes lost through perspiration. Assess skin integrity for patients who are perspiring profusely. Keep the skin clean and dry, and change the patient's gown and bed linen as needed. Preoperative teaching is extremely important for this patient, and should include instructions on how to properly support the head while turning in bed or rising to a sitting or standing position. The nurse (or patient) should place both hands behind the head and maintain anatomic position while the rest of the body is being moved. The patient is also taught to deep breathe, but the physician will determine whether coughing is to be done postoperatively, because coughing puts a strain on the suture line. The nurse should inform the patient that a period of "voice rest" may be enforced for 48 hours postoperatively and that pencil and paper will be provided for writing notes instead of talking. Voice checks may be done every 2 to 4 hours, as ordered by the physician. The nurse will ask the patient to say "ah" and check for excessive hoarseness or voice change. Slight hoarseness is to be expected and should not be cause for alarm. Approximately 12.4% of patients suffer some damage to the laryngeal nerve during surgery, but this is not always permanent.

Postoperative management of this patient includes keeping the bed in semi-Fowler's position, with pillows supporting the head and shoulders. The patient should be cautioned to avoid hyperextending the head to prevent excess tension on the incision, which is usually made in a naturally appearing horizontal crease in the anterior neck. There should be a suction apparatus and tracheotomy tray available for emergency use. A cool-mist humidifier at the bedside may help soothe the throat and prevent coughing. Vital signs should be checked frequently, with special attention paid to the rate and depth of respirations and observations for any dyspnea (shortness of breath or difficulty in breathing) related to edema in the operative site. Before any liquid is given orally, the nurse must be sure the swallowing and cough reflexes have returned. The nurse must be alert for signs of internal or external bleeding; early internal bleeding may be evidenced by restlessness, apprehension, increased pulse rate, decreased blood pressure, and a feeling of fullness in the neck. Later, cyanosis may develop, signaling an obstructed airway, and the surgeon must be notified immediately. The dressing on the neck should be inspected frequently for obvious external bleeding. The nurse should also check for bleeding at the sides and back of the neck and on top of the patient's shoulders, because oozing blood may pool there as a result of gravity. Most surgeons will allow a dressing to be reinforced as needed and loosened slightly if the patient complains that it is too tight.

Postoperatively, the diet will initially consist of clear, cool liquids, progressing to soft food as tolerated. This is followed by a regular diet as soon as possible in an effort to help the patient regain lost weight and correct any nutritional deficiencies.

In addition to hemorrhage, two significant postoperative complications exist after thyroidectomy, for which the nurse must be ever watchful. The first is tetany. One possible cause of tetany is the inadvertent removal of one or more of the parathyroid glands during surgery. Another is edema in the operative area, which causes an occlusion of parathyroid release into the bloodstream, resulting in a low serum calcium level, the symptoms of which include numbness and tingling in the fingertips and toes and around the mouth. There may be **carpopedal spasms** (muscle spasms in the wrists and feet) and increased pulse, respirations, and blood pressure, accompanied by anxiety and agitation. Laryngeal spasm and stridor may occur. Chvostek's sign will be positive (an abnormal spasm of the facial muscles elicited by light taps on the facial nerve in patients who are hypocalcemic), and Trousseau's sign may also be positive (assesses for latent tetany; carpal spasm is induced by inflating a sphygmomanometer cuff on the upper arm to a pressure exceeding systolic blood pressure for 3 minutes; a positive result may be seen in hypocalcemia and hypomagnesemia). The condition may, if untreated, progress to convulsions or lethal cardiac dysrhythmias. Emergency treatment of tetany is the intravenous administration of calcium gluconate, which should always be available postoperatively.

The other serious complication after thyroidectomy is thyroid crisis, or thyroid storm. Fortunately, it occurs rarely and can usually be attributed to manipulation of the thyroid during surgery, which causes the release of large amounts of thyroid hormones into the bloodstream. If thyroid crisis occurs, it usually does so within the first 12 hours postoperatively. In thyroid crisis, all the signs and symptoms of hyperthyroidism are exaggerated. Additionally, the patient may develop nausea, vomiting, severe tachycardia, severe hypertension, and occasionally hyperthermia up to 41° C (106° F). Extreme restlessness, cardiac dysrhythmia, and delirium may also occur. The patient may develop heart failure and die. Diagnostic tests indicate increased free thyroxine (FT_4) and decreased TSH. The three goals of thyroid storm management are (1) to induce a normal thyroid state, (2) prevent cardiovascular collapse, and (3) prevent excessive hyperthermia. Emergency treatment of thyroid crisis includes intravenous administration of fluids, sodium iodide, corticosteroids, antipyretics, and administer an antithyroid drug (such as propylthiouracil (PKU) or methimazole [Tapazole]) and oxygen as needed. Prompt, adequate treatment usually results in dramatic improvement within 12 to 24 hours.

Nursing diagnoses and interventions for the patient having a thyroidectomy include but are not limited to the following:

NURSING DIAGNOSES	NURSING INTERVENTIONS
Preoperative	
Risk for hyperthermia, related to increased metabolism	Assess body temperature at regular intervals.
	Regulate environment (room temperature, linens, clothing) to help keep patient comfortable.
	Administer acetaminophen as prescribed
Imbalanced nutrition: less than body requirements, related to increased metabolism	Encourage patient to eat prescribed diet, avoiding caffeine.
	Assess daily weight and food intake.
Postoperative	
Impaired swallowing, related to postoperative edema	Ensure swallowing and cough reflexes present before oral intake.
	Encourage patient to drink slowly and chew food thoroughly.
Ineffective breathing pattern, risk for, related to post-operative edema and pain	Monitor rate and depth of respirations.
	Assess breath sounds and skin color.
	Encourage slow, deep breaths at least once an hour.
	Position to maximize respiratory effort.

Patient education after thyroidectomy includes stressing the importance of follow-up medical supervision. Thyroid function tests are done periodically to determine resolution of the hyperthyroid condition, as well as the possible development of hypothyroidism, a se-

quela that occurs in approximately 43% of surgical cases. Before leaving the hospital, the patient should be taught proper care of the incision site and symptoms that might indicate development of an infection, in which case the surgeon must be notified immediately. Discuss with the patient the need for a high-calorie, high-protein, high-carbohydrate diet until weight is stable.

Prognosis

With adequate, appropriate medical or surgical treatment, these patients usually have a normal life expectancy. However, exophthalmos, if present, may remain to a lesser degree in some unfortunate patients.

HYPOTHYROIDISM
Etiology/Pathophysiology

Hypothyroidism is one of the most common medical disorders in the United States, affecting 8% of women and 2% of men older than 50 years of age. It occurs most often in women 30 to 60 years of age and is more common in the older adult than previously thought. Hypothyroidism is the clinical state that occurs when the thyroid fails to secrete sufficient hormones, resulting in a slowing of all the body's metabolic processes. It may be caused by a condition of the thyroid itself or by a failure of the pituitary gland to furnish sufficient TSH for proper stimulation of thyroid secretion. It is sometimes an unfortunate sequela of the medical or surgical treatment of hyperthyroidism. Severe hypothyroidism in adults is called **myxedema** (Figure 11-8). Congenital hypothyroidism is called **cretinism** (Figure 11-9) and is estimated to occur in 1 of every 4000 to 5000 newborns.

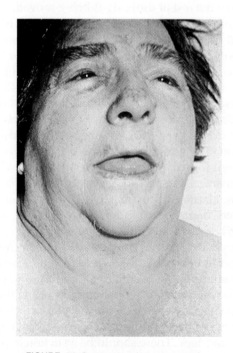

FIGURE **11-8** Person with myxedema.

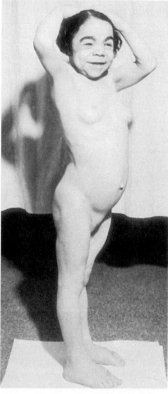
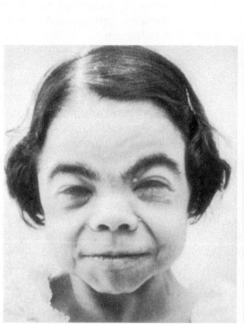

FIGURE **11-9** Adult cretin (33 years old, untreated). Note characteristic cretinoid features: dwarfism (44 inches in height), absent axillary and scant pubic hair, poorly developed breasts, protruding abdomen, and small umbilical hernia.

Clinical Manifestations

Clinical manifestations range from mild to severe and depend on the degree of thyroid hormone deficiency present. There is a slowing of all the body's metabolic processes, resulting in decreased production of body heat, intolerance to cold, and weight gain. Atherosclerotic changes may result in coronary artery disease.

Assessment

Collection of **subjective data** includes the patient's mental and emotional status, because he or she may display depression or paranoia, impaired memory, and general slowing of thought processes. Speech and hearing may be deficient. The patient is lethargic, forgetful, and irritable. Because of the body's slowed metabolism, anorexia and constipation may develop. Both sexes may experience decreased libido and reproductive difficulty. Female patients suffer from menstrual irregularities and may have difficulty conceiving or completing a pregnancy. Many experience spontaneous abortion, and this contributes to emotional distress and anxiety. The nurse should assess the patient's adaptive coping methods.

Collection of **objective data** includes assessment of the skin and hair. The hair thins and may fall out; the skin becomes thickened and dry. Facial features may enlarge to give the patient an edematous appearance. A masklike facial expression is common. The voice is characteristically low and hoarse. Decreased metabolism usually causes bradycardia, decreased blood pressure and respirations, and exercise intolerance. The patient's ability to perform activities may decrease because of weakness, clumsiness, and ataxia. The respiratory rate must be closely assessed after administration of any central nervous system depressant. The abdomen should be evaluated for distention, because **myxedema ileus** may occur.

Diagnostic Tests

The diagnosis of hypothyroidism is based on the physical examination and history and on appropriate laboratory tests, such as TSH, T_3, T_4, free T_4 (FT_4) levels. Low levels of T_3, T_4, and FT_4 are the underlying stimuli for TSH. Therefore a compensatory elevation of TSH occurs in patients with primary hypothyroid states, and low levels of T_3, T_4, and FT_4 are present. Subclinical cases may go undiagnosed for years, so the nurse should be aware of subtle clues while interviewing and caring for the patient. Recent research has suggested that mild hypothyroidism exists in approximately 5% of the population, more often in women. In children, when T_4 replacement begins before epiphy-

MEDICATIONS | *Endocrine Disorders*

MEDICATION	TRADE NAME	ACTION	SIDE EFFECTS	NURSING IMPLICATIONS
Bromocriptine	Parlodel	Inhibits prolactin secretion, lowers serum levels of growth hormone, dopamine receptor agonist	Nausea, headache, dizziness, abdominal cramping, orthostatic hypotension	Give with meals to prevent GI effects; change positions carefully to prevent orthostatic hypotension; contraindicated with hypersensitivity to ergot derivatives.
Calcium salts (gluconate, lactate, chloride gluceptate)	Many	Calcium electrolyte replacement	Hypercalcemia, phlebitis, necrosis, and burning at IV site; bradycardia, hypotension, and dysrhythmias with rapid IV administration	Monitor cardiac status and BP and for extravasation when giving IV.
Fludrocortisone	Florinef	Adrenol cortical steroid with mineralocorticoid activity; promotes sodium and water retention	Hypertension, edema, sweating, rash, hypokalemia	Monitor for hypokalemia and fluid retention/depletion; do not discontinue abruptly; patient should carry identification signaling use.
Levothyroxine (T_4)	Synthroid, Levothroid, others	Thyroid hormone replacement	Most are due to therapeutic overdose and include anxiety, insomnia, headache, hypertension, tremors, angina, dysrhythmias, tachycardia, menstrual irregularities	Give in morning to minimize insomnia; use caution in older adult or patients with coronary artery disease; monitor for signs of overdose; do not switch brands unless instructed.
Mitotane	Lysodren	Adrenal cytotoxic agent; reduces production of adrenal steroids	Anorexia, nausea, vomiting, diarrhea, lethargy, somnolence, vertigo, rash	Tell patient to use contraception; instruct patient to use caution when driving or performing tasks requiring alertness, monitor for dehydration.
Potassium iodide (SSKI)	Many	Blocks release of thyroid hormone in thyroid storm and hyperthyroidism; also used as an expectorant	Hypersensitivity reactions, rash, metallic taste, burning in mouth or throat, GI irritation, headache, parotitis, hyperkalemia	Should not be used in pregnant women; mix with fruit juice to mask taste.
Somatostatin analogs (octreotide)	Sandostatin	A secretory inhibitory growth hormone suppressant that suppresses secretion of serotonin, gastroenteropancreatic peptides. Enhances fluid and electrolyte absorption from the gastrointestinal (GI) tract; used for carcinoid tumors, vipomas, and high-output fistulas	Nausea, diarrhea, abdominal pain, headache, injection site discomfort, hyperglycemia, hypoglycemia	subQ is the preferred route of administration, but may also be given IV.

MEDICATIONS | *Endocrine Disorders—cont'd*

MEDICATION	TRADE NAME	ACTION	SIDE EFFECTS	NURSING IMPLICATIONS
Vasopressin (antidiuretic hormone)	Pitressin	Synthetic pituitary hormone with antidiuretic effects on the kidney (used to treat diabetes insipidus); also a potent vasoconstrictor (used to treat bleeding esophageal varices)	Nasal irritation and congestion with nasal preparations; hypertension; ischemia to heart, mesenteric organs, and kidneys; angina; myocardial infarction; water retention; hyponatremia	Use with caution in older patients or patients with coronary artery disease; use caution with heart failure; discontinue if chest pain develops; monitor urine output and serum sodium.

seal fusion, the chance for normal growth is greatly improved.

Medical Management

The treatment for hypothyroidism is replacement therapy, with desiccated animal thyroid (Armour Thyroid); thyroglobulin (Proloid); or synthetic products, such as levothyroxine sodium (Levothroid) or liothyronine sodium (Cytomel) by mouth (see Table 11-1). These drugs are usually given in the morning to enhance utilization of nutrients ingested during the daily meals. The patient initially is given a low dose, with increases as necessary until the desired effect is achieved. A maintenance dose will then be established. Early in treatment, monitoring of hormone levels occurs about every 6 to 8 weeks until the patient's TSH level is normal and at least yearly once normalized. The nurse should watch the patient for adverse effects of drug therapy, which mimic the signs and symptoms of hyperthyroidism. There is usually a dramatic change in the patient within a short time after replacement therapy begins (Medications table). Lifelong thyroid replacement therapy is usually required.

Nursing Interventions and Patient Teaching

Nursing interventions for the hospitalized severely hypothyroid patient center mainly on symptomatic relief. The room must be kept at least 20° to 23° C (68° to 74° F), and the patient should not be chilled during the bath or other procedures. Extra time should be allowed for physical care, so that the patient does not feel rushed. Accurate records of bowel elimination must be kept, because constipation may be severe. Stool softeners and bulk laxatives may be ordered. A high-protein, high-fiber, low-calorie diet is given and fluids are encouraged. Concentrated carbohydrates, such as sweets, should be avoided to help prevent excess weight gain. The patient should be encouraged to take increased oral fluids. The

nurse should watch for chest pain or dyspnea, accompanied by changes in the rate or rhythm of the heart, because this may indicate development of cardiac involvement. The patient should be taught not to stop taking the thyroid hormone without consulting a physician. This medication must be taken for the rest of the patient's life. Because most hypothyroid patients are more susceptible to the effects of sedatives, hypnotics, and anesthetics, the nurse must be alert for possible adverse effects if these agents are given for this condition.

Nursing diagnoses and interventions for the patient with hypothyroidism include but are not limited to the following:

NURSING DIAGNOSES	NURSING INTERVENTIONS
Decreased cardiac output, related to decreased metabolism	Assess pulse, blood pressure, skin color, and temperature. Schedule nursing activities around patient's activity cycle, with rest periods as needed to conserve energy.
Constipation, related to decreased peristaltic action	Assess frequency and character of stools. Encourage oral fluid intake and high-fiber food intake.

Regular checkups are essential because drug dosage may have to be adjusted from time to time. The patient and significant other should understand the desired effects of the medication as well as major adverse effects. The patient should be instructed to eat well-balanced meals of high-fiber foods, such as fruits, vegetables, and whole-grain cereals and breads; there should be adequate intake of iodine, in foods such as saltwater fish, milk, and eggs; and fluids should be increased to help prevent constipation. The patient and family should be told that mental and physical slowness may still be present but should improve with thyroid replacement therapy.

Prognosis

Most hypothyroid patients do well with proper medical supervision, although they will probably have to take medication for the rest of their lives.

SIMPLE (COLLOID) GOITER
Etiology/Pathophysiology

A simple, or colloid, goiter develops when the thyroid gland enlarges in response to low iodine levels in the bloodstream or when it is unable to utilize iodine properly. When the blood level of T_3 is too low to signal the pituitary to decrease TSH secretion, the thyroid gland then responds by increasing the formation of thyroglobulin (colloid), which accumulates in the thyroid follicles and causes enlargement of the gland (Figure 11-10). Most cases of simple goiter can be attributed to insufficient dietary intake of iodine, leading to this overgrowth of thyroid tissue.

Clinical Manifestations

There are usually no manifestations of overt thyroid dysfunction, and the diagnosis is essentially made using the patient's physical manifestations.

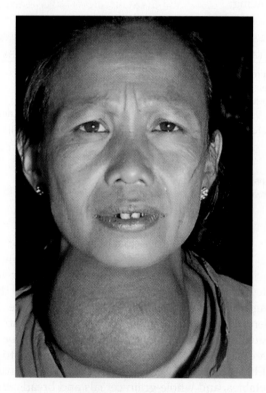

FIGURE **11-10** Simple goiter.

Assessment

Collection of **subjective data** focuses on assessing the patient's emotional response to the unsightly enlargement of the thyroid, and the patient should be encouraged to verbalize emotional responses. The patient may complain only of symptoms of dysphagia, hoarseness, or dyspnea related to the pressure of the enlarged gland against the esophagus and trachea. Dysphagia may contribute to difficulty ingesting adequate food and fluids. The patient should be assessed for increasing dyspnea. The patient's understanding of the need for medication, diet therapy, and medical follow-up should be determined.

Collection of **objective data** includes assessment of increased goiter size, voice changes, and adequacy of food and fluid intake. The thyroid may be only slightly enlarged, or it may be so enlarged that surgery must be done to improve respiration or swallowing.

Medical Management

Surgery may sometimes be performed for cosmetic effect, because this type of goiter can be very unsightly and damaging to the patient's self-image and self-esteem. If thyroidectomy is done, most of the gland is removed. Medical treatment consists of oral administration of potassium iodide, as well as foods high in iodine.

Nursing Interventions and Patient Teaching

Nursing interventions after thyroidectomy (previously discussed) are aimed at prevention of complications such as bleeding, tetany, and thyroid crisis. Nursing diagnoses and interventions for the patient with simple (colloid) goiter include but are not limited to the following:

NURSING DIAGNOSES	NURSING INTERVENTIONS
Risk for noncompliance, related to therapeutic regimen	Provide opportunities for patient to express feelings about treatment plan. Correct misconceptions and reinforce previous medical instructions. Stress importance of taking prescribed medications, having regular checkups, and avoiding any identified goitrogenic foods.
Risk for disturbed body image, related to altered physical appearance	Develop open and trusting relationship so that the patient will express his or her feelings. Discuss ways to disguise thyroid enlargement (scarves, high collars, makeup).

The nurse should stress the importance of adequate dietary intake of iodine by the patient. Medical supervision is recommended at regular intervals.

Prognosis

Most patients can expect to live a normal life after adequate treatment of goiter.

CANCER OF THE THYROID
Etiology/Pathophysiology

Cancer of the thyroid is a relatively rare malignancy, affecting approximately 25 of each 1 million people in the United States each year. However, more cases are expected, because between 1949 and 1960, many infants and children through adolescence were irradiated to shrink enlarged thymus tissue, tonsils, or adenoids and to treat severe cases of acne vulgaris. Cancer of the thyroid occurs more frequently in females and in whites. The incidence rises as age increases. Most malignancies of the thyroid are papillary, well-differentiated adenocarcinomas, a type of cancer that grows slowly, is usually contained, and does not spread beyond the adjacent lymph nodes. Cure rates after thyroidectomy in these cases are excellent. Other cancers, follicular and anaplastic, although much more rare, have extremely low cure rates.

Clinical Manifestations

The principal clinical manifestation of thyroid cancer is the presence of a firm, fixed, small, rounded mass or **nodule** that is felt during palpation of the gland. This nodule is painless. Only in rare instances have the symptoms of hyperthyroidism been seen.

Assessment

The collection of **subjective data** includes an assessment of the patient's use of adaptive coping methods to deal with the diagnosis, as well as an observation of the support system composed of the patient's significant others. The patient's understanding of the importance of medical follow-up should be assessed also.

Collection of **objective data** to be assessed includes progression of enlargement of the tumor area preoperatively, response to ^{131}I therapy, and skin involvement in the neck and torso after radiation therapy.

Diagnostic Tests

Diagnosis of papillary thyroid cancer is suspected when a thyroid scan shows a "cold" nodule, indicating decreased uptake of ^{131}I. Benign adenomas and follicular cancers are usually visualized as "hot" nodules because of their increased uptake of the isotope. Thyroid function tests usually yield normal results. To confirm the diagnosis, a thyroid needle biopsy may be done, but this should be attempted only by a skilled practitioner, because seeding of adjacent tissues may occur during the procedure. Metastasis can then result, with the prognosis becoming much more grave.

Medical Management

Treatment of thyroid cancer is a total thyroidectomy, with subsequent lifelong thyroid hormone replacement therapy. If metastasis is present at the time of the initial surgery, a radical neck dissection may be performed. In addition, radiation therapy, chemotherapy, and administration of ^{131}I may be done.

Nursing Interventions and Patient Teaching

Nursing interventions like those for the patient who has undergone thyroidectomy are instituted. Nursing diagnoses and interventions for the patient with cancer of the thyroid include but are not limited to the following:

NURSING DIAGNOSES	NURSING INTERVENTIONS
Anxiety, related to situational crisis	Encourage patient to discuss feelings about upcoming surgery. Monitor level of anxiety. Maintain a calm environment; try to decrease stressors.
Ineffective coping, related to personal vulnerability in crisis	Help patient identify previously successful coping methods. Teach new coping methods as needed.

The patient should be aware of the importance of proper medical follow-up to monitor thyroid hormone replacement therapy and to help ensure prompt diagnosis of any future metastatic lesions. Before discharge from the hospital, the patient should be taught proper care of the surgical incision.

Prognosis

The prognosis after treatment for thyroid cancer depends on the type of tumor involved. For papillary carcinoma the prognosis is excellent; for follicular and anaplastic carcinomas, the prognosis is much less favorable.

HYPERPARATHYROIDISM
Etiology/Pathophysiology

Hyperparathyroidism involves overactivity of the parathyroid glands, with increased production of parathormone. The cause of this condition may be a primary hypertrophy of one or more of the tiny parathyroid glands, usually in the form of an adenoma. It may also result from chronic renal failure, pyelonephritis, or glomerulonephritis. Parathyroid carcinoma is a rare condition, with rapid progress and a very grave prognosis. Hyperparathyroidism usually occurs in adults between 30 and 70 years of age, and it occurs twice as often in women.

Clinical Manifestations

The primary clinical manifestation is hypercalcemia. This occurs as calcium leaves the bones and accumulates in the bloodstream. As a result the bones become demineralized, causing skeletal pain, pain on weight bearing, and pathologic fractures (fractures that result from slight or no trauma to diseased bone). The high level of calcium in the blood may lead to the formation of kidney stones.

Assessment

Collection of **subjective data** includes assessment of the severity of skeletal pain, the degree of muscle weakness, and the effectiveness of analgesics. It is important to determine nursing measures that contribute to the patient's comfort and mobility. As neuromuscular function decreases, there is generalized fatigue, drowsiness, apathy, nausea, and anorexia; the degree of anorexia and nausea should be assessed. There may be constipation, personality changes, disorientation, and even paranoia. Symptoms that may indicate calculus formation are renal colic and dull back pain.

Collection of **objective data** includes careful observation for any skeletal deformity or abnormal movement of bone that might indicate a pathologic fracture. The urine should be observed for quantity and the presence of hematuria and stones. There may be vomiting and weight loss. Hypertension and cardiac dysrhythmias may present significant problems. Changes in the serum calcium level may cause bradycardia and other cardiac irregularities. The level of consciousness may decrease, resulting in stupor or coma.

Diagnostic Tests

Radiographic examination may reveal skeletal decalcification. Blood parathyroid hormone (PTH) levels are increased, as are alkaline phosphate levels. The patient should receive nothing by mouth for 8 to 12 hours before these tests. The serum calcium level is elevated, while the serum phosphorus level is decreased. Bone density measurements may also be used to detect bone loss. Imaging, such as MRI, CT, and ultrasound, may be used to localize the adenoma. A differential diagnosis should be made to rule out multiple myeloma, Cushing syndrome, vitamin D excess, and other causes of hypercalcemia.

Medical Management

The treatment for hyperparathyroidism is surgical removal of an existing tumor or of one or more parathyroid glands.

Nursing Interventions and Patient Teaching

Preoperative nursing interventions include helping restore fluid and electrolyte balance by encouraging increased oral fluid intake and by carefully monitoring the IV fluid therapy. The patient's intake and output

should be monitored, because diuretics may be used. Furosemide (Lasix) is the diuretic of choice. Thiazide diuretics are not used, because they decrease renal excretion of calcium and thus increase the hypercalcemic state. Urine may be strained because development of kidney calculi is not uncommon. Daily serum calcium levels may be ordered. The diet should be low in calcium, eliminating milk and other dairy products. Cranberry juice may be helpful in promoting acidic urine, thereby lessening the possibility of calculus formation. Some antacids are high in calcium and should not be used. The patient's pain should be accurately assessed, and prescribed analgesics should be administered as needed. Postoperatively, the patient will be cared for in the same manner as after a thyroidectomy, with careful monitoring of I&O. These patients commonly retain fluid in the tissues after surgery and will often have decreased urinary output. It is important to avoid overhydration at this point. The patient should be assessed frequently for signs of hypocalcemia (a deficiency of calcium in the blood serum), such as tetany, cardiac dysrhythmias, and carpopedal spasms. In the event that tetany does occur, calcium gluconate is usually administered intravenously.

Nursing diagnoses and interventions for the patient with hyperparathyroidism include but are not limited to the following:

NURSING DIAGNOSES	NURSING INTERVENTIONS
Activity intolerance, related to neuromuscular dysfunction	Assist patient to identify factors that increase or decrease activity tolerance and to eliminate or reduce painful, fatiguing activities. Encourage the patient to follow prescribed, individualized activity or exercise program.
Acute pain: skeletal, joint; renal colic, related to physiologic variables	Assess factors that cause or worsen, and help patient adjust body mechanics or activity. Encourage adequate fluid intake while assessing cardiac and renal output.

The patient should be taught the principles of good body mechanics so that pathologic fractures may be prevented during ambulation. The patient is reassured that bone pain should gradually decrease as electrolyte balance is restored and the condition is alleviated. The patient should be encouraged to participate in mild exercise as prescribed by the physician to regain muscle strength and a feeling of normal well-being. The nurse should teach the patient how to check the urine for the presence of stones or blood and how to monitor the pulse for any changes. The home environment should be evaluated and a plan developed for changes that may be necessary to prevent accidents.

Prognosis

With proper medical or surgical treatment, the patient can lead a fairly normal life. In patients with parathyroid carcinoma, the prognosis is very grave.

HYPOPARATHYROIDISM
Etiology/Pathophysiology

Hypoparathyroidism occurs when there is decreased parathyroid hormone, resulting in decreased levels of serum calcium. Idiopathic hypoparathyroidism is a rare condition, thought to be either autoimmune or familial in origin. The most common cause is the inadvertent removal or destruction of one or more of the tiny parathyroid glands during thyroidectomy.

Clinical Manifestations

Decreased parathyroid hormone levels in the bloodstream cause an increased serum phosphorus level and a decreased serum calcium level, resulting in neuromuscular hyperexcitability, involuntary and uncontrollable muscle spasms, and hypocalcemic tetany. Severe hypocalcemia may result in laryngeal spasm, stridor, cyanosis, and an increased possibility of asphyxia. In some patients there is calcification of the basal ganglia in the brain, causing a parkinsonian-like syndrome with bizarre posturing and spastic movements.

Assessment

Collection of **subjective data** includes assessment of neuromuscular activity for symptoms such as dysphagia and numbness or tingling in areas of the skin. The patient may feel anxious, irritable, or depressed. The patient may experience headaches and nausea. Abdominal or flank pain may occur if a renal calculus attempts to pass down the ureter into the bladder. The effectiveness of narcotics used to relieve renal colic must be assessed.

Collection of **objective data** to be assessed includes the appearance of positive Chvostek's sign or Trousseau's sign. If laryngeal spasm and stridor should occur, cyanosis may appear. Cardiac output may decrease as a result of hypocalcemia, and the patient may develop dysrhythmias. Tetanic spasms of the extremities may be observed.

Diagnostic Tests

Diagnostic laboratory studies confirm the presence of decreased serum calcium with increased urinary calcium, and increased serum phosphorus with decreased urinary phosphorus. Other possible causes of hypocalcemia—such as vitamin D deficiency, kidney failure, and acute pancreatitis—should be ruled out.

Medical Management

The immediate treatment of hypoparathyroid tetany is IV administration of calcium gluconate or calcium chloride (10%). This drug is very irritating to the vessel wall and should always be given very slowly, with a rate not to exceed 1 mL/minute. The patient may complain of a hot feeling of the skin or tongue. If given too rapidly, IV calcium can precipitate cardiac arrest. Care should be taken that none of the drug escapes the vein and extravasates into the tissues, because sloughing may occur. After the initial IV dose, calcium may be continued in a slow IV infusion until tetany is controlled; then it is given orally. Vitamin D is usually also given orally to help increase the absorption and blood level of calcium.

Nursing Interventions and Patient Teaching

Any patient receiving calcium, especially intravenously, must be monitored for signs of hypercalcemia. The most common clinical manifestations of this are vomiting, disorientation, anorexia, abdominal pain, and weakness. The nurse should assess the patient for respiratory distress; renal involvement; and adverse reactions to calcium therapy, such as bradycardia, syncope, and hypotension. Calcium should be used cautiously in digitalized patients, because it may cause digitalis toxicity. Cimetidine (Tagamet) interferes with normal parathyroid functioning and should be used carefully in these patients. The diet should contain foods high in calcium, such as dairy products, dark green vegetables, soybeans, and canned fish with the bones included. High-calcium snacks should be offered.

Nursing diagnoses and interventions for the patient with hypoparathyroidism include but are not limited to the following:

NURSING DIAGNOSES	NURSING INTERVENTIONS
Risk for injury, related to postoperative hypocalcemia	Assess for signs and symptoms of hypocalcemia (muscle spasms, laryngeal stridor, convulsion). Institute prescribed calcium therapy if need arises.
Imbalanced nutrition: less than body requirements, related to calcium intake	Give calcium replacement agents as scheduled. Monitor for Chvostek's and Trousseau's signs. Arrange for dietitian to discuss dietary sources of calcium. Assess patient's intake of high-calcium foods.

The patient should be taught the early symptoms of hypocalcemia and instructed to notify the nurse or physician if they occur. It is important that blood levels of calcium and phosphorus be drawn periodically while the patient is hospitalized. The patient should be taught to monitor the pulse for changes, as well as the proper maintenance of fluid balance and the use of calcium supplements at home.

Prognosis

For most patients, a fairly normal lifestyle and life expectancy are possible.

DISORDERS OF THE ADRENAL GLANDS

ADRENAL HYPERFUNCTION (CUSHING SYNDROME)

Etiology/Pathophysiology

Cushing syndrome is a spectrum of clinical abnormalities caused by excess corticosteroids, particularly glucocorticoids. This syndrome may be caused by hyperplasia of adrenal tissue resulting from overstimulation by the pituitary hormone ACTH, by a tumor of the adrenal cortex, by ACTH-secreting neoplasms outside the pituitary (such as small-cell carcinoma of the lung), and by prolonged administration of high doses of corticosteroids. The body's protective feedback mechanism fails, resulting in excess secretion of the adrenal hormones: glucocorticoids, mineralocorticoids, and sex hormones.

Clinical Manifestations

This overabundance of hormones produces the signs and symptoms commonly associated with Cushing syndrome, including moonface and buffalo hump. The arms and legs become thin as a result of muscle wasting. Hypokalemia (a condition in which an inadequate amount of potassium, the major intracellular cation, is found in the circulating bloodstream) is usually present. Hyperglycemia occurs because of glucose intolerance (associated with cortisol-induced insulin resistance) and increased glucose release by the liver. There is usually protein in the urine, as well as increased urinary calcium excretion, which may lead to the development of renal calculi. Osteoporosis results from abnormal calcium absorption, and kyphosis may develop. The patient is very susceptible to all kinds of infections, but the symptoms of these may be masked and not detected until the infection has progressed to a point that may be life threatening.

Assessment

Collection of **subjective data** includes assessment of the patient's ability to concentrate. Patients may feel irritable, and mental changes may develop. Some patients experience emotional instability, with severe mood swings and occasionally psychosis. Depression is very common, and the possibility of suicide is an ever present concern for the nurse, who must be alert to subtle changes in the patient's affect and keep the environment free from objects with which the patient may inflict self-harm. Patients of both sexes may experience loss of libido and alterations in self-esteem; there may be concerns about sexual dysfunction. The patient should be encouraged to verbalize concerns about altered body image. Severe backache is often present and may signal a compression fracture of a vertebral body. The severity of back pain should be assessed, as well as nursing measures that contribute to the patient's comfort. Appetite usually increases, so the patient's understanding of special dietary restrictions should be assessed, as well as his or her understanding of the importance of medical follow-up.

Collection of **objective data** includes observation of the skin for the presence of ecchymoses and petechiae. The skin becomes thin and fragile and wound healing is delayed. There may be weight gain and abdominal enlargement, with development of **striae** (a streak or linear scar that often results from stretching of the skin), and this increased girth may contribute to difficulty with mobility. Weight should be monitored, because peripheral edema and associated hypertension are common. Impaired carbohydrate metabolism results in hyperglycemia. Women may experience hirsutism (excessive body hair in a masculine distribution), menstrual irregularities, and deepening of the voice. Elevated body temperature may signal the presence of an undetected infection.

Diagnostic Tests

Diagnosis is usually based on the clinical appearance of the patient and on the results of laboratory tests. Plasma cortisol levels are usually elevated. Plasma ACTH levels may be increased or decreased, depending on the location of a tumor. Skull radiographic evaluation may detect erosion of the sella turcica in the presence of a pituitary tumor. Adrenal angiography will aid in diagnosing an adrenal tumor. A 24-hour urine test for 17-ketosteroids and 17-hydroxysteroids shows increased levels present. Blood glucose for hyperglycemia and urinalysis for glycosuria are other diagnostic tests associated with but not diagnostic of Cushing syndrome. Abdominal CT scan and ultrasound may help localize an abdominal tumor.

Medical Management

Treatment is directed toward the causative factor. If an adrenal tumor is present, adrenalectomy is usually indicated for its removal. Pituitary tumors may be irradiated or removed surgically by transsphenoidal microsurgery. If the patient is unable to undergo surgery because of inoperable cancer elsewhere in the body or another preexisting serious condition, mitotane (Lysodren) therapy may be used. This cytotoxic agent is toxic to the adrenal glands and is given for at least 3 months, during which time the patient must be monitored for symptoms of hepatotoxicity, such as jaundice, gastrointestinal upset, and pruritus. The diet should be lowered in sodium to help decrease edema. Reduced calories and carbohydrates will help control hyperglycemia, and foods high in potassium will help correct hypokalemia. If Cushing syndrome has developed during the course of prolonged administration of corticosteroids (e.g., prednisone), one or more of the following alternatives may be tried: (1) gradually discontinuing corticosteroid therapy, (2) reducing the corticosteroid dose, and (3) converting to an alternate-day regimen. Gradually tapering the corticosteroids is necessary to avoid potentially life-threatening adrenal insufficiency.

Nursing Interventions and Patient Teaching

Important nursing interventions include gentle handling to prevent skin impairment or excessive ecchymosis, as well as frequent assessment for areas of erythema, edema, or early signs of infection. The patient should be encouraged to turn frequently and ambulate as tolerated to eliminate undue pressure on bony prominences. Elbow and heel protectors and an eggcrate mattress pad may help prevent decubitus ulcers in the bedridden patient. The patient should be encouraged to participate as fully as possible in normal ADLs, interspersing personal hygiene tasks with rest periods to prevent overtiring.

Nursing diagnoses and interventions for the patient with Cushing syndrome include but are not limited to the following:

Nursing Diagnoses	Nursing Interventions
Deficient knowledge, related to therapeutic regimen	Assess patient's understanding of prescribed medication and diet. Encourage patient to wear medical-alert jewelry and carry wallet identification cards.
Activity intolerance, related to weakness and immobility	Assess patient's current activity tolerance and identify priorities for energy expenditures. Plan activity and rest periods with patient.

The patient's mental attitude is extremely important. The nurse should encourage verbalization of concerns and be watchful for the development of depression and the presence of suicidal thoughts. Patients should be helped to understand their prescribed medication, such as mitotane (Lysodren), as well as possible side effects. It is important for the patient to wear a medical alert bracelet or necklace and to carry a wallet card stating the diagnosis of Cushing syndrome. There may be a major lifestyle change to which the patient must adjust, and the aid of a social worker may be enlisted. Before adrenalectomy, the patient should be taught the importance of avoiding stress and avoiding infections. Postoperative teaching includes proper wound care and the symptoms of Addison's disease, which is sometimes an unavoidable sequela after this type of surgery.

Prognosis

Depending upon whether the etiology of the disease was benign or malignant, and whether the treatment was successful or unsuccessful, the patient with Cushing syndrome can expect to have major lifestyle changes, possibly with many complications and a shortened life expectancy.

ADRENAL HYPOFUNCTION (ADDISON'S DISEASE)
Etiology/Pathophysiology

Adrenocortical insufficiency occurs when the adrenal glands do not secrete adequate amount of glucocorticoids and mineralocorticoids. It may initially be seen as Addison's disease, a rather rare primary condition; it may result from adrenalectomy, pituitary hypofunction, or long-standing steroid therapy. The most common cause of Addison's disease is an autoimmune response. Adrenal tissue is destroyed by antibodies against the patient's own adrenal cortex. Addison's disease can result from idiopathic adrenal atrophy or cancer of the adrenal cortex. Tuberculosis can cause Addison's disease but this is now rare. Other causes include infarction, fungal infections (e.g., histoplasmosis), acquired immunodeficiency syndrome (AIDS), and metastatic cancer. Deficiencies in aldosterone and cortisol produce disturbances of the metabolism of carbohydrates, fats, and proteins, as well as sodium, potassium, and water. This results in electrolyte and fluid imbalance, dehydration, water loss, and hypovolemia.

Clinical Manifestations

Because manifestations do not tend to become evident until 90% of the adrenal cortex is destroyed, the disease is often advanced before it is diagnosed. Clinical manifestations are directly related to imbalances in adrenal hormones, nutrients, and electrolytes.

Assessment

Collection of **subjective data** to be assessed includes the presence of nausea, anorexia, and craving for salt. Postural hypotension may be associated with vertigo, weakness, and syncope, resulting in reluctance to attempt normal activities. The patient may complain of severe headache, disorientation, abdominal pain, or lower back pain, which could represent early symptoms of adrenal crisis. This patient tolerates stress poorly, feels anxious and apprehensive, and may thus suffer under emotional trauma more easily than a normal person would. It is important to assess emotional status and allow the patient to ventilate feelings about altered self-image. The nurse should also assess the patient's overall understanding of the disease process and the importance of medical treatment and follow-up.

Collection of **objective data** includes observation of changes in the color of the mucous membranes and the skin, with the appearance of darkly pigmented areas commonly observed. Skin hyperpigmentation, a striking feature, is seen primarily in sun-exposed areas of the body, at pressure points, over joints, and in creases, especially in palmar creases. There is usually weight loss, which may be accompanied by vomiting and diarrhea. Hypoglycemia may contribute to the patient's fatigue; the nurse should assess the patient's ability to perform ADLs. An abnormally low or abnormally high body temperature, hyponatremia, and hyperkalemia are signs of impending adrenal crisis, a life-threatening emergency caused by insufficient adrenocortical hormones or a sudden sharp decrease in these hormones. See Table 11-2 for a nursing assessment comparison of Cushing syndrome and Addison's disease.

Diagnostic Tests

Laboratory studies show decreased serum sodium, increased serum potassium, and decreased serum glucose. A 24-hour urine specimen shows decreased levels of 17-ketosteroids and 17-hydroxysteroids. Fasting plasma cortisol levels and aldosterone levels are low with an ACTH stimulation test. A glucose tolerance test may yield abnormal results.

Medical Management

Medical treatment involves the prompt restoration of fluid and electrolyte balance, as well as replacement of the deficient adrenal hormones. Fludrocortisone (Florinef) (a mineralocorticoid) is usually the drug of choice with glucocorticoids such as hydrocortisone (Hydrocortone). The diet should be high in sodium and low in potassium.

Nursing Interventions and Patient Teaching

The nurse should carefully assess the circulatory status of the patient, keep accurate I&O records, and record daily weight. Skin turgor should be checked and fluids offered frequently. Vital signs are monitored at regular intervals, with particular attention paid to the temperature and blood pressure. The patient is also monitored for response to prescribed steroid drugs, and any adverse effects should be promptly reported to the physician. The environment must be kept as free from stressors as possible. Visitors and hospital personnel should be screened for the presence of infectious disease and excluded from the patient's room. This patient should be continually assessed for signs of developing adrenal (addisonian) crisis, in which there may be a sudden, severe drop in blood pressure; nausea and vomiting; an extremely high temperature; and cyanosis, progressing to vasomotor collapse and possibly to death. Emergency treatment is intravenous administration of corticosteroids in a solution of saline and glucose. The patient should carry an emergency kit at all times. The kit should consist of 100 mg of IM hydrocortisone, syringes, and instructions for use. The patient and significant others should be taught how to give an IM injection in case replacement therapy cannot be taken orally.

Nursing diagnoses and interventions for the patient with Addison's disease include but are not limited to the following:

Table 11-2 | *Nursing Assessment of Patients with Cushing Syndrome or Addison's Disease*

AREA OF ASSESSMENT	CLINICAL MANIFESTATIONS IN CUSHING SYNDROME	CLINICAL MANIFESTATIONS IN ADDISON'S DISEASE
Cardiovascular	Mild to moderate hypertension	Postural hypotension, vertigo, syncope
Neurological	Impaired memory and concentration, insomnia, irritability	Lethargy, headache
Musculoskeletal	Muscle weakness, muscle wasting in extremities, back and rib pain, kyphosis	Muscle weakness, fatigue, muscle aches, muscle wasting
Integumentary	Thin skin; red cheeks, acne, frequent petechiae and ecchymoses, hyperpigmentation, poor wound healing	Hyperpigmentation, decreased body hair
Self-care and self-concept	Tires easily; insomnia, malaise, negative feelings regarding changes in body	Tires easily; very susceptible to infections of all kinds, profound weakness, lack of interest in usual activities and relationships
Nutrition/fluid balance	Increased appetite, moderate weight gain, edema, buffalo hump, moonface, obesity of trunk, hyperglycemia; need for decreased salt intake, reduced calories and carbohydrate intake, increased potassium intake	Nausea and vomiting, fluid and electrolyte imbalance, dehydration, weight loss, hypoglycemia; need for increased salt and decreased potassium intake

NURSING DIAGNOSES	NURSING INTERVENTIONS
Risk for infection, related to altered metabolic processes	Assess environment for stressors. Screen visitors and personnel for contagious disease. Monitor temperature routinely. Stress the importance of taking prescribed medications.
Ineffective tissue perfusion, peripheral, related to electrolyte imbalance	Monitor vital signs and I&O. Have patient make position changes slowly; monitor for vertigo, visual changes.

Before discharge from the hospital, the patient must be taught the importance of adhering to the prescribed drug therapy; having regular medical checkups; and immediately reporting all illnesses, even a cold, to the physician. The patient should understand the importance of avoiding stress, one of the major precipitating factors in adrenal crisis, and should be encouraged to eliminate excess stress. Other factors include overexertion, diarrhea, infection, decreased intake of salt, exposure to cold, and surgery. It is critical that the patient wear an identification bracelet (medical alert) and carry a wallet card stating that the patient has Addison's disease so that appropriate therapy be initiated in case of an unexpected trauma, accident, or crisis.

Prognosis

With long-term steroid therapy, adequate medical care, and follow-up, this patient has a fair prognosis.

PHEOCHROMOCYTOMA
Etiology/Pathophysiology

A pheochromocytoma is a chromaffin cell tumor, usually found in the adrenal medulla, that causes excessive secretion of catecholamines (epinephrine and norepinephrine). These tumors occur most often in adults between 20 and 60 years of age and are almost always benign; only about 10% are malignant.

Clinical Manifestations

The principal manifestation of pheochromocytoma is hypertension, which may be intermittent but is usually persistent. Hypertensive crisis episodes may occur, during which the blood pressure may fluctuate widely, sometimes as high as 300/175. Signs and symptoms may be triggered by an identifiable factor, such as overexertion or emotional trauma, or they may occur for no apparent reason. Extreme hypertension may result in stroke, kidney damage, and retinopathy. Cardiac damage may occur, resulting in heart failure.

Assessment

Collection of **subjective data** to be assessed during hypertensive crisis includes the presence of severe headache and palpitations. The patient may feel nervous, dizzy, and dyspneic and may experience paresthesias. There may be nausea and intolerance to heat. Anxiety is common, and the patient may have trouble sleeping. The nurse should question the patient about the occurrence of symptoms in relation to identifiable factors, such as excess stress or overexertion, and should assess the coping methods identified.

Collection of **objective data** includes frequent measurement of blood pressure and respiratory rate for increases and of pulse for tachycardia. There may be tremors, diaphoresis, dilated pupils, glycosuria, and hyperglycemia. The nurse should assess responses to prescribed medications.

Diagnostic Tests

The measurement of urinary metanephrines (catecholamine metabolites), usually performed as a 24-hour urine collection, is the simplest and most reliable test. Values are elevated in at least 90% of those with pheochromocytoma. Vanillylmandelic acid (VMA) may also be measured in a 24-hour urine sample. However, this test has more false negatives than urine metanephrines. Plasma catecholamines are also elevated. It is preferable to measure serum catecholamines during an "attack." CT scan and MRI of the adrenal glands may help in locating the tumor. Oral intake is restricted for 8 hours before IVP, and laxatives are usually administered the evening before the test.

Medical Management

Treatment is usually the surgical removal of the tumor, if possible, and sometimes the removal of the adrenal gland as well. Preoperatively, the patient may be given alpha-adrenergic blocking agents such as phentolamine mesylate (Regitine) or phenoxybenzamine HCl (Dibenzyline) in an effort to control hypertension. Metyrosine (Demser) may be given to help inhibit catecholamine production, and the drug must be continued on a long-term basis if the tumor is inoperable.

Nursing Interventions and Patient Teaching

Postoperative care is carried out in the same manner as for any major abdominal surgery, with the following special concerns. If the patient has undergone adrenalectomy, large amounts of hydrocortisone will be given. The patient must be watched carefully for fluctuations in blood pressure caused by adrenal manipulation during surgery, with subsequent release of epinephrine and norepinephrine. These fluctuations may be severe and life threatening if cardiovascular collapse occurs. The patient should avoid excess stress and must be allowed adequate time to rest; sedatives may be given to ensure this. A careful I&O record should be kept and IV solutions administered exactly as ordered. Vasopressors and corticosteroids may be given. The diet should be free from stimulants, such as coffee, tea, and soft drinks containing caffeine.

Nursing diagnoses and interventions for the patient with pheochromocytoma include but are not limited to the following:

NURSING DIAGNOSES	NURSING INTERVENTIONS
Ineffective tissue perfusion, cardiopulmonary, renal, related to hypertension	Monitor BP and pulse and record I&O. Eliminate smoking and caffeine-containing beverages.
Activity intolerance, related to hypertension	Assist with gradual position changes from lying to sitting or standing. Limit activity, as needed, to prevent increased hypertension.

Follow-up 24-hour urine tests (catecholamine metabolites or VMA) may determine return to normal levels. When this goal is achieved, the patient is pronounced cured and may resume normal activities. If the tumor is inoperable, it is important that the patient remain under lifelong medical supervision, and the importance of compliance with prescribed treatment must be stressed. Medical-alert jewelry should be worn and a wallet card carried. The patient should be taught self-monitoring of blood pressure and instructed when to call the physician if elevation occurs.

Prognosis

The prognosis after successful removal of the causative tumor is good; for an inoperable tumor, the prognosis depends on adequate medical management of hypertension.

DISORDERS OF THE PANCREAS

DIABETES MELLITUS
Etiology

Diabetes mellitus (DM) (*diabetes:* "like a sieve or siphon"; *mellitus:* "sweet or related to honey") is a systemic metabolic disorder that involves improper metabolism of carbohydrates, fats, and proteins. This condition may be caused by a decrease or absolute lack of insulin production by the beta cells of the islets of Langerhans in the pancreas or by the decreased activity of the insulin that is secreted. In nondiabetic people the beta cells are stimulated by increased blood glucose levels; insulin secretion reaches peak levels about 30 minutes after meals and returns to normal in 2 to 3 hours. Between meals or during a period of fasting, insulin levels remain low, and the body uses its supply of stored glucose and amino acids to provide energy for the tissues. In people with diabetes, the body's insulin supply is either absent or deficient, or target cells resist the action of insulin. There are several types of DM, but in each type, hyperglycemia is present as the principal clinical manifestation. Although the exact cause of DM is unknown, a number of factors have been demonstrated as contributing to its development: genetic predisposition, viruses (such as coxsackievirus B, rubella, and mumps), the aging process, diet and lifestyle, and ethnicity. Obesity is felt to be a major factor. Recent research has suggested that the T lymphocytes may play a role in the development of autoimmune destruction of the pancreatic insulin-producing cells.

Types of Diabetes Mellitus

There are two main types of DM: **type 1 (insulin-dependent) diabetes mellitus** (IDDM) and **type 2 (non–insulin-dependent) diabetes mellitus** (NIDDM). Type 1 was formerly called juvenile diabetes, or juvenile-onset diabetes. Type 2 was formerly called adult-onset diabetes, or maturity-onset diabetes. Other types of DM patients include those diagnosed with such conditions as pancreatitis, genetic syndromes, malnutrition, chemical- or drug-induced disease, and pregnancy. There are some distinct differences between type 1 and type 2 diabetes (Table 11-3). In type 1 (IDDM)—an autoimmune disease (probably stimulated by a virus) that eventually results in destruction of beta cells in the pancreatic islets and results in deficient insulin **production**—the patient retains normal sensitivity to insulin action. Within 5 years of diagnosis, all the patient's beta cells have been destroyed and no insulin is produced (Moshang, 2004). In type 2 (NIDDM), the main problem seems to be an abnormal resistance to insulin **action.**

Type 1 diabetes mellitus. Type 1 diabetes mellitus results from progressive destruction of beta-cell function as a result of an autoimmune process in a susceptible individual. The pancreatic islets of Langerhans cell antibodies and insulin autoantibodies cause a reduction in beta cells of 80% to 90% of normal before hyperglycemia and symptoms occur. Type 1 diabetes mellitus is characterized by autoimmune beta-cell destruction, which is attributed to a genetic predisposition. Genetics plus infection of one or more viral agents and possibly chemical agents are believed to cause type 1 diabetes. It is not known that these are the only factors involved. The onset and progression of hyperglycemic signs and symptoms are usually more rapid and acute in type 1 diabetes mellitus than in type 2. Type 1 diabetes may occur at any age. The patient is usually thin, and has an abrupt onset of signs and symptoms before 30 years of age. The patient often has strongly positive urine ketone tests with hyperglycemia and depends on insulin therapy to prevent ketoacidosis and to sustain life (Lewis et al, 2004).

Type 2 diabetes mellitus. The pathophysiologic factors that have been identified in type 2 diabetes mellitus include (1) decreased tissue (e.g., fat, muscle) responsiveness to insulin as a result of a receptor or postreceptor defects; (2) overproduction of insulin early in the disease, but eventual decreased secretion of insulin from beta-cell exhaustion; and (3) abnormal hepatic glucose regulation. These factors result in what is often referred to as peripheral insulin resistance. This resistance stim-

| Table 11-3 | *Comparison of Diabetes Mellitus Type 1 (IDDM) and Diabetes Mellitus Type 2 (NIDDM)* |

FACTOR	TYPE 1	TYPE 2
Age at onset	Usually 30 years or younger	Usually older than 30 years
Body weight	Normal or underweight	80% are overweight
Symptoms at onset	Sudden; polyphagia, polydipsia, polyuria, weight loss, weakness, fatigue; glycosuria, hyperglycemia; acidosis, progressing to DKA	Gradual; may be asymptomatic at onset; later, may develop signs and symptoms of type 1; others include slow wound healing, blurred vision, pruritus, boils or other skin infections; vaginal infections in women
Treatment	Diet, exercise, and insulin	Diet and exercise; or diet, exercise, and oral hypoglycemic agents; or diet, exercise, oral hypoglycemic agents, and insulin during times of illness or stress
Incidence of complications	Frequent	Frequent
Psychosocial and sexual concerns	Irritability; altered body image; mood swings, depression; menstrual irregularities; hirsutism; decreased libido	Altered body image; amenorrhea; decreased libido; poor tolerance to stress

ulates increased insulin production as a compensatory response, which may also predispose the patient to weight gain. A reduced-calorie diet for the obese patient with type 2 diabetes tends to reverse this problem. The patient with type 2 diabetes may benefit from oral antidiabetic agents, which have been found effective in several ways, including increasing insulin production, improving cell receptor binding, regulating hepatic glucose production, and delaying carbohydrate absorption from the small intestine. Type 2 usually occurs in people who are older than 30 years of age at diagnosis, are often obese, and have few classic symptoms. The patient is usually not prone to ketoacidosis except during periods of stress. Individuals with type 2 diabetes are not dependent on exogenous insulin for survival, but the patient may require it for adequate control of hyperglycemia (Lewis et al, 2004).

Regardless of the type of DM, all these patients have impaired glucose tolerance. Only 5% to 10% of all people with diabetes have type 1, but because they do not produce adequate amounts of endogenous (produced by the body) insulin, they must take regular injections of exogenous (from outside the body) insulin or they will die.

About 90% of people with diabetes in the United States have type 2, with a high incidence among African-Americans; Hispanic-Americans; and American Indians, especially members of the Pima tribe.

The American Diabetes Association (ADA) estimates that as many as 5.2 million of the 18.2 million Americans who have diabetes mellitus do not know they have it (ADA, 2002). It is estimated that, counting both diagnosed and undiagnosed DM, as much as 5.9% of the U.S. population have DM. Cases of type 2 diabetes are usually diagnosed after age 30, and 80% of these patients are overweight, with a familial history of diabetes. They are usually able to secrete suffi-

cient amounts of insulin, but their body tissues are unable to properly utilize it. These patients can usually achieve good control of their disease by diet and oral hypoglycemics, using insulin only when first diagnosed and during times of illness, surgery, or other periods when the body's insulin level is out of control. Most newly diagnosed type 2 diabetic patients have had the disease for as long as 10 years without treatment and have therefore been at risk for serious complications prior to diagnosis (Seley, 2004).

Pathophysiology

In normal metabolism the end products of digestion (glucose, fatty acids and glycerol, and amino acids) are absorbed into the venous circulation and carried to the liver, where they may be either used immediately or stored for later use. The liver can change glycerol and fatty acids into glucose, and glucose into triglycerides, as needed. Fatty acids may also be changed into ketone bodies (normal metabolic products, such as β-hydroxybutyric acid and aminoacetic acid, from which acetone may arise spontaneously), which serve as fuel for the muscles of the body and as an energy source for the brain. Glucose storage takes place in the form of glycogen in the liver. Free glucose in the bloodstream can always be used by the brain and kidney, because it is not necessary for insulin to be present to enable glucose molecules to enter the brain cells or the glomeruli. But insulin must be present for muscle cells and other body cells to be able to utilize glucose. Glycogen can be changed back into glucose as needed by the body for energy. In the patient with diabetes, lack of proper amounts of insulin, or its inadequate utilization, impairs the use of glucose by the body. Thus the excess glucose accumulates in the bloodstream, and hyperglycemia, (greater than normal amounts of glucose in the blood) exists. To rid the body of this abnormal amount of glucose, the kidneys will excrete it in the urine. This is called glycosuria (abnormal presence of a sugar, especially glucose, in the urine), a condition that necessitates an extra amount of water for proper dilution of the urine. The patient then develops polyuria (excretion of an abnormally large quantity of urine), and also experiences polydipsia (excessive thirst). Often the patient is unable to drink enough fluid to compensate for polyuria and may become dehydrated. Even though there is excess glucose available in the blood stream, it cannot be utilized by the body tissues without the help of insulin. Thus the cells are not properly nourished, and polyphagia (eating to the point of gluttony) develops. In spite of increased food intake, metabolism remains faulty, and the patient loses weight. Because carbohydrates cannot be utilized properly, proteins and fats are broken down and ketone bodies are used excessively for heat and energy. Because ketone bodies are acid substances, the patient may develop acidosis. Diabetic ketoacidosis (DKA) (acidosis accompanied by an accumulation of ketones in the blood), formerly called **diabetic coma,** may develop, and the patient could die. DKA is a severe metabolic disturbance caused by an acute insulin deficiency, decreased peripheral glucose utilization, and increased fat mobilization and ketogenesis.

Clinical Manifestations

The clinical manifestations of type 1 DM include the three classic "polys": polyuria, polydipsia, and polyphagia. These are the hallmark symptoms of type 1 DM. As ketone bodies accumulate in the bloodstream, imbalances of sodium, potassium, and bicarbonate result. Type 2 diabetic people, most of whom are more than 30 years of age, experience very different signs and symptoms. In the early stages of the disease, the patient may be asymptomatic but later may complain of symptoms associated with type 1, plus a number of others. These patients may not seek medical care until a severe complication such as kidney involvement, retinopathy, or gangrene occurs.

Assessment

Collection of **subjective data** to be assessed includes hunger, thirst, and nausea. In addition to frequent urination of large amounts, the patient may complain of nocturia, weakness, and fatigue. There may be blurred vision, the appearance of halos around lights, and headache. Symptoms such as cold extremities, cramping pain in the calves and feet during exercise or walking, decreased sensation to pain and temperature in the feet, and numbness and tingling of the lower extremities may occur. Symptoms of delayed stomach emptying such as nausea, vomiting, and early satiety (feeling of being full after eating) may develop. There may be pruritus. Male patients may become impotent. The patient may verbalize negative feelings about his or her body and the ability to cope with the illness. The nurse should assess coping methods, as well as the pa-

tient's knowledge about the disease process. Misunderstandings and lack of interest may result in inadequate skills—such as diet planning, injections, and exercise programs—to manage the necessary diabetic lifestyle. The patient's understanding of the importance of compliance with prescribed medical treatment should be assessed, as should the patient's willingness to obtain adequate follow-up.

Collection of **objective data** includes assessment of the skin, because slow wound healing, boils, carbuncles, and ulcerations are common. Women with DM may experience frequent vaginal infections, and vaginal discharge is often bothersome. In type 1 patients, weight loss and muscle wasting may be seen, but many type 2 patients remain obese. The skin on the lower extremities may appear shiny and thin, with less hair present. The legs and feet may feel cold to the touch, and there may be ulcerated areas. Gangrene of the toes is a dreaded sign. The nurse should assess the patient's ability to perform blood glucose testing and proper injection of insulin.

Diagnostic Tests

Diagnosis of DM is made on the basis of clinical manifestations, plus the patient's history and laboratory findings. The patient with random blood glucose greater than 200 mg/dL, a fasting plasma glucose level greater than 126 mg/dL or a glucose 2-hour postload (75 g anhydrous) level greater than 200 mg/dL should be further evaluated (Seley, 2004). Blood tests commonly performed include those in Box 11-2.

The ADA recommends self-monitoring of blood glucose (SMBG) instead of urine testing in any patient with IDDM. This is accomplished in a number of ways. Blood from a fingerstick may be placed on a reagent strip and compared with a color chart, or it may be placed into a reflectance meter. Another type of meter uses a glucose sensor instead of a meter, and test strips are not used; instead, a drop of blood is placed directly into the machine. SMBG is the monitoring tool of choice because it provides an accurate picture of current blood glucose levels.

The frequency of monitoring depends on the glycemic goals the patient and health care provider set and the intensity of the treatment regimen. The patient receiving two or more injections of insulin per day may want to test before meals and at bedtime every day. If the glycemic control is relatively stable, the patient may elect to test two or more times a day on certain days of the week. Testing is usually done before meals, but it can be done any time the patient needs to know the way a factor, such as stress, is affecting the blood glucose levels. The frequency of recording SMBG results to guide therapy decision should be jointly determined by the health care provider and the patient.

The technology of SMBG using the capillary blood glucose monitoring changes rapidly, with newer and more convenient systems being introduced every year.

Box 11-2 *Diagnostic Tests for Diabetes Mellitus*

Fasting blood sugar (FBS): After an 8-hour fast, blood is drawn. The normal is 60 to 110 mg/dL of venous blood; 126 mg/dL or greater is considered abnormal.

Oral glucose tolerance test (OGTT): When overt signs and symptoms of hyperglycemia, polyuria, polydipsia, and polyphagia, together with fasting blood glucose levels of 126 mg/dL or greater, are present, further oral glucose tolerance tests are usually not warranted. However, whenever glucose tolerance tests are used, the accuracy of test results depends on adequate patient preparation and attention to the many factors that may influence the outcome of such tests.

Serum insulin: Absent in IDDM; normal to high in NIDDM.

Postprandial (after a meal) blood sugar (PPBS): A fasting patient is given a measured amount of carbohydrate solution orally. An alternate method is to have the patient eat a measured amount of foods containing carbohydrates, fats, and proteins. A blood sample will be drawn 2 hours after completion of the meal. Elevated plasma glucose over 160 mg/dL may indicate the presence of DM.

Patient self-monitoring of blood glucose (SMBG): A blood sample is obtained by the fingerstick method, by either the patient or the nurse, and tested using a blood glucose-monitoring device.

Glycosylated hemoglobin (Hb A$_{lc}$): This blood test measures the amount of glucose that has become incorporated into the hemoglobin within an erythrocyte; these levels are reported as a percentage of the total hemoglobin. Because glycosylation occurs constantly during the 120-day life span of the erythrocyte, this test reveals the effectiveness of diabetes therapy for the preceding 8 to 12 weeks. Glycosylated hemoglobin levels remain more stable than plasma glucose levels and are evaluated by a venipuncture every 6 to 8 weeks. Normal Hb A$_{lc}$ is approximately 4% to 6% of the total. There is an urgent need to reduce Hb A$_{lc}$ values to below 7% to reduce complications. A result greater than 8% represents an average blood glucose level of approximately 200 mg/dL and signals a need for changes in treatment.

C-peptide test: In the production of insulin by the beta cells of the pancreas, there is first proinsulin with an A chain of amino acids and a B chain of amino acids with a connecting peptide or (C-peptide). The C-peptide allows the A and B proinsulin to fold and cleave together, creating the structure of insulin. After the connection has been made, the fusion occurs, creating insulin and a C-peptide by-product. C-peptide then gets secreted into the bloodstream by the pancreas along with insulin. The C-peptide level may be measured in a patient with type 2 diabetes mellitus to see if any insulin is being produced by the body. A newly diagnosed diabetic patient will often have C-peptide levels measured to determine if they are type 1 or type 2 diabetes. Normal values are: 0.5 to 2 ng/mL (nanograms per milliliter). The patient of type 1 diabetes is unable to produce insulin and will therefore have decreased levels of C-peptide; C-peptide levels in type 2 diabetic patients is normal or higher than normal. In type 2 diabetics, the problem seems to be an abnormal resistance to insulin action.

Blood glucose monitoring technology using a noninvasive spectroscopy—or a laser light on a skin surface such as the forearm or space between finger and thumb—is being researched for possible use in the future. Implantable sensors for continuous glucose monitoring are also being considered in research trials.

Urine testing for ketonuria is a valuable aid in determining the advent of DKA and is recommended for every patient with type 1 diabetes when the patient is experiencing hyperglycemia or acute illness. The amount of acetone is represented by a color change in shades of pink to purple. Acetone testing products include Ketostix and Acetest tablets.

Medical Management

Medical treatment for DM, no matter what type, consists mainly of education, monitoring, meal planning, medication, and exercise.

The overall goal is to assist people with diabetes in making changes in nutrition and exercise habits leading to improved metabolic control. Additional goals include the following:

- Maintenance of as near-normal blood glucose levels as possible by balancing food intake with insulin or oral glucose-lowering medications and activity levels.
- Achievement of optimal serum lipid levels.
- Provision of adequate calories for maintaining or attaining reasonable weight for adults, normal growth and development rates for children and adolescents, increased metabolic needs during pregnancy and lactation, or recovery from illnesses. Reasonable weight is defined as the weight the individual and health care provider acknowledge as achievable and maintainable in both the short term and the long term. This may not be the same as the usually defined desirable or ideal body weight.
- Prevention and treatment of acute complications such as hypoglycemia, and long-term complications such as renal disease, neuropathy, hypertension, and cardiovascular disease.
- Improvement of overall health through optimal nutrition. Dietary guidelines for Americans are

given in the U.S. Department of Agriculture's MyPyramid food planning tool (www.mypyramid.gov), which summarizes and illustrates nutritional guidelines and nutrient needs for all healthy Americans and can be used by the patient with diabetes.

It is hoped that the patient will assume a large part of the responsibility for self-care, with emphasis on optimal wellness instead of illness. Since 1921, when Charles Best and Frederick Banting first isolated insulin, medical science has made many dramatic strides in the care of the patient with diabetes, but physicians depend on the help obtained from other members of the health care team, especially nurses. Every newly diagnosed patient must undergo an intensive and extensive education program to learn proper diet, medication routines, home testing of blood glucose, and the role of exercise. The importance of the nurse as a teacher cannot be overemphasized.

Diet. Nutritional therapy for the patient with diabetes is aimed at helping to achieve a normal blood glucose level of less than 126 mg/dL and at attaining or maintaining a reasonable body weight, while ensuring proper growth and body maintenance. Nutritional therapy is the cornerstone of care for the person with diabetes. A nutritionally adequate meal plan with a reduction of total fat, especially saturated fat, is important. Monitoring of blood glucose levels, glycosylated hemoglobin, and lipids is essential. The services of a dietitian should be enlisted for each newly diagnosed diabetic. The menu must be individualized, taking into consideration the patient's age, weight, activity level, lifestyle, ethnic background, and food preferences. The ability to choose and pay for groceries, prepare food, and properly store leftovers must be assessed. After discharge from the hospital, detailed dietary instructions will be of no use to the patient who does not have money, cooking skills, and appliances necessary to comply with them. If the patient is living with the family, the person who will be planning and preparing the meals must be educated along with the patient, and this person should be taught how to fit the patient's dietary needs into the family menus. The physician and dietitian will decide the proper amounts of each nutrient in the dietary prescription. Dietary treatment, also called **medical nutrition therapy for diabetes,** involves individualized meal plans. Diets are based on ADA recommendations, and patients may obtain additional information and menus from that organization at no cost.

Quantitative diabetic diets, following the food choices and number of servings recommended by the U.S. Department of Agriculture's MyPyramid food planning tool (www.mypyramid.gov), include 45% to 50% of total kilocalories from carbohydrates, 10% to 20% of total kilocalories from proteins, and no more than 30% of total kilocalories from fats.

Rigid rules on carbohydrates have softened. Now the emphasis is on the total amount of carbohydrates consumed, rather than on the type. Recent research has debunked an old assumption. Once it was believed that a simple carbohydrate (sugar) would drive up blood glucose levels, so patients were advised to consume only complex carbohydrates. Two surprise findings, though, have made this rule obsolete:

1. Some complex carbohydrates (rice, potatoes, and bread) produce a glycemic response similar to that caused by sucrose (table sugar).
2. Milk and fruit have less effect on blood glucose than most starches.

As a result of these findings, sugars and complex carbohydrates are counted together as total carbohydrates.

Results of studies have shown that different carbohydrate foods affect the blood glucose level in different ways; this varying effect is termed the **glycemic index.** So, for the person with diabetes, emphasis may be placed not only on the amount of carbohydrate eaten but also on the glycemic index of those foods.

The **qualitative** diet is unmeasured and more unrestricted, stressing moderation when selecting foods from the MyPyramid food planning tool (www.mypyramid.gov) and reducing the use of simple carbohydrates, saturated fats, and alcohol. This diet may be used for the patient whose blood glucose levels are not extremely high, for the pediatric patient, or for the patient who is noncompliant with the ADA diet.

Insulin-dependent patients are usually given midafternoon and bedtime snacks in addition to their regular three meals a day. It is important that food intake be evenly distributed throughout the day, taking insulin dosage and exercise into consideration. The patient who plans to engage in strenuous exercise should be encouraged to eat more food, because exercise increases the absorption rate of insulin, thereby enabling muscles to use glucose more effectively.

Self-monitoring of blood glucose. Diabetic patients should do a fingerstick blood glucose level test before each meal and at bedtime each day until their disease is under control. A patient on a stable treatment regimen may find four checks a day on 2 or 3 days per week sufficient. If the treatment plan changes or the patient becomes ill, checks will need to be made four or more times every day (Bartol, 2002).

The patient may need follow-up visits with a dietitian as well as with the physician. Obese patients with NIDDM are encouraged to lose weight because many are then able to control their diabetes with only diet and exercise, eliminating the need for medication. The patient with IDDM should try to attain and maintain reasonable weight, because better control of the condition usually results. Good control of DM is desirable in helping to prevent complications.

Exercise. The patient with diabetes should exercise regularly. The physician will help determine the best type of exercise for each patient. Exercise is beneficial, not only because it aids in promoting proper utilization of glucose, but also because it is important to the overall functioning of the cardiovascular system and will increase the patient's feeling of well-being. Of all the therapies available for treating type 2 diabetes, exercise is probably the least expensive and most cost effective. Exercise can reduce insulin resistance and increase glucose uptake for as long as 72 hours as well as reduce blood pressure and lipid levels. However, it can carry some risks, including hypoglycemia. Patients older than age 40 should have a complete physical examination before beginning a rigorous exercise program. Like medications, exercise can be adjusted to improve blood glucose control. With exercise, motivation is more important than facts and information Encourage the patient in the benefits of exercise (Bartol, 2002).

Stress of acute illness and surgery. Both emotional and physical stress can increase the blood glucose level and result in hyperglycemia. However, it is impossible to avoid stress totally in life situations such as death in the family, job, interviews, and final examinations. These situations may require extra insulin to avoid hyperglycemia.

Common stress-evoking situations include acute illness and the controlled stress of surgery. The patient with diabetes who has a minor illness such as a cold or the flu should continue drug therapy and food intake. A carbohydrate liquid substitution such as regular soft drinks, gelatin dessert, or beverages such as Gatorade may be necessary. The patient should understand that food intake is important during this time because the body requires extra energy to deal with the stress of the illness. Extra insulin may be necessary to meet this demand without DKA concurrently developing.

Blood glucose monitoring should be done every 1 to 2 hours by either the patient or a person who can assume responsibility for care during the illness. Urine output and the presence and degree of ketonuria should be monitored, particularly when fever is present. Fluid intake should be increased to prevent dehydration, with a minimum of 4 ounces/hour for an adult.

The patient should be instructed to contact the health care provider when a blood glucose level exceeds 250 mg/dL; in such cases, fever, ketonuria, and nausea and vomiting may occur. The health care provider should supervise the necessary adjustments in the treatment regimen during times of stress. Eventually the well-informed patient will be able to make most adjustments independently on the basis of past successful experiences.

Surgery is controlled stress, and adjustments in the diabetes regimen can be planned to ensure glycemic control. The patient is given IV fluids and insulin immediately before, during, and after surgery when there is no oral intake. The type 2 diabetic patient receiving oral antidiabetics (OAs) usually has the OAs discontinued 48 hours before surgery and is treated with insulin during the surgical period. The patient should understand that this is a temporary measure

and is not to be interpreted as a worsening of diabetes.

Medications. Insulin and oral hypoglycemics are the drugs of choice for patients with diabetes. **Insulin administration** is necessary for all patients with type 1 and in patients with type 2 whose condition cannot be controlled by diet, exercise, or oral hypoglycemics alone.

Today, biosynthetic insulin is used almost exclusively, replacing insulin obtained from the pancreases of cows and pigs. Biosynthetic insulin is produced by genetically altering common bacteria or yeast using deoxyribonucleic acid (DNA) technology. This insulin exhibits chemical and biological properties identical to human insulin produced by human B cells in the pancreas (Figure 11-11). Insulin is a hormone and is absorbed into the patient's bloodstream. Insulin is given subcutaneously, and in rare instances, such as in DKA, is given intramuscularly to some patients.

Insulins differ in regard to onset, peak, action, and duration. The specific preparation of each type of insulin is matched with the patient's diet and activity.

By adding zinc, acetate buffers, and protamine to insulin in various ways, the onset of activity, peak, and duration times can be manipulated. Different combinations of these insulins can be used to tailor treatment to the patient's specific pattern of blood glucose levels. Formulas are classified as rapid-acting (insulin lispro [Humalog], insulin aspart [NovoLog]), short acting (regular insulin [Humulin R, Novolin R]), intermediate acting (NPH insulin [Humulin N, Novalin N], Lente), and long acting (ultralente insulin [Humulin U]). A recent insulin called Lantus is a long-acting synthetic (recombinant DNA origin, human-made) human insulin. It is used once a day at bedtime and works around the clock for 24 hours. Lantus is a "peakless" insulin glargine that provides a continuous insulin level similar to the slow, steady (basal) secretion of insulin from a normal pancreas. Lantus is very acidic and must not be mixed in the same syringe with other insulins because it will interfere with their action (Figure 11-12). If hyperglycemia occurs, elevated blood glucose is covered with sliding-scale regular insulin. Premixed combinations are 70/30 (70% NPH and 30% regular) (Box 11-3; see Figure 11-11) and 50/50 (50%

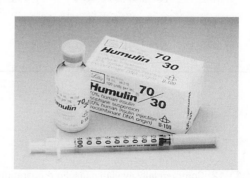

FIGURE **11-11** U/100 insulin and disposable U/100 insulin syringe.

NPH and 50% regular). Two recent combinations, 75/25 (75% lispro protamine [NPH] and 25% lispro Humalog [rapid acting] called Humalog mix 75/25) and 70/30 aspart protamine (70% protamin [NPH] and 30% aspart [rapid acting] called Novolog mix 70/30), are now available. The premixed insulins are most helpful for those who have stable insulin needs. Trying to get the timing of insulin action to match food intake can be a challenge, and it tends to be more difficult for people with type 1 diabetes because their only source of insulin is by injection. Regular insulin is prescribed when a rapid onset of glucose-lowering action is needed, such as before meals and during periods of acute illness, surgery, or stress. Only regular insulin can be administered IV; thus it is used in emergencies.

A recent human insulin formula called insulin lispro (Humalog) was approved in June 1996 by the U.S. Food and Drug Administration (FDA). Humalog begins to take effect in less than half the time of regular, fast-acting insulin. The products previously on the market must be taken subcutaneously 30 to 60 minutes before a meal; the new formula can be injected 15 minutes before a meal. This timing more closely mimics the body's own hormone activity. Lispro (Humalog) will bring the most benefit to people with type 1 diabetes who take short-acting insulin before meals combined with a longer-acting insulin once or twice a day. Another rapid-acting insulin aspart (Novolog) with similar onset of action as Humalog is also now available (Fain, 2004). Insulins are commonly used in combination to mimic the normal pancreatic insulin secretion.

The timing of insulin administration in relation to meals is important. When giving insulin, the nurse must be careful to inject into the **subcutaneous pocket** (space between the fat and muscle layers) only, avoiding depositing the medication directly into the fat or muscle (Figure 11-13).

Insulin administration requires the appropriate syringe. Most commercial insulin is available as U/100, indicating that each milliliter contains 100 units of insulin. U/100 insulin must be used with a U/100-marked syringe. For a user taking smaller doses of insulin, insulin syringes with larger black lines are marked for 25, 30, or 50 units and are available for use with U/100 syringes. One important distinction regarding the different sizes of syringes is that the 100-unit syringe is marked in 2-unit increments, whereas the 50-unit and 30-unit syringes are marked in 1-unit increments. It is important that the patient gets the correct size of syringe and does not switch syringes, thus avoiding serious dosing errors. Before the development of U/100 insulin, insulin was available in concentrations of U/40 and U/80. JCAHO now recommends using units instead of abbreviation U on medication orders and medication administration records to decrease errors in dosing.

Needles are very fine, usually 25 to 32 gauge, to be as atraumatic to the tissue as possible. Needles and syringes now used in the hospital and in the home are of the disposable type. An open bottle of insulin currently being used does not have to be kept in the refrigerator. In fact, it is now believed that insulin should be administered at room temperature, not straight

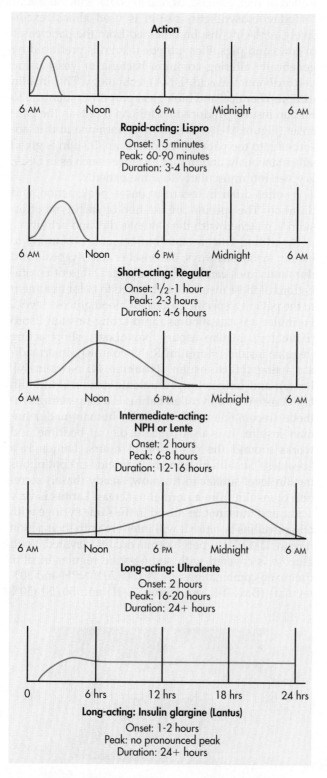

FIGURE **11-12** Commercially available insulin preparations, including onset, peak, and duration of action.

Box 11-3 *Types of Insulin*

Type of Insulin	Source and Color	Injection Time (Before Meal)	Risk Time for Hypoglycemic Reaction	Action	Start of Action	Peak Action	Duration
RAPID/SHORT ACTING							
Humalog (Lispro)	Human Clear	5-15 min	No meal within 30 min	Rapid	15-30 min	1-2 hr	3-4 hr
NovoLog (Aspart)	Human Clear	5-15 min	No meal within 30 min	Rapid	15-30 min	1-3 hr	3-5 hr
Regular Humulin R NovolinR	Human or pork Clear	30 min	Delayed meal or 3-4 hr after injection	Short	30-60 min	2-4 hr	6-8 hr
MIXED INSULINS							
Novolog Mix 70/30 (neutral protamine Aspart/Aspart)	Human Cloudy	15 min	No meal within 30 min	Rapid and intermediate	15-30 min	2-10 hr	12-16 hr
Humalog Mix 72/25 (neutral protamine Lispro/Lispro)	Human Cloudy	15 min	No meal within 30 min	Rapid and intermediate	15-30 min	2-10 hr	12-16 hr
70/30 or 50/50 (NPH/regular ratio)	Human Cloudy	30-60 min	Delayed meal or 3-4 hr after injection	Rapid and intermediate	30-60 min	6-12 hr	18-24 hr
INTERMEDIATE ACTING							
NPH	Human or pork Milky when mixed	30 min	4-6 hr after injection	Intermediate acting	2-4 hr	6-10 hr	12-16 hr
Lente	Human or pork Milky when mixed	30 min	3-6 hr after injection	Intermediate acting	1-3 hr	6-12 hr	18-26 hr
LONG LASTING							
Lantus (Glargine)	Clear. **Do not mix with others**	Usually take at 9 PM. Once daily.*	Starting dose should be 20% less than total daily dose of NPH	Long lasting	1-2 hr	No pronounced peak	24 hr†
Ultralente	Human or pork Milky when mixed	30 min	6 hr after injection	Long lasting	4-6 hr	18 hr	24 hr

Proper timing of insulin and eating if on regular or 70/30 in relationship with blood glucose	Insulin	Primarily covers
below 50 mg/dL = when meal is complete	AM: Rapid and short acting	Breakfast to lunch
50-70 mg/dL = at mealtime	AM: NPH or Lente	Lunch to evening meal
70-120 mg/dL = 15 min before meal	Noon: Rapid and short	Lunch to midafternoon
120-180 mg/dL = 30 min before meal	PM: Rapid and short acting	Evening meal to bedtime
over 180 mg/dL = 45 min before meal	PM: NPH and Lente	Late evening to early morning
	Bedtime: NPH or Lente	Midnight to following morning
	Bedtime: Lantus or Ultralente	Provides continuous coverage

From Lewis, S.M. et al. (2004). *Medical-surgical nursing: assessment and management of clinical problems.* (6th ed.). St. Louis: Mosby.
*May take at other times.
†Type 1, once or twice daily; type 2, once daily.

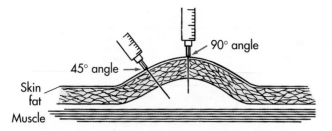

FIGURE **11-13** Insulin is injected into the pocket between subcutaneous fat and muscle occurring when the skin is pinched up. The angle of injection may be 45 or 90 degrees.

from the refrigerator, to help prevent insulin **lipodystrophy** (abnormality in the metabolism or deposition of fats; insulin lipodystrophy is the loss of local fat deposits). Extra bottles are stored in the refrigerator. Box 11-4 offers guidelines for preparation of a dose of insulin, one or two types at a time.

Patients who self-inject insulin at home may want to have a family member oversee the procedure. Nurses administering insulin injections must always have the dose drawn up in the syringe checked and documented by another licensed person to prevent medication errors. The patient with diabetes should ideally be taught self-injection technique before discharge from the hospital. However, some patients are unable to perform this because of physical problems or intellectual incapacity, visual disturbances, or age. In these cases, family members or others have to administer the injections. Before discharge, either the patient or the significant other, or both, must display the ability to correctly draw up and inject insulin. In a newly diagnosed patient, regular insulin may be injected before each meal.

After reasonable control of hyperglycemia is achieved, the dosage schedule may be changed to once a day, in the morning before breakfast, with the type of insulin being intermediate- or long-acting. See Figure 11-12 and Box 11-3 for types of insulin. Sometimes diabetic patients take two doses of insulin, in divided doses given before breakfast and before the evening meal. The nurse should be alert for signs of **hypoglycemia** (a less than normal amount of glucose in the blood, usually caused by administration of too much insulin, excessive secretion of insulin by the islet cells of the pancreas, or dietary deficiency) at the peak of action of whatever type of insulin the patient is taking. The patient should be instructed to notify a member of the nursing staff if any of the following signs of hypoglycemic (insulin) reaction occur: faintness, sudden weakness, excessive perspiration, irritability, hunger, palpitations, trembling, or drowsiness. After appropriate blood glucose testing, the patient will choose an injection site. The subcutaneous pocket is the desired layer into which insulin should be injected. Insulin should not be injected into the muscle, because it en-

Box 11-4 *Preparation of Insulin*

1. Thoroughly wash hands with warm water and soap. Bring the insulin to room temperature because an injection of cold insulin can be painful.
2. Assemble all equipment needed, such as properly calibrated insulin syringe with a prefitted needle, prep sponge, and insulin.
3. Turn the insulin vial onto its side and gently rotate between the hands several times to be sure it is mixed. The precipitate should be evenly blended. This does not need to be done with regular insulin, because it has no precipitate. Never shake insulin vigorously because this creates air bubbles.
4. Clean the rubber stopper on the vial with a prep sponge.
5. Remove the needle cover and draw in the same amount of air as units of insulin to be injected.
6. Insert the needle into the rubber stopper of the vial and then inject air. Invert the bottle with the syringe unit attached, making sure the tip of the needle is below the level of the insulin so that air will not be drawn into the syringe.
7. Pull back slowly on the plunger, a few units past the desired dose of insulin.
8. Inspect for air bubbles in the syringe; if any are seen, gently tap the barrel until they rise to the top, then push back into the vial with plunger to the level of the desired dose of insulin.
9. Holding on to the barrel and plunger, remove the syringe unit and put the needle cover back on. **Always** check insulin dose with a second licensed nurse. Proceed with injection procedure.

TWO INSULINS

1. Follow steps 1 through 5 above.
2. Insert the desired amount of air into the vial of the longer-acting insulin first. Insulins should not be mixed if they differ in purity or species origin. Example: Lantus is a long acting insulin which can **never** be mixed with regular insulin.
3. Inject the desired amount of air into the shorter-acting insulin vial; leave the syringe unit in this vial; invert, and proceed through steps 6 through 9, but do not inject yet. Set the vial of shorter-acting insulin out of reach to prevent accidental reuse.
4. Insert the needle into the vial of longer-acting insulin, being careful to hold on to the plunger so that none of the insulin in the syringe enters that vial.
5. Slowly pull the plunger to the level of the combined total of both types of insulin desired (such as regular 10 units, NPH 30 units, totaling 40 units). Do not pull extra units into the syringe. Take special care not to get any air bubbles into the syringe because they will displace some of the insulin and make the dose incorrect. If this happens, you will have to discard the whole syringe and start all over again. Check insulin dose with a second licensed nurse.
6. If the dose is correct, proceed with the injection procedure.

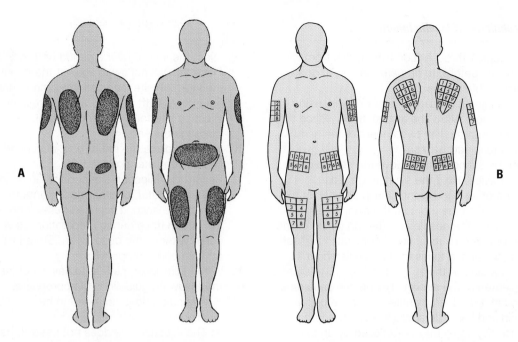

FIGURE **11-14** **A,** Rotation of sites for insulin injections. **B,** Injection diagram to track rotation of injection sites.

ters the bloodstream too quickly and could cause hypoglycemia. Site selection is crucial, as is site rotation. The patient may choose sites at the abdomen (except for 2 inches [5 cm] around the navel), the upper arms, the anterior or lateral aspects of the thighs, and the hips or buttocks. The abdomen provides the fastest, least variable absorption, followed by the arms, thighs, and buttocks. Patients may find it easier to keep track of their injection sites by recording each injection on a numbered chart (Figure 11-14).

Because of differing anatomic absorption rates of insulin, it is currently recommended that injections should be given in all the available areas in a site, such as the thigh, before moving to another site. In this way the diabetic may take eight or more injections, spaced 1 to 1½ inches apart, thus allowing the tissues in other sites to recover more fully before being used again. This technique helps prevent lipodystrophy and lipoatrophy, conditions that can lead to unsightly lumps under the skin and the inhibition of insulin absorption. If the patient engages in heavy exercise, an injection site may be chosen where movement will not be as great, because exercise may increase insulin absorption. The technique for insulin injection is described in Box 11-5.

Several new delivery systems are available to the person who finds injections emotionally and physically uncomfortable. These include automatic injectors, the jet stream (needleless) injector, the Insuflon indwelling insulin delivery service, and the button infuser.

Another method of insulin administration is continuous subcutaneous insulin infusion (CSII) using the external infusion pump. This small, battery-powered computerized device is worn on the user's body, usually in a pocket or on a belt. It is attached to a thin tube with a needle on the end, which is inserted into the subcutaneous tissue. A continuous, or basal, rate of regular insulin (such as Humulin BR) delivery can be programmed, with bolus doses administered as needed. The insulin pump is as close a substitute as available to a healthy, working pancreas. It mimics the pancreas by releasing small amounts of rapid-acting insulin every few minutes. Buffered regular insulin may be substituted in patients unable to use rapid-acting insulin to improve postprandial blood glucose levels and long-term glucose control (Bode et al, 2002). The basal rate is designed to keep the blood glucose level steady between meals and during sleep. When food is eaten, the pump is programmed (at the touch of a button) to deliver a larger quantity of insulin right away to cover the carbohydrate in the meal. This is called a bolus of insulin. The bolus can also be adjusted based on the blood glucose level and amount of planned physical activity. For carefully selected and properly educated patients, the pump offers improved flexibility in lifestyle, improved control of blood glucose and glycosylated hemoglobin (Hb A$_{1c}$) levels (see Box 11-2), as well as freedom from multiple daily injections. Properly disassembled insulin pumps such as the H-Tron V100 (Disetronic) can even be worn during bathing or while swimming. The insertion site is usually the abdomen, but the buttocks, thighs, arms, and sections of the back may be used, with the insertion site covered by a clear occlusive dressing, which is usually changed every other day.

Oral hypoglycemics are compounds used to treat type 2 diabetes, each having a different mechanism of action. Oral hypoglycemic agents are not oral insulin or a substitute for insulin. The patient must have some

Box 11-5 *Technique for Insulin Injection*

1. Follow steps 1 through 9 or 1 through 6 from Box 11-4, as before, to prepare the insulin dose.
2. Don disposable gloves.
3. Clean the injection site with a prep swab, using a circular motion. Allow the alcohol to dry. Place the swab between the last two fingers of the hand not used to inject the insulin.
4. Pick up the syringe and remove the needle cover and lay it aside. Hold the syringe like a dart.
5. Using the other hand, gently pinch up at least a 2-inch fold of tissue (not just the skin).
6. Quickly insert the needle into the top (apex) of the fold, entering the subcutaneous pocket. The "soft spot" technique is to insert the needle about 1 inch to the side of the apex of the fold, into softer tissue, entering the pocket. The needle should be inserted at a 90-degree angle unless the patient is very thin and has little subcutaneous tissue. In that case the angle may be reduced by up to 45 degrees to avoid IM injection.
7. Release the skinfold and use that hand to steady the barrel of the syringe. If blood appears in the syringe after needle is inserted, remove the syringe unit and start over with a second dose of insulin (Lewis et al, 2004).
8. Inject the insulin over a period of 3 to 5 seconds.
9. Place the alcohol swab against the needle hub, at the injection site, and pull the syringe unit straight out in one swift motion. Gently press on the injection site for a few seconds, but do not massage the site.
10. Carefully place the entire unit, uncapped, into the sharps container provided.
11. Record the injection site and insulin dose on a chart, computer, or other documentation sheet. Include the second licensed nurse who witnessed the insulin dose during preparation. Have the nurse witness the dose given. Store insulin and other supplies properly.
12. When instructing patient to self-inject insulin, use the following guidelines (if appropriate):
    - Aspiration does not need to be done before injection.
    - The injection site does not need to be cleansed with alcohol. The use of an alcohol swab on the site before self-injection is no longer recommended. Routine hygiene such as washing with soap and rinsing with water is adequate (Lewis et al, 2004).

functioning insulin production for oral hypoglycemics to be effective.

Five classes of oral drugs—sulfonylureas, meglitinides, alpha-glucosidase inhibitors, thiazolidinediones, and biguanide—are available for patients whose insulin production or utilization is inadequate due to type 2 diabetes mellitus (Table 11-4).

Sulfonylureas have blood glucose–lowering effects. They stimulate the pancreas to release insulin. They are classified as first generation or second generation, depending on when they were introduced into clinical use in the United States. The first generation of these drugs used in the treatment of DM includes tolbutamide (Orinase), tolazamide (Tolinase), and chlorpropamide (Diabinese). They are rarely prescribed today because they depend on renal excretion and stress the kidneys. A second generation of sulfonylureas, approved for use in the United States more recently includes glipizide (Glucotrol XL), glyburide (Micronase, DiaBeta, Glynase), and glimepiride (Amaryl). They are more potent and do not require renal excretion. The main disadvantage of second-generation drugs is their increased expense.

A class of oral hypoglycemics that stimulates increased insulin release in the pancreas is the **meglitinides,** which includes repaglinide (Prandin) and nateglinide (Starlix).

Another class of oral hypoglycemics lowers blood glucose by inhibiting delay of carbohydrate absorption from the small intestine; these are called **alpha-glucosidase inhibitors.** This drug class includes acarbose (Precose) and miglitol (Glycet). The best way to gauge effectiveness of therapy with acarbose and miglitol is to monitor the patient's 2-hour postprandial blood glucose level.

Thiazolidinediones are the class of oral hypoglycemics that lowers blood glucose by increasing insulin sensitivity at the insulin receptor sites on the cells. The two drugs currently available in this class are rosiglitazone (Avandia) and pioglitazone (Actos). They are most appropriate for adults whose bodies produce insulin but cannot use it because of inadequate or ineffective insulin receptor sites.

Metformin (Glucophage) is a **biguanide** glucose-lowering agent. It works primarily by reducing hepatic glucose production and lowers fasting blood glucose levels. It also enhances tissue response to insulin and improves glucose transport into cells. Metformin usually does not promote weight gain and may help improve lipid levels. Metformin is widely used by itself and in combination with sulfonylurea. Use of combined glyburide/metformin (Glucovance) has recently been approved by the FDA.

Once an oral drug becomes ineffective, simply substituting rarely works. But combination therapy can be

| Table 11-4 | *Five Classes of Oral Hypoglycemics* |

GENERIC AND BRAND NAME	MECHANICS OF ACTION
CLASSIFICATION: SULFONYLUREAS	
Chlorpropamide (Diabinese)—1st generation (rarely used)	Insulin secretagogues, primarily stimulate the beta cells of the pancreas to release insulin, particularly in the early course of type 2 diabetes mellitus. Sulfonylureas increase the sensitivity to insulin at receptor sites.
Tolazamide (Tolinase)—1st generation (rarely used)	
Tolbutamide (Orinase)—1st generation (rarely used)	
Glipizide (Glucotrol)—2nd generation	
Glyburide (DiaBeta, Micronase, Glynase)— 2nd generation	
Gllimepiride (Amaryl)—2nd generation	
CLASSIFICATION: MEGLITINIDES	
Repaglinide (Prandin)	Insulin secretagogues, like the sulfonylureas, stimulate the beta cells in the pancreas to increase insulin release. Their effects, which are glucose dependent, decrease when the patient's blood glucose level decreases. Requires functioning pancreatic beta cells.
Nateglinide (Starlix)	
CLASSIFICATION: BIGUANIDE	
Metformin (Glucophage, Glucophage XR)	It works primarily by reducing hepatic glucose production and lowers fasting blood glucose levels. It also enhances tissue response to insulin and improves glucose transport into the cells. It also decreases intestinal glucose absorption.
CLASSIFICATION: ALPHA-GLUCOSIDASE INHIBITORS	
Acarbose (Precose)	Metabolized by intestinal bacteria and digestive enzymes, alpha-glucosidase inhibitors delay carbohydrate absorption from the small intestine.
Miglitol (Glyset)	
CLASSIFICATION: THIAZOLIDINEDIONES	
Rosiglitazone (Avandia)	Combat type 2 diabetes mellitus by increasing insulin sensitivity at insulin receptor sites on the cell.
Pioglitazone (Actos)	Thiazolidinediones are most appropriate for adults whose bodies produce insulin but cannot use it because of inadequate or ineffective insulin receptor sites.

Data from Funnel, M. & Barlage, D. Managing diabetes with "agent oral." *Nursing*, 34(3):36, 2002.

highly effective. For example, oral drugs from two or more classes may be combined, or an oral drug may be combined with a bedtime dose of NPH or glargine insulin (Lantus). Metformin and insulin are commonly chosen for combination therapy with sulfonylureas (Funnel & Barlage, 2004).

Another drug that may be used in the treatment of hypoglycemic reactions occurring in DM is glucagon, a hormone normally secreted by the alpha cells of the pancreas. It stimulates the liver to change stored glycogen into glucose, which is then released into the blood stream. Glucagon is available in a purified, crystallized form for reconstruction and subcutaneous, intramuscular (IM), or IV administration in the event of loss of consciousness as a result of hypoglycemic reaction. The usual dose is 0.5 to 1 mg for adults, with smaller doses for children. Some form of oral protein and carbohy-

drate, such as milk and crackers, should be given after the patient regains consciousness. A commercially prepared kit containing glucagon is carried by many people with diabetes, along with concentrated carbohydrate such as candy or glucose gel. (See also Complementary & Alternative Therapies box.)

The surgical treatment of DM, type 1 (IDDM), is still an experimental area. Two procedures are now available to selected patients. One is pancreas transplant; the other is implantation of an insulin-infusion pump under the skin. Today many people have benefited from pancreatic transplant as well as the subcutaneously implanted insulin infusion method (Figure 11-15).

The pump devices are able to deliver insulin continuously in titrated amounts through tubing attached to a small pump device on one end and to a needle on the other end, which is placed subcutaneously in the

Endocrine Disorders

- Herbal medicines used in the treatment of non–insulin-dependent diabetes include aloe vera juice, beans *(Phaseolus species)*, bitter gourd, karela *(Momordica charantia)*, black tea *(Camellia sinensis)*, fenugreek *(Trigonella foenum-graecum)*, gumar *(Gymnema sylvestre)*, macadamia nut, and Madagascar periwinkle *(Catharanthus roseus)*. Effects of these herbs include lowering of blood pressure *(fenugreek)*, a boosting of insulin production *(gumar)*, and increased use of available insulin *(black tea)*.
- Kelp *(Fucus vesiculosus)* may help with weight loss in hypothyroid disorders. Milk thistle *(Silybum marianum)* is used for treatment and prohylaxis of chronic hepatotoxicity, inflammatory liver disorders, and certain types of cirrhosis.
- Yoga may aid the diabetic patient with diet control and may improve pancreatic function.

skin (see Figure 11-15). The pump delivers a preprogrammed dose of insulin that is designed to match the patient's basal profile to achieve a nearly normal insulin delivery on a continuous basis. The patient can also regulate meal coverage with bolus doses of insulin given at the patient's discretion.

Nursing Interventions and Patient Teaching

People with diabetes may be hospitalized as a direct result of their disease process, or they may have a different primary diagnosis. The main focus of nursing interventions must always be on the primary diagnosis, but the nurse must remember that the patient is also diabetic and is susceptible to a number of complications in addition to all those experienced by nondiabetic patients.

Daily routine for the patient with diabetes includes accurate monitoring of blood glucose levels, either by fingerstick specimens or by laboratory testing. Careful attention to diet is important, and the nurse should note the amount of food eaten at each meal and record it accurately.

If the patient with type 1 DM is ill, nauseated, or cannot eat for any reason, consult with the physician or primary care provider. Physiologic and psychological stress will raise the patient's blood glucose level. Do not withhold insulin in a type 1 diabetic patient. Without insulin to promote glucose to enter the cells, the body must seek an alternative source for energy. Fats and protein are used. When these cells break down, ketones are formed. Accumulation of ketones results in ketosis and acidosis. If this situation is not corrected, the patient may develop diabetic ketoacidosis (DKA).

Often the primary care provider will recommend substituting Popsicles or apple juice, which can compensate for a decrease in calories that may occur when a regular diet cannot be consumed. (Mohang, 2004). If the patient does not like the types of food on the meal tray, the dietitian should be consulted and a visit arranged.

Good skin care is essential for the person with diabetes, because poor circulation, so common in diabetes, can lead to the development of skin problems. Compromised skin integrity makes a diabetic person more susceptible to infection. In diabetes, elevated glycosylated hemoglobin in the RBCs impedes the release of oxygen to the tissues. Elevated blood glucose levels also make some pathogens thrive and proliferate rapidly. Vascular changes decrease blood, oxygen, and nutrient supply to the tissues and affect the supply of WBCs in the area, because if WBCs do not function properly, phagocytosis is defective (Mosby's Coping with Multisystem Complications, 1998).

Any abnormalities such as cuts, scratches, or lesions anywhere on the body should be reported to the physician and treated before infection develops. Special foot care is crucial for this patient, because poor circulation and decreased nerve sensation neuropathy (any abnormal condition characterized by inflammation and degeneration of the peripheral nerves) increase the danger of ulcers or other abnormal lesions developing into gangrene. Many patients seek the services of a podiatrist for their foot care. The patient should thoroughly wash the feet with soap and water every day, dry them thoroughly, and inspect them carefully for cracks, blisters, or foreign objects, paying special attention to the area between the toes. Foot soaks or powders are not recommended. Clean socks should be worn daily, and tight garters should be avoided. The toenails should be clipped straight across

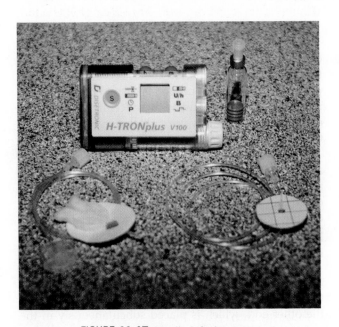

FIGURE **11-15** Insulin infusion pump.

so that the edges do not become ingrown. The nurse should never trim the toenails of a patient with diabetes without a physician's written order. No hot water bottles or heating pads should be put on the feet, because burns may occur and not be felt. Sturdy, properly fitting shoes should be worn. The nurse should suggest the patient wear shoes with wide toe boxes or molded shoes that are less constrictive. Medicare now reimburses diabetic patients who have certain conditions for the cost of specially molded shoes. The patient should not go barefoot at any time. The physician should be notified immediately of any injury to the toes or feet (Health Promotion Considerations box).

The patient who is receiving insulin should be watched very carefully for development of hypoglycemia, especially when the particular kind of insulin being injected is at its peak of action. Hypoglycemia is seen much less frequently in patients receiving oral hypoglycemics, but it can occur.

The emotional aspects of diabetes are numerous, and many patients experience a period of denial after the initial diagnosis. Some patients become very depressed. Because this disease affects all age groups, nursing interventions must be tailored to fit the needs of each patient (Older Adult Considerations box). Patients with diabetes must have help in working through their feelings, so the nurse must be a good listener and supportive at all times. The patient who does not satisfactorily resolve any major problems in accepting the diagnosis of DM may be noncompliant with the treatment plan.

The nurse who supervises the patient in a home setting must encourage the patient to take the prescribed medication faithfully, eat the right kinds of food, test blood or urine correctly, and exercise regularly. If a family member is going to be responsible for the patient's care, the nurse must make sure that the caregiver

---

Health Promotion Considerations

Foot Care for the Patient with Diabetes Mellitus

- Wash feet daily with a mild soap and *warm* water. Test water temperature with hands first.
- Pat feet dry gently, especially between toes.
- Examine feet daily for cuts, blisters, edema, erythema, and tender areas. If patient's eyesight is poor, have others inspect feet.
- Use lanolin on feet to prevent skin from drying and cracking. Do not apply between toes.
- Use mild foot powder on feet if perspiring.
- Do not use commercial remedies to remove calluses or corns.
- Cleanse cuts with *warm* water and mild soap, covering with clean dressing. Do not use iodine, rubbing alcohol, or strong adhesives.
- Report skin infections or nonhealing lesions to health care provider immediately.
- Cut toenails even with rounded contour of toes. Do not cut down corners. The best time to trim nails is after a shower or bath.
- Separate overlapping toes with cotton or lamb's wool.
- Avoid open-toe, open-heel and high-heel shoes. Leather shoes are preferred to plastic ones. Wear slippers with soles. Do not go barefoot. Shake out shoes before putting on.
- Wear clean, absorbent (cotton or wool) socks or stockings that have not been mended. Colored socks must be colorfast.
- Do not wear clothing that leaves impressions or constricts circulation.
- Do not use hot water bottles or heating pads to warm feet. Wear socks for warmth.
- Guard against frostbite.
- Exercise feet daily either by walking or by flexing and extending feet in suspended position. Avoid prolonged sitting, standing, and crossing of legs.

Older Adult Considerations

Endocrine Disorder

- Diabetes mellitus is more prevalent in older adults. A major reason for this is that the process of aging involves insulin resistance and glucose intolerance, which are believed to be precursors to type 2 diabetes.
- The classic signs and symptoms of diabetes may not be obvious in older adults.
- Dietary management may be complicated by a variety of functional, social, economic, and financial factors.
- Hormone supplements must be administered with caution because side effects are more likely.
- Older adult diabetic patients are at increased risk for infection and should be counseled to receive proper immunizations and seek regular medical attention for even minor symptoms. The older adult often has considerable difficulty in managing diabetes.
- Some symptoms of hypothyroidism in the older adult are similar to those in a younger person but are more likely to be overlooked because the symptoms— fatigue, mental impairment, sluggishness, and constipation—are often attributed solely to aging. The older person with hypothyroidism has symptoms unique to the age set, including more disturbances of the central nervous system, such as syncope, convulsions, dementia, and coma. There is often pitting edema and deafness.
- The older patient with hyperthyroidism frequently has manifestations related only to the cardiovascular system, such as palpitations, angina, atrial fibrillation, and breathlessness. The older adult may also have depression, anorexia, and constipation (apathetic hypothyroidism). Thus signs and symptoms often attributed to "aging" may actually indicate an endocrine problem.

NURSING CARE PLAN

The Patient with Diabetes Mellitus

Ms. T. is an obese, 52-year-old married patient with NIDDM diagnosed 3 years ago. She was referred to a short-term ambulatory diabetes education program by her physician for instruction on insulin administration because blood glucose control has not been achieved with dietary measures.

The nursing history identified the following:

She sees referral as necessary but perceives it, and inability to control weight and blood glucose, as a personal failure.

She maintains inconsistent sleep/activity schedule. (Works 8 PM to 8 AM Saturday and Sunday with 2 to 4 hours sleep during day; rises at 8 AM and retires at 11 PM on other days.)

She has accurate knowledge about dietary modifications and has participated successfully in several weight-reduction programs with 20- to 40-pound weight loss each time.

She does not exercise consistently.

She has monitored blood glucose once or twice on self (SMBG).

She states that work is important to her; satisfactions are derived from work and group socialization, and it "keeps me busy."

She fears that her husband will die suddenly at home. Two years ago she performed CPR when he had a cardiac arrest at home. Realizes that she maintains work schedule "to keep me from worrying about my husband."

Objective data included blood glucose, 220 mg/dL; weight, 200 lb; BP 134/84. Collaborative nursing actions include teaching Ms. T. those measures that will help her achieve control of blood glucose (insulin, diet, and exercise) and how to detect, prevent, and treat hypoglycemic reactions. The nurse reported Ms. T.'s work schedule to the physician and asked for insulin dosage alterations on weekends. The physician was unaware of her work schedule and stated that blood glucose control could not be optimum with this schedule.

NURSING DIAGNOSIS *Deficient knowledge: self-injections, self-blood glucose monitoring, related to lack of exposure*

Patient Goals/Expected Outcomes	Nursing Intervention	Evaluation
Patient will independently self-administer insulin.	Support patient as necessary to self-inject insulin.	Patient demonstrates safety in drawing up and self-administering insulin.
Patient will perform SMBG accurately.	Observe patient's skill in SMBG; correct as necessary.	Patient demonstrates accuracy in SMBG.
Patient will use measurements obtained by SMBG to achieve blood glucose less than 126 mg/dL.	Review with patient the effect of activity, dietary intake, and insulin on blood glucose.	Patient can verbalize the effect of activity, diet, and insulin on blood glucose.
Patient will be able to detect and treat hypoglycemia.	Instruct patient on frequency and timing of SMBG.	
	Review with patient signs and symptoms and treatment measures.	Patient can recite signs and symptoms of hypoglycemia and the correct immediate treatment to pursue.
	Refer to dietitian for modification of diet necessary with insulin and for verification of diet knowledge.	

NURSING DIAGNOSIS *Ineffective health maintenance, related to ineffective coping skills*

Patient Goals/Expected Outcomes	Nursing Intervention	Evaluation
Patient will state at least one change that will improve blood glucose control.	Teach patient effects of stress, lack of exercise, and activity pattern on blood glucose.	Patient has enrolled in an exercise and weight-reduction program to assist in achieving a reasonable weight and beneficial exercise.
	Explore with patient willingness and ability to change behaviors: sleep/activity, coping, and exercise.	
	Engage patient in mutual problem solving; refrain from prescribing.	
	Explore sources for long-term support in learning more effective coping skills; suggest support groups: 1. For patients with DM 2. For weight loss and maintaining weight loss 3. Available at work in health service program	
	Suggest to patient that she seek a trial period on day shift on weekends.	

NURSING CARE PLAN

The Patient with Diabetes Mellitus—cont'd

? CRITICAL THINKING QUESTIONS

1. Ms. T. has received Humalog 75/25, 25 units subcutaneously at 7:30 AM. She has eaten her ADA diet at breakfast and lunch. At 3:00 PM, she complains of being hungry, nervous, and tremulous. The immediate nursing intervention would include:

2. Ms. T. states, "I need to lose about 40 pounds, and I'm considering joining a weight-reduction club." Helpful suggestions by the nurse for Ms. T. would include:

3. In discharge planning, the nurse notes that Ms. T. has poorly fitting shoes. Important discharge teaching for foot care for Ms. T. would include:

---

is functioning adequately in this role. Some patients live alone and do very well caring for themselves, with occasional visits from a home health or public health nurse. Others who have visual disturbances, circulatory problems, or other conditions may need daily visits and more actual nursing intervention, such as help with hygiene, arrangements for meals, and administration of insulin injections (Nursing Care Plan box).

Acute complications. One of the acute complications of DM is coma, which may be attributed to three different causes. The first type of coma can occur during DKA, which results from inadequate amounts of insulin or from inadequate insulin utilization. The second type, Hyperglycemic Hyperosmolar Nonketotic Coma (HHNC), involves no acidosis or ketonemia, but results from excess glucose presence, diuresis, and dehydration without adequate fluid replacement. The third type may occur during hypoglycemic reaction, which results from an excess amount of insulin, with an inadequate amount of glucose present. These three complications are compared and contrasted in Table 11-5. (See also Safety Considerations: Emergency Care for Hyperglycemic Reaction and Safety Considerations: Emergency Care for Hypoglycemic Reaction boxes.)

Another acute complication faced by the patient with diabetes is the development of infections of any kind. The presence of hyperglycemia and ketonemia hinders the phagocytic action of leukocytes. An infection can therefore become more severe and last longer, with poor wound healing taking place. The possibility of DKA increases in the presence of infection, and control of the disease is harder to achieve. Patients with diabetes are often hospitalized for treatment of infections that might be handled on an outpatient basis for the nondiabetic patient.

Long-term complications. Long-term complications of diabetes include blindness, cardiovascular problems, and renal failure. Diabetes causes more cases of blindness in the United States than any other disease. Diabetic retinopathy involves progressive changes in the microcirculation of the retina, resulting in hemorrhages, scar tissue formation, and various degrees of retinal detachment. Surgical techniques such as laser beam coagulation of retinal vessels may improve vision for selected patients with early diagnosis. Vascular changes in patients with diabetes, especially capillary changes, contribute to the development of renal sclerosis, often progressing to end-stage renal disease (ESRD). Many of these patients have to undergo either peritoneal dialysis or hemodialysis as a result. Diabetes contributes to accelerated atherosclerotic changes in the blood vessels, resulting in myocardial infarction, stroke, and the development of gangrene in the lower extremities. Many people with diabetes have to undergo amputation as a result of this. Additionally, nervous system manifestations (diabetic neuropathy) are commonly seen, which cause pain and decreased sensation in the extremities and contribute to the development of diabetic gangrene. The patient has pain and paresthesias. The pain—described as burning, cramping, itching, or crushing—is usually worse at night and may occur only at that time. It may be relieved by walking. Complete or partial loss of sensitivity to touch and temperature is common. Foot injury and ulcerations may occur without the patient ever having pain. At times the skin becomes so sensitive (hyperesthesia) that even light pressure from bed sheets cannot be tolerated. Many men with diabetes experience problems with impotence or premature ejaculation. Reports of prevalence of impotence among men with diabetes vary from 30% to 60%. Impotence associated with DM is believed to result from damage to the sacral parasympathetic nerves. Patients of either gender may have orthostatic hypotension and bladder or bowel dysfunction.

Neuropathy affecting the autonomic nervous system may also result in gastropathy, a delayed gastric emptying that can produce anorexia, nausea, vomiting, early satiety, and a persistent feeling of fullness. These problems had been referred to as gastroparesis, but now the term *gastroparesis* is reserved for the condition in which the stomach is severely affected and is very slow to empty solid foods. Metoclopramide (Reglan) stimulates gastric emptying and has been used in the treatment of gastroparesis.

Table 11-5 *Comparison of Hyperglycemic Reaction, Diabetic Ketoacidosis, Hypoglycemic Reaction, and Hyperglycemic Hyperosmolar Nonketotic Coma*

ASSESSMENT	HYPERGLYCEMIC REACTION, DIABETIC KETOACIDOSIS (DKA)	HYPOGLYCEMIC REACTION	HYPERGLYCEMIC HYPEROSMOLAR NONKETOTIC COMA (HHNC)
Type of diabetes	Type 1 (IDDM)	Type 1 (IDDM) or type 2 (NIDDM)	Type 2 (NIDDM)
Cause	Inadequate insulin present	Too much insulin or oral hypoglycemic agent present	Inadequate insulin or oral hypoglycemic agent present
Patient history	Omitted or insufficient dose of insulin, physical or emotional stress, GI upsets, dietary noncompliance	Reduced food intake, delayed meal, too much exercise	Reduced fluid/food intake with increased urine output, resulting in severe dehydration
Onset of symptoms	Hours to days	Minutes to hours	Days
Previous diagnosis of having diabetes	Almost always	Yes; on medication	Usually type 2, on hypoglycemic agent
Age of patient	Usually younger patient	Usually younger patient	Usually elderly patient
Appearance of skin	Hot, dry, flushed	Cool, moist	Hot, dry; body temperature elevated
Breath	Fruity (from ketones)	Normal	Normal
Mucous membranes	Dry	Moist	Very dry
Respirations	Deep; may have Kussmaul respirations (air hunger) as a result of metabolic acidosis	Rapid, shallow	Normal
Neurosensory	Drowsiness to coma	Irritability, tremors, Impaired consciousness, personality changes; may lose consciousness	Lethargy, decreased consciousness; may lose consciousness
Blood pressure	Low	Normal	Decreased
Glycosuria and ketonuria	Present	Absent	Glycosuria present; no ketonuria
Polyuria and polydipsia	Present	Absent	Present
Hunger	Absent; may have nausea and vomiting	Present; may be nauseated	Absent
Blood glucose level	Usually 300-800 mg/dL	Usually less than 50 mg/dL	600-2000 mg/dL; serum osmolality very increased
Emergency treatment	Insulin, usually regular	Glucose (oral or IV) or glucagon (subQ, IM, or IV)	Large amounts of intravenous fluids; regular insulin

Nursing diagnoses and interventions for the patient with DM include but are not limited to the following:

NURSING DIAGNOSES	NURSING INTERVENTIONS
Ineffective therapeutic regimen management, related to health beliefs	Instruct in proper self-injection of insulin; have patient perform return demonstration. Reinforce instructions regarding availability of glucose and glycogen sources. Remove potentially hazardous objects from environment.
Noncompliance (diabetic management, high risk for), related to patient's value system	Establish therapeutic relationship so patient can express negative feelings. Correct misconceptions about treatment regimen. Assist patient in setting long-term goals for lifetime optimal disease management. Involve significant others whenever possible, and encourage communication between them and the patient. Refer patient to appropriate agencies and services (local support groups, ADA).

Safety Considerations

Emergency Care for Hypoglycemic Reaction
IMMEDIATE TREATMENT: IF CONSCIOUS

Give patient 10 to 20 g of quick-acting carbohydrate in some form, such as 4 to 6 oz orange juice or a regular soft drink (not a diet drink); half of any kind of candy bar; commercially prepared concentrated dextrose tablets or glucose paste; 1 tube Cake Mate icing gel (small); 2 tsp sugar or honey; 6 jelly beans or gumdrops; 5 or 6 Lifesavers or other roll candy; 4 animal crackers; 1 granola bar. Proceed with offering another 5 to 20 g of quick acting carbohydrate in 15 minutes if no relief is obtained.

Administration of additional food of longer-acting carbohydrate (e.g., slice of bread, crackers) after symptoms subside.

IMMEDIATE TREATMENT: IF UNCONSCIOUS

Squeeze one tube of glucagon gel between teeth and gums, in buccal space, or give glucagon 0.5 to 1 mg subcutaneously or intramuscularly; get patient to hospital. Hospitalized patients may receive IV bolus of 20 mL of 50% glucose or 50 mL of 20% glucose; glucagon may be given intravenously. May need IV 10% or 20% glucose at 100 mL/hr to follow.

NURSING INTERVENTIONS DURING AND AFTER HYPOGLYCEMIC EPISODE

- Stay with the patient; check vital signs and do fingerstick blood glucose levels.
- Monitor for worsening of condition, or relief of symptoms.
- If patient becomes unconscious, administer glucagon buccally, subcutaneously, intramuscularly, or intravenously.
- Be sure patient ingests food such as milk, crackers with peanut butter (6), or 1 slice cheese and 6 crackers after symptoms terminate.
- Observe closely for 1 to 2 hours after cessation of symptoms.
- Notify physician about the hypoglycemic reaction.
- Assess reason the reaction may have occurred.

Safety Considerations

Emergency Care for Hyperglycemic Reaction (Diabetic Ketoacidosis)
USUAL TREATMENT DURING ACUTE STAGE

- An IV is started, using an 18-gauge needle, and fluid replacement is begun, usually with 0.9% NaCl (normal saline), 1L/hr until BP stabilized and urine output 30 to 60 mL/hr. When blood glucose levels approach 250 mg/dL, 5% dextrose is added to the fluid regimen to prevent hypoglycemia.
- Regular insulin (the only kind that can be given IV) as a piggyback infusion, using 100 units regular insulin in 500 mL normal saline. The infusion is administered with a pump controller. The infusion rate is adjusted to obtain and maintain desired blood glucose levels.
- Hourly determination of blood glucose level (Accu-check method or venous sample)
- IV replacement of potassium to help move insulin into cells; monitor serum potassium
- Oxygen administration via nasal cannula or nonrebreather mask
- Cardiac monitoring; central venous pressure (CVP) and Swan-Ganz monitoring if available
- Foley catheter usually inserted with intake and output monitored hourly
- Vital signs and neurological status assessed frequently

NURSING INTERVENTIONS DURING AND AFTER DKA

- Keep airway patent.
- Maintain patent intravenous infusion at prescribed rate.
- Keep accurate intake and output record.
- Do accurate blood testing for glucose and urine testing for acetone.
- Monitor vital signs frequently, and assess cardiac status on monitor.
- Assess breath sounds for fluid overload.
- Assess level of consciousness frequently, and perform neurological checks as ordered.
- Assess the cause of DKA.

There are many important areas of education for the person with diabetes, including the importance of proper administration of insulin or oral hypoglycemics, as well as their side effects (Therapeutic Dialogue box); the signs and symptoms of hyperglycemia and hypoglycemia; methods of testing blood glucose levels and of urine testing for acetone; planning and preparing the prescribed diet; and personal hygiene, emphasizing skin and foot care. The nurse should stress the interrelationships of diet, medication, and exercise. The patient should be instructed to visit the dentist regularly and have an annual examination by an ophthalmologist. Because infections and illnesses of any kind could result in loss of diabetic control, the patient should be instructed to notify the physician at the first sign of any illness. Special plans for travel include providing extra insulin vials and syringes, carrying food and some form of concentrated carbohydrate, and arranging for SMBG or urine testing. Provisions for adequate rest time must be made,

Therapeutic Dialogue

Mr. G. is a 67-year-old Hispanic-American who was diagnosed 18 months ago with NIDDM. He has done well on a regimen of diet, exercise, and oral hypoglycemic medication (DiaBeta, 2.5 mg daily). Three days ago he dropped a brick on his right foot while remodeling his fireplace and was treated in the emergency department. He is being seen today for a follow-up visit with his internist. The office nurse, Mrs. B., will first talk with him and assess his condition.

NURSE: *Good morning, Mr. G. How are you doing this morning?*

PATIENT: *Much better, thank you. My foot still gives me a little trouble when I walk very far, but the swelling is down. I've been watching for red streaks, like they told me to in the emergency department, but so far there is only this scraped place and a bruise on the top of my foot (shows nurse the area).*

NURSE: *That's good. What kind of treatment are you using for your injured foot?*

PATIENT: *I'm washing my foot twice a day with soap and water, putting Neosporin ointment on the scrape, and then putting on a bandage.*

NURSE: *That sounds as if that should be adequate. Now let me get a close look at both feet (thoroughly examines the injured area, as well as the rest of the right foot, then examines the left foot.) The skin on your feet looks a little dry, Mr. G., and your toenails are getting quite thick and long. Do you have any problems cutting them?*

PATIENT: *I sure do! It's pretty hard for me to see exactly where I need to clip them sometimes, and I'm afraid I'll cut my toe, so I usually just let them go until my wife can help me. She's scared of cutting me, so she usually doesn't get them short enough.*

NURSE: *I understand. Proper foot care is very important for any patient with diabetes to prevent complications such as infection or tissue injury that could become very serious. Dr. M. usually refers his patients to a podiatrist when they are having problems such as yours. A podiatrist specializes in care of the feet, and can properly trim your toenails as needed, as well as care for any corns or calluses that may develop.*

PATIENT: *That sounds like a really good idea. I sure don't want to wind up like my cousin and some other people I've seen, having to have a toe or my whole foot amputated! Can you give me the name of a good podiatrist?*

NURSE: *Yes, I can (hands pamphlet to Mr. G.). This pamphlet stresses the importance of foot care, and on the back page has the names of four podiatrists Dr. M. recommends. You can choose the one you prefer. Now, I'm going to get Dr. M. so that he can examine you.*

PATIENT: *Thanks, Mrs. B. It's really good not to have to worry about cutting those toenails anymore!*

because exhaustion may lead to changes in the overall condition.

Before discharge from the hospital, the patient should verbalize an understanding of how complications may be prevented and display an interest in maintaining optimal wellness (Cultural and Ethnic Considerations box). The nurse should stress the importance of regular medical checkups. The social aspects of DM cannot be ignored. Patients need to learn about lifestyle adjustment and should wear medic-alert jewelry and carry medical information wallet cards at all times. Decisions such as whether to attempt pregnancy should be thoroughly explored by women with diabetes. Above all, the patient must accept the responsibility for self-care and recognize that making the right choices can affect life expectancy as well as the quality of life. A current trend is for hospitals to employ a diabetes nurse specialist to develop and implement patient and staff education (Home Health Considerations box).

Cultural and Ethnic Considerations

Chronic Conditions

- When dealing with a patient with a chronic condition, identification of the patient's cultural background and value-belief patterns can assist the health care team to identify appropriate regimens. This is particularly important in a condition such as DM, which may require major lifestyle changes for successful management.
- In assessing patients, it is important for the nurse to consider communicating across cultures. For example, Asian and Mexican cultures consider asking a direct question and expecting a direct answer to be ill mannered and rude. If the nurse is aware of this cultural difference, phrasing questions in a more indirect way will foster more effective communication.

Home Health Considerations

Diabetes Mellitus

- Considering the day of short hospitalization or no hospitalization and the overwhelming amount of information to be learned, home care is a high priority for people with DM.
- Frequently, the ability to be mobile is hindered, and changes in vision may hamper the drawing up of insulin.
- Often there is a missing link as to why control cannot be obtained; often that missing link can be found during a home visit.
- Diabetes caregivers and home care agencies often team up to provide good care for the older adult.
- Home care personnel network with other community resources to help increase the older adult's quality of life or help deal with economic issues.
- Diabetic management should include education in:
  1. Motivation
  2. Self-monitoring of blood glucose
  3. Exercise
  4. Nutrition therapy
  5. Medications
  6. Written treatment plan

Prognosis

Although the life expectancy for the person with diabetes is usually decreased, current research and recent advances have led to the hope of a much better prognosis. Early diagnosis and prompt, accurate treatment are essential in promoting longevity. Quality of life has been enhanced by better ways to control hyperglycemia and by earlier recognition of developing complications.

NURSING PROCESS *for the Patient with an Endocrine Disorder*

The role of the licensed practical nurse/licensed vocational nurse (LPN/LVN) in the nursing process as stated is that the LPN/LVN will:

- Participate in planning care for patients based on patient needs
- Review patient plan of care and recommend revisions as needed
- Review and follow defined prioritzation for patient care
- Use clinical pathways/care maps/care plans to guide and review patient care

Assessment

Hormones affect every body tissue and system, causing great diversity in the signs and symptoms of endocrine dysfunction. Endocrine disorders may have nonspecific or specific clinical manifestations. Some specific signs of endocrine dysfunction are the classic "polys" (**polyuria, polydipsia,** and **polyphagia**) in diabetes mellitus and exophthalmus in hyperthyroidism. Specific signs make the assessment easier, whereas nonspecific signs and symptoms—such as tachycardia, fatigue, and depression—are more problematic.

Nursing Diagnosis

Nursing diagnoses are determined from careful examination of patient data. Nursing diagnoses for the patient with an endocrine disorder may include but are not limited to the following:

  Deficient knowledge
  Risk for situational low self-esteem
  Disturbed sensory perception
  Risk for deficient fluid volume
  Risk for infection
  Risk for injury
  Sexual dysfunction
  Disturbed body image
  Ineffective coping
  Impaired home maintenance
  Noncompliance
  Imbalanced nutrition: less than body requirements
  Imbalanced nutrition: more than body requirements
  Activity intolerance

Expected Outcomes/Planning

The plan for management of patients with endocrine disorders must center on education to enable the patients to understand their endocrine disorders and develop a healthy lifestyle, which will assist them in preventing complications of their disease.

The plan of care focuses on accomplishing individual goals and outcomes that relate to the identified nursing diagnoses. Examples of these include the following:

Goal #1: Patient will demonstrate safety in self-injections of insulin.
Evaluation: Patient independently administers insulin injection to self safely and accurately.
Goal #2: Patient will demonstrate SMBG.
Evaluation: Patient performs SMBG accurately.

Patient uses measurements obtained by SMBG to achieve fasting blood glucose below 126 mg/dL.

Implementation

A major responsibility of the nurse is to help patients gain self-management skills for their chronic endocrine disorder through teaching and counseling. Self-management skills are probably the major factor in how well the health problem is controlled and how well the quality of life is maintained. The implementation of self-management skills is made through education in the disease process, the management of medications, and the management of nutrition; the provision of exercise knowledge; SMBG; hygiene; the prevention of complications; and assistance with psychological adjustment.

Evaluation

During and after patient educational teaching on self-management skills, the nurse assists in evaluating the success of the teaching by noting patient progress based on stated goals and outcomes. For example, when the patient performs SMBG, the nurse should observe the patient's skill, correct him or her as necessary, and evaluate the patient's technique to ensure accuracy. When patients are unable to meet expected outcomes, the nurse must be ready to revise the care plan to promote outcome success.

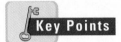
Key Points

- Endocrine glands are ductless glands that release chemicals (hormones) into the bloodstream to regulate body activities.
- The pituitary gland, located in the brain, is the master gland of the endocrine system.
- Hormones have a generalized effect on metabolism, growth and development, and reproduction.
- The endocrine glands regulate themselves by a series of negative feedback messages.
- The hormones secreted by the endocrine glands affect tissues of the entire body, and an imbalance in their levels may contribute to pathologic changes in many different systems.
- Acromegaly and gigantism, disorders of the pituitary gland, result in growth changes that may lead to negative effect on the patient's self-image and self-esteem.
- Diabetes insipidus is a disorder of the posterior pituitary and must not be confused with diabetes mellitus, a disorder of the pancreas.
- Clinically, SIADH is characterized by hyponatremia and water retention that progresses to water intoxication. When caring for the hyperthyroid patient, the nurse must provide for adequate rest periods and be sure that fluid and food intake meets the patient's nutritional needs.
- The emotions of the hyperthyroid patient are very labile, so the nurse must try to eliminate sources of stress from the environment, to help prevent emotional trauma.
- [131]I should not be administered to a pregnant patient because of the risk of danger to the fetus; pregnant nurses should not care for these patients.
- Three postoperative complications may be life threatening to the thyroidectomy patient: hemorrhage, tetany, and thyroid crisis.
- The hypothyroid patient may experience sluggish mental and physical functioning, so the nurse must be patient and allow adequate time for nursing routines.

- The prognosis for papillary adenocarcinoma of the thyroid is excellent, because few of these tumors metastasize.
- When administering intravenous calcium chloride to any patient, the nurse must be careful that none of the drug extravasates, because tissue sloughing may result.
- The extreme hypertension often seen in patients with pheochromocytoma may result in CVA.
- Depression is very common in the patient who suffers from Cushing syndrome; the nurse must be alert for suicidal thoughts and suicide attempts by this patient.
- The four main facets of medical treatment for the patient with diabetes mellitus are diet, blood glucose self-monitoring, exercise, and medication.
- IDDM is usually first diagnosed in people younger than 30 years of age; NIDDM is more commonly found after age 30, and the incidence increases with the aging process.
- As insulin resistance progresses, the pancreas secretes greater amounts of insulin to compensate. This in turn leads to progressive beta-cell failure and a lessening of insulin production. Both beta-cell dysfunction and insulin resistance are required for the development of hyperglycemia, the central metabolic characteristic of NIDDM.
- The older person with diabetes may have a very high blood glucose level before excreting any into the urine because of an increased renal threshold for glucose.
- The diabetic diet must be individualized, taking many factors into consideration, such as age, lifestyle, food preferences, and the ability to cook and store food.
- The person with IDDM must have access to a source of quick glucose at all times, in the event of a hypoglycemic reaction.
- The nurse must become familiar with the clinical manifestations of DKA/HHNC, and hypoglycemic reaction to properly assess diabetic patients, respond therapeutically, as well as educate them in self-care.
- Patients on insulin therapy and oral hypoglycemics must be observed carefully during the time of peak action of the medication, and treatment must be initiated promptly if hypoglycemia develops.
- The nurse must be knowledgeable about the various insulin types and characteristics.
- There are five classes of oral hypoglycemic drugs: sulfonylureas, meglitinides, biguanide, alpha-glucosidase inhibitors, and thiazolidinediones.
- DKA can result in seizures, brain damage, or death for the diabetic patient.

Go to your free CD-ROM for an Audio Glossary, animations, video clips, and Review Questions for the NCLEX-PN® Examination.

evolve Be sure to visit the companion Evolve site at http://evolve.elsevier.com/Christensen/adult/ for WebLinks and additional online resources.

CHAPTER CHALLENGE

1. The hormones responsible for "flight or fight" are:
   1. estrogen and testosterone.
   2. FSH and LH.
   3. epinephrine and norepinephrine.
   4. calcitonin and parathormone.

2. The hormones responsible for blood calcium levels are:
   1. calcitonin and parathormone.
   2. estrogen and progesterone.
   3. melatonin and follicle-stimulating hormone (FSH).
   4. thyroxine and parathormone.

3. The master gland of the body is the:
   1. thyroid gland.
   2. adrenal gland.
   3. pineal gland.
   4. pituitary gland.

4. What hormone is responsible for male secondary sex characteristics?
   1. Estrogen
   2. Progesterone
   3. Testosterone
   4. Adrenaline

5. Ms. P. is a 29-year-old secretary who received ^{131}I yesterday in an attempt to slow the progression of her hyperthyroid condition. For which of the following personnel would participating in her direct bedside care be dangerous?
   1. A 19-year-old first-semester nursing student
   2. A 34-year-old staff nurse who is new to the unit
   3. A 22-year-old aide who is 6 weeks pregnant
   4. A 49-year-old RN just returning from sick leave

6. Ms. C. is a 35-year-old patient who is the first night postoperative from having had a thyroidectomy. She experiences signs and symptoms of postoperative tetany. The nurse should implement the physician's order and immediately administer:
   1. sodium iodide po.
   2. potassium chloride IV.
   3. magnesium sulfate IM.
   4. calcium gluconate IV.

7. Ms. H. is a 47-year-old mother of three who had cranial surgery to remove a pituitary tumor 3 days ago, leaving her with partial left hemiparesis and diabetes insipidus. Which of the following nursing diagnoses is of the greatest priority postoperatively?
   1. Risk for deficient fluid volume, related to excessive loss via the urinary system
   2. Hopelessness, related to development of chronic illness (hemiparesis and diabetes insipidus)
   3. Risk for impaired oral mucous membrane, related to dehydration
   4. Coping, ineffective family: compromised, risk for, related to chronic illness

8. Mr. J. is a 34-year-old construction worker recently diagnosed as having acromegaly. Because of the pathophysiology of his condition, Mr. J.'s laboratory data will probably show elevated levels of:
   1. FSH
   2. LH
   3. TSH
   4. GH

9. While assessing Ms. C., a postoperative thyroidectomy patient, the nurse should check for damage to the laryngeal nerve. Which of the following is most likely to suggest that damage may have occurred?
   1. The patient complains of a slight sore throat
   2. The patient's voice tone has changed slightly
   3. The patient is unable to swallow fluids
   4. The patient is becoming increasingly hoarse

10. To help Mr. R., a newly diagnosed patient with IDDM, meet the goal of maintaining blood glucose control, which of the following is of greatest priority in the plan of care?
    1. Teach the patient the effect of diet, exercise, and insulin on the blood glucose level
    2. Refer the patient to the hospital dietitian for intense education about his dietary needs
    3. Instruct the patient on SMBG, observe return demonstrations, and correct his technique as needed
    4. Review with the patient the desired effects of his medication, as well as possible side effects

11. J.T. is a 22-year-old male who has had type 1 diabetes for the past year. Which of the following statements demonstrates his need for more teaching?
    1. "If I want to lose weight, all I have to do is increase my dose of insulin."
    2. "I can have an occasional beer if it's calculated into my diet."
    3. "I will maintain better control of my blood sugar if I eat regular meals."
    4. "It is important that I eat properly, exercise regularly, and take my insulin injections."

12. To meet the goal of prevention of injury to Mr. C., an IDDM patient, which of the following nursing interventions is most important to include in the care plan?
    1. Assess peripheral pulses and capillary refill in the lower extremities
    2. Instruct the patient in the proper technique for self-injection of insulin
    3. Stress the importance of keeping the skin on the feet soft and supple
    4. Remove potentially hazardous objects from the patient's environment

CHAPTER CHALLENGE—cont'd

13. Mr. A., age 45, has been admitted to your hospital unit with the primary medical diagnosis of Addison's disease (adrenal hypofunction). Assessment reveals the presence of postural hypotension, fatigue, nausea, vomiting, and poor skin turgor. Which of these nursing diagnoses is of greatest priority at this time?
    1. Risk for infection
    2. Risk for imbalanced body temperature
    3. Risk for injury
    4. Risk for deficient fluid volume

14. A human insulin formula that begins to take effect in less than half the time of regular, fast-acting insulin and more closely mimics the body's own hormone action is:
    1. Humulin R, Novolin R
    2. lispro (Humalog), aspart (Novolog)
    3. Humulin N, Novolin N
    4. Humulin 70/30, Novolin 70/30

15. The polydipsia and polyuria related to diabetes are caused primarily by:
    1. the release of ketones from cells during fat metabolism.
    2. fluid shifts resulting from the osmotic effect of hyperglycemia.
    3. damage to the kidneys from exposure to high levels of glucose.
    4. changes in RBCs resulting from attachment of excessive glucose to hemoglobin.

16. In planning care for a patient with type 2 diabetes admitted to the hospital with pneumonia, the nurse recognizes that the patient:
    1. must receive insulin therapy to prevent the development of ketoacidosis.
    2. has islet cell antibodies that have destroyed the ability of the pancreas to produce insulin.
    3. has minimal or absent endogenous insulin secretion and requires daily insulin injections.
    4. may have sufficient endogenous insulin to prevent ketosis but is at risk for development of hyperosmolar coma.

17. A diabetic patient takes a combination of regular and NPH insulin twice a day for glucose control. The nurse teaches the patient to be alert for hypoglycemia:
    1. immediately after breakfast and dinner.
    2. immediately after lunch and dinner.
    3. in the late afternoon and at bedtime.
    4. immediately after dinner and at bedtime.

18. The nurse assists the patient with dietary management of diabetes with the knowledge that a diabetic diet is designed:
    1. to be used only for type 1 diabetes.
    2. for use during periods of high stress.
    3. to normalize blood glucose by elimination of sugar.
    4. to help normalize blood glucose through a balanced diet.

19. In teaching a newly diagnosed type 1 diabetic "survival skills," the nurse includes information about:
    1. weight-loss measures.
    2. elimination of sugar from the diet.
    3. need to reduce physical activity.
    4. capillary blood glucose monitoring.

20. An appropriate instruction for the patient with diabetes related to care of the feet is:
    1. use heat to increase blood supply.
    2. avoid softening lotions and creams.
    3. inspect all surfaces of the feet daily.
    4. use iodine to disinfect cuts and abrasions.

21. The oral hypoglycemic that works primarily by reducing hepatic glucose production and lowers fasting blood glucose levels is:
    1. repaglinide (Prandin).
    2. acarbose (Precose).
    3. metformin (Glucophage).
    4. rosiglitazone (Avandia).

22. Fill in the blanks.
    The types of insulin used in an insulin pump are _____ or _____ insulin.

23. Circle all correct statements.
    1. Regular insulin (Humulin R) has an onset of action of 30 minutes to 1 hour.
    2. Lispro (Humalog) has an onset of action of 15 minutes.
    3. NPH (Humulin N) has an onset of action of 2 hours.
    4. Glargine (Lantus) has an onset of action of 6 to 10 hours.

CHAPTER 12

Care of the Patient with a Reproductive Disorder

BARBARA LAURITSEN CHRISTENSEN

Objectives

After reading this chapter, the student should be able to do the following:

Anatomy and Physiology

1. List and describe the functions of the organs of the male and female reproductive tracts.
2. Discuss menstruation and the hormones necessary for a complete menstrual cycle.

Medical-Surgical

3. Define the key terms as listed.
4. Discuss the impact of illness on the patient's sexuality.
5. List nursing interventions for patients with menstrual disturbances.
6. Discuss nursing interventions for the patient undergoing diagnostic studies related to the reproductive system.
7. Discuss the importance of the Papanicolaou smear test in early detection of cervical cancer and mammography as a screening procedure for breast cancer.
8. Discuss the etiology/pathophysiology, clinical manifestations, assessment, diagnostic tests, medical management, nursing interventions, and patient teaching for infections of the female reproductive tract.
9. Discuss four important points to be addressed in discharge planning for the patient with pelvic inflammatory disease (PID).
10. List four nursing diagnoses pertinent to the patient with endometriosis.
11. Identify the clinical manifestations of a vaginal fistula.
12. Describe the preoperative and postoperative nursing interventions for the patient requiring major surgery of the female reproductive system.
13. Describe the common problems with cystocele, rectocele, and the related medical management and nursing interventions.
14. Discuss the etiology/pathophysiology, clinical manifestations, assessment, diagnostic tests, medical management, nursing interventions, and patient teaching for cancers of the female reproductive system.
15. Identify four nursing diagnoses pertinent to ovarian cancer.
16. Describe six important points to emphasize in the teaching of breast self-examination.
17. Compare four surgical approaches for cancer of the breast.
18. Discuss adjuvant therapies for breast cancer.
19. Discuss nursing interventions for the patient who has had a modified radical mastectomy.
20. List several discharge planning instructions for the patient who has undergone a modified radical mastectomy.
21. Discuss the etiology/pathophysiology, clinical manifestations, assessment, diagnostic tests, medical management, nursing interventions, and patient teaching for inflammatory disorders of the male reproductive system.
22. Distinguish between hydrocele and varicocele.
23. Discuss the importance of monthly testicular self-examination beginning at 15 years of age.
24. Discuss patient education related to prevention of sexually transmitted diseases.

Key Terms

Be sure to check out the bonus material on the free CD-ROM, including selected audio pronunciations.

amenorrhea (ă-měn-ō-RĒ-ă, p. 579)
candidiasis (kăn-dĭ-DĪ-ă-sĭs, p. 624)
carcinoma in situ (kăr-sĭ-NŌ-mă ĭn SĪ-tū, p. 598)
chancre (SHANG-kĕr, p. 621)
Chlamydia trachomatis (klă-MĬD-ē-ă tră-KŌ-mă-tĭs, p. 624)
circumcision (sĭr-kŭm-SĬZH-ŭn, p. 617)
climacteric (klī-MĂK-tĕr-ĭk, p. 584)
colporrhaphy (kŏl-PŌR-ă-fē, p. 595)
colposcopy (kŏl-PŎS-kŏ-pē, p. 575)
cryptorchidism (krĭp-TŎR-kĭ-dĭz-ĕm, p. 618)
culdoscopy (kŭl-DŎS-kŏ-pē, p. 575)
curettage (KŪ-rĕ-tăhzh, p. 576)
dysmenorrhea (dĭs-měn-ō-RĒ-ă, p. 579)
endometriosis (ĕn-dō-mē-trē-Ō-sĭs, p. 593)
epididymitis (ĕp-ĭ-dĭd-ē-MĪ-tĭs, p. 617)
fistula (FĬS-tū-lă, p. 594)
introitus (ĭn-TRŌ-ĭ-tŭs, p. 595)
laparoscopy (lă-pă-RŎS-kŏ-pē, p. 575)
mammography (măm-MŎG-ră-fē, p. 577)
menorrhagia (měn-ō-RĀ-jă, p. 579)
metrorrhagia (mě-trō-RĀ-jă, p. 579)
panhysterosalpingo-oophorectomy (păn-HĬS-tĕr-ō-SĂL-ping-gō-oof-ō-RĔK-tō-mē, p. 601)
Papanicolaou (PAP) test (smear) (pă-pě-NĬ-kō-lōōz tĕst, směr, p. 575)
phimosis (fĭ-MŌ-sĭs, p. 617)
procidentia (prō-sĭ-DĔN-shă, p. 595)
sentinel lymph node mapping (SĔN-tĭ-nĕl lĭmf nōd MĂP-ing, p. 606)
trichomoniasis (trĭk-ō-mō-NĪ-ă-sĭs, p. 623)

Conception and birth are made possible through the dynamics of the normally functioning male and female reproductive systems. Reproduction of like individuals is necessary for the continuation of the species. The male and female sex glands (gonads) produce the gametes (sperm, ova) that unite to form a fertilized egg (zygote), the beginning of a new life.

OVERVIEW OF ANATOMY AND PHYSIOLOGY

MALE REPRODUCTIVE SYSTEM

The organs of the male reproductive system include the testes, the ductal system, the accessory glands, and the penis (Figure 12-1). These structures have various functions: (1) producing and storing sperm, (2) depositing sperm for fertilization, and (3) developing the male secondary sex characteristics.

Testes (Testicles)

The two oval **testes** (gonads) are enclosed in the **scrotum,** a saclike structure that lies suspended from the exterior abdominal wall. This position keeps the temperature in the testes below normal body temperature, which is necessary for viable sperm production and storage. Each testis contains one to three coiled seminiferous tubules that produce the sperm cells. After puberty, millions of sperm cells are produced daily.

The testes also produce the hormone testosterone. Testosterone is responsible for the development of male secondary sex characteristics.

Ductal System

Epididymis. Sperm (Figure 12-2) produced in the seminiferous tubules immediately travel through a network of ducts called the **rete testis.** These passageways contain cilia that sweep sperm out of the testes into the **epididymis,** a tightly coiled tube structure that lies superior to the testes and extends posteriorly. With sexual stimulation the walls of the epididymis contract, forcing the sperm along the seminiferous tubules of the testes to the vas deferens.

Ductus deferens (vas deferens). The **ductus deferens** is approximately 18 inches (46 cm) long and rises along the posterior wall of the testes. As it moves upward it passes through the inguinal canal into the pelvic cavity and loops over the urinary bladder. The ductus deferens, nerves, and blood vessels are enclosed in a connective tissue sheath called the **spermatic cord.** If a man elects to be sterilized for birth control management, it is a simple procedure to make small slits on either side of the scrotum and sever the ductus deferens. This procedure is called a **vasectomy.** It renders the man sterile because sperm can no longer be expelled.

Ejaculatory duct and urethra. Behind the urinary bladder, the ejaculatory duct connects with the ductus

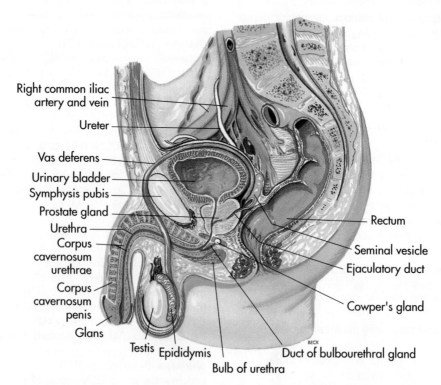

Right common iliac artery and vein

Ureter

Vas deferens

Urinary bladder

Symphysis pubis

Prostate gland

Urethra

Corpus cavernosum urethrae

Corpus cavernosum penis

Glans

Testis Epididymis

Bulb of urethra

Rectum

Seminal vesicle

Ejaculatory duct

Cowper's gland

Duct of bulbourethral gland

FIGURE **12-1** Longitudinal section of the male pelvis showing the location of the male reproductive organs.

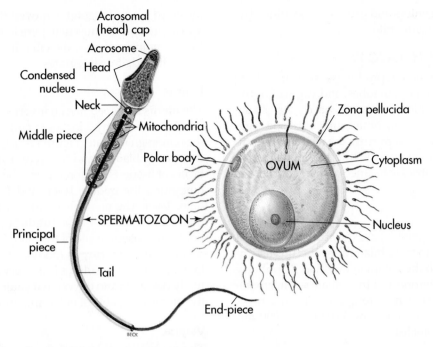

FIGURE **12-2** Male sex cell (spermatozoon) greatly enlarged *(left).* Female sex cell (ovum) surrounded by sperm at time of fertilization *(right).*

deferens. The ejaculatory duct is only 1 inch (2.5 cm) long. It unites with the urethra to pass through the prostate gland. The urethra extends the length of the penis with the urinary meatus. The urethra carries both sperm and urine, but, because of the urethral sphincter, it does not do so at the same time.

Accessory Glands

The ductal system transports and stores sperm. The accessory glands, which produce seminal fluid (semen), include the seminal vesicles, prostate gland, and Cowper's glands. With each ejaculation (2 to 5 mL of fluid), approximately 200 to 500 million sperm are released.

Seminal vesicles. The **seminal vesicles** are paired structures that lie at the base of the bladder and produce 60% of the volume of semen. The fluid is released into the ejaculatory ducts to meet with the sperm.

Prostate gland. The single, doughnut-shaped **prostate gland** surrounds the neck of the bladder and urethra. It is a firm structure, about the size of a chestnut, composed of muscular and glandular tissue. The ejaculatory duct passes obliquely through the posterior part of the gland. The prostate gland often hypertrophies with age, expanding to surround the urethra and making voiding difficult.

Cowper's glands. **Cowper's glands** are two pea-sized glands under the male urethra. They correspond to the Bartholin's glands in women and provide lubrication during sexual intercourse.

Urethra and Penis

The male **urethra** serves the twofold purpose of conveying urine from the bladder and carrying sperm to the outside. The cylindrical **penis** is the organ of copulation. The shaft of the penis ends with an enlarged tip called the **glans penis.** The skin covering the penis, called the **prepuce,** or foreskin, lies in folds around the glans. This excess tissue is sometimes removed in a surgical procedure called circumcision to prevent **phimosis** (tightness of the prepuce of the penis that prevents retraction of the foreskin over the glands).

Three masses of erectile tissue containing numerous sinuses fill the shaft of the penis. With sexual stimulation the sinuses fill with blood, causing the penis to become erect. After ejaculation, it returns to a flaccid state.

Sperm

At puberty, **spermatogenesis** (the process of development of spermatozoa) begins, continuing throughout life. Mature sperm consist of three distinct parts: (1) the head; (2) the midpiece; and (3) the tail, which propels the sperm. Once deposited in the female reproductive system, mature sperm live approximately 48 hours. If they come in contact with a mature egg, the enzyme on the head of each sperm bombards the egg in an attempt to break down its coating (see Figure 12-2). It takes thousands of sperm to break the coating, but only one sperm enters and causes fertilization. The remaining sperm disintegrate.

FEMALE REPRODUCTIVE SYSTEM

The organs of the female reproductive system include the ovaries, uterus, fallopian tubes, and vagina (Figure 12-3). These organs, along with a few accessory structures, produce the ovum, house the fertilized egg, maintain the embryo, and nurture the newborn infant. The ability to conceive and nurture this new human being requires the intricate balance of many hormones and the menstrual cycle.

Ovaries

The paired **ovaries** (gonads) are the size and shape of almonds. They are located bilateral to the uterus immediately inferior to the fallopian fimbriae. At puberty they release progesterone and the female sex hormone estrogen, and release a mature egg during the menstrual cycle. Each ovary contains 30,000 to 40,000 microscopic ovarian follicles.

Fallopian Tubes (Oviducts)

The **fallopian tubes** are a pair of ducts opening at one end into the **fundus** (upper portion of the uterus) and at the other end into the peritoneal cavity, over the ovary. They are approximately 4 inches (10 cm) long with the fimbriae at the distal ends. The entire inner surface of the tubes is lined with cilia. When the graafian follicle of the ovary ruptures and releases the mature ovum, the fimbriae sweep the ovum into the fallopian tube. Fertilization takes place in the outer third of this tube, and the

fertilized ovum **(zygote)** is moved through the tube by a combination of muscular peristaltic movements and the sweeping action of the cilia. If the mature ovum is not fertilized, it disintegrates.

Uterus

The **uterus** is shaped like an inverted pear and measures 3 inches (7.5 cm) by 2 inches (5 cm) by 1 inch (2.5 cm) in the nonpregnant state (Figure 12-4). It is situated between the urinary bladder and the rectum and consists of three layers of tissue: (1) endometrium, the inner layer; (2) myometrium, the middle layer; and (3) perimetrium, the outer layer. The uterus is divided into three major portions (see Figure 12-4). The **fundus** (upper, rounded portion) is the insertion site of the fallopian tubes. The larger midsection is the **corpus** (body). The smaller, narrower lower portion of the uterus is the **cervix,** part of which actually descends into the vaginal vault. During pregnancy the uterus is capable of enlarging up to 500 times.

Vagina

The **vagina** is a thin-walled, muscular, tubelike structure of the female genitalia, approximately 3 inches (7.5 cm) long. It is located between the urinary bladder and the rectum. The superior portion articulates the cervix of the uterus; the inferior portion opens to the outside of the body. The vagina is lined with mucous membrane, responsible for lubrication during sexual activity. The walls of the vagina normally lie in folds called **rugae.** This enables the vagina to stretch to receive the penis during intercourse and to allow passage of the infant during the birth process.

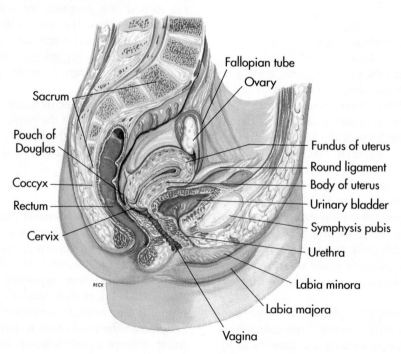

FIGURE **12-3** Longitudinal section of the female pelvis showing the location of the female reproductive organs.

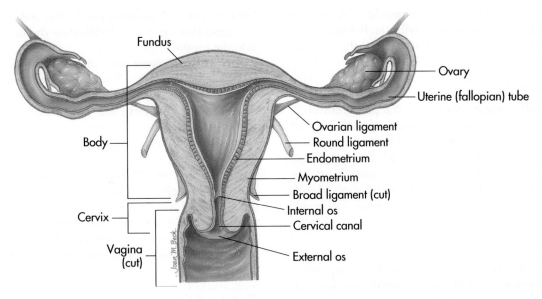

FIGURE **12-4** Sectioned view of the uterus showing relationship to the ovaries and vagina.

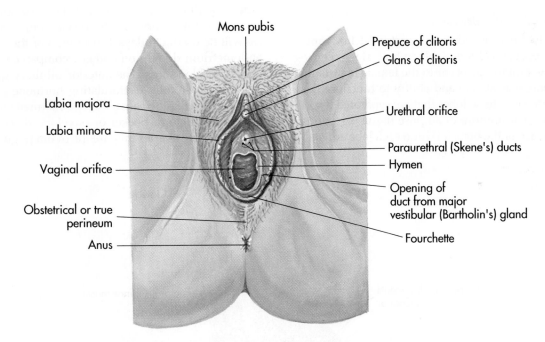

FIGURE **12-5** External female genitals (the vulva).

The external opening of the vagina is covered by a fold of mucous membrane, skin and fibrous tissue called the **hymen.** For centuries the hymen was a symbol of virginity, but it is now known that rigorous exercise or the insertion of a tampon may tear the hymen. If the hymen does remain intact, it will be ruptured by **coitus** (intercourse).

External Genitalia

The reproductive structures located outside the body are the external genitalia, or **vulva.** These structures include the mons pubis, labia majora, labia minora, clitoris, and vestibule (Figure 12-5).

Located superior to the symphysis pubis is a mound of fatty tissue, covered with coarse hair. This structure is the **mons pubis.** Extending from the mons pubis to the perineal floor are two large folds called the **labia majora** (large lips). These protect the inner structures and contain sensory nerve endings and an assortment of sebaceous (oil) and sudoriferous (sweat) glands. Directly under the labia majora lie the **labia minora** (small lips). These are smaller folds of tissue, devoid of hair, that merge anteriorly to form the prepuce of the clitoris. The **clitoris** is comparable to the male penis and is composed of erectile tissue that becomes engorged with blood during sexual stimulation.

The space enclosing the structures located beneath the labia minora is called the **vestibule.** It contains the **clitoris, urinary meatus, hymen,** and the **vaginal opening.**

Accessory Glands

Bilateral to the urinary meatus lie the **paraurethral,** or **Skene's, glands,** the largest glands opening into the urethra. These glands are responsible for the secretion of mucus and are similar to the male prostate gland. Bilateral to the vaginal opening are two small, mucus-secreting glands called the greater **Bartholin's glands (vestibular),** which lubricate the vagina for sexual intercourse.

Perineum

The area enclosing the region containing the reproductive structures is referred to as the **perineum.** The perineum is diamond shaped and starts at the symphysis pubis and extends to the anus.

Mammary Glands (Breasts)

The breasts are attached to the pectoral (chest) muscles. Breast tissue is identifiable in both sexes. During puberty, several things occur to the female breasts that change their size, shape, and ability to function. Each breast contains 15 to 20 lobes that are separated by adipose tissue. The amount of adipose tissue is responsible for the size of the breast. Within each lobe are many lobules that contain milk-producing cells; these lobules lead directly to the **lactiferous ducts** that empty into the nipple (Figure 12-6).

The nipple is composed of smooth muscle that allows it to become erect. The dark pink or brown tissue surrounding the nipple is called the **areola.** Milk production does not start until a woman gives birth. At this time, under the influence of prolactin, the milk is formed. The hormone oxytocin allows milk to be released.

Menarche, the first menstrual cycle, usually begins at approximately 12 years of age. Each month, for the next 30 to 40 years, an ovum matures and is released about 14 days before the next menstrual flow, which occurs on average every 28 days. If fertilization occurs, menstrual cycling subsides and the body adapts to the developing fetus.

Menstrual Cycle

Generally speaking the menstruation cycle can be divided into three phases: (1) menstrual, (2) preovulatory, and (3) postovulatory. For this discussion, a 28-day cycle will be used. On days 1 through 5 of the cycle, the endometrium sloughs off and is accompanied by 1 to 2 ounces of blood loss. The anterior pituitary gland begins to release follicle-stimulating hormone (FSH); as the level of FSH increases, the egg matures within the **graafian follicle** (a pocket or envelope-shaped structure where the ovaries prepare the ovum [Figure 12-7]).

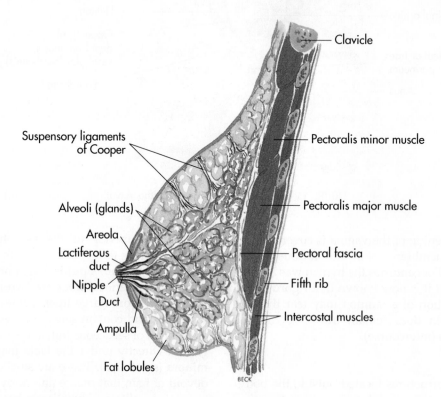

FIGURE **12-6** Lateral view of the breast (sagittal section). The gland is fixed to the overlying skin and pectoral muscles by the suspensory ligaments of Cooper. Each lobule of secretory tissue is drained by a lactiferous duct that opens through the nipple.

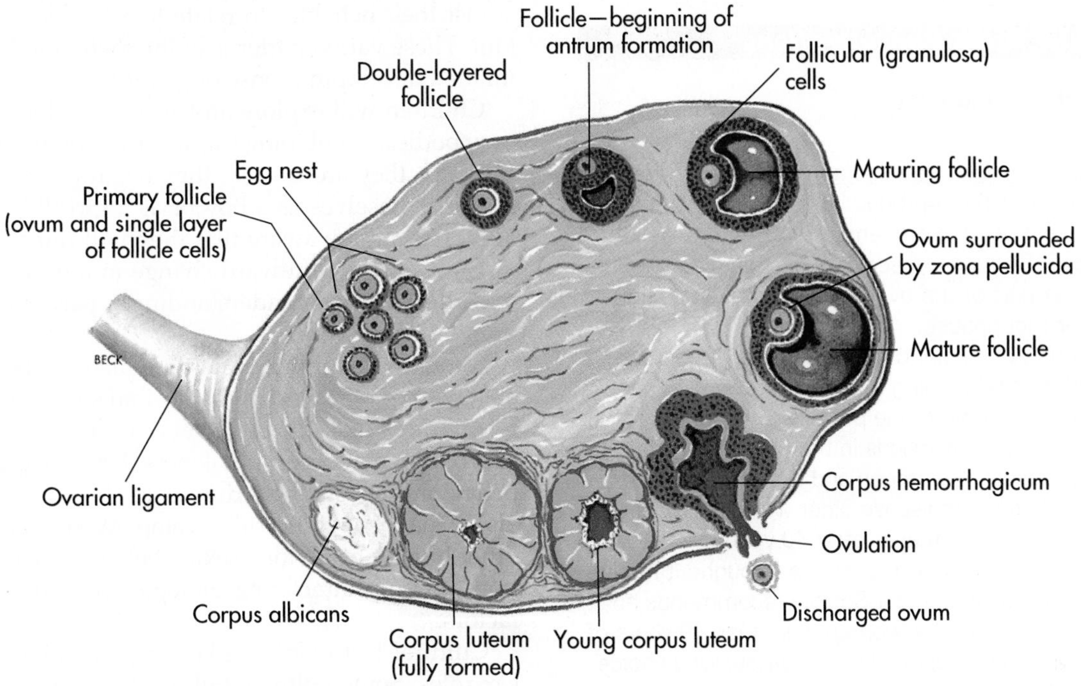

FIGURE **12-7** Mammalian ovary showing successive stages of ovarian (graafian) follicle and ovum development. Begin with the first stage (egg nest) and follow around clockwise to the final stage (corpus albicans).

From days 6 through 13 (preovulatory phase), estrogen is released from the maturing graafian follicle. This estrogen causes vascularization of the uterine lining. On day 14, the anterior pituitary gland releases luteinizing hormone (LH), which causes the rupture of the graafian follicle and release of the mature ovum. The fingerlike projections of the fallopian tubes, fimbriae, sweep the ovum into the fallopian tube. Once this mature ovum has been expelled, the follicle is transformed into a glandular mass called the **corpus luteum.** This structure secretes both estrogen and progesterone. During days 15 through 28 (postovulatory phase), the developing corpus luteum releases estrogen and progesterone, which maintains the vascularization of the uterus if pregnancy does occur. If this is the case, the corpus luteum continues to release estrogen and progesterone to maintain the uterine lining until the placenta is formed, which then takes over the job of hormonal release. If pregnancy does not occur, the corpus luteum lasts 8 days and then disintegrates. Normally the corpus luteum shrinks and is replaced by scar tissue called **corpus albicans.** At this point the hormone level decreases over several days and menstruation starts again.

EFFECTS OF NORMAL AGING ON THE REPRODUCTIVE SYSTEM

Menopause occurs in the normal woman between 35 and 60 years of age. The average age is 51. Whether it occurs earlier or later, menopause should not be considered abnormal. Cigarette smoking and living at high altitudes are associated with early menopause. During menopause the menstrual flow ceases and hormonal levels decrease. This is the period when a woman may experience "hot flashes" (sudden warm feelings), which are caused by the decrease in estrogen production. Changes also occur in the reproductive organs. The vagina loses some of its elasticity, and the breasts and vulva lose some adipose tissue, resulting in decreased tissue turgor. The bones may also become brittle and prone to osteoporosis.

In the man there is no menopausal period. Sperm production decreases but does not cease. In later years, testosterone production decreases, but not dramatically.

Basically, as long as the older individual is healthy, there is nothing in the aging process that prohibits normal sexual function (Older Adult Considerations box).

HUMAN SEXUALITY

Sexuality and sex are two different things. **Sexuality** is often described as the sense of being a woman or a man. It has biologic, psychological, social, and ethical segments.

Sexuality influences life experiences, and sexuality is influenced by life experiences. The term **sex** has a more limited meaning. It usually describes the biologic aspects of sexuality such as genital sexual activity. Sex may be used for pleasure or reproduction. As a result

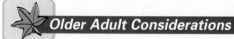

Reproductive Disorders

WOMEN

- Many older women are reluctant to seek medical care for problems of the reproductive system. This may be related to cultural factors, embarrassment, or lack of knowledge. Routine gynecologic examination should continue as part of the overall physical examination even after menopause.
- Certain forms of cancer of the reproductive tract are more common with aging. Any vaginal bleeding should be promptly reported to the physician, as should pelvic pain, pruritus, or skin lesions in the genital region.
- Decreased levels of estrogen and systemic diseases, such as diabetes, predispose older women to vaginitis.
- Breast cancer risk increases after 40 years of age. Breast examination should continue throughout the life span. The American Cancer Society recommends an annual mammogram for women older than 40 years of age. Each woman must make an individualized choice in consultation with her physician.

MEN

- Decreased production of testosterone results in changes in the male reproductive system, but the ability to procreate can continue until the eighth decade. Sexual interest often continues late into life.
- Chronic health problems, such as diabetes mellitus or hypertension, and many kinds of medication result in impotence in older men.
- Prostate enlargement is increasingly common with each decade after 40 years of age. Although this enlargement is most often benign, cancer of the prostate is a serious condition seen in older men. Ultrasonography of the prostate, when combined with rectal examination and prostate-specific antigen (PSA), is particularly useful in diagnosing prostatic cancer.

of life's changes or by personal choice, sexual activity may be absent from a person's life for brief or prolonged periods.

The process by which people come to know themselves as women or men is not clearly understood. Being born with female or male genitalia and subsequently learning female or male social roles seem to be factors, though these do not explain differences of sexuality and sexual behavior. Such variations are more understandable if the nurse remembers that sexuality is intertwined with all aspects of self.

SEXUAL IDENTITY

Biologic identity, or the differences between men and women, is established at conception and further influenced at puberty by the effects of hormones. Gender identity is the sense of being feminine or masculine. As soon as the infant is born (and sometimes before), the outside world labels the child as a girl or boy. Adults adjust their behavior to relate to a female or male infant. These varied patterns of interaction influence the infant's developing sense of gender identity.

Children will explore and seek to understand their own bodies. Combining this information with the way in which they are treated, they begin to create an image of themselves as a boy or as a girl. By 3 years of age, children are aware that they will remain boys or girls and that no outward change in their appearance will alter this. This understanding is part of the development of self-concept.

Gender role is the manner in which a person acts as a woman or man. Many believe that society influences female and male behavior and is thus the primary source of femaleness or maleness. Because gender role behavior is encouraged, differences between individuals' sexual behaviors will develop. Most likely, as with other human behaviors, sexual behavior is a combination of many interacting biologic and environmental factors.

Cultural factors can be key ingredients in defining sex roles. Some cultures tightly dictate roles as feminine or masculine (for example, the man is the breadwinner, and the woman is the caregiver). Other groups may be more flexible in role definition and encourage men or women to explore a variety of roles without labeling the behavior as feminine or masculine.

Sexual orientation is the clear and persistent erotic desire of a person for one sex or the other. There are heterosexual, homosexual, lesbian, and bisexual individuals, but the origins of sexual orientation are still not understood. Biologic theorists describe orientation in genetic terms, meaning it is determined at conception. Psychological theorists attribute orientation to early learning experiences, believing that cognitive processes are the determining factor. Still other theorists state that genetics and environment are the major influences in the development of sexual preference.

For some people the inward sense of sexual identity does not match the biologic body. These people are known as transsexuals. Researchers do not clearly understand how this mismatch occurs. Transsexuals do not see their sexual identity as a choice; it is a clear and persistent orientation dating back to early childhood. In contrast, most homosexual men and women define themselves as satisfied with their gender and social roles; they simply have a persistent desire for their same sex.

A transvestite is most often a heterosexual man who periodically dresses like a woman. This is usually done in private and kept secret even from those who are closest to him.

Because sexuality is linked to every aspect of living, any sexual choice involves personal, family, cultural, religious, and social standards of conduct. Ideas about ethical sexual conduct and emotions related to sexuality form the basis for sexual decision making. The range of attitudes about sexuality extends from a traditional view of sex only within marriage to a point of view that allows individuals to determine what is right. Sexual choices that overstep a person's ethical standard may result in internal conflicts.

Some people may judge sexual decisions as moral or immoral solely on religious standards; others view any private sexual act between consenting adults as moral. People will always differ in beliefs about sexual ethics. The debate over sexuality-related issues such as abortion, contraception, sex education, sexual variations, and premarital or extramarital intercourse will continue.

INFLUENCES ON SEXUAL HEALTH

Because overall wellness includes sexual health, sexuality should be a part of the health care program. Yet sexual assessment and interventions are not always included in health care services. The area of sexuality can be an emotional one for nurses and patients (Health Promotion Considerations box).

Nurses can best deal with personal attitudes by accepting their existence, exploring their sources, and finding ways to work with them. Professional behavior does not have to compromise the personal sexual ethics of nurses or patients. Professional behavior must guarantee that patients receive the best health care possible without diminishing their self-worth. Promotion of self-education and honest examination of sexual beliefs and values can help in reducing sexual bias.

Giving patients information about sexuality does not imply agreement with specific beliefs. Patients need accurate, honest information about the effects of illness on sexuality and the ways that it contributes to wellness. Nurses need to provide this information.

Although there is no single approach to taking a sexual history, application of certain principles contributes to both the patient's and the nurse's comfort (Box 12-1).

Health Promotion Considerations

Factors that Can Interfere with the Promotion of Sexual Health

- Lack of information
- Conflicting values system—attitudes and beliefs
- Anxiety (Are specific attitudes, feelings, and actions "normal"?)
- Guilt
- Lack of comfort with sexuality
- Invasion of privacy
- Lack of regard for hospitalized patient's need for time alone with significant other
- Manner in which the patient is touched
- Fear of being judged
- Lack of understanding of the effects of illness and treatment on sexual functioning

---

Box 12-1 *Requirements for Taking a Sexual History*

- Provision of privacy—a closed room
- An atmosphere of trust—ensure confidentiality
- Comfort on the part of nurses with their own sexuality

Box 12-2 *Brief Sexual History*

1. Has your (illness, pregnancy, hospitalization) interfered with your being a (husband, wife, significant other, father, mother)?
2. Has your (abortion, heart attack) changed the way you see yourself as a (woman, man)?
3. Has your (colostomy, mastectomy, hysterectomy) changed your ability to function sexually (or altered your sex life)?

Some principles to follow that contribute to a comfortable atmosphere for nurse and patient are:

- Obtain the sexual history early in the nurse-patient relationship, which indicates permission for patients to discuss sexual concerns.
- Avoid overreacting or underreacting to a patient's comments, which aids in truthful data collection.
- Use language that the patient understands; both the patient and the nurse may need to define their terms to ensure accurate data gathering.
- Move from the less sensitive to the more sensitive areas. This will promote nurse-patient comfort.
- Terminate the sexual history by inquiring if the patient has additional questions or concerns.

A brief history assessment may be made and included in the nursing history through the use of three questions (Box 12-2). The questions may be adapted to address illness, hospitalization, life events, or any other relevant matter that may influence or interfere with sexual health.

The questions may also be adjusted to draw out the patient's expectations of changes resulting from procedures, medications, or surgery. It is often unnecessary for the nurse to ask the last two questions because many patients voice their concerns about masculinity, femininity, and sexual functioning without further encouragement.

Nurses may intervene in sexual problems among patient populations through four strategies: (1) educating patient groups likely to have sexual concerns, (2) providing anticipatory guidance throughout the life cycle, (3) promoting a milieu conducive to sexual health, and (4) validating normalcy about sexual concerns.

Several self-help groups and other organizations publish easy-to-read pamphlets on sexuality (Health Promotion Considerations box). These pamphlets can

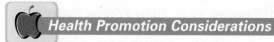

Self-Help Organizations that Publish Sexuality Pamphlets

- National Multiple Sclerosis Society: *Sexuality and MS*
- American Arthritis Foundation: *Living and Loving*
- American Cancer Society: *Sexuality for the Man with Cancer; Sexuality for the Woman with Cancer*
- American Diabetes Association: several pamphlets and articles for men and women with diabetes mellitus

---

often be purchased for a nominal fee and given to patients. Most pamphlets can be obtained directly from state or local chapters. Chapters of other self-help groups can be contacted about the availability of sexuality resources for patients. Some groups even publish newsletters that address sexuality.

Nurses can also write their own pamphlets for patients. Although this requires some effort, it may provide additional incentive for staff to address sexuality. Once developed, these pamphlets can be made available to others.

ILLNESS AND SEXUALITY

Illness may cause changes in a patient's self-concept and result in an inability to function sexually. Medications, stress, fatigue, and depression also affect sexual functioning. Alcohol abuse can lead to a reduced sex drive and inadequate sexual functioning.

Disinterest or lack of desire for sexual activity generally occurs with patients at a time when they are preoccupied with symptoms of illness. Most often these sexual symptoms disappear as patients recover from the acute phase of illness and sexual activity is resumed. However, some illnesses—such as diabetes mellitus, end-stage renal disease, spinal cord injuries, and heart disease—may cause patients concern or may result in actual inabilities with sexual function.

Changes in the nervous system, circulatory system, or genital organs may lead to sexual health problems. The patient with spinal cord injuries can experience an interruption of the peripheral nerves and spinal cord reflexes that involve sexual responses. But spinal cord–injured men and women also have reported orgasm in spite of complete denervation of all pelvic structures. They reported that the orgasm was satisfying and for many of them led to a comfortable resolution stage of sexual excitement.

Sexual dysfunction of a patient with diabetes mellitus can occur when the disease is not well controlled, but the dysfunction generally disappears when the lack of control is diagnosed and treated. Impotence is found in approximately half of the men who have diabetes mellitus and is generally related to poor control. Sexual counseling is important to (1) provide accurate information about the sexual aspects of the disorder, (2) dispel the patient's faulty assumptions and expectations, and (3) give advice designed to optimize the level of sexual self-esteem and dispel the guilt frequently found in both partners.

A mastectomy results in both physical and emotional trauma, and the resultant disfigurement is only one of multiple problems to be faced. A patient must also grapple with (1) how to cope with cancer, (2) how the operation will affect her relationship with her spouse or significant other, (3) how to relate to the strangeness of her own body, and (4) how her sexual life will be affected. Problems that arise with pelvic irradiation for cancer of the cervix are much harder to treat than those of mastectomy; the entire physiology of the vagina is altered by the radiation, causing a true loss of function. With a mastectomy the only function that is lost is the ability to nurse an infant. The goal for the patient and her partner is to face the issue in a straightforward manner, acknowledging the diagnosis and discussing their true feelings. If feelings are repressed—not verbalized or shared—both the patient and her significant other may suffer.

For the patient undergoing a mastectomy, sexual self-concept and intimate physical interactions can and will be affected. Two variables that influence a woman's sexual function are (1) sufficient self-love and acceptance, and (2) positive attitudes and feelings about sexuality. The male partner should be persuaded to face his own feelings so that he is able to offer support to his partner. Therapeutic counseling before surgery can aid the patient's and partner's acceptance and recovery after surgery.

LABORATORY AND DIAGNOSTIC EXAMINATIONS

DIAGNOSTIC TESTS FOR THE FEMALE

The pelvic examination is performed by a physician and is advantageous for visualization and palpation of the vulva, perineum, vagina, cervix, ovaries, and uterine surfaces. During the pelvic examination, specimens are frequently obtained for diagnostic purposes. The pelvic examination progresses from the visualization and palpation of the external genital organs for edema and irritations to an inspection for abnormalities of the internal organs. To visualize internal organs the physician inserts a vaginal speculum. The physician may perform a rectovaginal examination to evaluate abnormalities or problems of the rectal area and the posterior internal organs (Box 12-3).

Box 12-3 **Endoscopic Procedures for Visualization of Pelvic Organs**

Colposcopy   Visualization of vagina and cervix under low-power magnification
Culdoscopy   Insertion of a culdoscope through posterior vaginal vault into Douglas's cul-de-sac for visualization of fallopian tubes and ovaries
Laparoscopy   Insertion of a laparoscope (under general anesthesia) through small incision in abdominal wall (inferior margin of umbilicus); abdomen is then insufflated with carbon dioxide; permits visualization of all pelvic organs

Colposcopy

Colposcopy (*colpo*, a combining form meaning or pertaining to the vagina, *scopy*, a combining form meaning "observation") provides direct visualization of the cervix and vagina. The patient is prepared for a pelvic examination. The vaginal speculum is inserted, followed by the insertion of the colposcope for inspection of the area. The color of the tissue, presence of growths and lesions, and condition of the vascularity are observed and specimens are obtained as necessary.

Culdoscopy

Culdoscopy is a diagnostic procedure that provides visualization of the uterus and adnexa (uterine appendages, which are the ovaries and fallopian tubes). The patient is given a local, spinal, or general anesthetic. After the anesthetic is administered, the patient is assisted to a knee-chest position. The culdoscope is passed through the vaginal wall in back of the cervix. The area is examined for tumors, cysts, and endometriosis. During the procedure, **conization** (removal of eroded or infected tissue) may be done. This procedure is generally done on an outpatient basis.

Laparoscopy

Laparoscopy (the examination of the abdominal cavity with a laparoscope through a small incision made beneath the umbilicus) provides direct visualization of the uterus and adnexa. Preparation of the patient includes insertion of a Foley catheter to maintain bladder decompression for an open view. The procedure is done with a general anesthetic. The cervix is grasped by forceps and a lighted laparoscope is inserted through the incision. Carbon dioxide may be introduced to distend the abdomen for easier visualization. If a biopsy is to be done or organs are to be manipulated, a second incision may be made in the lower abdomen to allow for instrument insertion. The ovaries and fallopian tubes may be observed for masses, ectopic pregnancy, adhesions, and pelvic inflammatory disease (PID). Tubal ligations may be done using this procedure.

Papanicolaou (Pap) Test (Smear)

Papanicolaou (Pap) test (smear) (a simple smear method of examining stained exfoliative peeling and sloughed-off tissue or cells) is most widely known for its use in the early detection of cervical cancer. Scrapings of secretions and cells are taken from the cervix and spread on a glass slide. The slide is sprayed with a fixative and sent to the laboratory for analysis. It is important that slides be properly labeled. The label should give the date, time of the last menstrual period, and whether the woman is taking estrogens or birth control pills.

The American Cancer Society recommends that all women who are or have been sexually active or who are at least 18 years of age have an annual Pap test for 3 consecutive years and then every 2 to 3 years until middle age. More frequent testing may be recommended at the discretion of the physician for women with a history of multiple sexual partners or sexually transmitted diseases (STDs), a family history of cervical cancer, or those whose mothers used diethylstilbestrol (DES) during pregnancy.

Box 12-4 provides a classification of the cytologic findings. The results of Pap tests have been reclassified in recent years. Several classification systems were used in the past, including the Numerical System, the Dysplasia Cytologic Classification, and the Cervical Intraepithelial Neoplasia System (see Box 12-4 for interpretation and comparison of Pap test classifications and treatment recommendations). The Bethesda System is preferred because it provides better communication between the cytologist and the clinician. The Bethesda System evaluates the adequacy of the sample (e.g., satisfactory or not satisfactory for interpretation) and provides a general classification of normal or abnormal and a descriptive diagnosis of the Pap smear. Although the classification system may vary, all clinicians agree it is important to monitor Pap smears and ensure proper follow-up including treatment of vaginal infections and colposcopy if necessary.

Biopsy

Biopsies are procedures in which samples of tissue are taken for evaluation to confirm or locate a lesion. Tissue is aspirated by special needles or removed by forceps or through an incision.

A **breast biopsy** is performed to differentiate benign or malignant tumors. Breast biopsy is indicated for patients with palpable masses; suspicious areas appearing through mammography; and persistent, encrusted, purulent, inflamed, or sanguineous discharge from the nipples. The procedure is performed by needle biopsy, under local anesthetic, or by open biopsy, with general or local anesthetic. In a needle biopsy, fluid is aspirated from the breast and expelled into a specimen bottle. Pressure is placed on the site to stop

Box 12-4 | *Pap Test Interpretation Classifications and Action*

Interpretation	Numerical System	Dysplasia Cytologic Classification	Cervical Intraepithelial Neoplasia (CIN) Classification	Bethesda System*	Action
Negative (Normal)	Class I	Negative squamous metaplasia	No designation	Negative (Normal)	Repeat annually
Probably negative, may indicate infection	Class II	Atypical squamous cells	No designation	Infection Atypical squamous cells Reactive changes	Treat infection, repeat Pap
Suspicious, but not conclusive for malignancy	Class III	Mild dysplasia Moderate dysplasia	CIN I CIN II	Low-grade squamous intraepithelial lesion†	Treat infection, repeat Pap in 8-12 weeks; colposcopy
More suspicious, strongly suggestive of malignancy	Class IV	Severe dysplasia Carcinoma in situ	CIN III	High-grade squamous intraepithelial lesion*	Colposcopy, biopsy, treatment
Conclusive for malignancy	Class V	Invasive carcinoma	Invasive carcinoma	Invasive squamous cell carcinoma	Colposcopy, biopsy, treat with conization, hysterectomy

*The Bethesda system is the preferred system.
†The Bethesda Working Group suggests that "these two new terms encompass the spectrum of terms currently used to delineate the squamous cell precursors to invasive squamous carcinoma, including the grades of CIN, the degree of dysplasia, and carcinoma in situ."

bleeding. When bleeding has ceased, an adhesive bandage is applied. In an open biopsy an incision is made in a portion of the breast to expose the mass; tissue portions are incised, or the whole mass may be incised. Specimens of selected tissue may be frozen and stained for rapid diagnosis. The wound is sutured and a bandage is applied. The incision site should be observed for bleeding, tenderness, and erythema.

A **cervical biopsy** is done to evaluate cervical lesions and to diagnose cervical cancer. The biopsy is generally done without anesthesia. The colposcope is inserted through the vaginal speculum for direct visualization, the cervical site is selected and cleansed, and tissue is removed. The area is then packed with gauze or a tampon to check the blood flow.

An **endometrial biopsy** is performed to collect tissue for diagnosis of endometrial cancer and analysis for infertility studies. The procedure is generally performed at the time of menstruation when the cervix is dilated and cells are more easily obtained. The cervix is locally anesthetized, a curette is inserted, and tissue is obtained from selected sites of the endometrium.

Other Diagnostic Studies

Conization of the cervix is indicated when eroded or infected tissue is to be removed or when there is a need for confirmation of cervical cancer. A cone-shaped section is removed when the mass is confined to the epithelial tissue. After surgery the area is packed

with gauze to control bleeding. The patient is observed for bleeding and is generally discharged from the hospital the same day.

Dilation and curettage (D&C) (scraping of material from the wall of a cavity or other surface; performed to remove tumors or other abnormal tissue for microscopic study) is a procedure used to obtain tissue for biopsy, to correct cervical stricture, and to treat dysmenorrhea. The patient is placed under general anesthesia. While the patient is anesthetized, the cervix is dilated and the inside of the uterus scraped with a curette. A packing may be inserted for hemostasis, and a perineal pad is applied for absorption of drainage.

Cultures and **smears** are collected to examine and identify infectious processes, presence of abnormal cells, and hormonal changes of the reproductive tissue. Specimens collected for smears are prepared by spreading the collected smear on a glass slide and covering it with a second slide or spraying it with a fixative. Specimens should be handled with aseptic techniques, and caution should be observed to avoid the transfer and spread of organisms. Cultures are taken from exudates of the breast, vagina, rectum, and urethra. STDs and mastitis are diagnosed by isolation of the causative organisms.

Schiller's iodine test is used for the early detection of cancer cells and to guide the physician in doing a biopsy. An iodine preparation, applied to the cervix, produces a brown stain for normal vaginal cells.

Glycogen, which is present in normal cells, stains brown when the iodine solution is applied. Abnormal or immature cells do not absorb the stain. This method of detection is valuable but not entirely reliable, because normal cells sometimes lack glycogen, and malignant tissue sometimes contains glycogen. After the procedure the patient should wear a perineal pad to avoid stains on the clothing.

Radiographic examinations are performed to detect abnormal tissue, locate abnormal structures, and observe patency of ducts.

Hysterograms and **hysterosalpingograms** are studies for visualizing the uterine cavity to confirm (1) tubal abnormalities (adhesions and occlusions), (2) the presence of foreign bodies, (3) congenital malformations and leiomyomas (fibroids), and (4) traumatic injuries. The patient is placed in the lithotomy position. A speculum is inserted into the vagina, a cannula is inserted through the speculum into the cervical cavity, and a contrast medium is injected through the cannula. As the contrast medium progresses through the cavity, the uterus and fallopian tubes are viewed by a fluoroscope and films are taken.

Mammography is radiography of the soft tissue of the breast to allow identification of various benign and neoplastic processes, especially those not palpable on physical examination. It is believed that the average breast tumor is present for 9 years before it is palpable. Mammography is helpful as a screening procedure. The American Cancer Society recommends that baseline mammograms be performed on women between the ages of 35 and 39, and annually for women 40 years of age and older.

At the time the procedure is scheduled, the nurse advises the patient to refrain from using body powders, deodorants, and ointments on the breast areas, because this could cause false-positive results. Before the procedure the patient is provided with a patient gown and asked to remove jewelry and upper garments. The patient is asked to sit or stand in an upright position and rest one breast on the radiographic table. A compressor is placed on the breast, and the patient is asked to hold her breath as an anterior view is taken. The machine is rotated, the breast is again compressed, and a lateral view is taken. This procedure is repeated on the other breast. The patient may be asked to remain until the radiographic films are read.

In **pelvic ultrasonography**, high-frequency sound waves are passed into the area to be examined, and images are viewed on a screen; this is similar to a radiographic film. Ultrasound is useful in detecting foreign bodies (such as intrauterine contraceptive devices [IUDs]), distinguishing between cystic and solid tumor bodies, evaluating fetal growth and viability, detecting fetal abnormalities, and detecting ectopic pregnancy. Generally it is noninvasive, safe, and painless. The drinking of fluids beforehand is encouraged. The

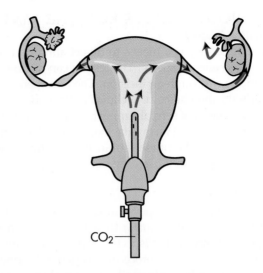

FIGURE **12-8** Rubin's test. Carbon dioxide escapes into abdominal cavity through patent left uterine tube.

nurse should explain that a full bladder is essential to the accuracy of the test.

Tubal insufflation (Rubin's test) involves transuterine insufflation of the fallopian tubes with carbon dioxide (Figure 12-8). The procedure enables evaluation of the patency of the fallopian tubes and may be part of a fertility study. Tubal insufflation takes approximately 30 minutes and is usually performed on an outpatient basis. If the tubes are open, the gas enters the abdominal cavity. A high-pitched bubbling can be heard through the abdominal wall with a stethoscope as the gas escapes from the tubes. The patient may complain of shoulder pain from diaphragmatic irritation. In this case a radiographic film will show free gas under the diaphragm. If the tubes are occluded, gas cannot pass from the tubes, and pain will not be reported.

All **pregnancy tests,** regardless of method, are based on detection of **human chorionic gonadotropin (HCG),** which is secreted in the urine after the fertilization of the ovum. Regardless of method, it is important to know that the tests do not indicate whether the pregnancy is normal. False-positive results may occur.

Serum CA-125 is a tumor antigen associated with ovarian cancer, since it is positive in 80% of women with epithelial ovarian cancer. CA-125 antigen levels in the blood will decrease as the cancer cells decrease. CA-125 has been touted as a way to detect primary ovarian cancer. Although a detection test for ovarian cancer is desirable, unfortunately, CA-125 does not fit this category. CA-125 is useful mainly to signal a recurrence of ovarian cancer and in following the response to treatment. Other conditions—such as endometriosis, PID, pregnancy, gynecologic cancers, and cancer of the pancreas—may result in an elevation of serum CA-125.

DIAGNOSTIC TESTS FOR THE MALE

Testicular Biopsy

Testicular biopsy is a means to detect abnormal cells and the presence of sperm. The testing can be done by aspiration or through an incision. The anesthetic used depends on the choice of technique. Postbiopsy care measures consist of scrotal support, ice pack, and analgesic medications. Warm sitz baths for edema may also be helpful. The nurse should instruct the patient to call the physician if bleeding occurs.

Semen Analysis

Semen analysis can be performed to substantiate the effectiveness of a vasectomy, to detect semen on the body or clothing of a suspected rape victim, and to rule out paternity. The procedure is generally one of the first tests to be performed on the male patient to evaluate fertility. Collection of semen for evaluation of fertility may be performed by manual stimulation, coitus interruptus, or the use of a condom.

Prostatic Smears

Prostatic smears are obtained to detect and identify microorganisms and tumor cells in the prostate. The physician massages the prostate by way of the rectum, and the patient voids into a sterile container prepared with additive preservative. The specimen is collected and a smear is prepared in the laboratory. It is possible to detect some cases of cancer and even tuberculosis of the prostate gland by this method.

Cystoscopy

In **cystoscopy** a man's prostate and bladder can be examined by passing a lighted cystoscope through the urethra to the bladder. It is usually performed without anesthesia, but a local anesthetic may be instilled into the bladder. Cytoscopy can be done for both men and women to detect bladder infections and tumors.

Other Diagnostic Studies

Other diagnostic studies for men include the rectal digital examination and the **prostate specific antigen** (PSA), a highly sensitive blood test. PSA, which is normally secreted and disposed of by the prostate, shows up in the bloodstream in cancer of the prostate and in a harmless condition called **benign prostatic hyperplasia** (BPH) or **prostate enlargement.** Elevated PSA levels in the bloodstream mean something needs to be checked. Even a slight increase in PSA level needs to be closely monitored. Still another study is the alkaline phosphatase (ALP) test. These specific tests are useful in diagnosing benign prostatic hypertrophy, prostatic cancer, bone metastasis in prostatic cancer, and other disease conditions (Box 12-5).

Box 12-5 | *Nursing Interventions for the Patient Undergoing Diagnostic Studies*

1. Explain the examination carefully.
2. Provide privacy.
3. Obtain a signed consent when necessary.
4. Prepare the skin for surgery according to agency protocol.
5. Assess the patient for allergies.
6. If appropriate, request that the patient partially or completely disrobe and remove all jewelry. Provide gown or drape.
7. Give preexamination instructions; instruct the patient to avoid food or drink, if appropriate.
8. Encourage verbalization and discussion of fears.
9. Administer preexamination medication as ordered by the physician.
10. If necessary, advise patients to go without medications for 24 hours. Obtain a medication history.
11. If the specimen is to be collected at home, stress the importance of handling all specimens precisely as directed.
12. It may be necessary to monitor vital signs.
13. Be attentive during examination. Offer support as necessary.
14. If appropriate, relay any immediate concerns to the physician.
15. Guide patients to follow any postexamination instructions.
16. Inform the patient that some discomfort can be expected. Minor discomfort can be relieved by mild analgesics such as aspirin or Tylenol, but if pain becomes more intense, the physician should be notified. Most discomfort is temporary.
17. When pertinent, tell the patient to rest and to avoid any heavy lifting for 24 hours after the examination as directed by the physician.
18. If relevant, advise the patient to avoid douching or intercourse until the site is healed. Consult the physician.
19. Caution the patient to report any bleeding from an incisional area.
20. Advise the patient to avoid the use of tampons as directed by the physician.
21. Inform the patient how test results may be obtained.

THE REPRODUCTIVE CYCLE

MENARCHE

Menarche, the beginning of menses, designates the first menstrual cycle. Menarche is a sign of puberty in a young woman and indicates that the body is capable of supporting pregnancy.

Menarche occurs from 9 to 17 years of age, the average age being 12½ years. The cycle length varies from 24 to 32 days, the average cycle lasting 28 days. The duration of the flow is from 1 to 8 days, the average being 3 to 5 days. The amount of flow is from 10 to 75 mL, the average being 35 mL per cycle.

The nurse should help patients promote reproductive and sexual health. Nurses may have the opportunity to instruct or counsel women about personal hygiene. Personal cleanliness is a health habit that should be promoted for all patients and implemented in each care plan. Cleanliness is especially meaningful during menstruation (Health Promotion Considerations box).

DISTURBANCES OF MENSTRUATION

Because of the relationship between the menstrual cycle and the body's mechanisms of hormonal secretion, a decrease or increase in the activity of the hormonal glands can disturb menstruation. The most common disturbances include the following:

Amenorrhea: absence of menstrual flow
Dysmenorrhea: painful menstruation
Abnormal uterine bleeding
Menorrhagia: excessive bleeding in amount and duration
Metrorrhagia: bleeding between menstrual periods
Another disturbance of the menstrual cycle is premenstrual syndrome (PMS), which will be discussed later.

Suggested nursing diagnoses are anxiety, ineffective coping, fear, pain, deficient knowledge, and low self-esteem. Nursing interventions are based on specific behaviors, symptoms, and treatments.

AMENORRHEA

Amenorrhea (absence of menstrual flow) is normal before puberty, after menopause, during pregnancy, and sometimes during lactation. Menstrual flow may also be absent or suppressed as a result of hormonal abnormalities or surgical interventions such as a hysterectomy (surgical removal of the uterus).

Etiology/Pathophysiology

Amenorrhea is classified as primary when menarche has not occurred by the age of 17 to 18 years. The cause may be a congenital defect. Secondary amenorrhea means menarche has occurred but flow has ceased for at least 3 months or there has been an absence of vagi-

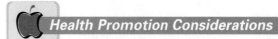
Health Promotion Considerations

Health Teaching for Menstruation

1. Knowledge of the physiologic process
2. Factors that may alter the menstrual cycle: stress, fatigue, exercise, acute or chronic illness, changes in climate or working hours, and pregnancy
3. Personal hygiene
   a. Wear pads during early period of heavy flow.
   b. Change tampons frequently to decrease risk of toxic shock syndrome.
   c. Consult physician if tampons cause discomfort.
   d. Take a daily shower for comfort; warm baths may relieve slight pelvic discomfort.
   e. Keep perineal area clean and dry; cleanse from anterior to posterior.
   f. Try to wear cotton underwear; remember that nylon pantyhose and tight-fitting slacks cause retention of moisture and should not be used for extended periods.
   g. Feminine hygiene products, such as vaginal sprays and suppositories, may contribute to a feeling of cleanliness.
   h. A daily douche is not recommended because it changes the protective bacterial flora of the vagina and predisposes the woman to infection.
4. Exercise
   a. Exercise is not contraindicated and may help prevent discomfort.
   b. Modify exercise if fatigue occurs.
5. Diet
   a. Restrict salt intake if fluid retention is present.
   b. Consult a physician if fluid retention persists after menstruation.
6. Discomfort
   a. For mild discomfort, take aspirin, acetaminophen (Tylenol), or ibuprofen (Motrin); apply warmth; and rest.
   b. For prolonged, severe discomfort, consult a physician.

nal fluid for 12 months, coupled with a history of irregular bleeding. Causes for secondary amenorrhea may be normal pregnancy; frequent, vigorous exercise, as in female athletes; or an emotional disorder such as depression, anorexia (lack of appetite), or bulimia (an insatiable craving for food, often resulting in episodes of continuous eating followed by purging).

Assessment

Early diagnosis and prompt management are necessary if more serious reproductive and genital problems are to be prevented. The nurse should urge the sexually active woman to see a physician as soon as a menstrual period is missed. Maintaining health during pregnancy is vital for both the mother and the fetus. Women who suspect their amenorrhea is caused by menopause can be examined by a physician to confirm this.

Obtaining a family history is important. Emotional factors or behaviors that may influence the menstrual cycle should be assessed. A menstrual history should include (1) the number of periods missed, and (2) whether amenorrhea was previously present. Recent use of medications and drugs needs to be determined.

Diagnostic Tests

Beyond the preliminary workup and when pregnancy is not a possibility, the diagnostic study for primary and secondary amenorrhea is the same. This study includes the following:

Pelvic examination
Blood, urine, and hormonal analysis
Determination of existing tumors
Pap test

Medical Management

Treatment is based on the underlying cause and must be determined on an individual basis. It may mean hormonal therapy will be needed.

Nursing Interventions and Patient Teaching

Nursing diagnosis and interventions for women with amenorrhea include but are not limited to the following:

Nursing Diagnosis	Nursing Interventions
Ineffective coping, related to lack of menstrual flow	Acknowledge patient's feelings. Provide emotional support. Refer to counseling as necessary. Explain diagnostic procedures. Provide information, privacy, consultation as indicated for sexual concerns.

The nurse should encourage compliance with treatment and emphasize the importance of follow-up visits with the physician for treatment, therapy, and further evaluation of treatment efficacy.

DYSMENORRHEA

Uterine pain with menstruation, commonly called "menstrual cramps," is dysmenorrhea. Primary dysmenorrhea that is not associated with pelvic disorders usually develops when ovulatory function is established (less than 20 years of age) and there is no underlying organic disease. Often it will disappear or decline after pregnancy or by a woman's late 20s. Secondary dysmenorrhea is painful menstruation caused by organic disease such as PID or endometriosis and most often occurs in women older than 20 years of age.

Studies in industries and schools have shown dysmenorrhea to be the greatest single cause of absenteeism among women. It is one of the most common health problems for which women seek treatment.

Etiology/Pathophysiology

The causes of dysmenorrhea can be related to endocrine imbalance; an increase in prostaglandin secretions; or chronic illnesses, fatigue, and anemia.

A recent theory proposes that hypercontractility of the uterus resulting from higher-than-normal levels of prostaglandins may be the cause of dysmenorrhea. Whatever the cause, the symptoms and pain are real. Conditions that cause general debilitation—such as inadequate diet and exercise, anemia, and fatigue—are often related to dysmenorrhea.

Assessment

Many women have systemic symptoms of breast tenderness, abdominal distention, nausea and vomiting, headache, vertigo, palpitations, and excessive perspiration.

The nurse should assess the woman for colicky and cyclic pain and, infrequently, dull pain in the lower pelvis that radiates toward the perineum and back. This pain may be experienced 24 to 48 hours before menses or at the onset of menses.

The family history is important, because dysmenorrhea has been reported to be significantly more common among mothers and sisters of women with dysmenorrhea.

Secondary dysmenorrhea is suspected if the symptoms begin after 20 years of age. It has been described as a steady or cramping pain and may be specific to the site of pelvic disorder.

Diagnostic Tests

Diagnostic studies to rule out organic causes for dysmenorrhea include pelvic examination, laparoscopy, D&C, and hysterosalpingography.

Medical Management

Treatment of secondary dysmenorrhea is aimed at the cause. Surgical and medication intervention may be appropriate, depending on the severity and type of pathologic condition.

If no organic cause is found, the nurse should instruct the woman to exercise and eat nutritious foods, especially those high in fiber, to avoid constipation.

Local applications of heat and mild analgesics are prescribed. Medications for dysmenorrhea include aspirin, which causes vasodilation of blood vessels, and prostaglandin inhibitors, such as ibuprofen (Motrin) and naproxen sodium (Anaprox). Oral contraceptives may be used to suppress ovulation by inhibiting prostaglandin levels (Medications table).

MEDICATIONS | *Reproductive Disorders*

MEDICATION	TRADE NAME	ACTION	SIDE EFFECTS	NURSING IMPLICATIONS
Oral contraceptives (estrogen-progesterone combinations)	Ortho Novum, Norlestrin, Ovral, Triphasil	Inhibits ovulation by suppressing gonadotropins, FSH and LH; alters genital tract to inhibit sperm penetration and inhibit implantation	Nausea, cramps, diarrhea, appetite change, acne, rash, increased BP, thrombophlebitis, edema, dysmenorrhea, bleeding irregularities, depression, fatigue, breast changes, cholestatic jaundice, optic neuritis	Monitor glucose, thyroid function, and liver function tests; check Homans' sign for clot detection; monitor BP, discontinue if patient is pregnant.
Conjugated equine estrogen	Premarin	Needed for proper functioning of female reproductive systems; affects release of gonadotropins; inhibits ovulation; is involved in adequate calcium use in bone structure	Nausea, peripheral edema, enlargement of breasts, breast tenderness, anorexia, vomiting, diarrhea, headache, thrombophlebitis, dizziness, depression	Notify physician of weight gain of 5 pounds or greater per week (patient may need diuretic); monitor BP; check liver function test; check Homans' sign for possible clots; give IV product slowly to prevent flushing.
Butoconazole Clotrimazole	Femstat Cream Mycelex-7, Gyne-Lotrimin, Femcare	Same as clotrimazole Interferes with fungal DNA replication; binds sterols in fungal cell membrane	Same as terconazole Rash, urticaria, stinging, burning, peeling, blistering skin fissures, abdominal cramps, bloating, urinary frequency	Same as clotrimazole. Watch for allergic reactions; note therapeutic response (decrease in size and number of lesions); use gloves for application; know that it can be used through menstrual cycle; avoid use of other vaginal creams or suppositories during therapy.
Miconazole nitrate	Monistat-3, Monistat-7	Same as clotrimazole	Vulvovaginal burning, itching, pelvic cramps, rash, urticaria, stinging, burning, contact dermatitis	Same as clotrimazole.
Tioconazole ointment	Vagistat-1	Same as miconazole but two to eight times more potent	Vulvovaginal burning, itching, soreness, swelling	Same as clotrimazole.
Metronidazole	Flagyl, Protostat	Direct-acting amebicide/trichomonacide binds, degrades DNA in organism	Rash, headache, dizziness, fatigue, convulsions, blurred vision, nausea, vomiting, diarrhea, pseudomembranous colitis, albuminuria, neurotoxicity, metallic taste, disulfiram type of reaction with alcohol	Watch for allergic reactions and super infection; check stool for parasites; give oral form with food; watch for vision problems; tell patient not to drink alcohol during therapy.
Nystatin	Mycostatin	Same as clotrimazole	Rash, urticaria, stinging, burning	Same as clotrimazole.

Continued

MEDICATIONS | *Reproductive Disorders—cont'd*

MEDICATION	TRADE NAME	ACTION	SIDE EFFECTS	NURSING IMPLICATIONS
Terconazole	Terazol-7, Terazol-3	Same as clotrimazole	Vulvovaginal burning, itching, pelvic cramps, rash, urticaria, stinging, burning	Same as clotrimazole.
Topical Nystatin	Nilstat, Mycostatin, O-V Statin	Interferes with fungal DNA replication; causes fungal cell membrane permeability	Rash, stinging, burning, urticaria, nausea, vomiting, anorexia, diarrhea	Watch for allergic reaction; use gloves for topical application; for vaginal preparation, tell patient that she may need lightday pads.
Topical amphotericin B	Fungizone—cream, lotion, ointment	Binds to ergosterol, altering cell membrane permeability in susceptible fungi	Urticaria, stinging, burning, dry skin, pruritis, contact dermatitis, staining of nail lesions	Cover lesions completely after cleansing and drying well; use gloves to prevent further infection; watch for allergic reactions; tell patient that it may cause skin and clothing discoloration.
Medroxyprogesterone acetate	Provera Amen, Cycrin, Depo-Provera	Inhibits secretion of pituitary gonadotropins, which acts to prevent follicular maturation and ovulation; stimulates growth in mammary tissue	Irregular bleeding, breast tenderness, masculinization of fetus, edema, cholestatic jaundice, thrombophlebitis, anorexia, acne, mental depression, weight gain or loss	Notify physician of weight gain of 5 pounds or greater per week; monitor BP at beginning of treatment and periodically thereafter check liver function test; discontinue if patient is pregnant.
Transdermal estrogen system	Estraderm	Same as conjugated equine estrogen	Same as conjugated equine estrogen	Same as conjugated equine estrogen.
Testosterone propionate	Testosterone Propionate	Increases weight by building body tissue; increases potassium, phosphorus, chloride, and nitrogen levels; increases bone development	Acne, flushing, gynecomastia, edema, hypercalcemia, nausea, cholestatic hepatitis, aggressive behavior, headache, anxiety, mental depression, androgenic and anabolic activity	Check weight daily; monitor blood pressure; monitor growth rate in children; check electrolyte (potassium-sodium, chloride, calcium) and cholesterol levels; monitor liver function test.
Danazol	Danocrine	Synthetic androgen, causes atrophy of endometrial tissue; decreases FSH and LH, which leads to amenorrhea and anovulation	Fluid retention, virilization, androgenic effects, weight gain, amenorrhea, dizziness, headache, rashes, hepatic impairment	Check weight; monitor I&O; check for edema; give with food or milk to decrease gastrointestinal upset.
Acyclovir ointment	Zovirax	Antiviral agent, interferes with DNA synthesis needed for viral replication	Mild pain with transient burning; stinging, pruritus, rash, vulvitis	Apply ointment every 3 hours or six times daily around the clock; cover all lesions; use gloves when applying for self-protection.

Nursing Interventions and Patient Teaching

Nursing diagnoses and interventions for women with dysmenorrhea include but are not limited to the following:

NURSING DIAGNOSES	NURSING INTERVENTIONS
Deficient knowledge, related to lack of education concerning disease process and treatment	Present information on disease process, procedures to be performed, medications, and treatments. Prepare for informational question and answer sessions according to patient needs. Teach procedures patient must know how to perform. Obtain feedback. Be certain learning has taken place; reinforce teaching as needed. Develop a trusting relationship. Involve patient in care.
Pain, related to biologic agent	Assess nature of pain. Observe nonverbal cues. Encourage pain reduction techniques as appropriate. Explore best method for controlling pain (medication, positioning, comfort measures such as back rub or use of heat or cold). Monitor vital signs. Provide quiet environment, calm activities. Promote wellness; discuss with significant other ways in which he or she can assist patient.

The nurse should encourage a positive attitude and instruct women to maintain good posture, exercise, and practice good nutrition. Women who are unable to engage in normal activities because of dysmenorrhea should be urged to seek health care.

ABNORMAL UTERINE BLEEDING

Abnormal uterine bleeding may take many forms. Two of these, menorrhagia and metrorrhagia, will be discussed.

Menorrhagia is excessive bleeding at the time of the regular menstrual flow. In younger women it may be attributed to endocrine disturbances, but in older women it is usually indicative of inflammatory disturbances or uterine tumors. Emotional or psychological problems may also affect uterine bleeding. The severity of menorrhagia is usually estimated in terms of the number of pads or tampons used in excess of those used for regular menstrual flow.

Metrorrhagia is the appearance of uterine bleeding between regular menstrual periods or after menopause. It merits early diagnosis and treatment because it may be indicative of cancer or benign tumors of the uterus.

Diagnosis is made through a routine speculum and pelvic examination. Endometrial biopsy and D&C are also used to diagnose gynecologic causes of menorrhagia and metrorrhagia.

The nurse should (1) assess for bleeding, pain, vaginal secretions, and psychosocial concerns; (2) encourage the woman to express her feelings; (3) explain the importance of recording dates, type of flow, and number of sanitary pads or tampons used; (4) teach the patient pain-relieving techniques; and (5) explain to the patient the importance of sharing her concerns with her partner.

Women of all ages need to be educated about the importance of follow-up care when abnormal uterine bleeding is initially detected.

PREMENSTRUAL SYNDROME (PMS)

PMS occurs in 30% to 50% of women between 25 and 45 years of age. It differs from dysmenorrhea because it has no relation to ovulation.

Etiology/Pathophysiology

The etiology and pathophysiology are not well understood. It is believed that PMS is related to the neuroendocrine events occurring within the anterior pituitary gland. It is known that there is a loss of intravascular fluid into the body tissues, which causes water retention, bloating, and weight gain. PMS is thought to have a biologic trigger with compounding psychosocial issues. Some women have a genetic predisposition to PMS. Other proposed causes of PMS include estrogen and progesterone imbalances and nutritional deficiencies of pyridoxine (vitamin B_6) or magnesium. **Premenstrual dysphoric disorder** (PMD-D) is the term applied to a type of PMS. Women with PMD-D have a severe mood disorder in addition to PMS.

PMS occurs 7 to 10 days before the menstrual period and usually subsides within the first 3 days after the onset of the menstrual flow.

Sodium intake and the use of alcohol, tobacco, and caffeine should be evaluated as possible causes.

Clinical Manifestations

Symptoms are multiple and vary among individuals. Behavioral symptoms include anxiety, mood swings, irritability, lethargy (inactivity), fatigue, sleep disturbances, and depression. Physical symptoms—such as headache, vertigo, backache, breast tenderness, abdominal distention, acne, paresthesia (burning or tingling) of hands and feet, and allergies—appear or may become worse. Many symptoms appear alone or in combination with other symptoms. Some women accept the symptoms as being normal and only after the symptoms become severe do they seek medical help.

Assessment

Collection of **subjective data** needs to be specific as to the symptoms and combination of symptoms that occur with each woman. Each patient is asked to maintain a log for three consecutive menstrual cycles and to note symptoms and activities that relate to the menstrual period. The collected information can be analyzed and symptoms treated accordingly.

Collection of **objective data** pertinent to the syndrome—especially the inability to perform activities of daily living (ADLs) in the multiple roles of being a wife, mother, and career person—should be assessed by the nurse.

Diagnostic Tests

PMS can be diagnosed only when other possible causes for the symptoms have been eliminated. A focused health history and physical examination are done to identify any underlying conditions, such as thyroid dysfunction, uterine fibroids, or depression, that may account for the symptoms. No definitive diagnostic test is available for PMS. When PMS or PMD-D is a possible diagnosis, a woman is given a symptom diary to record her symptoms for two or three menstrual cycles (Lewis et al, 2004). Tests include evaluation of estrogen and progesterone levels to rule out hormonal imbalances and determination of glucose levels; low levels may lead to irritability.

Medical Management

PMS has no single treatment and no specific medication. Some physicians prescribe analgesics, diuretics, and progesterone. The patient's diet should be reviewed. A diet high in complex carbohydrates, moderate in protein, and low in refined sugar and sodium should be eaten, especially during the premenstrual interval. Supplements of vitamin B$_6$, calcium, and magnesium may be administered as prescribed. The consumption of caffeine (in tea, coffee, or other beverages), chocolate, and alcohol and smoking should be reduced or eliminated. Regular exercise three or four times a week for 30 minutes is encouraged, especially during the premenstrual interval. Techniques for stress reduction include yoga, meditation, imagery, and biofeedback training. Because fatigue may exaggerate PMS symptoms, adequate rest, sleep, and relaxation are helpful. For anxiety, buspirone (BuSpar) taken during the luteal phase of the menstrual cycle has helped some women. Women with PMD-D may benefit from antidepressants, including fluoxetine (Sarafem) and tricyclic antidepressants such as amitriptyline (Elavil). Selective serotonin reuptake inhibitors (SSRIs) such as sertraline (Zoloft) have provided significant relief to women with severe PMS (Lewis et al, 2004).

Nursing Interventions and Patient Teaching

Nursing diagnosis and interventions for the woman with PMS include but are not limited to the following:

NURSING DIAGNOSIS	NURSING INTERVENTIONS
Anxiety, related to PMS	Encourage verbalization of feelings.
	Acknowledge existence of syndrome and its symptoms.
	Encourage patient to keep a menstrual symptom calendar to document the cycle and nature of the symptoms.
	Encourage patient to plan activities during the symptom-free part of her cycle.
	Administer supplements of vitamin B$_6$, calcium, and magnesium as prescribed.
	Encourage daily exercise and relaxation.
	Encourage self-help groups and the reading of self-help literature; group support tends to reduce stress.
	Provide emotional support in a nonjudgmental and caring manner.
	Assist in identifying possible sources of anxiety.
	Assist in identifying coping mechanisms.

The patient should take responsibility for following a dietary plan of eating small meals and restricting or eliminating sugar, alcohol, caffeine, and nicotine; this may minimize the symptoms of PMS or PMD-D.

MENOPAUSE

The climacteric is the phase of the aging process of women and men who are making a transition from a reproductive phase to a nonreproductive stage of life. This phase occurs in middle adulthood and marks the onset of physical changes, a decrease in hormone secretion, and the cessation of ovulation and menses. The female climacteric is called **menopause**. Female menopause is the normal cessation of menses; menstrual flow will appear on an infrequent cycle for a period of time that does not usually exceed 2 years. However, as long as the menstrual cycle occurs, no matter how infrequently, ovulation continues and the potential for conception exists.

Etiology/Pathophysiology

Menopause is the normal decline of ovarian function resulting from the aging process. Menopause begins in most women between 35 and 60 years of age (the average age being 51) and is characterized by infrequent ovulation, decreased menstrual function, and eventual cessation of the menstrual flow.

Menopause may be artificially induced by such procedures as irradiation of the ovaries or surgical removal of both ovaries. Both cause menstruation to cease. Surgical removal or irradiation of the ovaries results in menopause with all its physiologic changes, whereas ovaries left intact after a hysterectomy will continue to function provided the age of the climacteric has not yet been reached.

Decline in ovarian function produces a variety of symptoms, including a decrease in the frequency, amount, and duration of the menstrual flow, spotting, amenorrhea, and **polymenorrhea** (increased number of menstrual periods). Symptoms can last from a few months to several years before menstruation ceases permanently. Menopause is not considered to be complete until 1 year after the last menstrual period.

Clinical Manifestations

Physical changes that occur in the body do not generally develop until after permanent cessation of menstruation. Changes of the reproductive system include shrinkage of vulval structures, atrophic vulvitis, shortening of the vagina, and dryness of the vaginal wall. A pelvic relaxation of supporting structures is the result of the decrease in estrogen. Cystitis and urinary frequency and urgency may appear as a result of changes in the urinary system. There is loss of skin turgor and elasticity, increased subcutaneous fat, decreased breast tissue, and thinning of hair of the axilla, head, and pubis. About 25% of postmenopausal women develop osteoporosis.

Assessment

Collection of **subjective data** should include a family history. The nurse should determine whether family members and significant others are aware of the transition and if they are supportive. Emotional illness, if present, should be noted. Hot flashes caused by glandular imbalances may become prominent. Other symptoms may include fatigue, vertigo, headache, nausea, **dyspareunia** (painful intercourse), palpitations, and chest and neck pain. Some experience a feeling of being unwanted, and some may fear growing old; both feelings could cause depression.

Collection of **objective data** includes an awareness that some patients may display frequent crying spells or outbursts of anger. The use of contraceptives should be explored. Frequency, amount, and duration of the menstrual flow need to be assessed. Diaphoresis,

weight gain, and vomiting, as well as tachycardia, may occur. The nurse can note many of these disturbances.

Diagnostic Tests

Tests include analysis of hormonal levels. Other diagnostic testing may be indicated by specific symptoms. Some examinations are performed to rule out conditions such as cancer.

Medical Management

The status of hormone replacement therapy for postmenopausal women has undergone a radical reversal in the past several years. The Women's Health Initiative (WHI), sponsored by the National Institutes of Health, has conducted extensive research on the effects of hormone replacement therapy (HRT) on women's health. The findings of the WHI demonstrated that long-term use of an HRT estrogen-progestin combination heightened the risk of ischemic stroke, coronary heart disease, a higher incidence of breast cancer that is at a more advanced stage at the time of diagnosis, a greater risk of ovarian cancer, and a higher incidence of thromboembolism than for women in the control group. In 2003, further analysis of WHI data found hormone use to increase the risk of cognitive decline in a small percentage of those who receive it.

As a result of these studies, the American College of Obstetricians and Gynecologists (ACOG), the National Institutes of Health (the study's sponsor), and the U.S. Food and Drug Administration (FDA) recommend that women take the lowest effective dose of HRT for the shortest possible time to relieve menopause symptoms (Akert, 2003).

Nurses are in a good position to apprise their patients of the benefits, risks, and appropriate uses of HRT, which include its short-term use for the treatment of moderate to severe symptoms of menopause, such as hot flashes, night sweats, and vaginal dryness. At present, there are no data that might indicate how long HRT can be taken without the risk of cardiovascular or other adverse effects, and it is not known whether lower dosages lessen the risk of complications. In women with moderate to severe menopausal symptoms, it is reasonable to assume that such risk can be minimized by limiting the duration of therapy to the point at which the severe symptoms have dissipated and using the lowest effective dosage. Low-dose alternatives in HRT include low-dose Prempro, containing either 0.45 mg conjugated estrogens and 1.5 mg medroxyprogesterone, or 0.3 mg conjugated estrogens and 1.5 mg medroxyprogesterone, or low-dose intravaginal estrogen products, such as estrogen topical vaginal cream (Premarin vaginal cream or Estrace), and low-dose vaginal rings. Because of the later diagnosis of breast cancer and colon cancer in women receiving combination HRT, these women need to be closely screened and monitored for these complications. Any abnormal mammogram while a woman is taking combination HRT should be closely scrutinized, and screening for colon cancer should be part of the follow-up for these women.

Some physicians recommend calcium supplements, which are available in many forms; the generic calcium carbonate products are the most cost effective.

Nursing Interventions and Patient Teaching

Education regarding menopause should occur before its onset. Many women appreciate opportunities offered by nurses to discuss menopause. An exercise program should be set up that includes both movement and weight bearing. Walking is an excellent weight-bearing exercise. Other exercises include bicycling, stationary cycling, and aerobic dancing.

Nursing diagnoses and interventions for the menopausal patient include but are not limited to the following:

NURSING DIAGNOSES	NURSING INTERVENTIONS
Situational low self-esteem, related to concerns about femininity, sexuality, and aging	Encourage patient and significant others to verbalize concerns. Confirm accurate information. Correct information related to self-concept issues. Avoid value judgments. Refer patient to couple, family, and sex therapy as appropriate. Provide understanding and support as appropriate.
Deficient knowledge, regarding patient's physiologic and psychological changes, related to climacteric and menopause	Explain the process of climacteric and menopause, depending on the patient's ability to comprehend. Explain importance of keeping fit, eating a well-balanced diet, getting adequate rest and sleep, avoiding stress and fatigue, and continuing contraception until indicated by physician. If estrogen replacement therapy is ordered, inform patient about side effects. Instruct patient to report any vaginal bleeding occurring 6 months or more after last menstrual period. Inform patient of the availability of water-soluble lubricants if needed before coitus.

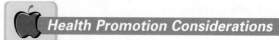

Health Promotion Considerations

Kegel Exercises

Kegel exercises are performed to help strengthen and tighten muscles that support the pelvic organs. These muscles (pelvic floor) are used to stop the flow of urine. To perform Kegel exercises while standing or sitting, tighten the pelvic floor muscles as hard as you can. Hold for 5 seconds, then release. Repeat at least 10 times. This exercise can initially be done many times throughout the day. Practice initially while urinating; try to stop the flow of urine by tightening the pelvic muscles.

For patient teaching, the nurse should emphasize that the climacteric is normal and self-limiting and that menopause is not the end of the patient's sex life. A nutritious diet and weight control will improve physical condition, and an exercise program will promote vitality. Interest and participation in various activities will help decrease anxiety and tension. Skin creams and lotions can be used to prevent drying, pruritus, and cracking skin. The nurse should encourage the woman to perform breast self-examination (BSE) monthly and monitor calcium intake. Contraceptives should be used for 1 year after the last menstrual period. The patient can obtain a prescription for treatment of pruritus or burning of the vulva. Women can practice Kegel exercises daily (Health Promotion Considerations box) to strengthen pelvic muscles. A water-soluble lubricant, such as KY jelly, can be used to prevent dyspareunia. The side effects of any medications or hormonal therapy should be explained. The nurse should emphasize that an annual physical examination is important for maintaining good health.

MALE CLIMACTERIC

The climacteric is less pronounced in men and often may not even be apparent in many men.

Etiology/Pathophysiology

The appearance of the climacteric phase is gradual and occurs between 55 and 70 years of age. There is a gradual decrease of testosterone levels and seminal fluid production. The impact is largely psychological, possibly because of the recognition of some reduction of sexual activity and interests.

Clinical Manifestations

Manifestations are mostly physiologic changes. Erections require more time and are not as full or firm. The prostate gland enlarges, and secretions diminish; seminal fluid decreases. The physical changes occur as the man grows older, and the most noticeable signs are loss or thinning of hair from the head, chest, axillae, and pubis. There may be some flushing and chilling. Muscle tone is decreased.

Assessment

Collection of **subjective data** reveals that the man is generally at the peak of his career or possibly considering retirement. He interprets his decreased sexual needs as a loss of productivity and sexual power. Therefore the assessment should invite verbalization of emotions with coping mechanisms.

Collection of **objective data** includes assessment of behaviors that may be causing the man stress and concern. Changes he has noted regarding his lifestyle and feelings of loss of self-worth should be expressed.

Diagnostic Tests

Diagnostic tests include a complete physical examination to rule out abnormalities of structure and function.

Nursing Interventions and Patient Teaching

Nursing diagnosis and interventions for men experiencing male climacteric include but are not limited to the following:

NURSING DIAGNOSIS	NURSING INTERVENTIONS
Ineffective coping, related to situational crisis (climacteric)	Show understanding and concern. Assist patient in identifying how the problem affects his life and future, his family, and significant others. Encourage patient to verbalize whether factors could be influencing the way he sees the problem. Assist patient in identifying strengths and coping skills and the nature and strength of situational support Collect data about current and potential sources of support. Assist patient in planning alternative solutions. Give positive reinforcement.

The patient should be informed that the climacteric is normal. The nurse should encourage patients to verbalize their fears and to seek counseling if stress increases.

IMPOTENCE

Impotence is the inability of an adult man to achieve penile erection. Several forms are recognized: (1) functional impotence, which has a psychological basis; (2) anatomical impotence, which results from a physical defect of genital structures; and (3) atonic impotence, which involves disturbed neuromuscular function. Some neuro-logical abnormalities that affect erectile function are tabes dorsalis, caused by advanced syphilis; congenital spinal cord anomalies, such as spina bifida; spinal cord tumors; amyotrophic lateral sclerosis (Lou Gehrig's disease); multiple sclerosis; or cord compression caused by a herniated disk. Radical prostatectomy often leads to impotence. The nurse can best understand impotence by developing a broad understanding of the factors that contribute to the condition.

Medical Management

Medical treatment is based on careful assessment of the causative factors. It is known that medications such as antihypertensive, antidepressive, and antianxiety agents, as well as some cardiac agents, may cause impotence. Illicit or abused substances such as alcohol, cocaine, and nicotine are also known to cause impotence. Disease conditions—such as diabetes mellitus or end-stage renal, heart, and chronic obstructive pulmonary disease—may also be causative factors in impotence.

A drug named sildenafil citrate (Viagra) is being prescribed as an oral therapy for erectile dysfunction. The physiologic mechanism of erection of the penis involves release of nitric oxide in the corpus cavernosum during sexual stimulation. The drug enhances smooth muscle relaxation and the inflow of blood in the corpus cavernosum during sexual stimulation, thus allowing erection to occur. For most patients, the recommended dosage is 50 mg taken as needed approximately 1 hour before engaging in sexual activity. However, Viagra may be taken anywhere from a half hour to 4 hours before sexual activity. Viagra has been shown to potentiate the hypotensive effects of nitrates; therefore its administration to patients who are using nitrates (either regularly or intermittently) in any form is contraindicated. Tadalafil (Cialis) is another anti-impotence agent for erectile dysfunction contraindicated for concurrent use with nitrates, nitric oxide, or alpha adrenergic blockers. Its use is contraindicated in patients who have unstable angina, recent history of stroke, life-threatening heart failure, uncontrolled hypertension, or myocardial infarction (MI) within 90 days. For most patients, the recommended dosage is 10 mg before sexual activity (range 5 to 20 mg; not to exceed one dose in 24 hours).

There are mechanical devices available for the patient with impotence. Surgical implantation of a penile prosthesis may be performed as a "same-day" procedure or may require hospitalization for 5 or more days, depending on the patient and the type of device used (Figure 12-9).

Nursing Interventions and Patient Teaching

The nurse is responsible for teaching the patient to administer hormonal medication (testosterone) and to watch for side effects. The nurse should advise the pa-

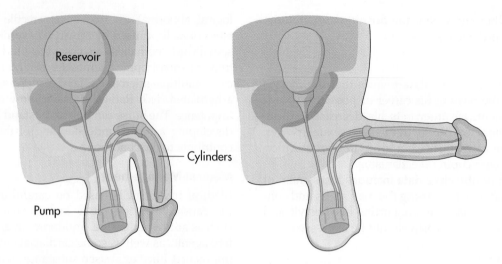

FIGURE **12-9** The Scott inflatable prosthesis has erect and flaccid positions designed to mimic normal erectile function.

tient to take oral hormonal replacement drugs with meals to prevent nausea.

The nurse should advise the patient about signs and symptoms of infection of the implant, including tenderness of the penis, fever, dysuria, and signs of urinary tract infection. The nurse should educate the patient to seek medical attention promptly if infection occurs.

INFERTILITY
Etiology/Pathophysiology

Infertility is defined as the inability to conceive after 1 year of sexual intercourse without birth control measures. Primary infertility refers to couples who have never conceived. Secondary infertility refers to couples who have conceived but are now unable to do so.

A woman's age has a significant bearing on her ability to conceive. The most fertile time of a woman's life is between 20 and 29 years of age. The most fertile time of a man's life is in his late teens and early 20s. A man's fertility does not decrease much as he grows older, but a woman's fertility drops dramatically.

Infertility may be caused by impaired sperm or ovum production or an occlusion in the reproductive system that prevents the sperm and ova from meeting. Infections of the reproductive tract (such as PID) and STDs (such as syphilis) are frequently associated with infertility. Because the man may be the infertile partner in 40% of the cases of infertility, the quality and quantity of his sperm must be analyzed. The primary causes of infertility in women are tubal insufficiency and ovarian and uterine conditions, such as endometriosis or congenital defects.

Assessment

Collection of **subjective** and **objective data** includes physical examination and health histories for both partners in order to make the infertility assessment and prepare a plan of treatment.

Diagnostic Tests

Specific testing is necessary to rule out systemic diseases such as diabetes mellitus, neoplasms, hepatic and renal diseases, and viral conditions. Genetic defects and disorders of the testes are explored. Diagnostic testing can produce a great deal of anxiety and stress. This testing may continue for fairly long periods with or without favorable results. Male testing is somewhat simpler and usually less expensive than female testing. If there is reason to suspect infertility or sterility of the man, it is appropriate to test him first. Male infertility testing includes semen analysis, which measures the quantity and quality of semen, volume of sperm cells, sperm motility, and sperm density; and endocrine imbalance testing, which explores possible disruption of the pituitary gonadotropins and testosterone production.

Female testing focuses on the ovulation process and reliability of the reproductive organs. The testing includes (1) basal body temperature to assess ovulation; (2) endometrial biopsy, which confirms ovulation and endometrial cyclic changes; (3) endocrine studies to detect the nature of the functioning of the adrenal and thyroid glands with anovulation cycles; (4) Rubin's insufflation test, which determines tubal patency; and (5) hysterosalpingography and hysterography to assess the position and alignment of the reproductive organs.

Male and female interaction studies include (1) Huhner's test, which examines the cervical mucus for motile sperm cells after intercourse, at midmenstrual cycle; (2) immunologic or immunoglobulin (antibody) testing for detection of spermicidal antibodies in the sera of the woman; and (3) testing both the man and woman for normalcy of their sex chromosomes.

Medical Management

The management of infertility problems depends on the cause. If infertility is secondary to an alteration in ovarian function, supplemental hormone therapy may be attempted to restore and maintain ovulation. Drugs used to induce ovulation include clomiphene citrate (Clomid), human menopausal gonadotropin (Pergonal), and bromocriptine (Parlodel). When an actual mechanical tubal blockage exists, a reparative microsurgical procedure can be done.

Poor cervical mucus may be a result of chronic cervicitis or inadequate estrogenic stimulation. Careful cauterization of the cervix may eradicate the chronic cervicitis, and the administration of estrogens can improve the quantity and quality of the cervical mucus.

Improving the patient's general health may help, especially when a debilitating or chronic illness is present. Removing or reducing psychological stress can improve the emotional climate, making it more conducive to achieving a pregnancy. Education of the couple regarding the probable time of ovulation and appropriate coital technique may also be indicated.

When a couple has not succeeded in conceiving while under infertility management, another option is intrauterine insemination with the partner's or donor's sperm. If this technique does not succeed, **in vitro fertilization** (IVF) may be used. IVF is the removal of mature oocytes from the woman's ovarian follicle via laparoscopy, followed by fertilization of the ova with the partner's sperm in a Petri dish. When fertilization and cleavage have occurred, the resulting embryos are transferred into the woman's uterus. The procedure requires 2 to 3 days to complete and is used in cases of fallopian tube obstruction, decreased sperm count, and unexplained infertility. IVF is costly and emotionally stressful, but it has become a recognized and an accepted method of therapy for infertile couples.

Assisted reproductive technologies (ARTs) have developed rapidly since the first IVF baby was born in 1978. ARTs consist of IVF, gamete intrafallopian transfer (GIFT), zygote intrafallopian transfer (ZIFT), cryopreserved embryo transfer (CPE), and donor oocyte programs (DOP). Current research predicts a rapid expansion of these techniques in the next decade. With the increased knowledge of freezing techniques for embryos (CPE), couples will have increased pregnancy potential. Research is also investigating the replication of normal tubal secretions. This important tubal factor is recognized because there is a higher pregnancy rate with GIFT and ZIFT than with IVF. Finally, the development of embryo biopsy and genetic engineering may allow for preconception techniques for those couples with identified genetic abnormalities. It also raises the possibility of gender selection. Noncoital reproduction poses many ethical, legal, and social concerns. All decisions related to infertility are influenced by the age of the couple, their wishes, and the length of time they have been attempting to conceive.

Nursing Interventions

The nurse has a major responsibility for teaching and providing emotional support throughout the infertility testing and treatment period. Feelings of anger, frustration, sadness, and helplessness between partners and between the couple and health care providers may heighten as more and more tests are performed. Infertility can generate great tension in a marriage as the couple exhausts their financial and emotional resources. Few insurance carriers cover the cost of infertility testing or the therapeutic measures associated with infertility. Shame and guilt may be precipitated when other people become involved in such an intimate area of a relationship. Recognizing and taking steps to deal with the psychological and emotional factors that surface can assist the couple in coping with the situation. Couples should be encouraged to participate in a support group for infertile couples and in individual therapy.

Provisions for providing information and emotional support by the nurse continue as therapeutic measures are attempted. Couples should be given ample opportunity to plan what is financially realistic—each GIFT and ZIFT attempt can exceed $10,000. Pergonal treatment costs about $3000 per month, and each IVF treatment costs $4500 to $6000.

Prognosis

Approximately 50% of couples who undergo assessment and treatment for infertility are likely to conceive.

INFECTIONS OF THE FEMALE REPRODUCTIVE TRACT

Infections of the female reproductive tract are most commonly found in the vagina, the cervix, the fallopian tubes, and their adjacent areas. The vagina is lubricated and protected by flora containing Döderlein's bacilli, acid pH, and secretions from the vaginal and cervical cells.

Causative organisms of vaginal infections are multiple. The most common organisms that cause infection are *Escherichia coli*, *Candida albicans*, and *Trichomonas vaginalis*. Infections are more likely to occur when the flora and the acidity of the vagina are disturbed by medications (birth control pills, antibiotics), stress, malnutrition, douching, aging, and disease. Yeast organisms grow best in an acid pH (−4.7), whereas *Trichomonas* and organisms causing nonspecific vaginitis flourish on a pH that is more alkaline (5+).

Organisms are often introduced from external sources by way of unclean douche nozzles, poor hygiene, inadequate handwashing, neglected nail care, soiled clothing, and intercourse. Vaginal infections can be sexually transmitted, and unless both partners are treated, the infection will return.

SIMPLE VAGINITIS

Etiology/Pathophysiology

Vaginitis is a common vaginal infection. It is usually caused by *E. coli*, an organism found in feces and the rectum. It may be caused by staphylococcal and streptococcal organisms, *T. vaginalis* (a flagellated protozoan), *C. albicans* (a yeastlike fungus), and *Gardnerella* bacillus.

Vaginitis is an inflammation of the vagina. If the patient changes perineal pads or tampons infrequently, an irritation of the vaginal tract and inner groin occurs. This creates a medium suitable for organism growth. Examination of the vaginal walls will show a profuse foamy (bubbly) exudate if the cause of the vaginitis is *T. vaginalis*. If *C. albicans* is the causative agent, a thick, cheeselike discharge results. Bacterial vaginitis produces a malodorous milklike discharge.

Clinical Manifestations

The exudate in vaginitis is yellow, white, or grayish white; curdlike; and generally accompanied by pruritus, burning, and edema of the surrounding tissue. Voiding and defecation generally intensify the symptoms.

Assessment

Collection of **subjective data** includes assessment of menstrual history, age at menarche, length of cycles, duration and nature of flow, dysfunctions, birth control methods, medications taken, family history of diabetes mellitus, previous vaginal infections, and STDs. Sexual practices and information about signs of infection in the sex partner should be elicited. Dysuria may occur as a consequence of local irritation of the urinary meatus.

Collection of **objective data** includes observation for excoriations of the skin caused by scratching, in which case secondary infection may result. The specific type of exudate is observed.

Diagnostic Tests

Diagnostic tests include direct visual examination of the vagina, culture of the organism, and bimanual examination to assess for inflammation of the vagina and its surrounding tissues.

Medical Management

Vaginal infection can be treated by a variety of methods. The major goals of treatment are to (1) cure the infection, (2) prevent reinfection, (3) prevent complications, and (4) prevent infection of the sexual partner or partners. Douching is frequently prescribed for treatment, as are local applications of vaginal suppositories, ointments, and creams. The patient should be advised to use the medication at bedtime; the patient should remain recumbent for more than 30 minutes after insertion to allow for absorption and to prevent loss of any medication from the vagina. During treatment the patient should refrain from intercourse or request that her partner use a condom (see Medications table).

Nursing Interventions and Patient Teaching

The nurse should advise the patient of the importance of handwashing before and after vaginal application of medications. Applications of heat in the form of douches, perineal irrigations, or sitz baths may be administered. Douching too frequently can alter normal vaginal flora.

Nursing diagnoses and interventions for the patient with vaginitis include but are not limited to the following:

NURSING DIAGNOSES	NURSING INTERVENTIONS
Pain, related to vaginal discharge	Flush vaginal flora with acid douche (15 mL white vinegar with 1000 mL water) as ordered. Apply antibiotic creams after douche as ordered. Provide sitz bath for edema.
Risk for infection, related to sexually transmitted diseases	Administer medication and treatments as ordered. Teach preventive methods, such as use of condoms. Recommend that partner be checked for infection and treated as necessary to avoid reinfection.

Most patients with vaginal infections are directed to abstain from sexual intercourse during treatment. The male partner's use of a condom until the symptoms of infection disappear may be advised. The patient is also informed that her sexual partner should be treated.

Prognosis

With proper treatment, the prognosis is good.

SENILE VAGINITIS OR ATROPHIC VAGINITIS

This condition occurs in women after menopause and upon aging. Low estrogen levels cause the vulva and vagina to atrophy and become susceptible to the invasion of bacteria. The exudate causes pruritus, edema, and skin irritations. Estrogen, vaginal suppositories, and ointments may be prescribed.

CERVICITIS

Cervicitis (infection of the cervix) is one of the most common diseases of the reproductive system. The infection is caused by vaginal infection or STDs, such as *Chlamydia trachomatis* infection, gonorrhea, herpes II, or trichomoniasis. The infection often follows childbirths or abortions in which lacerations occur. Therapy is specific to the causative organisms. Symptoms are backaches, whitish exudate, and menstrual irregularities. If cervicitis remains untreated, the tissues are continually irritated and the infection may spread to other pelvic organs. Personal hygiene and frequent warm tub baths can minimize odor and discomfort. Local applications of vaginal suppositories, ointments, and creams are usually prescribed.

PELVIC INFLAMMATORY DISEASE

PID is any acute, subacute, recurrent, or chronic infection of the cervix (cervicitis), uterus (endometritis), fallopian tubes (salpingitis), and ovaries (oophoritis) that has extended to the connective tissues lying between the broad ligaments.

Etiology/Pathophysiology

The most common causative organisms are *Neisseria gonorrhoeae, Streptococcus, Staphylococcus, Chlamydia,* and tubercle bacilli. PID can follow the insertion of a biopsy curette or an irrigation catheter, abortion, pelvic surgery, sexual intercourse, or infection during pregnancy. The condition may occur with or without gonorrheal infection and may be mild or severe.

When conditions or procedures alter or destroy the cervical mucus, bacteria ascend into the uterine cavity. Pelvic examination and movement of the reproductive organs become painful. PID is very serious, because it may cause adhesions and sterility. Sexually active women with more than one partner are at increased risk for PID.

Clinical Manifestations

The patient is usually hospitalized to isolate the organism and plan the treatment. The patient and those assisting with the care should be informed of all specific precautions and observe universal precautions. The use of goggles is recommended if any splashing is likely. Signs and symptoms are temperature elevation, chills, severe abdominal pain, malaise, nausea and vomiting, and malodorous purulent vaginal exudate.

Assessment

Collection of **subjective data** relates to the severity of the disorder, pain, time of onset, and frequency (primary infection or continuous reinfection). Sexual history, pelvic examinations, and pelvic procedures are important, because they may reveal the origin of the pathogen.

Collection of **objective data** invites assessment of the patient's knowledge, level of discomfort, and coping mechanisms used. The patient should be assessed for fever and the amount and characteristics of vaginal discharge.

Diagnostic Tests

Diagnostic tests include Gram stains of secretions from the endocervix, urethra, and rectum. Culture and sensitivity testing identifies organisms and is helpful in selection of antibiotics for treatment. Laparoscopy visualization of the pelvic inflammation may be necessary to confirm the extent of infection. Vaginal ultrasonic examinations can aid in diagnosing abscesses and following the treatment and healing process. The leukocyte count and erythrocyte sedimentation rate are also assessed to confirm an infectious process.

Medical Management

The goal of treatment is to control and eradicate the infection by preventing it from spreading to other body systems. Treatment includes systemic antibiotics administered intravenously or intramuscularly.

Nursing Interventions and Patient Teaching

Nursing interventions include (1) following the medical plan of treatment; (2) monitoring vital signs and progress of treatment; (3) providing fluids to avoid dehydration; (4) performing palliative measures for comfort in bathing, changing of perineal pads, personal hygiene, and warm douches; (5) providing patient support with a positive, nonjudgmental attitude; and (6) positioning the patient in Fowler's position to facilitate drainage.

Nursing diagnoses and interventions for the patient with PID include but are not limited to the following:

NURSING DIAGNOSES	NURSING INTERVENTIONS
Pain, related to infection process	Manage pain with analgesics as ordered; assess effectiveness of pain relief measures. Provide comfort measures.
Ineffective coping, related to condition	Provide emotional support. Encourage verbalization of feelings. Provide therapeutic environment for patient.
Ineffective health maintenance, related to insufficient knowledge of condition and complication	Patient teaching includes understanding of the significance of pelvic inflammatory disease and the importance of complying with medication therapy.

Discharge planning should include patient teaching and instructions for (1) contacting the physician if a low-grade fever persists or purulent vaginal discharge occurs; (2) understanding the significance of the pelvic inflammatory condition; (3) complying with medication therapy; (4) observing handwashing technique and practices of personal hygiene, such as bathing, avoidance of tampons, frequent changing of perineal pads, and clean clothing; (5) understanding the importance for the sexual partner to be examined and treated to avoid recurrence of the PID; and (6) recognizing that intercourse is sometimes very painful after an occurrence of PID and that sexual activity should be avoided until advised by a physician.

Prognosis

Women with PID are usually of childbearing age. If severe or chronic PID is present, infertility may result from adhesions in the fallopian tubes. With adequate treatment, the prognosis is good.

TOXIC SHOCK SYNDROME
Etiology/Pathophysiology

Toxic shock syndrome (TSS) is an acute bacterial infection caused by *Staphylococcus aureus* and usually occurs in women who are menstruating and using tampons (particularly superabsorbent tampons). If the tampon is left in place too long, the bacteria may proliferate and release toxins into the bloodstream, causing TSS. Women at the greatest risk are those who insert tampons with their fingers instead of with inserters, women with chronic vaginal infections, and women with genital herpes. TSS can also occur in non-menstruating women.

Clinical Manifestations

Often the patient will have flulike symptoms for the first 24 hours. Between days 2 and 4 of the menstrual period, the patient may have an elevated temperature (up to 102° F [39° C]), vomiting, diarrhea, myalgia, hypotension, and signs suggesting the onset of septic shock. Sore throat, headache, and a red macular palmar or diffuse rash followed by desquamation of the skin, hands, and feet may develop; urinary output is decreased, and the blood urea nitrogen (BUN) level is elevated. Disorientation may occur from dehydration and the release of toxins. Pulmonary edema and inflammation of mucous membranes may occur.

Assessment

Collection of **subjective data** includes determining whether the patient has recently used tampons, and how long she used a single tampon before changing it. Information should be obtained about myalgia, sore throat, headache, and fatigue.

Collection of **objective data** includes assessing for edema. The palms and soles should be assessed for the presence of an erythematous rash. Desquamation and sloughing occur within 1 to 2 weeks after the rash. The patient's level of consciousness should be noted. The presence of hypotension is a sign of TSS, as are non-purulent inflammation of the conjunctiva and hyperemia of the oropharynx and vagina.

Diagnostic Tests

There is no definitive test for TSS. However, cervical-vaginal isolates of *S. aureus* are present 90% of the time with TSS. Blood tests will demonstrate leukocytosis, thrombocytopenia, and elevated levels of bilirubin, BUN, creatinine, serum glutamic-pyruvic transaminase (SGPT or alanine aminotransferase [ALT]), serum glutamic-oxaloacetic transaminase (SGOT or aspartate aminotransferase [AST]), and creatine phosphokinase (CPK). Blood and urine cultures should be taken along with throat cultures when appropriate.

Medical Management

Treatment of TSS varies because of the range in types and severity of symptoms. Antibiotic therapy is given according to the results of a culture and sensitivity tests. Parenteral therapy is given to maintain proper fluid balance. Laboratory data are evaluated for electrolyte imbalance caused by vomiting and diarrhea, elevated BUN suggesting renal involvement, and elevated enzymes suggesting liver dysfunction.

Nursing Interventions and Patient Teaching

When the patient is hospitalized, bed rest is prescribed and antibiotics are administered. Close monitoring of vital signs and fluid status is important. If there is respiratory distress, oxygen therapy is instituted.

Nursing diagnoses and interventions for the patient with TSS include but are not limited to the following:

NURSING DIAGNOSES	NURSING INTERVENTIONS
Anxiety, related to TSS	Encourage patient to verbalize fears.
	Provide quiet, therapeutic environment.
	Provide support and understanding.
Deficient fluid volume, related to vomiting and diarrhea	Monitor amount, frequency, and characteristics of vomitus and diarrhea.
	Assess tissue turgor for evidence of dehydration.
	Assess patient for dry mucous membranes, and monitor parenteral fluids with electrolytes as ordered.
	Monitor I&O.

Because the use of tampons during menstruation has been linked to TSS, it is recommended that superabsorbent tampons not be used. If tampons are used, they should be alternated with the use of pads. Before using a tampon, it should be inspected for shedding and other flaws and discarded if any are noted. Tampons should be changed frequently (every 4 hours) and should be inserted carefully to avoid abrasions. Patients who have had TSS should not use tampons. The patient should be taught to wash hands thoroughly before inserting a tampon. Women who are menstruating and develop a sudden high fever accompanied by vomiting and diarrhea should be counseled by the nurse to seek immediate medical attention. If the woman is wearing a tampon, she should remove it immediately.

Prognosis

TSS is a rare and sometimes fatal disease. Prognosis depends on the severity of the disease and how quickly therapeutic measures to combat shock and renal failure, if present, are instituted.

DISORDERS OF THE FEMALE REPRODUCTIVE SYSTEM

ENDOMETRIOSIS

Endometriosis is a condition in which endometrial tissue appears outside the uterus.

Etiology/Pathophysiology

Endometrial tissue can be found on the ovaries, fallopian tubes, and uterus; within the abdominal cavity; and in the vagina (Figure 12-10). The spread of the tissue is believed to be through lymphatic circulation, by menstrual backflow to the fallopian tubes and pelvic cavity, or through congenital displacement of the endometrial cells.

The tissue responds to the normal stimulation of the ovaries, bleeds each month, and forms an endometrial crust, which causes an endometrial cyst. This cyst may rupture and cause further reproduction of tissue.

Clinical Manifestations

Symptoms are lower abdominal and pelvic pain with or without pain in the rectum. It may be unilateral or bilateral and may radiate to the lower back, legs, and groin. Symptoms are more acute during menstruation and subside after menstruation. There is some evidence that women have a greater chance (about seven times greater) of developing endometriosis if a sister

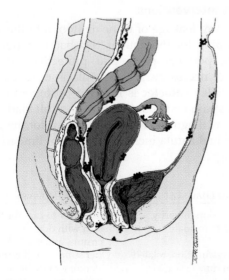

FIGURE **12-10** Common sites of endometriosis.

or mother has it. The highest incidence of endometriosis is among white women 25 to 35 years of age who are in the higher socioeconomic classes and who postpone childbearing until the later reproductive years. Women who have not conceived or lactated are at greater risk. Pregnancy is encouraged, because it is believed that an interruption of the menstrual cycle will slow the progress of the disorder. Pregnancy is also advised for women who want children, because one complication of endometriosis is infertility.

Assessment

Collection of **subjective data** includes obtaining a history of the patient's symptoms, including pelvic pain with menstruation, aching, cramping, a bearing-down sensation in the pelvis, or lower back dyspareunia. The type of pain may indicate the presence of ripe cysts that are about to rupture or may indicate the formation of infected tissue. The patient may reveal a history of menstrual irregularities such as amenorrhea.

Collection of **objective data** involves noting signs, which appear 5 to 7 days before menses and last 2 to 3 days. Signs may include abnormal uterine bleeding.

Diagnostic Tests

Laparoscopy with a biopsy of the lesions may confirm the diagnosis. Regular pelvic examinations are recommended to monitor progression.

Medical Management

Medical treatment consists of high-dose antiovulatory medications to inhibit ovulation and induce a state physiologically similar to pregnancy, thus suppressing menstruation. Synthetic androgens such as danazol may be prescribed to arrest proliferation of the endometrium and prevent ovulation, producing atrophy of the displaced endometrium. Occasionally women have spontaneous disappearance of endometriosis. Some women who become pregnant are asymptomatic after pregnancy. When involvement is severe, surgery may be necessary. A laparoscopy may be performed to remove endometrial implants and adhesions. Lasers may be used to vaporize the small implants of endometrial tissue. A total hysterectomy, oophorectomy, and salpingectomy may also be done.

Nursing Interventions and Patient Teaching

The nurse should reinforce the physician's explanation of the expected results of treatment; instruct the patient regarding the dosage, frequency, and side effects of prescribed medications; and emphasize the importance of regular checkups and of reporting abnormal vaginal bleeding. The nurse should also encourage the patient to verbalize her concerns. The nurse should assist the patient with comfort measures and help her with adaptive responses to self-concept.

Nursing diagnoses and interventions for the patient with endometriosis include but are not limited to the following:

NURSING DIAGNOSES	NURSING INTERVENTIONS
Pain, related to displaced endometrial tissue	Institute comfort measures to cope with pain, such as medications and warm compresses to abdomen. Maintain bed rest when pain is most severe.
Sexual dysfunction, related to painful intercourse or infertility	Emphasize importance of communicating fears and concerns that lead to anxiety.

The nurse caring for a patient who has endometriosis should reinforce the physician's explanation of the expected results of treatment; teach pain-relieving techniques to the patient; instruct the patient regarding the dosage, frequency, and possible side effects of any prescribed medications; and emphasize the importance of regular checkups and of reporting any abnormal vaginal bleeding.

Prognosis

Approximately half of the women with endometriosis are infertile. If a young woman has endometriosis, she is usually advised to have a family early, because the fertility rate is low. Menopause stops the progress of endometriosis.

VAGINAL FISTULA

A fistula is defined as an abnormal opening between two organs.

Etiology/Pathophysiology

Vaginal fistulas are caused by an ulcerating process resulting from cancer, radiation, weakening of tissue by pregnancies, and surgical interventions.

Vaginal fistulas are named for the organs involved (Figure 12-11):

Urethrovaginal fistula: opening between the urethra and vagina

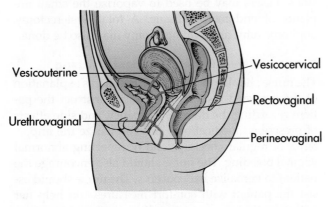

Vesicovaginal fistula: opening between the bladder and vagina

Rectovaginal fistula: opening between the rectum and vagina

Clinical Manifestations

Fistulas are recognized by their exudate, which has a distinct odor of urine or feces. Generally a bladder infection is present. The vesicovaginal fistula causes a constant trickling of urine into the vagina; a rectovaginal fistula allows feces and flatus to enter the vagina.

Assessment

Collection of **subjective data** includes the patient's understanding of the exudate that occurs as well as of any causative factors. The patient will report the presence of urine or feces from the vagina.

Collection of **objective data** includes noting any behaviors that indicate stress, anxiety, and pain. The patient may express feelings of disturbance in self-esteem because of the condition. The nurse should observe for urine or feces on the perineal pad.

Diagnostic Tests

Diagnostic testing includes a methylene blue instillation in the bladder, and an intravenous pyelogram or cystoscopy to assist in locating the fistula. Pelvic examination is performed.

Medical Management

Healing is promoted by an increase in vitamin C and protein in the diet. The patient is given oral or parenteral antibiotics. If the organ tissue is healthy, a surgical approach is recommended. The surgical approach may be similar to anterior or posterior colporrhaphy, which will be discussed later in the chapter. Fistulas that are difficult to repair or very large may require urinary or fecal diversion.

Nursing Interventions

Soiling from leakage of urine or stool into the vagina is disturbing for the patient. Sitz baths, deodorizing douches, perineal pads, and protective undergarments are necessary. If the fistula is repaired surgically, a Foley catheter is inserted postoperatively to prevent strain on the suture line by a full bladder.

Nursing diagnoses and interventions for the patient with vaginal fistula include but are not limited to the following:

NURSING DIAGNOSES	NURSING INTERVENTIONS
Impaired skin integrity, related to exudate	Teach how to care for the skin with douches, creams, and sitz baths.
Sexual dysfunction, related to pain during sexual activity	Offer support and understanding of distress toward sexual activities and self-esteem.

FIGURE **12-11** Types of fistulas that may develop in the vagina and uterus.

Prognosis

Vaginal fistulas may close spontaneously but frequently need to be repaired surgically. If so, 4 to 6 months are required for the inflammation to subside before surgery can be attempted.

RELAXED PELVIC MUSCLES

The most common problems resulting from relaxed pelvic muscles are displaced uterus with prolapse (downward displacement) and procidentia, cystocele, urethrocele, rectocele, enterocele, and malpositions of the uterus.

Displaced Uterus

A displaced uterus is usually congenital, but may be caused by childbirth. Normally the uterus lies with the cervix at a right angle to the long axis of the vagina, and the body of the uterus is inclined slightly forward. Backward displacement may be retroversion or retroflexion. Retroversion position places the cervix at the normal axis, but the body of the uterus is directed toward the sacrum. In retroflexion the angle of the body of the uterus is on the cervix. The patient has backache, muscle strain, leukorrheal discharge, and heaviness in the pelvic area, and the patient tires easily. Treatment consists of a pessary (a rubber or plastic doughnut-shaped ring placed in the vagina) and possible uterine suspension.

Uterine Prolapse

Etiology/pathophysiology. **Prolapse** of the uterus through the pelvic floor and vaginal outlet is traditionally rated as first-degree (the cervix comes down to the introitus [an entrance to a cavity, as in the vaginal introitus]), second-degree (the cervix protrudes through the introitus), or third-degree (procidentia [the entire uterus protrudes through the introitus]) prolapse (Figure 12-12).

Obstetric trauma, overstretching of the uterine muscle support system, coughing, straining, and lifting heavy objects contribute to uterine prolapse.

Clinical manifestations. The patient complains of a feeling of "something coming down." She may have dyspareunia, a dragging or heavy feeling in the pelvis, backache, and bowel or bladder problems if cystocele or rectocele are also present. Stress incontinence is a common and troubling problem. When second-degree or third-degree uterine prolapse occurs, the protruding cervix and vaginal walls are subjected to constant irritation, and tissue changes may occur.

Medical management. Surgery generally involves a vaginal hysterectomy with anterior and posterior repair of the vagina and underlying fascia. It is also called an **anteroposterior** colporrhaphy (suture of the vagina).

In situations in which surgery is contraindicated, pessaries are used to correct the prolapse. A pessary will provide uterine support. Before insertion of the vaginal pessary, the uterus is manually replaced in its normal position. Once inserted, the pessary holds the cervix in a posterior position, thus allowing the uterus to be in an anteflexed position. When the pessary is properly positioned, the woman is unaware of its presence and experiences no difficulty in voiding or during intercourse. A variety of pessaries are available for the different degrees of prolapse. Every 3 to 4 months the

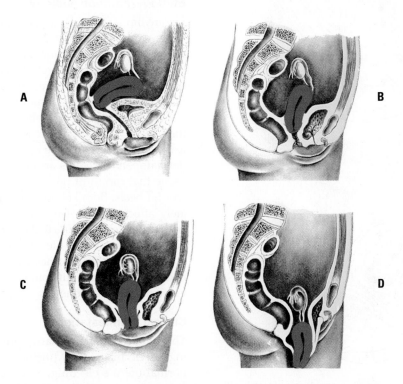

FIGURE **12-12** Uterine prolapse. **A,** Normal uterus. **B,** First-degree prolapse of the uterus.
C, Second-degree prolapse of the uterus. **D,** Third-degree prolapse of the uterus (procidentia).

pessary is cleaned and replaced by the woman, if possible, or by her health care provider. She is also checked for signs of excessive irritation. Pessaries that are unattended for long periods are associated with erosion, fistulas, and an increased incidence of vaginal carcinoma.

Cystocele and Rectocele

Etiology/pathophysiology. When the tissue, muscles, and ligaments that support the uterus and perineum have been stretched and weakened by childbearing, multiple births, or cervical tears, the organs gradually move into other positions. The relaxation of the tissues, muscles, and ligaments of the bladder causes a displacement of the bladder into the vagina. This is referred to as a **cystocele** (Figure 12-13, *A*).

Clinical manifestations. Clinical symptoms are urinary urgency, frequency, and incontinence; fatigue; and pelvic pressure. A large cystocele prevents complete emptying of the bladder, which leads to bacterial growth and infection.

The relaxation of the supporting tissues to the rectum causes the rectum to move toward the posterior vaginal wall and form a **rectocele** (see Figure 12-13, *B*). The rectocele causes constipation, rectal pressure, heaviness, and hemorrhoids.

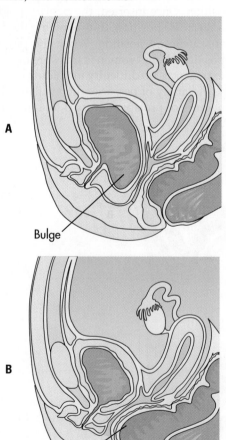

A

Bulge

B

Bulge

FIGURE **12-13 A,** Cystocele. **B,** Rectocele.

Medical management. Correction of cystocele and rectocele is a surgical repair involving shortening of the muscles that support the bladder and repair of the rectocele. This is known as anterior posterior or anteroposterior colporrhaphy. It is sometimes referred to as an A&P repair.

Nursing interventions and patient teaching. Preoperative care for colporrhaphy is especially important in ensuring as clean an operative area as possible. Patients may be given a cathartic followed by enemas to be sure the bowel is completely empty. A liquid diet for 48 hours before surgery will help keep the bowel empty. A cleansing vaginal douche is given the evening before and the morning of surgery. Postoperative care includes checking vital signs and observing for hemorrhage. A retention catheter is usually inserted into the bladder to keep it empty and prevent pressure on sutures. It is important to keep the fecal residue as soft as possible; some physicians order only liquids for several days, or they may order mineral oil to be given every night. An oil retention enema may be ordered, but cleansing enemas are not given. The patient's perineal area is cleansed carefully using surgical asepsis. Early ambulation is also encouraged.

The patient should be advised against standing for long periods or lifting heavy objects. Coitus must be avoided until healing occurs, usually after about 6 weeks.

Prognosis. With surgical correction, the prognosis is good.

LEIOMYOMAS OF THE UTERUS
Etiology/Pathophysiology

Leiomyomas (fibroids, myomas) are the most common benign tumors of the female genital tract (Figure 12-14). Fibroids are benign tumors arising from the muscle tissue of the uterus. Researchers have found that fibroid tumors lack the key protein dermatopontin, which plays a role in holding tissues together. Dermatopontin is a key component of the elastic meshwork of collagen that keeps cells in place. Moreover, the researchers learned that another type of growth, keloids, also lack dermatoponin. Keloids are an overgrowth of thick scar tissue that can form on the skin after a cut or another wound heals. Both keloids and fibroids disproportionately affect African-Americans (USUHS, 2004). It has been estimated that 20% to 25% of women older than 30 years of age develop uterine fibroid tumors. The size and number of leiomyomas vary. Most are found in the body of the uterus, but some occur in the cervix or involve the broad ligaments.

Clinical Manifestations

The symptoms are primarily pressure from an enlarging pelvic mass, pain (including dysmenorrhea), abnormal uterine bleeding, and menorrhagia with menstrual periods. If the fibroid tumor becomes large

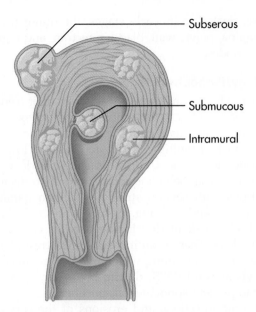

- Subserous
- Submucous
- Intramural

FIGURE **12-14** Leiomyomas. Uterine section showing whorl-like appearance and locations of leiomyomas, which are also called uterine fibroids.

enough to cause pressure on other structures, there may be backache, constipation, and urinary symptoms.

Assessment

Collection of **subjective data** includes asking the patient about the presence of pain with menstruation or abnormally heavy menstrual flow. The patient is asked to describe her symptoms, which may include pelvic fullness or heaviness, constipation, urinary frequency or urgency, and menorrhagia.

Collection of **objective data** includes assessing the patient for excessively heavy discharge of blood by observing the number and saturation of perineal pads.

Diagnostic Tests

Diagnostic studies may include a pregnancy test, D&C, laparoscopy, and ultrasonography.

Medical Management

The treatment of fibroid tumors depends on the symptoms and the age of the patient, whether or not more children are desired, and how near to menopause the woman is. **Myomectomy** (removal of uterine myomas while leaving the uterus in place) is the procedure of choice during childbearing years. If there is severe bleeding or an obstruction, a hysterectomy may be necessary.

Nursing Interventions and Patient Teaching

See the preoperative and postoperative nursing interventions for a patient who undergoes a hysterectomy. The nurse caring for a patient with fibroid tumors should reinforce the physician's explanation of the treatment plan—either a total hysterectomy or pelvic examination at regular intervals to monitor the status of the fibroid tumor. The nurse instructs the patient about the dosage, frequency, and possible side effects of prescribed medications. The patient with menorrhagia should be taught to include adequate iron in her diet to prevent iron deficiency anemia from the extra blood loss. The importance of regular checkups to monitor the status of the fibroid tumor should be emphasized, and the nurse can encourage the patient to express her feelings and assist her with coping mechanisms.

Nursing diagnoses and interventions for the patient with fibroid tumors include but are not limited to the following:

NURSING DIAGNOSES	NURSING INTERVENTIONS
Pain, related to fibroid tumors	Assess pain location, onset, and duration.
	Administer analgesics as ordered.
	Provide comfort measures as needed.
Risk for situational low self-esteem, related to the presence of fibroid tumors	Encourage verbalization of concerns.
	Be an active listener.

Prognosis

Fibroid tumors of the uterus tend to disappear spontaneously with menopause. They rarely become malignant. Infertility may result from a myoma that obstructs or distorts the uterus or fallopian tubes. Myomas in the body of the uterus may cause spontaneous abortions; those near the cervical opening may make the delivery of a fetus difficult and may contribute to postpartum hemorrhage.

OVARIAN CYSTS

Etiology/Pathophysiology

Ovarian cysts are benign tumors that arise from dermoid cells of the ovary or from a cystic corpus luteum or graafian follicle.

Clinical Manifestations

Ovarian cysts enlarge and are palpable on examination. They may cause no symptoms, or they may result in a disturbance of menstruation, a feeling of heaviness, and slight vaginal bleeding.

Medical Management

The cysts are usually removed by an ovarian cystectomy.

Nursing Interventions

Nursing interventions are similar to those for the patient having an abdominal hysterectomy.

Prognosis

The prognosis is good; ovarian cysts do not become malignant.

CANCER OF THE FEMALE REPRODUCTIVE TRACT

Cancer is the second most common cause of death in women, and malignant tumors of the reproductive tract represent a significant portion of the total number of deaths from cancer (Cultural and Ethnic Considerations box).

Uterine cancer, principally arising in the cervix, is the sixth most common cancer of women, ranking behind cancer of the (1) breast, (2) colon and rectum, (3) endometrium, (4) lung, and (5) ovary. Cervical cancer often affects women in their reproductive years. The cancer can be detected in its early stages with a diagnostic Pap test.

Endometrial cancer is primarily a disease of women older than 50 years of age, but the incidence among younger women is increasing. Most cases of ovarian cancer occur in women older than 50, but malignant neoplasms of the ovaries may occur at all ages.

CANCER OF THE CERVIX

Cancer of the cervix is a neoplasm that can be detected in the early, curable stage by Pap test. Cancer of the cervix is usually a squamous cell carcinoma. An estimated 10,520 cases of invasive cervical cancer were diagnosed in 2004. As Pap screening has become more prevalent, preinvasive lesions are detected far more frequently than invasive cancer. An estimated 3900 cervical cancer deaths occurred in 2004. Mortality rates have declined sharply over the past several decades.

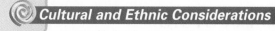

Cultural and Ethnic Considerations

Cancer of Female Reproductive System

- Ovarian cancer is seen more frequently among white women than among African-American women.
- Japanese women have a low incidence of ovarian cancer. However, second- and third-generation Japanese women in the United States have much higher rates, similar to white women born in the United States. Dietary practices may explain this difference.
- Endometrial cancer occurs more frequently among white women than among African-American women.
- Five-year survival rate for endometrial cancer (all stages combined) in 80% for white women and 55% for African-American women.
- Cervical cancer has a higher incidence among Hispanic, African-American, and American Indian women than among white women. The mortality rate for cervical cancer is more than twice as high among African-American women than among white women.
- There is a low incidence of cervical cancer among Jewish-American women.

Unless treated in its early stages, the tumor invades the vagina, pelvic wall, bladder, rectum, and regional lymph nodes.

Etiology/Pathophysiology

Women who become sexually active in their teens are at an increased risk for cancer of the cervix, as are those who have had multiple sexual partners, those who have had multiple births, and those of lower socioeconomic status. Cervical cancer risk is closely linked to sexual behavior and to sexually transmitted infections with several strains of human papilloma virus (HPV) and smoking. Women who smoke have a 50% higher risk of developing cervical cancer than nonsmokers. There is an increased incidence of cervical carcinoma in young women whose mothers took diethylstilbestrol (DES) during pregnancy as a treatment to prevent spontaneous abortion.

Chronic infections and erosions of the cervix are most likely significant in the development of cancer.

Carcinoma in situ is a preinvasive, asymptomatic carcinoma that can only be diagnosed by microscopic examination of cervical cells. Once diagnosed, it can be treated early without radical surgery. Carcinoma in situ of the cervix is essentially 100% curable.

Clinical Manifestations

Most cervical cancer is silent in the early stages and offers few symptoms. The two primary symptoms are leukorrhea and irregular vaginal bleeding or spotting between menses. Bleeding often occurs after coitus or after menopause. Bleeding is very slight at first, but as the disease progresses, the bleeding increases in amount. The vaginal exudate becomes watery, then increases and becomes a dark, bloody exudate with an offensive odor caused by necrosis (death of tissue) and infection of the tumor mass. As the cancer progresses, the bleeding may become constant and may increase in amount. With advanced stages there is severe pain in the back, upper thighs, and legs.

Assessment

Collection of **subjective data** includes the nurse urging women to have regular health appraisals and pelvic examinations, so that cancer of the cervix can be detected in its earliest stages. The patient will present no symptoms in the early stages of cancer of the cervix. If the tumor becomes more invasive, the patient will experience back and leg pain, weight loss, and malaise.

Collection of **objective data** includes assessing the patient for abnormal vaginal discharge by observing the sanitary pads. The vaginal exudate may be watery to dark red and malodorous. The number and saturation of the perineal pads should be noted. If the tumor becomes more invasive, the patient should be assessed for anemia, fever, and the presence of lymphedema.

Diagnostic Tests

The following tests are performed to determine the presence of cervical cancer: (1) Pap test; (2) Schiller's test; (3) physical examination; (4) cervical biopsy; and (5) additional diagnostic studies, such as a computed tomography (CT) scan, chest radiographic evaluation, intravenous pyelogram, cystoscopy, sigmoidoscopy, or liver function studies to determine the extent of invasion. The American Cancer Society recommends that cervical cancer screening begin approximately 3 years after a woman begins having vaginal intercourse, but no later than 21 years of age.

At or after age 30, women who have had three normal Pap test results in a row may get screened every 2 to 3 years. Some doctors may suggest getting the test done more often if a woman has certain risk factors, such as HIV infection or a weak immune system. Women 70 years of age and older who have had three or more normal Pap tests and no abnormal Pap tests in the past 10 years may choose to stop cervical cancer screening. Screening after a total hysterectomy (with removal of the cervix) is not necessary unless the surgery was done as a treatment for cervical cancer or precancer. Women who have had a hysterectomy without removal of the cervix should continue cervical cancer screening at least until age 70 (American Cancer Society, 2004).

Medical Management

Carcinoma in situ is treated by removal of the affected area. This removal can be accomplished through a variety of techniques, including electrocautery, cryosurgery (use of subfreezing temperature to destroy tissue), laser, conization, and hysterectomy. **Conization** is the surgical removal of a cone-shaped section of the cervix and is particularly useful in preserving childbearing function.

Early carcinoma of the cervix can be treated with a hysterectomy or intracavitary radiation (see Chapter 17).

A radical hysterectomy with pelvic lymph node dissection may be required for more extensive lesions. Invasive cervical cancers generally are treated by surgery, radiation, or both, as well as chemotherapy in some cases. Brachytherapy, or internally implanted radiation into the cervix, is often done. The patient is hospitalized for 48 hours for treatment. The treatment plan is tailored to each patient based on the extent of the disease.

Nursing Interventions and Patient Teaching

Nursing interventions should include verbal reassurance. In advanced cancer of the cervix, the nurse should position the patient comfortably; change her position slowly; maintain her body alignment; provide pain relief measures; change the patient's dressings and sanitary pads frequently; and assess color, odor, and amount of drainage. The skin is assessed for impairment. See the nursing interventions for a patient undergoing a hysterectomy.

Nursing diagnoses and interventions for the patient with cancer of the cervix include but are not limited to the following:

NURSING DIAGNOSES	NURSING INTERVENTIONS
Impaired urinary elimination related to post-surgical sensoriotor impairment	Connect indwelling catheter to closed gravity drainage. Give meticulous catheter care as indicated. Record color and amount of urinary output. Promote micturition at regular intervals when catheter is removed. Catheterize for residual urine as ordered.
Risk for situational low self-esteem, related to body image change and value of reproductive organs	Encourage verbalization with significant others. Relate importance of communicating anything that causes anxiety. Reinforce correct information and provide factual information to correct any misconceptions.
Ineffective tissue perfusion, peripheral, related to pelvic surgery, thrombophlebitis	Ensure that bed is not elevated in the knee gatch position. Assess proper placement of antiembolic stockings every 4 hours as ordered. Assist in passive and active leg exercises every shift. Encourage ambulation. Assess legs for erythema, increased tenderness, severe cramping, positive Homans' sign every shift.

The nurse can both educate and encourage patients to assume responsibility for their health by having a yearly Pap test. The nurse should encourage patients to seek prompt medical assistance for any abnormal vaginal exudate.

Prognosis

The prognosis is good if the cancer is treated in the early stages. It usually takes 2 to 10 years for squamous cell carcinoma to become invasive beyond the basement membrane and metastasize. Therefore early diagnosis and treatment are vital for survival. Survival for people with preinvasive lesions is nearly 100%. Ninety percent of cervical cancer patients survive 1 year after diagnosis, and 71% survive 5 years. When detected at an early stage, invasive cervical cancer is one of the most successfully treated cancers with a 5-year survival rate of 92% for localized cancers.

CANCER OF THE ENDOMETRIUM

Etiology/Pathophysiology

Cancer of the endometrium (uterine cancer) usually affects postmenopausal women. An estimated 40,320 cases of cancer of the uterine corpus (body of the uterus) were in 2004. An estimated 7090 deaths are expected for 2004. Endometrial cancer is usually an adenocarcinoma. The tumor is more likely to be localized, but may spread to the cervix, bladder, rectum, and surrounding lymph nodes. It is the most common malignancy of the female genital tract. Those groups at increased risk are those with a history of irregular menstruation, difficulties during menopause, obesity, hypertension, or diabetes mellitus; those who have not had children; and those with a family history of cancer of the uterus. Women who have used estrogen replacement therapy to treat menopausal symptoms have a greater likelihood of developing endometrial cancer. Progesterone plus estrogen replacement therapy (called hormone replacement therapy, or HRT) is believed to largely offset the increased risk related to using only estrogen. Women on tamoxifen are also at increased risk for developing uterine cancer.

The tumor in situ is slow growing. Invasion and metastasis occur later, with expansion to the cervix and myometrium and ultimately to the vagina, pelvis, and lungs.

Clinical Manifestations

About 50% of patients with postmenopausal bleeding have cancer of the uterus. In premenstrual or postmenopausal women, any abnormal bleeding or spotting should be reported.

Assessment

Collection of **subjective data** includes assisting the patient in identifying and reporting changes in reproductive or sexual health. The patient may report abdominal pressure and pelvic fullness. The patient will have a history of postmenopausal bleeding and leukorrhea. Pelvic and back pain and postcoital bleeding are late signs and symptoms.

Collection of **objective data** includes the nurse observing the patient for the color and amount of vaginal exudate on perineal pads. The nurse will assess the patient for complaints of pain and enlarged lymph nodes.

Diagnostic Tests

Pelvic and rectal examination and D&C are used to diagnose cancer of the endometrium.

Medical Management

Treatment of cancer of the endometrium depends on the stage of the tumor and the woman's health. Surgery, radiation, or chemotherapy may be used to remove the tumor and treat metastasis. For early cancer of the endometrium, total abdominal hysterectomy with bilateral salpingo-oophorectomy (TAH-BSO) is done. Intracavitary radiation followed by a hysterectomy and bilateral salpingo-oophorectomy may be done for the early stage of endometrial cancer (stage I). Patients with stage II disease may receive pelvic irradiation to cause shrinkage and help prevent spread. Afterward the patient will undergo a hysterectomy. Patients with stages III and IV disease are uncommon, and treatment is tailored for each patient based on the extent of the disease.

Nursing Interventions and Patient Teaching

See the section on interventions for the patient undergoing a hysterectomy; also see Chapter 17 for care of the patient through intracavitary radiation.

Health teaching and follow-up after discharge should emphasize the need for regular physical examination by the physician and the importance of compliance with the prescribed treatment plan.

Prognosis

Cancer of the endometrium is primarily a slow-growing adenocarcinoma. Metastasis occurs late, and the sign of irregular vaginal bleeding often appears early enough to allow for cure of the disease. Stage I tumors have the highest 5-year survival rate (about 94%).

CANCER OF THE OVARY

Etiology/Pathophysiology

Ovarian cancer, the fourth most common cause of cancer death in women, is the leading cause of gynecologic death in the United States, following cancer of the uterine corpus. Risk for ovarian cancer increases with age and peaks in the late 70s.

The American Cancer Society estimated that in 2004, 25,580 women would be diagnosed with ovarian cancer and nearly 16,090 would die of the disease.

In the early stages the tumors are asymptomatic and when detected usually have spread to other pelvic organs. Nothing alters the magnitude of risk for ovarian cancer more than genetics. Hereditary ovarian cancer accounts for 5% to 10% of ovarian cancers. In general, the closer the degree of relative, and the younger the relative at diagnosis, the higher the risk is. Women at increased risk are those who are infertile, anovulatory, nulliparous, and habitual aborters. Oral contraceptives taken for longer than 5 years may reduce the risk of ovarian cancer. Other risk factors include a high-fat diet and exposure to industrial chemicals such as asbestos and talc. Ovarian cancer commonly spreads by peritoneal seeding of the cancer cells. Common sites of metastasis are the peritoneum, omentum, and bowel surfaces.

Clinical Manifestations

In the early stages the symptoms may cause vague abdominal discomfort, flatulence, and mild gastric disturbances. As the tumor progresses, abdominal girth enlarges from the presence of ascites, and there is flatulence with distention. Other symptoms may include urinary frequency, nausea, vomiting, constipation, and weight loss.

Assessment

Collection of **subjective data** includes an awareness that cancer of the ovary is difficult to detect. The patient will report symptoms of abdominal discomfort, gastric disturbances (nausea, constipation), and urinary frequency.

Collection of **objective data** includes the nurse observing any increase in the abdominal girth. The patient may void at frequent intervals because of pressure on the bladder. The patient may be dyspneic due to ascites and pressure on the diaphragm.

Diagnostic Tests

Although detecting ovarian cancer early is difficult, an annual bimanual pelvic examination may help to identify pelvic masses. Because the ovaries are movable and therefore harder to assess, screening for ovarian tumors requires a thorough examination, including bimanual and rectovaginal examination. **Postmenopause palpable ovary syndrome** (a palpable ovary in a woman 3 to 5 years past menopause) may indicate an early tumor. CT scan of the pelvis and abdomen is indicated if palpable ovarian mass is present. Definitive diagnosis of ovarian cancer is usually established by a tumor biopsy at the time of exploratory laparotomy, when staging and tumor debulking take place.

Ovarian cancer is diagnosed by palpation of a pelvic mass and aspiration of ascitic fluid and detection of cancer cells in the fluid. A blood test to determine CA-125 is used to identify women with ovarian cancer.

High levels of CA-125 are found in the blood of 80% of women with epithelial ovarian cancer. But while the antigen test can help evaluate a woman's response to cancer treatment, it is controversial as an independent screening tool. Because of the test's lack of specificity and sensitivity, false-positive and false-negative results can occur. Many benign conditions, including endometriosis and fibroid tumors, can raise CA-125 levels above normal.

Vaginal ultrasonography, which also lacks specificity and sensitivity, may be used with pelvic examination and CA-125 antigen testing to follow a woman at increased risk.

Medical Management

Treatment often involves surgery alone or in conjunction with radiation or chemotherapy (see Chapter 17). Surgery may be a TAH-BSO and omentectomy (excision of portions of the peritoneal folds). In some very early tumors, only the involved ovary will be removed, especially in young women who wish to have children.

Nursing Interventions

Nursing interventions for any patient with ovarian cancer include management similar to that for patients undergoing abdominal hysterectomy and receiving chemotherapy and external radiation (see Chapter 17).

Because ovarian cancer is generally at an advanced stage when diagnosed, despite the woman's feeling well, support and encouragement to comply with the treatment regimen are important nursing interventions. As the disease progresses, the nurse will become involved in activities to increase the patient's comfort.

Nursing diagnoses and interventions for the patient with cancer of the ovaries include but are not limited to the following:

Nursing Diagnoses	Nursing Interventions
Fear, related to diagnosis of cancer	Assist patient with recognizing and clarifying fears and with developing coping strategies for those fears. Be an active listener.
Situational low self-esteem, related to body image change and value of reproductive organs	Encourage patient's comments and questions about condition. Encourage verbalization with significant others. Provide factual information to correct any misconceptions.

Prognosis

More than 60% of women with ovarian cancer are diagnosed with advanced disease. The 5-year survival rate for stage I tumors is 60% to 70%; for stage II tumors, the survival rate is 0% to 40%. For stages III and IV it is extremely poor. By the time most cases are diagnosed, the 5-year survival rate is below 20%.

HYSTERECTOMY

A hysterectomy involves the removal of the uterus, including the cervix. This procedure may be done for many conditions, such as dysfunctional uterine bleeding, endometriosis, malignant and nonmalignant tumors of the uterus and cervix, and disorders of pelvic relaxation and uterine prolapse.

Various terms are used to describe the removal of the uterus. A total hysterectomy is the removal of the entire uterus. The vagina remains intact, and intercourse is possible even though childbearing is not. Estrogens are still released. Menopause will occur naturally because the ovaries are still present. A total abdominal hysterectomy with bilateral salpingo-oophorectomy (TAH-BSO) is the removal of the uterus, fallopian tubes, and ovaries. It is sometimes called panhysterosalpingo-oophorectomy. A radical hysterectomy also includes the removal of the pelvic lymph nodes. If the ovaries are removed in these surgeries, the surgery will induce menopause.

VAGINAL HYSTERECTOMY

A vaginal hysterectomy may be done for a prolapsed uterus. It is not used nearly as often as the abdominal approach. The vaginal approach is selected for the patient who cannot tolerate abdominal surgery or prolonged anesthesia. There is no abdominal incision. The patient is placed in a lithotomy position, and the uterus is removed through the vagina. Advantages of the vaginal entrance are that (1) there is no wound dehiscence, (2) there is less pain, (3) complications are less likely, (4) hospitalization is shorter, and (5) there is no abdominal scar. The most important disadvantage is a limited view of the operative field for visualizing intrapelvic and intraabdominal organs. Vaginal hysterectomy is not used in cases of uterine fibroids or enlarged uterine size. Other disadvantages are risk of bleeding and postoperative infection.

ABDOMINAL HYSTERECTOMY

An abdominal hysterectomy is preferred when there is a need to explore the pelvic cavity and if the fallopian tubes and ovaries are to be removed. There are three procedures for an abdominal hysterectomy, named according to the extent of the surgery performed. A **subtotal hysterectomy** refers to the removal of the corpus (the midsection or body) of the uterus and leaves the cervical stump in place. A **total hysterectomy** is the removal of the entire uterus, including the cervix, but leaves the fallopian tubes and ovaries in place. TAH-BSO involves the removal of the entire uterus, the fallopian tubes, and the ovaries.

Nursing Interventions

Preoperative interventions. When the physician has explained the surgery to the patient, the nurse can reinforce the explanation and answer any questions the patient might have. The nurse should encourage verbalization of fears. Additional preoperative instructions are given to help the woman prepare for postoperative recovery. The nurse should instruct the patient how to turn, cough, and deep breathe.

Before a vaginal or abdominal hysterectomy, the colon is emptied to prevent postoperative distention. The patient may be on a low-residue diet for several days preoperatively. Enemas may be given the evening before surgery.

The bladder may be decompressed to prevent trauma during surgery. The indwelling catheter will generally remain in place for 1 or 2 days after surgery.

An antiseptic vaginal douche may be ordered to decrease microbial invasion of the surgical site.

If the surgeon anticipates excessive manipulation of the intestines, a nasogastric tube may be inserted to prevent abdominal distention. The patient should be instructed about the purpose of the tube and that it will be kept in place for a few days after surgery.

Surgical preparation of the skin includes the surgical prepping of the abdomen, pelvis, and perineum. The patient will sign a consent form, and oral intake after midnight will be restricted.

Postoperative interventions. Postoperative nursing interventions focus on monitoring vital signs and preventing urinary retention, intestinal distention, and venous thrombosis. If a retention catheter was inserted, it should be kept patent and connected to closed drainage. Meticulous catheter care is performed to prevent bladder infection. If no retention catheter is in place, the patient is checked frequently for bladder distention; an accurate urine output is recorded. The incidence of urinary retention after a hysterectomy is greater than after any other type of surgery, because some trauma to the bladder unavoidably occurs. If the patient does not have a catheter and is unable to void, catheterization every 8 hours may be necessary. Occasionally the patient will have residual urine. The physician often orders catheterization of the patient to check for residual urine; 50 mL or less is within the normal range.

A small up-and-down flush enema may be ordered to help relieve distention. Early ambulation is very helpful to return the bowel to normal function. When bowel sounds have returned and flatus is being expelled, the patient is allowed liquids by mouth and a gradual return to solid foods.

Patients undergoing pelvic surgery are more susceptible to venous stasis and thrombophlebitis because of trauma to blood vessels. The patient is usually permitted to be out of bed on the first postoperative day, but the nurse should encourage the patient to dangle her legs and to sit on the side of the bed before standing and walking to prevent the effects of postural hypotension. Antiembolic stockings may be used to prevent thrombus or embolus formation, and legs should be exercised frequently when the patient is in bed. Many physicians prescribe the use of intermittent pneumonic compression cuffs for the calves to prevent venous stasis. The patient should avoid bending her knees. This could cause pooling of blood in the pelvic cavity, resulting in stasis in the lower extremities. The patient at risk for thromboembolic disease may receive low-dose heparin to prevent thrombus formation.

Analgesics such as morphine may be ordered for relief of pain. Slight vaginal drainage may occur for 1 or 2 days, but any unusual bleeding should be reported to the physician.

The nurse will observe the abdominal dressing on the patient with an abdominal hysterectomy for evidence of hemorrhage. Surgical asepsis is carried out for the dressing change. The patient usually receives intravenous feedings for several days postoperatively. The rate of flow and the condition of the IV site are carefully monitored.

Nursing diagnoses and interventions for the patient who has had a hysterectomy include but are not limited to the following:

NURSING DIAGNOSES	NURSING INTERVENTIONS
Chronic pain, related to metastatic process	Establish trusting relationship with patient. Monitor and document pain characteristics. Administer prescribed analgesics every 3 to 4 hours to control pain. Provide environment conducive to comfort and rest.
Excess fluid volume, related to ascites	Monitor IV fluids. Maintain accurate I&O. Weigh patient daily. Observe for signs of edema. Measure abdominal girth daily.
Compromised family coping, related to poor prognosis	Assess present coping abilities. Encourage and allow time for verbalization of feelings. Support patient's coping strengths, and discuss alternative coping measures. Involve patient and significant others in nursing interventions and procedures.

Patient Teaching

Before the patient's discharge, the physician will explain to the woman and her partner that there should be no sexual intercourse for 4 to 6 weeks after surgery. If there has been an abdominal incision, there may be further restrictions on heavy lifting (nothing greater than 10 pounds), walking up and down stairs, and prolonged riding in the car. Riding in the car may cause pelvic pooling and development of a thrombus in the legs.

The patient should know that vaginal drainage is normal for about 2 to 4 weeks after an abdominal hysterectomy.

The patient should avoid wearing any tight clothing such as a girdle or knee-high hose, which might constrict circulation to the surgical site and cause venous stasis.

There are several signs and symptoms of infection that should be reported to the physician if they occur: (1) erythema, edema, exudate, or increased tenderness along the surgical incision; (2) increased malodorous vaginal exudate; (3) a temperature of 101° F (38.3° C) or more; and (4) any problems with urinating, such as difficulty in starting to void, voiding too often, voiding small amounts, or a burning sensation while urinating (indicative of a bladder infection).

DISORDERS OF THE FEMALE BREAST

FIBROCYSTIC BREAST CONDITION
Etiology/Pathophysiology

Fibrocystic breast condition involves benign tumors of the breasts, usually occurs in women 30 to 50 years of age, and is rare in postmenopausal women. This suggests that the occurrence is related to ovarian activity.

The cysts are characterized by numerous cellular changes, with an abnormal amount of epithelial hyperplasia and cystic formation within the mammary ducts. The cysts rarely become malignant, but the risk of breast cancer does increase for women who have fibrocystic breast condition; therefore the cysts are observed with great caution.

Clinical Manifestations

Cystic lesions are often bilateral and multiple. The cysts are soft, well-differentiated, tender, and freely movable. The lumpiness and tenderness are more apparent before menses.

Diagnostic Tests

The disorder is diagnosed by mammography or ultrasound and confirmed by biopsy. As a therapeutic measure, the cyst is aspirated by needle and syringe to empty the secretions, and the fluid is sent to the laboratory for cytologic examination. Aspiration produces a turbid, nonhemorrhagic, yellow, greenish, or brownish fluid.

Medical Management

When cysts recur in the same area and repeated aspirations are ineffective, surgical excision of the cyst may be done.

Conservative treatment is the usual approach to fibrocystic breast condition. The usefulness of eliminating methylxanthines (in coffee, tea, and cola) from the diet is still controversial, but it is the least expensive therapy. Many women have reported a lessening of symptoms after altering their diet, even though findings by palpation and mammogram were not significantly changed. Danazol (Danocrine) may be prescribed to inhibit FSH and LH production, thereby decreasing ovarian production of estrogen. Danocrine may cause weight gain, hot flashes, menstrual irregularities, hirsutism, and deepening of the voice. Vitamin E may also be prescribed, but its efficacy has not been proven.

Nursing Interventions and Patient Teaching

The nurse should instruct the patient to perform BSE 1 week after menses and be able to recognize the presence of cysts and note any changes.

ACUTE MASTITIS

Acute mastitis is an acute bacterial infection usually caused by *S. aureus* or streptococci. It is most often observed during lactation and late pregnancy. The infection may result from inadequate cleanliness of the breasts, a nipple fissure, or infection in the infant. The breasts are tender, inflamed, and engorged, causing the milk flow to be obstructed.

Treatment involves application of warm packs, support of the area with a well-fitting brassiere (which also supplies comfort), and systemic treatment with antibiotics.

CHRONIC MASTITIS

Chronic mastitis tends to develop in women between 30 and 50 years of age and is more common in those who have had children, have had difficulty with inverted and cracked nipples, and have had problems with nursing their infants. A traumatic blow to the breasts allows the fat to necrose in the area and form abscesses. There is an increased fibrosis of the tissue, which causes cysts to form. The cysts are tender, painful, and palpable on examination. The disorder is generally unilateral and benign and most frequently occurs in obese women. Treatment is the same as for acute mastitis.

BREAST CANCER

Breast cancer is the most common malignancy affecting women in the United States. Approximately 1 of every 8 women will develop breast cancer during her lifetime. The incidence of breast cancer in men is rare (less than 1%). Among men, there are about 1300 new cases of breast cancer and 400 deaths per year. The American Cancer Society predicted 215,990 women would be diagnosed with breast cancer in 2004 and that 40,580 would die. Breast cancer ranks second among cancer deaths in women (after lung cancer). Women consider this disease their most serious health problem. Older women (those older than 65 years of age) have twice the incidence of breast cancer as women ages 45 to 64. In women older than 55, 50% more patients have metastatic disease at presentation than do younger women. Vital to the process of detection are monthly BSE, breast imaging with mammography and other diagnostic studies to detect small tumors before they can be palpated, and periodic breast examinations by a physician.

Etiology/Pathophysiology

The cause of breast cancer is unknown. The high incidence occurring in women implies hormonal cause (Box 12-6).

The primary risk factors are female gender, age older than 50, North American or Northern European descent, a personal history of breast cancer, atypical hyperplasia or carcinoma in situ, having two or more first-

---

Box 12-6 *Predisposing Factors for Women at High Risk for Breast Cancer*

1. Gender: being a female introduces a high risk.
2. Age: higher incidence occurs with women older than 40 years of age and in the postmenopausal phase of life.
3. Race: white, in the middle or upper socioeconomic class.
4. Genetics: the inherited susceptibility genes *BRCA1* and *BRCA2*, account for approximately 5% of all cases and confer a lifetime risk in these women, ranging from 35% to 85%.
6. Parity (total number of pregnancies): decreased for women if birth is before 18 years; increased for women who are not sexually active, infertile women, and women who become pregnant after 35 years of age.
7. Menopause: menopause after 55 years of age.
8. Other cancer: had another cancer such as endometrial, ovarian, and colon; if cancer has appeared in one breast, it is more likely to occur in the other breast.

---

degree relatives with the disease, and having a first-degree relative with bilateral premenopausal breast cancer. Other risk factors include early menarche, a first pregnancy after age 30, natural menopause after age 55, and having one or more breast cancer genes. The inherited susceptibility genes, *BRCA1* and *BRCA2*, account for approximately 5% of all cases and confer a lifetime risk in these women ranging from 35% to 85% (American Cancer Society, 2004). Recent findings suggest that prophylactic removal of the breasts and/or ovaries in *BRCA1* and *BRCA2* carriers decreases the risk of breast cancer considerably, although not all women who choose this surgery would have developed cancer. Women who consider this option should have an opportunity to undergo counseling before reaching a decision (American Cancer Society, 2004). Whether or not estrogen therapy is a risk factor for the disease remains controversial. Results of a recent study are suggestive that women who are overweight are more likely to die from breast cancer. Current data indicate tamoxifen and raloxifene decrease breast cancer risk in women who are at increased risk (American Cancer Society, 2004). With the exception of advancing age and being female, though, most women who develop breast cancer do not have any risk factors for the disease. That is why it is so important to encourage even healthy women to undergo screening examinations.

Breast cancer is usually an adenocarcinoma, arising from the epithelium and developing in the lactiferous ducts; it infiltrates the parenchyma (the tissue of an organ other than the supporting or connective tissue). The cancer occurs most often in the upper outer quadrants of the breasts of women who have not given birth

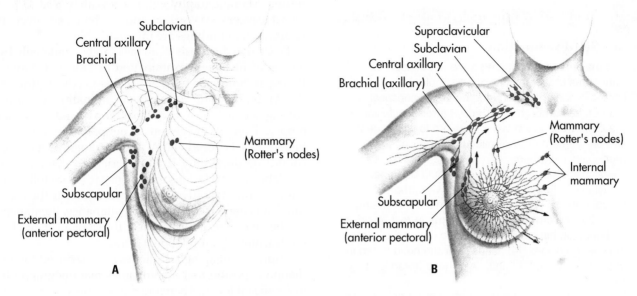

FIGURE **12-15 A,** Lymph nodes of the axilla. **B,** Lymphatic drainage of the breast.

or breastfed a child. A slow-growing breast cancer may take up to 8 or 9 years to become palpable or to have reached the size of a small pea. Metastasis is by the lymphatic system and bloodstream (Figure 12-15). The most common sites for metastasis are, in order: bones, lungs, pleura, breast site, central nervous system, and liver. When referring to estimated growth rate of breast cancer, the term "doubling time" indicates the time it takes malignant cells to double in number. Assuming that the doubling is constant and that the neoplasm originates in one cell, a carcinoma with a doubling time of 100 days may not reach clinically detectable size (1 cm) for 8 years. Rapid-growing cancers have a much shorter preclinical course and a greater tendency to metastasize to regional nodes or more distant sites by the time a breast mass is discovered.

Clinical Manifestations

Breast tumors are usually small, solitary, irregularly shaped, firm, nontender, and nonmobile. There may be a change in skin color, feelings of tenderness, puckering or dimpling (peau d'orange—skin appearance of an orange-peel) of tissue, nipple discharge, retraction of the nipple, and axillary tenderness.

More than 90% of breast cancers are detected by the patient. BSEs should be performed at monthly intervals, preferably 1 week after menses. BSE for postmenopausal women should be done on the same day each month (Figure 12-16). If there are questionable findings, the patient should immediately contact her physician (Health Promotion Considerations box).

Diagnostic Tests

The essential factors in the early detection of breast cancer are the regular performance of BSE, regular clinical breast examination (CBE), and routine mam-

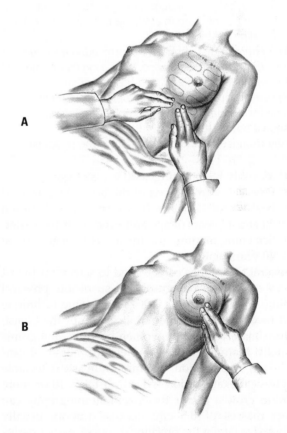

FIGURE **12-16** Methods for palpation. **A,** Back and forth. **B,** Concentric circles.

mography. The frequency of these examinations is determined by the woman's age, the presence of significant risk factors, and her past medical history. Current guidelines accepted by the American Cancer Society regarding breast surveillance practices include the following.

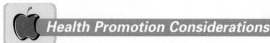

Breast Self-Examination

1. The majority of breast lumps are not cancer.
2. Cancerous breast lesions are treatable.
3. Breasts should be examined by premenopausal women each month, 7 or 8 days after conclusion of the menstrual period when they are least congested, and on the same day of each month for post-menopausal women.
4. Visual inspection and palpation should be done.
5. Visual inspection should be done when the woman is stripped to the waist and looking in a mirror, using the following arm positions: (1) arms at rest at sides, (2) hands on hips and pressed into hips, (3) contracting chest muscles, (4) hands over the head (torso in upright position), (5) hands over head (torso leaning forward).
6. Palpation may be done in the shower when the soap and water assist the hands to glide over the skin. However, the examination of large breasts and axillae is better done in a supine position rather than a standing position.
7. The entire breast should be examined in a systematic way, moving clockwise, with a circular motion. Always include the axillae in the examination.
8. Specific examination of the nipple, through compression for discharge, and the areola, through palpation, should not be forgotten.
9. Any changes should be reported to the physician.

- Monthly BSE starting at 20 years of age.
- Physical examinations of the breast by a trained health professional; CBE every 3 years between 20 and 40 years of age and every year thereafter.
- Screening mammography annually beginning at 40 years of age.

Several techniques can be used to screen for breast disease or provide a diagnosis of a suspicious physical finding. Mammography is a radiographic technique used to visualize the internal structure of the breast. Approximately 2 million women have mammograms annually. Mammography can detect tumors that cannot be felt by palpation. The minimum size detectable by physical examination is 1 cm. It takes 10 or more years to grow a tumor this size. Mammography can detect masses of 0.5 cm. Because tumors usually metastasize late in the preclinical course, earlier detection by mammography may prevent metastasis of these smaller lesions.

Comparative mammography may show early cancer tissue changes. The diagnostic accuracy of mammography in combination with physical examination has significantly improved early and accurate detection of breast malignancies. In younger women, mammography is less sensitive because of the greater density of breast tissue, resulting in more false-negative results. Mammography will not reveal 10% to 25% of breast cancers. Masses should be biopsied, even if mammogram findings are unremarkable.

Definitive diagnosis of a mass can be made only by means of histologic examination of biopsied tissues. Biopsy technique may be either fine-needle aspiration (FNA) biopsy and cytologic examination or core-cutting needle biopsy, excisional biopsy, and incisional biopsy. Even if the lesion is nonpalpable, an FNA biopsy can be used. FNA and cytologic evaluation should be done only if an experienced cytologist is available and all lesions read as negative are followed with a more definitive biopsy procedure. If the aspirated specimen is positive for malignancy, the patient can be given this information at the same visit and begin learning about treatment issues.

Improved imaging techniques have reduced the radiation exposure that accompanies mammography to insignificant levels. Therefore the benefits of mammography outweigh the risks from radiation exposure. Ultrasound (echogram, sonogram) is another diagnostic procedure that can be used to differentiate a benign cyst (fluid-filled) from a malignant mass (solid). An ultrasound will not detect microcalcifications, which are often the only indicators of very small tumors.

Other methods that are used to help diagnose and stage breast cancer include magnetic resonance imaging (MRI) and positron emission tomography (PET). MRI and PET scans are used to help differentiate between malignant and benign disease in select patients.

A relatively new diagnostic tool used prior to therapeutic surgery is sentinel lymph node mapping, which identifies the first lymph node most likely to drain the cancerous cells. During this procedure a radioactive substance is injected around the breast biopsy site. The patient is then sent to the operating room (OR), where a blue dye is injected as well. The area is then monitored to see which nodes take up the substances. The node that "lights up," containing the most radioactivity and blue dye, is considered the sentinel node and the one most likely to contain cancer cells. The identified node and at least two other nodes are then biopsied to see if they contain tumor cells. If they do not, it is likely that the more distant axillary nodes are cancer free and can be left intact. This reduces the threat of complications that can occur when all the axillary lymph nodes are removed—edema, infection, pain, and loss of function of the arm. Sentinel lymph node dissection has been associated with lower morbidity rates and greater accuracy as compared with complete axillary node dissection. National clinical research trials are evaluating whether standard lymph node dissection can be avoided if sentinel lymph node dissection is performed (Lewis et al, 2004).

Axillary lymph node involvement is one of the most important prognostic factors in early-stage breast cancer. The presence of metastasis in axillary nodes can be determined by pathologic examination of as few as 6 to 10 nodes. The more nodes involved, the greater the risk of recurrence. Patients with four or more positive nodes have the greatest risk of recurrence.

Another diagnostic test useful both for treatment decisions and prediction of prognosis is estrogen and progesterone receptor status. Receptor-positive tumors commonly (1) show evidence of being well differentiated (see Box 17-3); (2) frequently have a more normal DNA content and low proliferation; (3) have a lower chance for recurrence, and (4) are frequently hormone dependent and responsive to hormonal therapy. Receptor-negative tumors (1) are often poorly differentiated, (2) have a high incidence of abnormal DNA content and high proliferation, (3) frequently recur, and (4) are usually unresponsive to hormonal therapy (Lewis et al, 2004).

Medical Management

The intervention for treatment of breast cancer depends on the stage of the tumor, the age and health status of the patient, the hormonal status, and the presence of estrogen receptors in the tumor. Radiation, chemotherapy, and surgery alone or in combination are the most common modes of treatment of cancer of the breasts (see Chapter 17).

Staging. After breast surgery and axillary dissection, the staging process is completed. Axillary lymph node dissection is usually performed regardless of the treatment option selected. Examination of nodes provides the most powerful prognostic data currently available. Also, removal of axillary nodes is highly effective in preventing axillary recurrence, aids in decision making regarding adjuvant chemotherapy or hormonal therapy, and eliminates the need for axillary nodal radiation. Radiation of the axilla is equally effective in decreasing the incidence of axillary recurrence (see Figure 12-15).

The most widely accepted staging method for breast cancer is the American Joint Committee on Cancer's TNM system. This system uses tumor size (T), nodal involvement (N), and presence of metastasis (M) to determine the stage of disease (Box 12-7).

Staging depends on the size of the tumor, size and presence or absence of any nodal malignancy, and the presence or absence of distant metastasis. Tumors are classified from stage I to stage IV.

Surgical intervention. Surgery plays a vital role in the management of breast cancer. Tissue biopsy, inspection and biopsy of lymph nodes in the axillary areas, radiologic examinations, and laboratory reports are aids in making the decision that surgery should be performed.

Because estrogen can affect a tumor's invasive ability, some researchers suggest operating on premenopausal women during the menstrual phase, when estrogen levels are lower or opposed by progesterone.

Box 12-7 | *TNM System*

HOW BREAST CANCER IS STAGED

Breast cancer is staged using the TNM (tumor, node, metastasis) system which categorizes the disease by tumor size and spread, lymph node involvement and metastasis. The TNM system, which was developed by the American Joint Committee on Cancer (AJCC) and revised in 2003, works this way.

Tumor. A number from **0** to **4** indicates the tumor's size and whether it has spread to nearby tissue. (**Tis** indicates a carcinoma in situ.) Higher numbers indicate a larger tumor or wider spread. For example, a tumor labeled **T1** is 2 cm or smaller, **T4** indicates a tumor of any size that has spread to the chest wall or the skin.

Nodes. A number from **0** to **3** indicates whether the cancer has spread to surrounding lymph nodes and, if so, the number of nodes that are affected. For example, **N1** indicates a spread to 1, 2, or 3 lymph nodes under the arm on the same side as the breast cancer.

Metastasis. **M0** means the cancer has not spread to distant organs; **M1** means the cancer has metastasized to other organs.

All of this information is combined to determine an overall stage of **0** to **IV**.

Stage 0: Refers to carcinoma in situ, in which the tumor is confined to the milk duct or the lobule, no nodes have been affected, and no metastasis has occurred.

Stage I: The tumor is 2 cm or smaller. Lymph nodes are negative. There is no distant cancer spread.

Stage IIA: The tumor is 5 cm or smaller. It may have spread to 1, 2, or 3 axillary nodes. There is no distant cancer spread.

Stage IIB: The tumor can be larger than 5 cm. Up to three lymph nodes may be involved, but there is no metastasis to other organs.

Stage IIIA: The tumor may be more than 5 cm and has spread to more than 3 but fewer than 10 lymph nodes. No distant organs are involved.

Stage IIIB: The tumor, regardless of size, has spread to the chest wall or the skin. There is lymph node involvement but no distant metastasis.

Stage IIIC: Refers to any size tumor, including one that has spread to the chest wall or the skin. There is involvement of 10 or more lymph nodes, but no distant metastasis.

Stage IV: The tumor can be any size. There is nodal involvement and metastasis to distant organs.

American Cancer Society and National Comprehensive Cancer Network. "Breast Cancer. Treatment guidelines for patients." 2003. www.cancer.org/docroot/CRI/content/CRI_2_NCCN_Breast_Cancer_Treatment_Guidelines_for_Patients_2003.asp?sitearea=CRI (12 2003); Lewis, S.M. et al. (2004). *Medical-surgical nursing: assessment and management of clinical problems.* (6th ed.). St. Louis: Mosby.

Several surgical approaches may be selected for the removal of the breast carcinoma. Approaches may include the following:

- **Breast conservation surgery** (termed **lumpectomy),** which conserves the breast, is the removal of a circumscribed area along with the tumor. This surgery is usually done when the tumor is small and located on the peripheral area of the breast. The breast contour and muscle support are preserved if possible. Research has shown that there is no survival advantage in taking the whole breast when the malignancy is confined to just one area and its size is less than 2 cm—as long as adjunctive radiation to the surrounding region, ending with a radiation boost to the tumor bed, is done to destroy any remaining microscopic disease. Axillary nodes are often removed in these breast-sparing procedures as well. Contraindications to lumpectomy or excisional biopsy include two or more separate tumors in separate quadrants of the breast, diffuse microcalcifications, a history of previous radiation to the region, a large tumor-to-breast ratio, a history of collagen vascular disease, large breasts, and a tumor located underneath the nipple. One of the main advantages of breast conservation surgery and radiation is that it preserves the breast, including the nipple. The goal of the combined surgery and radiation is to maximize the benefits of both cancer treatment and cosmetic outcome while minimizing risks. Disadvantages of this surgery include the increased cost of the surgery plus radiation over surgery alone and the possible side effects of radiation. Lumpectomy is followed by 6 or 7 weeks of radiation (Greifzu, 2004).

- A **partial mastectomy** is another form of segmental mastectomy in which the quadrant of the breast in which the tumor is located is removed. In most instances, axillary nodes are dissected through a separate incision. Surgery aimed at augmentation may later be required, because partial mastectomies can be disfiguring.

- A **simple mastectomy** is the removal of the entire breast. The skin flap is retained to cover the incised area. Both pectoralis major and pectoralis minor muscles are left intact. The patient has the option of breast recontruction.

- A **modified radical mastectomy** may be performed when the tumor is 4 cm or larger, if it is invasive, or if the patient and physician decide this procedure is in the patient's best interest. In this operation all breast tissue, overlying skin, nipple, and pectoralis minor muscles are removed, as are samples of axillary lymph nodes, and fascia under the breast. The pectoralis major muscle remains intact. When a modified radical mastectomy is performed, the patient has the option of breast reconstruction. If the patient chooses to have reconstructive surgery, it can be performed immediately following the mastectomy or it can be delayed until postoperative recovery is complete (about 6 months). Most women diagnosed with early-stage breast cancer (tumors less than 5 cm) are candidates for either lumpectomy and radiation or modified radical mastectomy. Overall 10-year survival with lumpectomy and radiation is about the same as with modified radical mastectomy.

Adjuvant therapies

Radiation therapy. Depending on the size of the tumor, its regional spread, and its aggressiveness, lumpectomy or modified radical mastectomy will be followed by radiation therapy. The three situations in which radiation therapy may be used for breast cancer are (1) as the primary therapy to destroy the tumor or as a companion to surgery to prevent local recurrence; (2) to shrink a large tumor to operable size; and (3) as the palliative treatment for pain caused by local recurrence and metastasis. Lumpectomy is almost always followed by radiation. Radiation therapy is usually started 2 to 3 weeks after surgery, when the wound is completely healed and the patient can comfortably raise her arm over her head. Contraindications include a diagnosis of breast cancer during the first or second trimester of pregnancy, delayed wound healing, collagen vascular disease, and previous radiation to the same breast.

In *external beam radiation,* the actual radiation procedure uses an external beam of high-energy protons. The treatments are usually done 5 days a week for a total of 5 to 6 weeks. Adverse effects include fatigue and skin reactions such as burning, erythema, pruritus, dryness, infection, and pain.

Internal radiation, also known as implant radiation or *brachytherapy,* is now used in breast cancer. High-dose brachytherapy is a new procedure that is an alternative stage to traditional radiation treatment for early-stage breast cancer. The technique uses a balloon catheter to insert radioactive seeds into the breast after the tumor is removed. The seeds deliver a concentrated dose of radiation directly to the site where the cancer is most likely to recur. Traditional radiation treatment can take 6 weeks; in contrast, high-dose brachytherapy may require only 5 days (Greifzu, 2004; Lewis et al, 2004).

Chemotherapy. Patients who require postsurgical chemotherapy—typically those with lymph node involvement or metastasis to distant organs—will receive antineoplastic medications, hormones, a monoclonal antibody, or a combination of these medications. Regimens for node-negative disease (i.e., cancer that has not spread to the lymph nodes) include cyclophosphamide (Cytoxan, Neosar), methotrexate, and 5-fluorouracil

(Adrucil, Efudex), referred to as CMF; cyclophosphamide, doxorubicin (Adriamycin), and 5-fluorouracil, or CAF; and doxorubicin and cyclophosphamide, commonly called AC. For those with node-positive disease, the regimens include CAF, AC followed by paclitaxel (Taxol), doxorubicin followed by CMF, and CMF.

The most common adverse effects of traditional antineoplastic drugs are bone marrow suppression (which causes anemia, thrombocytopenia, and leukopenia), nausea and vomiting, alopecia, weight gain, mucositis, and fatigue. Agents such as filgrastim (Neupogen), which raise leukocyte counts, can combat the threat of infection that accompanies bone marrow suppressions. Epoetin alfa (Procrit) is helpful in raising erythrocyte counts to help correct anemia. Other drugs typically ordered for chemotherapy patients are phenothiazines, such as prochlorperazine (Compazine) and serotonin antagonists such as granisetron (Kytril) and ondansetron (Zofran). These drugs prevent or lessen nausea and vomiting (Greifzu, 2004).

Hormonal therapy. Estrogen can promote the growth of breast cancer cells if the cells are estrogen-receptor positive. Hormonal therapy removes or blocks the source of estrogen, thus promoting tumor regressions.

Two advances have increased the use of hormone therapy in breast cancer. First, hormone receptor assays, which are reliable diagnostic tests, have been developed to identify women who are likely to respond to hormone therapy. Both estrogen and progesterone receptor status of the tumor can be determined. The importance of these assays is their ability to predict whether hormonal therapy is a treatment option for women with breast cancer, either at the time of initial therapy or if the cancer recurs. Second, drugs have been developed that can inactivate the hormone-secreting glands as effectively as surgery or radiation. Premenopausal and perimenopausal women are more likely to have tumors that are not hormone dependent, whereas women who are postmenopausal are more likely to have hormone-dependent tumors. Chances of tumor regression are significantly greater in women whose tumors contain estrogen and progesterone receptors.

Estrogen deprivation can occur by destroying the ovaries by surgery or radiation or drug therapy. Hormonal therapy can block or destroy the estrogen receptors. Hormonal therapy is widely used to treat recurrent or metastatic cancer but may also be used as an adjuvant to primary treatment.

Tamoxifen (Nolvadex) is the hormonal agent of choice in postmenopausal, estrogen receptor–positive women with or without lymph node involvement. Tamoxifen, an antiestrogen drug, blocks the estrogen receptor sites of malignant cells and thus inhibits the growth-stimulating effects of estrogen. It is commonly used in advanced and early-stage breast cancer to pre-

vent or treat recurrent disease. Tamoxifen may also be used to prevent breast cancer in high-risk individuals. Side effects of tamoxifen are minimal but include hot flashes, nausea, vomiting, vaginal discharge, and other effects commonly associated with decreased estrogen. It also increases the risk of blood clots, cataracts, and endometrial cancer in postmenopausal women.

Toremifene (Fareston), an antiestrogen agent similar to tamoxifen, is indicated as first-line treatment for metastatic breast cancer in postmenopausal women with estrogen receptor–positive or estrogen receptor–unknown tumors.

Fulvestrant (Faslodex) may be given to women with advanced breast cancer who no longer respond to tamoxifen. This drug slows cancer progression by destroying estrogen receptors in the breast cancer cells. Fulvestrant is given intramuscularly on a monthly basis.

Aromatase inhibitor drugs, which interfere with the enzyme that synthesizes endogenous estrogen, are used to treat advanced breast cancer in postmenopausal women with disease progression. These drugs include anastrozole(Arimidex), letrozole (Femara), vorozole (Rizivor), exemestane (Aromasin), and aminogluthethimide (Cytadren).

Research has shown that letrozole (Femara) reduced the risk of recurrence of breast cancer among women by 43%. The women in the letrozole study had recently completed (after surgery) the standard 5-year course of tamoxifen, a powerful and widely used drug that eventually loses its effectiveness as, researchers believe, tumors become resistant to it. Until now, breast cancer patients who finished tamoxifen treatment could only wait and hope that their cancer wouldn't recur, which it does within 5 years, in up to 20% of such cases. Letrozole, previously approved by the FDA for advanced breast cancer, offers an exciting new option for extending treatment of early-stage disease. Letrozole, like tamoxifen, works by interfering with the hormone estrogen, which feeds breast cancer cells: tamoxifen blocks estrogen receptors on the cells, whereas letrozole inhibits the creation of estrogen. Bisphosphonates, such as pamidronate sodium (Aredia) are being used to delay bone metastases and reduce the occurrence of skeletal problems in patients with advanced breast cancer (Greifzu, 2004).

Raloxifen (Evista), used to prevent bone loss, may also reduce the risk of breast cancer without stimulating endometrial growth. Raloxifen acts as an estrogen antagonist at the hormone-sensitive tissues of breast cancer and bone. Additional drugs that may be used to suppress hormone-dependent tumors include megestrol (Megace), diethylstilbestrol (DES), and fluoxymesterone (Halotestin) (Lewis et al, 2004).

Monoclonal antibody therapy. A recent drug treatment for breast cancer is the monoclonal antibody trastuzumab (Herceptin). It is used to treat metastatic

NURSING CARE PLAN

The Patient Undergoing Modified Radical Mastectomy

Ms. C., age 52, was diagnosed with ductal cell carcinoma of the left breast. She has undergone a left modified radical mastectomy

NURSING DIAGNOSIS *Fear, related to the cancer diagnosis and surgical intervention.*

Patient Goals/Expected Outcomes	Nursing Intervention	Evaluation
Patient will be able to state fears. Patient will be able to state a positive improvement in coping.	Encourage patient to talk about specific fears and feelings about each fear. Provide a calm supportive environment. Provide information on coping mechanisms. Encourage consultation with resource persons (psychologist, clergy, nurse specialist, Reach to Recovery). Use support of family and significant others. Encourage use of comfort measures, such as music. Encourage patient's comments and questions about surgery and postoperative care.	Patient verbalizes fear, has support of significant others, and expresses confidence in ability to cope.

NURSING DIAGNOSIS *Infection, risk for, related to surgical incision and presence of drain.*

Patient Goals/Expected Outcomes	Nursing Intervention	Evaluation
Skin will remain free of signs and symptoms of infection. Vital signs and WBC values will be maintained within normal limits.	Assess skin integrity. Instruct on signs and symptoms of infection. Assess and report abnormal vital signs and elevated WBC; skin changes; and comfort level. Observe and record amount of exudate. Check drainage tubing for patency. Instruct patient to examine remaining breast once a month. Caution patient to avoid injections, vaccinations, taking of BP, taking of blood samples, or insertion of IV line in affected area.	Incision is without erythema or purulent drainage. Temperature remains within normal. WBC remains normal.

breast cancer in women who overexpress (i.e., have an excess amount of) a breast cancer cell antigen called HER2. Up to 30% of patients fall into this category.

Ovarian ablation. Another promising treatment option is **ovarian ablation** by means of a bilateral oophorectomy, which is used in combination with tamoxifen for metastatic disease.

Bone marrow and stem cell transplantation. Autologous (i.e., originating within self) bone marrow or stem cell transplantation combined with high-dose chemotherapy has been used to treat patients with advanced metastatic breast cancer. In this technique, patients donate their own bone marrow or peripheral blood, from which stem cells are harvested. Then they receive high doses of chemotherapy, which causes bone marrow suppression. The patient subsequently undergoes autologous bone marrow or stem cell transplantation to reconstitute or "rescue" their hematopoietic system to start producing hematopoietic blood cells.

Nursing Interventions

The physician will discuss with the patient and family the rationale for the specific surgical approach and the manner of coping with the cosmetic effects of and psychological response to the surgery. Patients will have questions about possible alternatives to standard or modified mastectomy.

The patient may be confused with so many options of therapy and surgical interventions. During this time the nurse plays an active role as listener and reinforcer of information provided by the physician and as a provider of responses that can encourage and assist the patient to verbalize her concerns and recognize her feelings about the surgery. The emotional preparation of the patient may be more important than the physical preparation. Often there is anticipatory grieving for the loss of a body part.

Preoperative preparation enlists the participation of patient, support group, and nursing staff so that progressive care can run continuously from admission

NURSING CARE PLAN

The Patient Undergoing Modified Radical Mastectomy—cont'd

NURSING DIAGNOSIS *Body image, disturbed, related to loss of breast through modified radical mastectomy.*

Patient Goals/Expected Outcomes	Nursing Intervention	Evaluation
Patient will verbalize acceptance of altered body image as evidenced by absence of weeping, irritability, verbalization of discomfort with present body, and the attempting of difficult physical or mental tasks despite limitations. Patient demonstrates interest in her personal appearance. Patient will verbalize plans to resume former activities.	Encourage patient's comments and questions about surgery, progress, and prognosis. Encourage patient to discuss change in her body with husband or significant other. Reinforce correct information, and provide factual information to correct any misconceptions. Relate importance of communicating anything that causes anxiety. Encourage patient to verbalize and explore feelings regarding impact missing body part might have on patient's functioning as a sexual partner and in ADLs. Encourage a patient to continue activities associated with femininity, such as fixing hair, using makeup, and wearing own apparel. Encourage patient to look at and touch the changed body part when she demonstrates readiness. Encourage use of rehabilitation services (Reach to Recovery, Wellness Community).	Patient verbalizes feelings about surgery and change in body image; indicates beginning resolution of negative feelings toward self; begins to accept altered body image.

? CRITICAL THINKING QUESTIONS

1. Ms. C. confides in her nurse that she feels ugly and unattractive and refuses to look at her incision. A helpful approach by the nurse could include:
2. In assessing Ms. C., the nurse notes her holding her left arm guardedly in an adducted position.

She does not use it for ADLs. Effective patient teaching would include:
3. Discharge teaching for Ms. C. to prevent trauma and infection of her left arm would include:

---

through surgery, recovery, and the postoperative period. The initial admission assessment provides data that are helpful in planning care by the nurse and patient. Nursing diagnoses can be developed and a plan of care individualized for the patient according to her needs (Nursing Care Plan box).

It is important for the nurse to assess and identify the members of the patient's support system to know their strengths and concerns about the pending treatment and interventions. Support does not always need to come from the immediate family and close circle of friends. Outside support and resources can come from coworkers, religious groups, oncology clinicians, psychologists, and Reach to Recovery support groups. It is important to openly discuss the patient's fears, and this is often done by the nurse who has established a therapeutic relationship with the patient and family.

Reach to Recovery volunteers have been a source of information, encouragement, and support for women with breast cancer. The organization is based on the premise that rehabilitation for a woman with breast cancer should include communication with and support from another who has shared a similar situation and who has learned to cope and resume her normal activities.

Nursing interventions for patients who undergo modified radical mastectomy include monitoring vital signs and observing for symptoms of shock or hemorrhage, since many large blood vessels are involved in the procedure. Drains such as Jackson-Pratt, Davol, or Hemovac may be placed in the axilla to facilitate drainage and prevent formation of a hematoma. Postoperative dressings are usually constrictive and bulky and may tend to embarrass respiratory effort as well as cause pain and discomfort. When the vital signs are stable, the patient is placed in a 45-degree Fowler's position to promote drainage. The position should be changed frequently, and deep breathing and coughing are encouraged.

Some patients may experience incisional pain for several days after surgery and when doing arm exercises. There may be complaints of numbness and referred pain in the arm of the operative area. The pain radiates to the shoulder and the back because of the severance of the peripheral nerves. Most of the nerves regenerate, but there are cases of residual numbness.

No matter what type of surgery the patient has, pain management and wound care will be priorities. Typically a patient will have a PCA pump with morphine for 12 to 24 hours. She will then receive oral analgesics as needed.

Patient Teaching

It is important for the patient to deep breathe and cough to prevent postoperative atelectasis.

Physicians differ in opinion about the best positioning of the affected arm. Some physicians place the affected arm in the dressing and place it in a sling for a couple of days postoperatively. Some physicians believe slings should be avoided. If the arm is not restricted by dressings, it may be elevated on a pillow with the hand and wrist higher than the elbow and the elbow higher than the shoulder joint. This will facilitate the flow of fluids through the lymph and venous routes and prevent lymphedema.

Usually the patient is allowed to ambulate on the first postoperative day. Assistance to move out of bed will be needed to have the patient learn to maintain balance because of breast removal and bulky dressings. If the surgical intervention was a modified radical mastectomy, defense mechanisms are lessened by the removal of lymph nodes.

Patients should be taught not to have any procedures involving the arm on the affected side—BP readings, injections, intravenous infusion of fluids, or the drawing of blood, which may cause edema or infection—and to guard against infections from burns, needle pricks (sewing), and gardening injuries. Removing lymph nodes and channels increases the risk of developing lymphedema, even years after surgery. Referral to physical therapy may be indicated to control lymphedema if it develops. An exercise regimen, built up gradually, can help decrease lymphedema. However, exercise should not be started until the incision has healed completely, which takes up to 2 weeks. Tell the patient to avoid lifting heavy objects with the affected arm for 6 to 8 weeks (Greifzu, 2004). The patient should be instructed to avoid sleeping on the involved arm. Clothing on the affected arm should be nonconstricting. Bracelets and watches should be worn on the unaffected arm (Box 12-8).

The longer the edema persists, the more difficult it is to manage. Diuretics and low-sodium diets are often prescribed. If the edema persists, an elastic stockinette is measured for precise fit to avoid venous flow constriction. The sleeve is applied from the wrist to the shoulder and worn when the patient is out of bed. When the patient is sleeping, the arm is positioned to aid venous flow. If the lymphedema is severe, the physician may order Jobst extremity therapy. There is an automatic inflation and deflation of a pneumomassage sleeve that can be placed on the arm. The compression pump is strictly contraindicated when there

---

Box 12-8   *Hand and Arm Care after Breast Surgery*

1. Prevention of infection:
   a. Wear gloves when cleaning with harsh detergent.
   b. Wear gloves when gardening.
   c. Avoid injections, vaccinations, and venipuncture in involved arm.
   d. Use cuticle remover in preference to cutting cuticles.
   e. Sew with a thimble.
   f. Avoid chapped hands; use lanolin cream daily.
   g. Take care when using equipment that might cut, scrape, or abrade.
   h. Shave underarms with an electric razor.
   i. Avoid insect bites; use insect repellent.
2. Prevention of constricting circulation:
   a. Do not take blood pressure in involved arm.
   b. Wear loose clothing; avoid tight bra straps or tight sleeves.
   c. Wear watch or jewelry on uninvolved arm.
   d. Carry purse on uninvolved arm or shoulder.
3. Prevention of burns:
   a. Wear padded mitts to reach into oven; use potholders.
   b. Prevent sunburn; use sunscreens with SPF of 15; cover arms during prolonged exposure.
4. Prevention of drag or pull:
   a. Carry heavy packages on uninvolved arm.
   b. Avoid motions that increase centrifugal force.
5. Immediately report any signs of erythema, edema, warmth, or pain.

---

is evidence of acute phlebitis, perivascular lymphangitis, or cellulitis.

Isometric exercises are helpful for increasing the circulation and development of the collateral lymph system. Opening and clenching fingers and squeezing a rubber ball can be started in the first few postoperative days. This activity provides extension and flexion of the wrist and elbow; it is equivalent to sewing, knitting, typing, and playing piano when at home.

Preventing muscle contractures. Specific exercises may be ordered to restore the muscle strength and full range of motion of the affected area. Gentle exercises started early in the postoperative course help to decrease muscle tension and to regain muscle function more quickly. The nurse or the therapist should instruct the patient and encourage the continuation of the exercises on discharge. Many of the exercises may be incorporated into ADLs as normal daily tasks are resumed (Figure 12-17; Box 12-9).

Exercising can be painful but can be accepted as a challenge by the patient with a support group encouraging her. The challenge can be met and the results of muscular strengthening achieved.

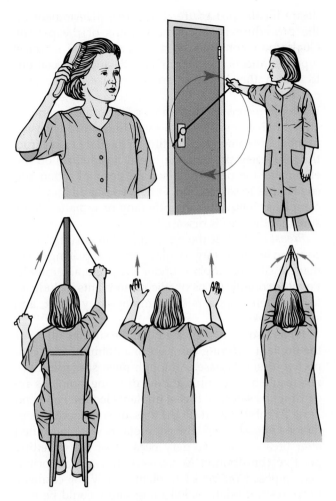

FIGURE **12-17** Exercises after mastectomy.

Body image acceptance. After losing a breast, many patients experience grief over the loss of a body part. This acute grief is like a crisis and may last 4 to 6 weeks or longer. Grief makes the fact of loss real. The process of grieving is essential for personal adaptation to the loss. The nurse can assist the patient to find helpful coping mechanisms.

Initial coping mechanisms often begin to lose effectiveness at about 3 months, and a period of depression ensues. It is important that the nurse provide anticipatory guidance for this eventuality. Special nursing interventions, in terms of both psychological support and self-care education, are necessary if a recurrence of cancer is found. Participation in a cancer support group is important and has been found to have a clinically significant impact on survival.

When deep breathing exercises are started immediately after surgery and the patient has been able to splint the area, as well as exercise her arm, the woman will recognize the absence of the breast through touch. Dressing changes and incision cleansing with patient involvement make the absence real. Being involved and responsible for the dressing and incision allows a more personal approach to the patient. At this time, support by the nurse is very important. The nurse can provide a mirror or seat the patient in front of the mirror so the patient can see the operative site being cleansed and dressed. The nurse must be very sensitive to the patient and be alert for signs of readiness by the patient to become involved in care and acceptance of the loss of the body part. The incisional area may be erythematous and edematous, but the discoloration

---

Box 12-9 | *Postmastectomy Arm Exercises*

EXERCISE: CLIMBING THE WALL

1. Stand facing wall with toes 6 to 12 inches from wall.
2. Bend elbows and place palms of hands against wall at shoulder level.
3. Move both hands parallel to each other up the wall as far as possible until incisional pull or pain occurs.
4. Move both hands down to starting position.
5. Goal is complete extension with elbows straight.
6. Activities that use the same action: reaching top shelves, hanging out clothes, washing windows, hanging curtains, setting hair.

EXERCISE: ELBOW PULL-IN

1. Extend arms sideways to shoulder level.
2. Clasp hands behind neck.
3. Pull elbows forward until they touch.
4. Return to position 2.
5. Unclasp hands and extend arms sideways at shoulder level.
6. Lower arms to side.

EXERCISE: BACK SCRATCH

1. Place hand of unoperated side on hip for balance.
2. Bend elbow of affected arm, placing back of hand on small of back.
3. Work hand up the back slowly until fingers reach opposite shoulder blade.
4. Lower arm and straighten both arms.

EXERCISE: ROPE PULL

1. Attach a rope over a shower rod, hook, or over top of an open door.
2. Sit on a chair (with door between legs if using a door) and grasp each end of rope.
3. Alternately pull on each end, raising affected arm to a point of incisional pull or pain.
4. The goal is to raise the affected arm almost directly overhead.

will gradually lessen and the site will become more comfortable. The patient should be encouraged to apply and massage in cocoa butter or a cream to make the incisional line softer. The patient should be counseled that it takes time to accept the loss and heal both emotionally and physically.

Prosthesis. A breast prosthesis should not be worn unless authorized by the physician. There are many breast forms available. Forms are made of gels, molded silicone, and saline solution. Most forms are covered with soft fabric, are lightweight, and feel like breast tissue. In selecting a breast form there is a shape for each type of breast, because each body is different and each surgery is different. Forms have been developed that can be fitted for a right or left breast, slanted for the breast that was slanted, or formed with an outer curve that simulates the extension of a full breast under the axilla and upward on the chest. It is advisable to have a skilled fitter from a reliable company fit the prosthesis.

A well-fitted brassiere is essential before choosing the shape form. If the woman is very active and desires a pocket or restraining cup, the brassiere needs to be equipped for it. Brassieres can be purchased with these adaptations. Some available forms can be worn against the skin with no underpadding or bra cups. Most forms can be washed with water and mild detergent to keep the form clean and supple. Many prostheses are waterproof and can be worn swimming; when wet they do not "weigh down" the wearer.

When the patient is being fitted with a prosthesis, the best assurance that the fit is right is when each of the following is observed:
- The brassiere fits snugly around the rib cage.
- The prosthesis fills the bottom of the bra cup.
- The prosthesis projects the same as the remaining breast, with form bulk and nipples in position.
- The breasts are separated when the bra is centered.
- The top of the bra cup is filled and appears like the other breast.

Breast Reconstruction

The patient whose disease is limited to the breast may benefit from reconstructive surgery. The benefits of breast reconstruction include avoidance of an external prosthesis that has potential for slipping, greater choice of clothing (including lower necklines), and loss of self-consciousness about appearance. For many women, breast reconstruction is beneficial in improving self-esteem. Breast reconstruction can produce psychological benefits and provide many women with a renewed sense of wholeness and a return to a normal state. The most important indicators for reconstruction are the patient's motivation and

desire for the procedure. The prime determinant for the procedure is the clinical status of the patient. Goals for reconstruction are to select the simplest type that meets the patient's needs and expectations to match the opposite breast in size, shape, and contour.

Breast reconstruction can be performed immediately after surgery or at a later time. An increasing number of women are electing immediate reconstruction; this may prolong the initial hospitalization but eliminates the need for a second hospitalization and contributes to self-esteem. Others wait until they have completed adjuvant chemotherapy or radiation to be sure that the area is disease free.

Breast implant. If the remaining skin is sufficient to cover an implant, surgery may consist of placing a permanent silicone implant under the pectoralis muscle. Possible complications of silicone implants include infection, deflation, a false mammography result, and silicone leaks.

It has also been suggested that the silicone filling or the implant covering can lead to autoimmune or connective tissue disease. Although most surgeries have not resulted in complications, differing opinions regarding the safety of breast implants led the Food and Drug Administration (FDA) to issue some recommendations in early 1992. Breast implants were permitted after breast cancer surgery because of the offsetting positive contribution to recovery, but a moratorium was imposed on breast implants solely for cosmetic purposes until data establishing safety could be provided. Many implants are now filled with saline or dextran instead of silicone.

Musculocutaneous flap procedure

Breast reconstruction. The myocutaneous flap has made reconstruction possible for most patients who have undergone mastectomy, even when the pectoralis muscles have been removed or when nerve damage has resulted in muscle atrophy. The flap receives its blood supply from muscle, but it can include an overlying layer of skin. At the same time that this procedure is performed, a silicone or saline breast implant may be inserted or, if enough pedicle tissue is available, no implant is needed.

Musculocutaneous flaps are most often taken from the back (latissimus dorsi muscle) or the abdomen (transverse rectus abdominis muscle). When the **latissimus dorsi musculocutaneous flap** is used for reconstruction, a block of skin and muscle from the patient's back is used to replace tissue removed during mastectomy (Figure 12-18, *E*). The **transverse rectus abdominis musculocutaneous (TRAM) flap** is the most frequently used flap operation for breast reconstruction. The rectus abdominis muscles are paired, flat muscles running from the rib cage down to the pubic bone. Arteries inside the muscle branch at many levels, and

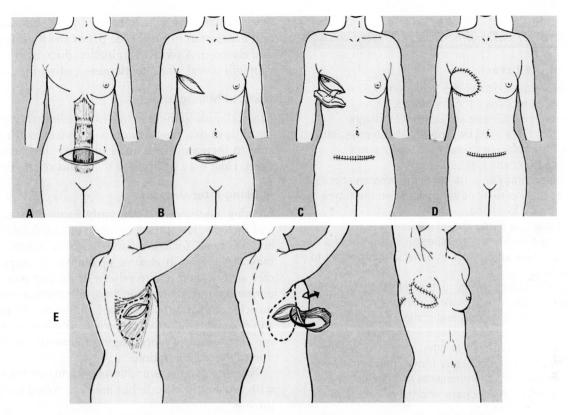

FIGURE **12-18** Transverse rectus abdominis musculocutaneous (TRAM) flap. **A,** TRAM flap is planned. **B,** The abdominal tissue, while attached to the rectus muscle, nerve, and blood supply, is tunneled beneath the abdomen to the chest. **C,** The flap is trimmed to shape the breast. The lower abdominal incision is closed. **D,** Nipple and areola are reconstructed after the breast has healed. **E,** In the latissimus dorsi musculocutaneous flap, a block of skin and muscle from the patient's back is used to replace tissue removed during mastectomy.

these branches supply blood to the fat and skin across a large expanse of the abdomen. In the TRAM technique, the surgeon elevates a large block of tissue from the lower abdominal area, but leaves it attached to the rectus muscle (see Figure 12-18, *A* to *D*). This tissue is then tunneled under the skin or detached and placed as a "free flap" at the site where the breast is to be reconstructed. The tissue is trimmed and shaped to form a breast mound similar to that of the opposite breast. An implant may be used in addition to the flap to achieve symmetry. The abdominal incision is closed in a fashion similar to that of an abdominal hysterectomy or a "tummy tuck." This surgical procedure can last 2 to 8 hours, with recovery taking 4 to 6 weeks. Complications include bleeding, hernia, and infection (Lewis et al, 2004).

Nipple reconstruction is usually performed as a separate procedure after the breast reconstruction has been completed. Nipple construction is generally from available tissue at the site or harvested tissue from the opposite breast. New techniques allow the nipple to be created from tissue and subcutaneous tissue of the breast mount. Areola reconstruction is provided by ob-

Table 12-1 | *Prognosis and Nodal Involvement in Breast Cancer*

LYMPH NODES INVOLVED	METASTATIC RECURRENCE
1 to 3 nodes	50% to 60% metastasis
4 to 10 nodes	75% to 85% metastasis
10 nodes	Even worse prognosis

taining pigmented skin from the upper thigh or by using skin from the lateral chest area.

Prognosis

The 5-year survival rate for localized breast cancer is 85% for white women and 79% for African-American women. After the disease spreads beyond the breast, the survival rate drops dramatically. Breast cancer is the leading cause of cancer deaths among women 15 to 54 years of age. The most important prognostic factor is the stage of the disease (see Box 12-7; see Table 12-1; Home Health Considerations box).

Cancer of the Breast

- The nurse should explain the follow-up routine to the patient and emphasize the importance of beginning and continuing BSE and annual mammography.
- Symptoms that should be reported to the physician include new back pain, weakness, constipation, shortness of breath, and confusion.
- If adjuvant therapy is to be used, the woman should have specific instructions about appointment times and treatment locations.
- If applicable, the nurse should stress the importance of wearing a well-fitting prosthesis. The return of a normal external appearance is especially important to most women.
- Often the husband, sexual partner, or family member may need assistance in dealing with their emotional reactions to the diagnosis and surgery for them to act as effective means of support for the patient.
- If difficulty in adjustment or other problems develop, counseling may be necessary for women with breast cancer to deal with the emotional component of a modified radical mastectomy and the diagnosis of cancer.

INFLAMMATORY DISORDERS OF THE MALE REPRODUCTIVE SYSTEM

PROSTATITIS

Etiology/Pathophysiology

Prostatitis is an acute or chronic infection of the prostate gland. It is commonly a result of bacterial invasion from the urethra. The causative organisms include *E. coli, Klebsiella, Proteus, Pseudomonas, Streptococcus,* and *Staphylococcus.* Bacterial invasion originates in the bloodstream or from a descending infection from the kidneys.

Clinical Manifestations

Symptoms include sudden onset of chills and fever. There is urgency and frequency of urination, dysuria (pain when urinating), cloudy urine, perineal fullness, lower back pain, arthralgia (pain in the joints), and myalgia (pain in the muscles). When the gland is palpated, there is tenderness, edema, and firmness. In chronic prostatitis, many patients may appear to be asymptomatic, but generally the same symptoms exist as in the acute phase with a lesser degree of intensity.

Diagnostic Tests

Diagnostic testing includes culture and sensitivity tests of the urethra, prostatic fluid, and urine for organism identification and appropriate antibiotic ther-

apy. Prostatic fluid is collected by prostate massage and expression of fluid. The pH of the fluid is generally elevated. A rectal examination done by the physician will reveal gland tenderness and edema.

Medical Management

Medical management includes antibiotic therapy and periodic digital massage of the prostate by the physician to increase the flow of infected prostatic secretions. Heat may be applied by means of sitz baths.

Nursing Interventions

Nursing interventions primarily focus on symptoms and include (1) a full explanation of antibiotic therapy and the need for compliance with treatment, which may be lengthy in chronic prostatitis; (2) supportive care such as bed rest to relieve strain and pain of the perineum and suprapubic area, sitz baths to promote muscle relaxation, and stool softeners to prevent straining on defecation; (3) monitoring intake and output (I&O); and (4) encouraging follow-up for evaluation of the inflammation.

Nursing diagnoses and interventions for the patient with prostatitis include but are not limited to the following:

Nursing Diagnoses	Nursing Interventions
Acute pain, related to disease process	Assess type and location of pain; provide analgesics as ordered. Encourage bed rest to promote comfort. Provide nonpharmacologic comfort measures: 1. Assist patient with assuming comfortable position. 2. Provide diversional activity. 3. Provide a restful environment. 4. Instruct patient in necessity of complying with taking prescribed antibiotics and following orders for activity level.
Risk for situational low self-esteem, related to fear of impotence and embarrassment	Encourage patient to express feelings. Actively listen. Encourage adaptive coping behaviors.

Prognosis

Recurrent episodes of acute prostatitis may cause fibrotic tissue to form; such fibrosis causes a hardening of the prostate gland that may initially be confused with carcinoma.

EPIDIDYMITIS

Etiology/Pathophysiology

Epididymitis is an infection of the cordlike excretory duct of the testicle. It is one of the common infections of the male reproductive tract. The causative organisms are *S. aureus*, *E. coli*, *Streptococcus* spp., and *N. gonorrhoeae*. The inflammation is associated with urethral strictures, cystitis, and prostatitis.

Symptoms can occur after trauma to the genital area, after instrumentation of the urethra and cystoscopy, and after physical exertion or prolonged sexual activity.

Clinical Manifestations

Severe pain appears suddenly in the scrotum and radiates along the spermatic tube. Edema appears and the patient develops a "duck walk" or "waddling gait" because of the sensitivity and pain that walking stimulates. The scrotal area becomes tender. Pyuria (pus in urine) is present. Chills and fever are noted.

Diagnostic Tests

Diagnostic testing includes examination of the first daily flow of urine and delivery of a midstream specimen to the laboratory to check for pyuria. The epididymis is massaged by the physician and a fluid expression specimen is sent to the laboratory. Physical examination of the scrotum is performed. The white blood count is monitored for leukocytosis.

Medical Management

Medical management includes a regimen of bed rest and support of the scrotum. Cold may be applied for relief of edema and discomfort, and the appropriate antibiotic is administered. If abscess formation occurs, incision and drainage (I&D) of the scrotum may be required.

Nursing Interventions

Nursing interventions for patients with epididymitis include (1) bed rest during the acute phase of illness; (2) support of the testicular area, with scrotal support by elevation of the scrotum on a folded towel during bed rest and athletic support when ambulatory; (3) ice compresses to the area in the initial phase to hasten recovery; and (4) explaining the need for compliance with antibiotic therapy until all signs of inflammation have disappeared.

Prognosis

The infection can be bilateral and may recur. Bilateral epididymitis can cause sterility. Untreated epididymitis leads to necrosis of testicular tissue; in addition, abscesses can form, and septicemia can develop, which can be fatal.

DISORDERS OF MALE GENITAL ORGANS

PHIMOSIS

Etiology/Pathophysiology

Phimosis is a condition in which the prepuce is too small to allow retraction of the foreskin over the glans. Phimosis is often congenital but may be acquired as a result of local inflammation or disease. The condition is rarely severe enough to obstruct the flow of urine but may contribute to local infection because it does not permit adequate cleansing treatment.

Medical Management

Circumcision may be performed in which a part of the foreskin is removed, leaving the glans penis uncovered.

Nursing Interventions

After a circumcision a sterile petrolatum gauze dressing is applied and changed after each voiding. The nurse should always observe the patient for unusual bleeding and obstruction of urine flow.

HYDROCELE

Etiology/Pathophysiology

A hydrocele is an accumulation of fluid between the membranes covering the testicle and the membrane enclosing the testicle. The scrotum slowly enlarges as the fluid accumulates. Pain occurs if the hydrocele develops suddenly. Most hydroceles occur in males older than 21 years of age. The actual cause is not known, but it may develop as a result of trauma in the area, orchitis (inflammation of the testes), or epididymitis.

Medical Management

Treatment includes aspiration of fluid from the sac or surgical removal of the sac to avoid constriction of the circulation of the testicles. After aspiration the pain is relieved and the scrotum can be examined more easily.

Nursing Interventions

Nursing interventions consist of maintaining bed rest, scrotal support with elevation, ice to edematous areas, and frequent changes of dressings to avoid skin impairment.

Prognosis

With treatment, prognosis is good.

VARICOCELE

Varicocele occurs when the veins within the scrotum become dilated. Obstruction and malfunctioning of the veins cause engorgement and elongation, which do not allow adequate drainage of the blood. The symptoms are a pulling sensation that causes a dull aching and pain accompanied by edema of the scrotal area. The treatment is surgical removal of the obstruction. Nursing interventions include bed rest with scrotal support, ice on the incisional site, and medication for discomfort as ordered.

Varicocele is often seen in men with low fertility. Ligation of the spermatic vein has been shown to improve semen quality.

CANCER OF THE MALE REPRODUCTIVE TRACT

The more common tumors of the male reproductive tract involve the testis, prostate gland, and penis. Most tumors of the male reproductive system are malignant. (See Chapter 10 for cancer of prostate gland.)

Men should be taught testicular self-examination (TSE). The examination takes 3 minutes and should be done monthly. The best time to perform a TSE is after the man has had a warm shower and the scrotal skin is relaxed. Each testicle should be rolled gently between the thumb and fingers of both hands, examining for lumps or nodules. If any lumps or nodules are found, a physician should be consulted promptly.

CANCER OF THE TESTIS (TESTICULAR CANCER)
Etiology/Pathophysiology

Testicular cancer is relatively rare, accounting for less than 1% of all cancers found in males. However, cancer of the testis is the most common malignancy in men 15 to 35 years of age and the most common cause of death in this age group. The causes are unknown. The incidence of this cancer is higher in men with cryptorchidism (failure of testes to descend into the scrotum). Other associated factors are testicular atrophy, orchitis, and scrotal trauma. Most testicular cancers develop from embryonic germ cells. The two types of germ cell cancers are seminomas and nonseminomas. Although seminomas are the most common, they are the least aggressive. Nonseminoma testicular germ cell tumors are rare, but are very aggressive.

Clinical Manifestations

Testicular cancer may have a slow or rapid onset, depending on the type of tumor. The signs and symptoms of early disease include an enlarged scrotum, and a firm, painless, smooth mass in the testicular area. Some patients complain of a dull ache or heavy sensation in the lower abdomen, perianal area, or scrotum. Acute pain is the presenting symptom in about 10% of patients.

Diagnostic Tests

Palpation of the scrotal contents is the first step in diagnosing testicular cancer. A cancerous mass is firm and does not transilluminate. Ultrasound of the testes is indicated whenever testicular cancer is suspected (e.g., palpable mass) or when persistent or painful tes-

ticular edema is present. If a testicular neoplasm is suspected, blood is obtained to determine the serum levels of α-fetoprotein (AFP) and human chorionic gonadotropin (hCG). A chest radiograph and CT scan of the abdomen and pelvis are obtained to detect metastasis.

Medical Management

Radical inguinal orchiectomy is usually the treatment of choice. This is the removal of the testis, epididymis, a portion of the gonadal lymphatics, and their blood supply. The remaining testis provides enough testosterone to maintain the man's sexual characteristics. He may have a lower sperm count and decreased sperm mobility. Surgery is generally followed by radiation or chemotherapy. Often a retroperitoneal lymph node dissection is performed to remove affected nodes and assist in determining the tumor stage. Staging a testicular tumor helps determine treatment.

Nursing Interventions and Patient Teaching

The priority for care of patients who have or are at risk for a tumor of the testis is early detection by TSE. Young men should be taught to perform TSE monthly beginning at 15 years of age. The scrotum is checked for color, contour, and skin breaks. The left side is usually longer because the left testicle is suspended from a longer spermatic cord. Each testicle is gently palpated by grasping the scrotum in the center with the thumb and index finger (Health Promotion Considerations box; Figure 12-19). Normal testicles are firm but somewhat resilient, smooth, and mobile. If a testicle is indurated (hardened), carcinoma is suspected.

Prognosis

With the advent of tumor markers (which indicate the presence of disease and enable the physician to monitor its response to treatment), early detection, refined surgery, and effective chemotherapy, 95% of the patients obtain complete remission.

CANCER OF THE PENIS
Etiology/Pathophysiology

Cancer of the penis is rare. It generally appears in men older than 50 years of age. Men who have not been circumcised, have not maintained good personal hygiene, or have had STDs are at risk.

Clinical Manifestations

The tumor is painless, and a wartlike growth or ulceration on the glans under the prepuce is present. It is common for metastasis to occur to the inguinal nodes and adjacent organs.

Diagnostic Tests

Biopsy confirms the diagnosis.

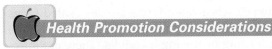

Health Promotion Considerations

Testicular Self-Examination

Perform TSE after a bath or shower when scrotum is warm and most relaxed.

Grasp testis with both hands and palpate gently between thumb and fingers. The testis should feel smooth and egg-shaped and be firm to touch.

The epididymis, found behind the testis, should feel like a soft tube (see Figure 12-1; see also Figure 12-19).

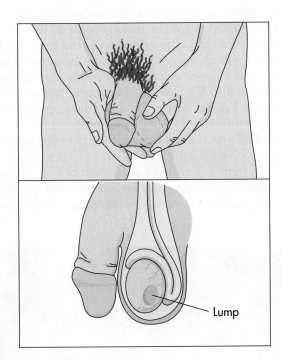

FIGURE **12-19** Testicular self-examination.

Medical Management

Surgical intervention requires removal of as little tissue as possible, but it may be necessary to do a partial or total amputation of the penis as well as remove the adjacent tissue and inguinal lymph nodes. When metastasis involves the bladder and rectum, more radical surgery may be needed, and outlets for urinary or fecal elimination are provided by creating an ileal conduit and a colostomy. The surgeon may place a suprapubic catheter into the bladder as a means of draining the urine from the bladder.

Nursing Interventions

Nursing interventions include providing emotional support. If amputation of the penis is required, the patient faces the psychological trauma associated with the loss of sexuality and the ability to urinate through the penis. Nursing interventions also include monitoring urine output by suprapubic catheter or, if an ileoconduit was performed, monitoring urine in the

urostomy bag. Elevation of the scrotum controls edema. The nurse will provide comfort measures to control pain.

See Chapters 10 and 17 for a discussion of cancer of the prostate.

SEXUALLY TRANSMITTED DISEASES

Today, despite sweeping advances in the diagnosis and treatment of communicable diseases, the incidence of infections transmitted through intimate or sexual activities continues to increase worldwide.

STDs, previously called venereal diseases, are infections that are usually transmitted during intimate sexual contact. They may have other routes of transmission (e.g., an infected mother to her newborn), occur with or without symptoms, and have long periods of asymptomatic infectivity.

Any sexually active person may be at risk for an STD. People who have frequent sexual contact with multiple partners are at increased risk. Common characteristics of these individuals are young, single, urban, poor, male, and homosexual. Because some STDs persist and are infectious for long periods (herpes genitalis, HIV-positive people), even people in mutually monogamous sexual relationships are at some risk. The proliferation of HIV since the late 1970s has produced an urgent reason to educate sexually active individuals about the risk of unprotected sexual contact.

As of 2001, the Centers for Disease Control and Prevention (CDC) reported over 810,000 cumulative cases of AIDS in the United States and estimated that more than 900,000 people were infected with human immunodeficiency virus (HIV), the causative organism of AIDS. It is difficult to determine with accuracy the number of confirmed HIV infections because only 27 states have laws or regulations requiring cases of HIV-positive people to be reported (see Chapter 16). These are sobering statistics indeed. The number of people contracting the traditionally defined STDs (e.g., syphilis, gonorrhea) is even greater. Gonorrhea is estimated to infect 250 million people worldwide and nearly 3 million in the United States each year. Annual syphilis incidence is about 50 million cases worldwide and 50,223 in the United States. No reliable statistics exist for the "new generation" STDs, such as trichomoniasis, herpes simplex virus (HSV), venereal warts, scabies, and others; these are probably even more prevalent. In addition, bowel pathogens such as *Salmonella*, amebae, hepatitis B, hepatitis C, and the herpesviruses may be sexually transmitted.

Despite the physical and emotional discomfort, the possibility of long-term disability (infertility, chronic infectivity), and advances in diagnosis and treatment that sharply decrease the period of infectivity, STDs continue to be among the world's most common communicable diseases. Four main factors are responsible: (1) unprotected sex, (2) antibiotic resistance, (3) treatment delay, and (4) sexual behavior patterns and permissiveness (Safety Considerations box). The following is a discussion of some of the more commonly diagnosed sexually transmitted diseases.

GENITAL HERPES
Etiology/Pathophysiology

Genital herpes, or HSV, is an infectious viral disease, characterized by recurrent episodes of acute, painful, erythematous, vesicular eruptions (blisters) on or in the genitalia or rectum.

Safety Considerations

Sexually Transmitted Disease

- Teach "safe" sex practices including abstinence, monogamy with an uninfected partner, avoidance of certain high-risk sexual practices, and use of condoms and other barriers to limit contact with potentially infectious body fluids or lesions.
- All sexually active women should be screened for cervical cancer. Women with a history of STDs are at greater risk for cervical cancer than women without this history.
- Instruct patient in hygiene measures, such as washing and urinating after intercourse to destroy many causative organisms.
- Explain the importance of taking all antibiotics as prescribed. Symptoms will improve after 1 to 2 days of therapy, but organisms may still be present.
- Teach patient about the need for treatment of sexual partners with antibiotics to prevent transmission of disease.
- Instruct patient to abstain from sexual intercourse during treatment and to use condoms when sexual activity is resumed to prevent spread of infection and prevent reinfection.
- Explain the importance of follow-up examination and reculture at least once after treatment if appropriate to confirm complete cure and prevent relapse.
- Allow patient and partner to verbalize concerns to clarify areas that need explanation.
- Instruct patient about symptoms of complications and need to report problems to ensure proper follow-up and early treatment of reinfection.
- Explain precautions to take, such as being monogamous; asking potential partners about sexual history; avoiding sex with partners who use IV drugs or who have visible oral, inguinal, genital, perineal, or anal lesions; using condoms; voiding and washing genitalia after coitus to reduce the occurrence of reinfection.
- Inform patient regarding state of infectivity to prevent a false sense of security, which might result in careless sexual practices and poor personal hygiene.

The two closely related forms are designated types I and II. Most people are infected in infancy with type I during feeding or kissing by adults. There are infrequent recurrences around the lips. A prior infection with HSV I confers relative immunity to HSV II. This immunity may enable people infected with HSV I to be completely resistant or have a less dramatic HSV II infection.

HSV II is usually acquired sexually after puberty in the genital or anal regions.

Clinical Manifestations

Signs appear as fluid-filled vesicles after the incubation period and in women usually occur on the cervix, which is considered the primary site, but may also be seen on the labia, rectum, vulva, vagina, and skin and on the glans penis, foreskin, and penile shaft of men (Figure 12-20). Other lesions may appear on the mouth and anus. Vesicles may rupture and develop into shallow, painful ulcers; they are erythematous with marked edema and tenderness. Lymph nodes may become involved. Initial lesions last from 3 to 10 days, and recurrent lesions have a duration of 7 to 10 days. The primary infection may be accompanied by fever; malaise; myalgia; dysuria; and, in women, leukorrhea.

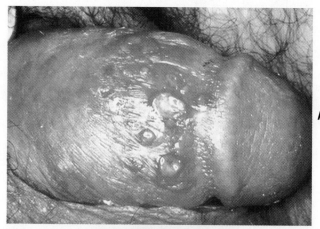

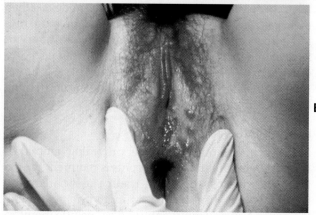

FIGURE **12-20** Herpes simplex virus type II in a male and female patient. Vesicular lesions on **A**, penis, and **B**, perineum.

Sites are painful in the presence of fever, stress, or emotional upset, or when exposed to intense heat. Urination may be painful from urine touching active lesions. Complications are rare.

Diagnostic Tests

Diagnosis is based on the physical examination and the patient history. The diagnosis is confirmed by appearance of the virus on tissue cultures.

Medical Management

The skin lesions of genital herpes heal spontaneously unless secondary infection occurs. Symptomatic treatment such as good genital hygiene and the wearing of loose-fitting cotton undergarments should be encouraged. The lesions should be kept clean and dry. Frequent sitz baths may soothe the area and reduce inflammation. Pain may require a local anesthetic such as lidocaine (Xylocaine) or systemic analgesics such as codeine and aspirin. Patients are advised to abstain from sexual contact while lesions are present. However, sexual transmission of HSV has been documented even in the absence of clinical lesions, and the use of condoms should be encouraged.

Currently, acyclovir (Zovirax), which inhibits herpetic viral replication, is being prescribed for primary infections or for suppression of frequent recurrences (more than 6 episodes per year). Although not a cure, acyclovir shortens the duration of viral shedding and the healing time of genital lesions and suppresses 75% of recurrences with daily use. Continued use of oral acyclovir for up to 5 years is safe and effective, but should be interrupted after 1 year to assess the patient's rate of recurrent episodes. Adverse reactions to acyclovir are mild and include headache, occasional nausea and vomiting, and diarrhea. The safety of systemic acyclovir for treatment of pregnant women has not been established. Acyclovir ointment appears to be of no clinical benefit in the treatment of recurrent lesions, either in speed of healing or in resolution of pain, and is not commonly recommended. Acyclovir is reserved for severe or life-threatening infections, because hospitalization is required and nephrotoxicity has been observed with its use.

Two other antiviral agents are also available for the treatment of HSV: valacyclovir (Valtrex) and famciclovir (Famvir). These purine analogues inhibit herpetic viral replication and are prescribed for primary and recurrent infections and are used to suppress frequent recurrences.

Nursing Interventions and Patient Teaching

The nurse should advise the patient to keep genital lesions clean and dry. Hands should be washed thoroughly after touching a lesion. Loose, absorbent underclothing is usually more comfortable than close-fitting clothing. Sitz baths decrease lesional discomfort and enhance urinary and bowel elimination. The patient should be taught that sexual intercourse during the active lesion phase increases the risk of transmission and may also be painful. Future sexual partners and health care providers should be advised of recurring or latent infections. The nurse should teach the role of stress, poor nutrition, and insufficient rest in recurrences of signs and symptoms. Women patients need a yearly Pap test and should inform their physician in the event of pregnancy so that the course of the disease can be monitored closely; there is a possibility of spontaneous abortion. The nurse should provide the patient with nonjudgmental support and with the contact number of the local herpes support group if one exists.

Prognosis

Genital herpes is a recurrent disease with no cure.

SYPHILIS
Etiology/Pathophysiology

The coiled spirochete *Treponema pallidum* causes syphilis. Congenital syphilis occurs in about 1 in 10,000 pregnancies, generally in minority populations. The age group with the highest incidence is 20 to 40 years. Data from the CDC show the number of reported syphilis cases in 1996 to be the lowest since 1959. However, the disease remains a significant problem among African Americans. This disease is occurring primarily among young, heterosexual, minority populations of a low educational and socioeconomic level and may be related to cocaine use and exchange of sex for drugs, especially crack cocaine.

Syphilis is the third most frequently reported communicable disease in the United States, exceeded only by varicella (chickenpox) and gonorrhea. Transmission occurs primarily through sexual contact during the primary, secondary, and latent stages of the disease. In addition to sexual contact, syphilis may be spread through contact with infectious lesions and sharing of needles among drug addicts. Prenatal infection from the mother to the fetus is possible. The organism thrives in the warm parts of the body and can be destroyed by soap and water. The spirochete penetrates intact skin as well as openings in the mucous membrane of the genital organs, rectum, and mouth.

Clinical Manifestations

Each stage of syphilis has its peculiar signs and symptoms: (1) primary, (2) secondary, (3) latent, and (4) tertiary. The signs and symptoms of syphilis range from the clean-based chancre (painless erosion or papule that ulcerates superficially with a scooped-out appearance) of primary syphilis to the skin rashes of secondary syphilis. Moist, raised, gray to pink lesions of the genital or perirectal skin; enlarged lymph nodes; fever; fatigue; or infections of the eyes, bones, liver, or meninges may occur. In the late stages of syphilis, dementia, pain or loss of sensation in the legs, and destruction of the aorta occur. Destructive inflammatory masses can appear in any organ. In tertiary or late-stage syphilis the heart and blood vessels (cardiovascular syphilis) and the central nervous system (neurosyphilis) are frequently involved. Tabes dorsalis, paresis, and various psychoses may result.

Diagnostic Tests

Diagnostic tests that are available include the Venereal Disease Research Laboratory (VDRL) slide test and rapid plasma reagin (RPR) test. All patients should be checked for gonorrhea as well.

Medical Management

Therapeutic management of syphilis is aimed at eradication of all syphilitic organisms. However, treatment cannot reverse damage that is already present in the late stage of the disease. Parenteral penicillin remains the treatment of choice for all stages of syphilis. To date, there is no evidence to suggest a decrease in the effectiveness of penicillin against *T. pallidum.* All stages of syphilis should be treated.

Appropriate antibiotic treatment of maternal syphilis before the 18th week of pregnancy prevents infection of the fetus. Appropriate treatment after 18 weeks of pregnancy cures both mother and fetus because the antibiotics can cross the placental barrier. Treatment administered in the second half of pregnancy may pose a risk of premature labor. Some authorities recommend hospitalization and fetal monitoring of women at 20 weeks of gestation or greater.

All patients with neurosyphilis must be carefully monitored, with periodic serologic testing, clinical evaluation at 6-month intervals, and repeated cerebrospinal fluid (CSF) examinations for at least 3 years. Specific therapeutic management is based on the specific symptoms.

Nursing Interventions

Other than the routine implications for patients with STDs, nursing interventions include monitoring for drug reaction to penicillin, stressing good handwashing technique to the patient, encouraging follow-up visits with the physician, and informing the patient that he or she should absolutely not engage in sexual intercourse until cured.

Prognosis

Syphilis can be successfully treated at any stage of the disease, but treatment may be prolonged in latent and late syphilis. Although syphilis can be cured in late stages, damage to the body is more difficult to manage. Untreated syphilis will go from primary to secondary, latent, and eventually tertiary stage.

GONORRHEA
Etiology/Pathophysiology

Gonorrhea is caused by *N. gonorrhoeae,* a gram-negative diplococcoid bacterium, and almost exclusively follows sexual contact. It is the most commonly reported communicable disease in the United States. It is estimated that at least 2 million unreported cases occur each year. The disease is most common in the 20-to-24 age group, closely followed by the 15-to-19 age group. Those at risk are sexually active individuals and women who use birth control pills or who are otherwise susceptible to infections. Gonorrhea is primarily an infection of the genital or rectal mucosa but is not limited to the genital organs; it can infect the mouth and throat through oral sex with an infected partner. It may also infect the eyes. Three times as many men are infected as women. The incubation period of gonorrhea is 3 to 5 days.

Clinical Manifestations

Some infected men may be asymptomatic after the incubation period but in a short time develop signs and symptoms of urethritis, dysuria, infection with a purulent discharge, and edema of the affected area. Most women remain asymptomatic but may show a greenish yellow discharge from the cervix. Other female signs and symptoms, which may vary depending on the infection site, are urinary frequency, purulent discharge from the urethra, pruritus, burning and pain of the vulva, vaginal engorgement and erythema, abdominal pain and distention, muscular rigidity, and tenderness. As the infection spreads, nausea, vomiting, fever, and tachycardia may develop. Other signs and symptoms may include pharyngitis, tonsillitis, rectal burning, pruritus, and purulent rectal discharge.

Diagnostic Tests

Diagnosis is determined by cultures from the site of infection. Cultures isolate the organism and establish an identification. Cultures of the discharge or secretion can provide a definitive diagnosis after incubation for 24 to 48 hours. An important concern in treatment for gonorrhea is coexisting chlamydial infection (see the discussion of chlamydia for more information). This infection has been documented in up to 45% of gonorrhea cases when adequate chlamydial cultures are performed. It is important to test for syphilis as well.

Medical Management

A history of sexual contact with a partner known to have gonorrhea is considered good evidence for the presence of gonorrhea. Because of the short incubation period and high infectivity, treatment is instituted without awaiting culture results, even in the absence of any signs or symptoms. The treatment of gonorrhea in the early stage is curative. Traditionally, the drug of choice for gonorrheal therapy had been penicillin, but changes have been made because of resistant strains of *N. gonorrhoeae* and the presence of coexisting chlamydial infection.

Recently, a rapid increase in the number of cases of gonorrhea caused by resistant strains of *N. gonorrhoeae* has been identified.

There is no clinical distinction between infections caused by resistant or sensitive strains of *N. gonorrhoeae*. As a result, ceftriaxone (Rocephin) a penicillinase-resistant cephalosporin, has become part of the treatment plan. Cefixine (Suprax) given orally one time is also effective. The high frequency of coexisting chlamydial and gonococcal infections has led to the addition of doxycycline (Vibramycin) or tetracycline (Tetracyn) to the treatment plan. The expense of diagnosing chlamydial infection and the sequelae of chlamydial infection make this strategy cost effective. Patients with coincubating syphilis are likely to be cured by the same drugs.

All sexual contacts of patients with gonorrhea must be treated to prevent reinfection after resumption of sexual relations. The "Ping-Pong" effect of reexposure, treatment, and reinfection will cease only when infected partners are treated simultaneously. Additionally, the patient should be counseled to abstain from sexual intercourse and alcohol for 2 to 4 weeks. Sexual intercourse allows the infection to spread and can retard complete healing as a result of vascular congestion. Alcohol has an irritant effect on the healing urethral walls. Men should be cautioned against squeezing the penis to look for further discharge. Follow-up examination and reculture should be done at least once after treatment, usually in 4 to 7 days. Relapse, reinfection, and complications should be treated appropriately.

Nurses need to be alert to changes in CDC recommendations. Report the disease to infection control authorities as prescribed by the local health agency.

Nursing Interventions and Patient Teaching

The nurse should advise patients that loose, absorbent underclothes, changed frequently after perineal or penile cleansing, will enhance comfort. Sitz baths decrease lower abdominal discomfort and dysuria. The patient should avoid infecting sexual partners and be taught that sterility may occur as a result of gonorrhea.

The nurse should obtain laboratory specimens as ordered. Alternative methods of birth control can be discussed as appropriate. The nurse should encourage notification of present and past sexual partners of the diagnosis and stress the need for them to promptly seek medical care.

Prognosis

With treatment, gonorrhea is curable, but recurrence is common. The inflammation may clear up without serious results, or it may become chronic and produce urethral stricture. It may produce complications such as prostatitis, epididymitis, orchitis, arthritis, and endocarditis. It can result in sterility in the female. No case of acute gonorrhea in the female should be considered cured until three consecutive negative smears of the cervix and Bartholin's and Skene's glands are obtained.

TRICHOMONIASIS
Etiology/Pathophysiology

Trichomoniasis is a sexually transmitted disease caused by the protozoan *T. vaginalis*, which affects about 15% of sexually active women and 10% of sexually active men. The incubation period is 4 to 28 days. Trichomoniasis is usually transmitted by sexual intercourse and, at times, by dirty douche nozzles, douche containers, and moist washcloths. Occasionally a newborn develops an infection from an infected mother. *T. vaginalis* thrives when the vaginal mucosa is more alkaline than normal. Frequent douching and use of oral contraceptives and antibiotics raise the normal pH of the vagina.

Clinical Manifestations

Most men and women are asymptomatic. The male signs and symptoms are mild to severe transient urethritis, dysuria, frequency of urination, pruritus, and purulent exudate. Approximately 70% of infected women are asymptomatic. When present, signs and symptoms include profuse, frothy, gray, green, or yellow, malodorous discharge; pruritus; edema; tenderness of vagina; dysuria; frequency of urination; spotting; menorrhagia; and dysmenorrhea. Signs and symptoms may persist for a week to several months and may be more pronounced after menstruation or during pregnancy.

Diagnostic Tests

Diagnosis is based on the microscopic examination of the vaginal discharge that identifies *T. vaginalis*.

Medical Management

Treatment for both men and women is oral metronidazole (Flagyl) in small doses for 7 days or a single large dose. The patient should avoid alcoholic beverages, because alcohol can cause reactions such as disorientation, headache, cramps, vomiting, and possibly convulsions. Metronidazole can cause the urine to turn dark brown (see the Medications table).

Nursing Interventions and Patient Teaching

The nurse should counsel the patient to avoid alcohol during treatment; inform patients that their urine may turn dark orange or brown; and counsel patients to avoid douches, sprays, and powders. The patient should be taught how to disinfect douche nozzles, applicators, diaphragms, and the toilet area. The nurse should encourage the patient to wear loose-fitting clothing and cotton underwear, encourage follow-up visits with the physician, and discuss the need to contact sex partners to encourage their treatment.

Prognosis

With treatment, trichomoniasis is curable. Reinfection is common if sexual partners are not treated simultaneously. Chronic infection may develop in untreated cases.

CANDIDIASIS
Etiology/Pathophysiology

Candidiasis (moniliasis) is a mild fungal infection that appears in men and women. Candidal infections are usually caused by *C. albicans* and *Candida tropicalis.* The fungi are a part of the normal flora of the gastrointestinal tract, mouth, vagina, and skin. The infection often occurs when the glucose level rises from diabetes mellitus or when resistance is lowered from diseases such as carcinoma. Radiation, immunosuppressant drugs, hyperalimentation, antibiotic therapy, and oral contraceptives may predispose individuals to candidiasis. Men and women display signs of scaly skin, erythematous rash, and occasional exudates that appear under the breasts, between the fingers, and in the axillae, groin, and umbilicus.

Clinical Manifestations

If the mother is infected, a newborn can contract thrush during delivery. The infant may display a diaper rash. Nails become edematous and have a darkened, erythematous nail base from which there is purulent exudate. Thrush may appear on the mucous membranes of the mouth and cause edema and engorgement. The infant may have an edematous tongue that can cause respiratory distress. The female patient may have a cheesy, tenacious white discharge accompanied by pruritus, and an inflamed vulva and vagina. The male patient presents signs of an infected penis with purulent exudate. Systemic infections are indicated by chills, fevers, and general malaise.

Diagnostic Tests

Diagnosis is based on evidence of the *Candida* species on a Gram stain of collected specimens from scraping of the vagina and penis, from pus, and from exudate from the mouth.

Medical Management

Treatment consists of treating and improving any underlying condition, such as controlling diabetes mellitus; discontinuing antibiotics and oral contraceptives; and catheter therapy. Nystatin (Mycostatin) is effective for superficial candidiasis; topical amphotericin B is effective for skin and nail infections.

Nursing Interventions and Patient Teaching

The nurse should emphasize the use of prescribed ointments, sprays, and creams as indicated for each part of the body affected. Teaching includes the method for inserting vaginal suppositories (to be inserted high into the vagina when in a dorsal recumbent position) and remaining on the back for 30 minutes to allow suppository absorption. Sexual partners should be encouraged to have an examination and treatment. Good handwashing techniques should be taught to avoid reinfection or the transfer of the fungi. The nurse should encourage pregnant women to accept treatment to prevent infection of the newborn at the time of delivery.

Prognosis

The condition of candidiasis is curable with the use of the prescribed treatment.

CHLAMYDIA
Etiology/Pathophysiology

Chlamydia trachomatis a gram-negative, intracellular bacterium, causes several commonly sexually transmitted diseases. Cervicitis and urethritis are most common, but like the gonococcus, chlamydial organisms also cause epididymitis in men and salpingitis in women. Chlamydial infections may be the most commonly occurring STD in the United States. Chlamydial infections are responsible for about 20% to 30% of diagnosed PID cases. It is estimated that about 11,000 women each year become involuntarily sterilized and 36,000 suffer ectopic pregnancies as a result of this organism. Chlamydia is highest in young, promiscuous, indigent, unmarried women who live in the inner city and in those who have a prior history of STDs. Because it is not a reportable disease, the actual number of cases is unknown. It is estimated that each year 3 to 4 million Americans suffer from epidemic chlamydial infections.

Although both men and women may have asymptomatic infection, women are more likely to be asymptomatic carriers despite deep pelvic infections, such as infection of the fallopian tubes and PID.

Clinical Manifestations

In men, signs and symptoms may include a scanty white or clear exudate, burning or pruritus around the urethral meatus, urinary frequency, and mild dysuria. Signs and symptoms of cervicitis in women may include one or more of the following: (1) vaginal pruritus or burning, (2) dull pelvic pain, (3) low-grade fever, (4) vaginal discharge, and (5) irregular bleeding.

Diagnostic Tests

The direct fluorescent antibody (DFA) test provides a ready basis for diagnosis. However, this test is less specific than a culture and may produce false-positive

Box 12-10   *Prevention of Sexually Transmitted Diseases*

- Reduce the number of sexual partners, preferably to one person.
- Avoid contact with individuals known to be infected or who are at risk of infection.
- Avoid contact with the genital area if signs and symptoms develop.
- Hands and the genital-rectal area should be washed before and immediately after having intercourse.
- Special attention must be given to washing the foreskin.
- A mouthwash or gargle with hydrogen peroxide (1 part peroxide to 3 parts of water) or Listerine antiseptic may slightly reduce the risk of oropharyngeal STD infection.
- Use barrier (condom) contraceptives with new partners.
- Use a water-based lubricant.
- Void after intercourse.
- Avoid excess douching.
- If an STD infection is suspected, seek medical help immediately.
- Individuals with multiple sexual partners should have an STD examination twice a year or more if needed.

results. Culturing for chlamydial organisms should be done if the laboratory facilities are available. New techniques using nucleic acid amplification promise to surpass culture as the gold standard of chlamydial testing. Treatment can be initiated promptly based on a confirmed diagnosis.

Medical Management

Chlamydial infections respond to treatment with tetracycline, doxycycline (Vibramycin), azithromycin (Zithromax), or ofloxacin (Floxin). For tetracycline, the dosage is 500 mg orally four times a day for at least 7 days. For doxycycline, the dosage is 100 mg two times a day. Doxycycline is more expensive than tetracycline. For ofloxacin, the dosage is 300 mg twice a day. Azithromycin (1 g in a single dose) offers the advantage of ease of administration, but safety for patients younger than 15 years of age has not been established. All of the above medications are contraindicated in pregnancy. Erythromycin is the drug of choice for use in pregnant patients. Follow-up care should include advising the patient to return if symptoms persist or recur, treatment of sex partners, and encouraging the use of condoms during all sexual contact.

Because chlamydial infections are closely associated with gonococcal infections, both infections are therefore usually treated concurrently even without diagnostic evidence.

Nursing Interventions and Patient Teaching

Patients' physical symptoms are commonly complicated by their emotional responses to STDs. Complaints of depression, anger, fear, and guilt are common and need to be addressed if education and treatment are to be effective. Outcome is also influenced by educational and income levels, primary language, health insurance coverage, and support network. The focus of patient education is on prevention (Box 12-10).

Prognosis

With treatment, chlamydial infection is curable. Reinfection occurs if sexual partners are not treated simultaneously. Chlamydial infections can be transmitted to infants during delivery, causing conjunctivitis and pneumonia.

ACQUIRED IMMUNODEFICIENCY SYNDROME

AIDS is the ultimately fatal, advanced stage of a chronic retroviral infection from the HIV virus that gradually destroys the cell-mediated immune system. (For a more detailed discussion on this STD, see Chapter 16.)

FAMILY PLANNING

Advances in drug therapy and family planning technology have made available a range of options for individuals wishing to prevent or plan conception. Birth control planning involves moral, religious, cultural, and personal values, and the nurse should be sensitive to these factors when discussing birth control with patients.

There are numerous types of birth control procedures or devices that can be employed. The selection of the particular method should be based on the health of the individual, effectiveness of the method, cost, ease of use, and age and parity (total number of pregnancies) of the patient. Willingness of the patient to comply with use and preference of the couple are two additional factors taken into consideration when selecting a method of contraception. The nurse can help by reinforcing information given by the physician and encouraging patients to seek more information, directing them to the source.

Contraceptive methods and products can be categorized as surgical (Figures 12-21 and 12-22), hormonal, barrier, and behavioral (Table 12-2).

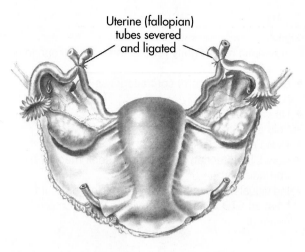

Uterine (fallopian) tubes severed and ligated

FIGURE 12-21 Tubal ligation. Oviduct ligated and severed.

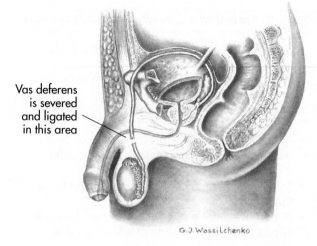

Vas deferens is severed and ligated in this area

G.J.Wassilchenko

FIGURE 12-22 Vasectomy. Sperm duct severed (and ligated).

Table 12-2 | *Methods of Birth Control*

DESCRIPTION	SIDE EFFECTS AND COMPLICATIONS	PATIENT EDUCATION
TEMPORARY METHODS		
Combined		
Combination pill contains both estrogen and progesterone (standard and low-dose). Usually taken on 5th through 25th day of each cycle. Prevents ovulation; causes changes in endometrium; alternations in cervical mucus and tubal transport. Simple and unobtrusive in use. 99% effective. Failure from irregular or incorrect use.	Side effects of weight gain, nausea and vomiting, spotting and break-through bleeding, postpill amenorrhea, breast tenderness, headache, chloasma, irritability, nervousness, depression, and decreased libido; complications of benign liver tumors, gallstones, myocardial infarction, thromboembolism, stroke (smokers older than 35 years of age at higher risk); contraindications of history of cardiovascular or liver disease, hypertension, breast or pelvic cancer and caution with diabetes mellitus, sickle cell anemia. Provides no protection against HIV transmission.	Instruct patient in correct use of pills. Tell patient to take pill same time each day; if forgotten one day, take two next day. Review side effects and contraindications. Explain that the patient should report cramps or edema of legs, chest pain. Discuss need for periodic (every 6-12 months), checkup that involves weight, BP, Pap smear, hematocrit. Review danger signs of drug. Take drug history, asking about use of phenytoin, phenobarbital, antibiotic (ampicillin), which decrease contraceptive action. Inform patient that method is usually not recommended for persons over 35 years of age. Discourage smoking.
Morning-after pill (Ovral) contains ethinyl estradiol 50 mcg and norgestrel 0.5 mg. Another use of combined hormonal contraception. 98.4% effective. Fewer side effects than DES. Creates hostile uterine lining and alters tubal transport.	Nausea for 1 or 2 days. Would not prevent an ectopic pregnancy. At risk for usual hormonal complications of abdominal pain, chest pain, cough, shortness of breath, headache, dizziness, weakness, leg pain.	Take two Ovral within 72 hours of coitus. Repeat if vomiting occurs. Take second dose 12 hours later. Menses should begin within 2 to 3 weeks. Start an ongoing method of contraception immediately after menses.
Progestin Only		
Progestin-only pills (POPs or Mini-pills) are taken daily, with no pill-free days. Preferred for women who are breastfeeding. Does not suppress lactation. Inhibits ovulation. Thickens cervical mucus. Alters uterine lining. Lower cardiovascular risk than combined pills.	Menstrual changes, breakthrough bleeding, prolonged cycles or amenorrhea. Increased in functional cysts of the ovary. Increase in ectopic pregnancy.	Use alternate contraception when starting POPs or if pill is missed. Take pill at same time every day. Keep record of menses and get pregnancy test if 2 weeks late.

Modified from Lewis, S.M. et al. (2004). *Medical-surgical nursing: assessment and management of clinical problems.* (5th ed.). St Louis: Mosby.

Table 12-2   *Methods of Birth Control—cont'd*

DESCRIPTION	SIDE EFFECTS AND COMPLICATIONS	PATIENT EDUCATION
Progestin Only—cont'd		
Depo-Provera (DMPA) is a progestin-only drug given by injection every 3 months. A private, convenient, and highly effective method. Efficacy similar to surgical sterilization.	May cause amenorrhea, headaches, bloating, and weight gain. Return of fertility may be delayed for several months.	Return every 3 months for injection. Discontinue method for several months before planning to conceive.
Norplant is a progestin-only subdermal implant. Six silicone capsules provide protection for 5 years. Continuous, long-term contraception. Failure rate is extremely low. Does not suppress lactation. Pregnancy rate 0.8 per 100 users over 5 years.	Surgical removal of capsules after 5 years. Menstrual irregularities, especially during the first year. Later may cause amenorrhea. May cause abdominal pain, headaches, weight gain.	Is effective after 24 hours. Keep arm dry for 48 hours after insertion. Report arm pain. Implants are soft and flexible and cannot break. Expect some irregular bleeding. Report any other changes. Remove implants in 5 years. Continue to protect against STDs.
Barrier Method		
Diaphragms are dome-shaped latex caps with flexible metal ring (varies in size) covering cervix. Inner surface coated with spermicide before insertion. Provides mechanical barrier to sperm. Prescription method. Fitted by professional. Recurrent motivation to use necessary. 87% effective. Failure from improper fitting or placement of device.	Allergy to latex or spermicide.	Demonstrate how to hold, insert, and remove device, using model. Allow for insertion and removal practice sessions. Advise patient that insertion may be any time before coitus, but removal should be 6 to 8 hours after coitus. Tell patient that bowel and bladder should be emptied before insertion. Give instructions for cleansing and storing, checking for holes or deterioration. Advise patient that diaphragm must be refitted following pregnancy, weight loss or weight gain. Advise patient that it is not suitable if severe pelvic relaxation is present.
Cervical caps are rubber thimble-shaped shields covering cervix held in place by suction. Spermicide in inner surface provides mechanical barrier to sperm. Fitted by professional. Effectiveness similar to diaphragm. Failure from dislodgement and improper fit.	Allergy to rubber or spermicide, possible cervical irritation or erosion from suction.	Provide sufficient time for practice with insertion and removal (more time than for diaphragm). Give instruction for cleaning, storing, and inspecting for damage. Inform patient that it can be used with abnormalities of vaginal canal but not with cervical inconsistencies or PID.
Condoms		
Male: Thin rubber sheath fitting over erect penis, providing mechanical barrier to sperm. Simple method to use. No prescription necessary. 85% effective. Failure from tearing or slipping during coitus. Used with spermicide. Affords some protection against STDs and HIV transmission.	Possible allergy to rubber, possible decrease in sensation and interference with foreplay.	Advise patient to roll sheath along entire penis, leaving slack at end to receive semen. Inform patient that sharp object (fingernails) may tear condom. Tell patient to hold sheath in place when penis is withdrawn to prevent emptying of sperm in or near vagina.

Continued

Table 12-2 | *Methods of Birth Control—cont'd*

DESCRIPTION	SIDE EFFECTS AND COMPLICATIONS	PATIENT EDUCATION
Female: Double-ring system fitted into vagina up to 8 hours before intercourse. No prescription necessary. Affords protection against HIV, cytomegalovirus, and hepatitis B.	No significant side effects; generally acceptable to couple.	Discuss insertion, lubrication, and method of removal. More expensive than male condoms.

Other Methods

Intrauterine devices (IUDs) are inserted into uterus and are flexible objects made of plastic or copper wire (nonmedicated or medicated with substance to alter uterine environment), usually with attached string that protrudes into vagina. Contraception probably prevented by inflammatory response in endometrium, preventing implantation. After insertion, no additional equipment necessary. 97% to 99% effective. Failure mainly from undetected expulsion. Most common type used today is Progestasert (contains progestins).	Increased menstrual flow, intramenstrual bleeding and cramping, especially during early months of use; possible complications of ectopic pregnancy, pelvic infection, perforation of uterus, infertility. Undetected expulsion of IUD resulting in pregnancy.	Discuss techniques and experience of insertion and removal. Inform patient that insertion may be more difficult and expulsion and complications greater in nulliparous patients. Instruct patient to check for string in vagina after each period; report to physician if unable to locate. Discuss need for annual pelvic examination and Pap test.
Rhythm method requires periodic abstinence during fertile portion of menstrual cycle. Requires strong motivation, self-control. Complies with all religious doctrines. 60% to 65% effective. Failure from difficulty in determining precise day of ovulation, irregularity of menses.	Inaccurate or incomplete knowledge of menstrual cycle.	Discuss methods to establish baseline menstrual patterns and identify ovulation. Give instructions in use of calendar or basal body temperature method to determine ovulation and fertile period.

PERMANENT
Tubal

Variety of abdominal and vaginal surgical procedures (laparotomy, laparoscopy, culdoscopy) that permanently prevent sperm and ovum from meeting. Crushing, ligating, clipping, or plugging of fallopian tubes (potentially reversible procedure). Nearly 100% (99.96%) effective. Failure due to recanalization of fallopian tubes, erroneous ligation (see Figure 12-21).	Bowel injury, hemorrhage, or infection.	Determine whether temporary contraceptives were used and reason for patient's dissatisfaction. Counsel regarding effects of procedure on physiology and sexual performance. Assist in obtaining written informed consent for procedure. Inform patient that procedure may require short-term hospitalization or can be done on outpatient basis.

Hysterectomy

Surgical removal of uterus. 100% effective.	Bladder infection, vascular disorders, infection, hemorrhage, pain, psychological adjustment.	Assess or counsel regarding understanding of extent of surgery, altered physiology, complications, and sexual performance. Hysterectomy only performed for other reasons; sterility is secondary benefit when desired.

Table 12-2 *Methods of Birth Control—cont'd*

DESCRIPTION	SIDE EFFECTS AND COMPLICATIONS	PATIENT EDUCATION
Vasectomy		
Bilateral surgical ligation and resection of ductus deferens.	Hematoma, edema, psychological adjustment (see Figure 12-22).	Inform patient that procedure is usually done as outpatient procedure and takes 15 to 30 minutes. Tell patient that alternative form of contraception is needed until no sperm are seen on examination. Explain that procedure does not affect masculinity.

NURSING PROCESS *for the Patient with a Reproductive Disorder*

The role of the licensed practical nurse/licensed vocational nurse (LPN/LVN) in the nursing process as stated is that the LPN/LVN will:

- Participate in planning care for patients based on patient needs.
- Review patient's plan of care and recommend revisions as needed.
- Review and follow defined prioritization for patient care.
- Use clinical pathways/care maps/care plans to guide and review patient care.

Assessment

People with reproductive disorders require skilled assessment by both the nurse and the physician. Assessment occurs through observation of the patient during the patient health history and while doing baseline and continuing assessment of the patient's objective and subjective data.

Health history data should be relevant to the developmental age of the patient. Information about reproductive health and sexuality can form a large portion of the collected data. This history is as important as the physical and mental information as a basis for determining appropriate nursing diagnoses and interventions. Data collected about sexual health, sexual relations, birth control methods, STDs, and the use of chemical substances provide an opportunity to clarify any misconceptions, myths, or hearsay revealed during history taking.

Data Collection for Females

Data collection for adolescent and adult women focuses on the reproductive tract and the menstrual, gynecologic, and obstetric history.

The menstrual history encompasses menarche (onset of menstrual flow) through the climacteric (cessation of menstrual cycle), including: (1) age of onset, (2) date of last menstrual flow, (3) usual amount and volume of flow (number of pads used per day), (4) presence of **dysmenorrhea** (painful menstruation), **menor-**rhagia (excessive flow), **amenorrhea** (absence of flow), or **metrorrhagia** (excessive spotting between cycles), and (5) other difficulties during menses.

The gynecologic assessment includes data on (1) vaginal discharge (odor, color, frequency, and duration), (2) vaginal pruritus (itching), (3) vaginal irritation with coital activity, (4) date and results of the last Pap test, (5) birth control methods or kinds of contraceptives used, and (6) any family history of cancer of the reproductive system.

If the adolescent or adult woman has conceived, information should be collected as to **gravidity** (number of pregnancies), **parity** (number of births), abortions, miscarriages, and stillbirths. Assessment of the breast includes (1) tenderness of the breast areas; (2) pain; (3) masses in any specific areas; (4) presence of nipple discharge; (5) knowledge and frequency of BSE; and (6) date of last mammogram, if applicable.

Data Collection for Males

The data collected from the male adolescent and the adult man include (1) urologic history of voiding difficulties and any discharge from the penis; (2) characteristics of the urine (odor, color, amount, and frequency); (3) information on prostate and testicular problems; (4) frequency of PSA testing, if applicable; (5) masses or lesions on genitalia; (6) frequency of TSE; (7) frequency of professional testicular examination; (8) nature of measures to prevent infections; and (9) birth control measures. In addition, the nurse should note concerns about sexual health voiced by the patient.

Nursing Diagnosis

Possible nursing diagnoses for the patient with a reproductive disorder include but are not limited to the following:

Anxiety
Disturbed body image
Ineffective coping
Fear
Deficient fluid volume
Ineffective health maintenance

Table 12-3 | *Planning and Setting Goals for the Patient with a Reproductive Disorder*

NURSING DIAGNOSIS	GOAL	OUTCOME
Coping, ineffective, related to fear of positive diagnosis of breast cancer	Patient will attend cancer support group weekly	Patient expresses fears of unfavorable outcome.
Knowledge, deficient, regarding postoperative care at home following modified radical mastectomy	Patient will state four postoperative risks before discharge	Patient verbalizes signs and symptoms of infection. Patient demonstrates exercises for affected arm. Patient verbalizes need to avoid injections, taking of blood, or BP in affected arm. Patient verbalizes need to examine remaining breast once a month.

Risk for infection
Deficient knowledge
Acute pain
Chronic pain
Chronic low self-esteem
Situational low self-esteem
Sexual dysfunction
Impaired skin integrity
Ineffective tissue perfusion
Impaired urinary elimination

Expected Outcomes/Planning

Planning is a category of nursing behaviors in which patient-centered goals are established and strategies designed to achieve the goals and outcomes that relate to the identified nursing diagnosis (Table 12-3).

Implementation

The implementation step for the patient with a reproductive disorder is the action-oriented phase of the nursing process in which the nurse initiates and carries out the objectives of the nursing care plan. See Complementary & Alternative Therapies box for additional treatment methods.

Evaluation

The evaluation phase of the nursing process determines the effectiveness of the nursing care plan, offering nurses the information needed to ensure optimum patient outcomes. A systematic process of evaluation requires the nurse to use critical thinking when comparing expected outcomes with the actual results of care. When patient goals are achieved, the patient has reached a level of health. If goals are unmet, the nurse analyzes the causes and establishes a more appropriate care plan. Examples of goals and their corresponding evaluative measures include the following:

Goal #1: Patient has ability for effective coping.
Evaluative measure: Patient able to verbalize fears

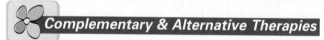
Complementary & Alternative Therapies

Male and Female Reproductive Disorders
PRIMARY DYSMENORRHEA
- It has been suggested that biofeedback, therapeutic touch, or acupuncture might be helpful

MALE REPRODUCTIVE SYSTEM
- *Pausinystalia yohimbe* has been used to treat erectile dysfunction and impotence

FEMALE REPRODUCTIVE SYSTEM
- Black cohosh *(Cimicifuga racemosa)* for menstrual irregularity, PMS, and menopausal problems
- Chamomile *(Marticaria recutita, Chamaemelum nobile)* for menstrual cramps
- Chaste tree *(Vitex agnuscastus)* for PMS
- Evening primrose *(Oenothera biennis)* for PMS
- Feverfew *(Tanacetum parthenium)* for menstrual problems
- Sage *(Salvia officinalis)* for menstrual irregularity
- Soybeans and other legumes for their phytoestrogens that may help prevent breast cancer

Modified from Back, J.M., et al. (2005). *Medical-surgical nursing.* (7th ed.). Philadelphia: Saunders.

and identify two strategies for dealing with fear, including questioning for clarification and relaxation breathing technique.

Goal #2: Patient has adequate knowledge regarding postoperative care at home after modified radical **mastectomy.**

Evaluative measure: Patient can state signs and symptoms of wound infection; list proper arm exercises; verbalize the need for BSE once per month; and state need to avoid blood pressure (BP) checks, injections, and blood draws in affected arm.

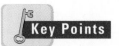
Key Points

- Sperm are produced in the seminiferous tubules and stored in the epididymis.
- Testosterone, the male sex hormone, is responsible for male secondary sex characteristics.
- Seminal fluid is produced in the seminal vesicles, prostate gland, and Cowper's glands.
- The male urethra serves the twofold purpose of conveying urine from the bladder and carrying the reproductive cells and secretions to the outside.
- The uterus consists of three layers of tissue: (1) endometrium, the inner layer; (2) myometrium, the middle layer; and (3) perimetrium, the outer layer.
- In the ovulating female, an egg matures each month in the graafian follicle, which is located in the ovary.
- The menstrual cycle prepares the uterus and causes ovulation to occur each month.
- Because of the relationship between the menstrual cycle and the body's mechanisms of hormonal secretion, a decrease or increase in the activity of the hormonal glands can disturb menstruation.
- Early diagnosis and prompt management are necessary if reproductive and genital problems of a more serious nature are to be prevented.
- Health teaching for patients with menstrual disturbances includes a knowledge of the physiologic process, factors that alter menstruation, personal hygiene, exercise, diet, and pain management.
- Discharge planning is vital to prevent reinfection after pelvic inflammatory disease.
- Pregnancy is encouraged in the patient with endometriosis, because it will slow the progress of the disorder; infertility is a complication as the condition continues.
- Menarche, the first menstrual cycle, usually begins around the age of 12 years.
- Serum CA-125 is useful mainly to signal a recurrence of ovarian cancer and in following the response to treatment.
- Prostate-specific antigen (PSA) is a highly sensitive blood test that is elevated in cancer of the prostate as well as in benign prostatic hyperplasia.
- There is no definitive test for toxic shock syndrome. However, cervical-vaginal isolates of *S. aureus* have been present 90% of the time with toxic shock syndrome.
- Vaginal fistulas are caused by an ulcerating process resulting from cancer, radiation, weakening of tissue from pregnancies, and surgical interventions.
- Correction of cystocele and rectocele is a surgical repair involving shortening of the muscles that support the

bladder and repair of the rectocele. This is known as anterior posterior colporrhaphy.
- A panhysterosalpingo-oophorectomy is the removal of the uterus, fallopian tubes, and ovaries.
- In breast cancer patients an axillary lymph node dissection is usually performed regardless of treatment option available. Examination of nodes provides the most powerful prognostic data currently available.
- A relatively new diagnostic tool used before therapeutic surgery for breast cancer is sentinel lymph node mapping, which identifies the first lymph node most likely to drain the cancerous cells.
- Overall 10-year survival with lumpectomy and radiation is about the same as with modified radical mastectomy.
- After losing a breast, many patients experience acute grief that may last 4 to 6 weeks or longer. Grief makes the fact of loss real.
- Caution patients who have undergone a modified radical mastectomy to avoid injections, vaccinations, taking of blood pressure or blood samples, or insertion of intravenous line in the affected arm.
- Phimosis is a condition in which the prepuce is too small to allow retraction of the foreskin over the glans penis.
- Young men should be taught to perform testicular self-examination monthly beginning at 15 years of age for detection of testicular carcinoma.
- Oral acyclovir (Zovirax) is being prescribed for primary herpes genitalis to shorten the duration of the healing of genital lesions and suppress 75% of recurrence with daily use.
- Parenteral penicillin remains the treatment of choice for all stages of syphilis. All stages of syphilis should be treated.
- Because of penicillin-resistant strains of *N. gonorrhoeae*, penicillin, the former drug of choice for treatment of gonorrhea, has been changed to ceftriaxone (Rocephin).
- Chlamydial infections respond to treatment with tetracycline (Tetracyn), doxycycline (Vibramycin), azithromycin (Zithromax), or ofloxacin (Floxin). Erythromycin is the drug of choice for use in pregnant patients.

Go to your free CD-ROM for an Audio Glossary, animations, video clips, and Review Questions for the NCLEX-PN® Examination.

evolve   Be sure to visit the companion Evolve site at http://evolve.elsevier.com/Christensen/adult/ for WebLinks and additional online resources.

CHAPTER CHALLENGE

1. Ms. M., a 61-year-old patient, visits her physician because of an increase in her abdominal girth and dyspnea during the past month as a result of pressure on her diaphragm. She is diagnosed as having cancer of the ovaries. These two clinical manifestations result from:
   1. development of ascites.
   2. metastasis to the bowel.
   3. dilation of the alveoli.
   4. bladder distention.

2. E.M. is a 30-year-old premenopausal female who is asking the nurse the most appropriate time of the month to do her self-examination of the breasts. The most appropriate reply by the nurse would be:
   1. during her menstruation.
   2. 7 to 8 days after conclusion of the menstrual period.
   3. the same day of each month.
   4. the 26th day of the menstrual cycle.

3. Ms. F. is a 52-year-old patient who has ductal cell carcinoma of the left breast. She is in the first postoperative day after having had a modified radical mastectomy. A Davol drain is in place in the left axillary region. The main purpose of this drain is to:
   1. control numbness of her left incisional site.
   2. improve her ability to perform range-of-motion exercises on her affected side.
   3. facilitate drainage and prevent formation of a hematoma.
   4. prevent postoperative phlebitis in her affected arm.

4. D.C. is a 35-year-old patient who has received a vasectomy. Teaching for this patient should include the following information:
   1. the procedure is reversible if he later changes his mind.
   2. he should abstain from sexual intercourse until the incision is completely healed.
   3. he should apply warm compresses to the scrotum four times a day.
   4. he should return to the physician at regular intervals for sperm counts.

5. Ms. B. is a 44-year-old patient who is admitted for an abdominal hysterectomy. She is instructed that she will have a Foley catheter in place postoperatively. She asks the nurse how many days she will have the catheter in place. The best response by the nurse would be that:
   1. the indwelling catheter will probably remain in place for 1 week.
   2. the indwelling catheter will be removed after you are fully awake from the anesthesia.
   3. the indwelling catheter will generally remain in place 1 to 2 days after surgery.
   4. the indwelling catheter will remain in place for a few days postdischarge.

6. Ms. P. is a 60-year-old patient who has had a vaginal hysterectomy for a prolapsed uterus. The nurse is very aware that patients undergoing pelvic surgery are more susceptible to certain postoperative complications, and thus adjusts postoperative interventions to prevent:
   1. wound dehiscence.
   2. wound infection.
   3. atelectasis and hypostatic pneumonia.
   4. venous stasis and thrombophlebitis.

7. Ms. L., 49 years of age, is an obese diabetic patient who has had a total abdominal hysterectomy. On the second postoperative day, Ms. L. complains of increased pain in the operative site. She states, "It feels like something suddenly popped." With the symptoms presented, it would be likely that when the nurse removes the abdominal dressing she may note that:
   1. the wound has purulent exudate.
   2. dehiscence has occurred.
   3. the wound is indurated and tender.
   4. the wound is well approximated.

8. Ms. B. is a 20-year-old patient who goes to the physician's office with vaginal pruritus, burning, dull pelvic pain, and purulent vaginal discharge. A diagnostic test reveals she has chlamydia. The nurse goes over the medication schedule carefully with Ms. B. Another very important nursing intervention to achieve satisfactory patient outcome would be to:
   1. encourage her to have her sexual partner(s) seek medical care as soon as possible to avoid reinfection of the patient.
   2. recommend she abstain from sexual contact while lesions are present.
   3. provide social and emotional support because the edematous, draining lymph nodes may be disturbing to Ms. B.'s self-image.
   4. educate Ms. B. that the causative organism is a spirochete that gains entrance into the body during intercourse.

9. Ms. M. is a 40-year-old patient with a right modified radical mastectomy with wide resection of the axillary lymph nodes. Which of the following are encouraged in the postoperative care for Ms. M.? (Choose all correct answers.)
   1. Encourage turning, coughing, and deep breathing, use of incentive spirometry.
   2. Take blood pressure readings on her right arm.
   3. Draw a circle around the drainage on the pressure dressing.
   4. Administer oxycodone (Percocet) tablets every 4 hours as needed for pain.

10. J.P. is a 23-year-old male who is diagnosed with gonorrhea. Because of statements made in his patient interview, the nurse has established a nursing diagnosis of noncompliance. Which is the most effective way to overcome noncompliance for this patient?
    1. Telephone follow-up
    2. Case finding
    3. Single-dose treatment of ceftriaxone (Rocephin) IM
    4. Extensive patient education program

11. The nurse is teaching a group of teenagers about contraception and sexually transmitted diseases. The nurse asks the students if they know which is the most prevalent of the sexually transmitted diseases. In a discussion they are surprised to learn it is:
    1. syphilis.
    2. chlamydial infections.
    3. gonorrhea.
    4. herpes genitalis.

12. Ms. T. is a 73-year-old patient who comes to the physician's office with the complaint of constant seepage of feces from her vagina, causing her embarrassment due to soilage and odor. She is presenting signs of:
    1. rectovaginal fistula.
    2. vesicovaginal fistula.
    3. urethrovaginal fistula.
    4. rectocele.

13. The American Cancer Society recommends that women have an annual screening mammography beginning at age:
    1. 21.
    2. 35.
    3. 40.
    4. 52.

14. The first lymph node most likely to drain the cancerous site in a breast cancer patient is known as the:
    1. axillary node.
    2. contaminated node.
    3. primary node.
    4. sentinal node.

15. While discussing risk factors for breast cancer with a group of women, the nurse stresses that the greatest risk factor for breast cancer is:
    1. being a female older than the age of 50.
    2. experiencing menstruation for 40 years or more.
    3. using estrogen replacement therapy during menopause.
    4. having a paternal grandmother with postmenopausal breast cancer.

16. A patient diagnosed with breast cancer has been offered the treatment choice of breast conservation surgery with radiation or a modified radical mastectomy. When questioned by the patient about these options, the nurse informs the patient that the lumpectomy with radiation:
    1. preserves the normal appearance and sensitivity of the breast.
    2. provides a shorter treatment period with fewer long-term complications.
    3. has about the same 10-year survival rate as the modified radical mastectomy.
    4. reduces the fear and anxiety that accompany the diagnosis and treatment of cancer.

17. Postoperatively the nurse teaches the patient with a modified radical mastectomy to prevent lymphedema by:
    1. using a sling to keep the arm flexed at the side.
    2. exposing the arm to sunlight to increase circulation.
    3. wrapping the arm with elastic bandages during the night.
    4. avoiding unnecessary trauma (e.g., venipuncture, BP) to the arm on the operative side.

18. The nurse plans early and frequent ambulation for the patient who has undergone an abdominal hysterectomy to:
    1. prevent urinary retention.
    2. prevent deep vein thrombosis.
    3. relieve abdominal distention.
    4. maintain a sense of normalcy.

13 Care of the Patient with a Visual or Auditory Disorder

PATRICIA HELMER OLES, KAREN H. RICHARDSON, and BARBARA LAURITSEN CHRISTENSEN

Objectives

After reading this chapter, the student should be able to do the following:

Anatomy and Physiology

1. List the major sense organs and discuss their anatomical position.
2. List the parts of the eye and define the function of each part.
3. List the three divisions of the ear, and discuss the function of each.

Medical-Surgical

4. Define the key terms as listed.
5. Describe two changes in the sensory system that occur as a result of the normal aging process.
6. Describe the purpose, significance of results, and nursing responsibilities related to diagnostic studies of the visual and auditory systems.
7. Describe age-related changes in the visual and auditory systems and differences in assessment findings.
8. Describe inflammatory conditions of the lid, conjunctiva, and cornea with etiology/pathophysiology, clinical manifestations, assessment, diagnostic tests, medical management, nursing interventions, patient teaching, and prognosis.
9. Compare the nature of cataracts, diabetic retinopathy, retinal detachment, glaucoma, and macular degeneration, and the etiology/pathophysiology, clinical manifestations, assessment, diagnostic tests, medical management, nursing interventions, patient teaching, and prognosis.
10. Discuss corneal injuries including etiology/pathophysiology, clinical manifestations, assessment, diagnostic tests, medical management, nursing interventions, patient teaching, and prognosis.
11. Differentiate between conductive and sensorineural hearing loss.
12. Describe major ear inflammatory and infectious disorders including etiology/pathophysiology, clinical manifestations, assessment, diagnostic tests, medical management, nursing interventions, patient teaching, and prognosis.
13. List tips for communicating with hearing- and sight-impaired people.
14. Give patient instructions regarding care of the eye and ear in accordance with written protocol.
15. Discuss noninfectious disorders of the ear, including etiology/pathophysiology, clinical manifestations, assessment, diagnostic tests, medical management, nursing interventions, patient teaching, and prognosis.
16. Describe the appropriate care of the hearing aid.
17. Identify communication resources for people with visual and/or hearing impairment.
18. Describe home health considerations for people with eye or ear disorders, surgery, or visual and hearing impairments.
19. Describe the various surgeries of the ear, including the nursing interventions, patient teaching, and prognosis.

Key Terms

Be sure to check out the bonus material on the free CD-ROM, including selected audio pronunciations.

astigmatism (ă-STĬG-mă-tĭsm, p. 645)
audiometry (ăw-dē-ŎM-ĕ-trē, p. 667)
cataract (KĂT-ă-răkt, p. 650)
conjunctivitis (kŏn-jŭnk-tĭ-VĪ-tĭs, p. 648)
cryotherapy (krī-ō-THĔR-ă-pē, p. 655)
diabetic retinopathy (dī-ă-BĔT-ĭk rĕ-tĭn-NŎP-ă-thē, p. 653)
enucleation (ē-nū-klē-Ā-shŭn, p. 664)
exophthalmos (ĕk-sŏf-THĂL-mŏs, p. 642)
glaucoma (glăw-KŌ-mă, p. 657)
hyperopia (hī-pĕr-Ō-pē-ă, p. 645)
keratitis (kĕr-ă-TĪ-tĭs, p. 648)
keratoplasty (kĕr-ă-tō-PLĂS-tē, p. 664)
labyrinthitis (lăb-ĭ-rĭnth-Ī-tĭs, p. 674)
mastoiditis (măs-toy-DĪ-tĭs, p. 671)
miotic (mī-ŎT-ĭk, p. 658)
mydriatic (mĭd-rē-ĂT-ĭk, p. 641)
myopia (mī-Ō-pē-ă, p. 645)
myringotomy (mĭr-ĭn-GŎT-ō-mē, p. 679)
radial keratotomy (RĀ-dē-ăl kĕ-ră-TŎT-ō-mē, p. 645)
retinal detachment (RĔ-tĭ-năl dē-TĂCH-mĕnt, p. 656)
Sjögren syndrome (SHĔR-grenz SĬN-drōm, p. 649)
Snellen's test (SNĔL-ĕnz tĕst, p. 641)
stapedectomy (stā-pĕ-DĔK-tō-mē, p. 678)
strabismus (stră-BĬZ-mŭs, p. 645)
tinnitus (TĬ-nĭ-tĭs, p. 671)
tympanoplasty (tĭm-pă-nō-PLĂS-tē, p. 679)
vertigo (VĔR-tĭ-gō, p. 674)

OVERVIEW OF ANATOMY AND PHYSIOLOGY

The sensory system constantly gathers information through millions of receptors scattered throughout the body and delivers it to the brain for interpretation. This process enables humans to survive safely by allowing appropriate responses to external stimuli. The five major senses are taste, touch, smell, sight, and hearing. The sense of balance (equilibrium) is linked with hearing, because the sensors are located within the ear.

ANATOMY OF THE EYE

The eye, which is only 1 inch (2.5 cm) in diameter, is a marvelous spherical structure that contains 70% of the sensory structures of the body. The optic tracts contain more than 1 million nerve fibers that carry messages from the eye to the brain, where they are interpreted. Only a small portion of the eye is visible externally; the remainder is enclosed in the skeletal bones of the face and cushioned layers of fat. The bones surrounding the eyeball include the frontal, zygomatic, ethmoid, sphenoid, and lacrimal bones.

ACCESSORY STRUCTURES OF THE EYE

The accessory structures of the eye—the eyebrows, eyelashes, eyelids, and lacrimal apparatus—function mainly as protective devices. In addition, six extrinsic eye muscles control gross eye movement and enable the eye to focus on any object in the visual field.

The structures of the **lacrimal apparatus** (Figure 13-1) manufacture and drain tears to keep the eyeball moist and sweep away debris that might enter the eye.

Tears are composed of a watery secretion that contains salt, mucus, and a bactericidal enzyme called **lysozyme.** The lacrimal glands are located superior and lateral to each eye. Blinking causes tears to flow medially to the lacrimal ducts, which empty into the nasolacrimal ducts and drain into the nasal cavity.

The six extrinsic eye muscles, which are attached to the sclera or white part of the eye, move the eye laterally, medially, superiorly, and inferiorly. Occasionally, children develop a condition commonly called **lazy eye,** which involves a weak or elongated eye muscle and is characterized by visual disturbances.

The **conjunctiva** (Figure 13-2) is a thin mucous membrane that lines the inner aspect of the eyelids and the anterior surface of the eyeball to the edge of the cornea. Sometimes the blood vessels of the conjunctiva become dilated because of irritation or congestion, and the individual is said to have "bloodshot" eyes.

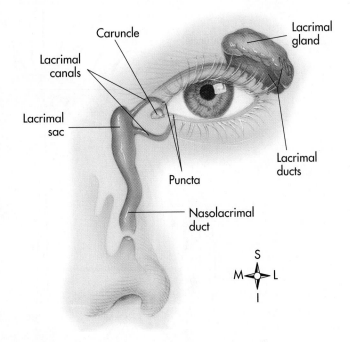

FIGURE **13-1** Lacrimal apparatus.

STRUCTURE OF THE EYEBALL

The eyeball is composed of three layers, or tunics (see Figure 13-2). The outermost layer of the eyeball is the fibrous tunic, composed of thick, white, opaque, connective tissue called the **sclera,** or white of the eye. The sclera gives shape to the eyeball and, because of its toughness, protects the inner eye structures. Posteriorly it is pierced by the optic nerve and, along with the transparent cornea, makes up the outermost of the three tunics covering the eyeball. The **cornea,** which is the central anterior portion of the sclera, is transparent and covers the iris, which is the colored portion of the eye. The cornea allows light rays to enter the inner portion of the eye. It is dense, uniform in thickness, nonvascular, and projects like a dome beyond the sclera. The cornea is one of the most highly developed, sensitive tissues in the body and is innervated by the trigeminal nerve (CNV). The avascular cornea obtains oxygen primarily through absorption from the tear film layer that bathes the epithelium. A small amount of oxygen is obtained from the aqueous humor through the endothelial layers. The degree of corneal curvature varies in different individuals and in the same person at different ages. The curvature is more pronounced in youth than in advanced age. Located at the junction of the sclera and cornea is a special structure called the canal of Schlemm. This tiny venous sinus at the angle of the anterior chamber of the eye drains the aqueous humor and

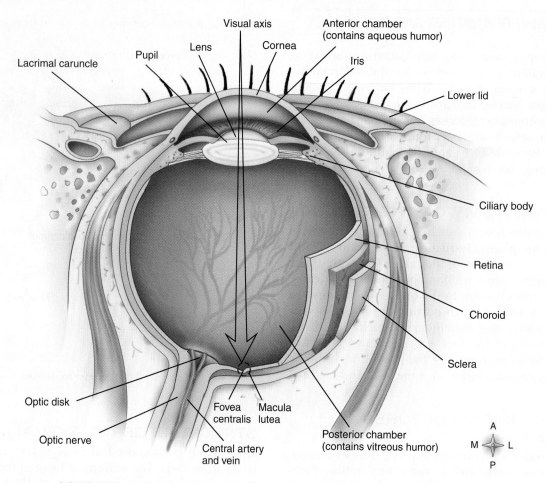

FIGURE **13-2** Horizontal section through the left eyeball. The eye is viewed from above.

funnels it into the bloodstream. This aids in controlling intraocular pressure (the pressure within the eyeball).

The middle layer of the eyeball is the vascular tunic. It contains the choroid, the ciliary body, and the iris. The posterior portion of the vascular tunic is the **choroid,** which is a thin dark brown membrane that lines most of the internal area of the sclera. It is highly vascular and supplies nutrients to the retina. The anterior portion of the vascular tunic forms the ciliary body, which is an intrinsic muscular ring that holds the lens in place and changes its shape for near or distant vision. The ciliary body also attaches to the iris, a pigmented intrinsic muscular ring that resembles a doughnut. Located slightly nasal to the center of the iris is a circular opening called the **pupil.** The iris lies between the cornea and the lens and regulates the amount of light entering the eye through the pupil, much like a camera lens. Two sets of smooth muscle control the iris, which in turn controls the pupil. In bright light the circular muscle fibers of the iris contract and the pupil contracts; in dim light the radial muscles contract and the pupil dilates.

The innermost tunic of the eye is the **retina,** a 10-layer, delicate, nervous-tissue membrane of the eye that receives images of external objects and transmits impulses through the optic nerve to the brain. It lies on the posterior portion of the eyeball. Located within the retina are specialized sensory cells called **rods** and **cones** (photoreceptors). The rods and cones are scattered throughout the retina except where the optic nerve exits the eye; this area is called the **optic disk** or **blind spot.** Rods are receptors for night vision and are also responsible for peripheral vision. Cones are responsible for day vision. There are three kinds of cones, each sensitive to a different color: red, green, or blue. Color pigments that are sensitive to light enable the rods and cones to function. The center of the retina is the fovea centralis, a pinpoint depression composed only of densely packed cones. This area of the retina provides the sharpest visual acuity. Surrounding the fovea is the macula, an area of less than 1 mm^2 that has a high concentration of cones and is relatively free of blood vessels. Vitamin A is responsible for the production of these color pigments. The absence of these three types of cones causes color blindness, which is an inherited condition found primarily in males.

CHAMBERS OF THE EYE

The eye is divided into two chambers by the **crystalline lens,** a transparent, colorless structure that is biconvex in shape, enclosed in a capsule, and held in place just behind the pupil by the suspensory ligament. The function of the crystalline lens is to focus light rays so that they form a perfect image on the retina. Anterior to the crystalline lens is the anterior chamber, which is filled with **aqueous humor,** a clear, watery fluid similar to blood plasma. It is continually secreted by the ciliary bodies of the choroid. It is constantly formed, drained, and replaced to maintain normal intraocular pressure. Aqueous humor also helps maintain the shape of the eyeball, keeps the retina attached to the choroid, and refracts light.

The posterior chamber is filled with **vitreous humor,** a transparent, jellylike substance that gives shape to the eyeball, keeps the retina attached to the choroid, and refracts light. It differs from the aqueous humor in that it is not continually replaced.

PHYSIOLOGY OF VISION

Light must travel through the cornea, aqueous humor, pupil, crystalline lens, vitreous humor, and finally to the rods and cones of the retina. The image is transported via the optic nerve to the visual center of the cerebral cortex in the brain.

Four basic processes are necessary to form an image:
1. **Refraction:** Light rays are bent as they pass through the colorless structures of the eye, enabling light from the environment to focus on the retina.
2. **Accommodation:** The eye is able to focus on objects at various distances. It is able to focus the image of an object on the retina by changing the curvature of the lens.
3. **Constriction:** The size of the pupil, which is controlled by the dilator and constrictor muscles of the iris, regulates the amount of light entering the eye.
4. **Convergence:** Medial movement of both eyes allows light rays from an object to hit the same point on both retinas.

ANATOMY AND PHYSIOLOGY OF THE EAR

The external ear (**pinna,** or **auricle**) reveals only a portion of the complex organ of hearing. Within the ear are many structures that enable hearing and interpretation of sound and assist in maintaining equilibrium (balance). Anatomically, from the external structures to the internal structures, there are three distinct divisions of the ear: the external ear, the middle ear, and the inner ear (Figure 13-3). The external ear and mid-

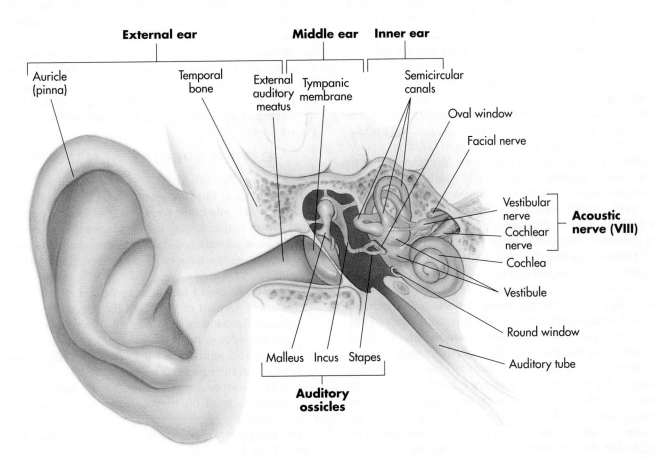

FIGURE **13-3** The ear. External, middle, and inner ear. (Not to scale.)

dle ear deal exclusively with sound waves, whereas the inner ear deals with sound waves and equilibrium.

EXTERNAL EAR

The external ear is composed of the auricle (pinna), the external auditory canal, and the **tympanic membrane** (eardrum)—a thin, semitransparent membrane. The tympanic membrane separates the external ear from the middle ear and transmits sound vibrations to the internal ear by means of the auditory ossicles. The external ear is designed to collect sound waves and channel them to the middle ear. The upper part of the pinna is composed of elastic cartilage, whereas the lower part—the lobe—is mainly fleshy tissue. The whole structure is attached to the head by ligaments and muscles.

The external auditory canal, or meatus, is a 1-inch (2.5-cm) tube that ends at the tympanic membrane. The walls of the canal are composed of cartilage-lined bone. The external auditory canal contains cilia (tiny hairs) and specialized sebaceous (oil) glands called **ceruminous glands.** They secrete **cerumen** (earwax), which protects the lining from infection. The cilia, in combination with the cerumen, also prevent foreign objects from entering the ear.

MIDDLE EAR

The middle ear, or tympanic cavity, is a small, air-filled chamber located within the temporal bone. The **eustachian tube,** or auditory canal, is lined with a mucous membrane that joins the nasopharynx and the middle-ear cavity. This tube equalizes the air pressure on either side of the tympanic membrane. During swallowing or yawning, the tube allows air to enter the middle ear, which equalizes the middle-ear and external-ear pressure. Because the pharynx, eustachian tube, and middle ear are all covered with a continuous mucous membrane, infection can travel very easily from the throat to the middle ear. This is often seen in young children. The posterior wall of the middle ear opens into the mastoid process, an area filled with air spaces, which also aids in equalization of air pressure. Infection of the middle ear, if untreated, can spread to the mastoid process.

Extending along the middle-ear chamber are three small bones (ossicles) that carry sound waves from the external ear to the inner ear. These ossicles are named according to their shape: the **malleus** (hammer), **incus** (anvil), and **stapes** (stirrup). The internal surface of the tympanic membrane is connected to the first of these three bones, the malleus. The malleus transfers sound waves to the incus, which in turn transfers them to the stapes. The stapes pushes against the oval window, a small membrane that marks the beginning of the inner ear. When sound waves cause the tympanic membrane to vibrate, that vibration is transmitted and amplified by the ear ossicles as it passes through the middle ear. Movement of the stapes against the oval window causes movements of fluid in the inner ear.

INTERNAL EAR

The most important portion of the ear, the inner ear or **labyrinth,** is a series of canals (Figure 13-4). Structurally, it contains the bony labyrinth, which is filled with a fluid called **perilymph** and contains three subdivisions called the **semicircular canal** (associated with the sense of balance), the **vestibule,** and the **cochlea.** The membranous labyrinth is a series of sacs and tubes that contain a thicker fluid called **endolymph.** Endolymph and perilymph conduct sound waves through the inner-ear system.

The **cochlea** resembles a snail's shell and contains the **organ of Corti,** the organ of hearing. It contains many hearing receptors or hair cells. These cells respond to sound waves by stimulating the cochlear nerve (a branch of the eighth cranial nerve—the vestibulocochlear nerve), which transmits the message to the brain. These hair cells may become damaged from noise pollution (i.e., high-intensity sounds such as those produced by jet engines, factory equipment, and rock bands). Once these cells are damaged or destroyed, hearing becomes permanently damaged.

Deeper in the inner ear, past the cochlea, is the **vestibule,** or the oval central portion of the bony labyrinth. The vestibule contains receptors that respond to gravity. They provide information on which way is up and which way is down, enabling an individual to remain in an upright position. Extending upward from the vestibule are three semicircular canals responsible for maintaining balance and equilibrium. They contain sensory hair cells and endolymph. The motion of the endolymph stimulates the hair cells, which stimulates the receptors; then the message is sent to the brain for interpretation (see Figure 13-4).

OTHER SPECIAL SENSES
TASTE AND SMELL

On the tongue of the average adult, there are approximately 10,000 taste buds; some are also located on the inner aspect of the cheeks. Taste buds are the receptors for four basic sensations. The four taste sensations and the locations of the taste buds that detect them are as follows:

1. **Sweet:** Respond to sugar and other sweet substances; located on the tip of the tongue
2. **Sour:** Respond to acid content of foods; located on the sides of the tongue
3. **Salty:** Respond to metal ions within foods; located on the tip of the tongue
4. **Bitter:** Respond to alkaline or basic ions within foods; located on the posterior portion of the tongue

The receptors for the sense of smell **(olfactory receptors)** are located in the roof or upper part of the nasal cavity. Upon inhalation an odor comes in contact with the olfactory receptors and the message is sent to

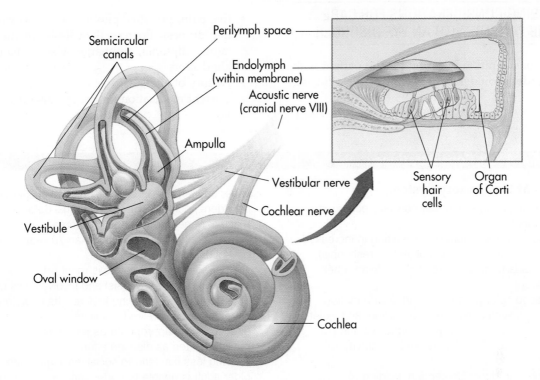

FIGURE **13-4** The inner ear. The bony labyrinth is the hard outer wall of the entire inner ear and includes semicircular canals, vestibule, and cochlea. Within the bony labyrinth is the membranous labyrinth (purple), which is surrounded by perilymph and filled with endolymph. Each ampulla in the vestibule contains a crista ampullaris that detects changes in head position and sends sensory impulses through the vestibular nerve to the brain. Inset shows a section of the membranous cochlea. Hair cells in the organ of Corti detect sound and send the information through the cochlear nerve. Then vestibular and cochlear nerves join to form the eighth cranial nerve.

the brain. Memory for certain odors is long standing and certain odors stimulate certain memories (e.g., pine scent reminds people of Christmas; talcum powder reminds people of infants). The body is not able to regenerate olfactory cells; once they are damaged, the sense of smell is impaired.

TOUCH

The receptors for touch **(tactile receptors)** are located throughout the integumentary system. They respond to touch, pressure, and vibration.

POSITION/MOVEMENT

Proprioception (sense of position) maintains the proper position of the body. **Proprioceptors** include any sensory nerve ending—such as those located in muscles, tendons, and joints—that responds to stimuli originating from within the body regarding movement and spatial position. They work in conjunction with the semicircular canals and vestibule of the inner ear to maintain proper coordination. They orchestrate the body for running, walking, dancing, and many other activities. Once they receive information from the environment, they send it to the cerebellum for interpre-

tation. Proprioceptors enable one to sense the position of the different parts of the body and be aware of the movement of each.

NORMAL AGING OF THE SENSORY SYSTEM

As an individual ages the crystalline lens of the eye hardens and becomes too large for the eye muscles, thus causing a loss of accommodation, which often results in a need for bifocals or trifocals. The crystalline lens loses some of its transparency and becomes more opaque, and glare begins to become a problem. Concurrently the pupil becomes smaller and decreases the amount of light that reaches the retina, causing one to need brighter light for reading.

The aging ear loses the ability to hear high frequencies and to distinguish consonant sounds, probably as a result of deterioration of the nerve fibers and breakdown of the cells in the organ of Corti.

The remaining senses undergo slight changes that decrease their reaction or threshold time, which results in slower response or diminished sensation (Older Adult Considerations box).

NURSING CONSIDERATIONS FOR CARE OF THE PATIENT WITH AN EYE DISORDER

An initial consideration in caring for the patient with an eye disorder should include review of the following items:

- Eye pain, pruritus, photophobia, excessive tearing, dryness, floaters, light flashes, halo around lights, diplopia, discharge, visual changes, or blind spots
- History of allergies
- Current medication for the eye disorder

 Older Adult Considerations

Disorders of the Sensory System

- Multiple changes in vision that normally occur with aging include:
  —Changes in accommodation, resulting in increased difficulty focusing on close objects (presbyopia), which leads to difficulty reading or doing other close work
  —Decreased color perception and discrimination, particularly with shades of blue, green, and violet
  —Poor adaptation to changes in light, resulting in "night blindness" and increased sensitivity to glare
  —Alterations in depth perception, leading to increased risk of falls
  —Decreased secretion of tears, resulting in complaints of dryness or pruritus, which leads to a high risk for irritation of the cornea
  —Increased incidence of moving particles or "floaters" that interfere with visually based tasks

- Older adults experience an increased incidence of eye disorders, including cataracts, retinal detachment, macular degeneration, and glaucoma.
- A third of all individuals older than 70 years of age have significant hearing loss.
- Hearing loss in older adults is most often sensorineural (presbycusis) and involves loss of the high frequencies. Hearing loss results in distortion of speech, which can lead to failure to respond to directions or inappropriate behaviors often misinterpreted as disorientation.
- Hearing loss can lead to social isolation when the older adult is unable to understand and participate in normal conversation.
- A decreased number of receptors in the nasal cavities and papillae of the tongue results in changes in smell and taste. Most affected are the sweet and salty tastes.
- Medications often affect the taste of food and can contribute to altered nutrition.

Table 13-1 | *Normal Findings of the Adult Eye*

AREA EXAMINED	FINDINGS
Eyelid	Blink reflex to light or touch intact. Lid margins just above the corneal borders.
Eyeball	Eyeball does not protrude beyond the supraorbital ridge of the frontal bone. The eyeball is usually moist; moisture may be diminished in the older adult.
Conjunctiva	**Palpebral** (eyelid): Pink, uniform blood vessels without discharge.
	Bulbar: Clear, tiny red vessels; in the older adult, the bulbar conjunctiva may lose luster.
Sclera	Generally white; may have yellow-tan dots in a dark-skinned individual.
Cornea	Transparent, smooth, convex. In the older adult, a gray ring around the cornea (*arcus senilis*) may be present as a result of lipid deposits.
Iris	Round, intact, bilateral coloration. In the older adult, color may be paler and shape less regular.
Pupil	Equal, round, reactive to light and accommodation. Response to light is equal bilaterally. In the older adult, constriction response may be slower.
Internal eye (including retina, vessels, and optic disk)	Retina is intact. Vessel structure is intact and bilaterally similar in pattern. Optic disk has well-defined border.
Visual acuity	
Distant vision	20/20 (able to read line 20 of eye chart at a distance of 20 feet).
Near vision	Able to read newspaper print at 14 inches.
Peripheral vision	Side vision is 90 degrees from central visual axis; upward 50 degrees; downward 70 degrees.
Eye movement	Coordinated eye movement bilaterally.
Color perception	Able to properly identify colors of major groups: red, blue, and green.

- Side effects of any medications
- Use of glasses or contact lenses
- Adequacy of current eyewear prescription
- Personal habits related to care of eyewear
- Any previous eye injuries or surgeries

Once the information has been gathered and communicated, the nurse assists with the eye examination. The results of the initial examination are compared with normal findings (Table 13-1).

LABORATORY AND DIAGNOSTIC EXAMINATIONS

Once the initial eye examination is completed, the patient may require additional diagnostic testing. The major diagnostic eye tests, including Snellen's test, are explained in Table 13-2.

Additional eye tests may be required to assist in the diagnosis. Amsler's grid test is used to detect a defect

Table 13-2 | *Major Diagnostic Eye Tests*

PURPOSE	EQUIPMENT	PROCEDURE	PATIENT TEACHING
Snellen's test* Assessment of visual acuity; used as screening test	Snellen's chart; eye patch/cover	1. Patient stands or sits 20 feet from chart. 2. Covers one eye. 3. Asked to read above or below the 20/20 line. 4. Repeats step 3 using the other eye. 5. Findings are documented.	1. Explain test. 2. If findings are abnormal (i.e., other than 20 feet required to read the chart line), encourage patient to seek further eye testing.
Color vision Prerequisite for driver's license	Color chart or machine	1. Color dots are reflected on a background of mixed colors. 2. Patient identifies color patterns on the test field. 3. Findings are documented.	1. Explain procedure. 2. Encourage patient to seek further testing when results indicate inaccurate recognition of color patterns.
Refraction Measurement of visual acuity to determine refractory errors such as: **myopia** (nearsightedness), **hyperopia** (farsightedness), **presbyopia** (inability to focus on close objects), and **astigmatism** (blurred vision)	Retinoscope or sample lenses	1. Ophthalmologist/ optometrist asks patient to indicate clear/blurred vision with each lens change in the retinoscope.	1. Explain procedure. 2. Examiner discusses results with patient and encourages appropriate corrective measures.
Ophthalmoscopy Evaluation of underlying structures of the eye; routine screening	Ophthalmoscope; **mydriatic** (causing pupillary dilation) drops to dilate the pupil	1. Mydriatic drops are applied. Mydriatic drops are contraindicated in patients with narrow angle glaucoma. 2. As pupil dilation occurs, the room is darkened. 3. Patient is instructed to remain still and focus on a stationary object. 4. Examiner uses ophthalmoscope to view internal eye structure. 5. Findings are documented.	1. Explain procedure. 2. Instruct patient that effects of the drops will last no longer than 1 hour. 3. Sunglasses are required when outside or in brightly lit room until pupils return to normal size. 4. Examiner discusses results with patient and encourages corrective measures.

*Eye chart test for visual acuity: letters, numbers, or symbols are arranged on the chart in decreasing size from top to bottom.

Continued

Table 13-2 *Major Diagnostic Eye Tests—cont'd*

PURPOSE	EQUIPMENT	PROCEDURE	PATIENT TEACHING
Tonometry (see Figures 13-11 and 13-12)			
Measurement of intraocular pressure to detect tumors and glaucoma; intraocular pressure can be measured by using a Schiøtz or Tono-Pen tonometer, but the most accurate readings are obtained by applanation tonometry	Tonometer (e.g., applanation, Schiøtz) (see Figure 13-12) Topical anesthetic may be used	1. Examiner places tonometer on cornea. 2. Pressure readings are obtained. 3. Findings are documented. 4. In applanation tonometry, the surface of the anesthetized cornea is applanated by the tonometer, and the cornea is observed through the biomicroscope (see Figure 13-12). The normal intraocular pressure ranges from 10 to 22 mm Hg.	1. Explain procedure. 2. Encourage patient to relax to avoid false high readings. 3. Eyes are not to be rubbed for approximately 30 minutes to avoid corneal irritation. 4. Contact lenses may be reinserted 2 hours after completion of test.
Amster grid test			
Used to diagnose and monitor macular problems	Handheld card printed with a grid of lines (similar to graph paper)	1. Patient fixates on center dot and records any abnormalities of the grid lines, such as wavy, missing, or distorted areas.	1. Explain test. 2. Regular testing is necessary to identify any changes in macular function.
Schirmer tear test			
Study measures tear volume produced throughout fixed time period. Useful in diagnosing keratoconjunctivitis sicca	Strip of lacrimal filter paper	1. One end of strip of filter paper is placed in lower culde-sac; area of tear saturation is measured after 5 minutes.	1. Explain test. 2. Test may be done with closed or open eyes. Normal results indicate 10-15 mm of wet paper. Less than 5 mm of wetting within 5 minutes is indicative of keratoconjunctivitis sicca.

of the macular area of the retina (see Table 13-2). The tangent screen evaluates central and peripheral fields of vision. The Goldmann perimetry test detects and evaluates the progression of glaucoma (an abnormal condition of elevated pressure within the eye because of obstruction of the outflow of aqueous humor), which affects peripheral vision. Exophthalmometry measures the degree of forward placement of the eye, known as exophthalmos (an abnormal condition characterized by a marked protrusion of the eyeballs). Slit-lamp examination is done to examine the conjunctiva, lens, vitreous humor, iris, and cornea. Schirmer's tear test evaluates the function of the major lacrimal glands (see Table 13-2). Fluorescein angiography is used to examine the microvascular structures of the eye and to assess patency of the lacrimal system.

DISORDERS OF THE EYE

BLINDNESS AND NEAR BLINDNESS
Etiology/Pathophysiology

Blindness is a loss of visual acuity that ranges from partial to total loss of sight. Total blindness is defined as no light perception and no usable vision. Functional blindness is present when the patient has some light perception but no usable vision. It may be congenital or acquired.

The World Health Organization (WHO) has determined that in the United States there are approximately 1 million people who are legally blind. The patient with either total or functional blindness is considered legally blind. Legal blindness refers to individuals with a maximum visual acuity of 20/200 with corrective eyewear and/or visual field sight capacity reduced to 20 degrees. (The normal visual field range is 180 degrees.)

Categories have been established to help determine the exact extent of the vision loss and what assistive measures are appropriate for the individual. These categories range from low vision loss (20/70 to 20/200) to three categories of blindness (20/400, 20/1200, and no light perception).

Congenital blindness results from various birth defects. Acquired blindness in adults occurs as a result of disorders such as diabetic retinopathy, glaucoma, cataracts, and retinal degeneration; acute trauma is also a common cause.

Clinical Manifestations

The degree of vision loss will depend on the extent of trauma or disease. Symptoms may include diplopia, pain, presence of floaters and light flashes, and pruritus or burning of the eyes. Additional physical manifestations of the visually impaired patient include loss of peripheral vision; halos (rainbow colors seen around lights); a sense of orbital pressure; bulging of the eye(s); and any difference in the appearance of an eye structure, such as the pupil.

The wide variety of emotional symptoms associated with blindness may range from fear, anxiety, disorientation, depression, helplessness, and hopelessness to acceptance.

Assessment

Collection of **subjective data** may include noting the patient complaint of blurred vision as an early symptom of an eye disorder. It is important to determine the onset, severity, and duration of the symptoms, as well as any factors that relieve symptoms.

Collection of **objective data** may include observations of squinting and rubbing of the eyes. It is important to note the patient's compensation measures, such as use of a magnifying glass. The use and effectiveness of assistive eyewear are also determined.

Emotionally the patient may experience poor interpersonal communication skills and coping mechanisms. Because self-care skills may be impaired, a blind individual may prefer isolation, causing additional physical and emotional difficulties.

Medical Management

Corrective eyewear (contact lenses and glasses) is the first method of medical management for a partially sighted individual. If the visual defect results from an inflammatory disorder, medication appropriate to the causative agent is prescribed.

Additional assistive devices for a visually impaired patient include canes, guide dogs, magnifying systems, and telescopic lenses. The patient should be evaluated by an eye specialist to determine which devices are best suited. Some of the more technologically complex devices are expensive and may not be covered by insurance.

Canes are the most frequently used device for the partially or totally blind person. They are lightweight and portable and allow the patient simple maneuvering. The drawback to their use is that overhead objects are not usually detected. The newer laser canes provide more information about objects in front and at head and foot levels, but these are not readily available and are expensive. Guide dogs allow the blind person mobility that would otherwise be difficult. Trained dogs steer the patient away from obstacles, both aerial and stationary.

Surgical correction of the visual defect may provide eyesight. New laser surgeries provide excellent results in selected cases.

Nursing Interventions and Patient Teaching

The nurse might falsely assume that patients should be in the acceptance phase if the blindness has been present for years. This is not necessarily the case. Complications of long-term blindness may result in physical and emotional problems. Physically the patient may be malnourished from diminished self-care cooking skills. The patient may also have secondary infections related to poor hygiene practices. Assistance with activities of daily living (ADLs) is a primary focus of patient care. Adequate time should be provided to allow the patient to assist in self-care. Emotional aspects of nursing interventions include appropriate communication (Box 13-1).

Vision loss affects not only the patient but also family, friends, and the community. Coping mechanisms differ between individuals. It is a nursing responsibility to educate, assist, counsel, and prevent complications. A comprehensive approach to patient care is essential with blind individuals. Home health care considerations include education on community resources. When a total approach is taken, the patient's successful adjustment to home, work, and society is possible. Blind individuals are capable of leading a full and active life and need to be treated in such a manner.

Box 13-1 *Guidelines for Communicating with Blind People*

- Talk in a normal tone of voice.
- Do not try to avoid common phrases in speech, such as "See what I mean?"
- Introduce yourself with each contact (unless well known to the person).
- Explain any activity occurring in the room.
- Announce when you are leaving the room so the blind person is not put in the position of talking to someone who is no longer there.

Nursing diagnoses and interventions for the patient with blindness or near blindness include but are not limited to the following:

NURSING DIAGNOSES	NURSING INTERVENTIONS
Fear, related to blindness	Determine the patient's level of fear.
Risk for injury, related to new environment	Orient the patient to use people and the environment. Use therapeutic touch. Avoid loud sounds that may startle the patient. Use protective devices, such as side rails and canes. Alter surroundings to afford safety—clear passageways, nonslip rugs, etc.

The patient will require instruction on ambulatory safety. Instructions to include are walking slowly, using verbal clues from the walking companion, and encouraging the patient to touch objects or borders.

The walking companion should precede the patient by about 1 foot, and the patient's hand should be on the companion's elbow to provide security (Figure 13-5). For both short-term and long-term blindness, if total vision is affected, a description of the surroundings is appropriate.

Prognosis

Blindness and near-blindness disorders have been reduced as a result of emphasis on early diagnosis and treatment. Laser surgery treatment has provided patients with advanced technology to reduce and limit complications.

Early childhood vision screening in schools has contributed to early diagnosis and treatment of refractory errors. Permanent visual loss may occur if strabismus and astigmatism are not treated at the preschool level. Physician monitoring of intermittent follow-up care is crucial until 10 years of age. New technology in eyewear significantly reduces refractory error problems in the adult. Radial keratotomy for myopia markedly improves vision and is under continued study for long-term complications.

REFRACTORY ERRORS
Astigmatism and Strabismus

Etiology/pathophysiology. Common refractory errors (astigmatism, strabismus, myopia, and hyperopia) are described in Table 13-3.

Clinical manifestations. See Table 13-3.

Assessment. See Table 13-3.

Diagnostic tests. Common tests used in the diagnosis of refractory errors include ophthalmoscopy, retinoscopy, visual acuity tests, and refraction tests.

Medical management. Many refractory errors are treated with corrective eyewear; however, the preferred treatment is surgical correction.

Nursing interventions and patient teaching. The hospitalized patient wearing corrective eyewear requires daily assistance in cleansing and maintenance. If eyeglasses are worn, the lenses are washed daily with a mild or diluted glass cleaner and rinsed before drying with a soft cloth. Screw fittings should be checked to make sure they are secure. Contact lenses are cared for based on the manufacturer's directions. Safety should be maintained when corrective eyewear is not worn.

Nursing diagnosis and interventions for the patient with astigmatism, strabismus, myopia, and hyperopia include but are not limited to the following:

NURSING DIAGNOSIS	NURSING INTERVENTIONS
Risk for injury, related to visual changes	Reinforce physician's instruction. Orient patient to the environment. Remove small, movable objects from the path of the visually impaired patient.

The patient should be encouraged to see an optometrist or ophthalmologist yearly to keep the eyewear prescription current. The patient should be instructed on the use and care of eyewear; complications may result if the patient does not follow use and care instructions.

Myopia

Etiology/pathophysiology. See Table 13-3.

Clinical manifestations. See Table 13-3.

Assessment. See Table 13-3.

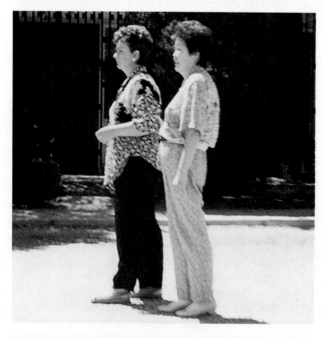

FIGURE **13-5** Sighted-guide technique. The walking companion serves as the sighted guide, walking slightly ahead of the patient with the patient holding the back of the companion's arm.

Table 13-3 | *Common Refractory Errors*

DESCRIPTION	ETIOLOGY/PATHOPHYSIOLOGY	CLINICAL MANIFESTATIONS	ASSESSMENT
Astigmatism			
Defect in the curvature of the eyeball surface	May be hereditary or a muscular deficit Occurs when the light rays cannot be focused clearly on a point on the retina, because the spherical curve of the cornea is not equal in all meridians	Blurring of vision	Collection of subjective data: complaints of eye discomfort, difficulty in focusing, blurred vision
Strabismus			
Inability of the eyes to focus in the same direction: commonly called **cross-eyed** Esotropia: eye turns in the direction of the nose Exotropia: eye turns outward	May result from neurological or muscular dysfunction or may be inherited Only one eye can fix on an object, because axes do not focus simultaneously	Eyeball position is not symmetrical	Collection of subjective data: states difficulty in following objects Collection of objective data: only one eye focuses or follows an object
Myopia			
Condition of nearsightedness	Elongation of the eyeball or an error in refraction so that parallel rays are focused in front of the retina	Inability to see objects at a distance	Collection of subjective data: difficulty seeing faraway objects Collection of objective data: Snellen's test
Hyperopia			
Condition of farsightedness	May result from error of refraction in which rays of light entering the eye are brought into focus behind the retina	Inability to see objects at close range	Collection of subjective data: difficulty seeing near objects Collection of objective data: Snellen's test

Diagnostic tests. Diagnosis of myopia commonly follows a visit to the physician because of the patient's inability to see distant objects clearly. After routine examinations (see Table 13-3) the patient will be assessed for corrective lenses or corrective refractory surgery.

Medical management. The majority of patients are prescribed corrective eyeglasses or contact lenses. Patients who are unable or unwilling to wear corrective eyewear for occupational or cosmetic reasons may elect surgical correction.

Surgical management. Refractory surgery is effective in treating the causes of visual problems instead of correcting symptoms. Patients are selected based on the degree of myopia; the shape of the cornea; and the absence of medical conditions such as severe diabetes, glaucoma, or pregnancy. The usual age for correction is between 20 to 60 years.

Keratorefractive surgery and photorefractive keratectomy. Keratorefractive surgery (surgery to alter the corneal curvature) is a new method of refractive correction. This surgical category includes a variety of procedures, including those in which the surgeon either makes cuts in the cornea or uses a laser and/or a special microsurgical knife to open and replace a flap of corneal tissue. Myopia is the refractive error most commonly corrected by refractive surgery. Currently it can be corrected by several methods.

Radial keratotomy (RK) is a technique in which the surgeon makes partial-thickness radial incisions in the patient's cornea, leaving an uncut optical zone in the center. The patient must evaluate the risk of serious complications, such as operative infection and corneal scarring, when considering this procedure.

Photorefractive keratectomy (PRK) is another procedure that uses an excimer laser to reshape the central corneal surface, primarily to correct myopia but is also used for hyperopia and astigmatism. There is evidence to suggest that final visual acuity with this procedure is more predictable than with radial keratotomy, at least in the short term. **Laser-in-situ-keratomileusis (LASIK)** is a procedure in which first a corneal flap is folded back, and then an excimer laser removes some of the internal layers of the cornea. Afterward, the flap is returned to normal position and allowed to heal in place. Evidence supports claims that LASIK creates earlier visual stability in patients with a high degree of myopia than with PRK. Unlike RK, both PRK and LASIK procedures affect the central zone of the cornea (Lewis et al, 2004).

Intacs, which are corneal ring segments, are the newest innovation in refractive procedures. Intacs are two tiny half rings of plastic that are placed between the layers of the cornea around the pupil after the surgeon makes a tunnel-like pathway with a specially designed surgical knife. They can also be removed if necessary, and the effects on refractive error are completely reversed (Lewis et al, 2004).

Nursing interventions and patient teaching. The postoperative patient will leave the hospital or clinic shortly after surgery. An eyepatch is placed on the operative site until the next morning. Patients can be up and around at home. Because of visual limitations, patients will need assistance. If the patient experiences pain, the physician will prescribe oral analgesics. The patient is seen the next day for physician follow-up. Postoperative physician checkups are scheduled at 1 week and then monthly for 1 year. A nursing diagnosis and interventions for the patient with myopia are the same as for astigmatism and strabismus errors.

Instruct the patient preoperatively to stop wearing hard contact lenses 1 to 2 days before the surgical evaluation. Encourage rest the first day postoperatively. Inform the patient that if pain persists after the first postoperative day, the physician should be notified. Instruct the patient that infection is a rare complication of the procedure. Teach the patient that vision is assessed regularly to evaluate functional vision without corrective eyewear. Patients are advised that postoperative visual acuity is not always 20/20 without glasses. The goals of operative interventions are improving ADLs and allowing the possibility of driving a vehicle without glasses during the day. As a result of a slightly dilated pupil, the patient may experience a glare or halos from lights, which may require that glasses be worn for night driving.

Hyperopia

Etiology/pathophysiology. Common refractory errors are included in Table 13-3.

Clinical manifestations. See Table 13-3.
Assessment. See Table 13-3.
Diagnostic tests. Common tests used in the diagnosis of hyperopia include ophthalmoscopy, retinoscopy, visual acuity tests, and refraction tests.

Medical management. The main treatment for farsightedness is corrective eyewear, either contact lenses or glasses. There are a variety of lenses available on the market, including hard, soft, and gas-permeable lenses.

Nursing interventions and patient teaching. The nurse should emphasize the importance of proper care of contact lenses (Health Promotion Considerations box). Eyeglasses should properly fit the bridge of the nose to eliminate slippage and an uneven level of each lens.

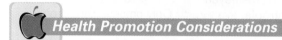
Health Promotion Considerations

Contact Lens Care

DO

- Wash and rinse hands thoroughly before handling a lens.
- Keep fingernails clean.
- Remove lenses from their storage case one at a time and place on the eye.
- Start with the same lens (left or right) at each insertion.
- Use lens-placement technique learned from eye specialist.
- Use proper lens-care products and clean the lenses as directed by the manufacturer.
- Keep the lens storage kit clean.
- Wear lenses daily and follow the prescribed wearing schedule.
- Remove a lens if it becomes uncomfortable.
- Avoid potential corneal abrasions.
- Report any signs of photophobia, dryness, excessive burning, or tearing.
- Keep regular appointments with the eye specialist.
- Remove lenses during sunbathing, showering, or swimming.

DO NOT

- Use soaps that contain cream or perfume for cleansing lenses.
- Let fingernails touch lenses.
- Mix up lenses.
- Exceed prescribed wearing time.
- Use saliva to wet lenses.
- Use homemade saline solution or tap water to wet or clean lenses.
- Borrow or mix lens-care solution.

A nursing diagnosis and interventions for the patient with hyperopia include but are not limited to the following:

NURSING DIAGNOSIS	NURSING INTERVENTIONS
Deficient knowledge, related to lack of experience with corrective eyewear	Answer all questions the patient may have on eyewear maintenance. Obtain literature on lens care. Encourage physician follow-up as directed.

INFLAMMATORY AND INFECTIOUS DISORDERS OF THE LID

Hordeolum, Chalazion, and Blepharitis

The most commonly seen infections and inflammatory disorders of the lid are listed in Table 13-4.

Clinical manifestations. See Table 13-4.

Assessment. See Table 13-4.

Diagnostic tests. The eyelid margin is examined. Culture and sensitivity tests of any drainage may be ordered. Visual disturbances are also noted.

Medical management. Antiinfective agents are prescribed. Localized incision and drainage of a cyst or stye may be performed under local anesthesia. Warm normal saline compresses are ordered for 10 to 20 minutes two to four times a day. Lid scrubs using no-tear baby shampoo may be ordered.

Nursing interventions and patient teaching. A primary objective of nursing care for the patient with an infectious or inflammatory process of the lids is prevention of the spread of infection. Care should be taken when applying compresses. Handwashing is essential before contact with the eye.

Instructions should be provided on the use of prescribed drops or ointments. The patient is taught the use of warm compresses and informed about specific hygiene practices, such as keeping hands clean and away from the eyes and replacing mascara after 3 to 6 months because the oils decompose and may harbor bacteria. The patient is cautioned to avoid irritating fumes or smoke, which may cause rubbing of the eyes, leading to further infection. The use of eye makeup is discouraged until all inflammation subsides.

Table 13-4 *Common Infections/Inflammatory Disorders of the Lid*

DESCRIPTION	ETIOLOGY/PATHOPHYSIOLOGY	CLINICAL MANIFESTATIONS	ASSESSMENT
Hordeolum (stye) Acute infection of eyelid margin or sebaceous glands of the eyelashes	Frequently caused by the *Staphylococcus* organism One or more pustules may form	Abscess localized to base of eyelashes, with edema of lid	**Collection of subjective data:** localized tenderness and pain resulting from edema; pain diminished after pustule ruptures **Collection of objective data:** raised, erythematous area on eyelid; pustule exudate
Chalazion Inflammatory cyst on the meibomian gland at the eyelid margin; may require weeks to develop into a cyst	May be caused by infection; associated with diabetes mellitus, gout, and anemia	Discomfort, mass on eyelid, edema, visual disturbance	**Collection of subjective data:** pressure felt as eyelid closes over cornea; patient may describe vision changes **Collection of objective data:** cyst formation; eyelid edema
Blepharitis Inflammation of eyelid margins	Ulcerative: caused by bacterial infection, usually staphylococcal organisms Nonulcerative: caused by psoriasis, seborrhea, or allergic response	Pruritus, erythema of eyelid, eyelid pain, photophobia Excessive tearing may occur in nonulcerative type	**Collection of subjective data:** eye pruritus; lids adhere together during sleep **Collection of objective data:** eyes erythematous; patient rubs eyes; sensitivity to light; tear spillage

Prognosis. In the majority of patients, the inflammatory and infectious phases of these conditions respond favorably to topical antimicrobials. Incision and drainage of cystlike formations results in minimal complications and risk to the patient.

Inflammation of the Conjunctiva

Etiology/pathophysiology. Conjunctivitis is an inflammation of the conjunctiva caused by bacterial or viral infection, allergy, or environmental factors. It is commonly called **pinkeye.**

Acute bacterial conjunctivitis is usually transmitted by direct contact with a contaminated object. Pneumococcal, staphylococcal, streptococcal, gonococcal, and chlamydial organisms are the major causative agents. The hands are the most common transmitter of bacteria from the contaminated object to the eye. Because of its warmth, moisture, and extensive vascularization, the eye provides the bacteria with an excellent medium for multiplication. Conjunctivitis represents about two thirds of the 1 million cases per year of eye inflammation and infection. The disease is usually self-limiting, leaving no permanent impairment.

Viruses of the respiratory or intestinal tract may result in a secondary infection of the eye. The two more common viral agents are *Chlamydia trachomatis* and type 1 herpes simplex. Trachoma, a highly contagious form of conjunctivitis, is caused by a strain of the *C. trachomatis* virus. Transmission is by direct contact with an ocular discharge. It is rare in the United States but is a major cause of blindness in the Far East and in Mediterranean countries.

Clinical manifestations. The inflammatory process that results from the contamination produces erythema of the conjunctiva, edema of the lid, and a crusting discharge on the lids and cornea. If untreated, this infection leaves the eyelid scarred with granulations that invade the cornea, resulting in loss of vision.

Assessment. Collection of **subjective data** includes an awareness that, during allergy seasons and because of exposure to environmental irritants, the patient may report pruritus, burning, and excessive tearing.

Collection of **objective data** includes observing eyes that are erythematous with edema of the lid. A dried exudate may be noted.

Diagnostic tests. The conjunctiva is scraped for bacteria and stained for microscopic examination.

Medical management. Medical treatment is similar to that for blepharitis.

Nursing interventions and patient teaching. The lid and lashes are cleansed of exudate with normal saline. Warm compresses are applied two to four times a day. When allergies are present, cold saline compresses may be ordered for control of edema and pruritus. Eye irrigations with normal saline or lactated Ringer's solution may be prescribed to remove secretions. Topical antibiotics and adrenocortical steroid medications are administered. Eye pads are contraindicated because they enhance bacterial growth.

Nursing diagnosis and interventions for the patient with conjunctivitis include but are not limited to the following:

NURSING DIAGNOSIS	NURSING INTERVENTIONS
Pain, related to pruritus, secondary to inflammatory process	Apply warm or cold compresses. Administer prescribed eye medications; ensure proper instillation of eyedrops and ointments; administer eye irrigation as prescribed. Administer analgesics as ordered. Assess patient's limitations in visual sensory perception. Implement safety measures as appropriate.

The patient and family should be instructed to avoid contact with the eyes or soiled materials when an infection is present. Individual washcloths and towels are to be used. The patient is instructed to wash hands if contact is made with the eyes and before any treatments and is also taught to perform and describe treatments such as irrigations, compresses, and medication administration. The patient should avoid noxious fumes or smoke and should not wear contact lenses during the suppuration period.

Prognosis. Conjunctivitis responds successfully to topical antimicrobials. Patient teaching reduces the risk of continued exposure and reinfection. Although highly contagious, the disease is self-limiting, leaving no chance of permanent visual impairment unless a chronic condition develops.

INFLAMMATION OF THE CORNEA
Etiology/Pathophysiology

Keratitis, an inflammation of the cornea, may result from injury; irritants; allergies; viral infection; or diseases such as congenital syphilis, smallpox, and some nervous disorders. It may be superficial and involve the epithelial layer only or may invade the subepithelial layer and the endothelial membrane. The layers of the eye are innervated, and thus, when inflammation is present, pain will be acute. Ulcers may form in the eye membrane layers, resulting in scattered scarring of the corneal surface.

Pneumococcus, Staphylococcus, Streptococcus, and *Pseudomonas* are the most common types of bacterial causes of keratitis. The viral agent most often responsible for corneal inflammation is the herpes simplex virus [HSV]). HSV keratitis is a growing problem, especially with immunocompromised patients. Keratitis can be triggered by stress, illness, and exposure to ultraviolet light. The condition may be associated with the use of ophthalmologic steroid medications. Overuse or abuse of topical steroids may injure epithelial cells.

Another form of keratitis is acanthamoebic keratitis. The *Acanthamoeba* organism is found in the soil, airborne dust, fresh water, and the noses and throats of healthy humans. This organism is often found to be resistant to antimicrobial agents. Contact lens wearers are more susceptible because traditional cleaning agents for lenses include rinsing with clean or distilled water. People who swim frequently are at greater risk because the amoeba is not killed by usual methods of disinfection, such as chlorine.

Clinical Manifestations

Severe eye pain is the most common symptom that differentiates this disease from other eye inflammatory diseases. If uncontrolled, keratitis may result in blepharospasms and vision loss. Other symptoms include photophobia, tearing, edema, and visual disturbances.

Assessment

Collection of **subjective data** includes noting the severity and duration of the pain, the extent of light sensitivity, and any vision loss.

Collection of **objective data** includes assessing the patient for facial grimacing, lacrimation, and photophobia.

Diagnostic Tests

Depending on the causative agent, a variety of diagnostic tests may be ordered, including culture and sensitivity tests, fluorescein staining, and Gram staining. Ophthalmoscopic examination is also performed.

Medical Management

Medical management includes topical antibiotic therapy. Systemic antibiotics may be prescribed for severe cases. Cycloplegic-mydriatic drugs may be ordered, which paralyze the ocular muscles of accommodation and dilate the pupil. For viral keratitis, therapy includes corneal debridement followed by topical therapy with vidarabine (Vira-A) or trifluridine (Viroptic) used for 2 to 3 weeks. Corticosteroids are contraindicated because they contribute to a longer course, possible deeper ulceration of the cornea, and systemic complications. Drug therapy may also include acyclovir (Zovirax). Analgesics are used to control pain associated with acute inflammation. Pressure dressings may be ordered to relax the eye muscle and decrease discomfort. These dressings are often applied to both eyes because the eyes move together. Warm or cold compresses two to four times daily are prescribed for symptomatic relief. Epithelial debridement of loose tissue may be performed. Surgical management involves a corneal transplant, known as **keratoplasty.**

Nursing Interventions and Patient Teaching

The focus of nursing interventions for keratitis includes control of pain, safety, and prevention of complications. Nursing diagnoses and interventions for the patient with keratitis are the same for conjunctivitis. The nurse should provide information on self-care of a corneal abrasion. The patient must also learn to wash the hands before instilling medication and to prevent infection by not rubbing the eyes. The patient is instructed to note any change in discharge or increase in pain and to notify the physician immediately.

Prognosis

Topical antibiotic, antiviral, or antifungal eyedrops when begun promptly after diagnosis by culture, result in rapid healing and minimal visual impairment. Chronic keratitis may develop if treatment is delayed. Tissue loss as a result of infection of the cornea produces corneal ulcer and vision loss as a result of opaque scarring of the cornea. Keratoplasty may then be indicated.

DRY EYE DISORDERS

Complaints of dry eye are caused by a variety of ocular disorders characterized by decreased tear secretion or increased tear film evaporation. Keratoconjunctivitis sicca is caused by lacrimal gland dysfunction from an autoimmune mechanism. If the patient with keratoconjunctivitis sicca has associated dry mouth, the patient has primary Sjögren syndrome. If the patient has associated rheumatoid arthritis, scleroderma, or systemic lupus erythematosus, the patient has secondary Sjögren syndrome. The patient complains of a sandy or gritty sensation that typically worsens during the day and is better in the morning after eye closure with sleep. Treatment is directed at the underlying cause (Lewis et al, 2004).

Diagnostic Tests

The definitive test for dry eye, a noninfectious disorder of the lacrimal gland, is **Schirmer's test** (see Table 13-2). Normal results should indicate 10 to 15 mm of wet paper.

Medical Management

Medical management for dry eye includes artificial tears replacement. Many nonprescription products are available for this purpose. They should be used sparingly because preservatives in the drops or overuse can cause further irritation. Punctal plugs (temporary or permanent) may be inserted to close the tear ducts. This in turn keeps the tears in the eyes longer.

Estrogen therapy may be prescribed for postmenopausal women. If possible, medications that may cause dry eye as a side effect should be limited. If an infection accompanies the dry-eye syndrome, antibiotic therapy will be prescribed.

As many environmental irritants as possible should be eliminated. If contact lenses cause local irritation and dry eye, a change in the prescription or type of lens is advised.

Results of the fluorescein staining test for excessive tear disorder are considered normal if the dye disappears from the lacrimal cul-de-sac within 1 minute.

When excessive tearing results from environmental irritants, the patient is encouraged to eliminate the noxious element. Filtering machines are available to control pollen and dust levels in the environment.

Surgical repair of an injured punctal sac by correctly aligning the eyelid margin or by probing an obstructed punctum (opening to the tear duct) to allow for tear reabsorption is the advised method of treatment.

Nursing Interventions and Patient Teaching

Pain related to lack of natural eye moisture would be the appropriate nursing diagnosis. Interventions are similar to those for conjunctivitis.

The patient should be instructed on instilling eye medications, and appropriate hygiene practices should be reinforced. Instructions are given on avoiding irritants.

Prognosis

Eyedrops alleviate the majority of symptoms caused by dry eye. Long-term use of artificial tears results in no adverse reactions. Control of medical conditions minimizes discomfort and complications. Surgical repair of the punctal sac is a safe procedure and has a good prognosis.

ECTROPION AND ENTROPION
Etiology/Pathophysiology

These two noninfectious disorders of the lid cause an abnormal turning of the eyelid margins: ectropion and entropion.

Ectropion is the outward turning of the eyelid margin. In the older patient it is common for the orbicularis oculi muscle to be relaxed. Paralytic ectropion occurs when orbicularis muscle function is disturbed, as with Bell's palsy. Other causes of ectropion are eyelid laceration and burns of the conjunctival tissue.

Entropion is an inward turning of the eyelid. The lower eyelid margin is the most frequently involved. The conjunctival membrane lining the eyelid and part of the eyeball are exposed. Entropion is caused by atrophy of the eyelid tissue, spasms of the orbicularis oculi muscle, or scarring of the tarsal plate (dense connective tissue that stiffens the eyelid) caused by congenital origin or trauma. Varying degrees of atonia exist in the older adult orbicularis; this is considered common.

Clinical Manifestations

Ectropion and entropion are characterized by abnormal direction of the eyelid with tear spillage and corneal dryness.

Assessment

Collection of **subjective data** includes noting the degree of vision loss and determination of tear loss and/or dryness of the cornea.

Collection of **objective data** includes observing the extent to which the patient can perform ADLs and the presence of any eyelid margin inflammation.

Diagnostic Tests

The physician determines these conditions through a visual and ophthalmologic examination.

Medical Management

Medical intervention consists of topical medications to reduce conjunctival and corneal inflammation or drying. Surgery is the preferred treatment. Resection of the tarsal plate, removal of the scarred tissue, or tightening of the orbicularis oculi muscle is the choice for permanent repair.

Nursing Interventions

Interventions for ectropion and entropion involve monitoring the medical treatment and reporting its progress. If the eyelid is surgically repaired, the patient should be monitored for safety considerations.

A nursing diagnosis and interventions for the patient with ectropion or entropion would focus on disturbed sensory perception related to edema and exudate. Interventions include assistance in self-care activities, safety measures, observation for infection/inflammation, and medication/dressing treatments as prescribed.

Prognosis

Early diagnosis and treatment of eyelid disorders reduces the risk of conjunctival and corneal inflammation and scarring. Monitoring treatment reduces the need for surgical intervention and minimizes visual disturbances.

DISORDER OF THE LENS
Cataracts

Etiology/pathophysiology. A cataract is a crystalline opacity or clouding of the lens. The patient may have a cataract in one or both eyes. If present in both eyes, one cataract may affect vision more than the other. The lens is normally clear and transparent. As a person ages, there is a gradual opacification of the lens. When a cataract develops, the lens becomes foggy, and vision decreases. If a large enough portion of the lens becomes opaque, light cannot reach the retina.

Cataracts may be congenital (e.g., exposure to maternal rubella) or acquired from systemic disease, trauma, toxins (e.g., radiation or ultraviolet [UV] light exposure, certain drugs such as systemic corticosteroids or long-term topical corticosteroids), intraocular inflammation. Most cataracts are age related (senile cataracts). The patient with diabetes mellitus tends to develop cataracts at a younger age than does the patient without diabetes. Smoking has been linked with the development of cataracts. Cataract development is mediated by a number of factors. In senile cataract formation, it appears that altered metabolic processes within the lens cause an accumulation of water and alterations in the fiber structure. These changes affect lens transparency, causing vision changes.

Clinical manifestations. Cataract symptoms include blurred vision, diplopia, photosensitivity, glare, abnormal color perception, and difficulty in driving at night. Glare is due to light scatter caused by the lens opacities, and it may be significantly worse at night when the pupil dilates. The visual decline is gradual, but the rate of cataract development varies from patient to patient. No pain is associated with cataract formation. There is an opacity in the center portion of the lens (Figure 13-6).

Assessment. Collection of **subjective data** includes noting blurred vision as often the first symptom to be expressed by the patient. The nurse should note any subjective complaints, such as "hazy" or "fuzzy" vision or abnormal color perception.

Collection of **objective data** involves observing the patient for difficulty in reading, noting whether the patient brings newsprint close to the eyes. Sensitivity to light should also be noted.

Diagnostic tests. Diagnosis is based on decreased visual acuity or other complaints of visual dysfunction. The opacity is directly observable by ophthalmoscopic or slit-lamp microscopic examination. A totally opaque lens creates the appearance of a white pupil.

Medical management. Medical intervention involves monitoring the patient for changes in vision associated with increasing size of the cataract. For many patients the diagnosis is made long before they actually decide to have surgery. Often, changing the patient's eyewear prescription can improve the level of visual acuity, at least temporarily. If glare makes it difficult to drive at night, a patient may elect to drive only during daylight hours or to have a family member drive at night. When palliative measures no longer provide an acceptable level of visual function, the patient is an appropriate candidate for surgery. Surgery is the only definitive method of treatment and can be performed at any age. It may be done using a local, topical, or general anesthesia. There are two methods of surgery: intracapsular and extracapsular extraction.

Intracapsular surgery involves removing the lens and its entire capsule. Although some surgeons still perform intracapsular extraction (and it may be necessary in instances of trauma), the intracapsular technique is rarely done and has been largely replaced by extracapsular extraction as the procedure of choice. In the extracapsular method, the most common form of treatment, the anterior capsule is opened and the lens nucleus and cortex are removed, leaving the remainder capsular bag intact. Healing is rapid with this method.

Phacoemulsification is the most common type of extracapsular cataract extraction (Figure 13-7). This technique uses ultrasound to break up and remove the cataract through a small incision, thereby reducing the healing time and decreasing the chance of complications.

During surgery the physician may implant a synthetic (not from a human donor) intraocular lens in the posterior chamber behind the iris. At the end of the procedure, the patient receives injections of subconjunctival corticosteroid and antibiotic medications. Then an antibiotic and corticosteroid ointment is applied and the patient's eye is covered with a patch and protective shield. The patch is usually worn overnight and removed during the first postoperative visit. When intraocular lenses are not implanted, the physician will instead prescribe external lenses or glasses. Special contact lenses provide the patient many options for comfort.

Nursing interventions and patient teaching. Preoperative and postoperative nursing care is a primary nursing responsibility (see Nursing Care Plan: The Patient with Cataracts).

Cataract symptoms usually develop slowly and can easily be detected. Annual examinations, especially for people 40 and older, should be encouraged. Surgery provides about a 90% success rate of acceptable levels of vision. Unless complications occur, the patient is usually ready to go home within a few hours after the surgery as soon as the effects of sedative agents have dissipated. Postoperative medications usually include

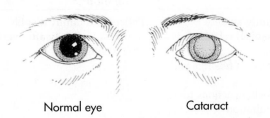

Normal eye   Cataract

FIGURE **13-6** Cataract, visible in the left eye as white opacity of the lens, is seen through the pupil.

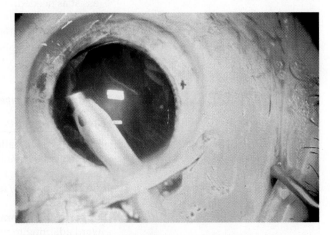

FIGURE **13-7** Phacoemulsification of a cataractous lens through a self-sealing, scleral-tunnel incision. Note the circular opening in the anterior lens capsule.

NURSING CARE PLAN
The Patient with Cataracts

Ms. J. is an 82-year-old who lives alone. She has developed bilateral cataracts and is admitted to same-day surgery for right cataract extracapsular procedure with intraocular lens implantation.

NURSING DIAGNOSIS *Risk for injury, related to altered visual acuity*

Patient Goals/Expected Outcomes	Nursing Interventions	Evaluation/Rationale
Patient will not have any evidence of injury. Patient will have a safe environment in which she will avoid injury.	**PREOPERATIVE** Instill eyedrops as prescribed wearing clean latex/vinyl gloves. Administer preoperative medications or sedatives as ordered. Explain postoperative procedures to expect, such as patches and eyedrops. **PREOPERATIVE** Instill mydriatic/cycloplegic and corticosteroid eyedrops as prescribed while wearing clean latex/vinyl gloves. Instruct patient to avoid sudden head movement, heavy lifting, bending over, coughing, sneezing, vomiting, and straining with elimination, which cause increased intraocular pressure. Maintain prescribed eyepatch/shield in position during specified hours. Remove environmental barriers to ensure safety. Keep side rails up at all times. Plan all care with patient: explain routines of what will happen and when. Visit frequently and announce yourself upon entering room. Assist with deep-breathing exercises every 1 to 2 hours while awake. Check with physician for any special positioning or precautions. (If turned, position patient on the unaffected side.) Elevate head of bed 30 degrees as ordered. Assist with and teach active and passive ROM exercises every 4 hours. Increased activities and ambulation as ordered; assist as needed. Teach self-care activities, and assist as needed. Instruct family to remove unnecessary furniture and pick up objects that may be blocking pathways.	Patient feels secure about upcoming surgery. Patient uses measures to control complications from surgery.

NURSING DIAGNOSIS *Anxiety/fear, related to visual impairment*

Patient Goals/Expected Outcomes	Nursing Intervention	Evaluation
Patient will experience less anxiety/fear.	Observe level of patient/family anxiety. Note patient's coping mechanism related to vision loss. Encourage patient/family to vent feelings and concerns. Support patient/family's positive actions toward adapting to visual limitations	Patient and family display trust and security after venting feelings.

NURSING CARE PLAN
The Patient with Cataracts—cont'd

❓CRITICAL THINKING QUESTIONS

1. Ms. J. puts her call light on and tells the nurse that she has severe pain and pressure in her right eye. The initial response by the nurse would include:

2. To minimize the risk of injury to Ms. J.'s operative eye, discharge planning would include:

3. In visiting with Ms. J., the nurse finds that she enjoys embroidery and knitting. Ms. J. states that she is looking forward to resuming her handiwork. Appropriate patient teaching would be:

---

antibiotic and corticosteroid drops to prevent infection and decrease the postoperative inflammatory response. There is some evidence that postoperative activity restrictions and nighttime eye shielding are unnecessary. However, many ophthalmologists still prefer that the patient avoid activities that increase intraocular pressure, such as bending or stooping, coughing, or lifting. Ophthalmologists may also recommend using an eye-shield over the operative eye at night for protection. Safety measures appropriate to vision alterations should be discussed, and the patient should be encouraged to notify the physician of any complications such as pain, erythema, drainage, or sudden visual changes. If sudden pain occurs, the nurse should call the physician (Therapeutic Dialogue; Clinical Pathway; Patient Teaching: After Eye Surgery).

Prognosis. Gradual loss of lens transparency can result in risk of injury to the patient because of vision loss. Patients must be carefully monitored for degeneration of the lens. The condition may be accompanied by secondary glaucoma, which further reduces visual acuity. Surgical intervention is advised to improve vision. Complications may recur years after cataract surgery and should be reported to the ophthalmologist.

DISORDERS OF THE RETINA
Diabetic Retinopathy

Etiology/pathophysiology. Diabetic retinopathy is a disorder of retinal blood vessels characterized by capillary microaneurysms, hemorrhage, exudates, and the formation of new vessels and connective tissue. After 15 years with diabetes mellitus, nearly all patients with type 1 diabetes mellitus and 80% with type 2 diabetes will have some degree of retinal disease accompanied by nephropathy. The incidence increases in relationship to the length of time the patient has had the disease. The disorder occurs more frequently in patients with long-standing, poorly controlled diabetes mellitus (Cultural and Ethnic Considerations box).

The initial stage of diabetic retinopathy may last for several years. The earliest and most treatable stages of diabetic retinopathy often produce no changes in vision. Because of this, the patient with diabetes must have regular dilated eye examinations by an ophthal-

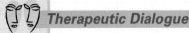 *Therapeutic Dialogue*

Mrs. B., age 71, has been experiencing decreasing vision for the past 5 years. She seeks medical attention and is told that surgery will be required to correct her condition. While talking to the patient, the nurse senses her reluctance to comply with postoperative treatment.

PATIENT: *I'm too old to go through all the routines that the doctor wants me to. It involves too much.*

NURSE: *I know that surgery is a concern for you. You must have many emotions that you are feeling right now. It's understandable that you have concerns about your recovery.*

PATIENT: *There's so much to think about and remember.*

NURSE: *The doctor and our staff are here to help make your recovery as easy as possible for you. Tell me what bothers you the most.*

PATIENT: *What if I go home and fall? I could reinjure my eye or break something, like my hip.*

NURSE: *There are several things that you and your family can do to prevent any injury to yourself. The doctor and staff will explain these things very carefully to you.*

PATIENT: *I'm afraid I'm too old to learn.*

---

mologist or specially trained optometrist for early detection and treatment. The blood vessels in the retina begin to widen and become tortuous. Microaneurysms then develop at the periphery and small hemorrhages develop. These may disappear, but they leave in their place scars that can decrease vision. Increased capillary permeability causes protein exudate.

As the disease progresses, new blood vessels form on the retina and into the vitreous. These new vessels rupture, causing decreased vision. Absorption of some of the blood can occur, which will improve vision until another hemorrhage occurs. Significant vision loss will eventually occur as these hemorrhages continue. Vitreous contraction and full detachment can occur as the vessels and surrounding tissue become fibrous.

Clinical manifestations. Symptoms include microaneurysms, which can only be identified by ophthalmoscopy in the initial stage. In the advanced stages the patient will have progressive vision loss and the presence of "floaters," which are minute products of the hemorrhage.

CLINICAL PATHWAY | *Home Health Care for Postoperative Cataract Surgery*

DAY 1	DAY 2	DAY 3	DAY 4
Pain control Initial immobilization of the eye Psychological support Infection control Discharge planning	Return follow-up visit with physician Pain control Dressing changes, if any dressing remaining Medication administration, as prescribed Reinforcement of previous precautions on activities Infection control Protection from environmental injury	Protection from environmental injury Medication therapy, as prescribed Infection control	Follow-up visit to physician Use of corrective eyewear, if permitted Protection from environmental injury Infection control Daily activity guidelines
Interventions include: Rigid eyeshield over 2 × 2 gauze pad Avoiding direct sunlight by wearing dark sunglasses Use medicated eyedrops as prescribed Limit activity to mainly bed rest except bathroom privileges (BRPs) Analgesics prn as prescribed Reinforcement of teaching to prevent bending down and straining Avoidance of sneezing, coughing, or nose blowing Obtain patient understanding of discharge teaching	Interventions include: Physician to assess eye pressure Reinforcement of discharge instructions Analgesic and eyedrop medications, as prescribed Reinforce handwashing technique Frequent rest periods during the day Wearing UV-blocking sunglasses when outside Eye protection, as ordered Encouraging diet with high fiber, if allowed Avoid jarring head movements Do not touch or rub eye	Interventions include: Eye protection, as ordered Medications, as ordered Stool softeners, as prescribed, if constipated Use of corrective eyewear, if permitted	Interventions include: Return visit to physician for eye pressure check Monitoring for infection Reinforcement of all discharge/activity instructions Instructions on activities such as driving

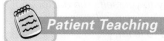 **Patient Teaching**

After Eye Surgery

- Teach patient and family proper hygiene and eye care techniques to ensure that medications, dressings, and/or surgical wound are not contaminated during necessary eye care.
- Teach patient and family about signs and symptoms of infection and when and how to report those to allow early recognition and treatment of possible infection.
- Instruct patient to comply with postoperative restrictions on head positioning, bending, coughing, and Valsalva's maneuver to optimize visual outcomes and prevent increased intraocular pressure.
- Instruct patient to instill eye medications using aseptic techniques and to comply with prescribed eye medication routine to prevent infection.
- Instruct patient to monitor pain and take prescribed medication for pain as directed and to report pain not relieved by prescribed medications.
- Instruct patient of the importance of continued follow-up as recommended to maximize potential visual outcomes.

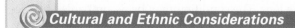 **Cultural and Ethnic Considerations**

Hearing and Visual Problems

- Whites have a higher incidence of hearing impairment than African-Americans or Asian-Americans.
- Incidence and severity of glaucoma are greater among African-Americans than among whites.
- Hispanics have an increased incidence of diabetic retinopathy.
- American Indians have an increased incidence of otitis media when compared with whites.
- Whites have a higher incidence of macular degeneration than Hispanics, African-Americans, and Asian-Americans.

Source: Lewis, S.M. et al. (2004). *Medical-surgical nursing.* (6th ed.). St. Louis: Mosby.

Assessment. Collection of **subjective data** must include assessment of the length and control of diabetes mellitus. The patient will have varying degrees of vision loss, from decreased vision to blindness. The patient's knowledge of therapy should be assessed.

Collection of **objective data** involves noting that in the early stages there are no symptoms; as the disease progresses, vision is diminished.

Diagnostic tests. Indirect ophthalmoscopy shows dilated and tortuous vessels and narrowing or obliteration of the arteries. Opacities, hemorrhages, and microaneurysms can be seen. Slit-lamp examination provides magnification of the lesions.

Medical management. Surgical intervention includes early photocoagulation, cryotherapy (cryopexy) and/or vitrectomy. Photocoagulation destroys new blood vessels, seals leaking vessels, and helps prevent retinal edema by use of a laser beam. A vitrectomy or cryotherapy may be performed when photocoagulation is not possible. Cryotherapy is a procedure in which a topical anesthetic is used so that a cryoprobe can be placed directly on the surface of the eye. When the probe is properly located, its tip creates a frozen area that extends through the external tissue, then through the eyeball until it reaches a specific point on the retina. Multiple points on the retina can be treated in this way (Lewis et al, 2004).

Nursing interventions and patient teaching. Nursing diagnosis and interventions for the patient with diabetic retinopathy include but are not limited to the following:

NURSING DIAGNOSIS	NURSING INTERVENTIONS
Fear, related to unfamiliarity with procedure	Determine patient's knowledge of purpose and procedures of photocoagulation, cryotherapy, or vitrectomy.

Home care after surgery for the patient with diabetic retinopathy is the same as for any eye surgery (see Clinical Pathway).

Prognosis. The best treatment of diabetic retinopathy is early detection. Frequent eye examinations reduce the complication of vision loss, and modern laser technology is a highly effective method of reducing further damage to the retina and improving vision.

Age-Related Macular Degeneration

Etiology/pathophysiology. Age-related macular degeneration (ARMD) is a condition of the aging retina characterized by slow, progressive loss of central and near vision. ARMD is the most common cause of vision loss in people older than 55. There are two types of macular degeneration. The first, called the **wet type** (also called neovascular macular degeneration) has new vessel growth in the macular region that occurs suddenly. The macula becomes displaced, and scarring occurs. Because scarred cells no longer register

light, vision loss is irreversible. Wet macular degeneration accounts for 10% of cases.

The second, known as the **dry type** (also called nonexudative or nonneovascular macular degeneration), is more common. It occurs in 90% of cases of macular degeneration. Degenerative changes are the cause: lipid deposits occur, followed by slow atrophy of the macular region, including the retina. People with dry ARMD notice that reading and other close-vision tasks become more difficult. In this form, the macular cells have wasted or atrophied and simply do not function as well as previously. Patients report that "sometimes I see the image and sometimes it sort of blinks at me, like I have a short circuit."

Clinical manifestations. The hallmark sign of ARMD is the appearance of drusen in the fundus found on ophthalmoscopic evaluation. Drusen appear as yellowish exudates beneath the retinal pigment of epithelium and represent localized or diffuse deposits of extracellular debris. The main symptom of macular degeneration is gradual and variable bilateral loss of central vision. One eye may have a greater loss than the other. Color perception may also be affected.

Assessment. Collection of **subjective data** includes noting that the patient may have difficulty distinguishing colors correctly. The nurse should assess for visual disturbances and coping mechanisms for the loss.

Macular degeneration develops differently in each person, so the symptoms may vary. However, some of the most common symptoms include the following:

- A gradual loss of ability to see objects clearly
- Distorted vision; objects appear to be the wrong size or shape or straight lines appear wavy or crooked
- A gradual loss of clear color vision
- Scotomas (blind spots in the visual field)
- A dark or empty area appearing in the center of vision.

Collection of **objective data** includes the nurse noting the degree to which the patient can centrally view objects.

Diagnostic tests. Indirect ophthalmoscopy is used to detect opacity, hemorrhage, and new blood vessel formation. In addition, retinal detachment or other abnormalities can be seen. The Amsler grid test may help define the involved area (see Table 13-2).

Medical management. Photocoagulation may be used, but only if the areas of new vessels have not grown into the macula. This procedure may be useful in the wet type if treatment is begun within the first few days after onset of symptoms. There is no treatment for the dry type.

Unfortunately, there is no way to restore central vision damaged by macular degeneration. However, since macular degeneration does not damage side vision, low vision aids such as telescopic and microscopic special lenses, as well as magnifying glasses and electronic magnifiers for close work, can be prescribed to help make the most of remaining vision. Often people, with adaptation, can cope well and continue to do most things they were accustomed to doing. The role of high-dose vitamin therapy, especially C, E, and beta-carotene, in slowing the progression of vision loss is under investigation.

Nursing interventions and patient teaching. The patient needs patience and understanding to cope with the continuing loss of sight. The nurse needs to assist the patient through the process of accepting loss of sight. Maintaining safety is important because only peripheral vision exists.

Nursing diagnosis and interventions for the patient with macular degeneration include but are not limited to the following:

NURSING DIAGNOSIS	NURSING INTERVENTIONS
Disturbed sensory perception, (visual), related to disease process	Note the extent of visual loss and the level of difficulty with ADLs; assist the patient in developing ways of performing these activities. Determine the patient's support systems and elicit help if available.

The nurse instructs the patient about the disease process, stressing that peripheral vision will be maintained. The patient is provided ways to maintain as much independence as possible, and family and friends can learn the areas in which to assist.

Prognosis. Early diagnosis of macular degeneration is critical to prevent blindness. Watchful waiting is the only approach to dry macular degeneration. Ophthalmic laser surgery is of limited benefit because of the gradual and progressive course of the disorder. Photocoagulation is preventive, not curative.

Retinal Detachment

Etiology/pathophysiology. Retinal detachment is a separation of the retina from the choroid in the posterior area of the eye (Figure 13-8). This usually results from a hole in the retina that allows vitreous humor to leak between the choroid and the retina.

The immediate cause may be severe trauma to the eye, such as contusion or a penetrating wound. In most cases, however, retinal detachment is the result of internal changes related to aging and sometimes inflammation of the eye. Retinal detachment may also occur in debilitated patients when there is sudden severe physical exertion.

As the detachment progresses, there is an interruption in the transmission of visual images from the retina to the optic nerve. The result is a progressive loss of vision to complete blindness.

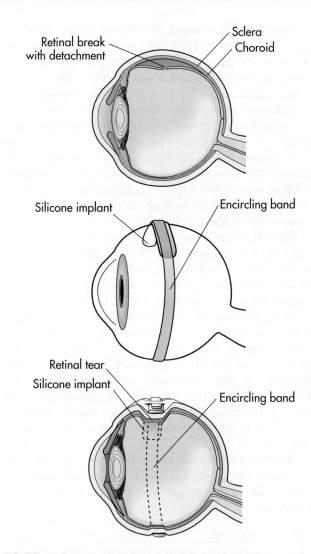

FIGURE **13-8** Retinal break with detachment: surgical repair by scleral buckling technique.

Clinical manifestations. Symptoms include a sudden or gradual development of flashes of light, followed by floating spots, a "cobweb," "hairnet," and loss of a specific field of vision.

Assessment. Collection of **subjective data** includes noting patient complaints of flashing lights unilaterally as well as floaters. There is a progressive vision restriction in one area. If the tear is acute and extensive, the patient will describe a sensation like a curtain being drawn across the eye. Because the retina does not contain sensory nerves that relay sensations of pain, the condition is painless.

Collection of **objective data** includes observing the patient for the ability to perform ADLs. The level of anxiety associated with coping is also assessed.

Diagnostic tests. Visual acuity measurements should be the first diagnostic procedure with any complaint of vision loss. Indirect and direct ophthalmoscopy is used to detect pallor of the retina as well as the detachment.

Three-mirror gonioscopy provides a magnified view of any retinal lesions. Slit-lamp examination magnifies the lesions. Ultrasound may be useful to identify a retinal detachment if the retina cannot be directly visualized (e.g., when the cornea, lens, or vitreous humor is hazy or opaque).

Medical management. The treatment of choice is early corrective intervention. One of four procedures may be performed.

Laser photocoagulation is used to burn localized tears or breaks that may have occurred in the posterior portion of the eyeball. This causes an eventual sealing of the tear or break.

Cryotherapy is used to freeze the borders of a retinal hole with a frozen-tipped probe. The probe is applied to the scleral surface directly over the retinal hole area. The hole seals when the resultant inflammatory process produces scarring.

Diathermy is used to burn a retina break using an ultrasonic probe. The probe is applied to the scleral surface directly over the retinal break. Sealing occurs from the resultant inflammatory and scarring process.

Scleral buckling is an extraocular surgical procedure that involves indenting the globe so the pigment epithelium, choroid, and sclera move toward the detached retina. This not only helps seal retinal breaks, but also helps relieve inward traction on the retina. The retinal surgeon sutures a silicone implant against the sclera, causing the sclera to buckle inward. The surgeon may place an encircling band over the implant if there are multiple retinal breaks, if the surgeon cannot locate suspected breaks, or if there is widespread inward traction on the retina (see Figure 13-8). If present, subretinal fluid may be drained by inserting a small-gauge needle to facilitate contact between the retina and the buckled sclera. Scleral buckling is usually accomplished under local anesthesia, and the patient may be discharged on the first postoperative day. Many surgeons now perform scleral buckling surgery as an outpatient procedure.

Nursing interventions and patient teaching. Postprocedure management includes cycloplegic, mydriatic, and antiinfective eyedrops. Eyepatches are applied over only the operative eye or both eyes, providing the required rest of the eye for 1 to 2 days. Safety measures are essential because the eyes are patched.

Depending on the procedures, the position of the head postoperatively may vary. If air is injected into the vitreous, the head will be positioned with the unaffected eye upward with the patient lying on the abdomen or sitting forward for 4 to 5 days.

Dark glasses are prescribed to decrease the discomfort of **photophobia** (abnormal sensitivity to light).

Nursing diagnosis and interventions for the patient with retinal detachment include but are not limited to the following:

NURSING DIAGNOSIS	NURSING INTERVENTIONS
Anxiety, related to visual alterations	Allow the patient the opportunity to discuss feelings and fears about the possible loss of vision. Answer questions honestly and correct any misunderstandings. Explain the reasons for restrictions of activities and for procedures.

Temporary restrictions of reaching, work, and activity should be discussed with the patient (see Patient Teaching: Retinal Detachment box).

Prognosis. Retinal detachment requires treatment; reattachment is successful in 90% of retinal attachments: the degree of sight restoration depends on the extent and duration of separation. Maximum vision is achieved within 3 months after surgery. Unless replaced, a detached retina slowly dies after several years of detachment. Blindness from retinal detachment is irreversible.

GLAUCOMA
Etiology/Pathophysiology

Glaucoma is not one disease, but rather a group of disorders characterized by (1) increased intraocular pressure and the consequences of elevated pressure, (2) optic nerve atrophy, and (3) peripheral visual field loss.

Glaucoma is an abnormal condition of elevated pressure within an eye because of obstruction of the outflow of aqueous humor. It is associated with a progressive loss of peripheral vision.

Glaucoma is found in people who are middle aged and older. Approximately 12% to 15% of all blindness

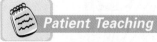

Patient Teaching

Retinal Detachment

- Return to sedentary activity in 2 weeks; no heavy lifting or active physical activity for 6 weeks, or as instructed by physician.
- Check with physician concerning shampooing of hair.
- Limit reading for 3 weeks or as instructed by physician.
- Use correct technique for administration of eye medications.
- Report to ophthalmologist any signs of further detachment (flashes of light, increase in floaters, blurred vision).
- Report for medical follow-up visits as instructed.

in the United States results from glaucoma. It is seldom seen in people younger than 35 years of age but may occur in infancy.

Glaucoma occurs when there is an obstruction of the aqueous humor drainage that increases the intraocular pressure (Figure 13-9). Damage to the optic nerve results.

Open-angle glaucoma, also known as **primary open-angle glaucoma,** represents 90% of the cases of primary glaucoma. In primary open-angle glaucoma, the outflow of aqueous humor is decreased in the trabecular meshwork. In essence, the drainage channels become occluded, like a clogged kitchen sink. The course of the disease is slowly progressive and results from degenerative changes. It is often bilateral.

Closed-angle glaucoma, also known as **primary closed-angle glaucoma (acute),** occurs if there is an abrupt angle change of the iris, causing rapid vision loss and dramatic symptoms. This type of glaucoma represents 10% of the total number of glaucoma cases in the United States.

Clinical Manifestations

In primary open-angle glaucoma the patient has no signs or symptoms during the early stages of the disease. As the symptoms become apparent, they include tunnel vision, eye pain, difficulty adjusting to darkness, halos around lights, and inability to detect colors. Intraocular pressures will be elevated.

Primary closed-angle (acute) glaucoma produces severe pain, decreased vision, and nausea and vomiting. The sclera is erythematous, and the pupil is enlarged and fixed. The patient sees colored halos around lights. There is an acute increase in the intraocular pressure.

As glaucoma progresses, **optic disk cupping occurs.** This is visible with direct or indirect ophthalmoscopy. The optic disk becomes wider, deeper, and paler (light gray or white). Optic disk cupping may be one of the first signs of chronic open-angle glaucoma. Optic disk photographs are useful for comparison over time to demonstrate an increase in the cup-to-disk ratio and progressive blanching (Figure 13-10).

Assessment

Collection of **subjective data** includes noting the time of day when the eye pain occurs. Frequency, intensity, and duration of the pain are also assessed. Complaints of peripheral vision loss, maladaptation to darkness, and halos seen around lights are noted. Severity of headaches and presence of nausea and vomiting are determined.

Collection of **objective data** includes noting a need for frequent eyeglass prescription changes. Elevated intraocular pressures are also present.

Diagnostic Tests

Schiøtz tonometry is used to test for intraocular pressure (Figure 13-11). A patient with glaucoma would test above the normal range of 10 to 22 mm Hg. Applanation tonometry is also used to measure intraocular pressure (Figure 13-12). Visual field studies will show a decline in the patient's peripheral vision.

Medical Management

Primary open-angle glaucoma is medically treated by the use of beta blockers, miotics, and carbonic anhydrase inhibitors (see the Medications table). A beta blocker, such as Betoptic, will reduce intraocular pressure. Miotics (agents that cause the pupil to contract), such as pilocarpine, constrict the pupil and draw the iris away from the cornea, allowing aqueous humor to drain out of the canal of Schlemm (see Figure 13-9). Carbonic anhydrase inhibitors, such as Diamox, decrease the production of aqueous humor. The result is

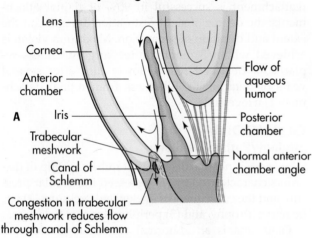

Slowly rising intraocular pressure

Lens
Cornea
Anterior chamber
A   Iris
Trabecular meshwork
Canal of Schlemm
Congestion in trabecular meshwork reduces flow through canal of Schlemm

Flow of aqueous humor
Posterior chamber
Normal anterior chamber angle

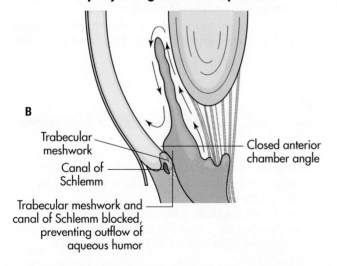

Rapidly rising intraocular pressure

B
Trabecular meshwork
Canal of Schlemm
Trabecular meshwork and canal of Schlemm blocked, preventing outflow of aqueous humor

Closed anterior chamber angle

FIGURE **13-9 A,** Primary open-angle glaucoma. Congestion in the trabecular meshwork reduces the outflow of aqueous humor. **B,** Primary closed-angle glaucoma (acute). Angle between the iris and the anterior chamber narrows, obstructing the outflow of aqueous humor.

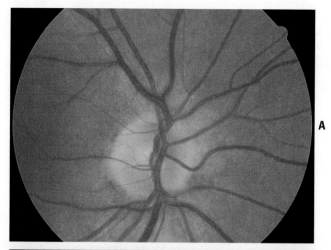

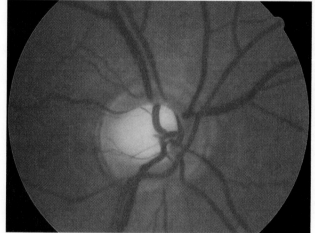

FIGURE **13-10 A,** In the normal eye, the optic cup is pink with little cupping. **B,** In the glaucomatous eye, the optic disk is bleached and optic cupping is present. (Note the appearance of the retinal vessels, which travel over the edge of the optic cup and appear to dip into it.)

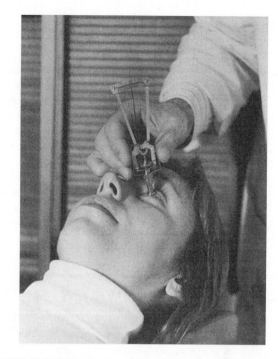

FIGURE **13-11** Measurement of intraocular pressure with the Schiøtz tonometer.

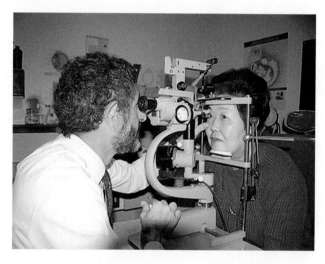

FIGURE **13-12** Applanation tonometry.

a lowering of intraocular pressure. Surgery, which consists of a trabeculectomy or laser trabeculoplasty, is done when medications do not control the pressure. **Trabeculectomy** is the removal of corneoscleral tissue, usually the canal of Schlemm and trabecular meshwork. This produces an increase in the outflow of aqueous humor. Laser trabeculoplasty produces openings in the trabecular meshwork.

Primary closed-angle glaucoma is medically treated with osmotic diuretics, such as mannitol, carbonic anhydrase inhibitors, and miotics. Surgical treatment includes a peripheral iridectomy or an iridotomy. A peripheral iridectomy is the removal of part of the iris. The procedure is performed with the patient under local anesthesia. This procedure often restores drainage of the aqueous humor. Postoperatively the patient is observed for signs and symptoms of local hemorrhage or excessive pain. An iridotomy is an incision into the iris of the eye to create an opening for aqueous flow. A

local or general anesthetic may be used. Postoperatively the dressing is observed for signs of drainage.

Nursing Interventions and Patient Teaching

Nursing interventions involve protecting the patient's safety, monitoring compliance to therapy, and reinforcing discharge instructions. The nurse has an important role in educating the patient and family about the risk of glaucoma. In addition, the nurse should stress the importance of early detection and treatment in preventing visual impairment. This knowledge should encourage the patient to seek appropriate ophthalmic health care. The nurse may fulfill this teaching role by educating individual patients and families,

MEDICATIONS | *Eye Disorders*

MEDICATION	TRADE NAME	ACTIONS/USES	SIDE EFFECTS	NURSING IMPLICATIONS
Sulfacetamide sodium	Sulamyd	Action: Broad-spectrum bacteriostatic anti-infective agent used in the treatment of ocular infections Uses: Conjunctivitis, corneal ulcers, trachoma, and chlamydial infections	Pruritus, edema, erythema, other eye irritations	Know that it is contraindicated in sulfonamide hypersensitivity and that purulent exudate may inactivate drug; do not use silver preparations concurrently; use proper ophthalmic technique; comply with full course of treatment, store properly; discard solution if it discolors; warn patient to avoid sharing washcloths and towels with family members.
Betaxolol hydrochloride	Betoptic	Action: Beta-adrenergic blocking agent that reduces formation of aqueous humor Use: Open-angle glaucoma	Insomnia, irritation of eyelids, stinging on installation, occasional tears, photophobia, systemic effects, possible disorientation, bradycardia, weakness, dyspnea	Know pregnancy cautions; do not touch dropper on eye; use proper administrative technique; give proper dosage; keep container tightly closed; determine intraocular pressure 4 weeks after treatment; use cautiously in patients with history of heart failure or with diabetes mellitus.
Timolol maleate	Timoptic	Action: Beta-adrenergic blocking agent that reduces aqueous humor formation Uses: Open-angle glaucoma and hypertension; used with caution for patients who have heart conditions	Ocular sensitivity, severe irritation of eye or eyelid, systemic effect of cardiac failure, chest pain, disorientation, diarrhea, dizziness, exacerbation of asthma	Know that it may mask hypoglycemia; measure intraocular pressure after 4 weeks of treatment; avoid abrupt cessation; used cautiously in bronchial asthma and heart conditions, know pregnancy and breast-feeding cautions; use proper administration technique; use correct amount; keep container tightly closed.
Dexamethasone	Decadron	Action: Decreases inflammation Use: Ocular inflammation	Local irritation, retardation of corneal healing, blurred vision, eye pain, secondary eye infection	Know that it may mask infection; use for only short term in children; tell patient not to wear contact lens during treatment; shake bottle before using; use proper administration technique; check with physician before using for future eye conditions; check with physician if condition does not improve in 5 to 7 days.

MEDICATIONS | *Eye Disorders—cont'd*

MEDICATION	TRADE NAME	ACTIONS/USES	SIDE EFFECTS	NURSING IMPLICATIONS
Acetazolamide	Diamox	Action: Lowers intra-ocular pressure Use: Open-angle glaucoma	Diarrhea, weakness, discomfort, urinary frequency, loss of appetite, nausea, vomiting, numbness in hands; contraindicated with severe renal hepatic or adrenocortical impairment	Know pregnancy and lactation cautions; give with food; give accurate dosage; in diabetes, know that it may increase blood and urine glucose levels; caution drowsiness; monitor I&O and weight daily.
Pilocarpine hydrochloride	Pilocar Isopto Carpine	Action: Reduces intraocular pressure Use: Open-angle glaucoma	Muscle tremors, nausea and vomiting, dyspnea, wheezing, bronchial spasms, local irritation	Encourage patient to have periodic intraocular pressure determinations; use proper administration technique; use exact dosage; monitor for blurred vision or changes in vision; use cautiously in bronchial asthma and hypertension; apply light finger pressure on lacrimal sac 1 minute after instillation of drops.
Cyclopentolate hydrochloride	Cyclogyl	Action: Anticholinergic drug that produces dilation of pupil and temporary paralysis of ciliary muscles Use: Glaucoma; a diagnostic agent for angle-closure glaucomas	Ataxia, behavioral disturbances, tachycardia, disorientation, fever	Prevent contamination of dropper; give proper dosage; warn patient of increased sensitivity to light and suggest sunglasses; know that it is contraindicated in narrow-angle glaucoma; use cautiously in older adults.
Osmitrol	Mannitol	Action: Osmotic diuretic that causes decrease in intraocular pressure Use: Glaucomas	Fluid and electrolyte imbalance, chest pain, tachycardia, chills and fever, difficult urination	Administer by intravenous infusion; know pregnancy caution; know that duration of action is 1 to 3 hours; monitor vital signs at least hourly and I&O, weight, and potassium levels daily.
Polyvinyl alcohol	Liquifilm Forte	Action: Tearlike lubricant Uses: Dry eyes and eye irritations	Headache, burning, blurred vision, eye pain	Teach patient to instill; warn patient not to touch dropper to eye; to avoid contamination of solution, warn patient not to touch tip of container to eye.
Gentamicin sulfate	Garamycin	Action: Bacteriocidal antibiotic Uses: Treatment of blepharitis and conjunctivitis	Pruritus, erythema, edema, ocular discomfort, blurred vision (may occur for few minutes after application)	Comply with full course of therapy; if no improvement occurs after a few days, check with physician.

groups of patients, or entire communities, depending on the nurse's practice setting. The patient should know that the incidence of glaucoma increases with age and that a comprehensive ophthalmic examination is invaluable in identifying people with glaucoma or those at risk of developing glaucoma. The current recommendation is for an ophthalmologic examination every 2 to 4 years for people between 40 and 64 years of age, and every 1 to 2 years for people 65 years of age or older. African Americans in every age category should have examinations more often because of the increased incidence and more aggressive course of glaucoma in these individuals.

Because of the chronic nature of glaucoma, the patient needs encouragement to follow the therapeutic regimen and follow-up recommendations prescribed by their ophthalmologist (Patient Teaching: Glaucoma box). The patient needs accurate information about the disease process and treatment options, including the rationale underlying each option. In addition, the patient needs information about the purpose, frequency, and technique for administration of prescribed antiglaucoma agents. In addition to verbal instructions, all patients should receive written instructions that contain the same information. This should be sufficiently detailed to provide all the necessary information without being so extensive that the patient becomes overwhelmed. The patient may be encouraged to comply with the medication regimen if the nurse

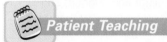

Patient Teaching

Glaucoma

* Medical supervision will be required for the rest of life.
* Eyedrops **must** be continued as long as prescribed even in the absence of symptoms; usually treatment is lifelong.
  —Blurred vision decreases with prolonged use.
  —Avoid driving for 1 to 2 hours after administration of miotics.
* To prevent complications:
  —Press lacrimal duct for 1 minute after eyedrop insertion to prevent rapid systemic absorption.
  —Have reserve bottle of eyedrops at home.
  —Carry eyedrops when away from home.
  —Carry card identifying glaucoma and the eyedrop solution prescribed.
* Bright lights and darkness are not harmful.
* There is no apparent relationship between vascular hypertension and ocular hypertension.
* Report any reappearance of symptoms immediately to ophthalmologist.
* If admitted to the hospital for a different medical condition, alert the staff of continued need for prescribed eyedrops.
* Avoid the use of mydriatic or cycloplegic drugs (e.g., atropine) that dilate the pupils.

promotes consideration of the sight-saving nature of the drops. The nurse can further encourage compliance by helping the patient identify the most convenient and appropriate times for medication administration or advocating a change in therapy if the patient reports unacceptable side effects (Lewis et al, 2004).

Prognosis

Today's method of medical and surgical management provides the patient with an excellent prognosis for a full recovery. Complications are few if care is early in the course of the condition. When glaucoma is ignored or noncompliance to therapy is noted, blindness may occur. Regular eye examinations are required to detect and monitor for increased intraocular pressure. Generally, once damage has occurred, the condition is irreversible. Surgery and medication help lessen the complications from glaucoma.

CORNEAL INJURIES
Etiology/Pathophysiology

Corneal injuries result from injuries to corneal layers of the eye. The cornea is the convex, transparent outermost layer of the eye. It is composed of five layers of tissue and is uniform in nature. The cornea is nonvascular; therefore no bleeding occurs from injury unless subcorneal structures are involved. The cornea is kept moist by tear production and is protected from daily insult by the eyelid.

Foreign bodies are the most common cause of corneal injury. Dust particles, propellants, and eyelashes may lodge in the conjunctiva or cornea. The eyes blink in response to the irritant, and further irritation occurs from the upper lid closing frequently, thus moving the foreign body into deeper layers or a wider area of the cornea.

Burns often occur in the home and workplace. When burns affect the eye, it is considered a medical emergency. Depending on the chemical causing the burn, the damage may be superficial or deep. Chemical irritants such as acids and alkalis and metal flashes from acetylene blowtorches cause significant pain, depending on the depth of chemical erosion.

Abrasions and lacerations are usually superficial scratches that occur from injuries to the eye, caused by fingernails or clothing. They may be painful, depending on the depth of the abrasion.

Penetrating wounds are the most serious corneal injuries. Eye structures may be injured permanently, resulting in total blindness. Infection may result from the introduction of microorganisms on the penetrating object.

Clinical Manifestations

Foreign bodies produce pain upon eyeball movement or when the eyelid moves over the eyeball during blinking. Excessive tearing, erythema of the conjunctiva, and pruritus may occur.

Acute pain and burning are the primary symptoms with any topical burn to the eye. Abrasions and lacerations produce mild to severe pain, depending on the depth of corneal involvement. The pain may be transitory and slight, or spasmodic and deep.

Penetrating wounds result in varying degrees of pain. If underlying structures are involved, pain may be absent because the nerves have been severed.

Assessment

Foreign bodies. Collection of **subjective data** includes noting the time and type of injury. The patient is assessed for the degree and severity of eye pain and vision loss. The patient should be asked about any first-aid treatment provided.

Collection of **objective data** includes observation of the foreign body and extent of damage. When the intracapsular area has been penetrated, fluid will be leaking from the eye.

Burns. Collection of **subjective data** includes determining the degree of pain. It is important to assess the substance causing the burn and any first aid treatment that has been provided. Vision loss is determined by the physician.

Collection of **objective data** includes noting the extent of the burn in and around the eye, including eyelashes and eyebrows, and assessing the condition of the eyeball.

Abrasions and lacerations. Collection of **subjective data** includes assessing the patient for the degree of pain after the incident and how the injury occurred. Treatments used at the time of injury are noted.

Collection of **objective data** includes assessing the degree of damage of the eyeball and surrounding structures, as well as noting any vision loss.

Penetrating wounds. Collection of **subjective data** includes noting the time and causative factors related to the injury. Presence and severity of pain are assessed. Determine if any first-aid treatment was rendered.

Collection of **objective data** includes determining the type and size of the penetrating object. Fluid leakage from the eye is noted. The damage to surrounding structures is assessed.

Diagnostic Tests

Tests include visual and ophthalmoscopic examination, fluorescein staining, peripheral vision tests, and slit-lamp examination.

Medical Management

Foreign bodies are medically treated with a flush of normal saline when the object is near the sclera and conjunctiva; it can then be removed by a clean swab or tissue. Cotton is not to be used, because it may scratch the cornea. If the object is not easily flushed away, the individual must see an ophthalmologist to have the object removed. Antibiotic topical eye ointments are ordered.

Burns are medically treated with a prolonged, 15- to 20-minute or longer tap water flush immediately after burn exposure. This will help prevent scar formation. The eyelids are separated during the flush procedure. The patient is then treated in a local emergency department or physician's office for follow-up care. Home remedy first-aid treatment should not be done. Topical antiinfective agents are ordered for the eye. Abrasions and lacerations of the eye are medically cleaned with a normal saline solution. Antibiotic therapy, usually topical, is prescribed. See Safety Considerations box for eye safety measures.

Immediately after a penetrating wound injury, both eyes should be covered while the patient is transported to the hospital because both eyes work in synchrony. Covering the eyes prevents the eye from involuntarily moving with the other eye. A shield reduces further injury but must not touch the foreign

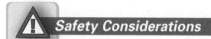

Safety Considerations

Eye Safety Measures

- Avoid frequent rinsing of eyes with unprescribed solutions.
- Discard any ophthalmic solution that is cloudy, discolored, has been open for longer than 3 months, or contains particles.
- Do not self-treat an eye inflammation with a medication prescribed for a previous eye disorder.
- To avoid eye strain:
  —Use a good light for reading or doing work that requires careful visual focus.
  —When reading or focusing eyes for long periods, look at distant objects for a few minutes at repeated intervals to rest eyes.
- Avoid rubbing eyes.
- Wash hands before and after touching eyes.
- Wear safety glasses when engaging in activities that could injure the eyes. If injury occurs, apply cool compress if no laceration is present; cover if laceration is present.
- Wear dark glasses for prolonged exposure to very bright light (such as sunlight or snow or water).
- Flush eyes immediately for 15 to 20 minutes or longer with cool water when any irritating substances are introduced.
- Do not attempt to remove foreign bodies from the cornea; cover the eye with an eyeshield (e.g., small paper cup) to prevent excessive movement or touching of the eye. Seek medical attention immediately.
- If a speck of dust blows in the eye, pull upper lid over lower lid and let the tears wash the speck to the inner canthus or lower lid, where it may be safely removed. Irrigate the eye with cool tap water, if necessary.
- Seek medical assistance immediately for eye injuries, chemical eye burns, and foreign bodies that remain in the eye.

object. A Styrofoam cup provides adequate coverage and is readily available. The foreign object should not be removed except by a trained physician.

Nursing Interventions and Patient Teaching

Foreign bodies. The nurse will assist with the required irrigation of the eye.

Burns. The nurse will assist with the flushing process and providing eye medications as ordered.

Abrasions and lacerations. The nurse will assist with cleaning the eye as ordered and providing general first-aid.

Penetrating wounds. The nurse should note whether the pupil on the affected side becomes irregular. This results when the iris of the affected eye moves to occlude the wound area. Infection potential is high; therefore topical and systemic antibiotics are ordered. If the wound is small, self-healing occurs. If the wound is large or deep, enucleation of the eye may be performed.

Effective and immediate therapy is crucial for any injury to the eye. If treatment is interrupted, ineffective, or not sustained, permanent eye damage will occur. The most frequent complications include infection, vision disturbances, and blindness. A nursing diagnosis for the patient with an eye injury would be **pain, acute, related to inflammatory process.** (See the discussion on conjunctivitis.)

The nurse should ensure that the patient can apply ointments and dressings, if ordered. The patient is instructed in the use of other therapy devices, such as warm or cool compresses. Proper handwashing techniques are taught. Dark sunglasses are to be worn by the patient if cycloplegic or mydriatic eyedrops are used. Instruct the patient to avoid future episodes of chemical or environmental hazards. The patient should understand discharge instructions, including the need for follow-up physician visits and symptoms to report. The nurse should determine the patient's knowledge about the progress of therapy.

Prognosis

Immediate and appropriate treatment reduces the severity and complications of eye injuries. The chosen treatment must be monitored to prevent permanent eye damage and vision problems. Superficial corneal abrasions usually heal without incident. Deeper abrasions or burns may result in permanent visual loss due to scarring.

SURGERIES OF THE EYE

ENUCLEATION

Eye enucleation is the surgical removal of the eyeball. It is often necessary after severe eye trauma but may be done for other reasons, such as malignant tumors. Surgical methods vary from removal of the entire eye-

ball or the eyeball contents to removal of the eyeball and all underlying structures.

Nursing Interventions

Preoperative care includes determining the patient's feelings about the surgical intervention. It may be a welcome relief from pain and pressure of a malignancy. For other patients it is a disfiguring surgery that leads to a drastic change in lifestyle. Other nursing responsibilities include therapeutic dialogue between the physician and patient regarding the exact nature of the surgery. If a prosthesis (commonly called a **glass eye**) is used, the nurse should ensure that the patient understands its care.

Postoperatively a pressure dressing is applied over the socket of the eye to control hemorrhage. The nurse observes the dressing at least every hour for the first 24 hours. The patient is questioned about any pain on the affected side of the head or any headache, which might indicate hemorrhage or infection. These findings should be reported to the physician immediately. Routine postoperative procedures of coughing and turning on the affected side are discouraged to prevent sutures from dislodging.

Prognosis

Patients who undergo enucleation surgery are excellent candidates for prosthetic replacements. A prosthetic eye may be worn once healing occurs, usually in 4 to 6 weeks.

KERATOPLASTY (CORNEAL TRANSPLANT)

Keratoplasty is the removal of the full thickness of the patient's cornea followed by surgical implantation of a cornea from another human donor. It is done to replace damaged cornea resulting from trauma, ulceration, or congenital deformities of the cornea. Improved methods of tissue procurement and preservation, refined surgical techniques, postoperative topical corticosteroids, and careful follow-up have decreased graft rejection. Medications to suppress rejection (e.g., cyclosporine) may be ordered.

Corneal grafts are usually taken within 4 hours after death from a donor who is ideally between 25 and 35 years of age. An appropriate donor is an individual who died of injury or acute disease. The corneas of people with chronic or communicable diseases—such as hepatitis, acquired immunodeficiency syndrome (AIDS), or cancer—are not appropriate for transplantation. The eye banks test donors for HIV and hepatitis B and C. The donor's eye should have normal light perception and projection. The donor's tissue is best used within a 5 days after removal.

The nurse is often the individual most accessible to the family when questions of organ donation occur.

Responsibilities would include notification of appropriate supervisory personnel. Keratoplasty is performed with the patient under local or general anesthesia. The transplanted tissue is sutured into place to maintain graft alignment and a watertight wound.

Nursing Interventions

Preoperatively the nurse encourages the patient to express fears related to surgery and gives instructions in the use of protective eyeglasses if dilation-causing eye medication is used. The nurse maintains safety in the environment by using safety devices and orienting the patient to each new environment. The surgical areas are cleansed and prepared as ordered, usually with an antiseptic solution. Preoperative teaching includes deep breathing and turning to reduce any complications associated with surgery. Coughing is discouraged, because sutures may break. Dietary restrictions, if ordered, should be maintained; a light breakfast may be allowed if the surgery is done with the patient under a local anesthesia. Prescribed medications are administered.

Postoperatively the nurse ensures that correct postoperative positioning is maintained; the patient is usually positioned on the back or nonoperated side until the physician allows turning to the operated side. Activity restrictions as ordered are reinforced to prevent injury to the eye. Safety measures are used until the patient is able to ambulate safely. Anyone coming into the room should announce his or her presence. The patient should avoid bending, lifting, and straining for approximately 1 month to prevent intraocular pressure or suture tension.

Progressive activity should be prescribed by the physician. Regular postoperative visits with the eye surgeon should be encouraged. The nurse should report any severe or progressive pain to the surgeon immediately, as well as any complaints of erythema, loss of vision, or photophobia that would occur with corneal rejection. Systemic and ophthalmic medications are administered. Strict surgical asepsis must be maintained during dressing changes. Staff, the patient, and the family must wash hands thoroughly before any contact with the eye area. The patient should be instructed to avoid the use of such irritants as powder, perfume, and propellants, which might cause sneezing and displacement of sutures. The patient should not rub the eye area, because contamination of the site or suture displacement may result. The patient's diversional activities should be assessed; television is usually permitted, but reading is limited because of the side-to-side movement of the eyes. The lateral motion of the eye may cause loosening of sutures. If an eyepatch or metal eyecup shield is ordered, the nurse can demonstrate care. The eyepatch is applied snugly to inhibit the blink reflex and allow the eye to rest. The metal eyeshield is used during the night to protect the eye from trauma. Discharge instructions should be obtained from the physician regarding use of eyewear.

Prognosis

The cornea is avascular; therefore, healing is slow. Incidence of infection is increased as a result. The transplanted donor tissue may be rejected. Incidence of rejection is reduced if the donor is a family member with similar tissue type.

PHOTOCOAGULATION

Using a laser, a small, intense beam of light is directed into a small spot on the retina. The light converts to heat energy, and coagulation of tissue protein occurs, which is called **photocoagulation.**

Photocoagulation is a nonsurgical procedure usually performed on an outpatient basis. Without surgical intervention, the structures of the eye remain undisturbed and only the sealing of leakage and offending tissue destruction occurs.

Photocoagulation is useful in diabetic retinopathy to cauterize hemorrhaging vessels. It cannot increase visual acuity but can prevent further loss. Usually no hospitalization or postoperative medical management is required.

Nursing Interventions

Postoperative assessment for patients who have undergone photocoagulation therapy includes assessment of vision. There may be a constriction of peripheral fields, and central vision may temporarily be decreased. A decrease in night vision and a headache resulting from the laser's bright light may also occur.

Prognosis

Photocoagulation is used to prevent eye damage and is not curative. Minimal destruction of tissue occurs with photocoagulation. The procedure is nonsurgical; therefore, infection risk is minimal.

VITRECTOMY

A vitrectomy is the removal of excess vitreous fluid caused by hemorrhage and replacement with normal saline. Any scar tissue may also be removed.

Postoperative management includes the prescription of topical eye medication for 4 to 6 weeks. Acetaminophen or acetaminophen with codeine is prescribed for pain management. A pressure patch to the operative eye is placed immediately after surgery. Ice packs to reduce inflammation are ordered.

Nursing Interventions and Patient Teaching

The patient is required to maintain a position on the abdomen or sitting forward resting the nonoperated side of the head on a table to allow air that is in the eye to float against the retina. These positions are maintained for 4 to 5 days.

Dark glasses are prescribed postoperatively to decrease the discomfort of photophobia. Postoperative assessment includes assessment of the eyepatch; ice packs; and abnormal vital signs, especially fever. The dressing should be assessed for bleeding.

Prognosis

The procedure has limited benefits and continues to be investigated as to its benefits versus complications.

NURSING CONSIDERATIONS FOR CARE OF THE PATIENT WITH AN EAR DISORDER

Once the history and general assessment have been done, the nurse should focus on aspects related to the ear. Additional information would include the following:

- Occurrence of ear drainage, tinnitus, vertigo, wax buildup, pressures, pain, and pruritus
- Behavioral clues indicating hearing loss (Box 13-2)
- History of medications used for ear disorders, specifically those known to be ototoxic
- Current medications for the ear disorder
- Side effects of medication, if any
- Associated speech pattern abnormalities
- Use of assistive hearing devices
- Home remedies that cause ear trauma

The nurse communicates the gathered data to the appropriate personnel and documents the findings in the patient record. The next step in the assessment process is to prepare the patient for the initial otoscopic diagnostic evaluation.

Box 13-2 | *Behavioral Clues Indicating Hearing Loss*

Any adult who:
- Is irritable, hostile, hypersensitive in interpersonal relations
- Has difficulty in hearing upper-frequency consonants
- Complains about people mumbling
- Turns up volume on television and radio
- Asks for frequent repetition and answers questions inappropriately
- Loses sense of humor, becomes grim
- Leans forward to hear better; face becomes serious and strained
- Shuns large- and small-group audience situations
- May appear aloof and uninterested
- Complains of ringing in the ears
- Has an unusually soft or loud voice
- Repeatedly asks, "What did you say?"

LABORATORY AND DIAGNOSTIC EXAMINATIONS

OTOSCOPY

With an otoscope the examiner can visualize the external auditory canal and the eardrum, or tympanic membrane. Normally the tympanic membrane is disk shaped and pearl gray or pale pink in color. This is the initial examination of the ear, performed before other testing. One responsibility of the nurse is to explain to the patient the purpose and procedure of otoscopy. The patient should be reassured that otoscopy is a painless test requiring only about 1 to 2 minutes, with slight pulling of the ear upward and backward for an adult and down and back for a child during the procedure.

TUNING FORK TESTS

The two most common tests using tuning forks are Weber's test and the Rinne test. These tests are used to determine hearing loss as well as data related to the type of loss.

Weber's test is a method of assessing auditory acuity, especially useful in determining whether defective hearing in an ear is a conductive loss caused by a middle ear problem or a sensorineural loss, resulting from a disorder in the inner ear or auditory nerve system. The test is performed by placing the stem of a vibrating tuning fork in the center of the patient's forehead or on the maxillary incisors. The loudness of the sound is equal in both ears if hearing is normal. If the person has a sensorineural loss in one ear, the unaffected ear perceives the sound as louder. When conductive hearing loss is present, the sound is louder in the affected ear, but it does not hear ordinary background noise conducted through the air and receives only vibrations by bone conduction (Figure 13-13).

The Rinne test is a method of distinguishing conductive from sensorineural hearing loss. The test is performed with tuning forks placed ½ inch (1.25 cm) from the external auditory meatus and the vibrating stem placed over the mastoid bone. While one ear is tested, the other is masked (Figure 13-14). In sensorineural loss the sound is heard longer by air conduction, whereas in conduction hearing loss the sound is heard longer by bone conduction.

Nursing responsibility in both Weber's test and the Rinne test includes explanation of the purpose and procedure of the tests. The nurse should stress that the patient will need to concentrate and indicate through the use of hand signals in which ear or ears the sound is heard in Weber's test and when it is no longer heard in the Rinne test. In addition, the nurse should assure the patient that the test is painless and requires only a few minutes.

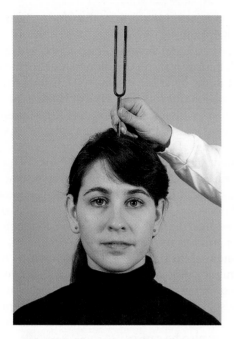

FIGURE **13-13** Weber tuning fork test.

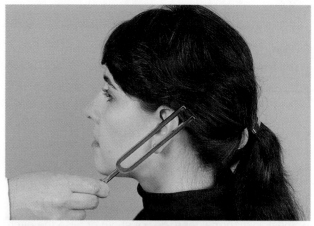

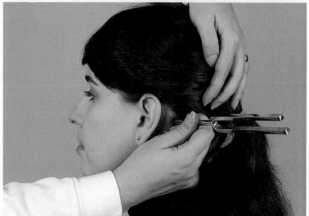

FIGURE **13-14** Rinne tuning fork test.

Audiometric Testing

Audiometry is a test of hearing acuity. Various audiometric tests determine the lowest intensity of sound at which an individual can perceive an auditory stimulus (hearing threshold), hear different frequencies, and distinguish different speech tones.

Nursing responsibilities include providing the patient with the purpose and procedure of each test. Any required responses by the patient should be reviewed.

Vestibular Testing

Vestibular testing measures balance and equilibrium. The Romberg and past-point tests are used for patients complaining of dizziness or disequilibrium.

The **Romberg test** measures the patient's ability to perform specific tasks with eyes open and then with eyes closed. The normal response is maintaining balance throughout the entire test. An abnormal response is indicative of loss of the sense of position (in which the patient loses balance when standing erect, feet together, eyes closed).

Past-point testing measures the patient's ability or inability to place a finger accurately on a selected point on the body. Inability to correctly perform the test indicates a lack of coordination in voluntary movements.

The nurse's responsibility is to explain the purpose and procedure of each test. Safety measures are taken to prevent patient injury during the Romberg test if the patient cannot maintain balance.

DISORDERS OF THE EAR

LOSS OF HEARING (DEAFNESS)

Hearing impairment is a state of decreased auditory acuity that ranges from partial to complete hearing loss. It is the most common disability in the United States: 28 million people have a hearing impairment. Among people older than 65 years of age, it is the third most common chronic condition. The quality of life for one third of the adults in the United States between 65 and 75 years of age is decreased because of hearing impairments. Recognition, diagnosis, and early treatment may help prevent further impairment and damage.

The implications of hearing loss are great. Hearing is needed to develop speech and conceptual ability; thus hearing loss may well affect personality development and intelligence-test responses when the hearing impairment is severe and congenital. This may have implications for the person's education and socialization. As hearing loss increases, the person may socially withdraw because of the inability to understand and be understood; this could lead to isolation and depression (Health Promotion Considerations box).

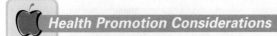

Health Promotion Considerations

Facilitating Communication for People with Impaired Hearing

- If patient wears a hearing aid, make certain it is in place, turned on, and functioning properly.
- Get the person's attention by raising an arm or hand.
- Ask permission to turn off the television or radio or turn down volume.
- Start with the light on your face; this will help the person speech read.
- Face the person when speaking.
- Speak clearly, but do not overaccentuate words.
- Speak in a normal tone; do not shout or raise the pitch of voice. Shouting overuses normal speaking movements and may cause distortion and be too loud for the person with sensorineural damage. If the person has conductive loss only, sometimes making the voice louder without shouting is helpful.
- If the person does not seem to understand what is said, express it differently. Some words are difficult to see in speech reading, such as **white** or **red**.
- Move closer to the person and toward the better ear if the person does not hear you.
- Write out proper names or any statement that you are not sure was understood.
- Do not chew gum or cover the mouth when talking to a person with limited hearing.
- Observe for inattention that may indicate tiredness or lack of understanding.
- Use phrases to convey meaning rather than one-word answers. State the major topic of the discussion first and then give details.
- Do not show annoyance by careless facial expression. People who are hard of hearing depend more on visual clues for acceptance.
- Encourage the use of a hearing aid if the person has one; allow the person to adjust it before speaking.
- If in a group, repeat important statements and avoid asides to others in the group.
- Avoid the use of the intercommunication system as this may distort sound and cause poor communication.
- Do not avoid conversation with a person who has hearing loss.

Modified from Conover, M., & Cober, J.: Understanding and caring for the hearing impaired. *Nursing Clinics of North America* 5:497, 1970.

Types of Hearing Loss

There are six types of hearing loss: conductive, sensorineural, mixed, congenital, functional (psycogenic), and central.

In **conductive hearing loss,** sound is inadequately conducted through the external or middle ear to the sensorineural apparatus of the inner ear. A common cause is buildup of cerumen. Sensitivity to sound is diminished, but clarity or interpretation of sound is not changed. When increased volume compensates for the loss, then hearing is normal; therefore a hearing aid can be helpful.

In **sensorineural hearing loss,** sound is conducted through the external and middle ear in a normal way, but a defect in the inner ear results in its distortion, making discrimination difficult. This type of hearing loss is usually caused by trauma, infectious processes, presbycusis (hearing loss caused by aging), congenital, or exposure to ototoxic drugs. Destruction of cochlear hair by intense noise may also cause sensorineural loss. Amplifying sound, such as with a hearing aid, will help some people with this type of loss. Many people have an intolerance to loud noise and would not be helped by a hearing aid.

Mixed hearing loss is a combined conductive and sensorineural hearing loss.

Congenital hearing loss is present from birth or early infancy. Anoxia or trauma during delivery may be causes. Rh incompatibility may also be a cause. The mother's exposure during pregnancy to syphilis or rubella and the use of ototoxic drugs during pregnancy may also be causes.

Functional hearing loss is a loss of hearing in which there is no organic cause. It is also known as **psychogenic** or **nonorganic hearing loss. Central hearing loss** occurs when the brain's auditory pathways are damaged, as in a stroke.

Clinical Manifestations

Clinical manifestations may vary, depending on the degree of deafness. Symptoms may range from subtle clues, such as requests for repeating information, to more obvious signs of nonresponse.

Assessment

Collection of **subjective data** includes noting the onset and progression of the condition, deficit in one or both ears, family history, history of head trauma, exposure to noise, current medications, visual or speech disorders, and any other ear symptoms.

Collection of **objective data** must include an assessment of behavioral clues that indicate a hearing difficulty. (See Box 13-2 for behavioral clues indicating difficulty hearing.)

Diagnostic Tests

Conductive hearing loss produces lateralization of sound to the deaf ear in Weber's test. Results of the Rinne test show that sounds transmitted through bone conduction are heard longer than or equal to sounds transmitted through air conduction.

Sensorineural hearing loss produces lateralization of sound to the better ear in Weber's test. Results of the Rinne test show that air-conducted sounds are heard longer than bone-conducted sounds, but not twice as long.

Audiometric testing determines the type of hearing loss and the degree of impairment.

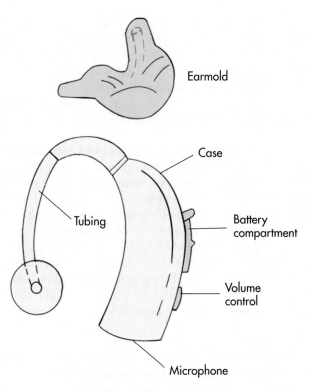

FIGURE **13-15** Parts of a hearing aid.

Medical Management

Medical management depends on the type of impairment. Surgical procedures may be required. Hearing aids or cochlear implants may be used when appropriate. Cochlear implantation is performed in individuals with profound bilateral sensorineural hearing loss who receive no measurable assistance from lip reading with a properly fitting hearing aid (see discussion of cochlear implants on p. 680 and Figure 13-16). The electrical activity of hearing is initiated by hair cells in the organ of Corti and sent to the brain along nerve fibers that make up the auditory nerve. In most deaf individuals, these hair cells are damaged. The goal of cochlear implantation is to bridge the gap created by the hair cell loss and directly stimulate the remaining neurons. Studies have shown that even when there is a complete loss of hair cells, a percentage of cochlear neurons remains. A small computer changes the spoken words into electrical impulses that are transmitted to an implanted cochlear coil.

Nursing Interventions

Patients with partial hearing loss may benefit from a hearing aid (Figure 13-15). The patient is assisted in caring for the hearing aid as detailed in Box 13-3.

The hearing aid can only be useful if it is worn. Factors leading to nonuse may include the patient seeing the hearing aid as a sign of disability. Also, the magnification of sound may cause discomfort or irritability. Therefore it is important to ensure that the hearing aid is used and works properly.

Box 13-3   *Care of the Hearing Aid*

DO
- Handle with care.
- Wash earmold or plug daily in mild soap and water, using a pipe cleaner to cleanse the cannula.
- Dry earmold or plug thoroughly before reconnecting it to the receiver.
- Always keep an extra battery and cord available.
- When hearing aid is not in use, turn aid off and open battery compartment.
- If hearing aid whistles, reinsert earmold.
- If hearing aid fails to work:
  —Check the on-off switch.
  —Inspect earmold for cleanliness.
  —Examine battery for tightness of fit.
  —Examine cord plug for tightness of insertion.
  —Examine cord for breaks.
  —Replace battery and/or cord.
- Check for cracks in tubing or earmold.
- Check to see that earmold and hearing aid are inserted in the correct ear.
- Check that earmold or hearing aid is properly inserted.
- Check that hearing aid is turned on.
- Check that volume control wheel is turned up to appropriate settings.
- If "whistling" occurs, check earmold and hearing aid fit.

DON'T
- Put hearing aid on heated surface.
- Wash hearing aid.
- Drop hearing aid.
- Wear hearing aid in bath or shower.
- Wear hearing aid overnight.
- Ignore a hearing aid that is "whistling."
- Use in contact with cream, oil, or hair spray when hearing aid is on.

Nursing diagnoses and interventions for the patient with hearing loss include but are not limited to the following:

NURSING DIAGNOSES	NURSING INTERVENTIONS
Disturbed sensory perception, (auditory), related to disease process	Facilitate communication with the patient by following the interventions provided in Health Promotion Considerations: Facilitating Communications for People with Impaired Hearing.
Social isolation, related to loss of hearing	Assess factors that contribute to social isolation. Identify support systems for patient. Identify patient concerns. Establish effective communication.

Patient Teaching

The nurse assists the patient in learning to care for a hearing aid, if prescribed. The patient can be instructed to request that others speak slowly or more clearly and repeat if necessary.

Prognosis

Surgical repair of the injured structures increases the likelihood of restoring partial or complete hearing, especially when implants are used. Complications of surgery are rare. Technical advances have also improved the quality of hearing. Microtechnology has reduced the size of hearing aids until they are almost undetectable.

INFLAMMATORY AND INFECTIOUS DISORDERS OF THE EAR

External Otitis

Etiology/pathophysiology. External otitis, or otitis externa, is an inflammation or infection of the external canal or the auricle of the external ear and is sometimes called **swimmer's ear.** External otitis may be acute or chronic.

External otitis can be caused by allergy, bacteria, fungi, viruses, and trauma. Allergic reaction can stem from nickel or chromium in earrings. In addition, chemicals in hair sprays, cosmetics, hearing aids, and medications (especially sulfonamides and neomycin) are common sources of allergy. Common bacterial agents are *Staphylococcus aureus*, *Pseudomonas aeruginosa*, and *Streptococcus pyogenes*. Frequently the viruses herpes simplex and herpes zoster are implicated. The external ear may also be affected by eczema, psoriasis, and seborrheic dermatitis. Fungi such as *Aspergillus* and *Candida* may also be causes. External otitis is more prevalent during hot, humid weather.

Trauma from cleaning or scratching the ear canal with a foreign object—such as a cotton swab, bobby pin, or finger—may result in irritation and possible introduction of infectious organisms.

Cerumen in the older person becomes dry and hard. Because the removal becomes more difficult, the cerumen may become impacted, causing discomfort and decreased hearing. Certain activities allow moisture to become trapped in the ear, creating a medium for infection; these include using earphones, hearing aids, earplugs, earmuffs, and stethoscopes. Excessive swimming may wash out the protective cerumen, remove skin lipids, and lead to secondary infection.

Malignant external otitis is a rare, lethal form caused by *Pseudomonas* and occurring mostly in patients with diabetes. It is a bone-destroying infection that quickly involves all surrounding ear structures.

Clinical manifestations. The acute inflammatory or infectious process produces pain with movement of the auricle or chewing, and often the entire side of the head aches. Erythema, scaling, pruritus, edema, watery discharge, and crusting of the external ear may occur.

Drainage may be purulent or serosanguineous. If the *Pseudomonas* organism is the cause of the infection, the drainage will be green and have a musty smell. Dizziness and decreased hearing may also be present if edema occludes the ear canal.

With chronic external otitis there is usually pruritus, but no pain with movement of the auricle. A discharge is also present.

Assessment. Collection of **subjective data** includes determining the onset, duration, and severity of pain, which is crucial to the assessment of inflammatory disease of the ear. The patient should be questioned about any home remedies used to treat infections. Knowledge of preventive measures is also assessed.

Collection of **objective data** includes noting a discharge, which may be watery or yellow and tenacious with a fetid odor. The discharge will be black if from a fungal infection. There may be a partial loss of hearing or the feeling that the ear is occluded if the ear canal is edematous or is obstructed by adenoids. Palpation of the external ear may produce pain.

Diagnostic tests. A culture of the exudate is obtained to identify bacterial, viral, or fungal organisms.

Medical management. Oral analgesics such as codeine may be used if the pain is severe. Corticosteroids (1% hydrocortisone) may be used to reduce edema to allow antibiotics to penetrate. A wick is inserted into the ear canal to prevent loss of medication from the canal and to maintain continuous absorption of the medicine. The physician orders the frequency of the wick change. Antimicrobial agents such as antibiotic or antifungal ear drops may be used. The most commonly used contain 0.5% neomycin or 10,000 units/mL of polymyxin B. Systemic antibiotics are used only if the infection is severe. The specific antibiotic used will be based on the results of the culture.

Nursing interventions and patient teaching. The ear canal is carefully cleansed. Heat may be applied to the external ear for pain relief. An adequate method of communication is implemented. Eardrops are instilled.

Acute external otitis may become a chronic problem. If the infection remains untreated and enters the brain, death can occur.

Nursing diagnosis and interventions for the patient with external otitis include but are not limited to the following:

Nursing Diagnosis	Nursing Interventions
Pain, related to inflammatory process	Apply warm compresses as ordered. Administer prescribed analgesics and instill ordered ear medications.

The nurse ensures that the patient has the knowledge to prevent further infection and can care for the infected ear.

Prognosis. External otitis responds favorably to topical antibiotic and corticosteroid ear drops. Systemic antibiotics are rarely required unless cellulitis is present. The rare malignant external otitis media has a mortality rate of 50% to 75% unless the condition is treated.

Acute Otitis Media

Etiology/pathophysiology. Acute otitis media, an inflammation or infection of the middle ear, is the most common disorder of the middle ear. Acute otitis media is most often caused by *Haemophilus influenzae* or *Streptococcus pneumoniae*. Chronic otitis media is usually caused by gram-negative bacteria, such as *Proteus, Klebsiella,* and *Pseudomonas.* In addition, allergy, exposure to cigarette smoke, mycoplasma, and several viruses may be factors.

Otitis media occurs more frequently in children, especially at 6 to 36 months of age, and in the winter and early spring. Children's shorter and straighter eustachian tubes provide easier access of the organisms from the nasopharynx to travel to the middle ear.

The patient usually has had a recent upper respiratory infection. The infection ascends via the eustachian tube and involves the lining of the entire middle ear. Usually only one ear is affected.

Viral infections frequently cause a serous otitis media. Retraction of the tympanic membrane occurs with a buildup of sterile serous exudate. If there is a secondary bacterial infection, purulent exudate collects behind the tympanic membrane, causing it to bulge. This is called **purulent otitis media.**

Clinical manifestations. The patient will experience a sense of fullness in the ear and also have severe, deep throbbing pain behind the tympanic membrane. This severe pain may disappear if the tympanic membrane ruptures. Hearing loss, tinnitus (a subjective noise sensation heard in one or both ears; ringing or tinkling sounds in the ear), and fever may also be present.

Assessment. For information on collection of **subjective data,** refer to the discussion of external otitis.

Collection of **objective data** is the same as for external otitis, with the exception of noting pain upon palpation of the external ear.

Diagnostic tests. A culture of the purulent drainage is obtained to identify the causative organisms.

Medical management. Antibiotic therapy is based on results of the culture. Amoxicillin for 10 days is the current therapy of choice in the United States. Analgesics are prescribed for severe pain. Sedatives may be prescribed for children to provide rest and pain relief. Local heat is used and nasal decongestants are ordered (Medications for Ear Disorders table).

Needle aspiration of secretions collected behind the tympanic membrane may be necessary. Myringotomy—a surgical incision of the tympanic membrane to relieve pressure and release purulent exudate from the middle ear—may be required to prevent spontaneous rupture. A tympanostomy tube may be placed for short- or long-term use. Prompt treatment of an episode of acute otitis media generally prevents spontaneous perforation of the tympanic membrane.

Nursing interventions and patient teaching. Inner-ear pressure may cause discomfort, requiring an analgesic to be prescribed. Sedatives may be ordered for young children.

Hearing loss may also occur. Effective communication is essential. Parents of young patients should be alerted to the fact, and their help enlisted in monitoring the level of loss.

Chronic otitis media caused by repeated attacks of acute otitis media may result in a permanent perforation of the tympanic membrane. The result is a slight to moderate conductive hearing loss.

A growth called **cholesteatoma** occurs when a tympanic membrane perforation allows keratinizing squamous epithelium of the external auditory canal to enter and grow in the middle ear. Enlargement is slow, but the mass can expand into the mastoid antrum and destroy adjacent structures. Unless removed surgically, a cholesteatoma can cause extensive damage to the structures of the middle ear, can erode the bony protection of the facial nerve, may create a labyrinthine fistula, or even invade the dura, threatening the brain.

Mastoiditis, which is an infection of one of the mastoid bones, may develop. It is usually an extension of a middle-ear infection that was untreated or inadequately treated. Signs of mastoiditis—including earache, fever, headache, malaise, and large amounts of purulent exudate—should be reported immediately.

Nursing diagnosis and interventions for the patient with otitis media include but are not limited to the following:

NURSING DIAGNOSIS	NURSING INTERVENTIONS
Impaired skin integrity, related to edema and exudate	Note and report any purulent outer ear exudate. Keep ear clean and dry; sterile cotton may be used to absorb drainage, if ordered. Monitor temperature and report changes.

The nurse should ensure that the patient and parents are aware of the necessity to complete the entire course of antibiotic therapy. Children are to be fed upright to prevent nasopharyngeal flora from entering the eustachian tube. The patient is instructed to blow the nose gently and not forcefully. If a myringotomy has been performed, the patient and parents are instructed to change the cotton in the outer ear at least twice a day (Patient Teaching: Ear Infection box).

Prognosis for otitis media. Middle-ear infections usually resolve completely with antibiotic therapy. Since the advent of treatment with antibiotics, the incidence of severe and prolonged infections of the middle ear

💊 MEDICATIONS | *Ear Disorders*

MEDICATION	TRADE NAME	ACTIONS/USES	SIDE EFFECTS	NURSING IMPLICATIONS
Carbamide peroxide	Debrox	Cerumen removal	Contact dermatitis	Do not use if eardrum is perforated or if there is ear discharge. Is not recommended for children. Avoid eyes. Reevaluate if edema, erythema, or pain persists. Use proper administration technique by allowing drops to enter ear canal; do not touch dropper.
Colistin/ neomycin/ hydrocortisone/ thonzonium	Coly-Mycin S otic	Antibiotic/steroid/ detergent used for susceptible disease of external auditory canal, mastoidectomy, and otitis media fenestration	Ototoxicity in prolonged use Contact dermatitis Hypersensitivity, including pruritus, skin rash, erythema, and edema	Do not heat bottle above body temperature. With herpes simplex, do not use if patient is infected. Do not use if eardrum is perforated. Use for 10 days only. Keep dropper from touching skin. Check with physician if signs and symptoms worsen or do not improve after 1 week. Shake well before using. Use cotton plug to keep moist; change plug daily.
Triethanolamine polypeptide oleate condensate	Cerumenex	Cerumen removal	Contact dermatitis	Fill ear canal. Insert cotton plug after 15 to 30 minutes. Irrigate ear canal with warm water.
Amoxicillin trihydrate	Amoxil	Systemic penicillin antibiotic used in acute otitis media	Anaphylaxis Skin rash Diarrhea	Use caution during pregnancy and lactation. Take for full treatment period. Consult with physician if no improvement occurs in a few days. Take on full or empty stomach. Check with physician about treating diarrhea. Do not give if patient has penicillin or cephalosporin allergy.
Cefaclor	Ceclor	Second-generation cephalosporin used to treat amoxicillin-resistant otitis media	Anaphylaxis Skin rash Joint pain Fever Diarrhea Abdominal cramping	Use proper administration technique if suspension is given. Store suspension in refrigerator. Give full course of therapy. Tell patient not to use alcohol. Give on full or empty stomach. Do not give if patient has penicillin or cephalosporin allergies.
Meclizine hydrochloride	Antivert	Anticholinergic antihistamine that acts as antiemetic, antivertigo agent Treatment and prophylaxis Possible effectiveness for diseases affecting vestibular system	Drowsiness Blurred vision Dry mouth	Use caution during pregnancy and breastfeeding. Give with food, water, or milk. Tell patient to avoid alcohol and CNS depressants. Not recommended for children under 12.

MEDICATIONS | *Ear Disorders—cont'd*

MEDICATION	TRADE NAME	ACTIONS/USES	SIDE EFFECTS	NURSING IMPLICATIONS
Dimenhydrinate	Dramamine	Anticholinergic antihistamine used in treatment of vertigo	Blurred vision Drowsiness Shortness of breath Painful urination Disorientation	Know that antihistamines may inhibit lactation. Give no CNS depressants. Give with food or milk. Use caution during pregnancy in early months.
Antipyrine/ benzocaine	Auralgan	Analgesic Local anesthetic Used for otitis media; adjunct to cerumen removal	Contact dermatitis	Use caution during pregnancy and lactation. Date bottle and discard after 6 months from first use. Do not use if eardrums are perforated. Warm bottle. Position patient on side and fill ear canal. Use cotton plug. Wash dropper before replacing in bottle.
Acetic acid	Vo Sol hydrochloride otic	Antibacterial Antifungal Astringent Used for superficial infections of external auditory canal	Contact dermatitis Transient stinging	Clean ear first. Use cotton plug for first 24 hours. Contact physician if condition worsens or no improvement occurs after 5 to 7 days. Do not wash dropper; doing so may dilute medication.
Trimethoprim-sulfamethoxazole	Bactrim	Systemic antibacterial Used for acute otitis media No sulfonamide allergy	Fever Itching Skin rash Photosensitivity Dizziness	Is not recommended when breastfeeding or during pregnancy. Emphasize importance of proper dental care. Know that blood glucose levels may be affected in patients using oral antidiabetic agents. Maintain adequate fluid intake. Advise patient to avoid sun exposure. Complete treatment. With pediatric suspension, shake well.
Polymyxin B/ neomycin/ hydrocortisone	Cortisporin	Antibiotic and steroid used in the same way as Coly-Mycin S Used to treat swimmer's ear	Ototoxicity in prolonged use Contact dermatitis pruritus Erythema Edema	Use caution during pregnancy and lactation. Do not use if eardrum is perforated. Keep dropper from touching skin. Shake well before using. Use cotton plug to keep moist; change plug daily.

has been greatly reduced. Chronic or untreated otitis media may lead to sound transmission hearing loss, which is successfully treated with tympanoplasty.

Prognosis for mastoiditis. The infection is difficult to treat and may require antibiotic therapy intravenously for several days. Because children are most often affected, immediate treatment of the infection is crucial. Residual hearing loss may follow the infection. If early decalcification is present, intense antibiotic therapy and myringotomy can usually cure mastoiditis; if it has progressed to further destruction, simple mastoidectomy is necessary.

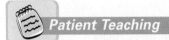
Patient Teaching

Ear Infection

PREVENTION OF FURTHER INFECTION

- Protect ear canal during showers (cotton with petrolatum in external canal; use a shower cap over ears).
- Avoid swimming during infection or after a perforated eardrum; avoid swimming in contaminated water when infection is healed.
- Continue antibiotic therapy for prescribed number of days, even when symptoms disappear.
- Get adequate and early treatment of upper respiratory tract infections and allergic conditions.

CARE OF INFECTED EAR

- Use correct eardrop insertion or ear irrigations, as prescribed.
- Wash hands before and after changing cotton plugs to prevent secondary infection.
- Keep external ear clean and dry to protect skin from drainage.

SIGNS REQUIRING MEDICAL ATTENTION

- Fever
- Return of ear pain or discharge

Labyrinthitis

Etiology/pathophysiology. Labyrinthitis is an inflammation of the labyrinthine canals of the inner ear. Labyrinthitis is the most common cause of vertigo (the sensation that the outer world is revolving about oneself or that one is moving in space). A common cause is a viral upper respiratory infection that spreads into the inner ear; other causes include certain drugs and foods. The vestibular portion of the inner ear may be destroyed by streptomycin. Tobacco and alcohol may also be causative factors. A rarer form of labyrinthitis is caused by bacteria. It is usually associated with middle-ear and mastoid infections. Since the advent of antibiotics, bacterial labyrinthitis occurs very infrequently.

Clinical manifestations. Severe and sudden vertigo is the most common symptom of labyrinthitis. Also present are nausea and vomiting, nystagmus, photophobia, headache, and ataxic gait.

Assessment. Collection of **subjective data** should include noting the frequency and duration of the vertigo, as well as any safety measures taken by the patient during an attack. Other symptoms—such as hearing ability, ringing in the ears, and nausea—are assessed. Because fear is associated with the attacks, the patient's feelings should be explored.

Collection of **objective data** includes noting vomiting as well as any jerking movement of the eyeballs, unilaterally or bilaterally. The color and moisture of skin are assessed to determine the extent of autonomic response.

Diagnostic tests. Electronystagmography may show a diminished or absent nystagmus with stimulation. Audiometric testing shows a low-tone sensorineural hearing loss.

Medical management. There is no specific treatment for labyrinthitis. Usually antibiotics and dimenhydrinate (Dramamine) or meclizine (Antivert) for vertigo are prescribed. If nausea and vomiting persist, parenteral fluids are administered.

Nursing interventions and patient teaching. It is important to note the frequency and degree of vertigo. Antibiotics and medications for vertigo are administered. Fluid intake is assessed to ensure that dehydration does not occur.

Nursing diagnoses and interventions for the patient with labyrinthitis include but are not limited to the following:

NURSING DIAGNOSES	NURSING INTERVENTIONS
Risk for injury, related to altered sensory perception (vertigo)	Keep side rails up. Note presence of vertigo before patient ambulates. Supervise ambulation. Caution the patient not to attempt ambulation alone and to call for assistance.
Fear, related to altered sensory perception (vertigo)	Explore patient's feelings about attack. Teach patient concerning actions during an attack (see Patient Teaching: Vertigo). Reinforce physician's treatment orders.

The nurse instructs the patient concerning vertigo (Patient Teaching: Vertigo box).

Prognosis. Labyrinthitis usually resolves itself, with little or no hearing impairment.

Obstructions of the Ear

Etiology/pathophysiology. Ear canal obstruction is usually caused by impaction or excessive secretion of cerumen or by foreign bodies, including insects. Children often place beans, beads, pebbles, and small toys in their ears. Usually those objects are found on routine examination.

Obstruction by cerumen can be caused when excessive amounts are produced by overactive glands or from impaction of cerumen in narrow or tortuous ear canals.

Clinical manifestations. The obstruction may cause the ear to feel occluded. There may be presence of tinnitus or buzzing, pain in the ear, and slight hearing loss.

Assessment. Collection of **subjective data** includes interviewing the patient about any possible foreign bodies being introduced into the ear and any home remedies used to remove the object. If the patient is a child, determination is made of risk factors causing ear obstructions, such as beads or nuts.

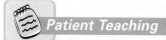
Patient Teaching

Vertigo

* Nature of the disorder
  —Physiologic basis for the vertigo
  —Avoidance of any known precipitating factors
  —Rationale for a low-salt diet
* Actions to take during an attack
  —Lie down immediately, and call for help if necessary at the first signs of an attack
  —If driving when an attack occurs, pull over immediately to the curb
  —Lie immobile, and hold head in one position until vertigo lessens
* Ask for assistance when ambulating if dizzy
* Take prescribed medications as instructed even if no recent attacks have occurred; check with physician before discontinuing any medication
* Symptoms requiring medical attention: changes in symptoms or nature of attacks

---

Collection of **objective data** involves the nurse noting any presence of a foreign body in the external ear canal. Children are observed for tugging of the pinna.

Diagnostic tests. Otoscopic examination provides visualization of the cause of the obstruction.

Medical management. Medical management includes removal of cerumen by irrigation or cerumen spoon. Foreign objects are removed with forceps, if possible. Insects are smothered with drops of an oily substance and removed with forceps. Medications, such as carbamide peroxide 6.5%, may be used to soften cerumen. Surgical removal of the foreign object may be necessary.

Nursing interventions and patient teaching. The nurse assists with the irrigation of the ear. Medications are instilled into the ear as ordered.

Nursing diagnosis and interventions for the patient with obstructions of the ear include but are not limited to the following:

NURSING DIAGNOSIS	NURSING INTERVENTIONS
Disturbed sensory perception, (auditory), related to presence of foreign body causing obstruction	Note the presence and amount of hearing impairment and tinnitus. Assure the patient or parents that once the obstruction is removed, any hearing loss or tinnitus should disappear.

The nurse informs the patient and parents about the danger of placing objects in the ears. The nurse also reinforces the method for preventing cerumen obstruction through the instilling of one or two drops of an oily substance at night. This is followed by hydrogen peroxide in the morning and cleaning with a soft cotton wick.

Prognosis. Ear canal obstructions caused by cerumen and foreign bodies resolve completely with treatment. Vertigo may be experienced temporarily until the ear canal dries. Disorientation in the older adult may occur from the cerumen impaction and temporary loss of hearing.

NONINFECTIOUS DISORDERS OF THE EAR
Otosclerosis

Etiology/pathophysiology. Otosclerosis is a condition characterized by chronic progressive deafness caused by the formation of spongy bone, especially around the oval window, with resulting ankylosis (immobility of a joint) of the stapes, causing tinnitus and then deafness. Otosclerosis is an autosomal dominant inheritance disease. Women are affected twice as often as men. Otosclerosis is bilateral in about 80% of patients. Frequently pregnancy triggers a rapid onset of this condition. Previous ear infections are not believed to be related to otosclerosis. Gradual replacement of normal bone in the otic capsule by highly vascular otosclerotic bone occurs. This replacement bone is described as spongy. Calcification of the area follows, and conductive hearing loss then results.

Clinical manifestations. The patient with otosclerosis will experience a slowly progressive conductive hearing loss and will describe a low- to medium-pitched tinnitus. The deafness is usually first noted between the ages of 11 and 20.

Assessment. Collection of **subjective data** includes noting the degree and progression of hearing loss or tinnitus as well as mild dizziness to vertigo. Family history for the disease is assessed.

Collection of **objective data** includes assessment of behavioral clues related to hearing loss as in Box 13-2.

Diagnostic tests. Otoscopy will reveal a normal eardrum. A pink blush called **Schwartz's sign** may be seen through the ear; this is indicative of a high degree of vascularity in active otosclerotic bone. The result of the Rinne test shows sounds transmitted by bone conduction lasting longer than by air conduction in the affected ear. Weber's test results are the reverse from normal hearing. Audiometric testing shows a lateralization of sound more to the affected ear. Weber's test in otosclerosis would result in a lateralization of sound to the affected ear. Audiometric testing may show minimal to total hearing loss. Tympanometry may reveal evidence of stiffness in the sound conduction system. Hearing loss ranges from mild in the early stages to total loss in the later stages.

Medical management. Otosclerosis is usually treated with a stapedectomy to restore hearing. The ear with poorer hearing is repaired first, and the other ear may be operated on 6 months to a year later. When a stapedectomy is not indicated, an air conduction hearing aid may be prescribed.

Nursing interventions and patient teaching. Nursing diagnoses and interventions of otosclerosis are specific to poststapedectomy care. For patient teaching, see the discussion on ear surgery.

Prognosis. Patients report varying degrees of success with hearing after stapedectomy surgery. For some patients, stapedectomy is successful in permanently restoring hearing. A hearing aid may further enhance sound conduction to more normal levels.

Ménière's Disease

Etiology/pathophysiology. **Ménière's disease** is a chronic disease of the inner ear characterized by recurrent episodes of vertigo, progressive unilateral nerve deafness, and tinnitus.

Ménière's disease is most common in women between 30 and 60 years of age. The cause is unknown, although occasionally the condition follows middle-ear infection or trauma to the head.

There is an increase in endolymph fluid, either from increased production or decreased absorption. This causes increased pressure in the inner-ear labyrinth. Attacks of severe vertigo, tinnitus, and progressive deafness result from this increased pressure. Usually one ear only is involved.

Clinical manifestations. The patient experiences recurrent episodes of vertigo with associated nausea and tinnitus, and hearing loss may be present. During an attack, nausea, vomiting, diaphoresis, tinnitus, and nystagmus may occur. These attacks last from a few minutes to several hours. Attacks may occur several times a year. Sudden movements often aggravate the symptoms.

Assessment. Collection of **subjective data** includes noting the frequency and severity of the vertigo attack. History and knowledge of the disorder and circumstances that precipitate an attack are noted. Assessment is made of actions taken by the patient during an attack and the degree of relief those actions provide.

Collection of **objective data** includes determining unilateral or bilateral hearing loss. The nurse observes the patient for associated signs during an attack.

Diagnostic tests. Diagnostic tests are ordered to rule out central nervous system disease. The audiogram demonstrates a mild low-frequency sensorineural hearing loss. Audiologic tuning fork tests show a sensorineural deficit. Vestibular testing shows lack of balance. Glycerol test determines the osmotic effect of glycerol that pulls fluid from the inner ear.

Medical management. There is no specific therapy for Ménière's disease. Fluid restriction, diuretics, and a low-salt diet are prescribed in an attempt to decrease fluid pressure. Avoidance of caffeine and nicotine are advised.

Dimenhydrinate (Dramamine), meclizine (Antivert), diazepam (Valium), and diphenhydramine (Benadryl) are prescribed for use between attacks. In acute attacks the medications may be given intravenously. Atropine is also given for its anticholinergic effect during these acute attacks.

For preservation of hearing, surgical procedures may be performed. Approximately 5% to 10% of the patients with Ménière's disease require surgery. These surgeries and subsequent nursing interventions are discussed in Table 13-5.

Table 13-5 | *Surgery for Ménière's Disease*

TYPE	DESCRIPTION	RESIDUAL	POSTOPERATIVE NURSING INTERVENTIONS
Surgical destruction of labyrinth	Extraction of membranous labyrinth by suction; access to inner ear through external canal (stapes and incus removed)	Destroys remaining hearing	Bed rest and NPO until vertigo subsides in 1 to 3 days Avoid sudden movement of head for 1 to 2 weeks Take action to prevent falls from unsteadiness for 1 to 3 weeks
Endolymphatic subarachnoid shunt	Insertion of drain tube from endolymphatic sac into subarachnoid space; access through mastoid	Preserves hearing in 60% to 70% of patients	Monitor for vertigo (rare)
Cryosurgery	Application of intense cold to lateral semicircular canals to decrease sensitivity or to create an otic-periotic shunt; access through mastoid	Preserves hearing in 80% of patients	Monitor for dizziness for 2 days Take action to prevent falls from unsteadiness for 2 to 3 weeks
Vestibular nerve section	Dissection of cranial nerve VIII (vestibular portion); access through mastoid or through cranial drilling over roof of internal auditory canal	Preserves hearing in 90% of patients	Same as for surgical destruction of labyrinth

Nursing interventions and patient teaching. The nurse should maintain the prescribed low-salt diet and administer diuretics as ordered. Acute vertigo is treated symptomatically with bed rest, sedation, and antiemetics or medications for motion sickness. During an acute attack the patient is kept in a quiet, darkened room in a comfortable position. The patient may have some auditory deficit, which will require alternate methods of communication. If the patient's tinnitus becomes distressing, an increase in background noise, such as music, may provide relief. Fluorescent or flickering lights or watching television may exacerbate symptoms and should be avoided. An emesis basin should be available because vomiting is common.

Nursing diagnoses and interventions for the patient with Ménière's disease include but are not limited to the following:

Nursing Diagnoses	Nursing Interventions
Risk for injury, related to sensory-perceptual alterations (vertigo)	Keep side rails up. Assist with ambulation and instruct the patient to call for assistance before attempting to ambulate. Have the patient sit or lie down when vertigo occurs. Have the patient move slowly and avoid turning the head suddenly.

Nursing Diagnoses	Nursing Interventions
	Administer medications as prescribed Position patient on unaffected side. Stand in front of patient and prevent head turning. Avoid bright or glaring lights around patient. Place all needed supplies so that patient does not have to turn head.
Social isolation, related to unpredictable vertigo attacks	Assess factors that contribute to social isolation. Assess feelings of loneliness and abandonment. Identify support systems for patient. Identify patient concerns. Establish effective communication.

The nurse provides information about a low-salt diet and taking diuretics. The patient should be warned to avoid reading when vertigo or tinnitus is present. The patient is instructed to avoid smoking to prevent vasoconstriction. The patient should learn to identify precipitating factors and the proper actions to take when an attack occurs: (1) sit or lie down immediately, (2) stop the car and pull over to the side of the road, and (3) keep medication available at all times (Nursing Care Plan: The Patient with Ménière's Disease).

NURSING CARE PLAN

The Patient with Ménière's Disease

Ms. L. is a 66-year-old patient admitted with Ménière's disease. She complains of severe dizziness, nausea, vomiting, ringing in the ears, hearing loss, and an unsteady gait. She is accompanied by her husband of 35 years.

NURSING DIAGNOSIS *Anxiety, related to effect of disorder*

Patient Goals/Expected Outcomes	*Nursing Interventions*	*Evaluation/Rationale*
Patient will experience decreased signs and symptoms of anxiety. Patient will experience anxiety control.	Encourage patient to explore concerns about decreased hearing and effects of vertigo attacks and to take action in relation to the concerns. Explore patient's knowledge of the disorder and correct misunderstandings. Educate patient on strategies that can give her back some control over her life. Suggest keeping an emesis basin, a pillow, a blanket, a car phone, and a large sign with the words "HELP, POLICE" in the car in case of a sudden Ménière's attack. Encourage realistic hope about expected hearing ability as described by physician. Refer patient to necessary support services, such as social worker or audiologist. Refer patient for more information to Vestibular Disorders Association or Ménière's Network.	Patient states that level of anxiety has decreased.

Continued

NURSING CARE PLAN

The Patient with Ménière's Disease—cont'd

NURSING DIAGNOSIS *Risk for injury, related to vestibular auditory alterations*

Patient Goals/Expected Outcomes	Nursing Interventions	Evaluation/Rationale
Patient will describe actions to avoid vertigo. Patient remains free of injury. Patient remains safe from fall occurrences.	Help patient identify avoidable actions that precipitate vertigo attacks. Encourage patient to move slowly and not turn head suddenly when vertigo is present. If tinnitus is distressing, increase background noises, such as music. If hearing is decreased: • Use measures to facilitate communication with hearing impaired. • Carry wax earplugs; even after losing some hearing, ears are often sensitive to loud noises and can trigger vertigo. • Refer patient to audiologist, if appropriate. Keep side rails up when patient with vertigo is in bed. Assist with ambulation as needed. Encourage patient to sit or lie down and to remain immobile if signs of dizziness occur. Teach patient to stop car at side of road immediately at first signs of dizziness while driving.	Patient avoids physical environment that could cause injury. Patient does not manifest evidence of injury.

? CRITICAL THINKING QUESTIONS

1. Ms. L. states that she would prefer going to the bathroom without the assistance of a nurse. The appropriate response by the nurse would be:
2. Ms. L. tells the nurse that she is very depressed because of her very unpleasant symptoms and wonders if she will ever feel well again. A therapeutic reply would be:
3. The nurse notes an unpleasant odor from Ms. L.; her hair is unkempt, and she has poor oral hygiene. The nurse is preparing to give her a warm, therapeutic bed bath. Ms. L. states, "I feel too dizzy to take a bath." To promote personal hygiene and patient compliance, the nurse would:

Prognosis. Approximately 75% to 85% of patients experience improvement with medical management and supportive therapy. The remainder of patients may, in time, require surgical intervention. There are usually several yearly attacks until the disease either resolves itself or progresses to complete deafness in the affected ear.

SURGERIES OF THE EAR

STAPEDECTOMY

Stapedectomy is the removal of the stapes of the middle ear and insertion of a graft and prosthesis. The stapes that has become fixed is replaced so that vibrations can again transmit sound waves through the oval window to the fluid of the inner ear. This is performed to restore hearing in the treatment of otosclerosis.

Using a local anesthetic and an operating microscope for visualization, the surgeon removes the stapes, and the opening into the inner ear is covered with a graft of body tissue. One end of a small plastic tube or piece of

stainless steel wire is attached to the graft, while the other end is attached to the two remaining bones of the middle ear, the malleus and the incus.

Nursing Interventions

Postoperative management consists of an external ear packing to ensure healing; the packing is left in place for 5 or 6 days. The patient should remain in bed for approximately 24 hours, depending on physician preference. Gradual activity, when allowed, is provided. The patient is kept flat with the operative side facing upward to maintain the position of the prosthesis and graft; therefore the nurse makes certain that the patient is not turned. Headache and dizziness are expected early in the postoperative period. The patient's hearing does not improve until the edema subsides and the packing is removed by the physician (Patient Teaching: Ear Surgery box).

Possible complications of the stapedectomy include infection of the external, middle, or inner ear. Displace-

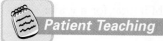
Patient Teaching

Ear Surgery

- Change cotton in ear daily as prescribed.
- Open mouth when sneezing or coughing and blow nose gently one side at a time for 1 week (to prevent increased ear pressure and infection).
- Keep ear dry for 6 weeks (to prevent infection).
  —Do not wash hair for 1 week.
  —Protect ear when outdoors using two pieces of cotton (use petrolatum jelly on outer ball).
  —Protect ear with shower cap when bathing.
- Wear ear protectors as necessary to prevent exposure to loud noises.
- Follow activity guidelines:
  —No physical activity for 1 week.
  —No exercises or active sports for 3 weeks.
  —Return to work in 1 week (3 weeks for strenuous work).
- Avoid exposure to people with upper respiratory tract infections.
- Avoid airplane flights for at least 1 week (to prevent effects of pressure changes).

ment or rejection of the prosthesis or graft may occur, or perilymph fluid may leak around the prosthesis into the middle ear, causing ringing in the ears and vertigo.

Prognosis

During surgery the patient will often report an immediate improvement in hearing in the operative ear. Because of the accumulation of blood and fluid in the middle ear, the hearing level decreases postoperatively but does return to near-normal levels. After stapedectomy, 90% of patients experience an improvement in hearing, in many instances to near-normal levels.

TYMPANOPLASTY

Tympanoplasty is any of several operative procedures on the eardrum or ossicles of the middle ear designed to restore or improve hearing in patients with conductive hearing loss. These operations may be used to repair a perforated eardrum, for otosclerosis, or for dislocation or necrosis of a small bone of the middle ear.

Nursing Interventions

Postoperative management consists of bed rest until the next morning. The head of the bed is elevated 40 degrees, and the operative side faces upward. Medications include opioid analgesics; tetracycline (Achromycin V) as an antiinfective agent; and meclizine (Antivert) for vertigo.

Postoperatively the presence of bleeding; the amount, color, and consistency of drainage; and temperature must be noted and reported. Complaints of vertigo when the patient is getting out of bed should

be noted; with sudden movements, nausea and vertigo may occur. Possible complications include infection and displacement of the graft.

Nursing diagnoses and interventions for the patient after a tympanoplasty include but are not limited to the following:

NURSING DIAGNOSES	NURSING INTERVENTIONS
Impaired physical mobility, related to surgical procedure	Note patient's ability to comply with bed rest order. Keep the patient's operative side up; do not allow the patient to be turned.
Risk for activity intolerance, related to pain and vertigo	Keep side rails up. When movement is allowed, begin gradually. Administer prescribed medications for pain and vertigo as needed. Assist with ambulation to prevent injury.

Prognosis

Improved hearing will be noted if there is no involvement of the ossicles.

MYRINGOTOMY

Myringotomy is a surgical incision of the eardrum. It is performed to relieve pressure and release purulent exudate from the middle ear. The procedure is done under either local or general anesthesia.

A myringotomy may be performed in one of two ways. Using a myringotomy knife, the surgeon makes a curved incision in the drumhead. In the second procedure, a heated wire loop is touched for about 1 second to the drumhead, producing a 2-mm hole.

Nursing Interventions and Patient Teaching

Pus and fluid may drain immediately, requiring suctioning. Cotton placed in the ear absorbs drainage, which may continue several days.

The incision usually heals quickly with little scarring. Disruption of hearing does not usually occur.

Postoperative management includes cotton in the ear for absorption of drainage. Cotton should be changed frequently to avoid recontamination of the surgical area. Medications commonly used are tetracycline (Achromycin V) and polymyxin B (Neosporin) ear drops as antiinfective agents. Tylenol with codeine may be used for pain.

Postoperatively the nurse monitors for signs of drainage and bleeding and reports any occurrence. Incisional pain or hearing impairment should be noted.

Patient teaching involves providing the information in Patient Teaching: Ear Surgery and ensuring understanding.

Prognosis

Once pressure is relieved, hearing is restored to more normal levels unless scarring is present.

COCHLEAR IMPLANT

The cochlear implant is used as a hearing device for the profoundly deaf. The system consists of a surgically implanted induction coil beneath the skin behind the ear and an electrode wire placed in the cochlea (Figure 13-16). The implanted parts interface with an externally worn speech processor. The system stimulates auditory nerve fibers by an electric current so that signals reach the brain stem's auditory nuclei and ultimately the auditory cortex. The implant is intended for the patient whose sensorineural hearing loss is either congenital or acquired. The ideal candidate is one who has become deaf after acquiring speech and language. The adult who was born deaf or became deaf before learning to speak may be considered a candidate for a cochlear implant if she or he has followed an aural/oral educational approach.

The implant offers the profoundly deaf the ability to hear environmental sounds, including speech, at comfortable loudness levels. Multichannel cochlear implants also serve as aids to speech production. Extensive training and rehabilitation are essential to receive maximum benefit from these implants. The positive aspects of a cochlear implant include providing sound to the person who heard none, improving the sense of security, and decreasing the feelings of isolation. With continued research, the cochlear implant may offer the possibility of hearing rehabilitation for a wider range of hearing-impaired individuals.

NURSING PROCESS *for the Patient with a Visual or Auditory Disorder*

The role of the licensed practical nurse/licensed vocational nurse (LPN/LVN) in the nursing process as stated is that the LPN/LVN will:
* Participate in planning care for patients based on patient needs.
* Review patient's plan of care and recommend revisions as needed.
* Review and follow defined prioritization for patient care.
* Use clinical pathways/care maps/care plans to guide and review patient care.

Assessment

The complexity of the assessment for eye and ear disorders is determined by the disease/problem that a patient has. Subjective data for both eye and ear disorders include the following:
* Health history, including any acute or chronic disease
* History of current complaint
* Medications, including prescription, over-the-counter (OTC), and home remedies or folk medicines
* Surgery and other treatments

Objective data includes the external and internal assessment of the eye and ear. Inspection and palpation are used to assess the external components of the eye and ear, noting any abnormalities. Results of the internal examination of the eye and ear by the primary care provider should be reviewed. Results of diagnostic tests should be noted. Because seeing and hearing are necessary for safety, communication, self-care, and psychosocial interaction, these areas should be assessed as well.

Nursing Diagnosis

Nursing assessment identifies the needs of the patient. Care of the patient is based on the nursing diagnoses that have been identified. Possible nursing diagnoses include the following:
* Ineffective health maintenance
* Anxiety
* Self-care deficit (specify)
* Fear
* Impaired environmental interpretation syndrome
* Impaired home maintenance
* Impaired social interaction
* Risk for injury
* Risk for loneliness
* Disturbed sensory perception: auditory
* Disturbed sensory perception: visual
* Social isolation

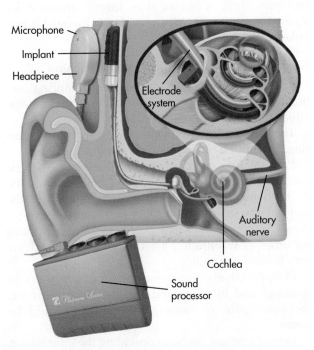

FIGURE **13-16** Cochlear implant.

Expected Outcomes/Planning

Impairment of vision or hearing will require a major adjustment in the life of an individual. Adjustment to the loss and changes in lifestyle must be dealt with, whether the loss is permanent or temporary. Assisting in the plan of care focuses on achieving specific goals and outcomes that relate to the identified nursing diagnoses. Examples of these include:

Goal #1: Patient remains free of injury.

Outcome: Patient/family inspects environment for potential hazards related to loss of vision or hearing.

Goal #2: Patient remains socially active.

Outcome: Patient displays interest in social and recreational activities.

Implementation

Measures used in the care of a patient with vision or hearing loss center around assisting the patient to remain physically and emotionally safe and secure and ensuring that the patient's needs are communicated and met while adjusting to the loss. Nursing interventions include the following:

- Promoting safety
- Assisting with ADLs
- Facilitating communication
- Encouraging diversional activity

The nurse also assesses readiness to learn and teaches health promotion practices (see Patient Teaching boxes). The nurse must consider the patient's culture, beliefs, values, and habits (Cultural and Ethnic Considerations box), as well as the special needs of the older adult (see Older Adult Considerations box).

Evaluation

Systematic evaluation requires the nurse to determine whether expected outcomes have been met. The nurse refers to the goals and outcomes identified when as-

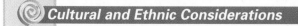

Cultural and Ethnic Considerations

Hearing and Visual Problems

- Eskimos are susceptible to primary, narrow-angle glaucoma, resulting from a thicker lens and a shallow chamber angle.
- Whites have a higher incidence of hearing impairment than African-Americans or Asian-Americans.
- Incidence and severity of glaucoma are greater among African-Americans than among whites.
- American Indians and African-Americans have a higher incidence of astigmatism than whites.
- American Indians have a higher incidence of otitis media than whites.
- Whites have a higher incidence of macular degeneration than Hispanics, African-Americans, and Asian-Americans.

sisting in the development of planning care and performing measures designed to specifically evaluate the achievement of the goals. Examples of goals and their evaluative measures include:

Goal #1: Patient remains free of injury.

Evaluative measure: Ask patient/family to describe what environmental changes need to be made to ensure safety.

Goal #2: Patient remains socially active.

Evaluative measure: Observe patient participating in social activities.

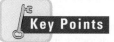

Key Points

- The five major senses are taste, touch, smell, sight, and hearing/balance.
- The accessory structures of the eye are the eyebrows, eyelids, eyelashes, and the lacrimal apparatus.
- The three tunics of the eyeball are the fibrous tunic (sclera), the vascular tunic (choroid), and the retina.
- The two chambers of the eye are the anterior chamber, which contains aqueous humor, and the posterior chamber, which contains vitreous humor.
- Image formation at the retina requires four basic processes: refraction, accommodation, constriction, and convergence.
- The photoreceptors of the retina are the rods and cones. The rods control vision in dim light and the cones control vision in bright light. The cones are also responsible for color vision.
- Light entering the eye must travel through the cornea, aqueous humor, pupil, crystalline lens, vitreous humor, and finally the retina.
- The ear is divided into external, middle, and inner ears.
- The external ear flap is called the pinna (auricle); it extends into the external ear canal.
- The middle ear contains the ossicles and the entrance of the eustachian tube and ends with the tympanic membrane.
- The internal ear contains the vestibule, cochlea, and semicircular canals.
- The organ of Corti is the organ of hearing; it is located within the cochlea.
- The semicircular canals are responsible for the sense of balance and equilibrium.
- The taste buds differentiate four basic tastes: sweet, sour, salty, and bitter. Food must be in solution for interpretation, because a chemical reaction occurs.
- Normal aging causes decreased hearing and sight as a result of normal changes of the structures.
- Individuals with chronic disease or individuals older than 40 years of age should be examined yearly to detect eye abnormalities or so that changes in therapy may be prescribed.
- Refractory errors include the conditions hyperopia (farsightedness), presbyopia (farsightedness related to the aging process), and astigmatism (objects waver).

- Ranges of 20/20 to 20/40 vision are considered normal, whereas 20/200 with correction is defined as legal blindness.
- Age-related macular degeneration (ARMD) is divided into two classic forms: dry (atrophic) and wet (exudative). In dry ARMD, which accounts for 90% of patients with ARMD, the macular cells have wasted or atrophied. Wet ARMD is characterized by the development of abnormal blood vessels in or near the macula.
- Cataracts are an opacity of the lens and may be removed by intracapsular or extracapsular extraction.
- Glaucoma is not one disease, but rather a group of disorders characterized by (1) increased intraocular pressure and the consequences of elevated pressure, (2) optic nerve atrophy, and (3) peripheral visual field loss.
- Loss of hearing may result from cerumen-buildup infection, trauma, or use of ototoxic drugs, or it may be a congenital condition.
- Conductive hearing loss is a decrease in amplification, whereas sensorineural hearing loss is interference within the inner ear.

- Prevention of serious complications of ear disorders—such as infections, mastoiditis, and brain abscess—requires early detection and treatment.
- Injury, risk for, is the primary nursing diagnosis for the patient experiencing vertigo, which occurs in labyrinthitis and Ménière's disease.
- An essential communication tip for speaking to the hearing impaired is to face the patient and to speak clearly without shouting.
- A cochlear implant is a hearing device for the profoundly deaf. The implanted device is intended for the patient with sensorineural hearing loss.

Go to your free CD-ROM for an Audio Glossary, animations, video clips, and Review Questions for the NCLEX-PN® Examination.

evolve Be sure to visit the companion Evolve site at http://evolve.elsevier.com/Christensen/adult/ for WebLinks and additional online resources.

CHAPTER CHALLENGE

1. Ms. R. is to have a laser treatment to cauterize hemorrhaging vessels caused by diabetic retinopathy. The name of the procedure is:

   1. enucleation.
   2. scleral buckle.
   3. photocoagulation.
   4. trabeculoplasty.

2. The parents of T., age 11 years, want to know more about T.'s conductive hearing loss. The nurse would explain that:

   1. sound is delivered through the external and middle ear, but a defect in the inner ear results in distortion of sound.
   2. sound is inadequately delivered through the external or middle ear to the inner ear.
   3. there is no organic cause, but a functional problem exists.
   4. the brain's auditory pathways are damaged.

3. Ms. J. has impaired hearing. To facilitate communication, the nurse would:

   1. face Ms. J. when speaking.
   2. overaccentuate words to make the communication more effective.
   3. shout to allow Ms. J. to hear.
   4. use one-word answers when speaking.

4. Mr. M. tells the nurse he has dizziness. He states that the doctor used another term. The medical term is:

   1. tinnitus.
   2. labyrinthitis.
   3. sensorineural.
   4. vertigo.

5. Ms. R. is diagnosed with an inner ear problem. The major symptom would be:

   1. echoing.
   2. intense pain.
   3. vertigo.
   4. loss of hearing.

6. Evaluation of the eye as it adjusts to seeing objects at various distances is called:

   1. PERRLA.
   2. refraction.
   3. focusing.
   4. accommodation.

7. Ms. O. has tunnel vision, eye pain, difficulty in adjusting to darkness, halos seen around lights, and failure to detect colors. These indicate:

   1. primary open-angle glaucoma.
   2. cataracts.
   3. entropion.
   4. detached retina.

8. Which of the following would be a safety hazard in the home of a patient who is visually impaired?

   1. Area rug
   2. Room carpeting
   3. Tile floor
   4. Concrete flooring

9. An older adult falls at home resulting in a blunt injury of an eyeball. The eye is tearing excessively, and the patient complains of a severe stabbing pain as if "something is in my eye!" First aid measures would include which of the following?

   1. Apply a cool compress three times a day (tid).
   2. Lightly cover the eye with a sterile gauze pad.
   3. Remove any particles that may be embedded in the eye.
   4. Irrigate the eye with tap water.

10. Ms. K. has just had cataract surgery. Important discharge instructions would include which of the following?

    1. Wear an eyeshield at night on the operative eye.
    2. Avoid bending, stooping, coughing, or lifting.
    3. Instill prescribed eyedrops into the conjunctival sac.
    4. All of the above.

11. Which of the assessment findings would indicate a need for possible glaucoma testing?

    1. Presence of "floaters"
    2. Colored halos around lights
    3. Intermittent loss of vision
    4. Pruritus and erythema of the conjunctiva

12. While communicating with a patient, you notice a possible hearing deficit in one ear. Which of the following would be an appropriate nursing intervention?

    1. Shout louder than usual in the affected ear
    2. Speak clearly and in a slightly louder voice toward the patient's face
    3. Plug the affected ear and shout in the unaffected ear
    4. Speak softer than usual in the affected ear

13. What is the most likely cause of hearing loss in the older adult?

    1. Cerumen buildup
    2. Ossification of the pinna
    3. Low batteries in the hearing aid
    4. Fluid in the ear

14. Patients with permanent visual impairment:

    1. feel most comfortable with other visually impaired people.
    2. may experience the same grieving process that is associated with other losses.
    3. may feel threatened when others make eye contact during a conversation.
    4. usually need others to speak louder so they can communicate appropriately.

15. Mr. H. is a 32-year-old construction worker who suffered a penetrating wound to the eye. The best intervention for anyone at the scene to take is:

    1. gently remove the object.
    2. wipe away the blood and tears.
    3. cover the object with a paper cup and tape.
    4. do nothing; rush to the hospital.

16. Mr. K., 71, complains of being severely dizzy. A nursing intervention to help Mr. K. includes which of the following activities?

    1. Avoid sudden movements.
    2. Avoid noises.
    3. Encourage fluid intake.
    4. Suggest patient lie on affected side.

17. Mr. P. has been blind for the past 10 years. He is hospitalized with heart failure. In the care of a long-term blind individual, it is important to:

    1. keep all items at a distance so he won't bump into them.
    2. schedule a consultation with an occupational therapist to teach activities of daily living.
    3. announce when you enter and leave the room.
    4. initiate a referral to the Department of Health and Human Services.

18. Mr. A. has a family history of cataracts. He asks what symptom would be present if he begins to develop them. The nurse might respond that the first symptoms of a cataract are usually:

    1. pain in the eyes.
    2. blurred vision.
    3. loss of peripheral vision.
    4. dry eyes.

19. Mr. H. has had cataract surgery. Discharge teaching would include:

    1. lifting light objects is acceptable.
    2. wearing eyepatches for the first 72 hours.
    3. bending at the knees and keeping the head straight.
    4. bending at the waist is acceptable if done slowly.

20. Mr. O. is scheduled for a stapedectomy. Appropriate postoperative teaching should include which of the following?

    1. Change cotton from external ear canal hourly
    2. Gently blowing both nares simultaneously
    3. Teaching patient to open mouth when sneezing or coughing
    4. Limiting activities for 3 weeks

21. M., a 15-year-old hearing-impaired patient, is having problems communicating with the staff. Which of the following behaviors would improve communication? (Choose all correct answers.)

    1. Overaccentuating words
    2. Facing M. when speaking
    3. Speaking in conversational tones
    4. Asking permission to turn off television or radio

22. Mr. T., 76, is partially blind. His physician has diagnosed primary open-angle glaucoma. The goal of treatment in glaucoma is to:

    1. decrease aqueous humor.
    2. increase aqueous humor.
    3. decrease discomfort.
    4. restore vision.

Continued

23. The priority nursing responsibility while caring for a patient with vertigo is:

    1. safety.
    2. comfort.
    3. hygiene.
    4. quiet.

24. Mr. W. is cleaning the garage and splashes a chemical in his eyes. The initial priority following the chemical burn is to:

    1. transport to a physician immediately.
    2. cover the eyes with a sterile gauze.
    3. irrigate with water for 15 minutes or longer.
    4. irrigate with normal saline for 1 to 5 minutes.

25. Ms. R. visits the physician for a routine physical examination that involves testing distance vision. As she faces the Snellen chart, the nurse is to instruct the patient to:

    1. use both eyes to read the chart.
    2. read the chart from right to left.
    3. cover one eye while testing the other.
    4. use any one eye because they will be the same.

26. Ms. P., 49, has recently been blinded as a result of an automobile accident. This is her initial ambulation to the bathroom. What precautions should the nurse take when ambulating the patient?

    1. Precede the patient with patient's hand on the nurse's elbow.
    2. Follow the patient with the patient's hand on the nurse's elbow.
    3. Walk in front of the patient telling of any obstacles.
    4. Walk behind the patient with the nurse's hand on the patient's shoulder.

27. Mr. J. comes into the clinic complaining of progressive loss of vision in the center of his visual field. His physician would probably diagnose this condition as:

    1. macular degeneration.
    2. primary open-angle glaucoma.
    3. color blindness.
    4. retinal degeneration.

28. Postoperatively, your cataract patient complains of sudden sharp pain in the operative eye. You should immediately:

    1. remove the metal eyeshield to relieve pressure.
    2. call the physician.
    3. administer an analgesic.
    4. document complaint of pain on chart.

29. A surgical procedure for the treatment of retinal detachment is:

    1. punctal sac repair.
    2. radial keratotomy.
    3. vitrectomy.
    4. scleral buckling.

30. The _____ _____ is a surgically implanted hearing device for the profoundly deaf person whose sensorineural hearing loss is either congenital or acquired.

31. Mr. E. is asked to sign a surgical consent for treatment of otosclerosis. Which of the following statements would indicate correct understanding of the procedure?

    1. "It involves surgical repair of the external ear."
    2. "It means cutting the nerve in my ear."
    3. "It cleans the ear canal of wax."
    4. "It will help me hear sounds again."

ELIZABETH SCHENK and BARBARA LAURITSEN CHRISTENSEN

Key Terms

Be sure to check out the bonus material on the free CD-ROM, including selected audio pronunciations.

agnosia (ăg-NŌ-zhă, p. 709)
aneurysm (ĂN-ūr-ĭ-zĭm, p. 692, 729)
aphasia (ă-FĀ-zē-ă, p. 692)
apraxia (ă-PRĂK-sē-ă, p. 723)
ataxia (ă-TĂK-sē-ă, p. 714)
aura (ĀW-ră, p. 712)
bradykinesia (brā-dē-kĭ-NĒ-zē-ă, p. 718)
diplopia (dĭ-PLŌ-pē-ă, p. 702)
dysarthria (dĭs-ĂHR-thrē-ă, p. 693)
dysphagia (dĭs-FĀ-jē-ă, p. 706)
flaccid (FLĂK-sĭd, p. 694)
Glasgow coma scale (GLĂS-gō KŌ-mă skāl, p. 692)
global cognitive dysfunction (GLŌ-băl KŎG-nĭ-tĭv dĭs-FŬNK-shŭn, p. 740)
hemianopia (hĕm-ē-ă-NŌ-pē-ă, p. 694)
hemiplegia (hĕm-ē-PLĒ-jă, p. 707)
hyperreflexia (hī-pĕr-rē-FLĔK-sē-ă, p. 743)
nystagmus (nĭs-TĂG-mŭs, p. 714)
paresis (pă-RĒ-sĭs, p. 693)
postictal period (pōst-ĬK-tăl PĒ-rē-ŏd, p. 711)
proprioception (prō-prē-ō-SĔP-shŭn, p. 694)
spastic (SPĂS-tĭk, p. 694)
stroke (strōk, p. 727)
unilateral neglect (ū-nī-LĂT-ĕr-ăl nĕ-GLĔCT, p. 694)

OVERVIEW OF ANATOMY AND PHYSIOLOGY

The nervous system is responsible for communication and control within the body. It interprets or processes the information received and sends it to the appropriate area of the brain or spinal cord, where the response is generated. The nervous system is the body's link with the environment. It works in conjunction with the endocrine system to maintain the body's homeostasis. The nervous system reacts in split seconds, whereas the hormones secreted by the endocrine glands work more slowly in initiating a response. The clinical picture for the patient with neurological problems is often complex. Understanding these conditions requires knowledge of the anatomy and physiology of the nervous system.

STRUCTURAL DIVISIONS

There are two main structural divisions of the nervous system. The first division, the central nervous system (CNS), comprises the brain and the spinal cord. It occupies a medial position in the body and is responsible for interpreting incoming sensory information and issuing instructions based on past experiences. The second component is the peripheral nervous system, which lies outside the CNS.

The peripheral nervous system contains two main divisions: the somatic nervous system and the autonomic nervous system. The somatic nervous system sends messages from the CNS to the skeletal muscles (voluntary muscles). The autonomic system transmits messages from the CNS to the smooth muscle, cardiac muscle, and certain glands. The autonomic system is sometimes called the **involuntary nervous system** because its action takes place without conscious control.

CELLS OF THE NERVOUS SYSTEM

There are two broad categories of cells within the nervous system. The first category, the neurons, are the transmitter cells (Figure 14-1). They carry messages to and from the brain and spinal cord. The second category, the neuroglial or glial cells, are the support cells to the neurons. They support and protect the neurons while producing cerebrospinal fluid (CSF), which continuously bathes the structures of the CNS.

Neuron

A neuron (nerve cell) is the basic nerve cell of the nervous system and is a separate unit composed of three main structures: the cell body, the axon and the dendrites. The cell body contains a nucleus surrounded by cytoplasm. The axon is a cylindric extension of a nerve cell that conducts impulses away from the neuron cell body. The dendrites are branching structures that extend from a cell body and receive impulses. Between each neuron is a gap (space) called the synapse, defined as the region surrounding the point of contact between two neurons or between a neuron and an effectors organ, across which nerve impulses are transmitted through the action of a neurotransmitter.

All neurons are governed by the "all or none law," which means there is never a partial transmission of a message—the impulse is either strong enough to elicit a response or too weak to generate the message.

Neuromuscular Junction

The area of contact between the ends of a large myelinated nerve fiber and a fiber of skeletal muscle is called the neuromuscular junction. This area of contact is necessary for functioning of the body. The neurotransmitters act to make sure that the neurological impulse passes from the nerve to the muscle.

Neurotransmitters

Numerous chemicals called neurotransmitters modify or result in the transmission of impulses between synapses. The best-known neurotransmitters are acetylcholine, norepinephrine, dopamine, and serotonin.

Acetylcholine plays a role in nerve impulse transmission; it spills into the synapse area and speeds the transmission of the impulse. The enzyme cholinesterase is then released to deactivate the acetylcholine once the message or impulse has been sent. This happens rapidly and continuously as each impulse is relayed.

Norepinephrine has an effect on maintaining arousal (awakening from a deep sleep), dreaming, and regulation of mood (e.g., happiness, sadness).

Dopamine primarily affects motor function; it is involved in gross subconscious movements of the skeletal muscles. It also plays a role in emotional responses. In Parkinson's disease there is a decrease in dopamine levels, and the individual suffers tremors, or involuntary, trembling muscle movements.

Serotonin, another neurotransmitter, induces sleep, affects sensory perception, controls temperature, and has a role in control of mood.

Neuron Coverings

Many neuron fibers (axons and dendrites) (see Figure 14-1) are covered with a white, waxy, fatty material called myelin. Myelin increases the rate of transmission of impulses and protects and insulates the fibers. Axons leaving the CNS are wrapped in layers of myelin with indentations called the nodes of Ranvier. These nodes further increase the rate of transmission, because the impulse can jump from node to node.

In the peripheral nervous system the myelin is produced by Schwann cells (see Figure 14-1). The outer membrane of the Schwann cells gives rise to another layer called the neurilemma. The neurilemma is a very important layer, because it helps to regenerate injured axons. Thus regeneration of nerve cells occurs only in the peripheral nervous system. Cells damaged in the

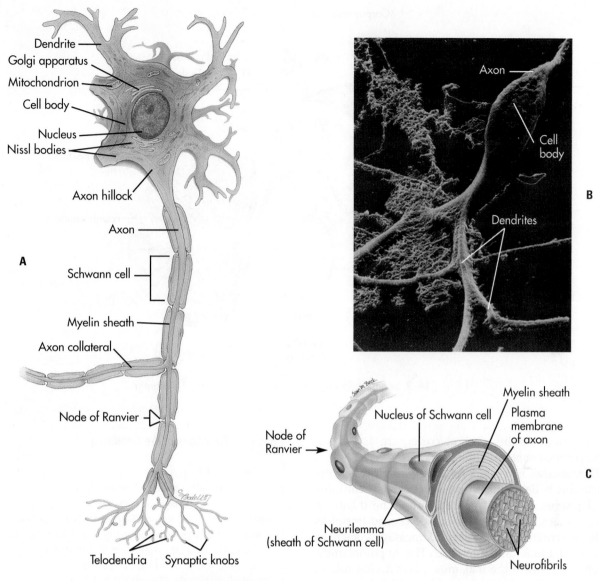

Dendrite
Golgi apparatus
Mitochondrion
Cell body
Nucleus
Nissl bodies
Axon hillock
Axon
Schwann cell
Myelin sheath
Axon collateral
Node of Ranvier
Telodendria   Synaptic knobs

A

Axon
Cell body
Dendrites

B

Myelin sheath
Plasma membrane of axon
Nucleus of Schwann cell
Node of Ranvier
Neurilemma (sheath of Schwann cell)
Neurofibrils

C

FIGURE **14-1 A,** Diagram of a typical neuron showing dendrites, cell body, and axon.
B, Scanning electron micrograph of a neuron. **C,** Myelinated axon, showing a cross-section of concentric layers of the Schwann cell filled with myelin.

CNS result in permanent damage (paralysis), because they do not have neurilemma and are not able to regenerate.

CENTRAL NERVOUS SYSTEM

The **central nervous system (CNS)**—one of the two main divisions of the nervous system and composed of the brain and spinal cord—functions somewhat like a computer but is much more complex. The cranium protects the brain and the vertebral column protects the spinal cord.

Brain

Specialized cells in the brain's mass of convoluted, soft, gray or white tissue coordinate and regulate the functions of the CNS. The brain is one of the largest or-gans weighing approximately 3 pounds (6.6 kg). It is divided into four principal parts: the cerebrum, the diencephalon, the cerebellum, and the brainstem.

Cerebrum. The cerebrum (Figure 14-2) is the largest part of the brain. It is divided into the left and right hemispheres. The outer portion of the cerebrum is composed of gray matter and is called the **cerebral cortex.** It is arranged in folds that are called **gyri** (convolutions); the grooves are called **sulci** (fissures). The connecting structure or bridge, the corpus callosum, divides the two hemispheres into four lobes that are named for the bones lying over them: the frontal lobe, parietal lobe, temporal lobe, and occipital lobe. The cerebrum controls initiation of movement on the opposite side of the body. The functions of the cerebrum are multiple and complex.

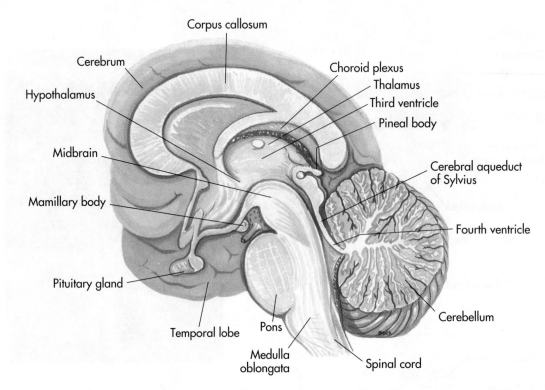

FIGURE **14-2** Sagittal section of the brain (note position of midbrain).

Specific areas of the cerebral cortex are associated with specific functions (Box 14-1).

Diencephalon. The diencephalon is often called the **interbrain: it lies beneath the cerebrum. It contains the thalamus** and the **hypothalamus.** The thalamus serves as a relay station for some sensory impulses while interpreting other sensory messages, such as pain, light touch, and pressure. The hypothalamus, which lies beneath the thalamus, plays a vital role in the control of body temperature; fluid balance; appetite; and certain emotions, such as fear, pleasure, and pain. Both the sympathetic and parasympathetic divisions of the autonomic system are under the control of the hypothalamus, as is the pituitary gland. Thus the hypothalamus influences the heartbeat, the contraction and relaxation of the walls of the blood vessels, hormone secretion, and other vital body functions (see Figure 14-2).

Cerebellum. The cerebellum lies posterior and inferior to the cerebrum and is the second largest portion of the brain. It contains two hemispheres with a convoluted surface much like the cerebrum. It is mainly responsible for coordination of voluntary movement and maintenance of balance, equilibrium, and muscle tone. Sensory messages from the semicircular canals in the inner ear send their messages to the cerebellum (see Figure 14-2).

Brainstem. The brainstem is located at the base of the brain and contains the **midbrain, pons,** and **medulla oblongata** (see Figure 14-2). These structures connect the spinal cord and the cerebrum. The brain-

Box 14-1 | *Functions of the Cerebrum*

FRONTAL LOBE

Written speech (ability to write)
Motor speech (ability to speak)
Motor ability—directs movements of body; the left side of the brain controls the right side of the body, and the right side of the brain controls the left side of the body
Intellectualization—the ability to form concepts
Judgment formation

PARIETAL LOBE

Interpretation of sensory impulses from the skin, such as touch, pain, and temperature
Recognition of body parts
Determination of left from right
Determination of shapes, sizes, and distances

TEMPORAL LOBE

Memory storage
Integration of auditory stimuli

OCCIPITAL LOBE

Interpretation of visual impulses from the retina
Understanding of the written word

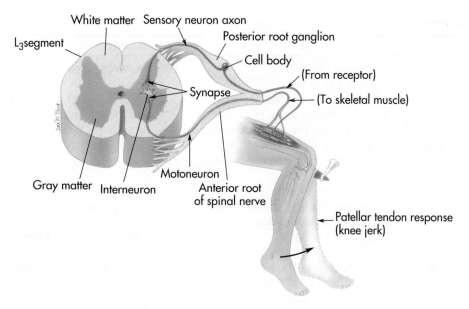

FIGURE **14-3** Neural pathway involved in the patellar reflex.

stem carries all nerve fibers between the spinal cord and the cerebrum.

Midbrain. The midbrain forms the superior portion of the brainstem. It is responsible for motor movement, relay of impulses, and auditory and visual reflexes. It is the origin of cranial nerves III and IV.

Pons. The pons connects the midbrain to the medulla oblongata; the word *pons* means "bridge." It is the origin of cranial nerves V through VIII. The pons is composed of myelinated nerve fibers and is responsible for sending impulses to the structures that are inferior and superior to it. It also contains a respiratory center that complements respiratory centers located in the medulla.

Medulla oblongata. The medulla oblongata is the distal portion of the brainstem. It is the origin of cranial nerves IX and XII. The medulla controls heartbeat, rhythm of breathing, swallowing, coughing, sneezing, vomiting, and hiccups (singultus). A vasomotor center regulates the diameter of the blood vessels, which aids in the control of the blood pressure.

Coverings of the brain and spinal cord. The brain and spinal cord are surrounded by three protective coverings called the meninges: (1) the dura mater, the outer most layer; (2) the arachnoid membrane, the second layer; and (3) the pia mater, the inner most layer, which provides oxygen and nourishment to the nervous tissue. These layers also bathe the spinal cord and brain in CSF.

Ventricles. The ventricles (there are four in all) are spaces or cavities located in the brain. The CSF, which is clear and resembles plasma, flows into the subarachnoid spaces around the brain and the spinal cord and cushions them. It contains protein, glucose, urea, and salts; it also contains certain substances that form a protective barrier (the blood-brain barrier) that prevents harmful substances from entering the brain and spinal cord.

Spinal Cord

The spinal cord is a 17- to 18-inch cord that extends from the brainstem to the second lumbar vertebra. It has two main functions: conducting impulses to and from the brain and serving as a center for reflex actions. The spinal cord is responsible for certain reflex activities, such as a knee jerk (Figure 14-3). A sensory neuron sends the information to the cord, a central neuron (located within the cord) interprets the impulse, and a motoneuron sends the message back to the muscle or organ involved. Thus a message is sent, interpreted, and acted upon without traveling to the brain.

PERIPHERAL NERVOUS SYSTEM

The **peripheral nervous system** comprises the motor nerves, sensory nerves, and ganglia outside the brain and spinal cord. It is composed of 31 pairs of spinal nerves, 12 pairs of cranial nerves, and the autonomic nervous system.

Spinal Nerves

The 31 pairs of spinal nerves are all mixed nerves. This means that they transmit sensory information to the spinal cord through afferent neurons and motor information from the CNS to the various areas of the body through efferent neurons. The spinal nerves are named according to the corresponding vertebra (e.g., C1, C2).

Cranial Nerves

There are 12 pairs of cranial nerves, which attach to the posterior surface of the brain, mainly the brainstem. All 12 pairs conduct impulses between the head, neck, and brain, excluding the vagus nerve (X), which also serves organs in the thoracic and abdominal cavities.

Table 14-1 | *Cranial Nerves*

NERVE*	CONDUCTS IMPULSES	FUNCTIONS
I Olfactory	From nose to brain	Sense of smell
II Optic	From eye to brain	Vision
III Oculomotor	From brain to eye muscles	Eye movements, pupillary control
IV Trochlear	From brain to external eye muscles	Eye movements
V Trigeminal ophthalmic branch maxillary branch mandibular branch	From skin and mucous membrane of head to brain; from teeth to brain; from brain to chewing muscles	Sensations of face, scalp, and teeth; chewing movements
VI Abducens	From brain to external eye muscles	Turning eyes outward
VII Facial	From taste buds of tongue to brain; from brain to facial muscles	Sense of taste; contraction of muscles of facial expression
VIII Acoustic (vestibulocochlear)	From ear to brain	Hearing; sense of balance
IX Glossopharyngeal	From throat and taste buds of tongue to brain; from brain to throat muscles and salivary glands	Sensations of throat, taste, swallowing movements, secretion of saliva
X Vagus	From throat, larynx, and organs in thoracic and abdominal cavities to brain; from brain to muscles of throat and to organs in thoracic and abdominal cavities	Sensations of throat, larynx, and of thoracic and abdominal organs; swallowing, voice production, slowing of heartbeat, acceleration of peristalsis
XI Spinal accessory	From brain to certain shoulder and neck muscles	Shoulder movements and turning movements of head
XII Hypoglossal	From brain to muscles of tongue	Tongue movements

*The first letter of the words in the following sentence are the first letters of the names of cranial nerves: "On Old Olympus's Towering Tops A Finn And German Viewed Some Hops." Many generations of students have used this or a similar sentence to help them remember the names of cranial nerves.

Table 14-1 lists the cranial nerves, their impulses, and functions.

Autonomic Nervous System

This portion of the nervous system controls the activities of the smooth muscle, cardiac muscle, and all glands. The autonomic nervous system is not a separate nervous system but a subdivision of the peripheral nervous system.

It is misleading to think of this system as the automatic system, although most activity is performed on an unconscious level. Its primary function is to maintain internal homeostasis; for example, it strives to maintain a normal heartbeat, a constant body temperature, and a normal respiratory pattern.

To maintain this homeostasis, the autonomic system has two divisions: the **sympathetic nervous system** and the **parasympathetic nervous system.** These two divisions are antagonistic—one slows an action, and the other accelerates the action. It is important to note that these systems function simultaneously, but they have the ability to dominate each other as the need arises. In times of stress, the sympathetic system takes over to prepare the body for "fight or flight." Heartbeat accelerates, blood pressure increases, and adrenal glands increase their secretions. To calm the body after a crisis, the parasympathetic system becomes domi-nate, slowing the heartbeat and decreasing the blood pressure and adrenal hormone output.

EFFECTS OF NORMAL AGING ON THE NERVOUS SYSTEM

The effects of aging on the nervous system are variable. The changes that occur include a loss of brain weight and a substantial loss of neurons (1% a year after age 50), with the cortex losing cells faster than the brainstem. The remaining cells undergo structural changes. There is also a general decline in interconnections of dendrites, a reduction in cerebral blood flow, and a decrease in brain metabolism and oxygen utilization. The neurons may contain senile plaques, neurofibrillary tangles, and the age pigment lipofuscin. There is often an altered sleep/wakefulness ratio, a decrease in the ability to regulate body temperature, and a decrease in the velocity of nerve impulses. The blood supply to the spinal cord is decreased, resulting in decreased reflexes.

Normal changes in the nervous system associated with aging are *not* the same as senility, organic brain disease, or Alzheimer's disease. Many older people reach old age with no functional deterioration of the nervous system. However, these normal changes may make care of the older patient a challenge. An example is the rehabilitation of older patients (Older Adult Considerations box).

Older Adult Considerations

Neurological Disorder

- As neurons are lost with aging, there is a deterioration in neurological function, resulting in slowed reflex and reaction time.
- Tremors that increase with fatigue are commonly observed in adults.
- The sense of touch and the ability for fine motor coordination diminish with aging.
- Most older people possess the ability to learn, but the speed of learning is slowed. Short-term memory is more affected by aging than long-term memory.
- The incidence of physiologic dementia or organic brain syndrome—including Alzheimer's disease, Pick's disease, and multiinfarct dementia—increases with aging.
- The incidence of stroke increases with age. The prognosis is affected by the location and extent of the cerebral damage. Rehabilitation potential after a stroke is often reduced by advanced age and coexisting medical problems.
- Nerve irritation resulting from arthritis, joint injuries, or spinal-cord compression can cause chronic pain or weakness.
- Dementia is not a normal consequence of aging but may be a result of many reversible conditions, including anemia, fluid and electrolyte imbalance, malnutrition, hypothyroidism, metabolic disturbances, drug toxicity, a drug reaction/idiosyncrasy, and hypotension.

PREVENTION OF NEUROLOGICAL PROBLEMS

Many conditions of the nervous system have no known cause. Other neurological problems can be prevented or their effects reduced by modifying lifestyle factors. Neurovascular diseases occur in part as a result of defined risk factors. These are the same factors that also increase the risk of cardiac disease and include high blood pressure, high blood cholesterol levels, cigarette smoking, obesity, stress, and lack of exercise.

The avoidance of cigarette smoking has been found to decrease the incidence of lung cancer. This is significant for the nervous system, because cancer of the lung often metastasizes to the brain.

Prevention of neurological problems resulting from trauma is a major challenge. These injuries include the fairly common diagnoses of spinal cord injury and head injury, which occur frequently in young people. Patient teaching regarding avoiding such injuries should include the following:

- Avoidance of drug and alcohol use
- Safe use of motor vehicles (e.g., use of automobile seat belts, helmets with motorcycles and snowmobiles)

 Safety Considerations

Preventing Neurological Injuries

- One of the best ways to prevent head injuries is to prevent car and motorcycle accidents.
- The nurse can be active in campaigns that promote driving safety and can speak to driver's education classes regarding the danger of unsafe driving and driving after drinking alcohol or taking drugs.
- The use of seat belts in cars and the use of helmets for riding on motorcycles are the most effective measures for increasing survival after accidents.
- Individual states are passing legislation requiring the use of automobile safety devices for both children and adults.
- The wearing of protective helmets by lumberjacks, construction workers, miners, horseback riders, bicycle riders, snowboarders, and skydivers is recommended.
- The nurse can encourage swimmers of all ages to refrain from diving into shallow water or areas in which water depth is unknown.

- Safe swimming practices (e.g., avoidance of diving in shallow water)
- Safe handling and storage of firearms
- Use of hardhats in dangerous construction areas
- Use of protective padding as needed for sports (Safety Considerations box)

Neurological diseases, such as meningitis or brain abscess, that occur as a result of infection can sometimes be prevented by prompt treatment of ear and sinus infections. The practice of safe and responsible sex is important, because some neurologically related diseases, such as syphilis and human immunodeficiency virus (HIV) disease, are spread by sexual contact. Safe practices include abstinence, monogamy, and the use of condoms. Treatment for drug abuse, especially intravenous use, is important, as in the prevention of HIV disease.

ASSESSMENT OF THE NEUROLOGICAL SYSTEM

HISTORY

A comprehensive history is essential for diagnosing neurological disease. This includes specifics about symptoms experienced, as well as the patient's understanding and perception of what is happening. Obtaining information from family members and/or significant others may also be helpful. The same format should be followed routinely to make sure information is complete.

For patients with suspected neurological conditions, the presence of many symptoms or subjective data may be significant. These include the following.

- Headaches, especially those that first occur after middle age or those that change in character; headaches that are worse in the morning or awaken a person from sleep are especially significant
- Clumsiness or loss of function in an extremity
- Change in visual acuity
- Any new or worsened seizure activity
- Numbness or tingling in one or more extremities
- Pain in an extremity or other part of the body
- Personality changes or mood swings
- Extreme fatigue or tiredness

MENTAL STATUS

Assessment of the neurological patient's mental status is important. An examination of mental status generally includes orientation (person, place, time, and purpose), mood and behavior, general knowledge (such as the names of U.S. presidents), and short- and long-term memory. The patient's attention span and ability to concentrate may also be assessed.

It is important to document mental status in specific terms. For instance, it is better to note "oriented to name, date, hospital, and purpose" than to note simply "oriented." Actual patient statements should be used. The nurse should vary orientation questions because some patients may learn the correct answers through repetition.

Level of Consciousness

Level of consciousness (LOC) is the earliest and most sensitive indicator that something is changing. A decreasing level of consciousness is the earliest sign of increased intracranial pressure. LOC has two components, *arousal* (or wakefulness) and *awareness*. Controlled by the brainstem, wakefulness is the most fundamental part of LOC. If the patient can open the eyes spontaneously to voice or to pain, it says that the wakefulness center in the brainstem is still functioning. Awareness, a higher function controlled by the reticular activating system in the brainstem, is the ability to interact with and interpret the environment. Awareness has four components:

1. Orientation: person, place, time, purpose
2. Memory: assess short-term memory; do not ask yes or no questions
3. Calculation: example, "If you had $2 and your apple costs $1.25, how many quarters would you get back?"
4. Fund of knowledge: Ask the patient to name the president and to tell you what's on the national news (Lower, 2002).

Restlessness, disorientation, and lethargy may be seen first. Observations are recorded in terms of behavior and signs—not labels such as "disoriented." See Table 14-2 for one method of classifying level of consciousness.

Table 14-2 *Levels of Consciousness*

LEVEL	DESCRIPTION
Alert	Responds appropriately to auditory, tactile, and visual stimuli
Disorientation	Disoriented; unable to follow simple commands; thinking slowed; inattentive, flat affect
Stupor	Responds to verbal commands with moaning or groaning, if at all
Semicomatose	Is in impaired state of consciousness, characterized by obtundation and stupor, from which a patient can be aroused only by energetic stimulation
Comatose	Unable to respond to painful stimuli; cornea and papillary reflexes are absent The patient cannot swallow or cough The patient is incontinent of urine and feces The EEG pattern demonstrates decreased or absent neuronal activity

Glasgow Coma Scale

The Glasgow coma scale (Figure 14-4) is a quick, practical, and standardized system for assessing the degree of consciousness impairment in the critically ill and for predicting the duration and ultimate outcome of coma, particularly with head injuries. The Glasgow coma scale was developed in 1974 and consists of assessment of three parts of the neurological assessment: eye opening, best motor response, and best verbal response.

The stronger the stimulus needed to obtain a response, the lower the patient's score. The number value assigned to each part of the scale is added to yield an objective score. The score for a patient who is not neurologically impaired is 14 to 16, depending on the system used. The lowest possible score is 3. Generally, any score of 8 or less is commonly accepted as a definition of coma. The scale has a high degree of consistency even when used by staff of varied experience.

LANGUAGE AND SPEECH

It is important to assess the language and speech capability of the neurological patient. Speech is a function of the dominant hemisphere, which is on the left side of the brain for all right-handed people and most left-handed people. Aphasia is an abnormal neurological condition in which the language function is defective or absent because of an injury to certain areas of the cerebral cortex—Broca's area in the frontal lobe and Wernicke's area in the posterior part of the temporal lobe.

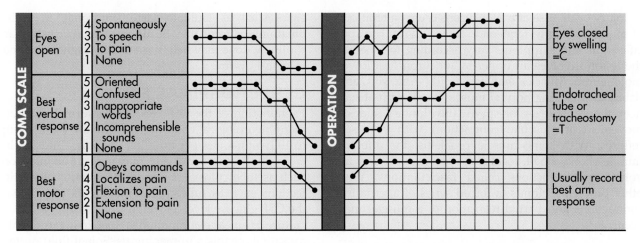

FIGURE **14-4** Glasgow coma scale, demonstrating measurement of level of consciousness. Record "C" if eyes are closed by edema; record "T" if endotracheal tube or tracheostomy tube is in place. Notice change in patient's condition just before and after surgery.

Aphasia includes all areas of language, including speech, reading, writing, and understanding. Aphasia has been subdivided as follows:

1. Sensory aphasia or receptive aphasia: inability to comprehend the spoken word or written word
2. Motor aphasia: inability to use symbols of speech (also called expressive aphasia)
3. Global aphasia: inability to understand the spoken word or to speak

Anomia is a form of aphasia characterized by the inability to name objects. Dysarthria is defined as difficult, poorly articulated speech that usually results from interference in the control over the muscles of speech. The general cause is damage to a central or peripheral nerve.

CRANIAL NERVES

Assessment of cranial nerve function is another important part of the neurological assessment. The 12 pairs of nerves emerge from the cranial cavity through openings in the skull (see Table 14-1 for specifics of cranial nerve classification and assessment).

The cranial nerves are tested in the following ways:

I (olfactory)	Identification of common odors
II (optic)	Testing of visual acuity and visual fields
III (oculomotor)	Testing of ability of eyes to move together in all directions, testing pupillary response
IV (trochlear)	Tested with oculomotor; testing eye movements
V (trigeminal)	Jaw strength and sensation of face, corneal reflex
VI (abducens)	Tested with oculomotor; testing eye movements
VII (facial)	Ability of face to move in symmetry, identification of tastes
VIII (acoustic, or vestibulocochlear)	Testing of hearing through whisper or other means and checking equilibrium and balance
IX (glossopharyngeal)	Identification of tastes
X (vagus)	Gag reflex, movement of uvula and soft palate
XI (spinal accessory)	Shoulder and neck movement
XII (hypoglossal)	Tongue motion

MOTOR FUNCTION

Evaluation of motor status of the neurological patient will detect abnormalities in the normal functioning of nerves and muscles. Motor function disturbances are the most commonly encountered neurological symptom. In general, the parts of the motor status examination include gait and stance, muscle tone, coordination, involuntary movements, and the muscle stretch reflexes.

Reflexes that are usually tested include the biceps, triceps, brachioradialis, quadriceps, gastrocnemius, and soleus muscles. The examiner taps briskly over the muscle with a reflex hammer. The response is noted and graded on a scale, usually from 0 to 4+, with 4+ being hyperreflexic. The most important feature of any reflex pattern is not the absolute value on the scale, but the comparison of one side of the body with the other. Stick figures are commonly used to record the bilateral values.

Damage to the nervous system often causes a serious problem in mobility. A loss of function is called **paralysis;** a lesser degree of movement deficit from partial or incomplete paralysis is called paresis.

Injury or disease of motoneurons causes alterations of muscle strength, tone, and reflex activity. The specific signs and symptoms vary according to whether the lesion involves an upper motoneuron or a lower motoneuron. Muscles may be flaccid (weak, soft, and flabby and lacking normal muscle tone), with absent deep tendon reflexes, or spastic (involuntary, sudden movement or muscular contraction), with increased reflexes. With some muscle problems, the affected muscle shows small, localized, spontaneous, and involuntary contractions called **fasciculations.** With other problems, clonus (a forced series of alternating contractions and partial relaxation of a muscle) may occur.

SENSORY AND PERCEPTUAL STATUS

The sensory examination is the most difficult part of the neurological evaluation. Specific alterations in sensation that should be assessed include pain; touch; temperature; and proprioception, the sensation pertaining to spatial-position and muscular-activity stimuli originating from within the body or to the sensory receptors that those stimuli activate. This sensation gives one the ability to know the position of the body without looking at it and the ability to know objects by the sense of touch.

Unilateral neglect, a condition in which an individual is perceptually unaware of and inattentive to one side of the body, may also occur. Another perceptual problem is hemianopia, which is characterized by defective vision or blindness in half of the visual field.

In most clinical settings it is usually not feasible or necessary to complete the total neurological examination during shift-to-shift assessments of the patient. However, in many settings, such as intensive care units, the neurological checks may be done as frequently as every 15 minutes. Factors that are the most important include orientation, level of consciousness, bilateral muscle strength, speech ability, involuntary movements, ability to follow commands, and any abnormal posturing.

LABORATORY AND DIAGNOSTIC EXAMINATIONS

BLOOD AND URINE TESTS

Assessment of the neurologically impaired patient includes a variety of blood and urine tests. A culture of the urine may rule out infection involving the urinary tract. Other urine testing may indicate the presence of diabetes insipidus. Urine drug screens may be done to rule out drug use as a cause of lethargy or to identify specific drugs ingested.

Arterial blood gas values may be an important diagnostic tool in monitoring the oxygen content of the blood. The gases may be altered with neurological dis-

eases such as Guillain-Barré syndrome, in which breathing patterns may be altered. Blood tests that are routinely done may help narrow the diagnosis of neurological disorder.

CEREBROSPINAL FLUID

Examination of the CSF can yield information about many neurological conditions. Normally there are up to 10 lymphocytes per milliliter of spinal fluid. An increase in the number of cells may indicate an infection, such as tuberculosis or a viral infection. Bacterial infections such as tuberculous meningitis often lower the CSF glucose level as well as the chloride levels. A culture or smear examination is done to determine the causative organism in meningitis. Spinal-fluid protein is elevated when degenerative diseases or a brain tumor is present. Blood in the spinal fluid indicates hemorrhage from somewhere in the ventricular system. A protein electrophoresis evaluation may give evidence of neurological diseases such as multiple sclerosis (MS) (Table 14-3).

OTHER TESTS

Routine skull radiographs of the head and vertebral column are useful in ruling out fractures of the skull and cervical vertebrae. Since the development of the computed tomography (CT) scan, skull radiographs are not used as extensively as before.

Computed Tomography (CT) Scan

The purpose of the CT scan, also called the **CAT scan,** is to detect pathologic conditions of the cerebrum and spinal cord using a technique of scanning without ra-

Table **14-3** *Normal Characteristics of Cerebrospinal Fluid (CSF)*

DETERMINATION	VALUE
Specific gravity	1.007
pH	7.35 to 7.45
Chloride	120 to 130 mEq/L
Glucose	50 to 75 mg/dL
Pressure	80 to 200 mm water
Total volume	80 to 200 mL (15 mL in ventricles)
Total protein	15 to 45 mg/dL (lumbar)
	10 to 25 mg/dL (cisternal)
	5 to 15 mg/dL (ventricular)
Gamma globulin	6% to 13% of total protein
Cell count	
RBC	None
WBC	0-10 cells (all lymphocytes and monocytes)
Culture and sensitivity	No organisms present
Serology for syphillis	Negative

dioisotopes. There is no special physical preparation of the patient for the test. A CT scan takes 20 to 30 minutes if done without contrast medium and about 60 minutes if the scan is also done with contrast. The procedure is painless, except for the slight discomfort that occurs when an intravenous line is started for the injection of the contrast dye. There is also some discomfort in lying still and possible feelings of claustrophobia as a result of the head being positioned in the head holder. If contrast medium is used, it is important for the nurse to document and report to the physician any history of allergy to iodine and seafood because iodine is present in the contrast medium.

During the procedure the patient lies supine with the head positioned within a rubber head holder to prevent air gaps between the machine and the scalp. The head is scanned in two planes simultaneously and at various angles. Each image that appears is a specific layer of brain tissue. The computer displays a printout that indicates areas of increased densities (e.g., tumors or thrombi).

Brain Scan

Like the CT scan, the brain scan's purpose is detecting pathologic conditions of the cerebrum. It uses radioactive isotopes and a scanner. There is no special physical preparation of the patient. The procedure takes approximately 45 minutes for the actual scan. The patient is injected with a radioisotope. While the patient lies still, a scanner passes over the brain area. Concentrated areas of uptake are reflected. There are generally no adverse effects from the procedure and only minimal discomfort associated with the intravenous administration of the radioactive isotopes. If mercury is used as the isotope indicator, a mercurial diuretic (meralluride [Mercuhydrin]) is administered several hours before the procedure to allow a greater concentration of the mercury to circulate to brain tissue because meralluride minimizes the uptake of mercury by the kidneys. Brain scan is being used less frequently than in the past because of the excellent results obtained from CT scan and magnetic resonance imaging (MRI).

Magnetic Resonance Imaging (MRI) Scan

MRI uses magnetic forces to image body structures. It has relevance in the nervous system as a way to detect pathologic conditions of the cerebrum and spinal cord, and is used in detection of stroke, multiple sclerosis, tumors, trauma, herniation, and seizure. Because MRI yields greater contrast in the images of soft-tissue structures than does the CT scan, it is the diagnostic test of choice for many neurological diseases. New advances in MRI techniques include diffusion-weighted imaging and magnetic resonance spectroscopy. Because the scan involves a magnetic force, the patient should be cautioned to remove watches, credit cards, and any metal from the clothing before entering the scanning room. The patient should also be questioned about the presence of any metal in the body that would preclude the use of the scan, such as orthopedic appliances, aneurysm clips, and pacemakers.

During the procedure the patient lies supine with the head positioned in a head holder. The test takes 45 to 60 minutes. The procedure is painless, except for the discomfort in lying still and possible feelings of claustrophobia. The patient should be warned that the machine makes different and somewhat loud noises during the scanning procedure.

Magnetic Resonance Angiography (MRA)

Magnetic resonance angiography (MRA) uses differential signal characteristic of flowing blood to evaluate extracranial and intracranial blood vessels. It provides both anatomic and hemodynamic information. It can be used in conjunction with contrast media (contrast-enhanced MRA [cMRA]). MRA is rapidly replacing cerebral angiography for use in diagnosing cerebrovascular diseases.

Positron Emission Tomography (PET) Scan

Another evaluative measure that is similar to the CT scan and MRI scan is the positron emission tomography (PET) scan. In this procedure the patient receives an injection of deoxyglucose with radioactive fluorine. The area in question is scanned, and a color composite picture is obtained. Shades of color give an indication of the level of glucose metabolism; this then can be translated into indications of a pathologic state. PET scanning provides a noninvasive means of determining biochemical processes that occur in the brain. There is increased clinical use of PET scan to monitor select patients following stroke, Alzheimer's disease, tumors, epilepsy, and Parkinson's disease. As with the CT scan, discomfort is minimal. The patient should be aware of the need to lie still for the duration of the scan, which is usually about 45 minutes.

Lumbar Puncture

A lumbar puncture is often performed as part of the diagnostic workup of the patient who may have a neurological problem. It is contraindicated in patients who might have increased intracranial pressure, because the withdrawal of fluid may cause the medulla oblongata to herniate downward into the foramen magnum.

A lumbar puncture is done to obtain CSF for examination, to relieve pressure, or to introduce dye or medication. It is a common procedure, done in the patient's room or in the diagnostic imaging department. The procedure takes 10 to 15 minutes. Slight pain and pressure may be felt as the dura is entered. A sharp, shooting pain down one leg may occur, caused by the needle coming close to a nerve.

The patient is usually positioned on the side with the knee and head flexed at an acute angle. This allows

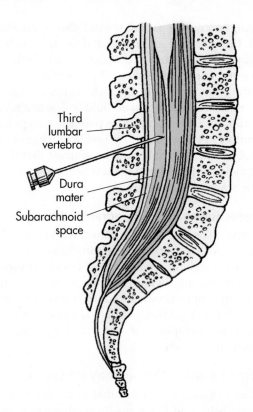

Third lumbar vertebra

Dura mater

Subarachnoid space

FIGURE 14-5 Position and angle of the needle when lumbar puncture is performed. Note that the needle is in the fourth lumbar interspace below the level of the spinal cord.

for maximal lumbar flexion and separation of the interspinous spaces. After anesthetizing the area with a local anesthetic, the physician inserts the needle below the level of the spinal cord, at the L4-L5 or L5-S1 interspace (Figure 14-5). The inner needle is removed to allow for drainage and measurement of spinal fluid. The level-of-fluid column in the manometer is used to measure the pressure. The first specimen of spinal fluid may contain blood from slight bleeding at the site of the puncture. This specimen should not be sent for cell count.

After the procedure the patient lies flat in bed for several hours. The site of the puncture should be assessed for any leakage, as evidenced by moisture on the bandage or around the puncture site. Headache is fairly common and is thought to be caused by the loss of spinal fluid through the dura mater. If a headache develops, bed rest, analgesics, and ice to the head may help. Opioids are usually not helpful.

Electroencephalogram

The electroencephalogram (EEG) is used to provide evidence of focal or generalized disturbances of brain function by measuring the electrical activity of the brain. Among the cerebral diseases assessed by EEG are epilepsy, mass lesions (e.g., tumors, abscess, hematoma), cerebrovascular lesions, and brain injury. There is no special preparation for this test, but the pa-

tient is encouraged to be quiet and rest before the procedure, unless it is to be a sleep-deprived EEG. With this the patient is kept awake the night before the test, and the EEG is usually done first thing in the morning. The EEG usually takes about 1 hour to complete. The hair and scalp of the patient should be clean. The electrodes are placed on the scalp with collodion in a set pattern to cover all scalp areas. There is no pain associated with an EEG.

The basic resting rhythm of the EEG is affected by opening the eyes or altering attention. Recordings are sometimes made while the patient is asleep or sleep deprived, when the seizure threshold may be lowered. Comparisons are made of different patterns of the recordings (Figure 14-6). After the test the patient should be allowed to rest. The patient should be assisted if necessary in washing the hair and removing the collodion from the scalp.

Myelogram

The myelogram is commonly used to identify lesions in the intradural or extradural compartments of the spinal canal by observing the flow of radiopaque dye through the subarachnoid space. The most common lesion for which this test is used is a herniated or protruding intervertebral disk. Other lesions include spinal tumors, adhesions, bony deformations, and arteriovenous malformations. Before the procedure the patient's baselines of lower-extremity strength and sensation are assessed and documented. The patient is informed that the procedure takes about 2 hours. The patient should also be told that there may be slight discomfort as the dura is entered and that he or she may be asked to assume a variety of positions during the procedure.

Water-soluble iodine dyes such as iopamidol (Isovue) are more often used because they are absorbed into the bloodstream and excreted by the kidneys. Preparation for this procedure is the same as for lumbar puncture. Before the dye is injected, patients must be asked whether they have any allergies, specifically whether they have had any anaphylactic or hypotensive episodes from other dyes. The patient is usually positioned on the side with both knees and the head flexed at an acute angle to allow maximal flexion of the lumbar area for ease in performing the lumbar puncture. After the puncture is performed, the inner needle is removed to allow drainage of CSF, measurement of pressure, and collection of specimens. The dye is instilled and the needle is removed. The patient is then turned to various positions so the spinal cord can be visualized while fluoroscopic and radiopaque films are taken. The patient usually undergoes a CT scan 4 to 6 hours after a myelogram.

The site of the puncture should be observed for any leakage of CSF, and the strength and sensation of the lower extremities should be assessed. Headache is fairly common after the procedure. It may be accompa-

Frontal motor

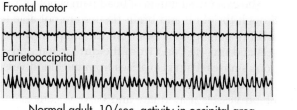

Parietooccipital

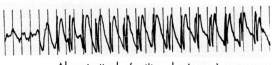

Normal adult, 10/sec. activity in occipital area.

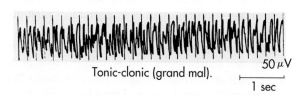

Absent attacks (petit mal seizures).
Synchronous 3/sec. spikes and waves.

Tonic-clonic (grand mal).

50 μV

1 sec

Right temporal

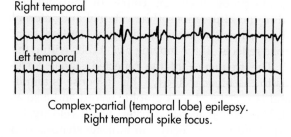

Left temporal

Complex-partial (temporal lobe) epilepsy.
Right temporal spike focus.

Right frontal

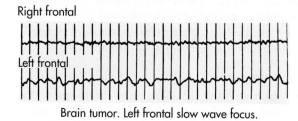

Left frontal

Brain tumor. Left frontal slow wave focus.

Right frontal

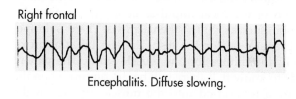

Encephalitis. Diffuse slowing.

FIGURE 14-6 Tracings of electroencephalogram. The normal tracing is demonstrated, as are several pathologic states.

nied by nausea and occasionally by vomiting. After myelography the patient should be flat for a few hours.

Angiogram

The angiogram (cerebral arteriography) is a procedure used to visualize the cerebral arterial system by injecting radiopaque material. It allows the detection of arterial aneurysms, vessel anomalies, ruptured vessels, and displacement of vessels by tumors or masses.

Before the procedure the patient is usually given clear liquids, although in some institutions all oral intake is restricted. The patient must be assessed for any allergy to iodine because the dye contains iodine. If the femoral approach is to be used, it is helpful to assess and mark the locations of the bilateral pedal pulses. If the carotid artery is used, the neck circumference is measured as part of the baseline data. Immediately before the procedure, baseline vital signs and pulses are measured, and a neurological check is performed and recorded.

The test takes approximately 2 to 3 hours. The patient may experience discomfort in lying still for that period of time. When the dye is injected, most patients complain of feeling extremely hot and seeing flashes of light.

The patient is positioned supine on the radiograph table. A local anesthetic agent is used to anesthetize the area of the puncture site. The catheter is introduced

percutaneously and introduced into the relevant vessels. At times the catheter may be inserted directly into the carotid or vertebral arteries. After all injections are done, the catheter is withdrawn and pressure is applied to the puncture site for at least 15 minutes.

After the procedure, bed rest is ordered for a specified time, usually 4 to 6 hours. Vital signs are checked frequently (at times as often as every 15 minutes), and a neurological check is performed with every vital sign check. The site of the puncture is assessed frequently for the presence of a hematoma. With a femoral stick, the pulses distal to the site are checked for evidence of arterial occlusion. With a carotid stick the patient is assessed for any difficulty in breathing or swallowing or an increase in the girth of the neck.

The patient undergoing this procedure is at risk for cerebral vascular accident as well as an increase in intracranial pressure. Any change in level of consciousness or other parts of the neurological assessment should be promptly reported.

MRA is replacing cerebral arteriography is some facilities.

Carotid Duplex

A carotid duplex study uses combined ultrasound and pulsed Doppler technology. A technician places a probe on the skin over the carotid artery and slowly moves the probe along the course of the common carotid to the bifurcation of the external and internal carotid arteries. The ultrasound signal emitted from the probe reflects off the moving blood cells within the vessel. The frequency of the reflected signal corresponds to the blood velocity. This response is amplified and is registered on a graphic record and also as sound. The graphic record registers blood velocity. Increased blood flow velocity can indicate stenosis of a vessel. Carotid duplex scanning is a noninvasive study that evaluates carotid occlusive disease. This study is often ordered when a patient has a transient ischemic attack to determine pathology of the carotids.

Electromyogram

An electromyogram (EMG) is used to measure the contraction of a muscle in response to electrical stimulation. It provides evidence of lower motoneuron disease; primary muscle disease; and defects in the transmission of electrical impulses at the neuromuscular junction, such as in myasthenia gravis. There is no special preparation for the test. The test takes approximately 45 minutes for one muscle study. The patient needs to know that there will be discomfort when the electrode is inserted into the muscle and when the electrical current is used. The muscle may ache for a short time after the procedure.

During the test an electrode is inserted into selected skeletal muscles. An electric current is passed through the electrode, and the machine graphs the variations of muscle potentials (voltage). After the procedure it is important to assess the patient for signs of bleeding at the site of the electrode insertion. The patient may need an analgesic for discomfort and a rest period.

Echoencephalogram

An echoencephalogram uses ultrasound to depict the intracranial structures of the brain. It is especially helpful in detecting ventricular dilation and a major shift of midline structures in the brain as a result of an expanding lesion. The preparation of the patient, the actual procedure, and aftercare are similar to those of the brain scan.

COMMON DISORDERS OF THE NEUROLOGICAL SYSTEM

HEADACHES
Etiology/Pathophysiology

Headache is a common neurological complaint; its significance is variable and it can result from many different causes. The source of recurring headache should be determined through careful physical examination with appropriate neurological assessment. Some tumors may produce no symptoms except for headache for a long period.

The exact mechanism of head pain is not known. Although the skull and brain tissues are not able to feel sensory pain, pain arises from the scalp, its blood vessels and muscles, and from the dura mater and its venous sinuses. Pain also arises from the blood vessels at the base of the brain and from cervical cranial nerves. Blood vessels may dilate and become congested with blood. Headaches can be classified as vascular, tension, and traction-inflammatory. Vascular headaches include migraine, cluster, and hypertensive headaches. Tension headaches may arise from psychological problems of tension or stress or from medical problems such as cervical arthritis. Traction-inflammatory headaches include those caused by infection, intracranial or extracranial causes, occlusive vascular structures, and temporal arteritis.

Clinical Manifestations

Headache pain may be made worse by stress or tension. Knowledge of the patient's perception of the effect of stress on the pain is important in planning effective interventions.

Migraine headaches are unusual in that there are prodromal (early signs and symptoms of a developing condition or disease) signs and symptoms that occur before the acute attack. These may include any of the following: visual field defects; experiencing unusual smells or sounds; disorientation; paresthesias; and, in rare cases, paralysis of a part of the body. During a migraine headache, signs and symptoms may include nausea, vomiting, sensitivity to light, chilliness, fatigue, irritability, diaphoresis, edema, and other signs of autonomic dysfunction. Abnormal metabolism of serotonin, a vasoactive neurotransmitter found in platelets and cells of the brain, plays a major role.

Assessment

Collection of **subjective data** includes the patient's understanding of the headache, possible causes, and any precipitating factors. It is important to determine what measures relieve the symptoms, as well as the location, frequency, pattern, and character of the pain. This includes the site of return of the headache, time of day, and intervals between the headaches. The initial onset of the headache, presence of any symptoms that occur before the headache or associated symptoms, the presence of allergies, and any family history of similar headache patterns are also important to assess.

Collection of **objective data** includes any behaviors indicating stress, anxiety, or pain. Changes in the ability to carry out activities of daily living (ADLs), an abnormally raised body temperature, and the presence of sinus drainage may be important. Abnormalities noted during the physical examination portion of the neurological assessment should also be documented (Therapeutic Dialogue box).

Therapeutic Dialogue

NURSE: *Can you describe your problem to me?*
PATIENT: *It's a pain in my head.*
NURSE: *When did this pain start?*
PATIENT: *About a month ago.*
NURSE: *Did anything else happen at that same time?*
PATIENT: *My daughter left home for college.*
NURSE: *How did you feel about that?*
PATIENT: *I was really upset. She was my baby. I can't believe that she's gone.*
NURSE: *Was there anything else that you noticed at the same time? Like an increased temperature or nasal drainage?*
PATIENT: *No, I don't think so.*
NURSE: *What made the headache worse?*
PATIENT: *Thinking about my loneliness.*
NURSE: *What made the headache better?*
PATIENT: *Sleeping or taking a Valium.*
NURSE: *Have you had trouble sleeping or noticed that your appetite was worse?*
PATIENT: *I wake up early in the morning. I don't feel much like eating.*
NURSE: *Have you lost weight?*
PATIENT: *About 10 pounds in the last month.*
NURSE: *Can you tell me what the pain feels like?*
PATIENT: *It's a pain that goes through my whole head. It throbs and gets worse in the evening.*
NURSE: *What do you think is the cause of the headache?*
PATIENT: *I guess maybe I'm upset that my daughter left.*

Diagnostic Tests

It is important to evaluate headaches that are not transient. Usual testing includes a neurological examination, a CT scan (MRI or PET scan may also be done), a brain scan, skull radiographs, and a lumbar puncture. A lumbar puncture is not done, however, if there is evidence of increased intracranial pressure or if a brain tumor is suspected because quick reduction of pressure produced by removal of the spinal fluid may cause brain herniation. In these situations a CT scan is done first.

Medical Management

Dietary counseling. Some foods may cause or worsen headaches. These include foods containing tyramine, nitrates, or glutamates. One example of this is monosodium glutamate (MSG), often used in the preparation of Chinese foods and on salad bars. Other substances that may provoke headaches include vinegar, chocolate, yogurt, alcohol, fermented or marinated foods, ripened cheese, cured sandwich meat, caffeine, and pork.

Psychotherapy. Patients with headaches may respond to psychotherapy. This is not to say that the headache pain is not physiological in nature, but counseling can help the patient develop awareness of stress factors and deal with the pain. The patient may need help in expressing feelings about intractable headache pain.

Medications. Medications are often used to treat headaches. These will be described in terms of their use for migraine, cluster, and tension headaches.

Migraine headaches. Acetylsalicylic acid (aspirin) may help relieve migraine pain. Ergotamine tartrate preparations taken early in the attack may prevent progression of the headache. These drugs are usually successful in treating migraines. Ergotamine tartrate preparations (which are serotonin receptor agonists) act by constricting cerebral blood vessel walls and reducing cerebral blood flow. They reduce inflammation and may reduce pain transmission. They can be given orally, sublingually, rectally, or by injection. These preparations are also available in combinations with other drugs, such as caffeine, phenobarbital, and belladonna. Side effects of ergot preparations include nausea, vomiting, numbness and tingling, muscle pain, and changes in heart rate. They cannot be taken by pregnant women because they stimulate contractions of the uterine smooth muscle.

Eletriptan (Relpax) is the seventh triptan to be marketed for treatment of migraine, joining almotriptan (Axert), frovatriptan (Frova), naratriptan (Amerge), rizatriptan (Maxalt), sumatriptan (Imitrex), and zolmitriptan (Zomig). Classified as selective serotonin receptor agonists, these drugs are all indicated to treat acute migraine (with or without aura) in adults.

Triptans are thought to act on receptors in the extracerebral, intracranial vessels that become dilated during a migraine attack. Stimulating these receptors constricts cranial vessels, inhibits neuropeptide release, and reduces nerve impulse transmission along trigeminal pain pathways.

Besides relieving headache pain, the triptans also relieve the nausea, vomiting, and photophobia associated with acute migraine attack (*Nursing*, 2004).

Other drugs that may be used include nonopioid analgesics such as phenacetin, acetaminophen, ibuprofen, or propoxyphene/acetaminophen (Darvocet N). Propranolol (Inderal) has been used in the prophylactic treatment of migraine and other vascular headaches. Intranasal lidocaine has been used with some relief.

Cluster headaches. Because the pain associated with vascular cluster headaches is often extremely severe, narcotic analgesics, sometimes given intramuscularly, are used. Patients with cluster headaches usually feel fine between attacks, so no analgesic is needed during these times.

Tension headaches. Nonnarcotic analgesics are often used to treat tension headaches. These include acetaminophen, propoxyphene, phenacetin, ibuprofen, and aspirin. Narcotics are avoided because these drugs are often subject to abuse; it is much better to counsel patients to develop other ways to relieve headaches.

Nursing Interventions and Patient Teaching

Because stress and emotional upsets may precipitate some headaches and worsen others, relaxation and rest should be facilitated. This includes relaxation techniques, planned sleeping hours, and regular rest periods. The patient may need the nurse to assist with this. Alcohol should not be used to relieve tension because it may become addicting and has been found to be a significant cause of cluster headaches. Regular physical exercise may also help prevent headaches, especially ones caused by tension.

If a patient is suffering from a severe headache, the nurse should plan nursing interventions so that only essential activities take place. Interventions should be grouped so that the patient has adequate time to rest.

Comfort measures. Other treatments that may be helpful for a patient with a headache include cold packs applied to the forehead or base of the skull. Pressure applied to the temporal arteries may be helpful. People with migraine headaches, especially, are usually most comfortable lying in a dark room with minimal auditory stimulation.

Identifying triggering factors. Triggering factors associated with severe and recurring headaches may include fatigue, alcohol, stress, seasonal climate changes, hunger, allergies, and menstruation. The nurse may need to help the patient identify these factors. They can be assessed through ongoing observation of the patient's personality, habits, and ADLs, as well as career plans, work habits, family relationships, coping mechanisms, and relaxation activities. A diary or journal kept by the patient may be helpful in determining these factors.

Nursing diagnoses and interventions for the patient with headache include but are not limited to the following:

NURSING DIAGNOSES	NURSING INTERVENTIONS
Anxiety, related to pain	Provide quiet environment. Encourage verbalization of concerns. Provide diversional activities.
Acute or chronic pain, related to disease process	Administer analgesics as ordered. Provide comfort measures. Maintain nonstressful environment. Encourage pain reduction techniques as appropriate: rocking movements, external warmth, breathing patterns.

Teaching is an important part of the nursing intervention of the patient with headaches. Topics include (1) avoidance of factors that trigger headaches, (2) relaxation techniques including biofeedback, (3) importance of maintaining regular sleep patterns, (4) medications to be used (including dose, actions, and side effects), and (5) the importance of follow-up care.

Prognosis

With proper treatment the person with headaches can expect to live a normal life. Changes in lifestyle may need to occur, especially during acute episodes of headache pain. The person may have to adjust to periodic headaches and will need to rest until the headache resolves.

NEUROLOGICAL PAIN
Etiology/Pathophysiology and Clinical Manifestations

Neurological pain other than headache is common. The transmission of pain is not fully understood, but patients may experience disabling pain either caused by a disorder within the nervous system or caused peripherally at a distant part of the body.

The transmission of pain impulses is not fully understood. Neurological pain may arise from lesions involving the peripheral cutaneous nerves, the sensory nerve roots, the thalamus, and the central pain tract (lateral spinothalamic) at some level. Each produces characteristic pain. Pain receptors are not adaptable, and pain impulses continue at the same rate as long as the stimulus is present. They are specific for pain only. Pain receptors can be activated by cellular damage, certain chemicals such as histamine, heat, ischemia, muscle spasm, and sensations of cold and pruritus that go beyond a specific level of intensity.

Pain that is described as unbearable and does not respond to treatment is classified as **intractable.** It is chronic and often debilitating, and may prevent the patient from functioning in ADLs.

Assessment

The perception of pain is highly subjective. Collection of **subjective data** includes the patient's understanding of the pain; any precipitating factors; and measures that relieve stress, including medication. The site, frequency, and nature of the pain are important, as well as the usual coping patterns of the patient when under stress. The presence of associated symptoms and measures that make the pain worse are important subjective data.

The quality of pain and its distribution are important factors to assess. Pain may vary from mild to excruciating.

Collection of **objective data** may be limited when assessing neurological pain. Objective factors that should be assessed are any behavioral signs indicating pain or stress, a change in the ability to carry out

ADLs, any muscle weakness or wasting, vasomotor responses (such as flushing), abnormalities of spinal reflexes, and abnormalities noted during the sensory examination.

Diagnostic Tests

Diagnostic tests for the patient in pain may include electrical stimulation used to define the pain to a greater degree. Psychological testing may be part of the workup. If back or neck pain is present, a myelogram is usually performed.

Medical Management

Nonsurgical methods of pain control. Neurological pain sometimes responds to other methods of pain control. These include transcutaneous electrical nerve stimulation (TENS) and spinal cord stimulation. Both techniques use electrodes applied near the site of pain or on or around the spine (see Chapter 2). The stimulator is used to modify the sensory input by blocking or changing the painful sensation with a stimulus that is perceived to be less painful or nonpainful. Acupuncture has also been used to treat patients with neurological pain.

Nerve block. A nerve block is used to control intractable pain. It involves injecting a local anesthetic, alcohol, or phenol close enough to a nerve to block the conduction of impulses. Sources of pain often treated with a nerve block include trigeminal neuralgia, cancer, or peripheral vascular disease. The duration of effect is from several months to several years. Pain and spasticity may also be controlled by means of an epidural catheter. Medication is usually administered continually.

Medications. Medications are often used to treat patients with neurological pain. Gabapentin (Neurontin) is often useful in controlling neurological pain. Medications include nonopioid analgesics such as acetaminophen, propoxyphene (Darvon), phenacetin, and acetylsalicylic acid. Opioids may be prescribed, as well as muscle relaxants, but these drugs may lead to abuse. The emphasis should be on helping the patient learn other measures to control the pain.

Surgical methods of pain control. In cases of intractable pain that does not respond to more conservative measures, surgery may be necessary to reduce or abolish pain. Neurosurgical procedures that may be done include neurectomy, rhizotomy, cordotomy, and percutaneous cordotomy.

These procedures all have potential complications that need to be considered before the decision is made to perform surgery. For example, a patient who undergoes a cordotomy may be expected to have difficulties with postural hypotension, ability to feel hot or cold, and possibly motor and bowel function. Temporary edema of the cord from the procedure may lead to temporary paralysis or leg weakness.

Nursing Interventions and Patient Teaching

Comfort measures. A patient with neurological pain may be very uncomfortable and should be assisted to assume a position of comfort. For example, the patient with back pain should avoid movements that cause direct or indirect movement of the spinal cord. The patient may find lying in a supine position uncomfortable. The nurse should help the patient find a comfortable position and may need to actively assist the patient in turning or moving. Straining when having a stool can intensify pain, and a stool softener may be needed. The nurse should offer prune juice and a high-fiber diet and encourage up to 2000 mL a day or more of fluids.

Promotion of rest and relaxation. As with headache, stress and emotional upsets may precipitate or exacerbate neurological pain. Rest and relaxation should be facilitated, with planned sleeping hours and rest periods as needed.

Some patients with pain, especially intractable pain, may respond well to psychotherapy. This does not mean that the pain does not have a physiological basis, but counseling can help the patient develop awareness of what makes the pain worse and how to cope with the discomfort.

Nursing diagnoses and interventions for neurological pain are the same as those listed previously for headache, with the addition of the following:

NURSING DIAGNOSES	NURSING INTERVENTIONS
Risk for disuse syndrome, related to lack of use of a body part as a result of pain	Explain need for regular exercise program to maintain joint mobility; ROM exercises to all body joints every 2 to 4 hours. Be positive and reassuring in approach.
Feeding, bathing/hygiene self-care deficit, related to pain	Provide basic ADL needs as necessary, but encourage patient to begin to participate at ability level. Provide sufficient time for ADLs. Facilitate use of self-help devices as needed. Provide for total hygiene as indicated.

Teaching is an important part of the nursing interventions of the patient with neurological pain. Teaching should include at least the factors that are taught to the patient with headache. Also important is the awareness of physical methods such as positioning the body to increase comfort and structuring the home and work setting to keep stressors at a minimum.

Prognosis

As with headache pain, neurological pain can in most cases be treated adequately. Lifestyle changes may be helpful in allowing the person to live a full life.

INCREASED INTRACRANIAL PRESSURE

Etiology/Pathophysiology and Clinical Manifestations

Increased intracranial pressure (ICP) is a complex grouping of events that occurs because of multiple neurological conditions. It often occurs suddenly, can progress rapidly, and often requires surgical intervention. It is a potential complication in many neurological conditions and can rapidly lead to death if not arrested and reversed.

Specific causes of increased intracranial pressure include space-occupying lesions that increase tissue volume, cerebrospinal problems, and cerebral edema. An increase in any one of the contents of the cranium is usually accompanied by a reciprocal change in the volume of one of the others. This is because the cranial vault is rigid and nonexpandable. The buildup of pressure may occur slowly over weeks or rapidly, depending on the cause. Usually one side of the brain will be more involved, but both sides of the brain will eventually be involved.

As the pressure increases within the cranial cavity, it is first compensated for by venous compression and cerebrospinal displacement. As the pressure continues to rise, the cerebral blood flow decreases and inadequate perfusion of the brain occurs. This inadequate perfusion starts a vicious cycle that causes the P_{CO_2} to increase and the P_{O_2} and pH to decrease. These changes cause vasodilation and cerebral edema. This edema leads to further increased intracranial pressure, which causes increased compression of neural tissue and an even greater increase in intracranial pressure.

When the pressure buildup is greater than the brain's ability to compensate, pressure is exerted on surrounding structures where the pressure is lower. This movement of pressure is called **supratentorial shift** and can result in herniation.

As a result of herniation of the brain, the brainstem is compressed at various levels, which in turn compresses the vasomotor center, the posterior cerebral artery, the oculomotor nerve, the corticospinal nerve pathway, and the fibers of the ascending reticular activating system. The life-sustaining mechanisms of consciousness, blood pressure, pulse, respiration, and temperature regulation are all impaired. A rise in systolic pressure and an unchanged diastolic pressure, resulting in a widening pulse pressure, bradycardia, and abnormal respiration, are late signs of increased ICP and indicate that the brain is about to herniate (Lower, 2004).

Assessment

The detection of increased intracranial pressure must occur early while it is still reversible. The ability to make accurate observations, interpret observations intelligently, and record observations carefully is most important for the nurse working with patients with increased intracranial pressure.

Collection of **subjective data** for a diagnosis of increased intracranial pressure includes the patient's understanding of the condition, presence of any visual changes such as diplopia or double vision, a change in the patient's personality, and a change in the ability to think. The diplopia usually results from paralysis or weakness of one of the muscles that controls eye movement. It often occurs fairly early in the process of increased intracranial pressure. The presence of nausea or pain, especially headache, is also important. The headache is thought to result from venous congestion and tension in the intracranial blood vessels as the cerebral pressure rises. Headache that occurs with increased intracranial pressure usually increases in intensity with coughing, straining at stool, or stooping. It is usually present in the early morning and may awaken the patient from sleep.

Collection of **objective data** includes a change in the level of consciousness, which is the earliest sign of increased ICP. When you assess the patient, you will find it takes more stimulation to get the same results. A change in the level of consciousness may include disorientation, restlessness, or lethargy. Observations are recorded in terms of behaviors and signs and symptoms, not in terms of labels. It is important to chart what is seen, not what is inferred. Pupillary signs may also change with increased intracranial pressure. Pupillary responses are controlled by cranial nerve III (oculomotor nerve). The pupils usually will change on the same side as the lesion. The first and most subtle clue to trouble is that the pupil reacts, but sluggishly. As the brain herniates, the nerve is compressed—with the top part of the nerve being affected first. The **ipsilateral** pupil (when the lesion is in one hemisphere) remains dilated and is incapable of constricting. The pupil appears larger than that of the affected side and does not react to light. As the intracranial pressure increases and both halves of the brain become affected, bilateral pupil dilation and fixation occur. Dilating pupils that respond slowly to light are a sign of impending herniation. A pupil that is fixed and dilated is sometimes called a **blown pupil** and is an ominous sign that *must* be reported to the physician immediately (Figure 14-7).

Changes in the blood pressure and pulse are seen with increasing intracranial pressure. Herniation causes ischemia of the vasomotor center, which excites the vasoconstrictor fibers, causing the systolic blood pressure to rise. If the intracranial pressure continues to increase, a widening pulse pressure will occur.

Pressure in the vasomotor center also increases the transmission of parasympathetic impulses through the vagus nerve to the heart, causing a slowing of the pulse. A widened pulse pressure, increased systolic blood pressure, and bradycardia are together called **Cushing's response.** It is considered an important diagnostic sign of late-stage brain herniation.

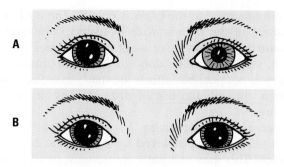

FIGURE **14-7 A,** Unequal pupils, also called anisocoria. **B,** Dilated and fixed pupils, indicative of severe neurological deficit.

Brain herniation produces respiratory problems that are variable and related to the level of the brainstem compression or failure. The breathing pattern may be deep and stertorous (snorelike) or periodic (Cheyne-Stokes) respirations. **Ataxic** breathing may also occur; this is an irregular and unpredictable breathing pattern with random, shallow, and deep breaths and occasional pauses. It is seen in patients with medulla oblongata damage. As intracranial pressure increases to fatal levels, respiratory paralysis occurs.

Failure of the thermoregulatory center because of compression occurs later with increased intracranial pressure. It results in high, uncontrolled temperatures. This hyperthermia increases the metabolism of brain tissue.

Compression of the upper motoneuron pathway (corticospinal tract) interrupts transmission of impulses to the lower motoneuron, and progressive muscle weakness occurs. The presence of Babinski's reflex, hyperreflexia, and rigidity are additional signs of decreased motor function. Seizures may occur. Herniation of the upper part of the brainstem may produce characteristic posturing when the patient is stimulated (Figure 14-8). The worsening of motor problems is significant, because it means that the intracranial pressure is continuing to increase.

Vomiting and singultus are two objective signs that may be seen with increased intracranial pressure. The vomiting is often projectile in nature and usually not preceded by nausea; this is called unexpected vomiting. Singultus is caused by compression of the vagus nerve (cranial nerve X) that occurs as brainstem herniation occurs.

One last objective sign is papilledema, which is detected with the use of an ophthalmoscope (usually a physician's function). As intracranial pressure increases, the pressure is transmitted to the eyes through the CSF and to the optic disk. As the optic disk becomes edematous, the retina is also compressed. The damaged retina cannot detect light rays. Visual acuity is lessened as the blind spot enlarges. **Papilledema** is also called a **choked disk.**

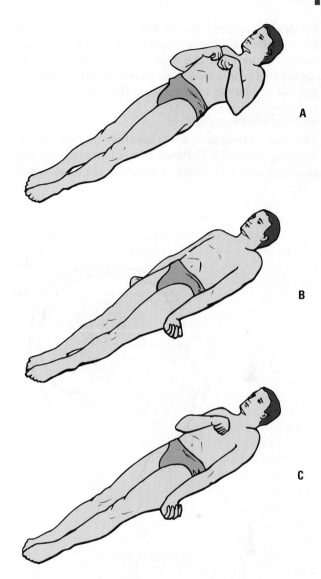

FIGURE **14-8** Decorticate and decerebrate responses. **A,** Decorticate response. Flexion of arms, wrists, and fingers with adduction in upper extremities. Extension, internal rotation, and plantar flexion in lower extremities. **B,** Decerebrate response. All four extremities in rigid extension, with hyperpronation of forearms and plantar extension of feet. **C,** Decorticate response on right side of body and decerebrate response on left side of body.

Diagnostic Tests

The diagnosis of increased intracranial pressure is usually made with a CT or MR scan, which can show actual structural herniation and shifting of the brain. However, most of the time, acute increased intracranial pressure is a medical emergency, and there is little time for diagnostic tests. The diagnosis must be made on the basis of frequent and careful observation and neurological testing. **The presence of even subtle changes can be very significant.**

In postoperative or critically ill patients, internal measuring devices are used to diagnose increased intracranial pressure. One of the most common measuring devices requires the placement of a hollow screw through the skull into the subarachnoid space. The device is connected to a transducer and oscilloscope for continuous monitoring. Waveforms are produced that indicate the intracranial pressure (Figure 14-9).

Medical Management

The goals of treatment are to identify and treat the underlying cause of ICP. Preventing ICP may not be possible, but preventing further increases in pressure with resulting damage to the brain is crucial. The medical treatment of the patient with increased intracranial pressure depends on the cause of the pressure. For example, surgery may be done to remove a tumor. If surgery is not possible, efforts are made to reduce the pressure through the use of drug therapy or other measures.

Mechanical decompression. Rapidly rising intracranial pressure can be relieved by mechanical decompression. This may include a craniotomy, in which a

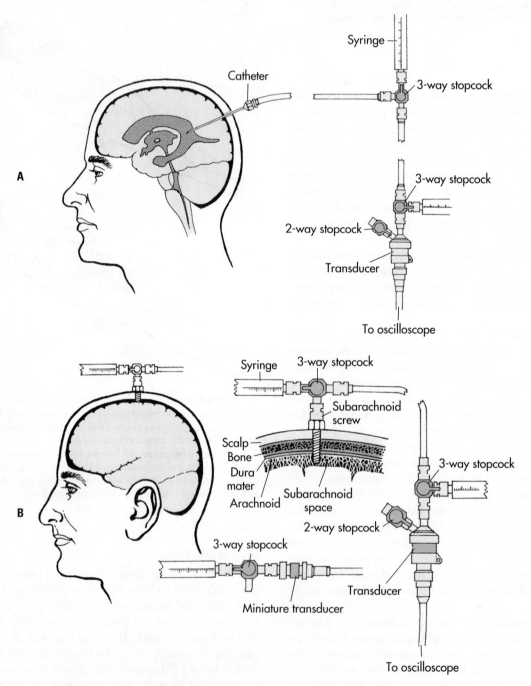

FIGURE **14-9** Equipment for intracranial pressure (ICP) monitoring. **A,** Ventricular pressure monitoring. Catheter is inserted through a burr hole in the skull into the lateral ventricle and attached to a transducer and oscilloscope to monitor ICP. **B,** Subarachnoid screw is inserted through a burr hole in the skull and attached to transducer and oscilloscope for continuous monitoring.

bone flap is removed and then replaced, or a craniectomy, in which the bone flap is removed and not replaced. The craniectomy is often done when pressure is high. Other means of decompression may include drainage of the ventricles or any subdural hematoma.

Ensuring adequate oxygenation to support brain function is the first step in management of ICP. Endotracheal intubation may be necessary. Arterial blood gas (ABG) analysis guides the oxygen therapy. With the use of controlled ventilation, the P_{CO_2} can be lowered to below normal, which causes a slightly alkalotic pH. The decrease in the P_{CO_2} and the increase in pH will decrease vasodilation and decrease intracranial pressure. The goal is to maintain the PaO_2 at 100 mm Hg.

Medications. Three types of medications are usually administered to patients with increased intracranial pressure: osmotic diuretics, corticosteroids, and anticonvulsants. Osmotic diuretics are also called hyperosmolar drugs. They draw water from the edematous brain tissue. An example of this type of medication is mannitol. It begins to reduce increased intracranial pressure within 15 minutes, and its effects last for 5 to 6 hours. Loop diuretics such as furosemide (Lasix), bumetanide (Bumex), and ethacrynic acid (Edecrin) may also be used in the management of ICP. Continuous midazolam (Versed), atracurium besylate (Tracrium) infusions are also used.

The corticosteroid that may be given is dexamethasone. Corticosteroids are thought to control edema surrounding cerebral tumors and abscesses but appear to have limited value in managing head-injured patients (Lewis et al, 2004). With this drug, monitoring of blood glucose levels is important because steroids can affect carbohydrate metabolism and glucose utilization and result in elevated blood glucose levels.

Anticonvulsants are given to prevent seizures. Phenytoin (Dilantin) is the most commonly given drug. It can be given intravenously but is usually not given intramuscularly because of poor absorption. Fosphenytoin (Cerebyx) is a short-term IV or IM anticonvulsant now being used also. Opioids and other drugs that cause respiratory depression are avoided.

Internal monitoring devices. Internal monitoring devices are being used more frequently to diagnose and monitor increased intracranial pressure. Three basic monitoring systems are used: the ventricular catheter, the subarachnoid bolt or screw, and the epidural sensor. These monitoring devices produce pressure waves that can be evaluated to indicate the status of increased intracranial pressure (see Figure 14-9).

Nursing Interventions and Patient Teaching

Therapeutic measures. Therapeutic measures to reduce venous volume may be implemented. These include the following:

1. Elevate the head of the bed to 30 to 45 degrees to promote venous return.
2. Place the neck in a neutral position (not flexed or extended) to promote venous drainage.
3. Position the patient to avoid flexion of the hips, waist, and neck as well as rotation of the head, especially to the right. Extreme hip flexion is avoided because this position causes an increase in intraabdominal and intrathoracic pressures, which can produce a rise in ICP.
4. Instruct the patient to avoid isometric or resistive exercises.
5. Restrict fluid intake.
6. Implement measures to help the patient avoid Valsalva's maneuver (any forced expiratory effort against a closed airway, such as straining to have a stool). Enemas and laxatives should be avoided if possible.
7. Have a Foley catheter in place if the patient is not alert because of the large amount of urine that is produced.
8. Perform suctioning only as necessary and for no longer than 10 seconds with administration of 100% oxygen before and after to prevent decreases in the PaO_2.
9. Administer oxygen via mask or cannula to improve cerebral perfusion.
10. Use a hypothermia blanket to control body temperature (increased body temperature increases brain damage).

Nursing diagnoses and interventions for the patient with increased intracranial pressure may include but are not limited to the following:

NURSING DIAGNOSES	NURSING INTERVENTIONS
Ineffective breathing pattern, related to neuromuscular impairment	Maintain patent airway; avoid flexion of neck. Administer oxygen and humidification as ordered. Provide oral nasopharyngeal airway as indicated for managing secretions; suction oropharynx prn.
Risk for injury, related to physiological effects of sustained elevations in intracranial pressure	Elevate head of bed 30 degrees. Maintain body position: avoid semiprone or prone position. Avoid compression of neck veins. Check blood pressure, pulse, and respiration every 30 minutes. Perform neurological check every 30 minutes using Glasgow coma scale; report any findings below 8 to physician.

The patient with increased intracranial pressure is often unresponsive. However, information about procedures that are being done should be shared with the patient and the family. This may help both be as cooperative as possible.

Prognosis

The prognosis for the patient with increased intracranial pressure depends on the cause and rapidness with which it is treated. The nurse assumes a very important role in monitoring the patient for signs and symptoms of increased pressure. After herniation of the brain has begun as a result of pressure, there is little chance for complete reversal without significant brain damage.

DISTURBANCES IN MUSCLE TONE AND MOTOR FUNCTION

Etiology/Pathophysiology

Motor function disturbances are the most commonly encountered neurological signs and symptoms. Damage to the nervous system often causes serious problems in mobility. An example of this is the patient with cerebral palsy.

Clinical Manifestations

Injury or disease of motoneurons results in alterations of muscle strength, tone, and reflex activity. Muscle tone may be described as **flaccid** (weak, soft, flabby, and lacking normal muscle tone) or **hyperreflexic** (increased reflex actions). The specific clinical manifestations differ according to the location of the neurological lesion.

Assessment

Collection of **subjective data** for patients with motor problems includes the patient's understanding of the problem and possible causes. The initial onset of the symptoms, measures that improve symptoms, and the presence of clumsiness or incoordination or abnormal sensation are important to assess. If the lesion occurs suddenly, as in spinal cord injury from trauma, subjective symptoms may be minimal. If the motor deficit develops slowly, subjective symptoms may be so subtle that they are at first ignored.

Collection of **objective data** includes coordination, muscle strength, muscle tone, and the presence of any muscle atrophy. Reflexes are often checked, as well as the presence of clonus or fasciculations and the ability to move muscles. Any abnormal gait is significant, as well as a change in the ability to carry out ADLs.

Diagnostic Tests

One of the most common procedures for detecting pathologic conditions of muscle is the electromyogram (EMG). It detects the various types of electrical activity and abnormal patterns that may appear in resting muscle in the presence of pathology.

Medical Management

Patients with motor problems may have problems with spasticity. Muscle relaxants may be used to decrease tone and involuntary movements. Some commonly prescribed medications include baclofen (Lioresal), dantrolene (Dantrium), and diazepam (Valium). Baclofen has been used intrathecally to reduce spasticity. Common side effects of these drugs include drowsiness and vertigo. These side effects are increased by the use of alcohol or other depressants.

Some patients may have severe swallowing difficulty (dysphagia). This commonly results from obstructive or motor disorders of the esophagus and is commonly associated with neurological problems. The patient with dysphagia often requires prefeeding and feeding exercises.

In patients at severe risk for aspiration, a video fluoroscopy with barium may be done to rule out aspiration. The procedure requires the patient to swallow a small amount of liquid or semisolid barium while a fluoroscopic examination is being done.

For patients with paralysis, the eye on the affected side of the body may need to be protected if the lid remains open and there is no blink reflex. The patient is at high risk for corneal scratches or irritation. Irrigation with a physiological solution of sodium chloride may be used, followed by eyedrops. An eye pad may be used to keep the eye closed, although an eyeshield is preferable.

Nursing Interventions

Safety needs. Patients with paralysis have significant safety needs. This includes protection from falling, including the use of side rails when the patient is in bed and a chair restraint when the patient is in a chair, especially if balance cannot be maintained. If the patient also has a sensory problem, which often accompanies paralysis, the danger to a part of the body may not be realized. An example is the patient with a stroke who is not aware that a hemiplegic arm is hanging over the side of the wheelchair arm.

The eye on the affected side of the body should be cleaned and assessed for signs of infection on a regular basis, usually at least three times a day. The patient must also learn to inspect affected body parts for injury.

Skin over bony prominences needs to be inspected regularly for signs of pressure. Paralyzed people are at risk for skin impairment and should be taught to turn themselves in bed and to reposition themselves in the bed or chair independently, if possible. If the patient is unable to turn independently, the nurse carries out this function. Usually the patient is turned from one side to another or from one side to the back to the other side. Repositioning also includes weight shifts, done by the patient or by staff. These weight shifts may include controlled leaning from one side to another or push-ups done by the patient. If the patient is not able to do the activity, she is taught to take the responsibility to remind the staff when it is time to do the weight shift.

Paralyzed or weakened areas should be inspected at least daily for any signs of skin impairment. A mirror is often used to assist in the assessment of skin by the patient. With this, the patient is able to visualize all skin areas and is not as dependent on staff or family.

Activity needs. The extremities of a person who has an acute motor problem may be flaccid at first. Spasticity of muscles develops gradually. The joints then become flexed and fixed in useless, deformed positions unless preventive measures are taken.

The nurse should carefully place the extremities in a normal anatomical position to prevent deformity. Counterpositioning may be helpful. In **hemiplegia** (paralysis of one side of the body) the affected upper extremity is pulled inward at the shoulder joint and the wrist drops; in the lower extremity the knee flexes and the foot drops. In counterpositioning the nurse positions the patient so that the shoulder and upper arm are in abduction, the elbow is flexed, the wrist is dorsiflexed, the knee is in neutral position, and the foot is dorsiflexed. If the person is supine, a pillow can be placed between the upper arm and body to hold the arm in abduction. Physical therapists and occupational therapists can provide splints and braces that can aid in positioning (Figure 14-10).

In positioning, footboards may be used to prevent footdrop, although some feel that these contribute to increased spasticity and should not be used routinely for patients who have muscle spasms. High-topped tennis shoes or other devices, such as splints or braces, can help prevent footdrop, if therapy is initi-

ated early. In some hospitals, casts are applied to patients' lower extremities to prevent footdrop or to reverse contractures. The presence of the cast impedes spasticity. A sling or hook hemiharness may be useful to support the affected arm to prevent shoulder subluxation.

The prone position is excellent for patients who are able to tolerate it. Not only is the chance of skin impairment decreased with this position, but it also causes extension of the hip and knee joints, and the ankles by means of gravity. A pillow placed under the chest may help patients comfortably assume this position.

Positioning of the paralyzed person is extremely important. Complications such as footdrop and flexion contractures of the knee seriously limit mobility. As a result, the level of self-care and independence is diminished. Most joint deformities in a paralyzed person are preventable with early and continuing nursing interventions.

In addition to positioning, interventions for the person with paralysis include range-of-motion (ROM) exercises to all joints. These may be passive (carried out by the nurse) or active (carried out by the patient). Passive ROM is indicated at least three times daily for all joints that the patient cannot voluntarily move.

Nutritional needs. Patience and persistence are often necessary in giving food and fluids to the patient with hemiplegia. Important nursing measures include avoiding foods that cause choking, checking the affected side of the mouth for accumulation of food and resultant poor hygiene, not mixing liquids and solid foods, and encouraging the patient to take small bites. If the patient has dentures, they should be worn. The patient should sit at a 90-degree angle with the head up and chin slightly tucked. The head should not be extended and the patient should be encouraged to tip the head toward the unaffected side while swallowing. Straws are to be avoided. Assistive devices for feeding include utensils with universal cuffs, covered plastic cups, scoop dishes, plate guards, and Asepto syringes. These enable the patient to be less dependent on the staff. These devices are usually available through therapists in most hospitals.

Activities of daily living. During the acute rehabilitative phases of a motor problem, patients with paralysis are taught how to carry out daily activities to the extent that they are able. A variety of devices are available to assist with dressing and grooming (Figures 14-11 and 14-12). The occupational therapist becomes involved in many of these activities, including homemaking. It is important to stress the concept of the rehabilitative team in managing these patients. The patient is taught to compensate for weakness or paralysis. It is important for the nurse to give the patient the time to do activities on her own if she is able.

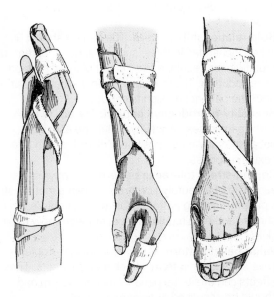

FIGURE **14-10** Volar resting splint provides support to wrist, thumb, and fingers of patient following cerebrovascular accident (stroke), maintaining them in position of extension.

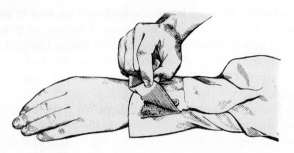

FIGURE **14-11** Velcro shirtsleeve to facilitate closure.

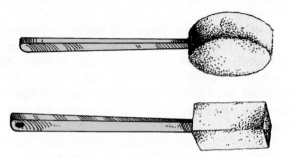

FIGURE **14-12** Long-handled bath sponges.

It is often easier and faster to do things for the patient, but this defeats the purpose of rehabilitation.

Psychological adjustments. The person with paralysis may need assistance in adjusting to body changes. The loss of the ability to function independently is traumatic, and the patient may have fears of rejection as well as loss of self-esteem and concerns about the future. A grief reaction similar to that described in the stages of dying and death may occur. At times the patient may relate to the paralyzed part of the body as though it were not a part of her and may have nicknames for the body part. Nursing interventions are essential in helping the patient cope with the loss of function and change in body image. This includes praising the patient for achievements, encouraging expression of fears and grief, and helping him see that there is life after disability. It might be helpful to have the patient visited by someone with the same disability who has been successfully rehabilitated (Health Promotion Considerations box).

Nursing diagnoses and interventions for the patient with alterations in muscle tone and motor function include but are not limited to the following:

Health Promotion Considerations

The Patient with a Neurological Disorder

- **Nutritional-metabolic pattern.** Neurological problems can result in problems of inadequate nutrition. Problems related to chewing, swallowing, facial nerve paralysis, and muscle coordination could make it difficult for the patient to ingest adequate nutrients.
- **Elimination pattern.** Bowel and bladder problems are often associated with neurological problems, such as stroke, head injury, spinal cord injury, multiple sclerosis, and dementia. It is important to determine if the bowel or bladder problem was present before or after the neurological event to plan appropriate interventions.
- **Activity-exercise pattern.** Many neurological disorders can cause problems in the patient's mobility, strength, and coordination. These problems can result in changes in the patient's usual activity and exercise patterns.
- **Sleep-rest pattern.** Sleep can be disrupted by many neurologically related factors. Discomfort from pain and inability to move and change to a position of comfort because of muscle weakness and paralysis could interfere with sound sleep.
- **Cognitive-perceptual pattern.** Because the nervous system controls cognition and sensory integration, many neurological disorders affect these functions.

The nurse should assess memory, language, calculation ability, problem-solving ability, insight, and judgment.
- **Self-perception–self-concept pattern.** Neurological disease can drastically alter control over one's life and create dependency on others for daily needs.
- **Role-relationship–pattern.** The patient should be asked if changes in roles, such as spouse, parent, or breadwinner, resulting from a neurological problem have occurred. These changes can dramatically affect both the patient and significant others.
- **Sexuality-reproductive pattern.** The ability to participate in sexual activity should be assessed because many nervous system disorders can affect sexual response.
- **Coping-stress tolerance pattern.** The physical sequelae of a neurological problem can seriously strain a patient's coping patterns. Often the problem is chronic and may require the patient learn new coping skills.
- **Value-belief pattern.** Many neurological problems have serious, long-term, life-changing effects. These effects can strain the patient's belief system and should be assessed. (Lewis et al, 2004)

Nursing Diagnoses	Nursing Interventions
Impaired physical mobility, related to neuromuscular impairment	Perform active or passive ROM exercises every 4 hours to all extremities, neck, hands, fingers, wrists, elbows, knees. Provide physical therapy as ordered: massage and stretching exercises. Maintain planned rest periods. Encourage ambulation to tolerance. Arrange for necessary assistive devices for home care needs.
Risk for disuse syndrome, related to impaired functioning of body part	Perform hand, finger, foot exercises; assist in active and passive ROM exercises every 2 to 4 hours. Assist patient with using supportive devices as indicated: overhead trapeze, braces, walker, cane. Encourage use of involved side when possible. Instruct patient to use unaffected extremity to support weaker side (e.g., lift involved left leg with right leg or lift involved left arm with right arm). Turn every 2 hours.

Patient Teaching

Teaching is an extremely important part of caring for the person with motor problems. Appropriate teaching activities include the following: safety needs, skin care, activity needs (ROM and positioning), medications (dosage, action, times, and side effects), the importance of good nutrition, ADLs, bowel and bladder care, and the importance of follow-up care. Written instructions are helpful to reinforce teaching and for the patient to refer to when he returns home. Family members should be prepared for when they will need to assume some of the care for the patient.

DISTURBED SENSORY AND PERCEPTUAL FUNCTION
Etiology/Pathophysiology

The presence of a lesion anywhere within the sensory system pathway, from the receptor to the sensory cortex, alters the transmission or perception of sensory information. The parietal cortex is of major importance in interpretation of sensation. Loss of, decrease in, or increase in sensation of pain, temperature, touch, and proprioception results in difficulty in daily functioning. Any alteration lessens the patient's ability to be completely protected from inadvertent injury.

One specific loss is proprioception, or the ability to know the position of the body and its parts without directly looking at the part. Agnosia is a total or partial loss of the ability to recognize familiar objects or people through sensory stimuli as a result of organic brain damage.

Assessment

Collection of **subjective data** includes the patient's understanding of the sensory disturbance, measures that relieve symptoms (including medications), and the presence of symptoms that occur with the sensory problem. An example is the person who experiences weakness of a hand and at the same time feels numbness and tingling. The onset of the sensory problem and the specific site in the body are important information to collect.

Collection of **objective data** includes noting the patient's ability to perform purposeful movements or to recognize familiar objects.

Medical Management

Refer to medical management for alterations in the patient's muscle tone and motor function.

Nursing Interventions and Patient Teaching

The most important nursing intervention for the patient with sensory dysfunction is teaching the patient protective measures in relation to the sensory deficit or alteration. This includes helping the patient learn to inspect parts of the body that have no feeling or protect sensitive body parts from the discomfort of linen rubbing over them. If a patient has a deficit in one sense, he should be taught to compensate with another (e.g., the patient who learns to lip read because of a hearing deficit; the patient with hemianopia who is taught to scan the printed page).

Nursing diagnosis and interventions for the patient with a sensory or perceptual problem are the same as those for the patient with a motor problem, with the addition of but not limited to the following:

Nursing Diagnosis	Nursing Interventions
Risk for injury, related to sensory/perceptual disturbances	Maintain safe environment. Teach patient to protect body parts that have decreased sensation. Teach patient to inspect body parts for possible injury. Protect patient from sustaining injury from hot liquid or heating pads.

The teaching for a patient with a sensory deficit is essentially the same as that for the patient with a motor deficit.

OTHER DISORDERS OF THE NEUROLOGICAL SYSTEM

Functioning of the neurological system can be interrupted for a variety of reasons. These include conduction abnormalities, degenerative diseases, vascular problems, infection, tumors, trauma, and cranial and peripheral nerve disorders. Selected disorders in each area will be discussed.

CONDUCTION ABNORMALITIES

EPILEPSY OR SEIZURES

Etiology/Pathophysiology

The incidence of epilepsy has been recorded throughout history. Seizures occur in all races and affect men and women equally. There is no apparent geographic distribution. In many the onset of seizures is before the age of 20, but it can begin at any age. The incidence is about 1 in every 200 to 300 people.

Clinical Manifestations

Seizures can be classified according to the varied features of the attack. This includes generalized tonic-clonic (grand mal), absence (petit mal), psychomotor (automatisms), jacksonian (focal), and miscellaneous (myoclonic and akinetic) seizures (Table 14-4).

Epilepsy can be defined as a transitory disturbance in consciousness or in motor, sensory, or autonomic function with or without a loss of consciousness. It is associated with paroxysmal, uncontrolled electrical discharges in the neurons of the brain that result in the sudden, violent, involuntary contraction of a group of muscles. The patterns or forms of seizures vary and depend on the area of the brain from which the seizure arises (see Figure 14-6). Seizures occur for a variety of reasons, including hypoglycemia, infection, electrolyte imbalance, alcohol, barbiturate withdrawal, and water intoxication.

Table 14-4 *Characteristics of Seizures*

INCIDENCE	CHARACTERISTICS	CLINICAL SIGNS	AURA	POSTICTAL PERIOD
GENERALIZED TONIC-CLONIC (GRAND MAL)				
Are most common	Generalized; characterized by loss of consciousness and falling to the floor or ground if patient is upright, followed by stiffening of the body (tonic phase) for 10 to 20 seconds and subsequent jerking of the extremities (clonic phase) for another 30 to 40 seconds	Aura Cry Loss of consciousness Fall Tonic-clonic movements Incontinence, cyanosis, excessive salivation, tongue or cheek biting	Yes Flashing lights Smells Spots before eyes (scotomata) Vertigo	Yes Need for 1 to 2 hours' sleep Headache, muscle soreness are common
ABSENCE (PETIT MAL)				
Usually occur during childhood and adolescence Frequency decreases as child gets older Rarely continues beyond adolescence	Sudden impairment in or loss of consciousness with little or no tonic-clonic movement Occurs without warning Has tendency to appear a few hours after arising or when person is quiet	Sudden vacant facial expression with eyes focused straight ahead that lasts only a few seconds All motor activity ceases except perhaps for slight symmetric twitching about eyelids Possible loss of muscle tone There may be an extremely brief loss of consciousness	No	No

The excessive neuronal discharges may result in a tonic convulsion, with alternate contraction and relaxation of opposing muscle groups. This gives the characteristic tonic-clonic jerking movements of the body. Seizures are followed by a rest period of variable length, called the postictal period. During this period the patient usually feels groggy and acts disoriented. Complaints of headache and muscle aches are common. Usually the patient sleeps after a seizure and may experience amnesia for the event.

When recurrent, generalized seizure activity occurs at such frequency that full consciousness is not regained between seizures, it is called **status epilepticus.**

This is a medical emergency and requires medical and nursing interventions to prevent death from brain damage resulting from prolonged hypoxia and exhaustion. The nursing interventions always involve ensuring that there is a patent airway and that the patient is protected from injury. Medications used to stop the seizure activity may be of such volume that the patient is rendered unconscious. The nurse must then assume total care of the patient's needs. A Foley catheter will usually be inserted and the patient will have an intravenous line. The patient may be intubated and receiving ventilatory support. The skin should be protected from injury. Care should be used with safety re-

Table 14-4 *Characteristics of Seizures—cont'd*

INCIDENCE	CHARACTERISTICS	CLINICAL SIGNS	AURA	POSTICTAL PERIOD
PSYCHOMOTOR (AUTOMATISMS)				
Occur at any age	Sudden change in awareness associated with complex distortion of feeling and thinking and partially coordinated motor activity Longer than absence seizures	Behaves as if partially conscious Often appears intoxicated May do antisocial things, such as exposing self or carrying out violent acts Autonomic complaints, such as shivering, lip smacking, repetitive movements that may not be appropriate may occur Urinary incontinence	Yes Complex hallucinations or illusions	Yes Confusion Amnesia Need for sleep
JACKSONIAN-FOCAL (LOCAL OR PARTIAL)				
Occur almost entirely in patients with structural brain disease	Depends on site of focus May or may not be progressive	Commonly begin in hand, foot, or face May end in tonic-clonic seizure	Yes Numbness Tingling Crawling feeling	Yes
MYOCLONIC				
May antedate tonic-clonic by months or years	May be very mild or may have rapid, forceful movements	Sudden, excess jerk of the body or extremities. The jerk may be forceful enough to hurl the person to the floor or ground. These seizures are brief and may occur in clusters. No loss of consciousness	No	
AKINETIC				
Not common	Peculiar generalized tonelessness	Person falls in flaccid state Unconscious for minute or two	Rarely	No

minder devices if the patient is awake and active so that they do not cause injury if she begins to have a seizure.

Assessment

Collection of **subjective data** includes the patient's awareness of the disorder and any precipitating factors. The presence of an aura preceding a seizure is important to consider. An aura occurs in about 50% of all patients with generalized tonic-clonic seizures. **Aura** is defined as a sensation, as of light or warmth, that may precede an attack of migraine or an epileptic seizure. An epileptic aura may be psychic, or it may be sensory with olfactory, visual, auditory, or taste hallucinations. The exact character of the aura varies from person to person and is specific to the individual. Awareness of

Table 14-5 *Antiseizure Medications Used to Prevent and Control Seizures*

DRUG	USE RELATED TO SEIZURE TYPE	TOXIC EFFECTS
Phenytoin sodium (Dilantin)	Generalized tonic-clonic, focal, psychomotor	Ataxia, vomiting, nystagmus, drowsiness, rash, fever, gum hypertrophy, lymphadenopathy
Phenobarbital (Luminal)	Generalized tonic-clonic, focal, psychomotor	Drowsiness, rash
Primidone (Mysoline)	Generalized tonic-clonic, focal, psychomotor	Drowsiness, ataxia
Ethosuximide (Zarontin)	Absence seizures, psychomotor, myoclonic, akinetic	Drowsiness, nausea, agranulocytosis
Trimethadione (Tridione)	Absence seizures	Rash, photophobia, agranulocytosis, nephrosis
Diazepam (Valium)	Generalized tonic-clonic and status epilepticus, mixed	Drowsiness, ataxia
Carbamazepine (Tegretol)	Generalized tonic-clonic, psychomotor	Rash, drowsiness, ataxia
Valproic acid (Depakene)	Absence seizures	Nausea, vomiting, indigestion, sedation, emotional disturbance, weakness, altered blood coagulation
Clonazepam (Clonopin)	Absence seizures, akinetic, myoclonic, generalized tonic-clonic seizures	Drowsiness, ataxia, hypotension, respiratory depression
Mephenytoin (Mesantoin)	Tonic-clonic, focal, psychomotor	Ataxia, nystagmus, pancytopenia, rash
Gabapentin (Neurontin)	Focal, generalized tonic-clonic in adults	Somnolence, fatigue, ataxia, dizziness, gastrointestinal upset
Lamotrigine (Lamictal)	Focal, generalized tonic-clonic in adults	Rash, dizziness, tremor, ataxia, diplopia, headache, gastrointestinal upset, Stevens-Johnson syndrome (rare)
Felbamate (Felbatol)	Seizures in children, generalized tonic-clonic seizures in adults. May be used to treat patients whose seizure disorders are refractory to other drugs.	Irritability, insomnia, anorexia, nausea, headache. Can cause aplastic anemia and hepatic failure
Fosphenytoin sodium (Cerebyx)	Short-term parenteral (IV or IM) in acute generalized tonic-clonic seizures; used for status epilepticus and for preventing and treating seizures occurring during neurosurgery	Dizziness, paresthesia, tinnitus, pruritus, headache, somnolence, ataxia, muscular incoordination, nystagmus, double vision, slurred speech, nausea, vomiting, and hypotension
Gabapentin (Neurontin), topiramate (Topamax), tiagabine (Gabitril) levetiracetam (Keppra) zonisamide (Zonegran)	Indicated for partial seizures and for secondary generalized seizures. These drugs are currently used as adjunctive therapy.	Neurontin: somnolence, dizziness, ataxia, nystagmus, fatigue; *Topamax:* somnolence, dizziness, ataxia, speech disorders and related speech problems, difficulty with memory, paresthesia, diplopia; *Gabitril:* dizziness/lightheadedness, asthenia/lack of energy, somnolence, nausea, nervousness, irritability, tremor, thinking abnormally/difficulty with concentration or attention

an aura allows the person to be aware of the impending seizure and seek safety and privacy.

Collection of **objective data** includes the number of seizures occurring within a specific time, the character of the seizure, and any behaviors noted and injuries suffered. The character of the seizure should be described as completely as possible, including duration, the nature of the patient's movements, whether the patient was incontinent, any cries or sounds that were made, and the level of alertness.

Diagnostic Test

The most common test used to evaluate seizures is the EEG. It allows a specific diagnosis of the nature of the seizure. This test was described on p. 696.

Medical Management

Medications. Treatment of patients with a seizure disorder almost always includes the use of one or more antiseizure drugs (Table 14-5). Therapy is aimed at preventing seizures because cure is not possible. Drugs generally act by stabilizing nerve cell membranes and preventing spread of the epileptic discharge. The choice of medication depends on the type of seizure. Failure to take the prescribed medication or an adequate dose is often the cause of treatment failure. Blood levels may be checked to provide an accurate check on the therapeutic level of the medications taken. In 70% of patients, seizure disorders are controlled by medication. The primary goal of antiseizure drug therapy is to obtain maximum seizure control with a minimum of toxic side effects. If medication is not effective, surgical removal of the brain tissue where the seizure occurs may be done.

Activities of daily living. Until seizures are controlled, activities such as driving a car, operating machinery, or swimming should be avoided. Maintaining adequate rest and good nutrition is also important. Alcohol use should be avoided. If the patient is receiving long-term phenytoin (Dilantin) therapy, good hygiene practices for the mouth and teeth are important because of the side effect of edematous and enlarged gums (gingival hyperplasia). The patient should wear a medical-alert bracelet or tag.

Nursing Interventions and Patient Teaching

Care during a seizure. The primary goals of the nurse and the family caring for a patient having a seizure are protection from aspiration and injury and observation and recording of the seizure activity. The patient should never be left alone. If the patient is sitting or standing, she should be lowered to the floor in an area away from furniture and equipment. Support and protect the head; if possible, turn the head to the side to maintain the airway. If there is time, clothing may be loosened around the neck. No effort should be made to restrain the patient during the seizure. The nurse

should *not* try to pry open the jaw to place a padded tongue blade. Padded side rails may be used, especially if seizures often occur during sleep.

When a seizure occurs, the nurse should carefully observe and record details of the event because the diagnosis and subsequent treatment often rests solely on the seizure description. All aspects of the seizure should be noted. What events preceded the seizure? When did the seizure occur? How long did each phase (aural [if any], ictal, postictal) last? What occurred during each phase?

Nursing diagnoses and interventions for the patient with seizures may include but are not limited to the following:

NURSING DIAGNOSES	NURSING INTERVENTIONS
Ineffective airway clearance, related to mucus accumulation in oropharyngeal area during seizure	Place patient in side-lying position to prevent aspiration and ensure airway patency. Suction secretions prn.
Risk for injury, related to rapid onset of altered state of consciousness and seizure activity	Pad side rails. If patient is out of bed during seizure activity, assist to the floor and remove objects that may harm him or her. Provide privacy. Maintain patent airway. Postictal, inform patient of seizure and reorient if necessary.

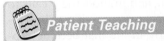

Patient Teaching

The Patient with Seizures

- Explain the need for the patient to continue taking medications even when seizure activity has stopped.
- Teach the patient about medications prescribed, including expected results, time and dosage, and side effects.
- The patient should be informed that medical alert bracelets, necklaces and identification cards are available. However, the use of these medical identification tags is optional. Some patients have found them beneficial, but others have found them to be more a burden than a help because they prefer not to be identified as having a seizure disorder.
- Caution the patient to avoid the use of alcohol if taking antiseizure medications.
- Explain the need for good oral hygiene for people taking phenytoin (Dilantin) (a side effect is gingival hyperplasia).
- Stress the importance of adequate rest and a balanced diet.
- Educate about available community resources.
- Explain restrictions concerning driving.
- Explain the importance of follow-up care.

Prognosis

The majority of patients with seizures are able to control them with medications and can lead a normal life. With most seizure disorders, the number and intensity of seizures stay constant. However, in patients who experience a first seizure as a result of a brain tumor or another brain pathology, the prognosis is more uncertain.

DEGENERATIVE DISEASES

The term **degenerative diseases** is used to refer to neurological disorders in which there is a premature aging of nerve cells, which is caused by suspected metabolic disturbance or for which the cause is unknown. Six diseases will be discussed: **multiple sclerosis (MS), Parkinson's disease, Alzheimer's disease, myasthenia gravis, amyotrophic lateral sclerosis,** and **Huntington's disease.**

MULTIPLE SCLEROSIS
Etiology/Pathophysiology

MS is a chronic, progressive degenerative neurological disease that affects many people. The cause is unknown, although genetics have been implicated, because there is a higher rate of the disease among relatives. Patients with the first signs and symptoms of MS have a proliferation of a certain type of immune cell called **gamma/delta T cells** in their spinal fluid in the initial phases of MS. These cells are not found in patients who have had the disease for a long time. T cells, the "field commanders" of the immune system, usually defend the body from outside attackers. In MS, however, something goes wrong and induces the T cells to attack the body. Myelin damage occurs—it may be a result of a viral infection early in life that becomes apparent as an immune process later in life. A viral infection may be the beginning mechanism, but a defective immune response seems to have an important role in the pathology of MS. People living in temperate climates have an increased risk of the disease.

The onset of signs and symptoms is usually between 15 and 50 years of age. Women are affected more often than men. The highest number of people with MS live in the Great Lakes area, the Pacific Northwest, and the North Atlantic states.

Multiple foci of **demyelination** are distributed randomly in the white matter of the brainstem, spinal cord, optic nerves, and cerebrum. During the demyelination process, the myelin sheath and the sheath cells are destroyed, causing an interruption or distortion of the nerve impulse so that it is slowed or blocked (Figure 14-13). There is evidence of partial healing in areas of degeneration, which explains the transitory nature of early signs and symptoms.

Clinical Manifestations

Because the onset is often insidious and gradual, with vague symptoms that occur intermittently over months or years, the disease may not be diagnosed un-

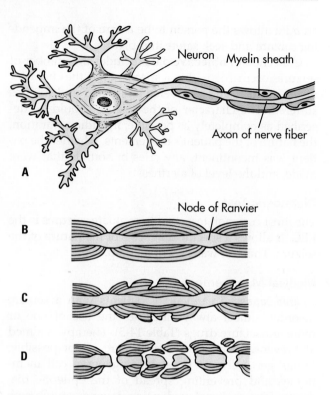

FIGURE **14-13** Pathogenesis of multiple sclerosis. **A,** Normal nerve cell with myelin sheath. **B,** Normal axon. **C,** Myelin breakdown. **D,** Myelin totally disrupted; axon not functioning.

til long after the onset of the first symptom. Because of the wide distribution of areas of degeneration, the variety of signs and symptoms in MS is greater than in other neurological diseases. These include visual problems, urinary incontinence, fatigue, weakness or incoordination of an extremity, sexual problems such as impotence in men, and swallowing difficulties. The majority of people have early remissions that may last for a year or more. Some patients have a benign course and they live a normal life span, with symptoms mild and requiring no specific treatment. Exacerbations may be aggravated or precipitated by fatigue, chilling, or emotional disturbances.

Assessment

Collection of **subjective data** includes the patient's understanding of the disease. The presence of eye problems such as diplopia, scotomata (spots before the eyes), and blindness is important. The patient may also talk about weakness or numbness of a part of the body, fatigue, emotional instability, bowel and bladder problems, vertigo, or loss of joint sensation. Involvement of the cerebellum can result in ataxia (impaired ability to coordinate movement) and tremor. In men, the presence of impotence is significant. Pain is not a common symptom.

Collection of **objective data** includes documented abnormalities in neurological testing that may include nystagmus (involuntary, rhythmic movements of the eye; the oscillations may be horizontal, vertical, rotary, or mixed); muscle weakness and spasms; changes in coordination; or a spastic, ataxic gait. Cerebellar signs include ataxia, dysarthria, and dysphagia. There may be evidence of behavior changes such as euphoria, emotional lability, or mild depression. Urinary incontinence and intention tremors of the upper extremities may be present.

Diagnostic Tests

Because there is no definitive diagnostic test for MS, diagnosis is based primarily on history and clinical manifestations. Examination of the CSF in patients with MS may show elevated gamma globulin and a proliferation of gamma/delta T cells in the initial phase as well as an increased number of lymphocytes and monocytes. A CT scan may show enlargement of the cerebral ventricles. MRI scanning has been very helpful in diagnosing MS over time in the presence of multiple lesions. MRI scanning may be helpful because sclerotic plaques as small as 3 to 4 mm in diameter can be detected.

Medical Management

Medications. There is no specific treatment for MS, although many different remedies have been tried. Favorable results often occur with the use of adrenocorticotropic hormone (ACTH) and corticosteroids such as prednisone (Deltasone) or dexamethasone (Decadron). These may be given orally, intramuscularly, or intravenously. The effects of ACTH and the steroids on the demyelinating process are unknown, although they probably are helpful by reducing edema and acute inflammation at the site of the demyelination. If steroids are used in high doses at the start of an exacerbation, the episode seems to resolve more rapidly. If spasticity is a problem, drugs such as diazepam (Valium), dantrolene (Dantrium), and baclofen (Lioresal) may be helpful in preventing or decreasing the spasms. Immunomodulating drugs modify the disease process. Interferon beta-1b (Betaseron) subcutaneously every other day is indicated for use in ambulatory patients with relapsing-remitting MS to reduce the frequency of clinical exacerbations. Interferon beta-1a (Avonex) treatment significantly decreases the frequency of exacerbations in selected patients and slows the progress of physical disability. It is recommended to be given intramuscularly once a week. Interferon beta-1a (Rebif) is administered subcutaneously three times weekly. Natalizumab (Antegren), a recombinant monoclonal antibody to a leukocyte adhesion molecule, is a promising new therapy for MS. It works by inhibiting the migration of lymphocytes, thus decreasing the inflammatory response. Mitoxantrone (Novantrone) is a new drug for the treatment of primary-progressive and progressive-relapsing MS. It is an immunosuppressant drug that reduces both B and T lymphocytes. It is given IV monthly. It has a lifetime dose limit because of cardiac toxicity; therefore, it can not be used for more than 2 to 3 years (Lewis et al, 2004). Many research studies are being conducted in the search for more effective medications to use in the treatment of MS.

Elimination. Urinary frequency and urgency may respond to propantheline (Pro-Banthīne). Cholinergic drugs such as bethanechol (Urecholine) can sometimes help the patient with a neurogenic bladder by exerting a direct antispasmodic effect on smooth muscles. Because urinary tract infections are a major problem in MS, some patients are given prophylactic doses of medications such as trimethoprim-sulfamethoxazole (Bactrim, Septra) or nitrofurantoin (Macrodantin). Cystometric studies can be helpful in defining the specific bladder problem.

The patient should be encouraged to drink adequate fluids (at least 2000 mL a day). If the patient suffers from constipation, a stool softener such as docusate sodium (Colace) may be used, as well as prune juice.

Nursing Interventions

Nutrition. A well-balanced diet with high-fiber foods and adequate fluids is important. Obesity will make it more difficult for the patient to meet daily needs and maintain mobility. The patient who is obese should be referred to the dietitian and be placed on a calorie-restricted diet that will help the patient lose weight slowly, while receiving adequate nutrition. Supplemental vitamins are usually advocated.

Skin care. It is important to teach the patient with MS and/or the caregiver frequent turning to avoid skin impairment. Devices to relieve pressure, such as eggcrate or air mattresses, may be helpful. Because of sensory involvement, the patient may not feel discomfort that signals the need to change position.

Activity. Patients with MS are encouraged to exercise regularly, but not to the point of fatigue. Daily rest periods may be helpful. During an acute exacerbation, patients are often kept as quiet as possible; this includes bed rest.

One side of the body is often more affected than the other. The patient must learn to stabilize the gait by leaning toward the less-involved side. If the foot slaps forward when he is walking, the patient should be taught to put the foot down in a pronounced fashion and roll the weight forward on the side of the foot.

Control of environment. Hot baths should be avoided because they often increase weakness. Traveling in hot weather should be planned so as to prevent travel during the warmest part of the day. If at all possible the patient should be in air-conditioned surroundings during the summer.

People with MS do best in a peaceful and relaxed environment. They may have slowness of speech and slowness in the ability to respond as well as sudden explosive emotional outbursts of crying or laughing. The patient and family will need support in terms of this behavior.

Nursing diagnoses and interventions for the patient with MS may include but are not limited to the following:

NURSING DIAGNOSES	NURSING INTERVENTIONS
Risk for powerlessness, related to physical limitations imposed by progressive physical deterioration, loss of body control, and threat to physical integrity	Provide emotional support, thorough explanations, and reassurance. Be alert to emotional changes and mood swings. Encourage patient's participation and expression of needs and feelings. Maintain planned rest periods. Encourage self-care as indicated. Provide physical care as indicated.
Bathing/hygiene, feeding, toileting self-care deficit, related to limitations in physical mobility imposed by disease process	Administer oral hygiene before meals. Assist with or provide physical hygiene as indicated by physical ability. Maintain appropriate bathing temperatures. Administer oral hygiene every 4 hours and prn. Catheterize intermittently as indicated; teach self-catheterization when possible. Plan bladder dysfunction program as appropriate for spasticity or flaccidity. Institute bowel control program (establish regular bowel routine, avoid constipation). Assist in dressing/grooming as indicated. Provide nutritious, attractive meals.

Patient Teaching

Teaching is important for both the patient with MS and significant others. In late stages of the disease, the care functions usually have to be assumed by someone other than the patient. Important points include those for the patient with motor and sensory problems (see pp. 706 to 710). In addition, it is important to teach about the importance of spacing activities and avoiding temperature extremes and the potential for emotional lability. The nurse should make sure that the patient and/or family has the address of the nearest MS society or support group.

Prognosis

The prognosis is variable. Some patients have MS for many years with few deficits, whereas other patients quickly become debilitated. The ability of the patient to conserve energy and avoid stress may help prevent exacerbations. Exacerbations are treated and may resolve. The average life expectancy after the onset of symptoms is more than 25 years.

PARKINSON'S DISEASE
Etiology/Pathophysiology

Parkinsonism is a syndrome that consists of a slowing down in the initiation and execution of movement (bradykinesia), increased muscle tone (rigidity), tremor, and impaired postural reflexes. Parkinson's disease, a form of parkinsonism, is named after James Parkinson, who, in 1817, wrote a classic essay on "shaking palsy," a disease whose cause is still unknown today. Many other disorders resemble this disease, but their causes are known. These include drug-induced parkinsonism, postencephalitic parkinsonism, and arteriosclerotic parkinsonism. The pathophysiology of these disorders, with the exception of drug-induced parkinsonism, is the same. Damage or loss of the dopamine-producing cells of the substantia nigra in the midbrain leads to depletion, in the basal ganglia, of dopamine that influences the initiation, modulation, and completion of movement and regulates unconscious autonomic movements. In cases of drug-induced parkinsonism, the dopamine receptors in the brain are blocked.

Parkinson's disease affects about 1.5% of the population in the United States more than 65 years of age. The disease shows no gender, socioeconomic, or cultural preference, and symptoms commonly occur after 50 years of age. The average age of the patient with Parkinson's disease is 65 years. There is apparent genetic cause and no known cure. The disease rarely occurs in African-Americans. Parkinson's disease is more common in men by a ratio of 3:2.

There are many causes of parkinsonism. Encephalitis lethargica, or type A encephalitis, has been clearly associated with the onset of parkinsonism. However, the incidence of postencephalitic parkinsonism has dwindled since the 1920s, when there was a large outbreak of this infectious illness. Parkinsonian-like symptoms have occurred after intoxication with a variety of chemicals, including carbon monoxide and manganese (among copper miners) and product of meperidine-analogue synthesis. Drug-induced parkinsonism can follow reserpine (Hydropres), methyldopa (Aldomet), (Haldol), and phenothiazine (Thorazine) therapy. Although patients with cerebrovascular disease may have parkinsonian-like symptoms, there is little evidence that parkinsonism is caused by arteriosclerosis. Distinguishing arteriosclerosis from true Parkinson's disease is important for prognostic purposes. Patients with arteriosclerosis do not respond as well to treatment and are more likely to experience side effects of drug therapy. Most patients with parkinsonism have the degenerative or idiopathic form, for which the term Parkinson's disease is usually reserved.

The pathology of Parkinson's disease is associated with the degeneration of the dopamine-producing neurons in the substantia nigra of the midbrain (Figure 14-14). Major signs and symptoms, such as tremors, muscle rigidity, slowed movements, and impaired balance and coordination, occur when approximately 70% of dopamine-producing cells have been destroyed. It is believed that there is normally a balance between acetylcholine (ACh) and dopamine (DA) in the basal ganglia. Any shift in the balance of activity (an increase in ACh or a decrease in DA) seems to lead to parkinsonism-like symptoms. Dopamine is a neurotransmitter that is essential for normal functioning of the extrapyramidal motor system, including control of posture, support, and voluntary motion. In Parkinson's disease the levels of DA-synthesizing enzymes and metabolites are reduced, and postmortem analysis of cross sections of the midbrain shows loss of the normal melanin pigment in the substantia nigra and loss of neurons. In addition, deficient amounts of gamma-aminobutyric acid (GABA), serotonin, and norepinephrine have been found in basal ganglia and in the substantia nigra.

Clinical Manifestations

The onset of Parkinson's disease is gradual and insidious, with a gradual progression and a prolonged course. In the beginning stages, only a mild tremor, handwriting changes, a slight limp, or a decreased arm swing may be evident. Later in the disease the patient

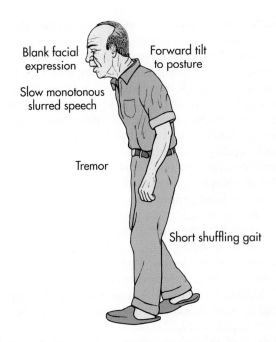

FIGURE **14-15** Characteristic appearance of a patient with Parkinson's disease.

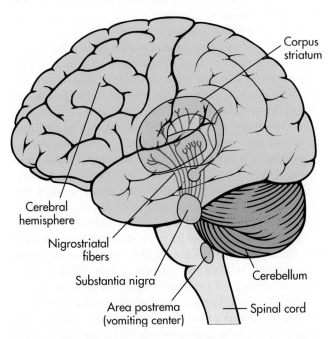

FIGURE **14-14** Nigrostriatal disorders produce parkinsonism. Left-sided view of the human brain showing the substantia nigra and the corpus striatum (*shaded area*) lying deep within the cerebral hemisphere. Nerve fibers extend upward from the substantia nigra, divide into many branches, and carry dopamine to all regions of the corpus striatum.

may have a shuffling, propulsive gait with arms flexed and loss of postural reflexes (Figure 14-15). In some patients there may be a slight change in speech patterns. None of these alone is sufficient evidence for a diagnosis of the disease.

Because there is no specific diagnostic test for Parkinson's disease, the diagnosis is based solely on the history, a thorough neurological examination, and clinical features. A firm diagnosis can be made only when there are at least two of the three characteristic signs of the classic triad: tremor, rigidity, and bradykinesia (slow or retarded movement). Dementia occurs in up to 40% of patients with Parkinson's disease. The ultimate confirmation of Parkinson's disease is a positive response to a low-dose trial of an antiparkinsonian medication, such as carbidopa-levodopa (Sinemet).

Tremor. Tremor, often the first sign, may be minimal initially, so the patient is the only one who notices it. This tremor can affect handwriting, causing it to trail off, particularly toward the ends of words. Parkinsonian tremor is more prominent at rest but disappears when one moves and is aggravated by emotional stress or increased concentration. The hand tremor is described as "pill rolling" because the thumb and forefinger appear to move in a rotary fashion, as if rolling a pill, coin, or other small object. Tremor can involve the hands, diaphragm, tongue, lips, and jaw but rarely causes shaking of the head. Eventually tremors can become so pronounced that one cannot hold a newspaper steady enough to read or make a telephone call using a push-button phone. Unfortunately, in many people a benign essential tremor has mistakenly been diagnosed as Parkinson's disease. Essential tremor occurs during voluntary movement, has a more rapid frequency than parkinsonian tremor, and is often familial.

Rigidity. Rigidity, the second sign of the triad, is the increased resistance to passive motion when the limbs are moved through their range of motion. Parkinsonian rigidity is typified by a jerky quality—as if there were intermittent catches in the movement of a cogwheel—when the joint is moved. This is termed **cogwheel rigidity.** The rigidity is caused by sustained muscle contraction and consequently elicits a complaint of muscle soreness; feeling tired and achy; or pain in the head, upper body, spine, or legs. Another consequence of rigidity is slowness of movement, because it inhibits the alternating of contraction and relaxation in opposing muscle groups (e.g., the biceps and triceps). Simple movements such as tying shoes and rising from a chair become a challenge.

Bradykinesia. Bradykinesia is particularly evident in the loss of automatic movements, which is secondary to physical and chemical alteration of the basal ganglia and related structures in the extrapyramidal portion of the CNS. In the unaffected patient, automatic movements are involuntary and occur subconsciously. They include blinking of the eyelids, swinging of the arms while walking, swallowing of saliva, self-expression with facial and hand movements, and minor movement of postural adjustment. The patient with Parkinson's disease does not execute these movements, and there is a lack of spontaneous activity. This accounts for the stoop posture, masked faces (deadpan expression), drooling saliva, and shuffling gait (festination) that are characteristic of a person with this disease (see Figure 14-15). There is often a shuffling, propulsive gait that the patient may not be able to stop until meeting an obstruction. In addition, there is difficulty initiating movement. Movements such as getting out of a chair cannot be executed unless they are consciously willed.

Assessment

Parkinson's disease starts with subtle symptoms and progresses slowly. Collection of **subjective data** includes symptoms of fatigue, presence of incoordination, judgment defects, emotional instability, and heat intolerance. The patient's understanding of the disease should be assessed.

Collection of **objective data** includes the presence of tremor, which is the outstanding sign of the disease. This has been described as a pill-rolling motion of the fingers or a resting tremor. Bradykinesia (an abnormal condition characterized by slowness of voluntary movements and speech) is present with rigidity and loss of postural reflexes. Muscle rigidity leads to a masklike appearance of the face and slowed, monotonous speech; and drooling. Swallowing may be abnormal, which poses the risk of choking and the potential for aspiration pneumonia. The patient may be constipated. There may be a scaly, erythematous

rash, particularly near the ears and eyebrows and in the scalp and nasolabial folds. Moist, oily skin is usually noted.

Diagnostic Tests

There is no specific diagnostic test for Parkinson's disease. A firm diagnosis can be made only when at least two of the three characteristic signs of the classic triad are present: **tremor, rigidity,** and **bradykinesia.** The clinical examination and history and the patient's response to medication confirm the diagnosis. The ultimate confirmation of Parkinson's disease is a positive response to antiparkinsonian drugs. If there is a history of chronic dementia, the CT scan may show cerebral atrophy. The EEG may show minimal slowing, and the upper GI evaluation may show decreased motility.

Medical Management

Medications. Treatment for Parkinson's disease is based on easing the signs and symptoms of the disease. There are several different drugs that may be used that have had a dramatic effect on the course of the disease:

Trihexyphenidyl HCl (Artane)
Benztropine mesylate (Cogentin)
Procyclidine HCl (Kemadrin)
Biperiden lactate (Akineton lactate; injection)
Levodopa (Dopar)
Amantadine HCl (Symmetrol)
Carbidopa-levodopa (Sinemet) (for 35 years, the cornerstone of therapy)
Selegiline HCl (Eldepryl)

After prolonged treatment with some of the drugs, side effects such as dyskinesia (abnormal involuntary movements) may occur, and the effectiveness of the medication may decrease. It may be helpful to admit the patient to the hospital, during which all drugs are withdrawn for a time. This is called a **drug holiday.** The medications are then restarted, and often smaller doses produce favorable results. To combat these problems, newer drug classes have been developed. Complications such as aspiration can occur during this time because withdrawal of the drugs causes immobility and rigidity (see Medications table).

Surgery. Surgery that involves destroying portions of the brain that control the rigidity or tremor has been found helpful with some patients. This is called ablation surgery. A surgical procedure called deep brain stimulation (DBS) involves placing an electrode in either the thalamus, globus pallidus, or subthalamic nucleus and connecting it to a generator placed in the upper chest (like a pacemaker). The device is programmed to deliver a specific current to the targeted brain location. DBS can be adjusted to control symptoms and is reversible (the device can be removed). The procedure is relatively safe and can improve motor performance and gait. This procedure is often reserved for patients

MEDICATIONS | *Disorders of the Neurological System*

MEDICATION	TRADE NAME	ACTION	SIDE EFFECTS	NURSING IMPLICATIONS
Amantadine hydrochloride	Symmetrel	Treats some Parkinson's disease and drug-induced extrapyramidal reactions, although its action in treatment of Parkinson's disease is unknown	Nausea, vomiting, vision changes, dysrhythmias, disorientation, orthostatic hypotension, depression, fatigue	Tell patient to drink no alcohol; administer no CNS depressants; know pregnancy cautions; tell patient not to cease taking medication without conferring with physician and not to deviate from prescribed dosage; for best absorption, instruct patient to take after meals if orthostatic hypotension occurs; instruct patient not to stand or change positions too quickly.
Baclofen	Lioresal	Reduces transmission of impulses from spinal cord to skeletal muscles; is antispasticity agent for treatment of spinal spasticity resulting from multiple sclerosis or spinal cord injury	Drowsiness, dizziness, disorientation, light-headedness, hypotension, urinary frequency, possible increase in blood glucose level	Be aware of pregnancy; give oral form with meals or milk to prevent gastrointestinal distress; watch for increased incidence of seizures in patients with epilepsy; tell patient to avoid activities that require alertness until CNS effects of drugs are known.
Trihexyphenidyl hydrochloride	Artane	Blocks central cholinergic receptors, helping to balance cholinergic activity of basal ganglia; is antidyskinetic and antiparkinsonian, controls some mild cases adjunct to more potent drugs; controls extrapyramidal reactions caused by drugs	Skin rash, eye pain, nervousness, headaches, tachycardia, urinary hesitancy, urine retention, dry mouth, disorientation	Do not give antacids or antidiarrheal agents within 1 hour of giving medication; give with food; caution patient to rise slowly; use cautiously in patients with narrow-angle glaucoma and hypertension; warn patient to avoid activities that require alertness until CNS effects of drugs are known; tell patient to relieve dry mouth with cool drinks, ice chips, and hard candy.
Pyridostigmine bromide	Mestinon	Inhibits destruction of acetylcholine released from parasympathetic and somatic efferent nerves; causes acetylcholine to accumulate, promoting increased stimulation of receptor; is used in myasthenia gravis and by the oral route for senility associated with Alzheimer's disease	Headache, seizures, bradycardia, hypotension, bronchospasm, increased bronchial secretions	Know that it is difficult to judge optimum dosage; monitor and document patient's response after each dose when using for myasthenia gravis; stress importance of taking drug exactly as ordered, on time, and in evenly spaced doses.

Continued

MEDICATIONS | *Disorders of the Neurological System—cont'd*

MEDICATION	TRADE NAME	ACTION	SIDE EFFECTS	NURSING IMPLICATIONS
Benztropine mesylate	Cogentin	Blocks central cholinergic receptors, helping to balance cholinergic activity in basal ganglia; is indicated in treatment of mild cases of Parkinson's disease and control of extrapyramidal reactions	Dizziness, drowsiness, depression, orthostatic hypotension, palpitation, tachycardia	Know importance of following prescribed dosage; discontinue drug slowly; tell patient not to drink alcohol, tell patient of breastfeeding warnings; give with food; tell patient to rise slowly and notify physician of severe allergic reactions; do not give with antacids.
Tacrine hydrochloride	Cognex	Is reversible cholinesterase inhibitor, used for treatment of mild to moderate dementia of Alzheimer's type	Bradycardia, nausea and vomiting, loose stools, ataxia, CNS disturbance, anorexia, agitation, increased serum transaminase levels, jaundice	Know risk of ulcers; monitor liver enzyme weekly for first 18 weeks; increase dosage at 6-week intervals; do not use NSAIDs concomitantly; know that it potentiates theophylline.
Levodopa	Dopar, Larodopa	Is antiparkinsonian agent (mechanism of action is unknown); increases balance between cholinergic and dopaminergic activity to allow more normal body movements and alleviate signs and symptoms	Aggressive behavior, involuntary grimacing, head and body movements, depression, suicidal tendencies, orthostatic hypotension, nausea, vomiting, darkened urine, excessive and inappropriate sexual behavior	Know that it is contraindicated in narrow-angle glaucoma; monitor patients receiving antihypertensive and hypoglycemic agents; advise patient to change positions slowly and dangle legs; protect drug from heat, light, moisture.
Carbidopa-levodopa	Sinemet	Increases levels of dopamine and levodopamine; is antiparkinsonian agent; improves modulation of voluntary nerve impulses transmitted to the motor cortex (lower dosage is needed than with single-dose therapy; efficiency may increase 75% when caridopa and levodopa are used in combination)	Mental depression, mental changes, nausea and vomiting, orthostatic hypotension, dizziness, uncontrollable body movements	Give with food; give only as directed, know that effectiveness may take months; warn patient of breastfeeding and pregnancy cautions; caution patient about drowsiness and getting up too fast; know that lying down may affect control of blood glucose and darken urine.

who are unresponsive to drug therapy or who have developed severe motor complications.

Medications are discontinued several days preoperatively so that signs and symptoms will be at their maximum at the time of surgery.

Another treatment approach for Parkinson's disease involves human fetal dopamine cell transplants in an attempt to provide viable dopamine-producing cells to the brain. The subject of using fetal tissue, however, is filled with controversy.

MEDICATIONS | *Disorders of the Neurological System—cont'd*

MEDICATION	TRADE NAME	ACTION	SIDE EFFECTS	NURSING IMPLICATIONS
Selegiline hydrochloride	Eldepryl	Is monoamine oxidase (MAO) inhibitor treatment adjunct to levodopa and levodopa-carbidopa; may slow Parkinson's disease and need for increased medication; may prolong life span of people with Parkinson's disease	Severe orthostatic hypotension, increased tremors, chorea, restlessness, grimacing, nausea and vomiting, slow urination, increased sweating, alopecia	Advise patient not to take more than 10 mg daily (there is no evidence that a greater amount improves effectiveness and it may increase adverse reactions); warn patient not to drink alcohol and drink only a little coffee; give with food; tell patient to rise slowly and notify physician of side effects; tell patient not to take over-the-counter cold remedies; monitor blood pressure and respirations.
Donepezil	Aricept	Improves cholinergic function by inhibiting acetylcholinesterase Anti-Alzheimer's agents may temporarily lessen some of the dementia associated with Alzheimer's disease. Does not alter the course	Diarrhea, nausea, vomiting, fatigue, headache, ecchymoses, atrial fibrillation, and vasodilation	Monitor heart rate (may cause bradycardia). Assess cognitive function periodically during therapy. Administer in the evening just before going to bed. May be taken without regard for food.
Memantine	Namenda	Believed to act as an N-methyl-D-aspartate (NMDA) receptor antagonist to decrease glutamate, which is an excitatory neurotransmitter in the CNS. Approved for the treatment of moderate to severe Alzheimer's disease. Memantine doesn't prevent or slow neurodegeneration, but it was found in clinical studies to slow symptom progression	Dizziness, headache, constipation, hypertension, urinary frequency	Provide I&O Contraindicated in severe renal impairment. Use cautiously in moderate renal impairment. Be aware conditions that increase urine pH, including severe urinary tract infections, lead to decreased excretion and increased serum levels.

Nursing Interventions

Activity needs. Special attention should be paid to posture. Lying on a firm bed without a pillow may help prevent the spine from bending forward. Holding the hands folded behind the back when walking may help keep the spine erect and prevent the arms from falling stiffly at the sides. Problems secondary to bradykinesia can be alleviated by relatively simple measures. The following are helpful hints for patients who tend to "freeze" while walking: consciously think about stepping over imaginary or real lines on floor, drop rice kernels and step over them, rock from side to side, lift the toes when stepping, take one step backward and two steps forward. The patient cannot be hurried, because it will make the bradykinesia worse.

Nutrition. Diet is of major importance to the patient with Parkinson's disease because malnutrition and constipation can be serious consequences of inadequate nutrition. Patients with dysphagia and bradykinesia need appetizing foods that can be easily chewed and swallowed. Food should be cut into bite-sized pieces before it is served. Eating six small meals a day may be less exhausting than eating three large meals. Ample time should be planned for eating to avoid frustration and encourage independence. When the disease is advanced, aspiration is a real concern. Care should be taken during feeding. Unless the disease is well controlled by medication, drooling can be a problem and increases with general excitement. When patients are dressed, garments with generous pockets for an ample supply of tissues will help them to be less conspicuous.

Elimination. The patient with Parkinson's disease may feel urgency and hesitancy in voiding. Measures appropriate for the patient with MS also apply to these patients.

Chronic constipation may be a real concern. The patient should be on a diet high in fiber and roughage for bulk. The nurse should encourage oral fluid intake, and stool softeners, suppositories, and prune juice are often helpful. Mild cathartics such as milk of magnesia are used if required.

Nursing diagnoses and interventions for the patient with Parkinson's disease are the same as those for the patient with MS, with the addition of, but not limited to, the following:

NURSING DIAGNOSES	NURSING INTERVENTIONS
Impaired physical mobility, related to rigidity, bradykinesia, and akinesia	Assist with ambulation to assess degree of impairment and to prevent injury. Perform active ROM exercises to all extremities to maintain joint ROM, prevent atrophy, and strengthen muscles. Consult physical therapist or occupational therapist for aids to facilitate ADLs and safe ambulation. Teach techniques to assist with mobility by instructing patient to step over imaginary line, rock from side to side to initiate leg movements because these are helpful in dealing with "freezing" (akinesia) while walking.

NURSING DIAGNOSES	NURSING INTERVENTIONS
Risk for aspiration, related to disease process	Ensure that when eating, the patient sits at 90-degree angle with head up and chin slightly tucked, avoiding extending the head. Provide soft-solid and thick-liquid diet because these consistencies are more easily swallowed. Consult speech therapist and dietitian because they can provide specific plans to improve swallowing. Encourage patient to take small bites. Avoid use of straws.

Patient Teaching

Education for the patient with Parkinson's disease should include the importance of taking medications on the prescribed time schedule. The importance of good skin care must be stressed, as well as the importance of keeping active so that the patient remains as mobile as possible. Proper ambulation and positioning should be demonstrated to the patient and family if they will be taking care of the patient. Proper feeding techniques to reduce the risk of aspiration should be taught to the family and patient (see Nursing Diagnoses box).

Prognosis

There is no cure for Parkinson's disease. Collaborative management is aimed at relieving the symptoms. Parkinson's disease is a chronic degenerative disorder with no acute exacerbations. If the patient takes medication as prescribed, signs and symptoms can be controlled for a long period.

ALZHEIMER'S DISEASE
Etiology/Pathophysiology

Alzheimer's disease (AD) is a chronic, progressive, degenerative disorder that affects the cells of the brain and causes impaired intellectual functioning. It is a common cause of dementia in the older person and affects men and women in equal numbers. Approximately 4 million Americans suffer from AD. It is estimated that 10% of people older than 65 and 50% of those older than age 85 have AD. Alzheimer's may strike people in their 40s and 50s. The cause is unknown, although research has shown a genetic link. The changes in the brain of patients with Alzheimer's disease include plaques in the cortex and neurofibrillary tangles (a tangled mass of nonfunctioning neurons). This neuronal damage occurs primarily in the cerebral cortex and causes a decrease in brain size. These changes were first discovered in 1907 by the German neurologist Alois Alzheimer. **Homocysteine** is a simple amino acid. Research is presenting evidence that in older adults, elevated plasma levels of homocysteine are associated with a significantly increased risk for Alzheimer's disease or another type of dementia. Put in practical terms, the investigators observed that a 5-mmol increment in the plasma homocysteine level increased the risk of Alzheimer's disease by 40% (Seshadri, 2002). Blood homocysteine levels may be lowered by eating foods rich in folic acid, such as fruits and green leafy vegetables.

Clinical Manifestations

The progression of Alzheimer's disease is commonly divided into four stages. In the early stage a person with Alzheimer's has relatively mild memory lapses and may have difficulty in using the correct word. The attention span is decreased, and there may be disinterest in surroundings. Depression may occur at this time. In the second stage the person has more obvious memory lapses, especially with short-term memory, and usually may be disoriented to time. Loss of personal belongings is common, as is confabulating (making up stories) to explain the loss of memory. Patients may lose their ability to recognize familiar faces, places, and objects and may get lost in a familiar environment. Loss of impulse control is common. Behavioral manifestations of AD (e.g., agitation) result from changes in the brain. They are neither intentional nor controllable by the individual with the disease. Some patients develop psychotic manifestations (i.e., delusions, illusions, hallucinations). By the time a person reaches the third stage, there is total disorientation to person, place, and time, and motor problems such as apraxia (an impairment in the ability to perform purposeful acts or to use objects properly) and **visual agnosia** (inability to recognize objects by sight) and **dysgraphia** (difficulty communicating via writing) interfere with the ability to carry out daily functions. Wandering is common. In the terminal stage, severe mental and physical deterioration is present. Total incontinence is common.

There may be some variations in these stages. However, all people with Alzheimer's disease experience a steady deterioration in their physical and mental status, usually lasting 5 to 20 years until death occurs.

Assessment

Memory loss is the first symptom usually noticed in AD, combined with the inability to carry out normal activities. Other evidence may be the presence of agitation and/or restlessness. It is important to rule out other conditions such as pernicious anemia, drug reactions, depression, or hormonal imbalances.

Diagnostic Tests

The diagnosis of AD is primarily a diagnosis of exclusion. There is no diagnostic test specific for Alzheimer's disease. A CT scan, EEG, MRI, and PET may be used to rule out other pathologic conditions. A family history of Alzheimer's disease is significant. At times the diagnosis can only be confirmed at the time of autopsy.

Medical Management

The care of the patient with Alzheimer's disease can be frustrating for the caregiver and the physician because the treatment options are so limited. Often medications make the condition worse. Lorazepam (Ativan) or haloperidol (Haldol) in small doses may be necessary to lessen agitation and unpredictable behavior. Tacrine (Cognex) is used to treat mild to moderate dementia of the Alzheimer's type with some benefit. Donepezil (Aricept) may have short-term benefit for mild cognitive impairment (MCI). Patients with MCI taking the drug are at reduced risk of progressing to AD for the first 18 months of a 3-year study, when compared with their counterparts on placebo. The reduced risk of progressing from MCI to a diagnosis of AD among participants on donepezil disappeared after 18 months and by the end of the study, the probability of progressing to AD was the same in the two groups (www.alzheimers.org, 2004). Memantine (Namenda) is the first drug approved for the treatment of moderate to severe AD. Memantine does not prevent or slow neurodegeneration, but it was found in clinical studies to slow symptom progression (www.fda.gov/bbs/tpics, 2003). Research shows that the simple addition to a normal diet of large doses of folic acid and vitamin B_{12} will substantially reduce homocysteine levels (Seshadri, 2002).

Nursing Interventions and Patient Teaching

Nursing interventions are directed toward maintaining adequate nutrition. This can be a challenge because often the patient will not sit still long enough to eat. Finger foods may be helpful, as well as letting the patient eat while walking. Frequent feedings with high nutritive value are important. Encouraging fluids up to at least 2000 mL a day is also helpful (Nursing Care Plan box).

Safety demands a special mention. Because of memory problems, patients with Alzheimer's disease often do dangerous things, such as walking outside while undressed, turning on stoves, wandering away, and setting fires. Measures that the family can take include removing burner controls from the stove at night, double-locking all doors and windows, and keeping the person under constant supervision. Disruptive behavior—including aggressive, agitated behavior—may occur. One very frustrating part of the disease is that many patients sleep for only short periods and are awake most of the night.

Most of the time, education is directed at the family, because by the time the condition is diagnosed there is usually serious mental impairment. The family should

NURSING CARE PLAN

The Patient with Alzheimer's Disease

Ms. A. is a 65-year-old who has been a seamstress. She has a history of progressive memory loss, paranoia, disorientation, and agitation. She was diagnosed as having Alzheimer's disease 2 years ago. Her family kept her at home until 6 months ago, when she was admitted to a long-term care institution. The nursing history indicates that she is incontinent of urine about 50% of the time and expresses a great deal of anxiety, especially around new situations or people. She cries frequently and at times attempts to hit the staff.

NURSING DIAGNOSIS *Anxiety, related to cognitive impairments*

Patient Goals/Expected Outcomes	Nursing Interventions	Evaluation/Rationale
Patient will demonstrate decreased anxiety as evidenced by decreased outbursts of agitation or crying, the ability to sleep through most of the night, and cooperation with care.	Continue to assess presence of anxiety. Comfort patient when crying. Provide simple explanation for all procedures. Use calm, undemanding, unhurried approach. Keep nursing interventions consistent and simple. Assist patient in doing relaxation techniques. Maintain consistency of caregiver when able. Minimize patient's choices in care. Encourage exercise. Offer snack at bedtime.	Patient sleeps 5 to 6 hours per night. Patient remains calm with care. Patient experiences decreased episodes of crying or striking out at others.

NURSING DIAGNOSIS *Functional urinary incontinence, related to condition and cognitive impairment*

Patient Goals/Expected Outcomes	Nursing Interventions	Evaluation/Rationale
Patient will be continent. Patient will be free of urinary tract infection.	Take patient to bathroom on regular schedule. Encourage adequate fluid intake (at least 2000 mL/day). Determine patient's preference for fluid. Place sign on door indicating "Toilet" or "Bathroom," or with a picture. If patient has urgency, ensure closeness to bathroom. Simplify closures on clothing. Avoid fluids just before bed. Use disposable protective perineal garments (Attends) only as needed.	Patient is free of episodes of incontinence. Patient is free of infection. Patient will void when taken to the bathroom.

❓ CRITICAL THINKING QUESTIONS

1. Ms. A. continually wanders about the long-term care facility. She is unable to sit at the table for an entire meal. She has lost approximately 20 pounds in the past 3 months. Helpful measures to improve her nutritional status would include:

2. To assist Ms. A. to obtain a better sleep pattern, helpful interventions include:

3. Ms. A. has difficulty in maintaining good personal hygiene. Methods for assisting Ms. A. to maintain personal hygiene would include:

be helped to set a realistic schedule that also allows them time for rest and relaxation. If necessary, the family may need to consider placing the patient in a long-term care facility. The family should be put in touch with the local support group for Alzheimer's disease.

Prognosis

There currently is no effective treatment to stop the progression of Alzheimer's disease, which progresses at a variable rate. The course of the disease can span 5 to 20 years. The economic costs of AD in the United States range from approximately $19,000 annually for the care of the person with early disease to $37,000 for the person with late disease. Ultimately, most patients die from complications such as pneumonia, malnutrition, and dehydration. Special Alzheimer's units and family and nursing approaches may help the patient stay as productive and safe as possible. The burden on the individual, family, caregivers, and society as a whole is staggering. Support groups for caregivers and family members have been formed throughout the United States to provide an atmosphere of understanding and to give current information about the disease itself and related topics such as safety, legal, ethical, and financial issues. Nurses often receive personal and professional satisfaction in participating in such support groups.

MYASTHENIA GRAVIS

Etiology/Pathophysiology

Myasthenia gravis (MG) is an autoimmune disease of the neuromuscular junction characterized by the fluctuating weakness of certain skeletal muscle groups. MG is an unpredictable neuromuscular disease with lower motoneuron characteristics. MG can occur at any age, but most commonly occurs between the ages of 10 and 65 years. The peak age of onset in women is 20 to 30 years. In young people, women are more affected than men, but among older people the distribution between the genders is about equal. Occurrence within families is rare; however, infants of affected mothers may have symptoms at birth. These symptoms usually disappear within several weeks. The incidence is about 14 in every 100,000 population.

With MG, no observable structural change occurs in the muscle or nerve. Nerve impulses fail to pass at the myoneural junction, resulting in muscle weakness. MG is caused by an autoimmune process. It is thought to be triggered by antibodies that attack acetylcholine (ACh) receptor sites at the neuromuscular junction, resulting in a decreased number of ACh receptor sites and interfering with impulse transmission to the muscles.

The fatigue and muscular symptoms of MG are caused by an antibody-mediated attack against the body's acetylcholine receptors at the neuromuscular junction—the space between the nerve ending and muscle fiber. This attack damages and reduces the number of receptor sites, preventing conduction along the normal pathway at normal conduction speeds. Studies show that patients with MG have only about one third as many acetylcholine receptors at the neuromuscular junction as is normal.

About 25% of the patients with MG have been found to have a thymoma, and almost 80% have changes in the cellular structure of the thymus gland.

Clinical Manifestations

MG occurs in both ocular and generalized terms. In ocular MG the signs and symptoms include ptosis (eyelid drooping) and diplopia (double vision). In about 15% of cases, MG remains confined to the eye muscles. The generalized variety may vary from mild to severe signs and symptoms. The patient may complain initially of ptosis and diplopia. Skeletal weakness involving the muscles of the extremities, neck, shoulders, hands, diaphragm; dysarthria; and dysphagia may follow. The vocal cords can become weak and the voice can sound nasal. As the disease progresses, the trunk and lower limbs are affected, leading to difficulty with walking, sustained sitting, and raising the arms over the head. Usually the distal muscles are not as affected as the proximal muscles. Muscle weakness may become so severe that the person cannot breathe without mechanical ventilation. Bowel and bladder sphincter weakness occurs with severe loss of muscle control. Exacerbations of the disease may be initiated by upper respiratory infections, emotional tension, and menstruation.

Assessment

Both subjective and objective data are important to collect from the patient with myasthenia gravis. **Subjective data** include the patient's understanding of the disease; complaints of weakness, double vision; difficulty in chewing or swallowing; and the presence of any bowel or bladder incontinence. Gathering **objective data** begins with any documented muscle weakness on neurological testing. Nasal-sounding speech may be noted; the voice often fades after a long conversation and breath sounds diminish. Ptosis of the eyelids may be noted, as well as weight loss if there are swallowing problems.

Diagnostic Tests

Because of the slow, insidious onset and occurrence of symptoms with stress, MG sometimes is misdiagnosed as hysteria or neurosis. The simplest diagnostic test for myasthenia gravis is to have the patient look upward for 2 to 3 minutes. If the problem is MG, there will be an increased droop of the eyelids so that the person can barely keep the eyes open. The diagnosis can be made partly on the basis of EMG. The intravenous (IV) anticholinesterase test is a reliable diagnostic test. Edrophonium (Tensilon), a short-acting cholinesterase inhibitor, which decreases the amount of cholinesterase at the neuromuscular junction while making acetylcholine available to muscles, is administered intravenously. The patient response is carefully evaluated. Muscle function improves dramatically in a short time with patients who have the illness. Another diagnostic test is serum testing for antibodies to acetylcholine receptors.

Acetylcholine receptor antibodies are present in 80% to 90% of patients with generalized myasthenia, so their presence can be used to diagnose the disease.

Medical Management

Medical management includes the use of medications. Anticholinesterase drugs such as neostigmine (Prostigmin) and pyridostigmine (Mestinon) may be administered. These medications promote nerve impulse transmission. They are quite effective at alleviating symptoms. Usually the patient is taught how to adjust the dosage depending on symptoms. Corticosteroids may be used as an adjunct therapy. Immunosuppressive medications including azathioprine (Imuran), cyclosporine (Sandimmune), and cyclophosphamide (Cytoxan) are being used because of MG's immune component. Many classes of drugs are contraindicated or must be used with caution in patients with MG, such as anesthetics, antidysrhythmics, antibiotics, quinine, antipsychotics, barbiturates, sedatives, hypnotics, opioids, tranquilizers, and thyroid preparations (Fisher, 2004).

Plasmapheresis as a therapy for MG was first reported in 1976. This procedure involves a separation of plasma from blood by a machine called a cell separator, which can be connected to the patient by a vascular cannula. This process removes the antibodies produced by the autoimmune response. Plasmapheresis can yield short-term improvement in symptoms and is indicated for patients in crisis or in preparation for surgery when corticosteroids need to be avoided.

Thymectomy is indicated for almost all patients with a thymoma and for some patients without thymoma with improvement in symptoms. Excision of the thymus reduces symptoms of MG in many patients. A thymectomy is a complex surgery, and patients with MG are at high risk for complications from anesthesia.

Another treatment option is the administration of intravenous immune globulin to reduce the production of acetylcholine antibodies. Intravenous immune globulin is used for a severe relapse of myasthenia gravis.

During exacerbations of the disease, and when the respiratory status is compromised, the patient may require intubation and mechanical ventilation. A tracheostomy may be necessary.

Nursing Interventions and Patient Teaching

Respiratory problems typically occur in patients with MG. Upper respiratory infections occur because the patient may not have the energy needed to cough effectively and pneumonia or airway obstruction may develop. Aspiration often occurs. During acute episodes of the disease, the patient may require hospitalization. Serial determination of vital capacity, minute volumes, and tidal volumes are made to assess the need for respiratory assistance. The patient may also be taught airway protective techniques during swallowing (e.g., chin tuck, double swallow). Suctioning is done as needed, and if swallowing becomes impaired, a feeding tube may be necessary.

People with MG may have to change daily patterns of activity. The nurse can help the patient and family plan so that minimal energy is used in activities that are essential to remaining relatively self-sufficient and yet allow for energy for activities in which the patient wishes to take part. Physical therapy such as ROM exercises may be beneficial for maintaining muscle function.

The patient with MG is usually able to adjust the medication depending on the symptoms. Also, the pa-

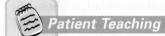
Patient Teaching

Myasthenia Gravis

- Teach the importance of taking medication at the time prescribed and to take it early enough before eating or engaging in activities to obtain maximum relief.
- Explain how to adjust medication dose to maintain muscle strength.
- Caution about medications to avoid.
- Teach importance of seeking medical attention at first sign of an upper respiratory infection.
- Explain importance of eating only when sitting up to prevent aspiration.
- Caution patient to avoid crowds in flu and cold season.
- Explain how to adjust to daily activities to allow for leisure activities and rest periods.
- Explain planning to use minimal energy in activities that are essential so that energy may be conserved for activities that patient enjoys.
- Advise patient to wear a medic-alert bracelet that identifies the patient as having MG.

tient can have much control over preventing respiratory complications. Therefore teaching is very important and should include those topics listed in Patient Teaching: Myasthenia Gravis.

Prognosis

MG is a chronic disease. The course is variable with periods of exacerbation and remission. Some cases are mild, but others are severe, with death resulting from respiratory failure. Patients with a thymoma may experience improvement after a thymectomy is performed.

AMYOTROPHIC LATERAL SCLEROSIS

Loss of motoneurons is the major pathologic change in **amyotrophic lateral sclerosis** (ALS), a rare progressive neurological disease that usually leads to death in 2 to 6 years. This disease became known as Lou Gehrig's disease when the famous baseball player was stricken with it in the early 1940s. The onset is between 40 and 70 years of age, and two times as many men as women are affected.

For unknown reasons, motoneurons in the brainstem and spinal cord gradually degenerate in ALS. The dead motoneuron cannot produce or transport vital signals to muscle. Consequently, electrical and chemical messages originating in the brain do not reach the muscles to activate them.

The primary symptoms are weakness of the upper extremities, dysarthria, and dysphagia. Muscle wasting and fasciculations result from the denervation of the muscles and lack of stimulation and use. Death usually results from respiratory infection secondary to compromised respiratory function. Unfortunately there is no cure for ALS.

A drug called riluzole (Rilutek) slows the progression of ALS. The drug helps protect motoneurons damaged by the disease, and can add 3 months or more to a patient's life.

Multidisciplinary ALS teams at large academic centers like Johns Hopkins Medical Center and Allegheny University Health Sciences are also offering renewed hope to these patients. Usually coordinated by a nurse, these programs provide experimental drugs; physical, occupational, and speech therapy; nutritional regimens; and psychological support. Outcome studies suggest that patients in these programs may live 15 years or more after diagnosis—three times the typical life expectancy.

This illness is devastating because the patient remains cognitively intact while wasting away. The challenge of nursing care is to support the patient's cognitive and emotional functions by facilitating communication, providing diversional activities such as reading and human companionship, and helping the patient and family with advance care planning and anticipatory grieving related to loss of motor function and ultimate death.

HUNTINGTON'S DISEASE

Huntington's disease is a genetically transmitted autosomal dominant disorder that affects both men and women of all races. The offspring of a person with this disease have a 50% risk of inheriting it. The diagnosis often occurs after the affected individual has had children. In the United States, approximately 25,000 people have Huntington's disease and another 150,000 have a 50-50 chance of developing it. Diagnosis is based on family history, clinical symptoms, and the detection of the characteristic DNA pattern from blood samples.

Like Parkinson's disease, the pathology of Huntington's disease involves the basal ganglia and the extrapyramidal motor system. However, instead of a deficiency of dopamine, Huntington's disease involves an overactivity of the dopamine pathway. The net effect is an excess of dopamine, which leads to symptoms that are the opposite of those of parkinsonism. The clinical manifestations, the onset of which is between 30 and 50 years of age, are characterized by abnormal and excessive involuntary movements (chorea). These are writhing, twisting movements of the face, limbs, and body. The movements get worse as the disease progresses. Facial movements involving speech, chewing, and swallowing are affected and may cause aspiration and malnutrition. The gait deteriorates and ambulation eventually becomes impossible. Perhaps the most devastating deterioration is in mental functions, which include intellectual decline, emotional lability, and psy-

chotic behavior. Death usually occurs 10 to 20 years after the onset of symptoms.

Because there is no cure, therapeutic management is palliative. Antipsychotic, antidepressant, and antichorea medications are prescribed and have some effect. However, they do not alter the course of the disease. This disease presents a great challenge to health care professionals. Transplantation of fetal striatal neural tissues into the brain is an experimental treatment that may be effective (Freeman, 2000). The goal of nursing management is to provide the most comfortable environment possible for the patient and the family by maintaining physical safety, treating the physical symptoms, and providing emotional and psychological support. Because of the choreic movements, caloric requirements are high. Patients may require as high as 4000 to 5000 calories per day to maintain body weight. As the disease progresses, meeting caloric needs becomes a greater challenge when the patient has difficulty swallowing and holding the head still. Depression and mental deterioration can also compromise nutritional intake. Genetic counseling is very important. DNA testing can be done on fetal cells obtained by amniocentesis or chorionic biopsy. Genetic testing can determine whether a person is a carrier. No test is available to predict when symptoms will develop.

VASCULAR PROBLEMS

Interference with function because of vascular conditions is a common cause of neurological impairment. Stroke is discussed in this section.

STROKE
Etiology/Pathophysiology

Stroke (or "brain attack") is an abnormal condition of the blood vessels of the brain, characterized by hemorrhage into the brain or the formation of an embolus or thrombus that occludes an artery, resulting in ischemia of the brain tissue normally perfused by the damaged vessels. Stroke is the most common disease of the nervous system. It is estimated that 700,000 people in the United States suffer a stroke annually, and is ranked as the third leading cause of death in the United States, with about 158,000 deaths annually. Strokes affect people in all age groups, but the greatest number of people are between 75 and 85 years of age. Strokes may leave many people with serious, long-term disability. Common long-term disabilities include hemiparesis, inability to walk, complete or partial dependence in ADLs, and aphasia (Cultural and Ethnic Considerations box).

Strokes are classified as ischemic or hemorrhagic, based on the underlying pathophysiologic findings. Ischemic strokes are thrombotic and embolic. These account for 85% of strokes. Hemorrhagic strokes account for 15% of all strokes and result from bleeding into the brain tissue itself (Figure 14-16). Many underlying factors are also contributing causes: atherosclerosis, heart disease, hypertension, kidney disease, peripheral vascular disease, and diabetes mellitus. Other risk factors include family history of stroke, obesity, high serum cholesterol, cigarette smoking, stress, cocaine use, and a sedentary lifestyle. Oral contraceptives also increase the risk of stroke. In 2002, data from the Women's Health Initiative (longitudinal intervention trial in middle-aged women) showed an increased risk of stroke in women taking estrogen plus progestin compared with those not receiving hormone replacement therapy. These data suggest that postmenopausal hormone replacement therapy does not protect against stroke (Women's Health Initiative, 2002).

Clinical Manifestations

A stroke can have an effect on many body functions, including motor activity, elimination, intellectual function, spatial-perceptual alterations, personality, affect, sensation, and communication. The functions affected are directly related to the artery involved and area of

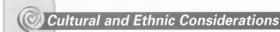

Cultural and Ethnic Considerations

Stroke

A high mortality rate from strokes exists among African-American men, possibly as a result of the high frequency of hypertension, obesity, and diabetes mellitus in this group. Thrombotic strokes are twice as common among African-Americans as among whites. Hemorrhagic strokes are three times more common among African-Americans than among whites. Hispanics, American Indians, and Asian-Americans have a higher stroke incidence than whites.

the brain it supplies. Permanent damage can result from a stroke because of anoxia of the brain. The vessel most commonly affected is the middle cerebral artery. The patient may be unconscious and may experience seizures. Both unconsciousness and seizures result from generalized ischemia and the brain's response to abrupt hypoxia.

Thrombotic stroke. Thrombosis is the most common cause of stroke, and the most common cause of cerebral thrombosis is atherosclerosis. Additional disease processes that cause thrombosis are hypertension or diabetes mellitus, both of which accelerate the arteriosclerotic process. Additional risk factors associated with thrombotic strokes include oral contraceptives, coagulation disorders, polycythemia vera, arteritis, chronic hypoxia, and dehydration. Stroke resulting from thrombosis is seen most often in the 60- to 90-year-old age group. Thrombosis occurs in relation to injury of a blood vessel wall and formation of a blood clot. The lumen of the blood vessel becomes narrowed, and if it becomes occluded, infarction occurs. Thrombosis develops readily where atherosclerotic plaques have already narrowed blood vessels. Thrombi usually occur in larger vessels. The internal carotid arteries are a common source of thrombi.

Symptoms of this type of stroke tend to occur during sleep or soon after arising. This is thought to result partly because recumbency causes a lowering of blood pressure, which can lead to brain ischemia. Postural hypotension may also be a factor. Neurological signs and symptoms frequently worsen for the first few hours after a stroke. The typical picture of the stroke is signs and symptoms that peak in severity within 72 hours as edema increases in the infarcted areas of the brain.

Emboli stroke. Embolism is the second most common cause of stroke. People who have a stroke resulting

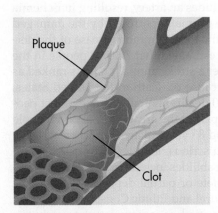

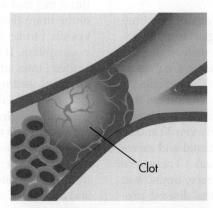

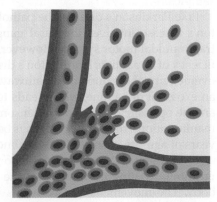

A Thrombotic stroke. Cerebral thrombosis is a narrowing of the artery by fatty deposits called *plaque.* Plaque can cause a clot to form, which blocks the passage of blood through the artery.

B Embolic stroke. An embolus is a blood clot or other debris circulating in the blood. When it reaches an artery in the brain that is too narrow to pass through, it lodges there and blocks the flow of blood.

C Hemorrhagic stroke. A burst blood vessel may allow blood to seep into and damage brain tissues until clotting shuts off the leak.

FIGURE **14-16** Three types of stroke.

from embolism are usually younger. The emboli most commonly originate from a thrombus in the endocardial (inside) layer of the heart, often caused by rheumatic heart disease, mitral stenosis and atrial fibrillation, myocardial infarction, infective endocarditis, valvular prostheses, and atrial-septal defects. Less common causes of emboli include air, fat from long bone (femur) fractures, amniotic fluid after childbirth, and tumors. The embolus travels upward to the cerebral circulation and lodges where a vessel narrows or bifurcates. They most frequently occur in the midcerebral artery.

Hemorrhagic stroke. Intracerebral or intracranial hemorrhages include bleeding into the brain itself or bleeding into the subarachnoid space. The bleed causes damage by destroying and replacing brain tissue. Intracranial hemorrhages are the third most common cause of strokes. The peak incidence of aneurysms occurs in people who are 35 to 60 years of age. Women are more frequently affected than men.

An aneurysm is often the cause of hemorrhage. An aneurysm is a localized dilation of the wall of a blood vessel usually caused by atherosclerosis and hypertension or, less frequently, by trauma, infection, or a congenital weakness in the vessel wall. It ruptures as a result of a small hole that occurs in a part of the aneurysm. The hemorrhage spreads rapidly, producing localized damage and irritation to the cerebral vessels. The bleeding usually stops when a plug of fibrin platelets is formed. The hemorrhage begins to absorb within 3 weeks. Recurrent rupture is a risk 7 to 10 days after the initial hemorrhage. The prognosis of intracerebral hemorrhage stroke is poor; 50% of patients die soon after the occurrence of the stroke. Only about 20% are functionally independent after 6 months. The patient with intracerebral hemorrhage has no forewarning; has rapid, severe symptoms; and has a poor prognosis for recovery.

Transient ischemic attack. Transient ischemic attack (TIA) refers to an episode of cerebrovascular insufficiency with temporary episodes of neurological dysfunction lasting less than 24 hours and often lasting less than 15 minutes. Most TIAs resolve within 3 hours. TIAs may be caused by microemboli that temporarily block the blood flow. The most common deficit is contralateral weakness of the lower face, hands, arms, and legs; transient dysphasia; numbness or loss of sensation; temporary loss of vision of one eye; or a sudden inability to speak. Other symptoms may include tinnitus, vertigo, blurred vision, diplopia, eyelid ptosis, and ataxia. Between attacks the neurological status is normal. Evaluation must be done to confirm that the signs and symptoms of a TIA are not related to other brain lesions, such as a developing subdural hematoma or an increasing tumor mass. CT of the brain without contrast media is the most important initial diagnostic study.

The major importance of TIAs is that they warn the patient of the existence of an underlying pathologic condition. At least one third of patients who experience TIAs will have a stroke in 2 to 5 years. Medications that prevent platelet aggregation—such as aspirin, ticlopidine (Ticlid), dipyridamole (Persantine), clopidogrel (Plavix), and anticoagulant medications (e.g., oral warfarin [Coumadin])—may be prescribed for long-term therapy after the TIA.

Surgical interventions for the patient with TIAs from carotid artery disease include carotid endarterectomy (CEA) or transluminal angioplasty. In CEA the atheromatous lesion is removed from the carotid artery to improve blood flow. CEA surgery causes a reduction in stroke and vascular death. This surgery is reserved for patients with occlusions of 70% to 99% of blood flow.

Transluminal angioplasty is the insertion of a balloon to open a stenosed artery to permit increased blood flow. This procedure has been used to treat patients with clinical manifestations related to stenosis in the vertebrobasilar or carotid arteries and their branches. The risk of the angioplasty procedure is the possibility of dislodging emboli, which can travel to the brain or retina.

Assessment

Collection of **subjective data** that are important with a patient experiencing a stroke includes the description of the onset of symptoms; the presence of headache; any sensory deficit, such as numbness or tingling; the inability to think clearly; and the presence of visual problems. In the case of a hemorrhage, the headache may be described as sudden and explosive. The patient's ability to understand the condition should be assessed.

Collection of **objective data** includes the presence of hemiparesis or hemiplegia, any change in the level of consciousness, signs of increased intracranial pressure, respiratory status, and the presence of aphasia. The exact clinical picture varies, depending on the area of the brain affected (Figure 14-17). When the middle cerebral artery is affected, as is most common, the signs and symptoms seen include contralateral paralysis or paresis, contralateral sensory loss, dysphasia or aphasia if the dominant hemisphere is involved, spatial-perceptual problems, changes in judgment and behavior if the nondominant hemisphere is involved, and **contralateral (homonymous) hemianopia** (Figure 14-18).

Diagnostic Tests

CT is the primary diagnostic test used to diagnose a stroke. CT can indicate the size and location of the lesion and differentiate between ischemic and hemorrhagic stroke. CT angiography (CTA) provides visualization of vasculature. MRI is used to determine the

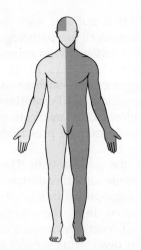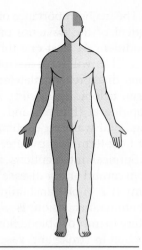

Right brain damage	**Left brain damage**
(Stroke on right side of the brain)	(Stroke on left side of the brain)
• Paralyzed left side: hemiplegia	• Paralyzed right side: hemiplegia
• Left-sided neglect	• Impaired speech/language aphasias
• Spatial-perceptual deficits	• Impaired right/left discrimination
• Tends to deny or minimize problems	• Slow performance, cautious
• Rapid performance, short attention span	• Impaired speech/language
• Impulsive, safety problems	• Aware of deficits: depression, anxiety
• Impaired judgment	• Impaired comprehension related to language, math
• Impaired time concepts	

FIGURE **14-17** Manifestations of right-sided and left-sided stroke.

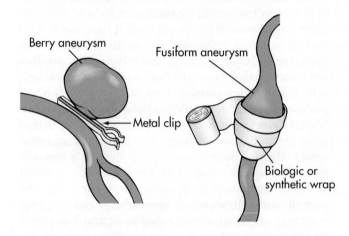

FIGURE **14-18** Spatial and perceptual deficits in stroke. Perception of a patient with homonymous hemianopsia shows that food on the left side is not seen and thus is ignored.

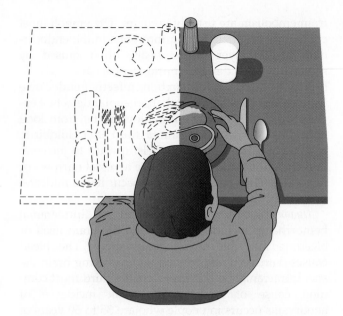

FIGURE **14-19** Clipping and wrapping of aneurysms.

extent of brain injury. MRI has greater specificity than CT. PET is also very useful in assessing the extent of tissue damage by showing the metabolic activity of the brain. After TIAs, a cerebral angiogram may be done. Doppler, computed tomographic angiography (CTA), or magnetic resonance angiography (MRA) studies of the carotid arteries may be performed. The results of these noninvasive carotid artery studies determine whether the more invasive cerebral angiogram is performed.

Medical Management

If the patient has had a hemorrhagic stroke as a result of an aneurysm, surgery may be necessary to prevent a rebleed. The surgery consists of a craniotomy; tying off or clipping of the aneurysm; and removing the clot to prevent rebleeding into the brain (Figure 14-19). An aneurysm often causes vasospasm in the brain. Vasospasm is caused by blood in the subarachnoid space that becomes an irritant. Vasospasm narrows blood vessels in the brain, decreasing perfusion to the areas they supply with blood. It can occur whether the pa-

tient has surgery or not. The amount of blood can directly affect the degree of vasospasm.

Typically occurring in 30% to 60% of cases between postoperative days 4 and 12, vasospasm has a mortality rate as high as 50%. If it is not treated rapidly, it can cause cerebral ischemia or cerebral anoxia, leading to severe mental and physical deficits or death. Any patient with subarachnoid hemorrhage should be started on the calcium channel blocker nimodipine (Nimotop) within 96 hours of bleeding and receive it for 21 days to prevent vasospasm.

The term *brain attack* is increasing being used to describe stroke and communicate the urgency of recognizing stroke signs and symptoms and treating their onset as a medical emergency, similar to what would be done with a myocardial infarction (heart attack). Research indicates that select patients with acute ischemic stroke can benefit from thrombolytics such as tissue plasminogen activator (t-PA, alteplase [Activase]), which digests fibrin and fibrinogen and thus lyses the clot. Because t-PA is clot specific in its activation of the fibrinolytic system, it is less likely to cause hemorrhage compared with streptokinase or urokinase. The results of one landmark study have revealed that selected patients who are treated within 3 hours of the onset of symptoms are at least 30% more likely than patients who do not receive timely treatment to recover with little or no disability after 3 months. Time lost is brain lost.

Patients with stroke symptoms need to be triaged, transported, and treated as rapidly as patients experiencing an acute myocardial infarction (MI). In administering thrombolytic drugs, the single most important factor is timing. Patients are screened carefully before treatment is initiated. This includes blood tests for coagulation disorders, recent history of GI bleeding, and a CT or MRI scan to rule out hemorrhagic stroke. In patients with acute ischemic stroke, thrombolytic therapy increases short-term mortality, increases (but not statistically significant) symptomatic or fatal intracranial hemorrhage, decreases long-term death rate, and decreases dependence in terms of ADLs. The use of thrombolytic therapy in an individual should be based on a discussion of the risks and benefits with the patient and family. Some patients would accept a high risk of death from hemorrhage in an attempt to improve their chances of escaping permanent aphasia or dependency. Others prefer to avoid interventions that carry significant risk (Lewis et al, 2004). Patients with stroke caused by thrombi and emboli (ischemic strokes) may also be treated with platelet inhibitors and anticoagulants (after the first 24 hours if treated with t-PA) to prevent the formation of more clots. Common anticoagulants include heparin, enoxaparin (Lovenox), and warfarin (Coumadin). Platelet inhibitors include aspirin, ticlopidine (Ticlid), clopidrogel (Plavix), and dipyridamole (Persantine).

Drugs to reduce intracranial pressure, such as dexamethasone (Decadron), may be given. Suppositories such as bisacodyl (Dulcolax) are generally prescribed to be given daily or every other day. However, some physicians order stool softeners, laxatives, or enemas.

Fluids may be restricted for the first few days after a stroke in an effort to prevent edema of the brain. The patient will be fed intravenous fluids, or a nasogastric or gastrostomy tube may be inserted and tube feedings begun.

The length of time the patient remains in bed depends entirely on the type of stroke suffered, deficits noted, and the judgment of the physician in regard to early mobilization. Some physicians prescribe fairly long periods of rest after strokes, whereas others believe in early mobilization—1 or 2 days after the accident has occurred.

Nursing Interventions

Goals in the initial phase are directed toward preventing neurological deficits. Neurological assessment is done at regular intervals but at least once each shift to detect changes in status and any complications such as worsening stroke. Some patients may be unconscious as a result of increased intracranial pressure and will need total care (Clinical Pathway box).

Because nutrition is a concern and the patient may have great difficulty in swallowing at first, tube feedings, as well as intravenous fluids, may be necessary, unless the patient is more alert. See the section on motor and sensory problems for a discussion of techniques to assist in feeding the patient with dysphagia.

If the patient is responsive after the onset of the stroke, the nurse needs to help the patient assume as much self-care as possible. This includes teaching the patient one-handed dressing techniques and one-handed feeding techniques if motor deficits have occurred. It is important to reinforce teaching by other members of the patient's health team.

The patient with a stroke may be incontinent at first. It is important to remove the urinary catheter (if there is one) as soon as possible to prevent urinary tract infection. The patient should be put on a bladder training program to assist in regaining continence. This usually includes taking the patient to the bathroom every few hours and encouraging fluids (at least 2000 mL per day). The patient's normal bowel pattern before the stroke needs to be assessed and included in the nursing care plan if possible. If the patient has difficulty with communication, the use of a picture of a bathroom or toilet can be useful.

Return of motor impulses and movement in involved extremities occurs in stages, lasting from hours to months. Recovery may also halt at a specific stage and progress no further. Return of function is significant for functional use of extremities but also increases the possibility of contractures. Appropriate nursing interventions to prevent contractures include passive exercise, active exercise, strength-building of the unaffected side, and early ambulation to promote the return of muscle function.

One approach to positioning the patient with a stroke is the **Bobath approach,** a treatment approach designed to normalize muscle tone by providing as many sensations of normal muscle tone, posture, and movement as possible. The goal of the treatment is to redirect short-term memory toward an appreciation of normal movement of the paralyzed side by incorporating techniques of weight bearing, counterrotation, and protraction of the shoulder girdle and pelvis. The reader is referred to a rehabilitation nursing text for further description of this technique. Nurses in rehabilitation settings are often taught this approach.

Patients may experience a loss of proprioception with a stroke. Neurological deficits of apraxia and ag-

CLINICAL PATHWAY | *Stroke*

DRG #: 014 EXPECTED LOS: 6

	DAY OF ADMISSION DAY 1	DAY 2	DAY 3	DAY 4	DAY 5	DISCHARGE TO HOME/ REHABILITATION DAY 6
Diagnostic Tests	CBC, UA, SMA/18,* ABGs, PT, INR/PTT, ECG, CT scan, MRI, chest film	PT, INR/PTT, ECHO, carotid Doppler	PT, INR/PTT, ?Arteriogram	PT, INR/PTT	SMA/6,† PT, INR/PTT, CT scan or MRI	PT, INR
Medications	IVs, thrombolytic (t-PA); when indicated; heparin; antihypertensive drugs if necessary	IVs, heparin	IV to saline lock; heparin	IV saline lock; heparin titrated; Coumadin	IV saline lock; Disc heparin; Coumadin	Disc saline lock; Coumadin
Treatment	I&O q8h; VS and neurological assessment q1h × 4, then q2h × 4, then q4h; telemetry, wt, O₂; assess skin and mouth and special care q2h; ROM to all extremities; assess for safety needs; ELS	I&O q8h including % of nutrition consumed; VS and neurological assessment q4h; telemetry, O₂; assess skin and mouth and special care q2h; ROM q2h; ELS; initiate bowel/bladder training if needed	I&O q8h including % of nutrition consumed; VS and neurological assessment q6h; telemetry, wt, O₂; assess skin and mouth q2h; ROM q4h; ELS	I&O q8h; VS and neurological assessment q8h; disc telemetry, disc O₂, ROM q4h; ELS	I&O q8h; VS and neurological assessments q8h; wt, ROM q4h; ELS	Disc I&O, VS and neurological assessment q8h; ROM q4h
Diet	NPO; assess swallowing ability, if unaffected clear liquids	Clear liquids; if tolerated, advance to full liquids	Full liquids; advance to soft diet as tolerated	Soft diet	Regular diet	Regular diet
Activity	Bed rest; HOB elevated 30 degrees while in bed; T & DB q2h	Bed rest, HOB elevated 30 degrees while in bed; T & DB q2h	Bed rest; up in chair with assistance × 1, HOB elevated 30 degrees; T & DB q2h	Up in chair with assistance × 2; HOB elevated 30 degrees; T & DB q2h	Ambulate with assistance × 2; up in chair × 4	Up ad lib
Consultations	Rehabilitation team	Physical therapy; occupational and speech therapy, dietary, social services	Continue with rehabilitation; SNU/ home health	Continue with rehabilitation	Continue with rehabilitation	Continue with rehabilitation

ABGs, Arterial blood gases; *disc,* discontinue; *ECHO,* echocardiography; *ELS,* elastic leg stockings; *HOB,* head of bed; *LOS,* length of stay; *PT,* prothrombin time; *INR,* International Normalized Ratio; *PTT,* partial thromboplastin time; *ROM,* range of motion; *SMA,* sequential multiple analysis; *SNU,* skilled nursing unit; *T & DB,* turn and deep breathe; *UA,* urinalysis; *VS,* vital signs; *wt,* weight.

*Serum calcium, phosphorus, triglycerides, uric acid, creatinine; BUN, total bilirubin, alkaline phosphate, aspartate aminotransferase (AST) (formerly serum glutamic-oxaloacetic transaminase [SGOT]), alanine aminotransferase (ALT) (formerly serum glutamate pyruvate transaminase [SGPT]), lactic dehydrogenase (LDH), total protein, albumin, sodium, potassium, chloride, total CO₂, glucose.

†Serum sodium, potassium, chloride, total CO₂, glucose, BUN.

nosia (a total or partial loss of the ability to recognize familiar objects or people) may also occur. The nurse can assist the patient with activities by repeating directions and demonstrating care. If the patient has hemianopia, which is common, the patient should be approached from the nonparalyzed side for care. The patient should be taught to scan past midline to the side where there is the deficit. These patients may also fail to recognize that they have a paralyzed side. This is called **unilateral neglect** (described earlier). This patient must be taught to inspect this side of the body for injury and to protect it from harm. These patients often show poor judgment and may move impulsively or unsafely. The need to be observed for this and safety precautions should be taken if needed until the patient can learn to compensate for this lack of judgment. Crying or emotional lability is common. Patients who have had a stroke may have difficulty controlling their emotions. Emotional responses may be exaggerated or unpredictable. Depression and feelings associated with changes in body image and loss of function can make this worse. Patients may also be frustrated by mobility and communication problems.

It is important to foster the patient's sense of self-esteem. The nurse must always treat the patient as an adult, not as a child. The patient's successful efforts and gains in self-care should be praised and reinforced.

Communication problems. Many stroke patients have speech problems, including dysarthria and aphasia. A speech pathologist will evaluate and treat the patient with language disorders. The patient may be frustrated and should be approached in an unhurried manner. Often the patient does much better with communication when not feeling pressured to speak. The nurse may find that giving the patient a communication board is helpful. The nurse should wait for the patient to communicate, rather than prompting or finishing the sentence before the patient has a chance to find the appropriate word. Inability to articulate does not mean that the patient has decreased cognitive abilities.

The nursing diagnoses and interventions for the patient who has had a stroke include but are not limited to the following:

NURSING DIAGNOSES	NURSING INTERVENTIONS
Impaired verbal communication, related to ischemic injury	Speak slowly and distinctly. Ask questions that can be answered by yes or no (or by signals). Try to anticipate patient needs. Provide call signal within reach of unaffected hand. Begin speech therapy as soon as possible.

NURSING DIAGNOSES	NURSING INTERVENTIONS
Imbalanced nutrition: less than body requirements, related to impaired ability to swallow	Provide IV fluids and tube feedings as prescribed during initial period. Assess ability to swallow before initiating feedings. Position patient with head elevated and turned to unaffected side when feeding patient. Provide foods initially that are easier to swallow (soft or pureed foods except for mashed potatoes). Use training cup or feeding syringe for fluids as necessary. Inspect mouth for food trapped in cheek pockets. Be patient when feeding patient and provide directions for swallowing as needed. Encourage patient to feed self as soon as possible; provide self-help devices as necessary.

Patient Teaching

Teaching for a patient with a stroke should include techniques to compensate for the deficits suffered as a result of the stroke. In this the nurse functions as part of the rehabilitation team. This rehabilitation must start at the time of admission to the acute care facility. The patient will probably be attending occupational and physical therapy and may need speech therapy. Depending on the patient's status, the patient's rehabilitation potential, and available resources, the patient may be transferred to a rehabilitation facility or unit.

If the patient is receiving medications (e.g., for hypertension or anticoagulation), it is important to teach the patient and/or family about side effects and the schedule for taking the medication. Plans for follow-up should be discussed. The patient and/or family may be referred to a stroke club for support.

The patient's family needs to be taught techniques to enhance safety and communication. If the patient has a problem with dysphagia, the family needs to be taught appropriate techniques. Because of the chronicity of caring for the stroke patient there is a high risk for caregiver stress. Referral to an appropriate stroke support group is needed. Instructions should be written out for the patient or family to refer to after discharge. Most rehabilitation centers will also include therapeutic leaves as a way to test the family's skills and knowledge. Each pass or leave has specific goals, and feedback is obtained from the family about additional teaching that may be needed. The family and patient should also be educated about the perceptual problems associated with stroke, along with techniques that compensate for these deficits (e.g., writing down instructions for the patient who has trouble carrying out an activity alone).

Prognosis

The prognosis for patients with a stroke depends on the size of the lesion in the brain as well as the patient's premorbid status. With therapy, significant functional gains can be made, even when paralysis or weakness continues. Many patients are able to return home and even remain independent after a stroke. With new medical treatment for selected patients, using tissue plasminogen activator for thrombolysis, the prognosis is greatly improved.

CRANIAL AND PERIPHERAL NERVE DISORDERS
TRIGEMINAL NEURALGIA
Etiology/Pathophysiology

Trigeminal neuralgia is one specific kind of peripheral nerve problem. It is caused by degeneration of or pressure on the fifth cranial nerve, and its etiology is unknown. It is also called **tic douloureux.** It usually affects people in middle or late adulthood and is slightly more common in women.

Clinical Manifestations

Trigeminal neuralgia is characterized by excruciating, knifelike, or lightninglike shock in the lips, upper or lower gums, cheek, forehead, or side of the nose. The pain radiates along one or more of the three divisions of the fifth cranial nerve (Figure 14-20). The fifth cranial nerve has both motor and sensory branches. In trigeminal neuralgia the sensory or afferent branches, primarily the maxillary and mandibular branches, are involved. The pain typically extends only to the midline of the face and head because this is the extent of the tissue supplied by the offending nerve. The attacks are usually brief, lasting only seconds to 2 to 3 minutes and are generally unilateral. Recurrences are unpredictable; they may occur several times a day or weeks or months apart. There are areas along the course of the nerve known as **trigger points,** and the slightest stimulation of these areas may initiate pain. People with trigeminal neuralgia try desperately to avoid triggering them. Precipitating stimuli include chewing, toothbrushing, a hot or cold blast of air on the face, washing the face, yawning, or even talking.

Medical Management

Carbamazepine (Tegretol), phenytoin (Dilantin), valproate (Depakene), and gabapentin (Neurontin) are the drugs of choice for the treatment of trigeminal neuralgia pain. Absolute alcohol may be injected into the peripheral branches of the trigeminal nerve. This provides relief for weeks to months.

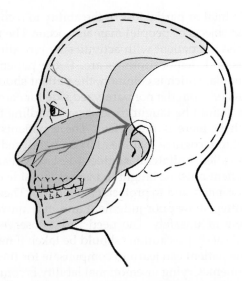

FIGURE **14-20** Pathway of trigeminal nerve and facial areas innervated by each of the three main divisions of this nerve.

Permanent relief of pain is obtained only by surgery that involves inserting a fine needle through the cheek and injecting an alcohol solution or surgically resecting the sensory root of the trigeminal nerve. This is not always successful. Within 24 hours after a fifth nerve resection, many patients develop herpes simplex of the lips (cold sores). Usually these lesions heal in approximately 1 week.

Nursing Interventions

It is common for patients with trigeminal neuralgia not to have eaten properly for some time because eating causes pain. They may be undernourished and dehydrated. They may not have washed, shaved, or combed the hair for some time. Oral hygiene often has been neglected. Measures to increase comfort for patients before surgery or for patients being treated nonsurgically are in Box 14-2.

Box 14-2 | *Comfort Measures for Patients with Trigeminal Neuralgia*

1. Keep room free of drafts.
2. Avoid walking briskly to bedside of patient.
3. Place bed out of traffic area to prevent jarring of bed.
4. Avoid touching the patient's face.
5. Do not urge patients to wash or shave the affected area or to comb the hair.
6. Avoid hot or cold liquids, which trigger pain.
7. Puree food and ensure that it is lukewarm. If necessary, suggest that food be taken through a straw.

Prognosis

The acute pain seldom lasts more than a few seconds or 2 or 3 minutes, but it is excruciating. The onset of pain can occur at any time during the day or night and may recur several times daily for weeks at a time. Some patients will have more or less continuous discomfort and sensitivity of the face. Although this condition is considered benign, the severity of the pain and the disruption of lifestyle can result in almost total physical and psychological dysfunction or even suicide. Permanent relief of pain is obtained only by surgery.

Another common type of peripheral nerve disorder is polyneuritis caused by alcoholism and vitamin deficiency.

BELL'S PALSY (PERIPHERAL FACIAL PARALYSIS)
Etiology/Pathophysiology

Bell's palsy is thought to be caused by an inflammatory process involving the facial nerve (VII) anywhere from the nucleus in the brain to the periphery. Although the exact etiology is not known, there is evidence that reactivated herpes simplex virus (HSV) may be involved in the majority of cases. The reactivation of the HSV causes inflammation, edema, ischemia, and eventual demyelination of the facial nerve VII, creating pain and disturbances in motor and sensory function. Any of the three branches of the facial nerve may be affected. The disorder can be unilateral or bilateral.

Clinical Manifestations

With Bell's palsy there is usually an abrupt onset of numbness or a feeling of stiffness or drawing sensation of the face. Unilateral weakness of the facial muscles usually occurs, resulting in inability to wrinkle the forehead, close the eyelid, pucker the lips, or retract the mouth on that side. The face appears asymmetric, with drooping of the mouth and cheek. Other symptoms that may occur include the following:

- Loss of taste
- Reduction of saliva on affected side
- Pain behind the ear
- Ringing in ear or other hearing loss

Medical Management

There is no specific therapy for Bell's palsy. Electrical stimulation or warm moist heat along the course of the nerve may be helpful. Stimulation may maintain muscle tone and prevent atrophy. Corticosteroids, especially prednisone, are started immediately, and the best results are obtained if corticosteroids are initiated before paralysis is complete. Because the herpes simplex virus is implicated in approximately 70% of cases of Bell's palsy, treatment with acyclovir (Zovirax), alone or in conjunction with prednisone, is used.

Newer drugs to treat HSV, including valacyclovir (Valtrex) and famciclovir (Famvir), have also been used in the management of Bell's palsy.

Nursing Interventions

Protection of the eye when the eyelid does not close is important. Massage of the affected areas is sometimes recommended. Exercises may be prescribed for 5 minutes 3 times a day. These include wrinkling the brow and forehead, closing the eyes, and puffing out the cheeks.

Prognosis

Some 85% of patients recover fully in weeks or months, although recovery may take as long as a year, with recovery of taste being the first sign of improvement. Recovery of taste within the first week signals a good chance for full recovery of motor function. This favorable prognostic sign also holds true if paralysis remains incomplete within the first 5 to 7 days. The remaining 15% of patients continue to be bothered by asymmetric movement of facial muscles.

INFECTION AND INFLAMMATION
Etiology/Pathophysiology

Interference with function because of infection or inflammation is a common occurrence. Some specific conditions include meningitis, encephalitis, brain abscess, Guillain-Barré syndrome, herpes zoster, neurosyphilis, poliomyelitis, and AIDS. Only Guillain-Barré syndrome, meningitis, encephalitis, brain abscess, and AIDS will be discussed in this chapter.

The nervous system may be affected by a variety of organisms and may suffer from toxins of bacteria and viruses. These toxins reach the nervous system from a variety of sources, including adjacent bones, blood, or lymph. Meningitis can occur as a result of an invasive procedure such as surgery.

Assessment

Subjective and objective assessments are important in any patient who has infection of the nervous system. Collection of **subjective data** includes a history of infection, such as an upper respiratory infection, and the presence of discomfort that may include headache or stiff neck. The initial onset of symptoms, any difficulty in thinking, and the presence of weakness may be important. The patient's understanding of the condition should be assessed.

Collection of **objective data** includes behavioral signs indicating discomfort or disorientation as well as an inability to carry out ADLs. The physical assessment part of the neurological assessment may reveal abnormalities; the presence of a fever, vomiting, abnormal CT results, seizures, altered respiratory patterns, tachycardia, or meningeal irritation is significant. The patient's level of consciousness and orientation should be assessed.

Diagnostic Tests

Many of the infections of the nervous system can be diagnosed by examining the CSE. A CT scan or an EEG may also be done.

Nursing Interventions and Patient Teaching

Nursing diagnoses and interventions for the patient with an infection or inflammation are the same as those for the patient who has had a stroke, with the addition of but not limited to the following:

NURSING DIAGNOSES	NURSING INTERVENTIONS
Hyperthermia, related to inflammatory response to CNS infection	Assess temperature every 2 hours and prn. Provide cooling measures prn; avoid cooling to point of shivering. Administer antipyretics as ordered. Administer antibiotics as ordered. Monitor parenteral fluids as ordered. Control exposure to extremes in temperature. Assess TPR every 2 hours as indicated.
Disturbed thought processes, related to neurophysiologic response to infection	Protect patient from self-injury. Provide soft safety reminder devices to prevent injury. Introduce self to patient and establish rapport to prevent agitation. Relate date, time of day, and recent activities. Speak in kind tone, using short, simple sentences. Maintain a therapeutic environment.

Education for the patient with an infection includes teaching about the disease process, the treatments involved, and the expected outcomes. If the patient is seriously ill, the initial teaching focuses on the family. Other aspects of teaching for motor and sensory problems may also be relevant for the patient with an infection or inflammation, depending on the signs and symptoms demonstrated.

GUILLAIN-BARRÉ SYNDROME (POLYNEURITIS)
Etiology/Pathophysiology

Guillain-Barré (GĒ-yă bă-RĀ) syndrome (GBS) is also called **acute inflammatory polyradiculopathy** or **postinfectious polyneuritis.** It results in widespread inflammation and demyelination of the peripheral nervous system.

The peripheral nervous system is composed of 31 pairs of spinal nerves, 12 pairs of cranial nerves, and various plexuses and ganglia. Each nerve cell, or neuron, is composed of several parts, including the axon.

Responsible for transmitting nerve impulses, axons are wrapped in segments of insulation called the myelin sheath, which is composed of Schwann cells.

In GBS the antibodies attack the Schwann cells, causing the sheath to break down—a process called demyelination—and the uninsulated portion of the nerve to become inflamed. Nerve conduction is interrupted, causing the classic signs of muscle weakness, tingling, and numbness, which begin in the legs or feet and work their way upward. It is possible that the signals to and from the legs are most vulnerable to interruption because they have to travel the longest distance. Perhaps that is why symptoms appear there first, and progress upward. The demyelination is self-limiting. Once it stops, the Schwann cells rebuild the lost insulation. Remyelination, and therefore recovery, occurs in reverse; it starts at the top of the body and proceeds downward.

The disease affects people of all ages and is seen equally in men and women. It affects 1.5 people in 100,000 each year. The cause is unknown but is thought to be a viral agent or an autoimmune reaction. More than half of the individuals affected have had a nonspecific infection 10 to 14 days before the onset of the disease. Many people developed the signs and symptoms after receiving swine flu vaccine in the early 1980s.

Clinical Manifestations

There is variation in the pattern of the onset of weakness as well as in the rate of progression of signs and symptoms. The progression may stop at any point. The patient may have difficulty swallowing, breathing, and speaking if cranial nerves VII, IX, and X are involved. Symmetrical muscle weakness and lower motoneuron paralysis are present. The paralysis usually starts in the lower extremities and moves upward to include the thorax, upper extremities, and face. Respiratory failure may occur if the intercostal muscles are affected. A fluctuating blood pressure may occur as a result of effects on the autonomic nervous system.

Diagnostic Tests

Guillain-Barré syndrome is diagnosed by elimination of other reasons for the signs and symptoms as well as by the characteristic muscle weakness. A CT scan may be ordered to rule out tumors or a stroke. Changes in the respiratory status may aid in the diagnosis. A lumbar puncture will be done.

Cerebrospinal fluid in patients with GBS commonly has elevated protein levels. The physician may order a nerve conduction velocity study to test for slow impulse transmission. An electromyography that records muscle activity is also helpful. A history of a recent infection is considered important.

Medical Management

Once GBS is suspected, hospitalization is essential. The patient's condition can rapidly deteriorate into paralysis that affects the respiratory muscles.

Adrenocortical steroids are used to treat the signs and symptoms of Guillain-Barré syndrome. It has also been found that therapeutic plasmapheresis (the removal of unwanted or pathologic components from the patient's blood serum by means of a continuous-flow separator) leads to decreased severity and length of symptoms. An alternative to plasmapheresis is intravenous immune globulin (Gamimune N).

Patients who develop respiratory failure require mechanical ventilation and may require a tracheostomy. Arterial blood gas monitoring and pulmonary function tests are used to assess the respiratory status. If the patient has severe paralysis and is expected to have a long recovery period, a gastrostomy tube may be placed to provide adequate nourishment.

Nursing Interventions

Close monitoring of respiratory function is important and necessary. If the patient requires mechanical ventilation, the nurse must be aware that cognition (the mental faculty or process by which knowledge is acquired) is not impaired and that the patient will require reassurance. The patient may also require nutritional maintenance intravenously or through a nasogastric tube. Attention to the prevention of complications, such as contractures, pressure ulcers, and loss of ROM is important to allow complete recovery. Physical therapy should be initiated early in the course of the disease to prevent contractures. Administer medication to help reduce neuropathic pain, such as gabapentin (Neurontin) or a tricyclic antidepressant such as amitriptyline (Elavil). Vital signs and the motor strength of the patient should be assessed frequently. The patient must be monitored for signs of hypoxia.

Prognosis

Of the people suffering from Guillain-Barré syndrome, 85% will regain complete function. Only 20% of patients will have weakness at 1 year and only 5% have severe permanent disability. The recovery period may vary from weeks to years. Those not recovering completely have some degree of permanent neurological deficit. Generally, recovery from the disease occurs in the reverse order of how the paralysis or weakness occurred.

MENINGITIS
Etiology/Pathophysiology

Meningitis is an acute infection of the meninges. It is usually caused by one of several organisms, including pneumococci, meningococci, staphylococci, streptococci, *Haemophilus influenzae,* and viral aseptic agents. The effect of the bacteria in the subarachnoid space is an inflammatory reaction in the pia mater and arachnoid and pus accumulates in the CSE, and the bacteria may injure nervous tissue.

Meningitis can be classified as bacterial or aseptic. The incidence of bacterial meningitis is higher in fall and winter when upper respiratory tract infections are common. Pathologic changes that can occur include hyperemia of the meningeal vessels, edema of brain tissue, increased intracranial pressure, a generalized inflammatory reaction with exudation of white blood cells into the subarachnoid spaces, and associated hydrocephalus (in infants) caused by exudate occluding the ventricles.

Clinical Manifestations

Two abnormal signs that occur with meningitis are **Kernig's sign** (the inability to extend the legs completely without extreme pain) and **Brudzinski's sign** (flexion of the hip and knee when the neck is flexed). The onset of meningitis is usually sudden and is characterized by severe headache, stiffness of the neck, irritability, malaise, and restlessness. Nausea, vomiting, and delirium develop, as well as increased temperature, pulse rate, and respirations.

Diagnostic Tests

Meningitis is diagnosed by examining the CSF. A culture and sensitivity test is done to ascertain the pathogenic organism. A CT scan of the head and an EEG are also ordered.

Medical Management

Treatment of meningitis consists of massive doses of antibiotics. Multiple antibiotics are often used. Ampicillin, penicillin, and a third-generation cephalosporin (usually ceftriaxone [Rocephin] or cefotaxime [Claforan]) are the drugs of choice for treating meningitis. These drugs are effective because of their ability to penetrate the blood-brain barrier. The medication is usually given intravenously or intrathecally. Hyperosmolar agents or steroids may be needed to decrease intracranial pressure. Anticonvulsants may be given to prevent seizures.

Nursing Interventions

Respiratory isolation is required until the pathogen can no longer be cultured from the nasopharynx. This is usually accomplished after 24 hours of effective antibiotic therapy. Other nursing interventions include the general care given a critically ill patient who may be irritable, disoriented, and unable to take fluids. Dehydration is common, and the patient almost always has an intravenous line. The room is kept darkened and noise is kept to a minimum because any increase in sensory stimulation may cause a seizure. If the patient is disoriented, safety precautions need to be taken, including safety reminder devices if needed.

Prognosis

With most cases of meningitis, the prognosis for complete recovery is good. The prognosis depends on the quickness with which antibiotics are administered. With severe cases of meningitis, there may be residual neurological damage or death.

ENCEPHALITIS

Encephalitis is an acute inflammation of the brain and is usually caused by a virus. Many different viruses have been implicated in encephalitis; some are associated with certain seasons of the year and endemic to certain geographic areas. Epidemic encephalitis is transmitted by ticks and mosquitoes. Nonepidemic encephalitis may occur as a complication of measles, chickenpox, or mumps.

Encephalitis is a serious, and sometimes fatal, disease. Overall mortality rate ranges from 5% to 20%, with the highest mortality rate in encephalitis caused by herpes simplex virus (HSV) and the eastern and Venezuelan equine viruses. Unfortunately, HSV encephalitis is the most common form of viral encephalitis. Cytomegalovirus encephalitis is one of the common complications in patients with acquired immunodeficiency syndrome.

Manifestations resemble those of meningitis, but they have a more gradual onset. They include headache, high fever, seizures, and a change in level of consciousness. Early diagnosis and treatment of viral encephalitis is essential for favorable outcomes. Brain imaging techniques such as MRI and PET, along with viral studies of cerebrospinal fluid, allow for earlier detection of viral encephalitis.

Medical management and nursing interventions are symptomatic and supportive. Cerebral edema is a major problem, and diuretics (mannitol) and corticosteroids (dexamethasone [Decadron]) are used to control it. The disease is characterized by diffuse damage to the nerve cells of the brain, perivascular cellular infiltration of glial cells, and increasing cerebral edema. The sequelae of encephalitis include mental deterioration, amnesia, personality changes, and hemiparesis.

Acyclovir (Zovirax) and vidarabine (Vira-A) are used to treat encephalitis caused by herpes simplex virus infection. Acyclovir has fewer side effects than vidarabine and is often the preferred treatment. Use of these antiviral agents has been shown to reduce mortality rates from 70% to 30%, although neurological complications may not be reduced. Long-term symptoms include memory impairment, epilepsy, anosmia, personality changes, behavioral abnormalities, and dysphasia. For maximal benefit, antiviral agents should be started before the onset of coma.

WEST NILE VIRUS

West Nile virus (WNV) has been commonly found in humans and birds and other vertebrates in Africa, Eastern Europe, western Asia, and the Middle East, but it was not documented in the United States until 1999. The virus can infect humans, birds, mosquitoes, horses, and some other animals.

The principal route of human infection with West Nile virus is through the bite of an infected female mosquito. Mosquitoes become infected when they feed on infected birds. When the virus is injected into humans by a mosquito, it can multiply and possibly cause illness. The incubation period ranges from 3 to 14 days. Most people who become infected with the virus will not have any type of illness. Those who develop West Nile fever have flulike manifestations of fever, headache, back pain, myalgias, and anorexia, lasting only a few days and without any long-term health effects. It is estimated that 1 in 150 people infected with West Nile virus will develop encephalitis or meningitis, a more severe form of the disease. **West Nile viral meningitis** is usually associated with a sudden onset of febrile illness, headache, chills, neck pain, and sometimes confusion. Patients with **West Nile viral encephalitis** often present with fever, headache, altered level of consciousness, disorientation, behavioral and speech disturbances, and other neurological signs such as hemiparesis, seizures, and coma. Advanced age is the most significant risk factor contributing to death from infection; conditions such as immunosuppression are also contributing factors (Bender, 2003). Even in areas where the virus is circulating, however, very few mosquitoes are infected with the virus. The chances of becoming severely ill from any one mosquito bite are extremely small.

The current standard for diagnosing WNV is by testing blood or cerebrospinal fluid with the IgM antibody capture enzyme-linked immunosorbent assay (ELISA) and IgG indirect ELISA. The IgM test may not be positive when symptoms first occur; however, it becomes positive in most infected people within days of symptom onset. Someone recently vaccinated against yellow fever or Japanese encephalitis also will have a positive IgM antibody test result.

West Nile virus cannot be transmitted through casual contact such as touching or kissing a person who has the disease. However, in a small number of cases, the virus has been transmitted through blood transfusion, organ transplantation, breastfeeding, and pregnancy (from mother to fetus).

One can reduce the risk of becoming infected with West Nile virus by applying insect repellent to exposed skin. Choose an insect repellent that contains *N,N*-diethyl-3-methylbenzamide (DEET) and one that provides protection for the amount of time to be spent outdoors. Also spray clothing, because mosquitoes can bite through thin clothing. Wearing long-sleeved shirts, long pants, and socks while outdoors can reduce the risk. Take special precautions from April to October, the months when mosquitoes are most active.

The ingredient *N,N*-diethyl-3-methylbenzamide (DEET) is the gold standard in currently available over-the-counter insect repellents. DEET was developed in 1946 by the U.S. Army for use by military personnel in insect-infested areas. It's been used worldwide for more than 40 years and has a remarkable safety profile. Toxic reactions can occur, and they're usually linked to misuse of the product, such as massive exposure to chronic use. Reports of greatest concern involve encephalopathy caused by DEET exposure. Most adverse reactions, though, are less serious, involving eye irritation and inhalation irritation (related to spraying repellent in the eyes or inhaling it).

DEET has been classified as a group D carcinogen (not classifiable as a human carcinogen). For casual use, a 10% to 35% concentration provides adequate protection. The American Academy of Pediatrics recommends limiting DEET repellents to a 30% maximum concentration when used on infants and children. DEET is not recommended for use in children younger than the age of 2 months. (Centers for Disease Control and Prevention. Division of Vector-Borne Infectious Disease, West Nile virus, http://www.cdc.gov/ncidod/dvbid/westnile/ga/testing_treating.htm; accessed January 22, 2004.)

Other means of decreasing the mosquito population and thus decreasing the possibility of transmission of the West Nile Virus includes:

* Limit outdoor activities between dusk and dawn.
* Place mosquito netting over infant carriers/strollers when outdoors.
* Keep swimming pools, outdoor saunas, and hot tubs clean and properly chlorinated. Remove standing water from pool covers.
* Turn plastic wading pools and wheelbarrows upside down when not in use.
* Change the water in birdbaths once a week.
* Make sure roof gutters drain properly and water doesn't stand in them.
* Drill holes in the bottom of recycling containers that are left outdoors.
* Store any containers that may become filled with standing water, such as cans, flowerpots, or trash cans, indoors.
* Install or repair window and door screens so that mosquitoes can't get indoors (Overstreet, 2003).

If WNV infection is confirmed, treatment is supportive, intended to manage symptoms, such as headache, fever, and nausea. In more severe cases, patients may need intensive therapy, often involving hospitalization for intravenous fluids, airway management, respiratory support, and prevention of secondary infections such as pneumonia. To manage WNV encephalitis, the patient may receive interferon alfa-2$_b$, steroids, antiseizure medications, or osmotic diuretics.

Approximately 80% of WNV infections are asymptomatic. Infected people have a transient viremia, making transmission of the virus via donated blood, organs, or tissue possible. As with many viruses, contact with the blood of an infected person could lead to transmission of the virus; therefore, use the same standard precautions as with all patients.

Since July 2003, more than 2.5 million blood donations have been screened for WNV. As of September 16, 2003, the Centers for Disease Control and Prevention's surveillance system reported that 601 viremic donations had been identified.

Two cases of blood transfusion–associated WNV infection were detected in the United States in 2003—one in Texas and one in Nebraska. Both people were receiving care, including blood transfusions, for other serious health conditions. They developed encephalitis from the WNV infection; both recovered (Goldrick, 2003).

BRAIN ABSCESS

Brain abscess is an accumulation of pus within the brain tissue that can result from a local or a systemic infection. Direct extension from ear, tooth, mastoid, or sinus infection is the primary cause. Other causes for brain abscess formation include septic venous thrombosis from a pulmonary infection, infective endocarditis, skull fracture, and a nonsterile neurological procedure. Streptococci and staphylococci are the primary infective organisms.

Clinical manifestations are similar to those of meningitis and encephalitis and include headache and fever. Signs of increased ICP may include drowsiness, confusion, and seizures. Focal symptoms may be present and reflect the local area of the abscess. For example, visual field defects or psychomotor seizures are common with a temporal lobe abscess, whereas an occipital abscess may be accompanied by visual impairment and hallucinations.

Antimicrobial therapy is the primary treatment for brain abscess. Other manifestations are treated symptomatically. If drug therapy is not effective, the abscess may need to be removed if it is encapsulated. In untreated cases the mortality rate approaches 100%. Seizures occur in approximately 30% of the cases. Nursing interventions are similar to those for management of meningitis or increased ICP. If surgical removal is the treatment of choice, nursing interventions are similar to those described under intracranial tumors.

Other infections of the brain include subdural empyema, osteomyelitis of the cranial bones, epidural abscess, and venous sinus thrombosis after periorbital cellulitis.

ACQUIRED IMMUNODEFICIENCY SYNDROME
Etiology/Pathophysiology

Acquired immunodeficiency syndrome (AIDS) is a disease that has serious implications for the nervous system, with more than 80% of advanced HIV disease patients having neurological signs and symptoms. Patients develop neurological signs and symptoms either as a result of infection with HIV itself or as a result of associated infections. See Chapter 16 for a discussion of advanced HIV disease (AIDS).

Clinical Manifestations

Patients with AIDS may have ADC (AIDS dementia complex), which is known as subacute encephalitis. This may be manifested as difficulty in concentrating or a recent memory loss, which may progress to a global cognitive dysfunction (generalized impairment of intellect, awareness, and judgment). Patients may also experience opportunistic infections such as meningitis, herpes simplex, cytomegalovirus, toxoplasmosis, and cryptococcal meningitis. Primary malignant lymphomas of the CNS may also develop.

Diagnostic Tests

The diagnostic tests used to determine whether a neurological problem is related to AIDS include serologic studies, analysis of CSF through a lumbar puncture, CT scan, and MRI. At times, a cerebral biopsy may be necessary to make the differential diagnosis.

Medical Management

Treatment of the patient with neurological problems related to AIDS depends on the nature of the infection. Various methods of treatment have included administration of antiviral, antifungal, and antibacterial agents. Radiation has been used on the affected part of the brain. Experimental therapies including iron dextran (DexFerrum) have been attempted. Dehydration or shock is treated with fluid volume expanders. Seizures are controlled with diazepam (Valium), phenytoin (Dilantin), or fosphenytoin (Cerebyx). Mortality remains high despite aggressive therapy.

Nursing Interventions

The patient is likely to be disoriented and may need to be reoriented frequently. Safety measures such as padded side rails may be necessary to prevent injury to the patient, who may have seizures.

The patient may experience pain and have difficulty sleeping. It is important to administer medications to patients as needed and to structure activities to avoid waking them. The patient may also have visual problems associated with the disease, and the nurse must be careful to orient the patient to nursing interventions.

Most patients with AIDS experience depression and powerlessness about the nature of the disease. They may isolate themselves from others. Patients should be encouraged to talk about their fears and concerns, be assisted to find emotional support, and be referred to a support group. The nurse needs to maintain a nonjudgmental attitude.

The patient may be incontinent of bowel and bladder. It is important to encourage an active bowel and bladder program. If the patient is experiencing diarrhea, it is important to keep the rectal area as clean and dry as possible and administer antidiarrheals if ordered. The patient may also have difficulty with nausea. Foods that the patient likes should be offered in small, frequent meals. Tube feedings or total parenteral nutrition may be needed if the patient agrees.

Prognosis

The prognosis for the patient with AIDS is terminal, often within a short time. Currently, there is little that can be done to substantially lengthen life. After a patient experiences neurological complications, AIDS is usually fairly well advanced.

INTRACRANIAL TUMORS
Etiology/Pathophysiology

Intracranial tumors include both benign and metastatic lesions. All areas and structures of the brain can be affected. Primary intracranial tumors, or **neoplasms,** arise from the cells of brain tissue and the primary and pineal glands. These tumors include gliomas, meningiomas, pituitary tumors, and neuromas. Metastatic tumors also occur frequently in the brain. Brain tumors are named for the tissues from which they arise.

Assessment

Collection of **subjective data** includes the patient's understanding of the diagnosis as well as changes in personality or judgment and the presence of abnormal sensations or visual problems. Complaints of unusual odors may be present with tumors of the temporal lobe. Headache, hearing loss, or the inability to carry out daily activities is also important to assess.

Collection of **objective data** includes motor strengths, gait, the level of alertness and consciousness, and orientation. The pupils are assessed for response and equality. The presence of seizures in an adult is significant. Speech abnormalities, cranial nerve abnormalities, and signs and symptoms of increased intracranial pressure are also significant.

Diagnostic Tests

No one procedure is entirely diagnostic of brain tumors, but a CT scan is often the basis for the diagnosis. Other tests that may be performed include the brain scan, MRI, PET scans, and the EEG. Arteriography may also be done.

Medical Management

The general method of treatment for intracranial tumors includes surgical removal when feasible, radiation, and chemotherapy. The choice of therapy is determined by the tumor type and site. A combination of methods is often used.

Surgery. A surgical opening through the skull is called a **craniotomy.** After removal of the bone, an incision is made into the meninges and the tumor is removed. The removed bone is carefully preserved and may be replaced at the end of surgery if there is no indication of infection or increased intracranial pressure. The removal of part of the skull without replacement is called **craniectomy.** Recent advances have been made in the use of intracranial endoscopy.

Nursing Interventions

Preoperative preparation of both the patient and the family is important. Specific fears may be related to a permanent change in appearance, dependency, and possible death. A baseline neurological assessment is important. Treatments and procedures, including the shaving of hair, are explained. Usually hair is shaved in the operating room. It is then given to the patient, who may choose to have it made into a wig. The family needs to be prepared for the appearance of the patient after surgery.

Postoperative care is determined by the patient's condition. Most patients spend one or two nights in an intensive care unit under close nursing observation with frequent neurological checks. The patient should be assessed carefully for indications of increased intracranial pressure. The patient may have residual motor or sensory problems as a result of the tumor or surgery.

Nursing diagnoses and interventions for the patient with a brain tumor are the same as those for the patient who has had a stroke, with the addition of but not limited to the following:

Nursing Diagnoses	Nursing Interventions
Disturbed sensory perception: visual, auditory, kinesthetic, tactile, related to compression/displacement of brain tissue	Maintain method of communication. Provide for social interaction. Maintain safe environment. Provide orientation and appropriate level of stimuli.
Disturbed thought processes, related to altered circulation or destruction of brain tissue	Protect patient from self-injury. Provide soft safety reminder devices as indicated. Assist patient in self-care activities. Speak in kind tone using short, simple sentences. Give one direction at a time. Relate date, time of day, and recent activities. Maintain a therapeutic environment. Keep equipment and personal possessions in same place. Encourage socialization.

Prognosis

The outlook for the patient with a brain tumor depends on whether the tumor is benign or malignant and on the size and location of the mass. Tumors that infiltrate the brain usually result in a decreased life span. With radiation and chemotherapy, patients with malignant tumors may be assisted in living longer.

TRAUMA

Interference with neurological function can occur as a result of trauma. Parts of the nervous system commonly subjected to trauma include the craniocere-brum, the spinal cord, and peripheral nerves. Only the first two will be discussed in this chapter.

CRANIOCEREBRAL TRAUMA
Etiology/Pathophysiology

Craniocerebral trauma, or head injury, causes death or serious disability in people of all ages. Head injury is the second most common cause of neurological injuries and the major cause of death between ages 1 and 35. Causes of head injury include motor vehicle and motorcycle accidents, falls, industrial accidents, assaults, and sports trauma.

Craniocerebral trauma may result in injury to the scalp, skull, and brain tissues. Injuries vary from minor scalp wounds to concussions and open fractures of the skull with severe damage to the brain. The amount of obvious damage is not indicative of the seriousness of the trouble. Effects of severe head injury include cerebral edema, sensory and motor deficits, and increased intracranial pressure.

Injuries to the brain can result from direct or indirect trauma to the head. Indirect trauma is caused by tension strains and shearing forces transmitted to the head by stretching of the neck. Direct trauma occurs when the head is directly injured. This results in an **acceleration-deceleration** injury, with rotation of the skull and its contents. Bruising or contusion of the occipital and frontal lobes and the brainstem and cerebellum may occur.

Clinical Manifestations

Head injuries may be open or closed. Open head injuries result from skull fractures or penetrating wounds. The amount of injury with this type of wound is determined by the velocity, mass, shape, and direction of the impact. A skull fracture (linear, comminuted, depressed, or compound) may also occur. Fractures of the base of the skull are more serious because of their location near the medulla.

Closed head injuries include concussions (a violent jarring of the brain against the skull), contusions, and lacerations. Lacerations of the scalp bleed profusely because of the large vascularity in the region. Hemorrhage resulting from craniocerebral trauma may occur in the following sites: scalp, epidural, subdural, intracerebral, and intraventricular. Epidural and subdural hematomas require careful and continuous observation by the nurse. Epidural hematomas resulting from arterial bleeding form as blood collects rapidly between the dura and skull. If lethargy or unconsciousness develops after the patient regains consciousness, an epidural hematoma may be suspected and needs immediate treatment.

A subdural hematoma forms as venous blood collects below the dura. Because the bleeding is under venous pressure, the hematoma formation is relatively slow. The clot will cause pressure on the brain surface and will displace brain tissue. If a patient who has been conscious for several days after head injury loses consciousness or develops neurological signs and symptoms, a subdural hematoma should be suspected. Subdural hematomas may be classified as acute, subacute, or chronic.

Assessment

Collection of **subjective data** includes the patient's understanding of the injury and the resulting pathologic processes. Determining how the injury happened and whether the patient has headache, nausea, or vomiting is important. Abnormal sensations and a history of a loss of consciousness and of bleeding from any orifice should be noted.

Collection of **objective data** includes the status of the respiratory system, level of alertness and consciousness, and size and reactivity of the pupils; these should be checked frequently. The nurse also assesses the patient's orientation, motor status, vital signs, the presence of bleeding or vomiting, and abnormal speech patterns. The presence of **Battle's sign** (a small hemorrhagic spot behind the ear) usually is indicative of a fracture of a bone of the lower skull (Figure 14-21, *B*).

Diagnostic Tests

CT, MRI, and PET scanning are the primary diagnostic imaging examinations in assessing soft tissue injuries.

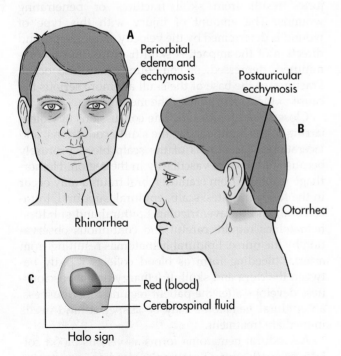

FIGURE **14-21** **A,** Raccoon eyes and rhinorrhea. **B,** Battle's sign (postauricular ecchymosis) with otorrhea. **C,** Halo or ring sign.

Medical Management

Immediate care of the patient with a head injury is directed toward life-saving measures and the maintenance of normal body function until recovery is ensured. It is extremely important to maintain a patent airway and ensure adequate oxygenation. Suctioning may be necessary (but never through the nose because of the possibility of a skull fracture), as well as the administration of oxygen. Arterial blood gas levels are checked.

Medications are used to reduce cerebral edema and increased intracranial pressure, which are common problems in patients with head injuries. Medications include mannitol and dexamethasone. Pegorgotein, a scavenger of oxygen-derived free radicals, has been used experimentally. Codeine or other analgesics that do not depress the respiratory system are used for pain control. Anticonvulsants may be given to prevent seizures. Measures to control elevated temperatures are taken because hyperthermia increases brain metabolism, resulting in brain damage.

Nursing Interventions

Prevention of infection. The patient's ears and nose are checked carefully for signs of blood and serous drainage, which indicate that the meninges are torn and spinal fluid is escaping. No attempt should be made to clean out the orifice. If there is evidence of drainage from the nose, the patient should not cough, sneeze, or blow the nose. If there is a question about whether drainage is CSF, a Tes-Tape will show a positive reaction for sugar. Meningitis is a possible complication when communication with the meninges and the nose or ears occurs.

Emotional support. It is not uncommon that the patient with a head injury shows a loss of memory and loss of initiative. Behavioral problems associated with a lack of judgment and restlessness may also occur. Restlessness in the head-injured patient may be caused by the need for a change of position, pain, or the need to empty the bladder. These patients need firm but gentle care, with specific guidelines for what behavior is allowed. Medications to decrease agitation may be needed. It is not helpful to argue with patients. It may be helpful to redirect their attention. Memory aids such as a log book or written schedule can be very useful in assisting with orientation.

The length of convalescence will depend on the amount of brain damage and how rapid the recovery is. Many patients with head injury will recover physically but will have behavioral and psychological problems that make it difficult for them to function independently.

Nursing diagnosis and interventions for the patient with a head injury are the same as for the patient who has had a stroke, with the addition of but not limited to the following:

NURSING DIAGNOSIS	NURSING INTERVENTIONS
Impaired social interaction, related to cognitive and affective deficits from neurophysiological trauma	Encourage and support verbalization about feelings, medical conditions, and current treatment; listen nonjudgmentally. Build trust through consistency and keep promises. Involve patient in plan of care. Give full attention to patient during verbal interactions and recognize qualities to promote self-esteem.

Patient Teaching

A patient with a mild head injury may be seen in the emergency department but not be admitted to the hospital. Such a patient needs to be taught about observations for complications such as increased drowsiness, nausea, vomiting, worsening headache or stiff neck, seizures, blurred vision, behavioral changes, motor problems, sensory disturbances, or decreased heart rate. Teaching for patients with a head injury and who have residual deficits severe enough to require rehabilitation is similar to that needed for patients with motor or sensory problems.

Prognosis

The outcome for a patient with a head injury is often unpredictable. The extent of damage or recovery is not positively correlated with the amount of damage seen in surgery or on CT scan. Even minor head injuries can result in residual effects. The person with a head injury is more prone to injuries and problems related to the brain damage.

SPINAL CORD TRAUMA
Etiology/Pathophysiology

Spinal cord injury from accidents is a common and increasing cause of serious disability and death. Approximately 10% of traumatic injuries to the nervous system involve the spinal cord. Most people involved with spinal cord injuries are males between 18 and 25 years of age. Automobile, motorcycle, diving, surfing, and other athletic accidents and gunshot wounds are major causes of spinal cord injury.

The soft tissue of the spinal cord is protected by the vertebral column. Injuries that occur to this column include a simple fracture, compressed or wedged fracture, comminuted or burst fractures, or dislocation of the vertebrae (Figure 14-22). As a result the cord is often damaged. Severe traumatic lesions of the spinal cord may result in total transection of the spinal cord or a tearing of the cord from side to side at a particular level, with a complete loss of spinal cord function. This total transection is also called a **complete cord injury.** With this type of injury, all voluntary movement below

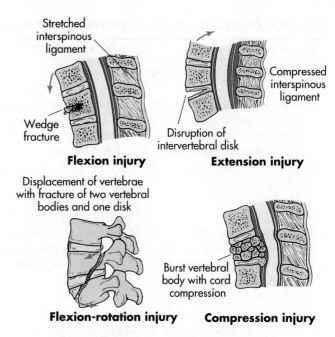

FIGURE **14-22** Mechanisms of spinal injury.

the level of the trauma is lost. A partial transection or **incomplete injury** involves a partial transection or injury of the cord. Quadriplegic patients (now referred to as tetraplegic) are those who sustain injuries to one of the cervical segments of the spinal cord. Paraplegic patients are those whose lesions are confined to the thoracic, lumbar, or sacral segments of the spinal cord. The signs and symptoms of an incomplete injury are variable (Table 14-6).

Clinical Manifestations

Spinal shock. Initially, in most spinal cord injuries, there is a period of flaccid paralysis and a complete loss of reflexes below the trauma. Sensory and autonomic functions are also lost. The loss of systemic sympathetic vasomotor tone may result in vasodilation, increased venous capacity, and hypotension. This is called **areflexia** or spinal shock and is temporary. During this time the patient may need temporary respiratory support.

Autonomic dysreflexia. One complication of spinal cord injury that is extremely important to understand is autonomic dysreflexia or hyperreflexia, a neurological condition characterized by increased reflex actions. It occurs in patients with cord injuries at the sixth thoracic vertebra or higher and most commonly in patients with cervical injuries. **Autonomic dysreflexia** occurs as a result of abnormal cardiovascular response to stimulation of the sympathetic division of the autonomic nervous system as a result of stimulation of the bladder, large intestine, or other visceral organs (Figure 14-23). The clinical signs include severe bradycardia, hypertension (systolic pressure up to 300 mm Hg), di-

Table 14-6 *Functional Level of Spinal Cord Injury and Rehabilitation Potential*

LEVEL OF INJURY	MOVEMENT REMAINING	REHABILITATION POTENTIAL
TETRAPLEGIA		
C1-C3		
Often fatal injury, vagus nerve domination of heart, respiration, blood vessels, and all organs below injury	Movement in neck and above, loss of innervation to diaphragm, absence of independent respiratory function	Ability to drive electric wheelchair equipped with portable ventilator by using chin control or mouth stick, headrest to stabilize head; computer use with mouth stick, head wand, or noise control; 24-hour attendant care, able to instruct others
C4		
Vagus nerve domination of heart, respirations, and all vessels and organs below injury	Sensation and movement in neck and above; may be able to breathe without a ventilator	Same as C1-C3
C5		
Vagus nerve domination of heart, respirations, and all vessels and organs below injury	Full neck, partial shoulder, back, biceps; gross elbow, inability to roll over or use hands; decreased respiratory reserve	Ability to drive electric wheelchair with mobile hand supports; indoor mobility in manual wheelchair; able to feed self with setup and adaptive equipment; attendant care 10 hours per day
C6		
Vagus nerve domination of heart, respirations, and all vessels and organs below injury	Shoulder and upper back abduction and rotation at shoulder, full biceps to elbow flexion, wrist extension, weak grasp of thumb, decreased respiratory reserve	Ability to assist with transfer and perform some self-care; feed self with hand devices; push wheelchair on smooth, flat surface; drive adapted van from wheelchair; independent computer use with adaptive equipment; attendant care 6 hours per day
C7-C8		
Vagus nerve domination of heart, respirations, and all vessels and organs below injury	All triceps to elbow extension, finger extensors and flexors, good grasp with some decreased strength, decreased respiratory reserve	Ability to transfer self to wheelchair; roll over and sit up in bed; push self on most surfaces; perform most self-care; independent use of wheelchair; ability to drive car with powered hand controls (in some patients); attendant care 0 to 6 hours per day
PARAPLEGIA		
T1-T6		
Sympathetic innervation to heart, vagus nerve domination of all vessels and organs below injury	Full innervation of upper extremities, back, essential intrinsic muscles of hand; full strength and dexterity of grasp; decreased trunk stability, decreased respiratory reserve	Full independence in self-care and in wheelchair; ability to drive car with hand controls (in most patients); independent standing in standing frame
T6-T12		
Vagus nerve domination only of leg vessels, GI and genitourinary organs	Full, stable thoracic muscles and upper back; functional intercostals, resulting in increased respiratory reserve	Full independent use of wheelchair; ability to stand erect with full leg brace, ambulate on crutches with swing (although gait difficult); inability to climb stairs

From Lewis, S.M. et al. (2004). *Medical-surgical nursing: assessment and management of clinical problems.* (7th ed.). St. Louis: Mosby.

Table 14-6	*Functional Level of Spinal Cord Injury and Rehabilitation Potential—cont'd*		
LEVEL OF INJURY	**MOVEMENT REMAINING**	**REHABILITATION POTENTIAL**
L1-L2 Vagus nerve domination of leg vessels	Varying control of legs and pelvis, instability of lower back	Good sitting balance; full use of wheelchair; ambulation with long leg braces
L3-L4 Partial vagus nerve domination of leg vessels, GI and genitourinary organs	Quadriceps and hip flexors, absence of hamstring function, flail ankles	Completely independent ambulation with short leg braces and canes; inability to stand for long periods

GI, Gastrointestinal.

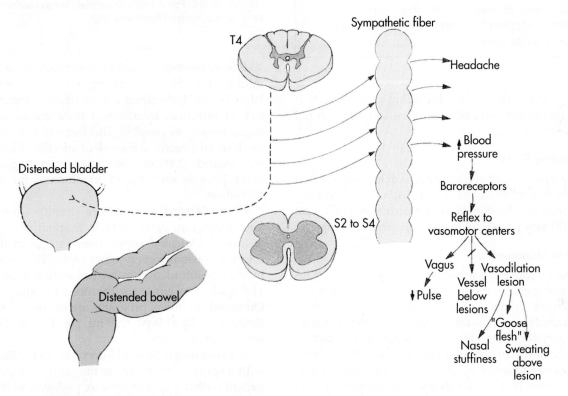

FIGURE **14-23** Pictorial diagram of cause of autonomic hyperreflexia (dysreflexia) and results.

aphoresis, "gooseflesh," flushing (above the level of the lesion), dilated pupils, blurred vision, restlessness, nausea, severe headache, and nasal stuffiness. Patients tend to develop individual signs and symptoms of this condition and are soon able to recognize them.

The most common causes of this condition include a distended bladder or a fecal impaction. It is a medical emergency that requires immediate treatment to prevent a stroke, blindness, or death (Box 14-3).

Sexual function. In most cases, men experience impotence, decreased sensation, and difficulties with ejaculation. Impairment of fertility is common. The experience of orgasm is described as different than be-

fore the injury. Women with spinal cord injury are able to continue to perform sexually, although perception of sexual pleasure is usually altered.

Assessment

Collection of **subjective data** includes information about the nature of the injury, presence of any dyspnea, and unusual sensations. The presence of pain, any loss of consciousness, and the absence of sensation on sensory examination are important to assess.

Collection of **objective data** includes the level of alertness and consciousness; orientation; pupil size and reactivity; motor strength; skin integrity; and

| Box 14-3 | *Emergency Care for Autonomic Dysreflexia or Hyperreflexia*

- Unless contraindicated, place patient in sitting position to decrease blood pressure.
- Check patency of catheter for kinking. If catheter is occluded, insert new catheter immediately.
- Check rectum for impaction.
- If it is necessary to remove impaction, an anesthetic ointment should be used.
- Administer ganglionic blocking agent such as hexamethonium or a vasodilator such as nitroprusside (Nipride) as ordered if conservative measures are not effective.
- Continue monitoring blood pressure.
- Send urine for culture if no other cause is found; urinary infection can lead to symptoms of autonomic dysreflexia.

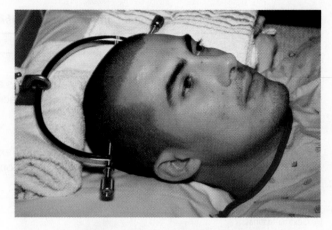

FIGURE **14-24** Patient with Crutchfield tongs inserted into skull to hyperextend head and neck.

bowel and bladder status, including distention. It is important to assess for other injuries, such as fractured bones or head injury.

Diagnostic Tests

Radiographs are often taken first to detect any cervical vertebra fracture or displacement. A spinal tap or myelogram may also be done to detect occlusion. A CT scan and MRI may be helpful to rule out spinal cord injury.

Medical Management

Immediate care after spinal cord injury is directed toward realignment of the bony column in the presence of fractures or dislocations. The measures involved may include simple immobilization, skeletal traction, or surgery for spinal decompression. Skeletal traction may include Crutchfield tongs (Figure 14-24), halo traction (see Chapter 4), or a Stryker or Foster frame. Bracing may be used for thoracic or lumbar injuries. Often a surgical decompression is not performed until after a period of skeletal traction if the injury involves the cervical region. In patients seen within 8 hours of injury, high-dose methylprednisolone is given.

Nursing Interventions and Patient Teaching

Mobility. Throughout all stages of hospitalization of the patient with a spinal cord injury, nursing and medical interventions are directed toward restoration of structural or body integrity. All efforts are taken to ensure that the skin is intact, that contractures do not develop, and that ROM is maintained. Early mobilization is important. When patients, especially quadriplegics, begin to sit up, it may be necessary to wrap the legs with thromboembolism stockings to encourage venous return. Slowly increasing the angle of sitting up is essential to prevent hypotension. A recliner wheelchair is usually necessary.

Urinary function. Usually a Foley catheter is inserted initially; later bladder training is started (see Chapter 10). Chronic indwelling catheterization increases the risk of infection. Intermittent catheterization should begin as early as possible. This helps to maintain bladder tone and decrease the risk of infection. Fluid intake that exceeds 2000 mL per day is encouraged. Cranberry juice is encouraged to decrease renal calculi formation.

Bowel function. Patients are usually started on a bowel program early in their hospital stay. At first, bisacodyl (Dulcolax) suppositories are given at regular intervals—usually every other night. This is followed by digital stimulation to further stimulate peristalsis. The goal is to eliminate the need for suppositories. Other aids to bowel programs are the use of adequate fluids (usually at least 2000 mL per day), stool softeners, and prune juice.

Nursing diagnoses and interventions for the patient with a spinal cord injury are the same as those for the patient with a motor or sensory problem, with the addition of but not limited to the following:

NURSING DIAGNOSES	NURSING INTERVENTIONS
Autonomic dysreflexia, related to neurophysiological trauma to spinal cord above sixth thoracic vertebra	See Box 14-3 for emergency interventions.
Impaired urinary elimination, related to sensory-motor impairment	Check carefully for voiding and for distention of bladder Teach patient intermittent self catheterization if indicated. Teach patient Credé's maneuver as indicated. Use Foley catheter if indicated; administer meticulous aseptic technique in changing catheters.

Nursing Diagnoses	Nursing Interventions
	Teach patients signs of infection.
	Encourage patient to have a genitourinary checkup at least yearly.
	Maintain fluid intake of 3 to 4 L daily unless contraindicated.
	Use adult perineal protector for incontinence, if necessary.

Teaching of the patient with a spinal cord injury includes education about autonomic dysreflexia and about sexual functioning after spinal cord injury. Other teaching points are found in the sections of this chapter dealing with the patient with motor or sensory problems.

Prognosis

In cases of a complete spinal cord injury, there is almost no chance of return of any function. However, the paraplegic or tetraplegic (quadriplegic) patient can live a satisfying life with adaptations and assistance. Today, with improved treatment strategies (specifically, intermittent catheterization), even the very young patient with a spinal cord injury can anticipate a long life. The prognosis for life is generally only about 5 years less than for people of the same age without spinal cord injury. Care will be necessary to prevent infections, such as urinary tract or respiratory infections. With patients with incomplete cord lesions, the amount of return of function is variable and often unpredictable.

NURSING PROCESS *for the Patient with a Neurological Disorder*

The role of the licensed practical nurse/licensed vocational nurse (LPN/LVN) in the nursing process as stated is that the LPN/LVN will:

- Participate in planning care for patients based on patient needs.
- Review patient's plan of care and recommend revisions as needed.
- Review and follow defined prioritization for patient care.
- Use clinical pathways/care maps/care plans to guide and review patient care.

Assessment

People with neurological deficits require skilled assessment by both a nurse and a physician. Assessment occurs by observing the patient during the patient history. Nursing assessment is an ongoing process and should be tailored to meet the needs of the patient. For example, hourly neurological checks will not be as detailed as the initial assessment.

While interviewing the patient, the nurse obtains data about subjective complaints, such as pain, dizziness, or vision difficulties. The ability to speak and reason can also be assessed. Observations may also include vital signs, data about gait, symmetry of body parts, evidence of pain, or seizure activity. During ongoing assessments, data is usually obtained about pupil size, level of alertness, ability to perform motor tasks, changes in level of consciousness, and ability to speak. Because subtle changes in neurological nursing can often be the first sign of a complication, the nurse must be able to detect small changes in the neurological assessment and report these to the proper person.

Nursing Diagnosis

Nursing assessment helps identify the patient's needs for care and observation. The actual care of the patient is then based on the nursing diagnoses that have been identified. Possible nursing diagnoses for a patient with a neurological disorder include, but are not limited to the following:

Autonomic dysreflexia
Impaired verbal communication
Compromised family coping
Risk for disuse syndrome
Risk for falls
Grieving
Risk for infection
Deficient knowledge
Impaired memory
Impaired physical mobility
Imbalanced nutrition: less than body requirement
Acute pain
Chronic pain
Bathing/hygiene self-care deficit
Feeding self-care deficit
Toileting self-care deficit
Impaired swallowing
Disturbed thought processes
Ineffective tissue perfusion (cerebral)

Expected Outcomes/Planning

The plan for providing neurological assessment and care should focus on the type of deficit the patient is experiencing as well as possible complications. Considering a patient's preferences and mental status is important. The type of care required determines the supplies and equipment needed. The nurse should schedule necessary care around tests and procedures and on the need of the patient for rest.

The plan of care focuses on achieving specific goals and outcomes that relate to the identified nursing diagnosis. Examples of these include the following:

Goal #1: Patient's cerebral perfusion is maintained.
   Outcome: Patient remains awake, alert, and oriented; coma scale score remains the same or improves.

Goal #2: Patient's optimal nutrition is maintained.

Outcome: Patient's optimal weight is maintained or attained, and lab values indicating nutritional health are within normal limits.

Implementation

Nursing interventions for the patient with a neurological disorder include those that maintain cerebral perfusion and other functioning, as well as those that prevent complications such as decubitus, falls, or contractures. Certain principles guide nurses in providing neurological care.

- The neurological system is a complex system that produces a wide variety of neurological signs and symptoms.
- Identical disorders may result in different sets of signs and symptoms in different patients.
- The maintenance of cerebral perfusion is of utmost importance.
- The patient with a neurological illness is very prone to complications.
- Disorders of the nervous system produce not only physical problems, but a wide variety of cognitive difficulties.

While providing specific care for the difficulties presented by the patient, the nurse should also assess the patient's readiness to learn. Ongoing teaching is important for the patient. At times the family must receive the primary teaching because the patient is unable to understand. The preferences and background of the patient are important in delivering care. The nurse encourages the patient to be as independent as possible and gives appropriate feedback. The dignity and privacy of the patient are preserved whenever possible. The special needs of older patients must also be taken into consideration (Older Adult Considerations box).

Evaluation

The nurse evaluates the success of planned interventions during and after care is given. The process is ongoing and dynamic because the patient's condition often changes. The nurse must always be ready to revise the care plan as needed. For example, if a patient is found to have new episodes of confusion after surgery, the doctor is notified, safety measures are increased, and assessment occurs more frequently. Ongoing systematic evaluation requires the nurse to determine whether specific outcomes have been met. The evaluation is specific to measure the goals identified. Examples of goals and their corresponding evaluative measures include the following:

Goal #1: Patient is free of infection.

Evaluative measure: Assess patient for any signs of infection such as increased temperature, frequency of urination, erythematous incision, elevated white blood count, or confusion.

Goal #2: Patient remains clear and oriented in thought processes.

Evaluative measure: Ask patient to respond to orientation questions. Observe ability to engage in conversation and to carry out care activities.

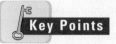 **Key Points**

- The nervous system is the body's link with the environment. It allows the interpretation of information and appropriate action to occur.
- The two main structural divisions of the nervous system are the central nervous system and the peripheral nervous system.
- The central nervous system is composed of the brain and the spinal cord.
- The peripheral nervous system is composed of the nerve cells lying outside of the central nervous system. It is composed of the somatic nervous system and the autonomic nervous system.
- A nerve cell is composed of three parts: the dendrite, the cell body, and the axon.
- The brain and spinal cord are protected by the bony coverings (skull and vertebral column), the cerebrospinal fluid, and the three meninges (pia mater, arachnoid, and dura mater).
- The cerebrum is the largest part of the brain and contains five major areas: motor, sensory, visual, speech, and auditory. The cerebrum governs the ability to reason and make judgments.
- The diencephalon lies beneath the cerebrum and contains the thalamus and hypothalamus. The thalamus serves as a relay station, while the hypothalamus has several roles, such as temperature control, water balance, and appetite.
- The cerebellum is the second largest portion of the brain and is responsible for coordination of skeletal muscles and maintenance of balance and equilibrium.
- The peripheral nervous system is composed of the cranial nerves, the spinal nerves, and the autonomic nervous system.
- The autonomic nervous system contains two subdivisions: the sympathetic nervous system and the parasympathetic nervous system. The sympathetic nervous system speeds things up and the parasympathetic nervous system slows things down.
- Normal changes of aging are not the same as senility, Alzheimer's disease, or organic brain damage.
- The source of any headache should be determined through neurological testing because it may be a symptom of a serious pathologic condition.
- A lumbar puncture should not be done if there is evidence of increased intracranial pressure because of the danger of brain herniation.
- Any increase in the volume of one of the contents of the cranium (brain, blood vessels, and cerebrospinal fluid) results in increased intracranial pressure because the cranial vault is rigid and does not expand.
- Classic signs of increased intracranial pressure include restlessness, disorientation, headache, contralateral

hemiparesis, an ipsilaterally dilated pupil, and visual changes that include blurring and diplopia.

- Nursing intervention measures can significantly influence intracranial pressure.
- Epilepsy is a transitory disturbance in consciousness or in motor, sensory, or autonomic functions with or without loss of consciousness, caused by sudden, excessive, and disorderly electrical discharges of the brain.
- Early signs and symptoms of MS are usually transitory.
- Stroke, or "brain attack," is the most common disease of the nervous system and can be caused by thrombus, embolus, or hemorrhage. The term *brain attack* is being used to describe stroke and communicate the urgency of recognizing stroke signs and symptoms and treating their onset as a medical emergency similar to what would be done with a myocardial infarction (heart attack).
- Helpful nursing interventions for the patient with Alzheimer's disease include using nonverbal clues or demonstrations as adjuncts to verbal cues, providing very few choices, and not hurrying the patient.
- Trigeminal neuralgia (tic douloureux) is characterized by excruciating, burning pain that radiates along one or more of the three divisions of the fifth cranial nerve.
- With Bell's palsy, there is usually an abrupt onset of numbness, a feeling of stiffness, or a drawing sensation of the face.
- Of the people suffering from Guillain-Barré syndrome, 85% will retain complete function.

- Approximately 80% of patients with advanced HIV disease (AIDS) have neurological symptoms that result from infection from HIV itself or from associated complications of advanced HIV disease.
- Many patients with head injury may recover physically, but they will have behavioral and psychological problems that make it difficult for them to function independently.
- The signs and symptoms of intracranial tumors result from both local and general effects of the tumor.
- Autonomic dysreflexia in the patient with spinal cord injury is a medical emergency that demands quick nursing interventions.
- The first sign of increased intracranial pressure may be a lessening of the state of consciousness.
- It is important to document patients' behaviors in terms of what is seen, not what is inferred.
- It is estimated that 1 in 150 people infected with West Nile virus will develop encephalitis or meningitis, a more severe form of the disease.

Go to your free CD-ROM for an Audio Glossary, animations, video clips, and Review Questions for the NCLEX-PN® Examination.

evolve Be sure to visit the companion Evolve site at http://evolve.elsevier.com/Christensen/adult/ for WebLinks and additional online resources.

CHAPTER CHALLENGE

1. Mr. J. is admitted to the hospital with the diagnosis of transient ischemic attack. What normal change of aging would the nurse expect to see with this 90-year-old man?

   1. Increased sense of touch
   2. Diminished long-term memory
   3. Increased reflex time
   4. Decreased fine motor coordination

2. Ms. S. is a 35-year-old patient being seen for complaints of headache, which she has experienced for the past month. Her physician wants to rule out a brain tumor. In this case, what diagnostic test is contraindicated?

   1. Brain scan
   2. PET scan
   3. Lumbar puncture
   4. Electroencephalography

3. Ms. F., a nurse in the emergency room of her community hospital, is asked to speak to a group of sixth graders about the prevention of head and spine injuries. Teaching about avoiding such injuries includes all but which of the following?

   1. Use of helmets for bicycles, motorcycles, and skate boarding
   2. Use of a lumbar support for sports activities
   3. Safe handling and storage of guns
   4. Use of seat belts and shoulder harnesses in a car

4. Mr. B. is a 70-year-old with the complaint of back pain. He is scheduled to have a myelogram in the morning to rule out pathology of the spine. In preparing him for the procedure, what information is important to share with the patient?

   1. That mental status will be assessed frequently
   2. That the patient will lie completely supine and still during the procedure
   3. That the patient will be able to ambulate immediately after the test
   4. That strengths of the lower extremities will be assessed frequently

Continued

CHAPTER CHALLENGE—cont'd

5. Ms. M. is an 80-year-old who has suffered a stroke. The nursing assessment found that she had difficulty with swallowing. A video fluoroscopy with barium was done to rule out aspiration. The rehabilitation team in the skilled nursing facility has determined that she can eat a soft diet with one-to-one supervision. Which of the following is important to prevent aspiration?
   1. Tipping the head toward the unaffected side while swallowing
   2. Extending the head during swallowing
   3. Mixing solids and liquids to facilitate swallowing
   4. Encouraging the patient to take large bites to make swallowing easier

6. S.S. is a 12-year-old student with a history of generalized tonic-clonic seizures. Your job as the school nurse is to educate his classmates about his seizure activity. What will be important to tell his classmates during this time?
   1. That he will be normal immediately after the seizure
   2. That it is important to place a tongue blade in his mouth during the seizure
   3. That his desk should be placed in a corner of the room by himself
   4. That he may cry out at the beginning of a seizure

7. Mr. E. is a 43-year-old involved in a snowmobile accident. On admission to the emergency department, he is receiving oxygen and is intubated. His Glasgow coma scale score is 6. About 10 minutes after arrival, he is noted to have a widened pulse pressure, increased systolic blood pressure, and bradycardia. These signs are considered an important diagnostic sign of late stage increased intracranial pressure. Together they are known as which of the following?
   1. Anisocoria
   2. Supratentorial shift
   3. Cushing's response
   4. Medullary reflex

8. Mr. J. is a 76-year-old who has had Parkinson's disease for the past 6 years. He has now been admitted to a nursing home. The nurse who is doing the admission interview and assessment notices a characteristic sign of the disease. This would be which of the following?
   1. Bradykinesia
   2. Increased postural reflexes
   3. Sensory loss
   4. Intention tremor

9. S.F. is a 13-year-old student admitted to the pediatric unit with possible meningitis. The nurse caring for S. finds that she cannot extend her legs completely without experiencing extreme pain. The nurse knows that this is an indication of the presence of meningitis and is called:
   1. Brudzinski's sign.
   2. Battle's sign.
   3. Kernig's sign.
   4. Cosgrow's sign.

10. Ms. D. is suffering from Bell's palsy as indicated by a feeling of stiffness and a drawing sensation of the face. In teaching her about the disease, what would be important to tell her?
   1. There is a heightened awareness of taste, so that foods must be bland
   2. There may be an increased sensitivity to sound
   3. The eye is susceptible to injury if the eyelid does not close
   4. Drooling from an increase of saliva on the affected side may occur

11. What is the *first* nursing intervention that is necessary if a patient has autonomic dysreflexia?
   1. Sit the patient upright, if permitted.
   2. Check for bowel impaction.
   3. Give medication as ordered.
   4. Place the patient in supine position.

12. In teaching the patient with Parkinson's disease, which response would indicate the need for further education?
   1. "If I miss an occasional dose of the medication, it is not of much significance."
   2. "I need to exercise at least some every day."
   3. "I need to be sitting straight up and my chin slightly tucked so I won't choke when I eat or drink."
   4. "I should eat a diet high in fiber and roughage to decrease my constipation."

13. Important nursing interventions for a patient with sensory dysfunction are: (Choose all correct answers.)
   1. Teaching the patient protective measures in relation to the sensory deficit
   2. Inspecting parts of the body that have no feeling to ascertain any impairment of skin integrity
   3. Having the patient practice scanning the printed page
   4. Keeping the patient warm with the use of heating pads

14. When injury to the spinal cord is in the cervical region, the resultant complication would be:

    1. quadriplegia.
    2. hemiplegia.
    3. paraplegia.
    4. paresthesia.

15. The nurse determines that a patient is unconscious when the patient:

    1. has cerebral ischemia.
    2. responds only to painful stimuli.
    3. is unaware of self or environment.
    4. does not respond to verbal stimuli.

16. The nurse plans care for the patient with increased intracranial pressure with the knowledge that the best way to position the patient is to:

    1. keep the head of the bed flat.
    2. maintain the head of the bed at 30 degrees.
    3. increase the head of the bed's angle to 30 degrees with patient on left side.
    4. use a continuous-rotation bed to continuously change patient position.

17. During admission of a patient with a severe head injury to the emergency department, the nurse places the highest priority on assessment for:

    1. patency of airway.
    2. presence of a neck injury.
    3. neurological status with the Glasgow coma scale.
    4. cerebrospinal fluid leakage from the ears or nose.

18. The primary goal of nursing interventions after a craniotomy is:

    1. prevention of infection.
    2. ensuring patient comfort.
    3. avoiding need for secondary surgery.
    4. preventing increased intracranial pressure.

19. A right-handed patient with right-sided hemiplegia and aphasia resulting from a stroke most likely has a lesion in the:

    1. left frontal lobe.
    2. right brainstem.
    3. motor areas of the right cerebrum.
    4. medial superior area of the temporal lobe.

20. A patient experiencing TIAs is scheduled for a carotid endarterectomy. The nurse explains that this procedure is done to:

    1. promote cerebral flow to decrease cerebral edema.
    2. reduce the brain damage that occurs during a stroke-in-evolution.
    3. prevent a stroke by removing atherosclerotic plaques obstructing cerebral blood flow.
    4. provide a circulatory bypass around thrombotic plaques obstructing cranial circulation.

21. Mr. S., 69 years of age, has been admitted to the medical floor with a diagnosis of Parkinson's disease. His nursing interventions will include which of the following (choose all correct answers):

    1. Encouraging activities to improve his ability to increase his speed for doing ADLs
    2. Care during feeding to prevent aspiration
    3. Providing means for disposal of facial tissues
    4. Diet high in fiber and generous fluid intake

Matching

22. _____ MRI

23. _____ Myelography

24. _____ Babinski's sign

25. _____ Nystagmus

26. _____ Papilledema

A. Optic disk is edematous "choked disk"

B. Involuntary rhythmic movement of the eyes; oscillations may be horizontal, vertical, or mixed

C. Use of magnetic forces to image body structures

D. Backward flexion of the great toe due to an abnormal CNS condition

E. Diagnostic procedure done to identify tumors of the spinal cord or herniated nucleus pulposus by observing flow of amipaque dye

27. Which of the following signs and symptoms of late-stage increased intracranial pressure should the LPN/LVN be aware of: (choose all correct answers):

    1. Increase in systolic blood pressure
    2. Widening of pulse pressure
    3. Bradycardia
    4. Unequal pupils that react slowly to light
    5. Tachycardia

28. The nursing interventions that would be appropriate and beneficial to Mr. L., who has had a stroke with right-sided hemiplegia and expressive aphasia, include which of the following (choose all correct answers):

    1. State questions so that Mr. L. can verbalize freely to articulate his needs.
    2. Encourage self-help, such as washing.
    3. Remain calm and converse in an intelligent manner.
    4. Perform ROM to all extremities every shift.

Continued

CHAPTER CHALLENGE—cont'd

29. The nurse has the responsibility to teach patients with potential aspiration problems airway protective techniques during swallowing. Which of the following procedures should be taught (choose all correct answers):

    1. Chin tuck
    2. Double swallow
    3. Full Fowler's position
    4. Use of a straw
    5. Soft or pureed foods

30. The pathophysiology of myasthenia gravis is caused by:

    1. myelin sheath breakdown.
    2. degeneration of the dopamine-producing neurons in the midbrain.
    3. antibodies attacking the acetylcholine receptors, damaging them and reducing their number.
    4. inflammation of cranial nerve VII.

31. A graphic recording of the electrical conduction activities of the brain that is a helpful diagnostic tool for a patient with seizures is called:

    1. ECG.
    2. MRI.
    3. PET.
    4. EEG.

32. The condition that involves cranial nerve VII that results in tenderness to the posterior ear, followed by paralysis of the facial muscles unilaterally with ptosis of the eyelid and mouth pulled to opposite side of the face, is:

    1. trigeminal neuralgia.
    2. Bell's palsy.
    3. Romberg.
    4. proprioception.

15 Care of the Patient with an Immune Disorder

BARBARA LAURITSEN CHRISTENSEN and ELAINE ODEN KOCKROW

Objectives

After reading this chapter, the student should be able to do the following:

1. Define the key terms as listed.
2. Differentiate between natural and acquired immunity.
3. Review the mechanisms of immune response.
4. Compare and contrast humoral and cell-mediated immunity.
5. Explain the concepts of immunocompetency, immunodeficiency, and autoimmunity.
6. Discuss five factors that influence the development of hypersensitivity.
7. Identify the clinical manifestations of anaphylaxis.
8. Outline the immediate aggressive treatment of systemic anaphylactic reaction.
9. Discuss the two types of latex allergies and recommendations for preventing allergic reactions to latex in the workplace.
10. Discuss selection of blood donors, typing and cross-matching, storage, and administration in preventing transfusion reaction.
11. Discuss the causation of autoimmune disorders; explain plasmapheresis in the treatment of autoimmune diseases.
12. Explain an immunodeficiency disease.

Key Terms

 Be sure to check out the bonus material on the free CD-ROM, including selected audio pronunciations.

adaptive immunity (ă-DĂP-tĭv ĭ-MŪ-nĭ-tē, p. 754)
allergen (ĂL-ĕr-jĕn, p. 756)
antigen (ĂN-tĭ-jĕn, p. 755)
attenuated (ă-TĔN-ū-āt-ĕd, p. 757)
autoimmune (aw-tō-ĭ-MŪN, p. 765)
autologous (aw-TŎL-ŏ-gŭs, p. 764)
cellular immunity (SĔL-ū-lăr ĭ-MŪ-nĭ-tē, p. 757)
humoral immunity (HŪ-mŏr-ăl ĭ-MŪ-nĭ-tē, p. 755)
hypersensitivity (hī-pĕr-sĕn-sĭ-TĬV-ĭ-tē, p. 758)
immunity (ĭ-MŪ-nĭ-tē, p. 754)
immunization (ĭm-ū-nĭ-ZĀ-shŭn, p. 755)
immunocompetence (ĭm-ū-nō-KŎM-pĕ-tĕns, p. 753)
immunodeficiency (ĭm-ū-nō-dĕ-FĬSH-ĕn-sē, p. 764)
immunogen (ĭm-Ū-nō-jĕn, p. 757)
immunology (ĭm-ū-NŎL-ŏ-jē, p. 754)
immunosuppressive (ĭm-ū-nō-sŭ-PRĔ-sĭv, p. 764)
immunotherapy (ĭm-ū-nō-THĔR-ă-pē, p. 758)

innate immunity (ĭ-NĀT ĭ-MŪ-nĭ-tē, p. 754)
lymphokine (LĬM-fō-kīn, p. 755)
plasmapheresis (plăz-mă-fĕ-RĒ-sĭs, p. 765)
proliferation (prō-lĭf-ĕ-RĀ-shŭn, p. 755)

NATURE OF IMMUNITY

The human body exists in an environment of antagonistic forces that are constantly attacking and threatening its integrity. In response to these onslaughts, the body exhibits a wide array of adaptations to protect against external and internal harmful agents. This chapter deals with those mechanisms.

The word *immune* is derived from the Latin word *immunis,* meaning "free from burden." Immunology is an evolving science that essentially deals with the body's ability to distinguish self from nonself. This distinction is accomplished through a complex network of highly specialized cells and tissues that are collectively called the **immune system.** The immune system (also called the **host defense system**) is critical to our survival.

The immune system has three main functions: (1) to protect the body's internal environment against invading organisms, (2) to maintain homeostasis by removing damaged cells from the circulation, and (3) to serve as a surveillance network for recognizing and guarding against the development and growth of abnormal cells. When the immune system responds appropriately to a foreign stimulus, the body's integrity is maintained; this is called immunocompetence.

Immunocompetence is the ability of the immune system to mobilize and use its antibodies and other responses to stimulation by an antigen. If the immune response is too weak or too vigorous, homeostasis is disrupted, causing a malfunction in the system, or immunoincompetence. Disruption of the homeostatic balance of the immune system can cause a number of diseases to manifest. Inappropriate responses of the immune system have been classified into four categories: (1) hyperactive responses against environmental antigens (e.g., allergy); (2) inability to protect the body, as in immunodeficiency disorders (e.g., acquired immunodeficiency syndrome [AIDS]); (3) failure to recognize the body as self, as in autoimmune disorders (e.g., systemic lupus erythematosus); and (4) attacks on beneficial foreign tissue (e.g., organ transplant rejection or transfusion reaction).

Immunity is the quality of being insusceptible to or unaffected by a particular disease or condition. There are two major subclassifications of immunity: innate (natural) and adaptive (acquired) (Figure 15-1). Innate immunity is nonspecific, whereas adaptive immunity is specific. The study of the immune system is **immunology.**

INNATE, OR NATURAL, IMMUNITY

The body's first line of defense, **innate immunity,** provides physical and chemical barriers to invading pathogens and protects against the external environment. The innate system is composed of the skin and mucous membranes, cilia, stomach acid, tears, saliva, sebaceous glands, and secretions and flora of the intestine and vagina. These organs, tissues, and secretions provide biochemical and physical barriers to disease. The first line of defense provides nonspecific immunity to the individual (Table 15-1).

ADAPTIVE, OR ACQUIRED, IMMUNITY

If the components of innate or natural immunity fail to prevent invasion or to destroy a foreign pathogen, the adaptive immune response is summoned to assist in the battle. This is the body's second line of defense against disease. **Adaptive immunity** provides a specific reaction to each invading antigen and has the unique ability to remember the antigen that caused the attack. Adaptive immunity protects the internal environment. The adaptive immune system is composed of highly specialized cells and tissues, including the thymus, spleen, bone marrow, blood, and lymph (Figure 15-2). Adaptive, or acquired, immunity includes both humoral and cell-mediated immunity. The characteristics of an adaptive immune system are specificity (i.e., being specific) and memory. This specific immunity results from the production of antibodies in the cells. Antibodies develop naturally after infection or artificially after vaccinations.

The cells of the immune system are the macrophages (any phagocytic cell involved in defense against infection) and the lymphocytes. When organisms pass the epithelial barriers, phagocytes become activated. Phagocytes also have the ability to migrate through the bloodstream to the tissues for the body's second line of defense against disease. Phagocytes engulf and destroy microorganisms that pass the skin and mucous membrane barriers. These cells also assist in the immune response by carrying antigens to the lymphocytes.

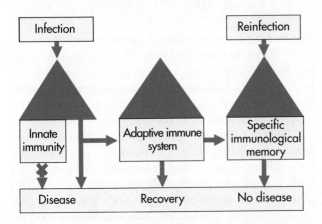

FIGURE 15-1 When an infectious agent enters the body, it first encounters elements of the innate immune system. These may be sufficient to prevent disease but, if not, a disease will result and the adaptive immune system is activated. The adaptive immune system produces recovery from the disease and establishes a specific immunologic memory, so after reinfection with the same agent, no disease results. The individual has acquired immunity to the infectious agent.

Table 15-1 | *Innate (Natural) and Adaptive (Acquired) Immunity*

CHARACTERISTICS	INNATE (NATURAL)	ADAPTIVE (ACQUIRED)
Physical barriers	Physical defense: skin and mucous membranes Mucous membranes line body cavities such as the mouth and stomach. These cavities secrete chemicals (saliva and hydrochloric acid) that destroy bacteria. Cilia, tears, and flora of the intestine and vagina also provide natural protection.	None
Response mechanisms	Nonspecific: mononuclear phagocytic system; inflammatory response	Specific immune response humoral immunity, cellular immunity
Soluble factors	Chemical defense: lysozyme, complement, acute phase proteins, interferon	Antibodies, lymphokines
Cells	Phagocytes, natural killer (NK) cells	T lymphocytes, B lymphocytes
Specificity	None	Present
Memory	None	Present

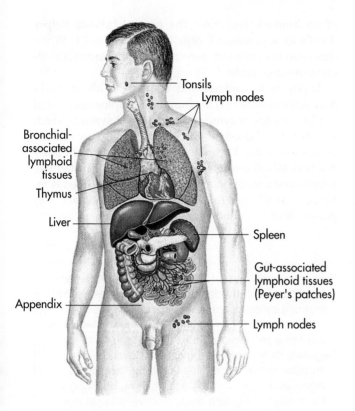

FIGURE **15-2** Organization of the immune system.

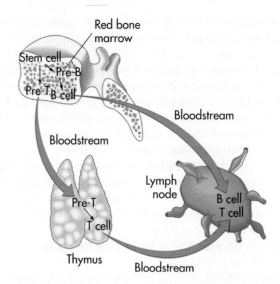

FIGURE **15-3** Origin and processing of B and T cells. B and T cells originate in red bone marrow. B cells are processed in the red marrow, whereas T cells are processed in the thymus. Both cell types circulate to other lymph tissues. B cells produce antibodies to destroy specific foreign antigens (humoral immunity). T cells attack and destroy antigens (cell-mediated immunity).

Lymphocytes include the T and B cells (Figure 15-3) and the large, granular lymphocytes also known as **natural killer,** or NK, cells. Approximately 70% to 80% of the lymphocytes are T-cell lymphocytes. When activated, T cells release a substance called lymphokine. **Lymphokine** is one of the chemical factors produced and released by T cells that attracts macrophages to the site of infection or inflammation and prepares them for attack. T cells cooperate with the B cells to produce antibodies but do not produce antibodies themselves. T cells are responsible for cell-mediated immunity and provide the body with protection against viruses, fungi, and parasites. T cells also provide protection in allograft (transfer of tissue between two genetically dissimilar individuals of the same species) and against malignant cells.

B cells make up approximately 20% to 30% of the lymphocyte population. B cells cause the production of antibodies and proliferate (increase in number) in response to a particular antigen (a substance recognized by the body as foreign that can trigger an immune response). An antigen is usually a protein that causes the formation of an antibody and reacts specifically with that antibody. B cells migrate to the peripheral circulation and tissues and eventually are filtered from the lymph and stored in the lymphoid tissue of the body.

The initial formation of B cells does not require antigen stimulation or any other environmental stimulus.

However, B-cell **proliferation** (reproduction or multiplication of similar forms) depends on antigen stimulation. B cells are responsible for humoral immunity. B cells produce antibodies and provide protection against bacteria, viruses, and soluble antigens. See Table 15-1 for innate and adaptive immunity presentation.

HUMORAL IMMUNITY

Humoral immunity (one of the two forms of immunity that respond to antigens, such as bacteria and foreign tissue) is mediated by the B cells. B cells produce antibodies in response to antigen challenge. On first exposure to a given antigen, a primary humoral response is initiated. This response is generally slow compared with subsequent antigen exposures. When a second exposure occurs, memory B cells cause a quick response, regardless of whether the first exposure was to an antigen or to immunization. **Immunization** is a process by which resistance to an infectious disease is induced or increased.

Antigen is presented to the T-cell helper population by the macrophage. T lymphocytes can be categorized into T-helper (CD_4) and T-suppressor (CD_8) cells. Most are then taken to the B cells and, assisted by helper T cells, the B cells initiate production of antibodies. Suppressor T cells maintain the humoral response at a level appropriate for the stimulus.

Antibodies produced by one's own body are said to provide active immunity. An example of active immunity is a person who has been vaccinated against rubeola (red measles). Antibodies formed by another in response to a specific antigen and administered to an individual provide only temporary, or passive, immunity. An example of passive immunity is hepatitis B immunoglobulin (HBIG). This contains a high titer of hepatitis B immune globin and is preferred for use after exposure to hepatitis B virus in a nonimmune person.

Even though humoral immunity is mediated by the B-cell population, helper T cells and suppressor T cells have a function and are vital to the immunocompetent person. **Immunocompetence** is the ability of an immune system to mobilize and deploy its antibodies and other responses to stimulation by an antigen. Both the number and functions of the helper and suppressor T cells help determine the strength and persistence of an immune response. The normal ratio of helper T cells to suppressor T cells in the body is 2:1. When this ratio is disrupted, autoimmune and immunodeficient diseases occur.

Exposure to antigen and response with antibody may activate either (1) the humoral complement (one of the 25 complex enzyme serum proteins) system, which results in breakdown of the bacteria and release of lysosomes to destroy bacteria; or (2) the antigen/antibody reaction, which results in mast cells releasing histamine, which produces the symptoms of allergy. Antigen is referred to as **allergen** (a substance that can produce a hypersensitive reaction in the body but is not necessarily

---

Box 15-1 *The Four "Rs" of the Immune Response*

Recognize self from nonself. Normally the body recognizes its own cells as nonantigenic; therefore an immune response generally is triggered only in response to agents that the body identifies as foreign. In autoimmune disorders the ability to differentiate self from nonself is disrupted, and the immune system attacks the body's own cells as if they were foreign antigens.

Respond to nonself invaders. The immune system responds in part by producing antibodies that target specific antigens for destruction. New antibodies are produced in response to new antigens. Deficits in the ability to respond can result in immunodeficiency disorders.

Remember the invader. The ability to remember antigens that have invaded the body in the past is the immune system's memory. This characteristic allows a quicker response if subsequent invasion by the same antigen occurs.

Regulate its action. Self-regulation allows the immune system to monitor itself by "turning on" when an antigen invades and "turning off" when the invasion has been eradicated. Regulation prevents the destruction of healthy or host tissue. The inability to regulate could result in a chronic inflammation and damage to the host tissue.

Box 15-2 *Review of the Mechanisms of Immune Response*

- The skin and mucous membranes are natural barriers to infectious agents. When these barriers are crossed, the immune response is begun in the immunocompetent host.
- The first time an antigen enters the body, the antigen is processed by macrophages and presented to lymphocytes. Responses of B cells to the antigen in humoral immunity require interaction with T helper cells, which assist B cells in responding to the antigen by proliferating, synthesizing, and secreting the appropriate antibody. Antigens are then neutralized by antibodies or can form immune complexes or be phagocytosed by macrophages or neutrophils.
- Humoral immunity responds to antigens such as bacteria and foreign tissue. Humoral immunity is the result of the development and continuing presence of circulating antibodies in the plasma. Humoral immunity consists of antibody-mediated immunity. **Humoral** means body fluid. Antibodies are proteins found in plasma; therefore the term is **humoral immunity.**
- Cellular immunity is the primary defense against intracellular organisms, including viruses and some bacteria (e.g., *Mycobacterium*).

- In cellular immunity the antigen is processed by macrophages and recognized by T cells. T cells produce lymphokines, which further attract macrophages and neutrophils to the site for phagocytosis, or cytotoxic killer T cells can respond directly.
- Immunodeficiency is an abnormal condition of the immune system in which cellular or humoral immunity is inadequate and resistance to infection is decreased. The immunodeficiency diseases are sometimes classified as B-cell (antibody) deficiencies, T-cell (cellular) deficiencies, and combined T- and B-cell deficiencies.
- Hypersensitivity reaction is an inappropriate and excessive response of the immune system to a sensitizing antigen. The antigen stimulant is an allergen. Humoral reactions, mediated by the circulating B lymphocytes, are immediate such as anaphylactic hypersensitivity. Cellular reactions, mediated by the T lymphocytes, are delayed cell-mediated hypersensitivity reactions.

inherently harmful) when symptoms of allergy occur. Antigen is referred to as immunogen (any agent or substance capable of provoking an immune response or producing immunity) when immunity results.

CELLULAR IMMUNITY

Cellular immunity, also called **cell-mediated immunity** (the mechanism of acquired immunity characterized by the dominant role of small T cells), results when T cells are activated by an antigen. Whole cells become sensitized in a process similar to that which stimulates the B cells to form antibodies. Once these T cells have been sensitized, they are released into the blood and body tissues, where they remain indefinitely. On contact with the antigen to which they are sensitized, they will attach to the organism and destroy it. Cellular immunity is involved in resistance to infectious diseases caused by viruses and some bacteria.

Cell-mediated immunity is of primary importance in (1) immunity against pathogens that survive inside cells, including viruses and some bacteria (e.g., *Mycobacterium*); (2) fungal infections; (3) rejection of transplanted tissues; (4) contact hypersensitivity reactions; (5) tumor immunity; and (6) certain autoimmune diseases (Box 15-1).

Hypersensitivity reactions are cell-mediated responses of the body (Box 15-2).

COMPLEMENT SYSTEM

The word *complement* became part of the terminology of immunology at the turn of the century, when researchers recognized that blood plasma contained a substance necessary to complete the destruction of bacteria. The complement system is a system of approximately 25 serum enzymatic proteins that interact with one another and with other components of the innate (natural) and adaptive (acquired) immune systems. Normally, complement enzymes are inactive in plasma and body fluids. When an antigen and antibody interact, the complement system is activated. Complement functions in a "step-by-step" series much like the clotting mechanism, but with a different purpose. The complement system can destroy the cell membrane of many bacterial species, and this action attracts phagocytes to the area.

GENETIC CONTROL OF IMMUNITY

More is being discovered about the genetic role in immunity. There is a genetic link to both well-developed immune systems and poorly developed or compromised immune systems.

The immune system develops at different rates and at different times in fetal and early life. For humans, bone marrow provides the continuous service of stem cells and all the other cells involved in the immune response.

EFFECTS OF NORMAL AGING ON THE IMMUNE SYSTEM

With advancing age, there is a decline in the immune system. The primary clinical evidence for this immunosenescence is the high incidence of tumors in older adults. A greater susceptibility also occurs to infections (such as influenza and pneumonia) from pathogens that an older person has been relatively immunocompetent against earlier in life.

Aging does not affect all aspects of the immune system. The bone marrow is relatively unaffected by increasing age. However, aging has a pronounced effect on the thymus, which decreases in size and activity with aging. These changes in the thymus are probably a primary cause of immunosenescence. Both T and B cells show deficiencies in activation, transit time through the cell cycle, and subsequent differentiation. However, the most significant alterations seem to involve T cells. As thymic output of T cells diminishes, the differentiation of T cells in peripheral lymphoid structures increases. Consequently, there is an accumulation of memory cells rather than new precursor cells responsive to previously unencountered antigens.

Delayed hypersensitivity response, as determined by skin testing with injected antigens, is frequently decreased or absent in older adults. The clinical consequences of a decline in cell-mediated immunity are evident. Diminished responses to delayed hypersensitivity skin tests in older adults are related to an increased risk of cancer mortality, as well as mortality in general (Older Adult Considerations box).

IMMUNE RESPONSE

There are two ways of assisting the body to develop immunity: **immunization** and **immunotherapy**. The theory behind immunization is that controlled exposure to a disease-producing pathogen develops antibody production while preventing disease. The first immunization is credited to Edward Jenner (1796), who observed that individuals who had had cowpox became immune to the disease. The idea of administering "attenuated [weakened] microbes" developed, and the scientific approach was applied by Louis Pasteur. Vaccines and toxoids are altered, or attenuated (the process of weakening the degree of virulence of a disease organism), in such a way as to reduce their degree of power without losing their ability to stimulate the production of antibodies. In immunization the immune system mounts a greater response to a second

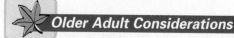

Older Adult Considerations

Immune Disorder

- Older adults are at increased risk for inflammation and infections resulting from changes in natural defense mechanisms.
- Pathogens are able to enter through breaks in fragile, dry skin, increasing the risk of skin infections.
- Decreased movement of respiratory secretions increases the risk of respiratory infections.
- Decreased production of saliva and gastric secretions increases the risk of gastrointestinal infections.
- Decreased tear production increases the risk of eye inflammation and infections.
- Structural changes in the urinary system that lead to urinary retention or stasis increase the risk of urinary tract infection.
- Signs and symptoms of infection tend to be more subtle than in younger individuals. Because older adults have decreased body temperature, fever may be more difficult to detect. Changes in behavior such as lethargy, fatigue, disorientation, irritability, and loss of appetite may be early signs of infection.
- Immune system functioning declines with advanced age. Research is continuing.
- The older adult's immune system continues to produce antibodies; therefore immunization for diseases such as pneumonia and influenza is recommended.
- Older individuals who have chronic illnesses are generally at increased risk for infection.

encounter with an antigen. The vaccine, or toxoid, stimulates humoral immunity, which provides protection from disease for months to years.

Immunotherapy (a special treatment of allergic responses that administers increasingly large doses of the offending allergens to gradually develop immunity) consists of injecting a person with a very diluted antigen (allergen) to which the patient has a type I hypersensitivity. The strength of the dilution is increased over a long period, and weekly injections are given over a 1- to 3-year period. The theory behind immunotherapy is to assist the individual to build a tolerance to the allergen without developing fever or increased signs and symptoms. *Desensitization* is another term used for immunotherapy. It is indicated for patients with clinically significant disease for whom avoidance of the allergen or treatment with medication is inadequate. It is considered safe in properly selected patients but does present problems, which include a lengthy, expensive process and a potential for severe anaphylaxis.

Immunotherapy may be co-seasonal, preseasonal, or perennial. Perennial therapy is most widely accepted because it allows for a higher cumulative dose, which produces a better effect. Perennial therapy usually be-

gins with 0.05 mL of a 1:10,000 dilution and increases to 0.5 mL in a 6-week period. The amount given again decreases to 0.05 mL while the dilution lessens to 1:1000 to begin the next series. The amount increases each week until a 0.5-mL dose is given. The next cycle begins with a 0.05-mL dose of 1:100 dilution. Over another 6-week period, the amount administered will increase to 0.5 mL. Perennial therapy is administered subcutaneously. The patient must always be observed for at least 20 minutes after administration because hypersensitivity reaction or anaphylaxis may occur.

The treatment protocol for anaphylaxis with immunotherapy is generally accepted to be 0.2 to 0.5 mL of 1:1000 epinephrine hydrochloride (Adrenalin Chloride) subcutaneously every 20 minutes for three doses.

Most patients begin immunotherapy at the physician's office, and subsequent weekly injections are given until the maintenance level is reached. Home administration by the patient or a family member is acceptable once maintenance level is reached. Interrupted regimens because of illness may place the patient at risk for reaction. The physician should be consulted before administering a dose of diluted allergen if illness or interruption of time schedule has occurred while the patient is on maintenance immunotherapy.

Failure of the immune system occurs in several ways and expresses itself in mild to severe form. The system can malfunction at many points while attempting to provide the body with protective defense.

It is thought that failures occur because of genetic factors, developmental defects, infection, malignancy, injury, drugs, or altered metabolic states.

Severity of altered immune response disorders ranges from mild to chronic to life threatening and is categorized as follows:

I **Hypersensitivity** disorder: involves allergic response and tissue rejection
II **Immunodeficiency** disease: involves altered and failed immune response
III **Autoimmune** disease: involves extensive tissue damage resulting from an immune system that seemingly reverses its function to one of self-destruction

(See Box 15-1 for the four Rs of the immune response.)

DISORDERS OF THE IMMUNE SYSTEM

HYPERSENSITIVITY DISORDERS
Etiology/Pathophysiology

Hypersensitivity is an abnormal condition characterized by an excessive reaction to a particular stimulus. **Hypersensitivity** reaction is an inappropriate and excessive response of the immune system to a sensitizing antigen. **Hypersensitivity disorders** arise when harmless substances—such as pollens, danders, foods, and chemicals—are recognized as foreign. The body mounts an immune response in much the same way it does to any foreign protein. The result, however, differs. The host becomes sensitive after first exposure, and on subsequent exposure the allergic individual exhibits a hypersensitivity reaction. Chronic exposure leads to chronic allergy response, which ranges from mild to incapacitating signs and symptoms.

Hypersensitivity disorders are believed to be a genetic defect that allows increased production of IgE (immunoglobulin E—a humoral antibody) with release of histamine and other mediators from mast cells and basophils. Humoral reactions, mediated by the circulating B lymphocytes, are immediate. Cellular reactions mediated by the T lymphocytes are delayed, cell-mediated hypersensitivity reactions. Exposure to antigen may occur by inhalation, ingestion, injection, or touch (contact). Signs and symptoms occur as a result of histamine release and cause vasodilation, edema, bronchoconstriction, mucus secretion, and pruritus. Reaction may be local (gastrointestinal, skin, respiratory, conjunctival) or systemic (anaphylaxis). The exact mechanism and pathway of these inflammatory responses are not clearly understood.

It is known that a combination of interrelated factors occurs with increased severity of symptoms (Box 15-3). The disorders that result from hypersensitivity, which will be discussed elsewhere in the text, are urticaria, angioedema, allergic rhinitis, allergic conjunctivitis (hay fever), and atopic dermatitis.

Assessment

Assessment should involve predominantly the integumentary, gastrointestinal, respiratory, and cardiovascular systems. The nurse should be aware of the seasonal nature of the complaints.

Collection of **subjective data** includes pruritus, nausea, and uneasiness.

Collection of **objective data** includes sneezing, excessive nasal secretions, lacrimation, inflamed nasal membranes, skin rash or areas of raised inflammation, diarrhea, cough, wheezes, impaired breathing, and hypotension.

Diagnostic Tests

Hypersensitivity illnesses are diagnosed largely through patient history and physical examination. Laboratory studies are supportive tools for diagnosis and therapy.

A thorough history is the most important diagnostic tool. A detailed history is taken, listing (1) onset, nature, and progression of signs and symptoms; (2) aggravating and alleviating factors; and (3) frequency and duration of signs and symptoms. Environmental, household, and occupational factors are assessed. Common offenders include pollens, spores, dusts, food, drugs, and insect venoms. Many but not all offenders are seasonal. Signs and symptoms generally vary from mild upper respiratory manifestations, such as sneezing and excessive nasal secretions, to watery, itching eyes. Skin signs and symptoms are often eczema-like or urticarial (hives). Diarrhea may be a gastrointestinal complaint in some individuals. More severe signs and symptoms include those of the lower respiratory tract, such as coughing, wheezing, chest discomfort, breathing difficulties, and shock, which could be followed by cardiovascular collapse and respiratory arrest. The complete history will assist in accurate diagnosis (Health Promotion Considerations box).

Health Promotion Considerations

Assessing the Patient with Allergies

- A comprehensive history that covers family allergies, past and present allergies, and social and environmental factors is essential.
- Identifying the allergens that may have triggered a reaction is essential to control allergic reactions.
- Determining the time of year that an allergic reaction occurs can be a clue to a seasonal allergen.
- Information should also be obtained about any over-the-counter or prescription medications used to treat allergies.
- In addition to identification of the allergen, information about the clinical manifestations and course of allergic reaction should be obtained.
- Social and environmental factors, especially the physical environment, are important.
- Questions about pets, trees, and plants on property; air pollutants; and floor coverings, house plants, and cooling and heating systems in the home and workplace can provide valuable information about allergens.
- A daily or weekly food diary with a description of any untoward reactions is important.
- Of particular interest is a screening for any reaction to mediation.
- Questions about the patient's lifestyle and stress level should be reviewed in connection with the appearance of allergic symptoms.

Box 15-3 *Factors Influencing Hypersensitivity*

Host response to allergen. The more sensitive the individual, the greater the allergic response is.

Exposure amount. Generally, the greater the amount of allergen the individual is exposed to, the greater the chance of severe reaction is.

Nature of the allergen. Most allergy reactions are precipitated by complex, high-molecular–weight protein substances.

Route of allergen entry. Most allergens enter the body via gastrointestinal and respiratory routes. Injections of venoms and medications hold a more severe threat of allergic response.

Repeated exposure. Generally, the more the individual is exposed, the greater the response is.

MEDICATIONS | *Immune Disorders*

MEDICATION	TRADE NAME	ACTION	SIDE EFFECTS	NURSING IMPLICATIONS
Diphenhydramine	Benadryl	Antihistamine	Drowsiness, confusion, nasal stuffiness, dry mouth, photosensitivity, urine retention	Use cautiously with CNS depressants, including alcohol; give with food; know that it is safe hypnotic for older adults; tell patient to avoid driving or hazardous activity due to drowsiness.
Astemizole	Hismanal	Nonsedating antihistamine	Dysuria, urinary retention, impotence, dry nose and throat, hemolytic anemia, pancytopenia, nausea, diarrhea, constipation, drowsiness, tremors, photosensitivity	I&O ratio, be alert for urinary retention, frequency, dysuria; assess respiratory status: note rhythm, wheezing. Administer on an empty stomach 1 hr before or 2 hr after meals. Instruct patient not to exceed prescribed dose.
Loratadine	Claritin	Nonsedating antihistamine	Slight sedation (more common with increased doses)	Store in tight container at room temperature. Teach patient/family to avoid driving, other hazardous activities if drowsiness occurs.
Fexofenadine	Allegra	Nonsedating antihistamine	The potential for Allegra to cause dysrhythmias has been carefully evaluated. It has not been observed to cause dysrhythmias. People receiving Allegra concurrently with erythromycin or ketoconazole had no difference in the incidence of cardiac problems when compared with those receiving Allegra alone	

The physical examination should include a thorough assessment of the skin, middle ear, conjunctiva, nasooropharynx, and lungs.

Laboratory studies are usually not necessary unless allergic signs and symptoms are severe and protracted. A complete blood count (CBC), skin testing, total serum IgE levels, and a specific IgE level for a particular allergen may be ordered. The latter test is called RAST (radioallergosorbent test).

Medical Management

Treatment of hypersensitivity disorders includes (1) symptom management with medications, (2) environmental control, and (3) immunotherapy. The most effective treatment is environmental control, which includes avoidance of the offending allergen.

Pollens are seasonal and can be avoided at season peaks with air conditioning and limiting time spent outdoors. Mold spores can be reduced by maintaining dry conditions and using air filters. House dust can be controlled by damp dusting, use of air filters, and decreased use of carpet and overstuffed furniture. Most other offending allergens can simply be avoided (food, drugs, chemicals, and stinging insects).

Medications are used to treat and alleviate signs and symptoms. Antihistamines compete with histamine by attaching to the cell surface receptors and blocking histamine release. Antihistamines therefore must be initiated soon after exposure or taken on a regular basis. Drowsiness, mucous membrane dryness, and occasionally central nervous system excitation are

MEDICATIONS | *Immune Disorders—cont'd*

MEDICATION	TRADE NAME	ACTION	SIDE EFFECTS	NURSING IMPLICATIONS
Dexamethasone	Decadron, Turbinaire	Corticosteroid (inhaled)	Nasal irritation, rebound congestion, hypertension, headache, seizure, fluid retention	Do not use for extended period; use cautiously with diabetes and peptic ulcers; know that it is not effective for acute episodes; tell mothers not to breastfeed while using.
Flunisolide	Nasalide, Rhinalar	Corticosteroid (inhaled)	Headache, transient nasal burning epistaxis, nausea, vomiting	Know that it is not effective for acute episodes; use regularly; teach care and cleaning of inhaler; if symptoms do not improve in 3 weeks, consult physician.
Epinephrine	Adrenalin, Sus-Phrine, EpiPen	Bronchodilator	Nervousness, tremor, headache, hypertension, tachycardia, ventricular fibrillation, stroke	Do not use with monoamine oxidase inhibitor; use cautiously in patients with hyperthyroid, hypertension, diabetes, and heart disease.

side effects of the earlier antihistamines. Examples of these include pseudoephedrine (Actifed), diphenhydramine (Benadryl) chlorpheniramine (Chlor-Trimeton), and brompheniramine (Dimetapp). Nonsedating antihistamines include astemizole (Hismanal), cetirizine (Zyrtec), loratadine (Claritin), and fexofenadine (Allegra). The nonsedating antihistamines are more desirable for those who experience drowsiness with antihistamine use (Medications table).

Leukotriene inhibitors are agents that contribute significantly to reducing symptoms of an allergic reaction caused by the release of leukotrienes from mast cells and basophils. Three are currently available in the United States: montelukast (Singulair) and zafirlukast (Accolate) act as leukotriene-receptor blockers, and zileuton (Zyflo) inhibits the production of leukotrienes.

Nursing Diagnoses

Nursing diagnoses for patients with hypersensitivity include (1) risk for injury, related to exposure to allergen; (2) activity intolerance, related to malaise; and (3) risk for infection, related to inflammation of protective mucous membranes.

Patient Teaching

Patient teaching should revolve around the specific diagnosis. The patient should be informed regarding seasonal avoidance of the offending allergens and should understand the therapeutic medication plan. The nurse will focus on health promotion and health teaching for self-care management (Safety Considerations box).

Safety Considerations

Treating the Patient with a Hypersensitivity Reaction

- It is extremely important that all of a patient's allergies be listed on the chart, the nursing care plan, and the medication record.
- After an allergic disorder is diagnosed, therapeutic treatment is aimed at reducing exposure to the offending allergen, treating the symptoms, and if necessary, desensitizing the person through immunotherapy.
- All health care workers must be prepared for the rare, but life-threatening anaphylactic reaction, which requires immediate medical and nursing interventions.
- The patient should be taught to wear a medical-alert bracelet listing the particular drug allergy.
- For a patient allergic to insect stings, commercial bee sting kits containing a preinjectable epinephrine and a tourniquet are available. The nurse has the responsibility to instruct the patient about the technique of applying the tourniquet and self-injecting the subcutaneous epinephrine. This patient should also wear a medical-alert bracelet and carry a bee sting kit whenever going outdoors.

ANAPHYLAXIS
Etiology/Pathophysiology

The most severe IgE-mediated allergic reaction is anaphylaxis, or systemic reaction to allergens. The antigens causing anaphylaxis include (1) venoms;

(2) drugs, such as penicillin and aspirin; (3) contrast media dyes; (4) insect stings; and (5) some foods.

Clinical Manifestations

In anaphylaxis the reaction occurs very rapidly after exposure, from seconds to a few minutes. Fatal reactions are associated with a fall in blood pressure, laryngeal edema, and bronchospasm, leading to cardiovascular collapse, myocardial infarction, and respiratory failure.

In anaphylaxis, massive release of mediators initiates events in target organs throughout the body. Skin and gastrointestinal (GI) signs and symptoms may occur, although respiratory and cardiovascular signs and symptoms predominate. Anaphylactic reactions are classified as mild, moderate, and severe.

Assessment

Early recognition of signs and symptoms and early treatment may prevent severe reactions and even death. Generally, the more rapid the onset, the more severe the outcome is. Overall, the individual may have a feeling of uneasiness that increases to a sense of foreboding and leads to a fear of impending death. The skin may or may not be involved. Urticaria and pruritus may be present in mild and moderate anaphylaxis, whereas cyanosis and pallor may be seen in severe reactions. Upper respiratory signs and symptoms range from congestion and sneezing to edema of the tongue and larynx with stridor and occlusion of the upper airways. Lower respiratory signs and symptoms will follow, including bronchospasm, wheezing, and severe dyspnea. GI signs and symptoms will increase from nausea, vomiting, and diarrhea to dysphagia and involuntary stools. The patient may have cardiovascular signs and symptoms, such as tachycardia and hypotension. Signs and symptoms may increase, and the patient may display coronary insufficiency, vascular collapse, dysrhythmias, shock, cardiac arrest, respiratory failure, and death.

Medical Management

Immediate aggressive treatment is the goal in anaphylaxis. At the first sign, 0.2 to 0.5 mL of epinephrine (Adrenalin Chloride) 1:1000 is given subcutaneously for mild symptoms. It may be repeated at 20-minute intervals as prescribed by the physician. Epinephrine 1:10,000, 0.5 mL IV at 5- to 10-minute intervals may be administered for severe reaction as prescribed by the physician. Benadryl 50 to 100 mg may be given IM or IV as indicated for allergic signs and symptoms. If moderate to severe signs and symptoms occur, IV therapy may be initiated to prevent vascular collapse, and the patient may be intubated to prevent airway obstruction. Oxygen may be administered by nonrebreather mask. Place the patient in recumbent position and elevate legs. Keep patient warm.

Nursing Interventions and Patient Teaching

These measures include the following:
1. Assess respiratory status, including dyspnea, wheezing, and decreased breath sounds.
2. Assess circulatory status, including dysrhythmias, tachycardia, and hypotension.
3. Assess vital signs continuously.
4. Assess intake and output (I&O).
5. Assess mental status, including anxiety, malaise, confusion, and coma.
6. Assess skin status, including erythema, urticaria, cyanosis, and pallor.
7. Assess GI status, including nausea, vomiting, diarrhea, and incontinence.

The diagnosis is most often made by a history of signs and symptoms. Looking at and listening to the anxious patient should be leading clues in suspecting anaphylaxis.

An alert diagnostician will question the patient about recent exposure to known antigens that cause anaphylaxis (Box 15-4). Most laboratory studies would not be beneficial.

Nursing diagnoses for the patient with anaphylaxis include but are not limited to the following:

Nursing Diagnoses	Nursing Interventions
Ineffective breathing pattern, related to edema, bronchospasm, and increased secretions	Maintain airway. Administer high-flow oxygen via nonrebreather mask. Administer prescribed medications. Keep warm. Monitor vital signs. Suction if necessary. Anticipate intubation with severe respirator distress.
Decreased cardiac output, related to increased capillary permeability and vascular dilation	Monitor IV fluid infusions as ordered. Monitor vital signs. Monitor I&O. Obtain complete allergy history. Document signs and symptoms, interventions, and response.

The nurse's responsibilities in patient education are as follows:
- Reassure patient during procedures.
- Teach patient avoidance of allergen.
- Teach the use of medic-alert identification.
- Teach patient preparation and administration of epinephrine subcutaneously.

Prognosis

If the signs and symptoms are left untreated, anaphylaxis can lead to death in a relatively short time.

Box 15-4 | *Common Allergens Causing Anaphylaxis*

Drugs	Venoms	Foods
Vaccines	Honeybees	Milk
Allergen extracts	Wasps	Peanuts
Enzymes	Hornets	Brazil nuts
Penicillins		Cashew nuts
Sulfonamides		Strawberries
Cephalosporins		Shellfish
Dextrans		Egg albumin
Hormones		Chocolate
Contrast media		
Anesthetic agents		

LATEX ALLERGIES

Allergies to latex products have become a problem of increasing proportion, affecting patients as well as health care professionals. The increase in allergic reactions have coincided with the sharp increase in glove use related to the introduction of universal precautions against infectious diseases in 1987. It is estimated that 8% to 17% of health care workers regularly exposed to latex are sensitized. The more frequent and prolonged the exposure to latex, the greater likelihood of developing a latex allergy. In addition to gloves, many latex-containing products are used in health care, such as blood pressure cuffs, stethoscopes, tourniquets, intravenous (IV) tubing, syringes, electrode pads, O_2 masks, tracheal tubes, colostomy and ileostomy pouches, urinary catheters, anesthetic masks, and adhesive tape. Latex proteins can become aerosolized through powder on gloves and can result in serious reactions when inhaled by sensitized individuals.

Types of Latex Allergies

Two types of latex allergies that can occur are **type IV allergic contact dermatitis and type I allergic reactions.** Type IV contact dermatitis is caused by the *chemicals used in the manufacturing process of latex gloves.* It is a delayed reaction that occurs within 6 to 48 hours. Typically the person first has dryness, pruritus, fissuring, and cracking of the skin, followed by erythema, edema, and crusting at 24 to 48 hours. Chronic exposure can lead to thickening and hardening of the skin, scaling, and hyperpigmentation. The dermatitis may extend beyond the area of physical contact with the allergen.

A type I allergic reaction is a response to the *natural rubber latex proteins* and occurs within minutes of contact with the proteins. These types of allergic reactions can manifest as various reactions ranging from skin erythema, urticaria, rhinitis, conjuctivitis, or asthma to full-blown anaphylactic shock. Systemic reactions to latex may result from exposure to protein via various routes, including the skin, mucous membranes, inhalation, or blood.

Nursing Interventions

The identification of patients and health care workers sensitive to latex is crucial in preventing adverse reactions. A thorough health history and history of any allergies should be collected, especially on patients with any complaints of latex contact symptoms. Not all latex-sensitive individuals can be identified, even with a careful and thorough history. Risk factors include long-term exposure to latex products (e.g., health care personnel, individuals who have had multiple surgeries, rubber industry workers). Additional risk factors include a patient history of hay fever, asthma, and allergies to certain foods (e.g., avocados, guava, kiwi, bananas, water chestnuts, hazelnuts, tomatoes, potatoes, peaches, grapes, apricots, peanuts).

The National Institute for Occupational Safety and Health (NIOSH) has published recommendations for preventing allergic reactions to latex in the workplace. This free publication (no. 97-135 can be obtained from NIOSH at 800-356-4674 or *www.cdc.gov/niosh*). In summary they include the following:

1. Use nonlatex gloves for activities that are not likely to involve contact with infectious materials (e.g., food preparation, housekeeping).
2. Use powder-free gloves with reduced protein content.
3. Do not use oil-based hand creams or lotions when wearing gloves.
4. After removing gloves, wash hands with mild soap and dry thoroughly.
5. Frequently clean work areas that are contaminated with latex-containing dust.
6. Know the signs and symptoms of latex allergy, including skin rash; hives; flushing; itching; nasal, eye, or sinus symptoms; asthma; and shock.
7. If symptoms of latex allergy develop, avoid direct contact with latex gloves and products.
8. Wear a medical-alert bracelet and carry an epinephrine pen.

Latex precaution protocols should be used for those patients identified as having a positive latex allergy test or a history of signs and symptoms related to latex exposure. Many health care facilities have created latex-free product carts that can be used for patients with latex allergies (Lewis et al, 2004).

TRANSFUSION REACTIONS

Transfusion reactions are a hypersensitivity disorder and are best illustrated by reactions that occur with mismatched blood.

Careful selection of blood donors is important in preventing transfusion reaction, followed by careful typing and cross-matching of blood from donor to recipient. Storage of blood and administration protocol are important in blood reaction prevention. Blood and blood components should be refrigerated at specific temperatures until $\frac{1}{2}$ hour before administration. Blood must be administered within 4 hours of refrigeration, and blood components within 6 hours of refrigeration. Donor and recipient numbers are specific and must be thoroughly checked and the patient identified with an armband. All blood and blood products are administered through microaggregate filters. The nurse should monitor for adverse effects.

Transfusion reactions are labeled mild, moderate, and severe. The most severe reactions occur within the first 15 minutes, moderate reactions within 30 to 90 minutes, and mild reactions may be delayed to late in the transfusion or hours to several days after transfusion.

Mild transfusion reaction signs and symptoms include dermatitis, diarrhea, fever, chills, urticaria, cough, and orthopnea. Treatment includes (1) stopping the transfusion; and (2) administering saline, steroids, and diuretics as ordered. Transfusion may continue at a slower rate. In moderate reactions—in which fever, chills, urticaria, and wheezing occur after the first 30 minutes of administration—the transfusion is stopped and saline is continued. Antihistamines and epinephrine may be given. The physician decides whether the transfusion is to continue. With severe reaction the transfusion is stopped and saline is given to provide venous access. It is recommended that the blood or blood product be returned to the laboratory for immediate testing if any type of reaction occurs. A urine specimen is sent to the laboratory if reaction occurs.

The best method for prevention of transfusion reaction is autologous (pertaining to a tissue occurring naturally and derived from the same individual) transfusion, or use of one's own blood, for replacement therapy. The blood can be frozen and stored for as long as 3 years. Usually the blood is stored without being frozen and is given to the person within a few weeks of donation.

DELAYED HYPERSENSITIVITY

Delayed hypersensitivity reactions occurring 24 to 72 hours after exposure are mediated by T cells accompanied by release of lymphokines. Delayed reaction contact dermatitis, such as after contact with poison ivy, is one example. Tissue transplant rejection is another example. Only transplant rejection is discussed here.

TRANSPLANT REJECTION

Transfer of healthy tissue or organs from a donor to a recipient has been done for many years. The immune process that protects the body from foreign protein is the same process at work in tissue transplant rejection. Knowledge of the function of the immune system enabled medical experts to find a way to control the re-

jection process. It is now possible to prepare the body before tissue transplant for grafting to be successful.

Autograft, or transplantation of tissue from one site to another on an individual, is successful. It is used after trauma, especially on full-thickness burns, and in reconstructive surgery. Isograft is transfer of tissue between genetically identical individuals, such as identical twins. Allograft is a term applied to the transplantation of tissue between members of the same species. Because few humans are born with an identical twin, allograft is the most common form of tissue transplant.

Antigenic determinants on the cells lead to graft rejection via the immune process. Therefore recipient tissue is as closely matched as possible to donor tissue antigenic determinants before transplantation. Tissue matching leads to a better chance of success.

Tissue rejection does not occur immediately after transplantation. It takes several days for vascularization to occur. Seven to 10 days after blood supply is adequately established, sensitized lymphocytes appear in sufficient numbers for sloughing to occur at the site.

Graft rejection is slowed through use of chemical agents that interfere with the immune response process. Included are corticosteroids, cyclosporine (Neoral, Sandimmune), and azathioprine (Imuran). This chemical therapy is referred to as immunosuppressive therapy (the administration of agents that significantly interfere with the ability of the immune system to respond to antigenic stimulation by inhibiting cellular and humoral immunity).

Infection is a threat to the immunosuppressed patient. Meticulous aseptic technique is required when caring for these individuals. Prophylactic antibiotic therapy may be advisable, and good skin care is necessary. Visits to the bedside are limited in frequency for both staff and family. People with infection are not allowed at the bedside.

IMMUNODEFICIENCY DISORDERS

The first evidence of immunodeficiency (an abnormal condition of the immune system in which cellular or humoral immunity is inadequate and resistance to infection is decreased) disease is an increased susceptibility to infection. The problem can manifest as recurrent infection or chronic infection. Unusually severe infection with complications or incomplete clearing of an infection may also indicate an underlying immunodeficiency.

Defects in genes leading to immunodeficiency provide a hereditary link to the diseases. Many diseases are believed to occur because of immunodeficiency. These diseases include AIDS, agammaglobulinemia, and multiple myeloma, which are discussed elsewhere in the text.

When the immune system does not adequately protect the body, an immunodeficient state exists. The immunodeficiency disorders involve an impairment of one or more immune mechanisms, which include (1) phagocytosis, (2) humoral response, (3) cell-mediated response, (4) complement, and (5) a combined humoral and cell-mediated deficiency. Immunodeficiency disorders are primary if the immune cells are improperly developed or absent and secondary if the deficiency is caused by illnesses or treatment. Primary immunodeficiency disorders are rare and often serious, whereas secondary disorders are more common and less severe.

PRIMARY IMMUNODEFICIENCY DISORDERS

The basic categories of primary immunodeficiency disorders include (1) phagocytic defects, (2) B-cell deficiency, (3) T-cell deficiency, and (4) a combined B-cell and T-cell deficiency.

SECONDARY IMMUNODEFICIENCY DISORDERS

Drug-induced immunosuppression is the most common type of secondary immunodeficiency disorder. Immunosuppressive therapy is prescribed for patients to treat autoimmune disorders and to prevent transplant rejection. In addition, immunosuppression is a serious side effect of cytotoxic drugs used in cancer chemotherapy. Generalized leukopenia often results, leading to a decreased humoral and cell-mediated response. Therefore secondary infections are common in immunosuppressed patients.

Stress may alter the immune response. This response involves interrelationships between the nervous, endocrine, and immune systems.

A hypofunctional state of the immune system exists in young children and older adults. Laboratory studies have demonstrated that immunoglobulin levels decrease with age and therefore lead to a suppressed humoral immune response in older adults. Thymic involution occurs with aging, along with decreased numbers of T cells. The incidence of malignancies and autoimmune diseases increases with aging and may be related to immunologic deterioration.

Malnutrition alters cell-mediated immune responses. When protein is deficient over a prolonged period, atrophy of the thymus gland occurs and lymphoid tissue decreases. In addition, an increased susceptibility to infections always exists.

Radiation destroys lymphocytes either directly or through depletion of stem cells. As the radiation dose is increased, more bone marrow atrophies, leading to severe pancytopenia and severe suppression of immune function.

Surgical removal of lymph nodes, thymus, or spleen can suppress the immune response. Splenectomy in children is especially dangerous and may lead to septicemia from simple respiratory infections.

Hodgkin's disease greatly impairs the cell-mediated immune response, and patients may die from severe viral or fungal infections. Viruses, especially rubella, may cause immunodeficiency by direct cytotoxic damage to lymphoid cells. Systemic infections can place such a demand on the immune system that resistance to a secondary or subsequent infection is impaired.

AUTOIMMUNE DISORDERS

Autoimmune (pertaining to the development of an immune response [autoantibodies or cellular immune response] to one's own tissues) disorders are failures of the tolerance to "self." Autoimmune disorders may be described as an immune attack on the self and result from the failure to distinguish "self" protein from "foreign" protein.

For some unknown reason, immune cells that are normally unresponsive (tolerant to self-antigens) are activated. Both T cells and B cells have the ability for tolerance to self-antigens. Therefore an alteration in T cells alone or in both B cells and T cells can produce autoantibodies and autosensitized T cells to cause pathophysiologic tissue damage. The particular autoimmune disease manifested depends on which self-antigen is involved.

Autoimmune diseases tend to cluster so that a given person may have more than one autoimmune disease (e.g., rheumatoid arthritis and Addison's disease), or the same or related autoimmune diseases may be found in other members of the same family. This observation has led to the concept of genetic predisposition to autoimmune disease.

As a person ages, the probability of failure in any system occurs. It is not clearly understood what happens when autoimmune responses occur.

Whatever the cause, autoimmune disorders exist. Many illnesses are now believed to be in this classification. Included are pernicious anemia, Guillain-Barré syndrome, scleroderma, Sjögren syndrome, rheumatic fever, rheumatoid arthritis, ulcerative colitis, male infertility, myasthenia gravis, multiple sclerosis, Addison's disease, autoimmune hemolytic anemia, immune thrombocytopenic purpura, type 1 diabetes mellitus, glomerulonephritis, and systemic lupus erythematosus. These conditions are discussed elsewhere in the text.

Plasmapheresis. Plasmapheresis is the removal of plasma that contains components causing, or thought to cause, disease. When plasma is removed, it is replaced by substitution fluids such as saline or albumin. Therefore the term *plasma exchange* more accurately describes this procedure.

Plasmapheresis has been used to treat autoimmune diseases such as systemic lupus erythematosus, glomerulonephritis, myasthenia gravis, thrombocytopenic purpura, rheumatoid arthritis, and Guillain-Barré syndrome.

The rationale for performing therapeutic plasmapheresis in autoimmune disorders is to remove pathologic substances present in plasma. Many disorders for which plasmapheresis is being used are characterized by circulating autoantibodies (usually of the IgG class) and antigen-antibody complexes. Immunosuppressive therapy has been used to prevent recovery of IgG production, and plasmapheresis has been used to prevent antibody rebound.

In addition to removing antinuclear antibodies and antigen-antibody complexes, plasmapheresis may also remove inflammatory mediators (e.g., complement) that are responsible for tissue damage. In the treatment of systemic lupus erythematosus, plasmapheresis is usually reserved for the patient in an acute attack who is unresponsive to conventional therapy.

Plasmapheresis involves the removal of whole blood through a needle inserted in one arm and circulation of the blood through a cell separator. Inside the separator the blood is divided into plasma and its cellular components by centrifugation or membrane filtration. A needle is inserted into the opposite arm for return of the blood to the patient. Plasma, platelets, white blood cells (WBCs), or red blood cells (RBCs) can be separated selectively. The undesirable component is removed, and the remainder is returned to the patient. The plasma is generally replaced with normal saline, lactated Ringer's solution, fresh frozen plasma, plasma protein fractions, or albumin. When blood is manually removed, only 500 mL may be taken at one time. However, with the use of apheresis procedures, more than 4 L of plasma can be pheresed in 2 to 3 hours.

As with administration of other blood products, nurses must be aware of side effects associated with plasmapheresis. The most common complications are hypotension and citrate toxicity. Hypotension is usually the result of vasovagal reaction or transient volume changes. Citrate is used as an anticoagulant and may cause hypocalcemia, which may manifest as headache, paresthesias, and dizziness. See text for complete coverage of various autoimmune disorders.

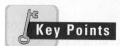

Key Points

- The two major forms of immunity are innate (natural) and acquired (adaptive).
- T lymphocytes, B lymphocytes, and macrophages are the three major cells active in acquired immunity.
- B lymphocytes produce antibodies.
- T lymphocytes do not produce antibodies, but assist the B cell.
- T lymphocytes release lymphokines.
- Macrophages trap, process, and present antigen to T lymphocytes.
- Autoimmune disorders are failures of the tolerance to "self."
- Plasmapheresis is used to treat autoimmune diseases such as systemic lupus erythematosus, glomerulonephritis, myasthenia gravis, thrombocytopenic purpura, rheumatoid arthritis, and Guillain-Barré syndrome.
- Infection is a primary threat to the immunosuppressed patient. Aseptic technique is required when caring for these patients. Good skin care is necessary.
- Careful selection of blood donors and careful typing and cross-matching of blood are important in prevention of transfusion reaction.
- Early recognition of signs followed by early treatment may decrease the severity of allergic reaction.
- The five factors influencing hypersensitivity response include host response to allergen, exposure amount, nature of the allergen, route of allergen entry, and repeated exposure.
- Two types of latex allergies are **type IV allergic contact dermatitis** and **type I allergic reactions.** Type IV is caused by the chemicals used in the manufacturing process of latex gloves, whereas type I allergic reaction is a response to the natural rubber latex proteins.

Go to your free CD-ROM for an Audio Glossary, animations, video clips, and Review Questions for the NCLEX-PN® Examination.

evolve Be sure to visit the companion Evolve site at http://evolve.elsevier.com/Christensen/adult/ for WebLinks and additional online resources.

CHAPTER CHALLENGE

1. Immune disorders that result from failure of the tolerance to "self" responding immunologically to one's own antigens are called:
   1. immunodeficiency disorders.
   2. hypersensitivity disorders.
   3. desensitization disorders.
   4. autoimmune disorders.

2. Mr. T. is recovering from having a kidney transplant. The nursing intervention of this immunosuppressed patient should include:
   1. prophylactic antibiotic therapy.
   2. meticulous aseptic technique.
   3. restriction of all visitors.
   4. antineoplastic medication administration.

3. Innate or natural immunity is:

   1. the body's first line of defense against disease, which protects locally against the external environment.
   2. the body's second line of defense against disease, which protects the internal environment.
   3. mediated by B cells to produce antibodies in response to antigenic challenge.
   4. an immunity that is specific.

4. Ms. K. is a 26-year-old patient with a history of numerous allergies. The nurse's most important teaching concept is:

   1. immunotherapy regimen.
   2. avoidance of the allergen.
   3. antihistamine administration.
   4. adrenaline administration.

5. Humoral immunity is mediated by:

   1. T cells.
   2. B cells.
   3. macrophages.
   4. myeloblasts.

6. Cellular immunity develops when which cells are activated by an antigen?

   1. T cells
   2. B cells
   3. Neutrophils
   4. Monoblasts

7. Desensitization is another term for:

   1. autoimmune disorders.
   2. adaptive immunity.
   3. immunotherapy.
   4. immunodeficiency disease.

8. After a bee sting, Ms. W.'s face becomes edematous and she begins to wheeze. Based on this assessment, the nurse would be prepared to administer:

   1. aminophylline.
   2. Benadryl.
   3. epinephrine.
   4. Valium.

9. The nurse gave an intramuscular penicillin injection to a patient. Which of the following would be a sign of a systemic anaphylactic response?

   1. Increased blood pressure
   2. Bradycardia
   3. Urticaria
   4. Wheezing

10. Ms. R. is a 38-year-old patient who is receiving two units of packed cells at 125 mL per hour. Fifteen minutes after the start of the transfusion, the nurse notes the following vital signs: pulse 110, respirations 28, BP 98/58, and temperature 101° F. The patient is shivering. The nurse's next action would be to:

    1. slow the infusion rate.
    2. stop the infusion.
    3. administer aspirin as ordered for elevated temperature.
    4. report the findings to the nurse manager.

11. Ms. H., 72, is admitted to the hospital with a diagnosis of immunodeficiency disease. For Ms. H. the primary nursing goals would be to:

    1. reduce the risk of her developing an infection.
    2. encourage Ms. H. to provide self-care.
    3. plan nutritious meals to provide adequate intake.
    4. encourage Ms. H. to interact with other patients.

12. Mr. K. tells the nurse he is overwhelmed. There is so much he must do to keep his new kidney functioning, and then rejection may still occur. Which of the following nursing diagnosis is appropriate at this time?

    1. Ineffective coping
    2. Disturbed body image
    3. Impaired adjustment
    4. Situational low self-esteem

13. Choose all of the correct nursing interventions for anaphylaxis:

    1. Assess vital signs every 4 hours.
    2. Assess respiratory status frequently.
    3. Maintain patent airway.
    4. Administer epinephrine 1:1000, 0.2 to 0.5 mL subcutaneously as ordered.

14. Mr. R. comes to the clinic for his weekly allergy injection. He missed his appointment the week before because of a family emergency. Which action by the nurse is appropriate in administering Mr. R.'s injection?

    1. Administer the usual dosage of the allergen.
    2. Double the dosage to account for the missed injection the previous week.
    3. Consult with the physician about decreasing the dosage for this injection.
    4. Reevaluate Mr. R.'s sensitivity to the allergen with a skin test.

15. The nurse advises a friend who asks him to administer his allergy injections that:

    1. it is illegal for nurses to administer injections outside of a medical setting.
    2. he is qualified to do it if the friend has epinephrine in an injectable syringe provided with his extract.
    3. avoiding the allergens is a more effective way of controlling allergies and allergy shots are not usually effective.
    4. immunotherapy should only be administered in a setting where emergency equipment and drugs are available.

Continued

CHAPTER CHALLENGE—cont'd

16. A female patient is undergoing plasmapheresis for treatment of systemic lupus erythematosus. The nurse explains that plasmapheresis is used in the treatment to:

   1. remove T lymphocytes in her blood that are producing antinuclear antibodies.
   2. remove normal particles in her blood that are being damaged by autoantibodies.
   3. exchange her plasma that contains antinuclear antibodies with a substitute fluid.
   4. replace viral-damaged cellular components of her blood with replacement whole blood.

17. Type I allergic reaction to latex is a response to the _____ _____ _____ _____.

16 Care of the Patient with HIV/AIDS

CRAIG E. NIELSEN

Objectives

After reading this chapter, the student should be able to do the following:

1. Define the key terms as listed.
2. Describe the agent that causes HIV disease.
3. Describe definition of AIDS given in January 1993 by the Centers for Disease Control and Prevention.
4. Explain the differences between HIV infection, HIV disease, and AIDS.
5. Describe the progression of HIV infection.
6. Discuss how HIV is and is not transmitted.
7. Discuss the pathophysiology of HIV disease.
8. Discuss the laboratory and diagnostic tests related to HIV disease.
9. Describe patients who are at risk for HIV infection.
10. Discuss the use of effective prevention messages in counseling patients.
11. Discuss the issues related to HIV antibody testing.
12. Define the nurse's role in the prevention of HIV infection.
13. Discuss the nurse's role in assisting the HIV-infected patient with coping, grieving, reducing anxiety, and minimizing social isolation.
14. Describe the multidisciplinary approach in caring for a patient with HIV disease.
15. Discuss the importance of adherence to HIV treatment.
16. List signs and symptoms that may be indicative of HIV disease.
17. List opportunistic infections associated with advanced HIV disease (AIDS).
18. Implement a care plan for the patient with AIDS.

Key Terms

Be sure to check out the bonus material on the free CD-ROM, including selected audio pronunciations.

acquired immunodeficiency syndrome (AIDS) (ĭm-ū-nō-dĕ-FĬSH-ĕn-sē, p. 780)
adherence (ăd-HĔR-ĕns, p. 796)
CD$_4$⁺ lymphocyte (LIM-fō-sīt, p. 779)
Centers for Disease Control and Prevention (p. 769)
enzyme-linked immunosorbent assay (ELISA) (ĭm-ū-nō-ăb-ZOR-bĕnt, p. 775)
HIV disease (p. 779)
HIV infection (p. 780)

human immunodeficiency virus (HIV) (p. 769)
Kaposi's sarcoma (kă-PŌS-sēz săr-KŌ-mă, p. 769)
opportunistic (ŏp-pŏr-tū-NĬS-tĭk, p. 770)
phagocytic (făg-ō-SĬT-ĭk, p. 779)
Pneumocystis jiroveci (formerly carinii) pneumonia (PCP) (nōō-mō-SĬS-tĭs kă-RĬN-ê-i, p. 769)
retrovirus (rĕ-trō-VĪ-rŭs, p. 777)
seroconversion (sĕr-ō-kŏn-VĔR-zhŭn, p. 775)
seronegative (sĕr-ō-NĔG-ă-tĭv, p. 782)
vertical transmission (p. 773)
viral load (p. 774)
virulent (VĬR-ū-lĕnt, p. 770)
Western blot (p. 775)

NURSING AND THE HISTORY OF HIV DISEASE

As early as 1979, physicians in New York and California were noting cases of *Pneumocystis jiroveci* (formerly *carinii*) pneumonia (PCP), an unusual pulmonary disease caused by a fungus and primarily associated with people who have suppressed immune systems. These physicians also noted an increase in the number of people with Kaposi's sarcoma (KS), a rare cancer of the skin and mucous membranes characterized by blue, red, or purple raised lesions seen mainly in Mediterranean men. The interesting thing was that these two diseases were occurring at alarming rates in clusters of young homosexual men whose immune systems were failing. The Centers for Disease Control and Prevention (CDC) (a division of the U.S. Public Health Service in Atlanta, Georgia, that investigates and controls various diseases, especially those that have epidemic potential) soon learned that this immune disorder was also affecting injecting drug users and hemophiliacs. They later learned that it also affected heterosexual men and women.

Although the origins of acquired immunodeficiency syndrome (AIDS) remain obscure, it is known that human immunodeficiency virus (HIV) (a retrovirus that causes HIV infection and HIV disease) occurred as long ago as the late 1950s in isolated individuals, with computerized analyses of HIV and its mutations indicating that it dated back as far as 1930 (Ungvarski, 2001). HIV is also known as "zoonotic," an organism that has been able to cross from an animal species to humans. In the case of HIV, a very similar virus was noted in primates, and most likely crossed into humans with the hunting and consumption of these animals. Other examples of zoonotic transmission include severe adult respiratory distress syndrome (SARS), anthrax, hantavirus, and West Nile virus (Galvani, 2004). It began to spread in the middle to late 1970s, but because of the long incubation period, the virus did not cause widespread disease until the 1980s. In most countries, in its early stages the viral epidemic progressed undetected. The advent of this new disorder provoked fear among laypeople and health care providers alike. It was also an exciting time for health care workers because they knew they were seeing a new pathogen with a route of transmission not completely understood. In spite of the stigmas and fears that emerged—which still exist in some form today—nurses were at the forefront providing care. Nurses met the challenges of providing and coordinating services, organizing community-based organizations, teaching about prevention, and helping patients deal with a terminal disease.

On June 5, 1981, a small communication appeared in the CDC publication *Morbidity and Mortality Weekly Report (MMWR)*; it described a handful of individuals with unusual opportunistic infections that would eventually become known as AIDS and be described as the most challenging infectious disease of the 20th century. Since then, nearly 22 million people worldwide have died of AIDS, and another 40 million have become infected with HIV (Joint United Nations Programme on HIV/AIDS [UNAIDS], 2004; Nielsen, 2001). In 2004 alone, it is estimated that 3.1 million individuals died from HIV disease and close to 5 million individuals have become infected with HIV. In 1982, concerned about the fact that blood or other body fluids may be implicated in the transmission of HIV, the CDC issued the first precautions to be followed by individuals who might have contact with these fluids.

In 1983, researchers in France isolated a virus, believed to be the agent responsible for AIDS, initially named **lymphadenopathy-associated virus** (LAV). One year later, an American scientist claimed the discovery of the etiologic agent and named it the human T-cell lymphotropic virus type III (HTLV-III). Others conducting research discovered viruses that appeared to be the same, or close members of the same family. In 1986 the International Society of the Taxonomy of Viruses renamed the virus, calling it the human immunodeficiency virus (HIV). In that same year, a second and distinctly different strain of the virus was discovered in Africa. Since that time, the scientific names to distinguish between the two viruses are HIV-1 and HIV-2 (Essex & Kanki, 1988; Ungvarski, 2001).

This discovery was both major and alarming because it was the first clue that indicated HIV could change its appearance and mutate very rapidly. The capability of HIV to mutate rapidly is often referred to as **genetic promiscuity,** and it has become the trademark of this virus because it represents an immense challenge for scientists as they search for treatment and vaccine strategies. HIV-1 is found worldwide, but is most prevalent in the United States and Europe. HIV-2 is prevalent in western Africa and countries with historical or commercial ties to that region (although there are increased reports of cases in the United States [Bartlett & Gallant, 2001]). HIV-2 also appears to be less **virulent** (toxic) (Zwolski, 2001). A study in Africa found that 33% of HIV-1 infected women progressed to AIDS within 5 years of infection, whereas none of the HIV-2 infected women developed AIDS during the same period (Bartlett & Gallant, 2001; Marlink et al, 1994).

In the time since the first cases of AIDS were reported in 1981, the CDC has revised the case definition three times in response to improved laboratory and diagnostic methods, increased knowledge of the natural history of HIV disease, and improved clinical management. The current definition, used by all states and U.S. territories, allows the disease to be consistently monitored for public health purposes (CDC, 2000). This definition, which was initially based on highly specific clinical signs and symptoms of disease, was expanded in 1985, 1987, and 1993 to include additional clinical conditions, HIV antibody test results, and laboratory measures concerning the effect of the virus on the immune system (CD_4^+ and viral test results) (Table 16-1). Because HIV selectively infects and destroys cells that display CD_4^+ molecules on their surface (primarily lymphocytes), the new definition includes all HIV-infected people who have CD_4 counts of 200 cells/mm^3 or fewer (as opposed to the normal 600 to 1200 cells/mm^3). These revisions to the AIDS surveillance case definition incorporated advances in diagnostic methods and medical practices in order to provide complete, consistent, and reliable information on the numbers of life-threatening opportunistic (caused by normally nonpathogenic organisms in a host whose resistance has been decreased by such disorders as HIV disease) illnesses and deaths among HIV-infected individuals.

It was not until 1987, after the CDC reported three cases of occupationally acquired HIV infection in health care providers, that guidelines called "Universal Blood and Body Fluid Precautions," or standard precautions, were developed for the prevention of occupational exposure. This forever changed the way health care personnel protected themselves and others from the spread of bloodborne pathogens. That same year, the Association of Nurses in AIDS Care (ANAC) was established to address the needs of individuals with HIV disease and to provide a professional forum for nurses who often faced discrimination for providing care to HIV-infected patients.

Table 16-1 *Diagnostic Criteria for AIDS*

1993 CLASSIFICATION SYSTEM FOR HIV INFECTION IN ADOLESCENTS AND ADULTS

	CLINICAL CATEGORIES		
CD₄ CELL CATEGORIES*	(A) ASYMPTOMATIC, PGL, ACUTE HIV INFECTION	(B) SYMPTOMATIC, NOT (A) OR (C) CONDITIONS	(C) AIDS-INDICATOR CONDITIONS
(1) ≥500/μL	A1	B1	C1
(2) 200-499/μL	A2	B2	C2
(3) <200/μL	A3	B3	C3

CLINICAL CATEGORY A CONDITIONS	CLINICAL CATEGORY B CONDITIONS	CLINICAL CATEGORY C CONDITIONS
• Asymptomatic HIV infection • Persistent generalized lymphadenopathy (PGL) • Acute primary HIV illness (acute retroviral or sero-conversion illness)	• Bacillary angiomatosis • Candidiasis, oropharyngeal (thrush) • Candidiasis, vulvovaginal; persistent, frequent, or poorly responsive to therapy • Cervical dysplasia (moderate or severe) or cervical carcinoma in situ • Constitutional symptoms, e.g., severe (38.5° C) or diarrhea lasting more than 1 month • Herpes zoster (shingles) involving at least two distinct episodes or more than one dermatome • Idiopathic thrombocytopenic purpura (ITP) • Listeriosis • Oral hairy leukoplakia (OHL) • Pelvic inflammatory disease (PID), particularly if complicated by tubo-ovarian abscess • Peripheral neuropathy	• Candidiasis of bronchi, trachea, or lungs • Candidiasis, esophageal • Cervical cancer, invasive • Coccidioidomycosis, disseminated or extrapulmonary • Cryptococcus, extrapulmonary • Cryptosporidiosis, chronic intestinal (>1 month's duration) • Cytomegalovirus disease (other than liver, spleen, or nodes) • Cytomegalovirus (CMV) retinitis • Encephalopathy, HIV-related • Herpes simplex; chronic ulcer(s) (>1 month's duration); or bronchitis, pneumonitis, or esophagitis • Histoplasmosis, disseminated or extrapulmonary • Isosporiasis, chronic intestinal (>1 month's duration) • Kaposi's sarcoma (KS) • Lymphoma, Burkitt's (or equivalent term) • Lymphoma, primary of brain • *Mycobacterium avium* complex (MAC) or *kansasii*, disseminated or extrapulmonary • *M. tuberculosis,* any site • Mycobacterium, other identified or unidentified species, disseminated or extrapulmonary • *Pneumocystis jiroveci* (formerly *carinii*) pneumonia (PCP) • Pneumonia, recurrent • Progressive multifocal leukoen-cephalopathy (PML) • Salmonella septicemia, recurrent • Toxoplasmosis of brain • Wasting due to HIV

People with AIDS-indicator conditions (A3, B3, C1, C2, and C3) are currently reportable to local health departments in every state and U.S. territory. The red categories incorporate the AIDS surveillance case definition; these categories are AIDS indicators.
*According to the lowest, most accurate count, not the most recent count.

By now, a broad spectrum of individuals, from children to adults, and crossing all socioeconomic strata, are affected by this disorder (Older Adult Considerations box). Nurses have been instrumental in establishing care standards, collaborating with community-based organizations to provide education and treatment standards. Today, nurses comprise the largest group of health care providers who care for individuals with HIV disease, stressing the importance of prevention and influencing policymakers. HIV nursing

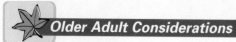

Older Adult Considerations

HIV Disease

- Approximately 6.2% of the total AIDS cases reported through the end of 2003 were in people age 55 or older at the time of diagnosis. This figure does not include individuals who are HIV positive. Although still relatively small, the number of individuals in the older adult population is increasing steadily.
- Improved treatments and prophylactic medications are contributing to individuals with HIV disease living longer, making the disease one of a chronic nature.
- A decrease in the ability of the immune system to fight infection as efficiently in the geriatric patient leads to faster progression of HIV disease and increased complications.

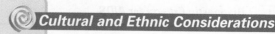

Cultural and Ethnic Considerations

HIV Disease

- Since 1990 there has been a 58% increase in the number of Hispanics living in the United States. This population increase is not the result of immigration, but of increases in fertility because the population is young. Future population growth is taking place in areas with the highest rates of HIV seroprevalence. Hispanics experience a higher seroprevalence rate than whites, and as a result, HIV prevention education is very important. Although Hispanics comprise only 14% of the total U.S. population, they represented 21.2% of the AIDS cases diagnosed in the year 2003, almost four times that of whites.
- Barriers to prevention have included difficulty in providing care in a nonthreatening environment where health care providers are viewed as authorities.
- There is reluctance to seek HIV care because this condition disqualifies one for U.S. legal residency, and undocumented residents fear deportation. Additionally, nearly 80% of Hispanics are members of the Catholic church, which has historically been opposed to sex outside marriage, men who have sex with men, and artificial birth control. These beliefs complicate prevention efforts that stress the use of condoms.
- The nurse should appreciate the deportation threat and recognize that Hispanic-American patients may not share important health information.
- Assessment and interventions should be sensitive to language and cultural differences.
- The nurse should provide a safe, supportive environment for assessment and treatment, and encourage advocacy for patients who need treatment—regardless of ability to pay for services or residency status.

has imparted lessons that can be useful in other patient populations as well: the importance of patient education, adherence to medical regimens, prevention, and health-promoting behaviors (Nielsen, 2001).

SIGNIFICANCE OF THE PROBLEM

By the end of 2003, reports by U.S. states, territories, and local health departments to the CDC indicated more than 929,985 cumulative cases of AIDS; of these, 524,060 (56%) patients are known to have died. Among the cumulative cases, 749,887 (80%) were men; 170,679 (18.3%) were women; and 9419 (1%) were children younger than 13 years of age (CDC, 2003).

African-Americans, Hispanics, and women continue to represent an increasing proportion of people with AIDS (Cultural and Ethnic Considerations box). Among the 43,171 new AIDS cases reported to the CDC in 2003, 49.4% were African-Americans, 20.3% were Hispanics, and 26.6% were females. Heterosexual contact accounted for 79% of all HIV/AIDS cases diagnosed in 2003. The percentage of new AIDS cases in African-Americans surpassed whites in 1996, and new cases of HIV infections have continued to grow steadily ever since (Bradley-Springer, 2001; CDC, 2003). In 2003 the rates of reported AIDS cases per 100,000 people were 58.2 for African-Americans, 20 for Hispanics, and 8.1 for American Indians/Alaska Natives. The rates were lowest among whites (6.1) and Asian-Americans/Pacific Islanders (4).

Although the proportion of AIDS cases in men who have sex with men (MSM) has declined to 41% of reported cases (CDC, 2003), MSM still account for the largest number of individuals with HIV and AIDS. Increases in AIDS cases in women and heterosexuals and a slowing of cases in the MSM category are a direct reflection of early educational efforts directed at the MSM population, who were believed to be the only population at risk. Recently, there has been a return to risky behaviors in the MSM population (*MMWR,*

1999), because prevention measures have been less focused on this population. Lack of education geared toward people of color, the shift toward treating HIV as a chronic disease (as opposed to fatal), and entirely new generations of people growing up without considering HIV a death sentence are contributing to increases in HIV incidence. It is just as important today to focus on prevention as a means to prevent new infections. New AIDS diagnoses among MSM are highest in the African-American population (55.5 per 100,000 people), whereas white MSMs have an incidence of 10.9 per 100,000 (CDC, 2001). Some researchers have suggested that there exists a greater stigma against homosexuality in communities of color, which may hinder prevention and treatment services they need (CDC, 2000).

There are an estimated 1 million individuals infected with HIV in the United States and its territories

(CDC, 2003). These data need to be interpreted with caution because only 34 states or territories have laws or regulations that require confidential reporting by name. Further, HIV surveillance reports are not representative of all individuals infected with HIV because not all infected people have been tested. Many HIV-reporting states offer anonymous testing as well as confidential testing, and home collection HIV test kits are widely available in the United States. Anonymous test results or those obtained from home test kits are not reported to regulatory agencies, such as the CDC or local and state health departments.

Worldwide, HIV disease has affected nearly 40 million individuals, with approximately 90% of these cases in the developing world (Laurence, 2001). This figure is more than 50% higher than what the World Health Organization (WHO) predicted in 1991 (UN-AIDS, 2000). Although HIV/AIDS is a serious threat to people in all areas of the world, sub-Saharan Africa is most at risk. Africa is home to 70% of the adults and 80% of the children living with HIV in the world. Of the 5.6 million people infected with HIV in 1999, 4 million live in this region, where there were an estimated 2.2 million deaths from HIV/AIDS during 1999 (85% of the global total), although only one tenth of the world's population lives there (UNAIDS, 2000). The effects of HIV infection in the developing world are far reaching—culturally, socially, and economically. For example, in South Africa, the epidemic is projected to reduce the economic growth rate by 0.3% to 0.4% annually, resulting by the year 2010 in a gross domestic product 17% lower than it would have been without AIDS, and wiping nearly $22 billion (U.S.) off the country's economy. This will result in eroded development gains, and reductions in the income of some of the world's poorest nations (UNAIDS, 2000). For the nearly 3.8 million adults and children newly infected in 2000, the cost for palliative care, pain control, treatment and prevention of opportunistic infections, and care for children orphaned was at least $1.5 billion (U.S.) annually. Updated statistical information is available from the CDC and local and state health departments, as well as the WHO.

TRANSMISSION OF HIV

Even though there has been significant research into the modes of transmission of HIV, considerable fear and misinformation about HIV transmission, perhaps more than for any other disease, still exists. It is imperative that health care providers and patients be knowledgeable about modes of transmission and behaviors that put them at risk for HIV infection. Modes of transmission have remained constant throughout the course of the HIV pandemic. It is also important for health care providers to remember that transmission of HIV occurs through sexual **practices,** not sexual **preferences.**

The patterns in the spread of HIV have changed considerably during the first 20 years of the epidemic in the United States. HIV does not discriminate. It is not who you are, but what you do that determines whether you can become infected with HIV. Worldwide, sexual intercourse is by far the most common mode of HIV transmission, but in the United States, as many as half of all new HIV infections are now associated either directly or indirectly with injection drug use—that is, using HIV-contaminated needles to inject drugs or having sexual contact with an HIV-infected drug user. Overall, compared to the 1980s, HIV infection is spreading fastest in the United States among young people, injecting drug users, women, African-Americans, and Hispanics. The number of estimated pediatric AIDS cases diagnosed each year has declined since 1992. The decline in pediatric AIDS incidence is associated with the increased compliance with universal counseling and testing of pregnant women and the use of zidovudine by HIV-infected pregnant women and their newborn infants (CDC, 2000).

HIV is an **obligate virus,** meaning it must have a host organism to survive. Without a host, the virus cannot live very long outside the human body. HIV transmission depends on the presence of the virus, the infectiousness of the virus, the susceptibility of the uninfected host, and any conditions that may help put the person at risk. HIV is transmitted from human to human through infected blood, semen, cervicovaginal secretions, and breast milk. If these infected fluids are introduced into an uninfected person, the potential for HIV transmission exists. In addition to the aforementioned body fluids, HIV is also found in pericardial, synovial, cerebrospinal, peritoneal, and amniotic fluids. Vertical transmission of HIV, or transmission from a mother to a fetus, can occur during pregnancy, during delivery, or through postpartum breastfeeding (transmitted in the breast milk). Conditions that affect the likelihood of infection include the duration and frequency of exposure, the amount of virus inoculated, the virulence of the organism, and the host's defense capability (immune system). Although HIV has been found in other body fluids such as saliva, urine, tears, and feces, there has been no evidence that these substances are capable of transmission, unless the fluids contain visible blood.

HIV is generally transmitted by **behaviors** and not by casual contacts, such as hugging, dry kissing, shaking hands, or sharing food and utensils. HIV is not transmitted by animals or insects, coughing, sneezing, or sharing objects such as pencils or computer keyboards. The three most common modes of HIV transmission are anal or vaginal intercourse, contaminated injecting drug equipment and paraphernalia, and transmission from mother to child.

Generalized virologic and immunologic course of HIV disease

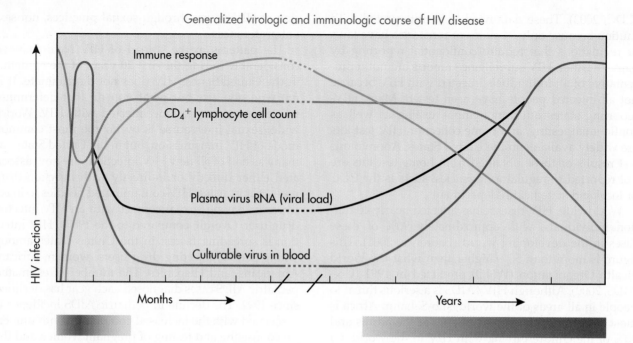

FIGURE **16-1** Viral load in the blood and the relationship to CD₄⁺ lymphocyte cell count over the spectrum of HIV disease.

Once infected, an individual is capable of transmitting HIV to others at any time throughout the disease spectrum, even when the host appears healthy and there are no obvious signs of immune destruction. In HIV infection the viral load (amount of measurable HIV virions) is highest immediately after infection and during the later stages of the disease (Figure 16-1). During these periods, unprotected exposure (through sexual behaviors or blood) to an infected individual increases the likelihood that transmission will occur. However, it is important to remember that HIV can be transmitted during the entire disease spectrum.

SEXUAL TRANSMISSION

Sexual transmission of HIV remains the most common mode of transmission in the world today and is responsible for the majority of the world's total AIDS cases. Sexual activity provides the potential for the exchange of semen, cervicovaginal secretions, and blood. Although the majority of HIV transmissions in the United States occur in the MSM category via receptive anal intercourse, heterosexual transmission via anal intercourse is becoming increasingly prevalent. Heterosexual couples may use this method of sexual expression because the risk of pregnancy is eliminated. Unfortunately, the risk of acquiring HIV and other sexually transmitted diseases (STDs) still exists. The sexual orientation or sexual practices of an individual are irrelevant in HIV transmission. Factors that are important are the presence of HIV in one or both partners

and the occurrence of behaviors that puts one or both partners at risk for transmission.

The most risky sexual activity is unprotected receptive anal intercourse. This type of sexual activity frequently results in trauma to the rectal mucosa. Because the rectum is generally tighter and less well lubricated than the vagina, mucosa may be torn; this increases the risk of HIV transmission. The compromised mucous membranes provide an excellent portal for the virus to enter the bloodstream. Still, some individuals become infected with HIV after a single unprotected sexual encounter, whereas others remain free from infection after hundreds of such encounters.

During any form of sexual intercourse (anal, vaginal, oral), the risk of infection is considerably higher for the receptive partner, although infection can be transmitted to an insertive partner. The receptive partner generally has a prolonged exposure to semen. Other factors that may increase the risk of sexual transmission include ulcerating genital diseases, such as herpes simplex virus (HSV) and syphilis; chancres secondary to STDs; intact (uncircumcised) foreskin; and immune suppression due to drug use, including the use of nicotine and alcohol. The transmission of HIV from an infected male to an uninfected female is estimated to be 18 times more likely than from an infected female to an uninfected male. Oral-genital transmissions have been reported but are considered rare, and there is varying expert opinion on whether this constitutes an actual mode of transmission.

PARENTERAL EXPOSURE

Injecting Drug Use

HIV may be transmitted by exposure to contaminated blood through the accidental or intentional sharing of injecting equipment and paraphernalia. Such equipment includes syringes, needles, cookers (spoons or bottle caps used for mixing the drug), and filtering devices (such as cotton balls). Injecting drug users represent the second highest exposure category, following the MSM category (CDC, 2003). Although typically seen in large metropolitan areas, injecting drug use (IDU) occurs in smaller cities and rural areas as well. IDU is not limited to illicit drugs; HIV can be transmitted via contaminated "works" used to inject steroids, vitamins, and insulin.

Injecting drug users confirm needle placement in a vein by drawing back blood into the syringe; the substance is then injected into the vein. They may also draw blood back into the syringe and inject numerous times, a procedure called "booting." This ensures that no substance remains in the syringe. Other factors that put injecting drug users at risk for HIV include poor nutritional status, poor hygiene, and impaired judgment due to mood-altering substances. The long-term effects of IDU put individuals at increased risk for other diseases, such as hepatitis B, hepatitis C, and other bloodborne illnesses.

Blood and Blood Products

In the United States, transfusion of infected blood and blood components and transplantation of infected tissues accounts for 1% of the total adult and adolescent AIDS cases and 2% of the total pediatric AIDS cases (CDC, 2003). The risk of contracting HIV from a blood transfusion is estimated to be 1 in 400,000. In 1985, blood banks implemented procedures to screen all donated units of blood and blood products for HIV as well as to screen donors who might be at risk for HIV infection. All blood collected in the United States is now screened for seven infectious agents: HIV-1, HIV-2, HTLV-1, HTLV-2, hepatitis B virus, hepatitis C virus, and syphilis. As a result of these changes, the risk of acquiring an HIV infection from a blood transfusion is extremely low. However, an infected donor who is not eliminated through the screening process may still have undetected HIV antibodies, because the infection was recent and seroconversion has not occurred. A person is said to have seroconverted when there is development of a detectable level of HIV antibodies found in the blood through the use of the enzyme-linked immunosorbent assay (ELISA) (a rapid enzyme immunochemical assay method to detect certain bacterial antigens and antibodies) and Western blot (technique for analyzing small amounts of antibodies) laboratory tests (Table 16-2). Seroconversion occurs in 95% of people within 3 months and 99% of people within 6 months of exposure to HIV.

| Table 16-2 | *Tests Used to Detect HIV Infection* |

ANTIBODY DETECTION TESTS

Screening Tests
- Enzyme-linked immunosorbent assay (ELISA)
- Agglutination assays
- Oral fluid test (Orasure, Epitope)
- Urine screening test

Confirmatory Test
- Western blot (interpretated by a pathologist)
- Indirect immunofluorescent antibody assay
- Radioimmunoprecipitation assay (RIPA)

ANTIGEN DETECTION TESTS

Nucleic Acid Determination Assays

Reverse transcriptase–polymerase chain reaction (RT-PCR)

Branched DNA (bDNA)

Nucleic acid sequence–based analysis (NASBA)

Viral Culture Method

HIV culture

ACTIVATED IMMUNE MARKERS

Neopterin

β_2-microglobulin

Absolute CD_4 cell count

CD_4 percentage

CD_8 percentage

CD_4/CD_8 ratio

Individuals with hemophilia and other coagulation disorders who received clotting factors before 1985 make up approximately 1% of the total AIDS cases in the United States (CDC, 2003). However, it is anticipated that there will be no new cases of HIV infection caused by the infusion of factor concentrates; these products are now produced using a recombinant technique or are treated with heat or chemicals to deactivate the HIV.

Occupational Exposure

Of the adults reported with AIDS in the United States through the end of December 31, 2000, 23,047 have been employed in health care. These cases represent 5.1% of the total AIDS cases reported to the CDC for whom occupational information was known. There have been 58 documented cases of occupationally acquired HIV or AIDS infection, with another 138 cases of possible occupational transmission (CDC, 2001). HIV has been transmitted to health care personnel after percutaneous injury, mucocutaneous exposure, and exposure via open wounds on the skin and mucous membranes. The majority of occupationally acquired HIV infections have occurred through puncture wounds after a needlestick injury. The overall risk of acquiring HIV after a percutaneous exposure is approximately 0.3% (CDC, 2001). The majority of occupationally acquired HIV infections occurred in nurses, followed by laboratory workers.

A percutaneous exposure is defined as a needlestick exposure to known HIV-infected blood. The risk of transmission is higher if the exposure is caused by a blood-filled, hollow-bore needle placed in an artery or vein; through deep injury; or through a source patient who dies as a result of HIV disease within 60 days of exposure (presuming there are higher concentrations of HIV in the blood). Needles used for intramuscular (IM) or subcutaneous (subQ) injections, as well as scalpels and suture needles, present less risk. The risk of seroconversion after a mucous membrane exposure is approximately 0.09% (CDC, 2001). Although episodes of HIV transmission after nonintact skin exposure have been documented, the average risk for transmission by this route has not been precisely quantified but is estimated to be less than the risk for mucous membrane exposures.

Perinatal (Vertical) Transmission

HIV infection can be transmitted from a mother to her infant during pregnancy, at the time of delivery, or after birth, through breastfeeding. In the United States, it is estimated that approximately 30% of infected mothers will transmit HIV to their infants, with approximately 50% to 70% of the transmissions occurring late in utero or intrapartum (Mofenson, 1997). For unknown reasons, the rate of vertical transmission varies around the world; the rate in France is around 11%, but it is nearly 50% in parts of Africa. In the United States, among children who are less than 13 years old and have AIDS, 93% were infected at birth (CDC, 2003). Factors such as the stage of maternal HIV disease (it is more likely to be transmitted during the initial and later stages of infection, when more of the virus is circulating in the mother's blood and body fluids), a decreased CD_4^+ count or high viral load, the presence or absence of STDs, and the nutritional status of the mother all play a role in vertical transmission. Factors that increase the risk of transmission during the actual delivery include extreme prematurity; complicated pregnancies leading to extended labor; the mixing of maternal and fetal blood; newborn ingestion of maternal blood, amniotic fluid, or vaginal secretions; skin excoriation in the newborn; and being the first child born in a multiple gestation.

In 1994 the AIDS Clinical Trials Group (ACTG) 076 study demonstrated that a plan of zidovudine (ZDV, AZT, Retrovir) therapy started after the 14th week of gestation, given intravenously to the mother during delivery and including ZDV syrup given to the infant after birth, reduces the risk of HIV transmission by 67% (Perinatal HIV Guidelines Working Group, 2001). The long-term effects of ZDV or combination therapy are not known, but anecdotal evidence suggests that polydactyly (the congenital presence of more than the normal number of fingers and toes) and ventricular

septal defect (VSD) may be caused by ZDV. It is difficult to determine whether the occurrences of these defects are caused by in utero exposure to ZDV or whether the incidence is the same as in the general population. Children who received ZDV in the womb and for the first 6 weeks of life are closely monitored by authorities to document any long-term side effects that appear later in life. In addition, substantial advances have been made in the understanding of the pathophysiology, treatment, and monitoring of HIV infection. These advances have resulted in changes in the standard of care for individuals, including pregnant women, with HIV infection. More aggressive combination drug regimens that provide maximal viral suppression are now recommended. Although pregnancy alone is not a reason to defer treatment, the use of anti-HIV drugs during pregnancy requires special consideration. The potential risks and benefits to both the mother and fetus, and the effectiveness of reducing perinatal transmission, must be discussed. Unfortunately, no long-term data regarding the long-term effects on the fetus exist. Because of this, offering antiretroviral therapy to HIV-infected women—whether to primarily treat HIV infection or to reduce the likelihood of perinatal transmission—should be accompanied by a discussion of the known and unknown short- and long-term benefits and potential risks. Because of the findings of ACTG 076, zidovudine (ZDV, AZT) should be a part of this treatment regimen.

An HIV-positive pregnant woman should be given this information in order to make an informed decision about treatment options. Current recommendations call for routine HIV counseling and voluntary HIV testing of pregnant women and those women considering pregnancy. There are no legal requirements that a woman must take ZDV during pregnancy or that she be tested for HIV antibodies. This information is helpful when counseling the HIV-infected person who is struggling with difficult decisions related to reproduction.

Infants born to HIV-infected mothers will have positive HIV antibody results as long as 15 to 18 months after birth. This is caused by maternal antibodies that cross the placenta during gestation and remain in the infant's circulatory system. An earlier diagnosis of HIV infection can be made by doing an HIV viral culture or by measuring the amount of HIV ribonucleic acid (RNA) or viral load through a technique called polymerase chain reaction (PCR) or branched chain DNA testing (bDNA).

TRENDS AND MOST AFFECTED POPULATIONS

Since the use of highly active antiretroviral therapy (HAART) became widespread during 1996, trends in AIDS incidence have become less reflective of underlying trends in HIV transmission. The distribution of

AIDS and HIV disease cases varies greatly among geographic areas, racial and ethnic groups, and other subpopulations. In December 2003, MSM accounted for only 47% of the total AIDS cases reported in the United States (CDC, 2003), a decrease from 90% reported through the end of 1989. Women and children constitute a quickly growing segment of the population with AIDS. The number of cases attributed to heterosexual contact has increased from the 120 reported in 1985 to 149,989 (16%) through the end of 2003 (CDC, 2003).

AIDS takes a disproportionate toll on African-American and Hispanic populations. African-Americans constitute approximately 13% of the total U.S. population, but they also constitute approximately 40% of the total AIDS cases reported to date. More than 59% of the total female cases are African-American women, and nearly 59% of the pediatric AIDS cases are African-American children. Although comprising only approximately 13% of the total U.S. population, 20% of AIDS cases reported through the year 2003 were in Hispanics. The incidence of HIV/AIDS in Hispanics is nearly four times greater than the incidence in whites. Hispanic children represent 23% of pediatric cases. Clearly, the population at greatest risk is women, especially women of color. The predominant mode of exposure among an estimated 9207 adult and adolescent women diagnosed with AIDS in 2003 was heterosexual contact. Adolescents and young adults are also a quickly emerging risk population, comprising 27% of all new HIV infections reported through 2003 (CDC, 2003). Fifty percent of all new HIV infections occurring in the United States each year are in individuals younger than the age of 25 (AmfAR, 2001).

PATHOPHYSIOLOGY

HIV, the etiological agent of AIDS, was discovered in 1983. It is a member of the lentivirus (slow virus) family of **retroviruses** (Figure 16-2). HIV carries its genetic material in RNA rather than deoxyribonucleic acid (DNA), and it replicates by converting RNA into DNA. Like all viruses, HIV is an obligate parasite, meaning it cannot replicate unless it is inside another living cell. HIV has an attraction for cells that have the CD_4^+ molecules on their surface, such as T-helper lymphocytes, monocytes, and macrophages. Researchers have identified at least two conditions HIV needs before it can attach itself to human cells. These conditions ordinarily function as receptors for cytokines, or chemokines (Marmor et al, 2001). These chemokines are produced by the CD_8^+ T cells in response to immune activation and block the entry of HIV-1 in some individuals (approximately 1% of whites). This finding appears to illustrate why certain individuals remain uninfected despite repeated exposure to HIV.

Research has shown that receptors other than CD_4 may also play a role in enabling HIV to infect human

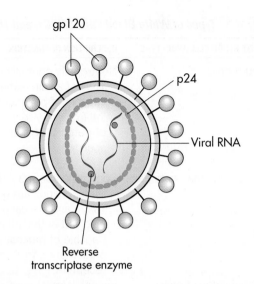

FIGURE **16-2** HIV is surrounded by an envelope of proteins (including gp 120) that contains a core of viral RNA and core proteins, such as p24.

cells. These other receptors are referred to as co-receptors, with three identified thus far: CCR-5, which is found on the surface of macrophages; CXCR4, also called fusin, which is found on the surface of T cells; and CCR3, which is found on the surface of microglia (monocyte-like cells of the central nervous system). Different strains of HIV may have different affinity, or attraction, to these co-receptors. These co-receptors normally recruit immune cells to the site of tissue damage or act as receptors for the binding of cytokines. Both cellular and humoral immune mechanisms play an important role in limiting HIV replication and slowing down disease progression. These responses are able to temporarily contain HIV but are not able to eliminate it (Table 16-3).

Initial infection with HIV results in a viremia during which large amounts of the virus can be isolated in the blood. Amounts as high as 10 million particles of HIV per milliliter of blood have been found during the early stage of infection, and up to 10 billion particles of HIV are produced and cleared daily in an infected individual Feng et al, 1996; Ungvarski, 1996). This dynamic equilibrium results in the continuous turnover of the virus, with approximately one half of the circulating virus being replaced with newly produced virus each day. The half-life of HIV in the blood plasma appears to be only 1 or 2 days. This massive production of HIV is coupled with the production and destruction of nearly 2 billion CD_4^+ lymphocytes each day. HIV infection is a dynamic process with production and clearance of massive quantities of virus each day. The amount of virus in the blood is directly linked to the rate of virus production, which determines the rate of CD_4^+ cell destruction. A prolonged period in which HIV is not readily detectable in the blood follows within a few weeks or months of the initial infection (Figure 16-3). This

Table 16-3 *Types of White Blood Cells (WBCs) and Their Involvement in HIV Disease*

WHITE BLOOD CELL (WBC) TYPE	DESCRIPTION OF FUNCTION	ROLE IN HIV DISEASE
Neutrophils	Neutrophils normally constitute 50% to 75% of all circulating leukocytes and are capable of phagocytosis. Important in the inflammatory response and the first line of defense against infection. Short life span.	Neutropenia (decreased WBC) commonly occurs in advanced HIV disease. Drug-induced neutropenia is common, especially with drugs used to treat PCP, toxoplasmosis, CMV retinitis or colitis, and with zidovudine (AZT) usage.
Monocytes/macrophages	Constitute about 3% to 7% of all WBCs. Macrophages are distributed throughout tissue and are capable of phagocytosis. Involved in the inflammatory response. Capable of processing antigens for presentation to T cells. They have CD_4 receptors.	Monocytes/macrophages serve as a reservoir for HIV. When activated by stimulation with interferon (inflammatory response), they produce neopterin. Neopterin levels are increased in HIV disease.
Basophils/mast cells	Basophils/mast cells are involved in acute inflammation; breakdown of mast cells releases histamine and other factors.	In HIV infection, may inhibit leukocyte migration.
Helper T cells (CD_4 or T_4 cells)	T-helper cells contain CD_4 receptors. They are considered the "conductor" of the immune system because of their secretion of cytokines, which control most aspects of the immune response.	Major target of HIV. Progressive infection gradually destroys the available pool of T-helper cells so that the overall CD_4 cell count drops. Lower CD_4 cell counts correspond with more immunodeficiency and the onset of opportunistic infections. Infection with HIV can impair T-helper cell function without killing the cell.
Cytotoxic T cells or cytotoxic T lymphocytes (CTL/CD_8 cell)	Cytotoxic T cells contain CD_8 receptors and produce cytokines in a more limited fashion than CD_4 cells. They regulate viral and bacterial infections and are involved in direct killing of target cells by binding to them and releasing a substance that can perforate the cell membrane.	Increase in HIV infection. Represent the cellular response to infection. The strength of this initial cellular response has been shown to predict progression to AIDS (i.e., better cell response equals slower disease progression). Cytotoxic T cells kill T-helper cells infected with HIV.
Natural killer (NK) cells	Large granular lymphocytes involved in cell-mediated immune response. Target cells are coated with antibody that binds to receptors on the surface of NK cells, allowing the NK cell to attach to the target cell and kill them. NK cells kill target cells by releasing a substance that triggers lysis (breakdown of cell wall) of cell.	Retain normal counts and normal structure in patients with HIV infection, but they are functionally defective.
B cells	B cells produce antibodies specific to an antigen. They are capable of being stimulated by T-helper cells.	B cells are involved in the humoral response to HIV infection and produce a variety of antibodies against HIV. Present throughout the course of HIV disease.

titer, or viral load, falls dramatically as the immune system responds and controls the HIV infection (Bartlett & Gallant, 2001; Nelson, 2001), and it may last 10 to 12 years. During this period, there are few clinical symptoms of HIV infection, although an individual is still capable of transmitting HIV to others. It was initially thought that this phase represented a period of biologic and clinical latency and that HIV replication was minimal. However, studies have demonstrated that this is not true; HIV continues to replicate in the lymph tissues, in areas such as the lymph nodes, the tonsils, and the spleen (Schacker et al, 2000).

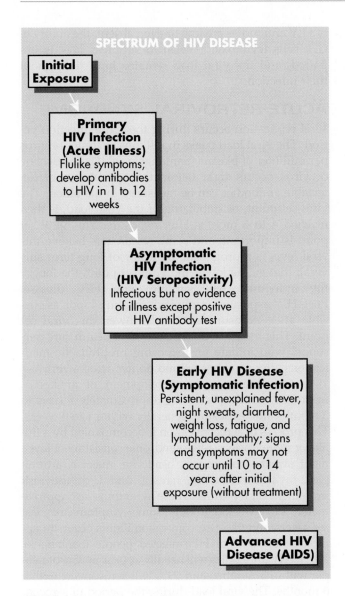

SPECTRUM OF HIV DISEASE

Initial Exposure

Primary HIV Infection (Acute Illness)
Flulike symptoms; develop antibodies to HIV in 1 to 12 weeks

Asymptomatic HIV Infection (HIV Seropositivity)
Infectious but no evidence of illness except positive HIV antibody test

Early HIV Disease (Symptomatic Infection)
Persistent, unexplained fever, night sweats, diarrhea, weight loss, fatigue, and lymphadenopathy; signs and symptoms may not occur until 10 to 14 years after initial exposure (without treatment)

Advanced HIV Disease (AIDS)

FIGURE **16-3** Spectrum of HIV disease and associated signs and symptoms at various stages of the disease process.

In a normal immune response, foreign antigens interact with B cells, which initiate the process of antibody development, and with T cells, which initiate a cellular immune response. In the initial stages of HIV infection, these cells respond and function normally. B cells make HIV-specific antibodies that are effective in reducing viral loads in the blood, and activated T cells respond to the site of viruses trapped in the lymph nodes. This immune response works better than any anti-HIV medication at keeping the virus under control (see Table 16-3).

Immune dysfunction results predominantly from the dysregulation and destruction of T-helper cells, or CD$_4^+$ lymphocytes. These cells are targeted because they have more CD$_4^+$ receptors on their surfaces than other cells. The CD$_4^+$ lymphocytes play a pivotal role in the ability of the immune system to recognize and

defend against foreign invaders. An adult normally has 600 to 1200 CD$_4^+$ lymphocytes per microliter (μL) of blood. Generally, the immune system remains healthy with CD$_4^+$ cells counts greater than 500 cells/μL. Minor immune problems occur when the CD$_4^+$ count falls from 200 to 499 cells/μL, and severe problems occur with CD$_4^+$ counts less than 200 μL. It has been estimated that 2% to 5% of the CD$_4^+$ cells in the body are replaced daily because of HIV infection.

Activated CD$_4^+$ lymphocytes are the perfect target for HIV. The CD$_4^+$ cells are attracted to the sites of HIV infection, such as the lymph tissue, whereupon they are exposed to and infected with additional HIV. Once infected, the activated cells support viral reproduction and assist in spreading or seeding the infection throughout the lymph system. Lymphoid tissue thus becomes a reservoir for HIV replication, with production occurring during the asymptomatic phase of infection. Eventually, HIV causes significant degenerative changes in the lymph system. At this point, viral particles spill over into the blood, a factor in disease progression, and significantly impair the immune system's ability to respond to new infections. Although HIV infection can lead to abnormal B-cell function, the predominant destruction and deficiency occurs in the cell-mediated immune response. Eventually, so many CD$_4^+$ lymphocytes are destroyed that there are not enough to regulate immune responses (see Figure 16-1). At this point, an HIV-infected individual is susceptible to many life-threatening infections.

HIV can also infect monocytes by attaching to CD$_4^+$ receptors that are present on certain subsets of the cells or by phagocytic (ingestion and digestion of bacteria) ingestion. Infected monocytes move into the body tissues, where they differentiate into macrophages. Although HIV replicates in infected macrophages, no external budding occurs. This allows the cell to remain intact and act as an "HIV factory." A local inflammatory process may cause the infected macrophage to rupture, distributing the newly formed HIV into surrounding tissues. Tissues in the skin, lymph nodes, lungs, central nervous system, and possibly the bone marrow have been directly infected in this manner.

SPECTRUM OF HIV INFECTION

HIV disease is a broad diagnostic term that includes the pathology and clinical illness caused by HIV infection. It replaces previous and inaccurate terms such as AIDS-related complex (ARC) and AIDS. HIV disease results from the progressive deterioration of the immune system over time; a diagnosis of AIDS is made in a later stage of this progression. Clinicians often talk about two phases of HIV disease—the **asymptomatic** and the **symptomatic** phases of infection. The term AIDS has been defined for surveillance and reporting purposes; it is not used alone to diagnose serious disease caused by HIV infection (Box 16-1).

Acquired immunodeficiency syndrome (AIDS) is defined as an acquired condition that impairs the body's ability to fight disease; it is the end stage of a continuum of HIV infection (the state in which HIV enters the body under favorable conditions and multiplies, producing injurious effects) (see Figure 16-3). AIDS occurs when the HIV-infected person has a CD_4^+ count of 200 or fewer cells per mm^3. HIV infection may exist for many years without symptoms before it progresses to **symptomatic HIV disease**—indicated by persistent unexplained fever, night sweats, diarrhea, weight loss, and fatigue—and then to the end-stage illness of AIDS. The course of HIV disease varies from person to person and can be influenced by several factors. Factors that have been linked to increased mortality and morbidity include lower socioeconomic status, lack of access to adequate care, receiving care in a hospital with limited HIV experience, and being treated by a physician with little experience in HIV care.

There is significant variation in the rate that HIV-infected individuals progress from early to late HIV infection (progressors versus nonprogressors). Three patterns have been identified: (1) typical progressors, (2) long-term nonprogressors, and (3) rapid progressors. About 80% to 90% of all infected people fit the pattern of typical progression. A typical progressor has a period of relative clinical latency—occurring immediately after the primary infection (seroconversion illness)—that can last for several years. Long-term nonprogressors remain free of symptoms for 10 years or more and account for about 5% of the total cases of HIV infection. Many studies focusing on this group of patients have demonstrated their tendency to have a vigorous immune response to HIV infection (both cellular and humoral), which results in a lower viral load. In addition, their CD_4^+ cell counts remain normal or show only slight declines. The lymph node system is well preserved and the number of absolute CD_8 cells is significantly and consistently higher when compared with other HIV-infected individuals.

In contrast, rapid progressors (about 5% to 10% of all individuals infected with HIV) advance to an AIDS diagnosis within 2 or 3 years after seroconversion. Several features distinguish rapid progressors: the levels

of HIV antibodies are low or even absent, the ability of CD_8 cells (cytotoxic T cells) to suppress HIV is impaired, and the viral load remains high throughout their infection.

ACUTE RETROVIRAL SYNDROME

Viral replication occurs during the acute infection period. The viral load peaks in millions of copies of virus per milliliter of plasma (Santangelo, 2001). The decline of virus occurs right before the appearance of detectable antibodies can be measured in the blood. The viral set point, or stabilizing of the viral load, is then reached 4 to 6 months after exposure. This viral set point is important, and some researchers believe this viral level is a prognostic indicator of long-term survival; that is, the lower the viral set point, the longer the individual will survive with HIV disease. Post–HIV exposure prophylaxis, begun as soon as possible after exposure, may help lower this viral set point. This theory is demonstrated in health care personnel who initiate postexposure prophylactic medications after an exposure and do not seroconvert.

Seroconversion is the development of antibodies from HIV, which takes place approximately 5 days to 3 months after exposure, generally within 1 to 3 weeks. This process of seroconversion is accompanied by a flu-like or mononucleosis-like syndrome consisting of fever, night sweats, pharyngitis, headache, malaise, arthralgias, myalgias, diarrhea, nausea, and a diffuse rash prominent on the trunk. These symptoms last approximately 1 to 2 weeks, although some symptoms may last for several months. Seroconversion illness occurs in approximately 89% of HIV-infected people (Santangelo, 2001). HIV antibodies will usually appear in 95% of people within 3 months, and 99% will seroconvert within 6 months. The viral load during the period of seroconversion is extremely high, with a short-term drop in CD_4^+ cells. The CD_4^+ level quickly returns to normal as the immune system mounts an attack against the viral infection, resulting in viral loads existing at nearly undetectable levels in the blood. In most people the acute retroviral illness is mild and may be mistaken for a cold or other minor viral infection (Table 16-4).

EARLY INFECTION

The median time between HIV infection and the development of end-stage HIV disease, or AIDS, in an untreated individual is anywhere from 10 to 14 years (Figure 16-4). This phase of HIV disease is sometimes called the asymptomatic phase, because the HIV-infected individual looks and feels healthy. Some individuals have vague symptoms indicative of a viral infection, including fatigue, headaches, low-grade fever, and night sweats. Because many of the symptoms of early infection are nondescript, a diagnosis of HIV infection might not be made. Consequently, individuals may continue to engage in risky sexual and drug-using behaviors. Although seemingly healthy, the

---

Box 16-1 *Proper Terms Related to HIV and AIDS*

Misleading Phrases	More Accurate Phrases
High-risk groups	High-risk behaviors
Infected with AIDS	HIV infection
AIDS test	HIV antibody test
AIDS positive	HIV positive
AIDS victim or patient	Person living with HIV or AIDS
AIDS carrier	HIV-infected person

HIV-infected individual is capable of transmitting HIV to others. Lack of knowledge of one's HIV antibody status puts one at risk for earlier development of more advanced disease, because changes in behaviors, such as those that promote health, are not instituted. Furthermore, if an individual is aware of the virus, early intervention with antiretroviral medications may prolong the asymptomatic phase and prevent progression to end-stage HIV disease (AIDS).

EARLY SYMPTOMATIC DISEASE

Historically, this phase of HIV infection had been called AIDS-related complex (ARC). This term is no longer used to describe the condition in which the CD_4^+ cell count drops below 500 cells/μl. Early symptoms include constitutional problems such as persistent, unexplained fevers, recurrent drenching night sweats, chronic diarrhea, headaches, and fatigue. These signs and symptoms become severe enough to affect activities of daily living (ADLs). A physical examination may reveal persistent generalized lymphadenopathy (PGL); recurrent or localized infections; and neurological manifestations, such as numbness and tingling or weakness in the extremities (Box 16-2).

One of the most common infections seen in individuals with early symptomatic disease is oral candidiasis (thrush), a fungal infection rarely seen in healthy adults (Figure 16-5). Other infections that signal immune dysfunction include varicella-zoster virus (VZV), or shingles, infection; persistent vaginal candidiasis (yeast infections); and increased frequency of oral or genital

Table 16-4 *Primary HIV Infection: Signs and Symptoms*

SIGNS/SYMPTOMS	% OF PATIENTS EXPERIENCING
Fever	96%
Adenopathy	74%
Pharyngitis	70%
Rash*	70%
Myalgias	54%
Diarrhea	32%
Headache	32%
Nausea and vomiting	27%
Hepatosplenomegaly	14%
Weight loss	13%
Thrush	12%
Neurological symptoms†	12%

*Erythematous maculopapular rash on face and trunk, sometimes extremities, including palms and soles. Some have mucocutaneous ulceration involving mouth, esophagus, or genitals.
†Aseptic meningitis, meningoencephalitis, peripheral neuropathy, facial palsy, Guillain-Barré syndrome, brachial neuritis, cognitive impairment, or psychosis.

Box 16-2 *Signs and Symptoms of HIV Infection*

Abdominal pain	Malaise
Chills and fever	Muscle or joint pain
Cough (dry or productive)	Night sweats
Diarrhea	Oral lesions
Disorientation	Shortness of breath
Dyspnea	Skin rash
Fatigue	Sore throat
Headache	Weight loss
Lymphadenopathy (any disorder of the lymph nodes or lymph vessels)	

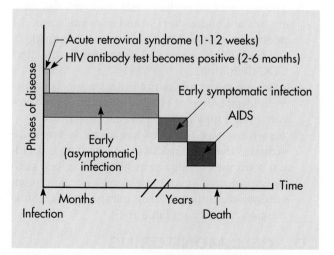

FIGURE **16-4** Timeline for the spectrum of HIV infection. This timeline represents the course of the illness from the time of infection to the clinical manifestations of it in an untreated individual.

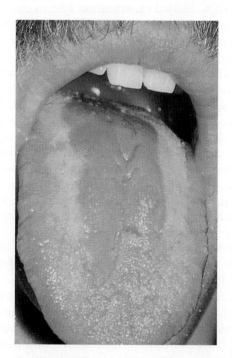

FIGURE **16-5** Oral candidiasis, or "thrush," manifests with a whitish, curdlike substance on the tongue or inside of the mouth.

HSV outbreaks. The appearance of oral hairy leuko-plakia (OHL), a condition related to the Epstein-Barr virus, and oral thrush are early indicators for HIV disease and are prognostic markers for disease progression. Because of this, dental health professionals are key individuals in case finding for early HIV disease.

PGL is defined as two or more enlarged lymph nodes (1 cm or greater), located in places other than the inguinal region, that persist for at least 3 months. PGL may be present for many years before an individual progresses to an AIDS diagnosis.

Neurological manifestations of HIV disease are common. Upwards of 90% of individuals who are infected will experience some type of neurological symptoms. These include peripheral neuropathies, headaches, aseptic meningitis, cranial nerve palsies, and myopathies. These conditions may be caused by the HIV infection itself, or may be side effects related to antiretroviral medications.

There are several cofactors that may influence a more rapid progression of HIV disease. Very young children and very old adults progress more quickly. Concurrent infections such as HSV, cytomegalovirus (CMV), or Epstein-Barr virus affect progression. Drug and alcohol use, including smoking, may suppress the immune system. Malnutrition is also known to affect immune function, but further study relative to HIV is needed.

AIDS

AIDS is used to describe the end-stage, or terminal, phase of the spectrum of HIV infection. There are specific diagnostic criteria, developed by the CDC, that must be applied to make this diagnosis (see Table 16-1 for the CDC revised classification system currently in use). These conditions are more likely to occur with severe immune suppression. As HIV disease progresses, the CD_4^+ lymphocyte cell count decreases, and the ratio of CD_4^+ to CD_8^+ cells (T-helper cells to T-suppressor cells), which is normally 2 to 1, gradually shifts, resulting in more T-suppressor cells (CD_8^+) than T-helper cells (CD_4^+). The amount of virus detectable in the blood increases rapidly and remains high despite pharmacological interventions. There may also be a decrease in the number of white blood cells (WBCs), and the person's reactivity to skin tests, such as purified protein derivative (PPD) tuberculin, is decreased or absent. An individual is said to be anergic if no skin response is noted.

Without treatment, the median time from an AIDS diagnosis to death averages 1.3 years (Bartlett et al, 2001), although this varies greatly. With the advent of more effective antiretroviral and opportunistic disease prophylaxis, the life span of an HIV-infected individual is unpredictable. There is a wide variation of morbidity in people with advanced HIV disease. Some people are severely ill and become terminal rather quickly, whereas others only have to make minor adjustments

in their lifestyle to cope with medical regimens or physical symptoms, such as fatigue or pain. Significant advances in the management of HIV disease have made it resemble a chronic illness. The effects of therapy on mortality have been significant, with a leveling off of new AIDS cases reported to the CDC every year. This can be attributed to effective prophylaxis for opportunistic infections, and to the development of a highly active antiretroviral therapy (HAART).

DIAGNOSTIC TESTS

There is strong evidence that early intervention postpones the onset of severe immune suppression. Individuals at risk for HIV infection should be encouraged to seek HIV antibody testing as well as receive education in decreasing the risk of HIV transmission (see Table 16-2).

HIV ANTIBODY TESTING

Individuals need to understand the implications of an HIV antibody test:

1. The individual's blood is tested with ELISA or enzyme immunoassay (EIA), antibody tests that detect the presence of HIV antibodies. If the EIA is positive for HIV, then the same blood is tested a second time. If the second EIA is positive, a more specific confirming test such as the Western blot is done. Blood that is reactive or positive in all three steps is reported to be HIV positive.

2. Tests with indeterminate results are repeated at a later date, generally 4 to 6 weeks. Consistently indeterminate results require the use of a viral culture or the measurement of viral load using a bDNA, a reverse transcriptase–polymerase chain reaction (RT-PCR), or nucleic acid sequence–based amplification (NASBA) laboratory measures.

3. The series of laboratory tests confirms the presence of antibodies to HIV and does not mean the person has AIDS. The tests are not diagnostic of AIDS. AIDS is diagnosed according to the 1993 CDC definition.

4. A seronegative test is not an assurance that the individual is free of HIV infection, because sero-conversion may not yet have occurred.

5. A seronegative test does not mean that an individual is free from risk of infection. If an individual continues to engage in risky behaviors, such as unprotected sexual intercourse or using contaminated needles or drug paraphernalia, transmission may occur (Table 16-5).

CD_4^+ CELL MONITORING

The monitoring of CD_4^+ cells is one of the laboratory parameters used to track the progression of HIV disease. As the disease progresses, there is a decrease in

Table 16-5 │ *Pretest and Posttest Counseling Associated with HIV-Antibody Testing*

GENERAL GUIDELINES

People who test for HIV are commonly fearful of the test results; therefore, the nurse should carry out the following:
- Establish rapport with the patient.
- Assess patient's ability to understand counseling.
- Determine the patient's ability to access support systems.

Explain the following benefits of testing:
- Testing provides an opportunity for education that can decrease the risk of new infections.
- Infected patient can be referred for early intervention and support programs.

Discuss the following negative aspects of testing:
- Breaches of confidentiality have led to discrimination.
- A positive test affects all aspects of the patient's life (personal, social, economic) and can raise difficult emotions (anger, anxiety, guilt, thoughts of suicide).

PRETEST COUNSELING

Determine the patient's risk factors and when the last exposure risk occurred. Counseling should be individualized according to these parameters.

Provide education to decrease future risk of exposure.

Provide education that will help the patient protect usual and drug-sharing partners.

Discuss problems related to the delay between infection and an accurate test:
- Testing will need to be repeated at intervals for 6 months after each possible exposure.
- Discuss the need to abstain from further risky behaviors during that interval.
- Discuss the need to protect partners during that interval.

Discuss the possibility of false-negative tests, which are most likely to occur during the window period.

Explain that a positive test shows HIV infection and not AIDS.

Explain that the test does not establish immunity, regardless of the results.

Assess support systems; provide telephone numbers and resources as needed.

Discuss patient's personally anticipated responses to test results (positive and negative).

Outline assistance that will be offered if the test is positive.

POSTTEST COUNSELING

If the test is negative, reinforce pretest counseling and prevention education. Remind patient that test needs to be repeated at intervals for 6 months after the most recent exposure risk.

If the test is positive, understand that the patient may be in shock and not hear what is said.
- Provide resources for medical and emotional support, and help the patient get immediate assistance.
- Evaluate suicide risk and follow up as needed.
- Determine need to test others who have had risky contact with the patient.
- Discuss retesting to verify results. This tactic supports hope for the patient, but more important it keeps the patient in the system. While waiting for the second test result, the patient has time to think about and adjust to the possibility of being HIV infected.
- Encourage optimism:
  —Remind patient that treatments are available.
  —Review health habits that can improve the immune system.
  —Arrange for patients to speak to HIV-infected people who are willing to share and assist the newly diagnosed patients during the transition period.
  —Reinforce that an HIV-positive test means that the patient is infected, but a positive test does not necessarily mean that the patient has AIDS.

Modified from Bradley-Springer, L.A. & Fendrick, R. (1994). *HIV instant instructor cards.* El Paso, Tex: Skidmore-Roth.

the number of CD_4^+ cells. The more significant the loss, the more severe immunosuppression becomes. The CD_4^+ count is the best marker for the immunodeficiency associated with HIV infection. As such, the CD_4^+ count is used in making decisions about antiretroviral and prophylactic drug therapy and in evaluating specific complaints relative to the risk for contracting particular opportunistic infections (OIs). For example, *Mycobacterium avium* complex (MAC) and CMV infections are rare in patients with CD_4^+ counts more than 50 cells/mm³. PCP and cryptococcosis are unusual in patients with CD_4^+ counts greater than 200 cells/mm³. The CD_4^+ count is not a perfect surrogate marker of immunodeficiency, and factors such as the patient's clinical status must always be taken into account.

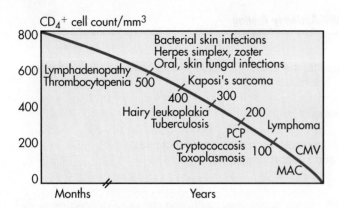

FIGURE **16-6** Common clinical conditions associated with various CD_4^+ lymphocyte counts as HIV disease progresses.

The CD_4^+ cell count reflects the number of CD_4^+ cells per cubic millimeter or per microliter (µl) of blood. It does not indicate the total number of CD_4^+ cells in the body. Millions of new CD_4^+ cells are produced daily and cleared by normal body processes (unrelated to the virus). Thus the CD_4^+ count is a marker of the net level of cells represented per mm³. The absolute CD_4^+ count can vary greatly in the same individual depending on what time of day the blood is drawn; which laboratory is used; and the presence of acute illness or other factors, such as alcohol. It is therefore necessary to continue to use the same lab, draw blood at the same time of day, and avoid testing on days when the patient is acutely ill or under abnormal stress. When the CD_4^+ count is being used to make important treatment decisions, such as initiating prophylaxis for OIs, it is advisable to draw two separate samples a few weeks apart (Figure 16-6).

VIRAL LOAD MONITORING

The ability to detect HIV viral load measurements in plasma is a significant advancement in the monitoring of HIV disease. Viral load or burden refers to a quantitative measure of HIV viral RNA in the peripheral circulation, or the level of virus in the blood. Important characteristics include the following (Sonza & Crowe, 2001):

- In all clinical stages of illness, HIV viral detection techniques identify measurable viral RNA copies in the plasma of most HIV-infected individuals.
- Viral load can provide significant information toward predicting the course of disease progression, initiating antiretroviral therapy, recognizing the degree of antiretroviral effect achieved, and noting the failure of a drug regimen.
- Plasma HIV RNA levels fall dramatically following effective antiretroviral therapy.

- Determinations of quantitative HIV RNA levels in plasma do not detect any virus present in lymphoid or other tissues.

Viral replication is rapid and continuous from the time of infection; billions of copies are produced daily. Viral load indicates both live infectious particles and dead virions in the blood. A stable level, or set point, occurs after primary infection and remains relatively constant in the absence of disease progression or therapeutic effects. It is believed that this set point is an accurate predictor of long-term progression. A lower viral set point indicates someone who might live longer than someone with a higher viral set point.

Viral load and CD_4^+ cell counts are distinct markers that provide different information. Viral load can predict disease progression and long-term clinical outcome; CD_4^+ cell measurements can indicate the damage sustained by the immune system (the loss of CD_4^+, or T cells) and the short-term risk for developing opportunistic infections. Each is an independent predictor of clinical outcome, and when used in combination they can give a more complete indication of clinical status, treatment response, and prognosis. Generally, a high viral load indicates an increased risk for disease progression, and lower levels indicate less risk for progression. A metaphor used by John Coffin describes the asymptomatic, infected patient as a train rushing along a track, heading for a bridge that has been destroyed. There are two variables that determine when the crash would occur: (1) where the train was at that instant (CD_4^+), and (2) how fast it was going (viral load) (Coffin, 1996).

A baseline determination of viral burden is recommended, with subsequent measurements every 3 to 4 months, in conjunction with CD_4^+ cell monitoring and clinical evaluations such as a history and physical examination. It is likely that guidelines will continue to be revised as the implications of viral measurement evolve and its interpretation and use become better understood. In the future, OI prophylaxis may be based on viral load as well as CD_4^+ cell counts.

OTHER LABORATORY PARAMETERS

Hematologic abnormalities are common in HIV infections and may be caused by the HIV itself, OIs, or by drug or radiation therapy. A decreased WBC count is often seen, usually in conjunction with lymphopenia (decreased lymphocytes). Thrombocytopenia (decreased platelet count) may be caused by antiplatelet antibodies. Anemia is related to the chronic disease process and to HIV invasion of the bone marrow; it is a common adverse effect of antiretroviral agents.

Alterations in liver function tests are not uncommon. Abnormalities may be caused by viral hepatitis, alcohol abuse, OIs, neoplasms, or medications. Early identification of hepatitis B and hepatitis C viral infections is important because these infections may follow a more serious course in the patient with HIV disease. It is not uncommon for individuals who are HIV positive to also be positive for hepatitis B, because both infections are bloodborne and sexually transmitted. In addition, about one fourth of HIV-infected people in the United States are co-infected with hepatitis C. Hepatitis C is one of the most important causes of chronic liver disease and progresses more rapidly in HIV-infected people (CDC, 1998).

Syphilis testing is important because syphilis is more complicated and aggressive in the HIV-infected individual. It is also more difficult to treat with standard therapies and more likely to advance quickly to neurosyphilis. If a person is positive for syphilis, assessment and treatment should begin immediately.

THERAPEUTIC MANAGEMENT

Therapeutic management of the HIV-infected patient focuses on monitoring HIV disease progression and immune function, preventing the development of opportunistic diseases, initiating and monitoring antiretroviral therapy, detecting and treating opportunistic diseases, managing symptoms, and preventing complications of treatment.

HIV-positive individuals need to be linked to various points of intervention, depending on their individual needs. Individuals often deny the infection, neglect their mental and physical health, and continue behaviors that put themselves and others at risk. Interventions need to be sustained and reinforced; the emotional impact of such devastating news ("you are HIV positive") can override any initial information or education provided. Providers need to stress safer behaviors and the need for medical and emotional support. Types of assistance may include family planning, treatment for substance abuse, treatment for STDs, treatment for tuberculosis (TB), and immunizations.

A transdisciplinary care approach is the most appropriate method of care for patients with HIV disease because of their complex medical and psychosocial needs. The HIV-infected individual should be the primary member of this team, working along with a physician who specializes in HIV and AIDS, a social worker, the case manager, a dietitian, and the nurse. Other team members may include a dentist, a primary care provider (medical doctor, doctor of osteopathy, nurse practitioner, or physician assistant), a mental health worker, a substance abuse counselor, a nontraditional therapist (such as a massage therapist or acupuncturist), and the individual's family and significant other.

PHARMACOLOGICAL MANAGEMENT
Opportunistic Diseases Associated with HIV

A number of opportunistic diseases and debilitating problems associated with HIV can be delayed or prevented through the use of antiretrovirals and prophylactic interventions. Prophylactic medications have contributed to the decreased morbidity and mortality associated with HIV infection during the past several years. Therefore they are recommended according to established parameters. Probably the most difficult aspect of the medical management of HIV is dealing with the many opportunistic diseases that develop as the immune system degenerates. Although it is usually impossible to totally eradicate opportunistic diseases, there are treatments that can control their emergence or progression. However, these regimens must continue throughout the patient's life, or the disease will return. Advances in the diagnosis and treatment of opportunistic diseases have contributed significantly to increased life expectancy. Table 16-6 lists common opportunistic diseases associated with HIV disease. Table 16-7 lists common treatments and prophylactic regimens in the HIV-infected individual.

Antiretroviral Therapy

Combination antiretroviral therapy is an important component in the management of HIV infection (Table 16-8). There are many antiretroviral medications approved by the U.S. Food and Drug Administration (FDA) for treatment of HIV disease (Medications: HIV Disease [Antiretrovirals] table on pp. 791 to 793 lists the most common). In 1987 zidovudine was the only medication available to treat patients with HIV disease. Today, there are 18 approved anti-HIV medications available, with significantly more in development.

Scientists have found that the most effective medication regimen is the use of **cocktails** (at least two, but generally three or more compounds given together). Utilizing medication combinations makes it much more difficult for the virus to develop resistance to the drugs. Such intervention may also slow the progression from asymptomatic or mildly symptomatic HIV infection to a more advanced disease. Recent developments include therapies that can dramatically reduce the quantity of circulating virus in the blood; in many cases, blood circulating levels become undetectable. Protease inhibitors directly reduce the ability of HIV to replicate, or make copies of itself inside cells. As increasing numbers of therapeutic agents and clinical trial results become available, decisions about antiretroviral therapy have become increasingly complex. For now, these combination therapies offer renewed optimism for successful disease management and improvements in the quality and duration of life. It is important for the nurse to administer anti-HIV medica-

Table 16-6 *Common Opportunistic Diseases Associated with HIV/AIDS*

ORGANISM OR DISEASE	CLINICAL MANIFESTATIONS	DIAGNOSTIC TESTS	TREATMENT
RESPIRATORY SYSTEM			
Pneumocystis jiroveci (formerly *carinii*) pneumonia (PCP)	Fever, night sweats, nonproductive cough, progressive shortness of breath	Chest radiograph, induced sputum for culture, bronchoalveolar lavage	Trimethoprim-sulfamethoxazole, dapsone + pyrimethamine + leucovorin, clindamycin, atovaquone, pentamidine, steroids, trimetrexate, and folinic acid
Cryptococcus species	Pneumonia, fever, cough, malaise	Sputum culture, serum antigen assay	Fluconazole, itraconazole, amphotericin B
Histoplasmosis	Pneumonia, fever, cough	Sputum culture, serum antigen assay	Amphotericin B, itraconazole, fluconazole
Mycobacterium tuberculosis	Productive cough, fever, night sweats, fatigue, weight loss	Chest radiograph, sputum for acid-fast bacteria (AFB) stain and culture, skin test	Isoniazid, ethambutol, rifampin pyrazinamide, streptomycin, azithromycin, clarithromycin
Coccidioidomycosis	Fever, weight loss, cough	Sputum culture, serology	Amphotericin B, fluconazole, itraconazole
HSV-I	Vesicular eruptions on tracheobronchial mucosa	Viral culture	Acyclovir, famciclovir, valacyclovir
Toxoplasma gondii	Fever, shortness of breath (SOB), nonproductive cough	Antibody test	See Neurological system section
Rhodococcus equi	Chest pain, productive cough, SOB, fever, hemoptysis	Culture from sputum or bronchoalveolar lavage	Vancomycin + imipenem + ciprofloxacin with or without rifampin, erythromycin
Aspergillosis	Fever, cough, SOB, chest pain, hemoptysis, occasional CNS	Stain of respiratory secretions of biopsy	Amphotericin-B, itraconazole
INTEGUMENTARY SYSTEM			
HSV-I	Vesicular eruptions on mouth	Viral culture	Acyclovir, foscarnet, famciclovir, valacyclovir
HSV-II	Vesicular eruptions around perianal area	Viral culture	Acyclovir, foscarnet, valacyclovir, famciclovir
Varicella zoster virus (VZV)	Shingles: erythematous macules, rash, pain, pruritus	Viral culture	Acyclovir, foscarnet, valacyclovir
KS	Firm, flat, raised, or nodular, hyperpigmented, multicentric lesions	Biopsy of lesions	Radiation, chemotherapy, alpha interferon, palliative, bleomycin, daunorubicin
Bacillary angiomatosis	Erythematous papules and nodules	Biopsy of lesions	Erythromicin, doxycycline, clarithromycin, azithromycin
EYE			
CMV retinitis	Lesions on the retina, blurred vision, loss of vision	Ophthalmoscopic examination	Ganciclovir, foscarnet, cidofovir
HSV-I	Blurred vision, corneal lesions, acute retinal necrosis	Ophthalmoscopic examination, culture	Acyclovir, foscarnet, famciclovir, valacyclovir
VZV	Ocular lesions, acute retinal necrosis	Ophthalmoscopic examination, culture	Acyclovir, foscarnet, valacyclovir, famciclovir
Toxoplasma gondii	Visual field defects	Antibody test	See Neurological system section

Table 16-6 *Common Opportunistic Diseases Associated with HIV/AIDS—cont'd*

ORGANISM OR DISEASE	CLINICAL MANIFESTATIONS	DIAGNOSTIC TESTS	TREATMENT
GASTROINTESTINAL SYSTEM			
Cryptosporidium muris	Watery diarrhea, abdominal pain, weight loss, nausea, fever	Stool examination	Antidiarrheals, paromomycin, azithromycin
CMV	Stomatitis, esophagitis, gastritis, colitis, bloody diarrhea, pain, weight loss	Endoscopic visualization, culture, biopsy; rule out other causes	Ganciclovir, foscarnet, cidofovir
HSV-I	Vesicular eruptions on tongue, buccal, pharyngeal, or perioral esophageal mucosa	Viral culture	Acyclovir, foscarnet, famciclovir, valacyclovir
Candida albicans	Whitish yellow patches in mouth, esophagus, gastrointestinal (GI) tract	Microscopic examination of scraping from lesion	Nystatin, clotrimazole, ketoconazole, fluconazole, itraconazole, amphotericin B
Mycobacterium avium complex (MAC)	Watery diarrhea, weight loss, fever, fatigue, night sweats, anemia, ↑ LDH, ↑ Alk phos	Small bowel biopsy with AFB stain and culture Blood cultures	Azithromycin or clarithromycin + rifabutin, ofloxacin rifampin, clofamizine, amikacin, ciprofloxacin, ethambutol
Isospora belli	Diarrhea, weight loss, nausea, abdominal pain	Stool examination	Trimethoprim-sulfamethoxazole, pyrimethamine + folic acid
Salmonella	Gastroenteritis, fever, diarrhea	Blood and stool culture	Ampicillin, amoxicillin, ciprofloxacin, trimethoprim-sulfamethoxazole
KS	Diarrhea, hyperpigmented lesions of mouth and GI tract, GI bleeding	GI series, biopsy	Radiation, chemotherapy, highly active antiretroviral therapy (HAART)
Non-Hodgkin's lymphoma	Abdominal pain, fever, night sweats, weight loss	Lymph node biopsy	Chemotherapy, HAART
NEUROLOGICAL SYSTEM			
Toxoplasma gondii	Cognitive dysfunction, motor impairment, fever, headache, seizures, ↓ LOC, hemiparesis	Magnetic resonance imaging (MRI), computed tomography (CT) scan, toxoplasma serology	Pyrimethamine + leucovorin + sulfadiazine, clindamycin, azithromcycin, clarithromycin
Jamestown Canyon (JC) virus	Progressive multifocal leukoencephalopathy, mental and motor declines	MRI, CT scan, brain biopsy, autopsy	No proven therapy, but HAART may help, IV interferon-α or cutosine arabinoside
Cryptococcal meningitis	Cognitive impairment, motor dysfunction, fever, seizures, stiff neck, nausea/vomiting	CT scan, serum antigen test, cerebrospinal fluid analysis	Amphotericin B + 5-flucytosine, fluconazole, itraconazole
Central nervous system lymphomas	Cognitive dysfunction, motor impairment, aphasia, seizures, personality changes, headache	MRI, CT scan	Radiation, chemotherapy
HIV-associated cognitive motor complex (dementia)	Triad of cognitive, motor, and behavioral dysfunction (progressive)	Neurological examination, CT or MRI, CSF analysis	Zidovudine may help, use of HAART

Table 16-7 *Opportunistic Illness Prophylaxis Guidelines*

		PREVENTIVE REGIMENS		
PROBLEM	INDICATION	FIRST CHOICE	ALTERNATIVE CHOICES	COMMENTS
STRONGLY RECOMMENDED AS STANDARD OF CARE				
Pneumocystis jiroveci (formerly *carinii*) pneumonia (PCP)	CD_4^+ cell count <200 μL or CD_4^+ % <14%, presence of oral thrush or other AIDS-defining illness	Trimethoprim-sulfamethoxazole (TMP-SMX), 1 DS tab every day; consider desensitization protocol for patients with non-life-threatening allergy	Dapsone, aerosolized pentamidine, atovaquone	May stop if CD_4^+ cell count >200 μL for 3 months; patients receiving dapsone should be checked for G6PD deficiency
Mycobacterium tuberculosis	Skin test (PPD) ≥5 mm or prior positive skin test	Isoniazid + pyridoxine for 9 months	Rifampin, 600 mg qid for 6 months	Rule out active or extrapulmonary disease which requires multidrug therapy; remember that a negative PPD in the presence of HIV does not exclude a diagnosis of tuberculosis
Toxoplasma gondii	CD_4^+ cell count <100 μL, and positive IgG antibody; check for antibodies soon after diagnosis	TMP-SMX, 1 DS tab qid	Dapsone + pyrimethamine	If using dapsone, check for G6PD deficiency. May stop if CD_4^+ cell count >200 μL for at least 3 months
Mycobacterium avium complex (MAC)	CD_4^+ cell count <50 μL	Azithromycin, 1200 mg once each week; or clarithromycin 500 mg po bid	Rifabutin, 300 mg PO every day or; azithromycin 1200 mg once weekly	
Varicella zoster virus (VZV)	Significant exposure to chickenpox or shingles for patients who have no history of either illness	Varicella zoster immune globulin (VZIG) IM ≤96 hours after exposure		
GENERALLY RECOMMENDED				
Streptococcus pneumoniae	CD_4^+ cell count ≥200 μL	Pneumovax		Provide as soon as possible during course of infection; antibody response is optimal with CD_4^+ cell count >200 μL
Hepatitis B virus (HBV)	All susceptible patients	Heptatitis B vaccine series		
Influenza	All patients before influenza season	Inactivated trivalent influenza vaccine, dosed each year	Oseltamivir 75 mg po qid; rimantidine 100 mg po bid, or amantadine 100 mg po bid (active against influenza A only)	

Table 16-7 *Opportunistic Illness Prophylaxis Guidelines—cont'd*

		PREVENTIVE REGIMENS		
PROBLEM	INDICATION	FIRST CHOICE	ALTERNATIVE CHOICES	COMMENTS
GENERALLY RECOMMENDED—cont'd				
Hepatitis A virus (HAV)	All susceptible patients at risk for HAV infection: illicit drug users, men who have sex with men, hemophiliacs, chronic liver disease	Hepatitis A vaccine (2 doses)		Combination vaccine available for hepatitis A and hepatitis B (Twinrix)

Table 16-8 *Pros and Cons of Highly Active Antiretroviral Therapy (HAART)*

PROS	CONS
• Minimize chance of emergence of resistant virus • May play a role in the reduction of HIV transmission • Slows disease progression • Improves quality of life	• Drugs can be toxic • Frequent side effect • Complexity of drug and dosing regimens • Impact of nonadherence on treatment failure • Expensive

tions around the clock. For example, a medication ordered three times per day (tid) should be given as close to every 8 hours as possible, not three times while the patient is awake. When medications are not given regularly, the drug levels in the blood fall low enough to allow HIV to develop resistance. This is a critical teaching point for nurses to communicate to patients.

Considerations for antiretroviral therapy include the following:

- Combination therapy is now the standard of care. A single drug (monotherapy) is no longer recommended due to the likelihood of the development of viral and therapeutic resistance. Cocktails are more effective than single-drug therapy. This is referred to as "highly active antiretroviral therapy" or HAART.
- Previous antiretroviral experience may affect the efficacy of a proposed therapy, because previous drug therapy may have allowed the HIV to become resistant to those medications taken by the patient in the past (e.g., AZT, 3TC).
- Certain combinations of antiretrovirals may reverse the resistance built up against a single drug. Recycling drugs previously taken can sometimes lead to improved viral suppression. Incorrect dosing (timing) or usage (missed doses) can cause drug resistance.

- Drug incompatibilities, similar side effect profiles, and toxicities must be considered when choosing a regimen.
- The individual's commitment and ability to adhere with complex drug regimens must be considered. Inadequate adherence can lead to drug resistance and, ultimately, to drug failure. This point must be stressed to the patient. Adherence is paramount to survival and success of treatment.

There is considerable difference of opinion as to when to initiate antiretroviral therapy. The availability of an increasing number of antiretroviral agents and the rapid evolution of new information has introduced extraordinary complexity into the treatment of HIV-infected people. A provider with expertise in HIV should supervise the care of the HIV-infected person. With regard to specific recommendations, treatment should be offered to all patients with acute HIV syndrome (seroconversion illness), those within 6 months of HIV seroconversion, and all patients with symptoms credited to HIV infection. In general, treatment should be offered to individuals with fewer than 350 CD_4^+ T cells/mm^3 or plasma HIV viral loads exceeding 30,000 copies/mL (bDNA method) or 55,000 copies/mL (PCR method).

The strength of the recommendation to treat an asymptomatic patient should be based on the willingness and readiness of the individual to begin therapy; the degree of existing immunodeficiency as determined by the CD_4^+ cell count; the risk of progression as determined by the CD_4^+ cell count and viral load; the potential benefits and risks of initiating therapy in asymptomatic individuals; and the likelihood, after counseling and education, of adherence to the prescribed treatment regimen. Once the decision has been made to begin antiretroviral therapy, the goal should be maximal and durable suppression of viral load, restoration or preservation of immunological function, improvement in the quality of life, and reduction of HIV-related morbidity and mortality.

Clinical trials being conducted by the AIDS Clinical Trials Group (ACTG) and the National Institutes of Health in conjunction with universities, pharmaceutical companies, and other agencies may be important

MEDICATIONS | *HIV Disease (Antiretrovirals)*

DRUG	SIDE EFFECTS	COMMENTS
NUCLEOSIDE REVERSE TRANSCRIPTASE INHIBITORS (NUCLEOSIDE ANALOGS, "NUKES")		
Zidovudine (ZDV, AZT, Retrovir) 300 mg po every 12 hours	Anemia, fever, malaise, headache, rash, nausea, insomnia, myalgia, confusion, agitation, seizures; bone marrow suppression, anemia, granulocytopenia, thrombocytopenia, hepatomegaly	Drug of choice to be used initially in combination therapy in antiretroviral-naive patients. Side effects, such as headache and nausea, typically resolve within 1 month. Bone marrow suppression side effects occur after long-term use (6 months to 2 years). Anemia can be treated with blood transfusions or erythropoietin (Procrit); consider treating granulocytopenia or neutropenia with colony-stimulating factor (G-CSF), such as Neupogen.
Didanosine (ddI, Videx) >60 kg: 400 mg every day <60 kg: 250 mg every day po	Pancreatitis, painful peripheral neuropathy (dose-related and reversible), nausea, abdominal pain, diarrhea, rash, hyperglycemia, hyperuricemia, hepatic failure, headache, insomnia, seizures, thrombocytopenia	Take on an empty stomach 2 hours apart from other drugs, such as dapsone, intraconazole, or ketoconazole. Need alkaline environment for absorption. Avoid use with H_2 blockers, alcohol, and omeprazole (Prilosec).
Zalcitabine (ddC, HIVID) >30 kg: 0.75 mg po every 8 hours <30 kg: 0.375 mg po every 8 hours	Painful peripheral neuropathy (dose-related and reversible), fever, rash, oral or esophageal ulcers, stomatitis, pancreatitis, seizures, nausea, diarrhea, fatigue, elevations in (LFTs) (AST/ALT), cardiomyopathy, headache	Not used in monotherapy; used in combination therapy. Take on an empty stomach.
Stavudine (Zerit) >60 kg: 40 mg po every 12 hours <60 kg: 30 mg po every 12 hours	Painful peripheral neuropathy, elevations in AST/ALT anemia, headache, rash, abdominal pain, diarrhea, nausea, vomiting, myalgia	Crosses the blood-brain barrier. Used in combination therapy for patients who are intolerant of zidovudine (AZT). Decrease dose in patients with impaired renal function.
Lamivudine (3TC, Epivir) 150 mg po every 12 hours	Neutropenia, rash, insomnia, fever, headache, fatigue, diarrhea, vasculitis, photophobia, paresthesias	Generally well tolerated, with most patients reporting no side effects. Pancreatitis has been reported in 15% of children taking lamivudine. Never used alone, because HIV develops resistance quite rapidly. Typically used with ZDV or d4T, ddC, or ddI.
Abacavir (Ziagen) 300 mg po every 12 hours	Nausea, vomiting, headache, fatigue, rash	About 3% of people develop a hypersensitivity, which results in flulike symptoms. Can be life-threatening development of Stevens-Johnson syndrome—stop drug immediately and do not rechallenge—death may occur. Avoid alcohol (increases abacavir levels in blood). No dietary restrictions.
COMBINATION MEDICATIONS		
Emtricitabine (FTC, Emtriva) 200-mg capsule once daily	Headache, diarrhea nausea, rash, lactic acidosis, "fatty liver"	No food restrictions, also active against hepatitis B virus infection, should not be combined with lamivudine/epivir (3TC).
Tenofovir (TDF, Viread) 300-mg tablet once daily	Mild side effects, some nausea, vomiting, loss of appetite, potential for renal failure, bone mineral density loss	Do not combine with lamivudine (3TC, Epivir) and abacavir (Ziagen): people taking ddI (didanosine, Videx) should take tenofovir 2 hours before or 1 hour after didanosine. No food restrictions.

MEDICATIONS | *HIV Disease (Antiretrovirals)—cont'd*

DRUG	SIDE EFFECTS	COMMENTS
COMBINATION MEDICATIONS—cont'd		
Combivir	See zidovudine and lamivudine	Combination of 300 mg zidovudine and 150 mg lamivudine in 1 tablet given every 12 hours, significantly reduces the number of pills a patient has to take in 1 day.
Trizivir 1 tablet po every 12 hours	See zidovudine, lamivudine, and abacavir	Combination of 300 mg zidovudine, 150 mg lamivudine, and 300 mg abacavir.
Truvada (tenofovir plus emtricitabine) 1 tablet once daily	See emtricitabine and tenofovir	No food restrictions.
Epzicom (abacavir plus lamivudine) 1 tablet once daily	See abacavir and lamivudine	No food restrictions. Blood levels may be increased by bactrim/septra; do not take with zalcitabine or stavudine.
Combivir (zidovudine plus lamivudine) 1 tablet every 12 hours	See zidovudine and lamivudine	Do not take with zalcitabine or stavudine.
Trizivir (zidovudine plus lamivudine plus abacavir) 1 tablet every 12 hours	See zidovudine, lamivudine, and abacavir	No food restrictions. Monitor for rash.
NUCLEOTIDE REVERSE TRANSCRIPTASE INHIBITORS (NTARTI)		
Tenofovir (Viread) 300 mg po once per day		
NONNUCLEOSIDE REVERSE TRANSCRIPTASE INHIBITORS (NNRTIS)		
Nevirapine (Viramune) 200 mg po every day for 14 days, then 200 mg po every 12 hours	Rash, thrombocytopenia, fever, headaches, nausea	Used in combination therapy. Report any new rash immediately; rash may progress to Stevens-Johnson syndrome, which may result in death.
Delavirdine (Rescriptor) 400 mg po every 8 hours	Rash, elevated (LFTs)	Used in combination therapy.
Efavirenz (Sustiva) 600 mg once daily (initially at bedtime)	Initial dizziness, insomnia, transient rash, vivid dreams, nightmares, difficulty concentrating	This drug may cause hyperlipidemia; monitor cholesterol and triglycerides regularly.
PROTEASE INHIBITORS		
Saquinavir (Fortovase) (soft gel capsule) 1800 mg po every 12 hours	Nausea, vomiting, neutropenia, elevated CPK, AST elevation, diarrhea	Generally well tolerated because of low absorption rate (4%-5%). Used in combination with nucleoside analogs, NNRTIs, and in combination with other protease inhibitors. Dose reduction made when given with ritonavir (400-600 mg po every 12 hours). Take within 2 hours of a high-fat meal (increases absorption).

Continued

considerations for people with HIV disease. Patients may be able to participate in clinical trials or may benefit from the results of such research studies. Benefits include access to new and potentially beneficial treatments for HIV disease before they are released to the public, and the chance to have physician visits and labwork paid for by the research study.

Alternative and Complementary Therapies

Nontraditional or complementary therapies are commonly used by people with HIV disease. Massage, acupuncture or acupressure, and biofeedback are examples of adjunctive activities. Some patients use nutritional supplements or herbal remedies with the hope of alleviating the side effects of the disease and

MEDICATIONS | *HIV Disease (Antiretrovirals)—cont'd*

DRUG	SIDE EFFECTS	COMMENTS
PROTEASE INHIBITORS		
Ritonavir (Norvir) 600 mg po every 12 hours	Nausea, vomiting, diarrhea, circumoral paresthesias (numbness and tingling), peripheral paresthesias, taste perversions, asthenia (weakness), increased liver enzymes, elevated cholesterol and triglyceride levels	Due to side effects, dose escalation should be instituted. Start with 300 mg po every 12 hours and increase by 100 mg every 3 to 4 days until at full dose of 600 mg po every 12 hours. Take with food to decrease GI side effects. Ritonavir has many drug interactions: benzodiazepines, opiates, long-acting nonsedating antihistamines (Seldane, Hismanal, Claritin), antidysrhythmics, calcium channel blockers, rifabutin, clarithromycin levels increased by 80%. Medication must be refrigerated. May be given in combination with saquinavir as "salvage therapy" for patients who are not responding to other combinations. Use 400 mg po every 12 hours per day when given with saquinavir.
Indinavir (Crixivan) 800 mg po every 8 hours, or 1200 mg po every 12 hours	Headache, nausea (for the first few weeks), kidney stones, (signs include kidney pain, fever, abdominal tenderness, and painful urination), asymptomatic elevation of bilirubin and liver enzymes	Must be taken on an empty stomach (1 hour before or 2 hours after meal); recommend 6 to 8 glasses of water per day; take 1 hour before or after didanosine (ddl): ketoconazole increases indinavir levels by 60%; should not be used with rifampin or terfendadine (Seldane). Taken in combination with nucleoside analogs of NNRTIs.
Nelfinavir (Viracept) 750 mg po every 8 hours	Diarrhea most common side effect	Can be taken without regard to food. Used in combination with nucleoside analogs or NNRTIs. Diarrhea can be managed with antidiarrheals (Lomotil or Immodium) and increased fiber in diet.
Amprenavir (Agenerase) 1200 mg po every 12 hours	Nausea, vomiting, diarrhea, rash, perioral paresthesias, altered mood	Drug is a sulfa drug; use caution in sulfa-allergic patients. May be taken with or without food; however, a high-fat meal decreases absorption. Drug contains vitamin E; patients should not take additional vitamin E supplements. Patients taking ddl or antacids should take these at least 1 hour before or after amprenavir. Contraindicated in children less than 4 years of age, pregnant women, and patients with liver or kidney impairment. Do not coadminister with disulfiram (Antabuse) or metronidazole (Flagyl).
Lopinavir/Ritonavir (Kaletra) 400 mg lopinavir/ 100 mg ritonavir, 3 pills every 12 hours	Diarrhea, nausea, headaches, loss of strength	Combination drug of lopinavir and ritonavir. Can be taken without regard to food. Dose of lopinavir should be increased to four capsules twice a day if taken with efavirenz or nevirapine.
Atazanavir (Reyataz, ATZ) 300 to 400 mg (2 capsules) orally each day	High levels of bilirubin. Nausea, headache, rash, stomach pain, vomiting, diarrhea, tingling in hands or feet, and depression. Changes in heart rhythm	Take with food. If taken with didanosine (ddl, Videx) take 2 hours before or after atazanavir. Efavirenz and tenofovir lower levels of atazanavir (take with ritonavir to compensate). Do NOT take proton pump inhibitors (Prilosec, Nexium, et al.). Take H$_2$ blockers such as Pepcid and Zantac 12 hours apart from atazanavir.
Saquinavir (Invirase, SQV) hard gel capsule 1000 mg (5 capsules) plus 100 mg ritonavir every 12 hours	Minimal nausea, diarrhea, vomiting, headache, fatigue	Take up to 2 hours after a full meal. Take with high-fat food. Refrigerate in hot climates.

MEDICATIONS | *HIV Disease (Antiretrovirals)—cont'd*

DRUG	SIDE EFFECTS	COMMENTS
PROTEASE INHIBITORS		
Fosamprenavir (Lexiva, FPV) 1400 mg (two 700-mg tablets), two times a day. May be combined with ritonavir and dosed as 1400 mg FPV plus 200 mg ritonavir once daily, or 700 mg FPV plus 100 mg ritonavir twice daily	Nausea, diarrhea, vomiting, rash, numbness around mouth, abdominal pain	No food restrictions. Less than 1% of people get serious skin reactions, including Stevens-Johnson syndrome. No other side effects seem to be very serious. The diarrhea in most cases can be controlled with over-the-counter medications. Fosamprenavir can increase triglycerides (a blood fat). However, fosamprenavir might cause less of an increase in cholestrerol than other protease inhibitors. Fosamprenavir is a sulfa drug. If you are allergic to sulfa drugs, be sure to tell your physician.
FUSION INHIBITORS		
Enfuvirtide (T-20, Fuzeon) 90 mg (1 mL) injected subcutaneously twice daily in the upper arm, thigh, or abdomen (for patients weighing >94 lb (42.6 kg)	Skin reactions where drug is injected, ranging from redness and itching to hard lumps. Other side effects include headache, pain and numbness in feet or legs, dizziness, and loss of sleep	Almost everybody who uses enfuvirtide gets these skin reactions. They can be very mild, such as slight redness. They can include itching, swelling, pain, hardened skin, or hard lumps. Each reaction might last up to a week. With two injections each day, people using enfuvirtide might have reactions at several spots on their body at the same time. Very few patients have stopped using it because of skin reactions.

the medications. Many patients prefer these therapies because of the limitations or side effects of approved drugs, mistrust of the health care system, easier access, lack of adequate insurance coverage, or the high cost of anti-HIV medications. These alternatives are best used in conjunction with approved therapeutic intervention. Patients should be encouraged to use complementary therapies as long as they do not cause undue harm and are not part of quackery medicine, which tends to drain financial resources. Patients should be warned about unproven drugs and the potential for fraud and quackery in a manner that does not discount their efforts at self-care. Patients may need guidance to avoid expensive and particularly dangerous forms of alternative treatments. However, it is important to remember that alternative forms of therapy may be beneficial and should always be thoroughly explored. An open relationship and good communication with the patient build trust, creating a positive atmosphere for addressing difficult issues. They also reinforce a philosophy of the patient as an important member of the health care team.

NURSING INTERVENTIONS

The nurse needs to establish a comfort level in interacting with people with HIV disease. Patients need to be treated in a nonjudgmental, empathic, and caring manner regardless of their sexual practices or history of drug use. The attitudes, values, and beliefs of the nurse should not interfere with the care a patient with HIV disease needs. Patients are very aware when their caregiver is not comfortable dealing with HIV disease. The nurse must see the patient as a unique individual with a need to be cared for with compassion, consideration, and dignity. Knowledge of HIV transmission and competence in standard precautions and body substance isolation will minimize the fear of caring for HIV-infected patients. Box 16-3 and Table 16-9 lists appropriate nursing assessments and activities specific to HIV disease. Box 16-4 lists nursing interventions for the patient with HIV infection and disease.

Nursing diagnoses and interventions for the patient with HIV disease include but are not limited to the following:

NURSING DIAGNOSES	NURSING INTERVENTIONS
Risk for caregiver role strain, related to advancing disease in care receiver and lack of caregiver coping patterns	Assess needs and capabilities of patient and caregiver. Assess factors that contribute to caregiver strain. Develop supportive and trusting relationship with caregiver. Enlist the help of family members, significant others, and friends to assist caregiver.

Continued

Box 16-3 *Nursing Assessment of the Patient with HIV Infection*

SUBJECTIVE DATA

Important Health Information

Past health history: Route of infection, risk factors, history of hepatitis or other STDs, frequent viral infections, parasitic infections, tuberculosis, alcohol and drug use, foreign travel

Medications: Use of immunosuppressive drugs

Functional Health Patterns

Health perception–health management: Chronic fatigue, malaise, weakness

Nutritional-metabolic: Unexplained weight loss, low-grade fevers, night sweats; anorexia, nausea, vomiting; oral lesions, bleeding, ulcerations; abdominal cramping; lesions of lips, mouth, tongue, throat; sensitivity to acidic, salty, or spicy foods, problems with teeth or bleeding gums, difficulty swallowing; skin rashes or color changes, lesions (painful or nonpainful), blisters; nonhealing wounds, pruritus

Elimination: Persistent diarrhea, constipation, painful urination

Activity-exercise: Muscle weakness, difficulty with ambulation; cough, shortness of breath

Cognitive-perceptual: Headaches, stiff neck, chest pain, rectal pain, retrosternal pain; blurred vision, photophobia, loss of vision, diplopia; confusion, forgetfulness, attention deficit, changes in mental status, memory loss; hearing impairment, personality changes, paresthesias; hypersensitivity in feet

Sexuality-reproductive: Lesions on genitalia (internal or external), pruritus, or burning in vagina or penis; painful sexual intercourse; changes in menstruation; vaginal or penile discharge

OBJECTIVE DATA

General: Vital signs, weight, general status, diaphoresis

Eyes: Presence of exudate, retinal lesions or hemorrhage, papilledema, pupillary response, extraocular muscle movements

Oral: Presence of a variety of mouth lesions, including blisters (herpes simplex virus–1 lesions), white-gray patches (Candida), painless white lesions on lateral aspects of tongue (oral hairy leukoplakia), discolorations (Kaposi's sarcoma), gingivitis, tooth decay or loosening

Neck: Enlarged lymph nodes, nuchal rigidity, enlarged thyroid

Throat: Redness or white patchy lesions

Integumentary: Observe integrity and skin turgor; general appearance; presence of lesions, eruptions, discolorations; enlarged lymph nodes, bruises, cyanosis, dryness, delayed wound healing, alopecia

Respiratory: Presence of crackles or rhonchi, dyspnea, cough (productive or nonproductive, color and amount of sputum), wheezing, tachypnea, intercostal retractions, use of accessory muscles

Lymphatic: Generalized lymphadenopathy

Abdominal: Tenderness, masses, enlarged liver or spleen, hyperactive bowel sounds

Genitourinary/rectal: Presence of lesions or discharge, abdominal pain denoting pelvic inflammatory disease (PID), difficult or painful urination

Neuromuscular: Aphasia, ataxia, lack of coordination, sensory loss, tremors, slurred speech, memory loss, apathy, agitation, social withdrawal/isolation, pain, inappropriate behavior, changes in level of consciousness, depression, seizures, paralysis, coma

NURSING DIAGNOSES	NURSING INTERVENTIONS
	Encourage interaction in support groups for caregivers.
	Teach stress reduction techniques to caregiver.
	Encourage caregiver to attend to own personal and health care needs.
Diarrhea, related to gastrointestinal infections, malabsorption, or medication side effects	Document quantity, quality, and frequency of stools.
	Monitor intake and output, vital signs, and daily weight.
	Assess for skin impairment.
	Administer antidiarrheals on a routine schedule.
	Encourage increased electrolyte-rich fluid intake (fruit juices, Gatorade, Pedialyte).
	Encourage high-protein, high-calorie, and low-residue diet.

Health care needs can be unpredictable and assessment difficult because of the clinical diversity of HIV infection. HIV disease may require alternating periods of long-term and acute care. The patient may fear isolation from the community or family and friends because of the social stigma associated with HIV disease.

The disease primarily affects young people who are at the most productive time in their lives, a time when they are expected to take control. For this reason, they often want to have an active role in the decision-making and planning stages of their care. Patients may experience bouts of serious, debilitating illness, then recover enough to function effectively for an unpredictable amount of time. People with HIV disease often prefer to stay at home as long as possible, and some prefer to die at home. But long-term care in an inpatient setting (e.g., long-term care facility) is not very compatible with the social needs of the young patient. Prolonged care is expensive, and many patients with HIV disease do not have health insurance; alternative care is an important consideration. Church and community-based organization volunteers, such as

Table 16-9   *Nursing Activities in Human Immunodeficiency Virus Disease*

LEVELS OF CARE AND GOALS	ASSESSMENT	INTERVENTIONS
HEALTH PROMOTION AND MAINTENANCE		
Prevention of HIV infection Early detection of HIV infection	Risk factors: What behaviors or social, physical, emotional, pathologic, and immune factors place patient at risk? Does patient need to be tested?	Educate, including knowledge, attitudes, and behaviors, with an emphasis on risk reduction to: <ul><li>General population (cover general information)</li><li>Individual patient (specific to assessed need)</li></ul>Empower patient to take control of prevention measures. Provide HIV-antibody testing with pretest and posttest counseling.
ACUTE INTERVENTION		
Promotion of health and limitation of disability Successful management of problems caused by HIV infection	Physical health: Is patient experiencing problems? Mental health status: How is the patient coping? Resources: Does the patient have family and social support? Is patient accessing community services? Is money and insurance a problem? Does patient have access to spiritual support?	Provide case management. Educate regarding HIV, the spectrum of infection, options for care, signs and symptoms to watch for. Educate regarding immune enhancement and harm reduction. Refer to needed resources. Establish long-term, trusting relationship with patient, family, and significant others. Provide emotional and spiritual support. Provide care during acute exacerbations: recognition of life-threatening developments, life support, rapid intervention with treatments and medications, patient and family emotional support during crisis, comfort and hygiene needs. Develop resources for legal needs: discrimination prevention, wills and powers of attorney, child care wishes. Empower patient to identify needs, direct care, seek services.
CHRONIC AND HOME MANAGEMENT		
Maximizing quality of life Resolution of life and death issues	Physical health: Are new symptoms developing? Is patient experiencing drug side effects or interactions? Mental health status: How is patient coping? What adjustments have been made? Finances: Can patient maintain health care and basic standards of living? Family, social, and community supports: Are these supports available? Is patient using supports in an effective manner? Spirituality issues: Does patient desire support from an established religious organization? Are spirituality issues private and personal? What assistance does patient need?	Continue case management. Educate regarding treatment options. Empower patient to continue to direct care and to make desires known to family members and significant others. Continue physical care for chronic disease process: treatments, medications, comfort and hygiene needs. Support patient and family and significant others in a trusting relationship. Refer to resources that will assist in identified needs. Promote health maintenance measures. Assist with end-of-life issues: resuscitation orders, funeral plans, estate planning, child care continuation.

Box 16-4 | *Nursing Interventions for the Patient with HIV Infection or HIV Disease*

PREVENT INFECTION

1. Wash hands frequently and use skin lubricants for patient and caregiver to prevent skin breakdown.
2. Use a gentle liquid soap (such as castile); avoid bar soaps, which may irritate skin.
3. Provide for daily showering or basin bath; avoid tub bath if rashes are present; avoid extremely hot temperatures.
4. Use a separate washcloth for lesions.
5. Use soft toothbrushes; nonabrasive toothpaste; and mouth rinses with sodium bicarbonate, saline, or lemon and hydrogen peroxide before meals and at bedtime.
6. Use measures to prevent skin impairment, such as turning sheets, air mattresses.
7. Elevate and support areas of edema.
8. Observe biopsy sites and IV insertion sites daily for signs of infection.
9. Change dressings at least every other day; avoid plastic occlusive dressings.
10. Avoid sources of microbes, such as plants or ingestion of uncooked fresh fruits and vegetables.
11. Carry out measures to prevent spread of infection: use gloves for contact with bodily secretions, double plastic bags to dispose of bodily secretions, use bleach and water (1:10) for cleaning contaminated areas.

MODIFY ALTERATIONS IN BODY TEMPERATURE

1. Administer prescribed antibiotics, IV fluids, or antipyretics.
2. Encourage fluid intake >2500 mL.
3. Maintain daily I&O records.
4. Weigh daily.
5. Provide tepid sponge baths and linen changes as necessary.
6. Instruct patient in deep-breathing and coughing exercises to prevent atelectasis and additional fever.

PROMOTE GOOD NUTRITION

1. Provide instruction for high-calorie, high-protein, high-potassium, low-residue diet.
2. Encourage high-calorie, high-potassium snacks.
3. Suggest foods that are easy to swallow (gelatin, yogurt, puddings) when dysphagia is present.
4. Avoid foods that are spicy or acidic, rare meats, and raw fruits and vegetables.
5. Provide oral care before patient eats.
6. Encourage patient to get out of bed and sit up for meals if possible.
7. Avoid odors by aerating room.
8. Make appropriate dietary consultations.

PROMOTE SELF-CARE

1. Assess realistic functional ability.
2. Plan, supervise, and assist with ADLs as necessary.
3. Encourage patient to be as active and independent as possible.
4. Assist patient with range-of-motion exercise to prevent contractures.
5. Provide equipment such as assistive eating devices, walkers, and commodes to promote patient independence.
6. Pace activities and schedule rest periods to prevent fatigue.

PROVIDE COUNSELING

1. Assess and support patient coping mechanisms.
2. Explore with patient and significant others normalcy of grief.
3. Assist patient and significant others in acknowledging and planning for anticipated losses.
4. Provide information as desired and necessary, depending on patient's ability to understand.
5. Suggest appropriate religious support.
6. Facilitate participation in support groups or individual counseling as pertinent.

AIDS project workers, are known to provide support and care services for patients and families. Friends, family, and significant others are also important resources to be considered when planning care for the patient with HIV disease.

ADHERENCE

As Dr. Margaret Chesney has noted, with regard to HIV disease, "There is no point in medical history where we have ever expected any patient to adhere to a regimen this complex, as an ambulatory patient, for an indefinite period of time." The maintenance of **adherence** to a prescribed regimen is of paramount importance to survival and the success of treatment. The nurse is in the unique position to help patients adapt

and maintain vigilance with their treatment. It is important for patients to understand that antiretroviral treatment is a lifelong, complex undertaking. Multiple factors affect the ability to incorporate anti-HIV treatment into a lifestyle. Factors such as treatment knowledge, underlying psychiatric or psychological pathology, physical status, family/caregiver support, health care views, culture, fear of side effects, misinformation about therapy, denial, and possessing skills (memory, impaired function) necessary to care out a medical regimen are all determinants of adherence.

Strategies the nurse can employ to increase adherence include assessing your level of comfort with HIV, learning to listen, having knowledge and skills, giving permission to grieve and allow sadness, acknowledging frustration and helplessness, providing a safe environment, and seeking expert assistance as needed. All of these can help patients incorporate this difficult treatment into their lifestyles (Table 16-10).

PALLIATIVE CARE

The WHO has defined palliative care as the active, total care of patients whose disease is not responsive to curative treatment (O'Neill & Alexander, 1997). Palliative care is not seen as hastening the dying process or postponing death. Nurses realize that death is a natural process of life, but there are others who feel that the death of a patient signifies the failure of medicine. The goal of palliative care is to address physical, psychological, social, spiritual, and existential needs of patients with progressive, life-threatening illnesses, with the overall goal of improving the quality of life. Most hospice programs use a palliative care approach, understanding that impending death means a shifting from curing to caring. The important concept to remember with palliative care is that the goal is to relieve suffering through pain and symptom management at *any* point in the patient's disease process. It comes as no surprise that care for dying people in the United States often does not meet the needs or expectations of the patient or family (Sherman, 2001).

Palliative care for the patient with HIV disease is different from the care provided to a patient with a cancer diagnosis. Patients are treated for the chronic debilitating conditions associated with HIV disease, but also for

superimposed acute exacerbations of opportunistic infections and related symptoms. Intravenous therapy, blood transfusions, and antibiotic usage may be considered palliative in the end stage of HIV disease because these interventions keep the patient comfortable and help maintain a relative quality of life. In AIDS care, short-term aggressive curative therapy is often important in treating acute infections, whereas the overall goal may remain palliation (Sherman, 2001). The complex needs of patients with HIV disease requires the nurse to participate in a multidisciplinary team comprising physicians, social workers, dietitians, physical therapists, and clergy; remember that the nurse is the "voice and advocate" for the patient who may or may not be able to communicate his or her treatment desires. Because of this unique role, it is important for the nurse to be comfortable discussing treatment issues and options with patients, as well as being respectful of those decisions. Families and significant others of patients with end-stage HIV disease can experience what is called **disenfranchised grief,** defined as the grief that people experience when they incur a loss that is not openly acknowledged, publicly mourned, or socially supported (Sherman, 2001). Symptoms such as pain, fatigue, anorexia, fever, shortness of breath, diarrhea, and insomnia are commonly experienced. The nurse must become familiar with the causes and interventions necessary to alleviate these symptoms. Remember that symptoms such as pain are a subjective experience, and must be treated appropriately until the patient has verbalized benefit. Although this phase of life is difficult for both patient and nurse to experience, many nurses express significant satisfaction with these interactions, relationships, and their outcomes.

PSYCHOSOCIAL ISSUES

The psychosocial implications for the patient with HIV disease are generally complex. Such patients have considerably more psychosocial problems than patients with other terminal illnesses. They face uncertainty, isolation, fear, and depression. The condition is contagious and incurable (though treatable) and attracts significant media attention. The stigma of the disease—because of its association with drug use, homosexuality, and sexual transmission—is a major concern. The fear of potential abandonment and isolation from family and friends is also very real; the patient may even have already experienced it. The patient is usually young and may have limited financial resources to handle the expensive treatment; the average annual cost for care is between $20,000 and $24,700 (Hellinger & Fleishman, 2000). The costs of providing care to HIV-infected individuals in 1996 was estimated to be between $6.7 billion and $7.8 billion. Data for 1998 show that about 55% of the total expenditure was for medications, 15% for outpatient services, and 30% for hospitalizations (Bozzette et al, 2001). The patient may be gay, struggling with issues of

Table 16-10 *Factors Related to Nonadherent Behavior*

FACTOR	EXAMPLES
Psychosocial factors	• Locus of control • Ineffective communication • Mental health problems • Trust • Internal conflict, social stress, stigma • Paternalistic behavior of the health care provider
Medications and treatments	• Complex regimens • Inconvenient dosing schedules • Skepticism about treatment effectiveness
Cultural issues	• Lack of understanding of cultural influences • Differing worldview
Substance use	• Continuing substance use • Lack of social support • Tenuous living arrangements • Negative view of addiction

Modified from Crespo-Fierro, M. Compliance/adherence and care management in HIV disease. *Journal of the Association of Nurses in AIDS Care (JANAC)*, 8(4):43-54, 1997.

sexuality and acceptance from family and community. The patient may be a single mother who has no financial resources or family support, and she may be more concerned about her children than her own physical or emotional needs. The patient may have, or previously had, issues with substance abuse. For all of these potential reasons, nurses need to offer their own feelings of sympathy in these difficult situations. Words are one way to convey caring; listening is another important tool. The nurse can develop a good therapeutic relationship with the patient by allowing the patient to assist with and participate in the planning and decision-making process of the care program. Nurses must remember that patients have a right to make decisions that may seem unwise, such as refusing lifesaving antibiotics or medications; the nurse should be supportive of these decisions.

ASSISTING WITH COPING

Individuals who are exposed to HIV infection, but who are without the symptoms or complications of infections or cancers, live with a great deal of uncertainty and anxiety interspersed with denial and hopefulness (Box 16-5). The role of the nurse in this stage of the disease process is to provide continued education about HIV disease and prevention, as well as to assist in realistic goal setting. Patients are encouraged to participate in their own care and to maintain positive relationships.

As HIV disease progresses through the clinical complications of infections and cancers, patients experience multiple losses, including the loss of energy; a self-care deficit requiring assistance with ADLs; and the loss of independence, employment, finances, and hope. The reality of death emerges. Nursing interventions should focus on a philosophy of facing life a day at a time and living each day to the fullest extent possible by resolving multiple conflicts. This may be a time for strengthening personal and spiritual relationships.

Empathetic listening and the ability to help patients find meaning in life become critical nursing interventions. Assisting families and significant others in providing support to the terminally ill patient despite their own anger and grief is a unique nursing challenge. Such care, although emotionally draining for the nurse, can provide positive feelings of professional accomplishment.

The diagnosis of HIV infection, with its social stigma, relatively poor prognosis, and chronic nature is indeed a catastrophic event for patients and caregivers. Patients experience a variety of intense emotions that threaten self-esteem and predispose them to depression and feelings of powerlessness. Anxiety is a response that pervades the entire HIV disease continuum. Denial often accompanies the initial diagnosis and intensifies with the subsequent physical decline and possible loss of independence, job, and finances. Anxiety may become incapacitating as death becomes a reality. Nursing interventions to promote effective coping focus on exploring and strengthening healthy coping strategies and maintaining sources of psychological support.

REDUCING ANXIETY

Individuals, families, and significant others experiencing the anxiety of HIV disease are often in a state of crisis. Continued clarification and education about HIV disease, complications, and treatment are critical. Every effort should be made to include the patient and his or her support system in the planning of medical and nursing interventions. An assessment of past coping styles and support systems should be made early in the care process and continually reevaluated. Healthy patterns of coping, such as talking or relaxation and meditation, are encouraged. Relationships with family, friends, and significant others should be maintained, and they may even be strengthened by the HIV crisis; conversely, past conflicts, especially among family members, may persist and intensify during the illness.

Occasionally, anxiety, denial, depression, and even grief may persist for extended periods, interfering with daily functioning, productive communication and relationships, and even the ability to make decisions. The nurse must be able to assess normal periods of anxiety, depression, and grief, as well as refer patients and significant others for psychological evaluation and counseling for ineffective coping patterns. Although reactions of anxiety and depression are normal, professional intervention is necessary whenever they preclude communication and daily functioning for an extended time (usually longer than 3 months). Patients with HIV disease and depression should be assessed regularly for suicidal ideation, because this phenomenon occasionally occurs in terminally ill patients who are experiencing fear of further pain and physical decline. Early recognition of depression is critical because many cases of depression and anxiety will respond to medications and psychotherapy.

Box 16-5 *Psychological Crisis Intervals in the Course of HIV Disease*

- Diagnosis of HIV infection
- Viral load testing
- Increases in viral load
- Initiation of antiretroviral therapy
- Signs of treatment failure
- Adding prophylaxis therapies (e.g., PCP)
- Occurrence of opportunistic illnesses (OIs)
- Change in antiretroviral treatment regimen
- Illness and/or death in support networks
- New treatment advances

Individuals with diffuse anxiety often feel they have little control over their daily existence. A schedule of activities developed by the patient with guidance from health care professionals may decrease anxiety and feelings of powerlessness. Opportunities for spiritual support and comfort should be explored. Community support groups for patients and significant others may offer additional sources of support and contribute to healthy coping. Planned, uninterrupted time with only the nurse, patient, and significant other may create a supportive environment that decreases anxiety and promotes healthy coping.

MINIMIZING SOCIAL ISOLATION

The psychosocial aspects of HIV disease are devastating. Because no cure currently exists, the diagnosis of HIV infection brings denial, fear, depression, and anger (much as a cancer diagnosis does). The social stigma of HIV disease based on associations with homosexuality, drug use, and sexual transmission cannot be minimized. One of the earliest issues that HIV-infected individuals face is sharing the diagnosis with other people. A tremendous fear of family, significant others, and friends reacting with anger, rejection, or abandonment is a real concern. Often families and friends who are struggling with their own anxieties and fears do abandon the patient. When this happens, the nurse should try to assist the patient to find other sources of social support. In some cities, there are support groups for patients and separate groups for significant others. HIV-infected individuals who have been exposed through contaminated blood or women from homosexual/heterosexual spouses may feel unique and experience intense anger and hostility. These patients are usually supported by their families and friends, but can be isolated by other people who do not understand that HIV is not unique to MSMs.

ASSISTING WITH GRIEVING

Like patients with other terminal illnesses, patients diagnosed with HIV disease experience strong emotions. Some patients benefit from individual empathic listening and exploring feelings, fears, and treatment options. Others may benefit from support groups consisting of patients experiencing similar feelings. Significant others and family members experience their own feelings of fear, anger, embarrassment, and shame; individual counseling and support groups may help loved ones be a source of support for the patient. Practical issues such as employment disability, housing, discrimination, insurance coverage, and preparation for death also need to be addressed. Referrals to social workers and appropriate community agencies can alleviate many concerns that plague acute or terminally ill patients. Continued participation in religious services and the support of fellow worshipers and clergy should not be overlooked as a source of healthy coping; many members of the clergy are experienced in grief counseling.

CONFIDENTIALITY

Respect for the patient's right to confidentiality is particularly important for the patient with HIV disease. The diagnosis needs to be carefully protected and shared only with caregivers who need to know for the purpose of assessment and treatment. Do all health care providers have a right to know a patient's HIV status? The answer to that depends upon why health care personnel need to know. If a phlebotomist needs to know so he or she can wear two pairs of latex gloves, then the answer is no. If an oncoming shift nurse needs to know so he or she may develop an appropriate plan of care, then the answer is yes. Ancillary personnel such as laboratory or radiograph technicians, dietary personnel, and housekeeping staff generally do not need to know this detail about the patient. The utilization of standard precautions by all staff members for all patients all the time simplifies this issue. Knowing a patient's HIV status merely provides a false sense of security; for every patient who is known to be HIV positive, there are an additional four to seven whose seroconversion status is unknown (perhaps even to the patient). The patient should be in control of who is told of the diagnosis. The nurse should have the utmost respect for the patient's right to confidentiality, meaning the patient or the diagnosis should *never* be discussed at mealtime, during breaks, or in the elevator with co-workers, friends, or family.

DUTY TO TREAT

A nurse's professional obligation to treat patients in need transcends concerns about the diseases or conditions of the patients. As infectious disease health care providers note, it is not the known HIV-infected patient who is of concern; it is the patient whose HIV or infectious status is not known who presents the greatest risk. If a nurse's primary concern is personal safety, the nurse needs to reexamine his or her commitment to the profession. The patient with HIV disease can provide valuable lessons in issues related to infectious disease control, the stereotyping of patients, and an understanding of the dedication of health care providers.

HIV disease has taught health care providers to be more aware of the human condition so that they can deal with their own prejudices, judgments, and concerns. Health care providers are challenged by the patient with HIV disease whose needs and suffering require more than nursing skill, education, and technology. A spirit of compassion stemming from a genuine willingness to serve the needs of others is essential in caring for the patient with HIV disease.

Ethical and Legal Principles

- The Rehabilitation Act of 1973 and the Americans with Disabilities Act (ADA) prohibit discrimination against the handicapped and the disabled. HIV-infected people or those with AIDS are included under these acts.
- Refusal to treat or care for people who are HIV-infected or have AIDS, when that refusal is not based on a medical judgment, is as unethical as discrimination based on race, gender, or other characteristics.
- Health care professionals may not pick and choose their patients, if they are true to their oaths to provide care to all those in need.

ACUTE INTERVENTION

Early intervention after detection of an HIV infection can promote health and limit or delay disability. Because the course of HIV is extremely variable, assessment is of primary importance. Nursing interventions will be based on and tailored to any patient needs noted during assessment. The nursing assessment of HIV disease should focus on the early detection of constitutional symptoms, opportunistic diseases, and psychosocial problems (Box 16-6).

HIV disease progression may be delayed by promoting a healthy immune system. Useful interventions for the HIV-infected patient include the following:

- Nutritional changes that maintain lean body mass, increase weight, and ensure appropriate levels of vitamins and micronutrients
- Elimination of smoking and drug use
- Elimination or moderation of alcohol intake
- Regular exercise
- Stress reduction
- Avoidance of exposure to new infectious agents
- Mental health counseling
- Involvement in support groups
- Safer sexual practices

The nurse needs to help patients gain control of the situation and their emotions. Facilitating empowerment is particularly important, because the individual with an HIV infection often experiences loss, including an overwhelming feeling of loss of control. Empowerment is facilitated through education and honest discussions about the patient's health status.

The patient should be taught to recognize clinical manifestations that may indicate progression of the disease; this will ensure that prompt medical care is initiated. Early manifestations that need to be reported include unexplained weight loss, night sweats, diarrhea, persistent fever, swollen lymph nodes, oral hairy leukoplakia (OHL), oral candidiasis (thrush), and persistent vaginal yeast infections. Additionally, the patient should report unusual headaches, changes in vision, nausea and vomiting, and numbness or tingling in the extremities. The patient should be given as much information as needed to make health care decisions. These decisions will dictate the appropriate medical and nursing interventions.

Nursing interventions become more complicated as the patient's immune system deteriorates and new problems arise to compound existing difficulties. The nursing focus should be on quality-of-life issues and symptom management, rather than on issues regarding a cure.

When opportunistic diseases develop, symptomatic nursing interventions, education, and emotional support are necessary. For example, an acute case of PCP requires intensive nursing intervention. Interventions include monitoring the respiratory status, administering medications and oxygen, positioning the patient to facilitate breathing, managing anxiety, promoting nutritional support, and helping the patient conserve energy to decrease oxygen demand. Because the potential for death is associated with advanced HIV disease, emotional support for the patient, caregiver, or significant other is particularly important (Nursing Care Plan box).

Diarrhea is often a long-term problem for HIV-infected people. Damage to the intestinal villi, malabsorption, infections of the gastrointestinal (GI) tract, and the side effects of medications all contribute to a large number of patients developing diarrhea. Nursing interventions include recommending dietary interventions (Table 16-11), encouraging adequate fluid intake to prevent dehydration, instructing the patient about skin care, and managing excoriation around the perianal area. In some cases the nurse must administer antidiarrheals to help control diarrhea and prevent further complications. The nurse can recommend the use of incontinence products to prevent soiling of the clothes and bed linens. In addition, the nurse should assess for factors that may trigger the diarrhea, such as anxiety, medications, or lactose intolerance.

Wasting and Lipodystrophy Syndromes

AIDS wasting has been a common clinical manifestation of HIV disease since early in the epidemic. Wasting is due to disturbances in metabolism, which interferes with the effective use of nutrients, resulting in the loss of lean (muscle) body mass (Winson, 2001). It is characterized by depletion of lean body mass, often without reduction of body fat. This loss of lean body mass is a primary cause of functional decline in wasting, resulting in increased risk of opportunistic infections, reduced quality of life, and reduced survival.

The causes of wasting are most likely multifactorial. Food intake may be inadequate because of mechanical difficulties (e.g., thrush or esophageal ulcers), loss of appetite (e.g., side effect of medications or neurological disease), or psychological factors such as depression and anxiety. There may also be decreased absorption in the intestine due to infections and a damaged

Box 16-6   *Conducting a Risk Assessment*

Risk assessment specific to HIV and sexually transmitted diseases (STDs), as well as bloodborne diseases, is crucial in health care delivery today. Risk assessment should be done on a regular basis with all patients and performed with the evaluation of any new patient. Sexual and drug use risks should be determined along with other risks during routine history taking.

KEY QUESTIONS TO ASK

Any "yes" responses require further assessment and evaluation
- Have you ever had a blood transfusion? Have you ever received any other kind of blood product? Before 1985?
- Do you now or have you ever shared injection equipment?
- Are you now or have you ever been sexually active?

KEY POINTS TO CONSIDER

Begin by assuring confidentiality and telling the patient why asking these questions is important:
- "I am going to ask some personal questions. I ask all of my patients these questions so I can provide better care. All of your responses will be kept confidential. Is it OK to proceed?
Ask direct questions about specific behaviors:
- "When was the last time you . . .?"
- "How often do you . . .?"
- "Have you ever exchanged sex for money or drugs?"
Exploratory questions may help (especially with adolescents and young adults):
- "Do your friends use condoms?"
- "What happens at parties?"
- "How easy is it to get drugs?"
Honest responses may be more forthcoming if the behaviors are normalized:
- "Some of my patients who use drugs inject them. Do you inject drugs or other substances?"
- "Sometimes people have anal intercourse. Have you ever had anal intercourse?"

DRUG USE ASSESSMENT

It is important to be nonjudgmental and nonmoralistic:
- Injection drug use is illegal in the U.S. and many patients are afraid to be honest unless trust is established.
Start with less threatening questions:
- "What over-the-counter or prescription medications are you taking?"
- "How often do you use alcohol? Tobacco?"
- "Have you ever used drugs from a nonmedical source?"
- "Have you ever injected any kind of drug?"

Do not assume anything.
- Drug use occurs in all socioeconomic strata. Do not forget that people inject substances such as insulin, steroids, and vitamins. Any sharing, even one time, can result in HIV exposure.
Look for other clues in the history and physical exam:
- Antisocial behavior, recurrent criminal arrests, needle tracks.
If there is a positive history of drug injection use, get more information:
- "Do/did you share needles/other equipment?"
- "Is/was the equipment you use(d) clean? How did you know it was clean?"
- "What drugs did you inject?"

SEXUAL RISK ASSESSMENT

Direct and nonjudgmental questions work best:
- "Do you have sex with men, women, or both?"
- "Do you have oral sex? Vaginal sex? Anal sex?"
- "What do you know about the sexual activities of your partners?"
- "What do you do to protect yourself during sex?"
- "Do you use condoms? How often?"
- "Have you ever had sex with someone you didn't know or just met?"
Ask for an explanation of sexual practices:
- "When you say you had sex, what exactly do you mean?"
- "I don't know what you mean; could you explain . . .?"
Do not assume anything.
- Marriage does not always mean an individual is monogamous or heterosexual.
- People who identify as homosexual may also have heterosexual sex.
Use specific terms:
- Use "men who have sex with men" or "women who have sex with women" instead of gay. Some men do not consider themselves "gay" if they practice anal insertive intercourse, but their receptive partners are considered to be gay (can be culturally related).

CLINICAL RISK ASSESSMENT

Assess the patient for constitutional signs, history of chronic infection and HIV, and associated problems:
- Headaches
- Diarrhea
- Fatigue
- Shingles
- History of STD, hepatitis, or TB
- Fever, chills, night sweats
- Skin lesions
- Weight loss
- Oral thrush
- Generalized lymphadenopathy

Modified from *HIV risk assessment, a quick reference guide.* Mountain Plains AIDS Education and Training Center, Denver, Colo.

NURSING CARE PLAN

The Patient Who Is HIV Positive

Ms. J. is a 20-year-old who presents to the emergency department, accompanied by her mother, with complaints of severe vomiting and recent weight loss of 10 pounds. Ms. J. went to the 24-hour clinic and learned that she is approximately 8 weeks pregnant, and due to risk factors for HIV exposure, gave informed consent for HIV antibody testing. It was later determined that she is HIV positive by ELISA and Western blot testing. Ms. J. is tearful and reluctant to answer questions about her recent HIV diagnosis and positive pregnancy test. She states it is not possible that she could be HIV positive because she has only had sexual intercourse with her boyfriend of 5 years. Additionally, Ms. J. is concerned about telling her mother about her HIV status and the pregnancy because she lives with her mother, who is also taking care of her sick elderly grandmother. Ms. J. does not have a job and is dependent upon family members to help her meet financial obligations and needs. Ms. J. feels the added burden to her mother would "be too much" and is considering leaving home to live in a shelter.

NURSING DIAGNOSIS *Risk for caregiver role strain, related to advancing disease in care receiver, lack of caregiver coping pattern*

Patient Goals/Expected Outcomes	Nursing Intervention	Evaluation
Caregiver will use available community and personal resources. Caregiver will have the ability to complete necessary caregiving tasks. Effective support for caregiver.	Assess needs and capabilities of patient and caregiver. Assess factors that contribute to caregiver strain (unrealistic expectations, poor insight, inability to use resources, unsatisfactory relationship with care receiver, insufficient financial and psychosocial resources). Develop supportive and trusting relationship with caregiver. Enlist help of other family members or friends to assist. Teach caregiver to perform care activities in a safe, efficient, and energy-conserving manner. Teach stress-reduction techniques. Encourage caregiver to attend to own personal and health needs.	**The caregiver:** • Provides safe, supportive care to the HIV-infected patient. • Acknowledges need for personal support and accesses resources in family and community. • Shares frustrations about difficulty of care for significant other. • Receives assistance from family members and/or professional caregivers.

NURSING DIAGNOSIS *Imbalanced nutrition: less than body requirements, related to chronic infections and/or malabsorption, nausea/vomiting/diarrhea, fatigue, or side effects of medications as evidenced by 10% or greater loss of ideal body mass*

Patient Goals/Expected Outcomes	Nursing Intervention	Evaluation
Patient's weight will remain stable. Patient's nutritional intake will exceed metabolic needs. Patient will regain lost weight.	Assist with diagnosis of underlying opportunistic infections. Assess patient's knowledge of optimal nutritional intake. Increase protein, calorie, and fat intake. Offer nutritional supplements (Carnation Instant Breakfast, Boost, Sustacal, etc.). Schedule procedures that are painful, stressful, or nauseating so they do not interfere with mealtimes. Eat several small meals throughout day as opposed to three large meals. Provide referrals to dietitians, social workers, and case managers. Weigh patient daily.	Weight will remain stable or increase. Patient reports increased energy level. Patient able to complete ADLs. Patient experiences increase in lean muscle mass.

NURSING CARE PLAN
The Patient Who Is HIV Positive—cont'd
? CRITICAL THINKING QUESTIONS

1. Ms. J. is very tearful and asks the nurse if there is any treatment to prevent her baby from becoming HIV positive. The nurse's information to Ms. J. would include:
2. Ms. J. asks the nurse if she can legally require her boyfriend to be tested for HIV. The most appropriate response would be:
3. Ms. J. asks the nurse when she will develop AIDS now that she is HIV positive. The correct answer would be:

Table 16-11 | *Nutritional Management: HIV Infection*

DIETARY RECOMMENDATION	INTERVENTION
DIARRHEA Lactose-free, low-fat, low-fiber, and high-potassium foods	Avoid dairy products, red meat, margarine, butter, eggs, dried beans, peas, raw fruits and vegetables. Cooked or canned fruits and vegetables will provide needed vitamins. Eat potassium-rich foods such as bananas and apricot nectar. Discontinue foods, nutritional supplements, and medications that may make diarrhea worse (Ensure, antacids, stool softeners). Avoid gas-producing foods. Serve warm, not hot, foods. Plan small, frequent meals. Drink plenty of fluids between meals.
CONSTIPATION High-fiber foods	Eat fruits and vegetables (beans, peas), cereal, and whole wheat breads. Gradually increase fiber. Drink plenty of fluids. Exercise.
NAUSEA AND VOMITING Low-fat foods	Avoid dairy products and red meat. Plan small, frequent meals. Prepare nonodorous foods. Eat dry, salty foods. Serve food cold or at room temperature. Drink liquids between meals. Avoid gas-producing, greasy, spicy foods. Eat slowly in a relaxed atmosphere. Rest after meals with head elevated. Take antiemetics 30 minutes before meals.
CANDIDIASIS Soft or pureed foods	Serve moist foods. Drink plenty of fluids. Avoid acidic and spicy foods. Use straw and tilt head back and forth when drinking. To decrease discomfort, eat soft foods, such as puddings and yogurt.
FEVER High-calorie, high-protein foods	Use nutritional supplements. Increase fluid intake.
ALTERED TASTE Diet as tolerated	Try herbs and spices. Marinate meat, poultry, and fish. Serve food cold or at room temperature. Drink plenty of fluids. Add salt or sugar. Introduce alternative protein sources.
ANEMIA High-iron foods	Eat organ meats and raisins. Drink orange juice when taking iron supplements to facilitate absorption.
FATIGUE High-calorie foods	Cook in large quantities and freeze in meal-size packets. Use microwave and convenience foods. Use easy-to-fix snack foods. Use social support system to assist with meal planning and preparation. Access in-home homemaker services. Access community Meals on Wheels programs.

mucosal barrier, which may lead to diarrhea. Some patients stop eating so as to decrease the number of bowel movements per day.

Wasting causes disturbances in self-concept and self-image, and patients report this weight loss as being one of the most difficult consequences of HIV infection to accept. Useful interventions for these disturbances include creating an atmosphere of acceptance and reassurance, encouraging a focus on past accomplishments and personal strengths, and facilitating the use of positive affirmations.

Decreased levels of testosterone have been reported in 35% to 50% of HIV-infected men (Winson, 2001). Testosterone has two distinct biologic properties: virilizing activity (androgenic effect) and protein building (anabolic effect). Because testosterone is an anabolic hormone, a deficiency may cause a loss of body cell mass, contributing to HIV wasting. The role of gonadotrophic hormones in women with wasting has not been studied sufficiently. Women who are wasted tend to lose a significant amount of body fat, but body cell mass is not significantly decreased. Conversely, men tend to lose a significant amount of lean body mass (e.g., skinny arms and legs), with preservation of fat.

With the advances in HIV treatment and opportunistic infection prophylaxis, serious malnutrition is less evident. However, nutrition does not return to normal after anti-HIV treatment begins, and a syndrome of increased truncal obesity (abdomen), and metabolic abnormalities are developing. Characteristic alterations in body composition, most notably the development of truncal (visceral, abdominal) obesity and subcutaneous fat loss on the extremities and face (also called lipoatrophy), as well as hyperlipidemia and insulin resistance have been reported in both men and women.

There are three hypotheses to explain the above-mentioned changes. The first is that the changes are a side effect of either protease inhibitors (Carr et al, 1998) or nucleoside reverse transcriptase inhibitors (NRTIs) (e.g, AZT, d4T). The second hypothesis is that the changes may represent an altered stress response, with mild chronic hypercortisolism in some patients (Carr et al, 1998). Finally, some researchers have suggested that these changes are part of long-term HIV disease and have only been noticed in recent years because of increased survival time.

The management of wasting and lipodystrophy is difficult, and generally requires multiple interventions. The nurse can assist by assessing for and documenting the presence of diminished appetite and weight. Nursing interventions include encouraging nutritional supplementation (see Table 16-9), increasing protein intake, providing enteral supplements (through nasogastric or gastric tubes if necessary), and assisting with total parenteral nutrition (TPN). Administering medications to stimulate appetite, such as megestrol (Megace) or dronabinol (Marinol) can help.

Unfortunately, these medications tend to increase body fat and not lean muscle mass. Testosterone (anabolic steroid) can be administered by mouth, intramuscularly, or transdermally to increase lean body mass and weight. The effect of testosterone can be enhanced by the addition of a low-weight resistance-training program (e.g., weightlifting) because it maintains muscle tone and improves appetite.

Nutrition counseling is vital to ensure that individuals with HIV disease maintain a well-balanced diet and include supplements if necessary. The dietitian can assist in this counseling, as well as provide the patient with high-protein and high-calorie diets, and suggest meal planning that fits the patient's lifestyle. Smaller, more frequent meals can be less overwhelming than larger meals. Of course, teaching about food safety is of paramount concern because enteric infections (e.g., cryptosporidiosis, microsporidiosis, and amebas) in HIV disease are often not treatable or are relapsing. In some cases, enteral or parenteral feeding becomes necessary.

Management of elevated triglycerides and lipids (cholesterol) is becoming common in HIV disease. As in other patient populations, these elevations can lead to cardiac and vascular disease and, in some cases, diabetes. Lipid-lowering agents such as the statins may be effective in treating this complication. However, because the liver metabolizes many of the antilipid agents, it is important to choose a statin that is safer than those that must pass through the liver to be activated. In the HIV-infected individual with elevated lipids and currently taking anti-HIV medications, safer anticholesterol drugs such as pravastatin (Pravachol), fluvastatin (Lescol) and possibly atorvastatin (Lipitor) should be considered. A program of diet control, exercise, and medications can safely lower lipids and reduce the chances of a cardiovascular event occurring.

Insulin resistance and/or diabetes sometimes responds to oral hypoglycemic agents (e.g., metformin or rosiglitazone [Avandia]). In some cases, the anti-HIV therapy needs to be changed to a protease-sparing combination. Managing diet, stopping smoking, weight loss, and exercise can help control the elevated blood sugars that can occur with the use of anti-HIV medications. Studies are being conducted to determine the appropriate interventions for HIV-infected individuals who are experiencing fat redistribution body changes.

Unfortunately, as with any overwhelming viral infection, the metabolic needs of the HIV-infected individual increase by as much as 40% (Winson, 2001). This hypermetabolism results in the need for a higher energy expenditure than is provided by the number of calories taken in by the patient. Malnutrition, weight loss, and generalized wasting are common problems in patients with HIV disease (Nursing Care Plan box). It is estimated that as many as 70% to 90% of patients with HIV disease will experience wasting. It is well documented that when a patient's weight is reduced to 60% of his or her ideal body weight, death can occur, regardless of the underlying condition (Winson, 2001). Malnutrition may influence morbidity and mortality in several ways. Malnutrition contributes to wasting, and wasting hastens the negative immune consequences of HIV infection. HIV wasting contributes to slower recovery from infection, impaired wound healing, increased risk of secondary infection, and decreased cardiac and respiratory function, and can lead to an earlier death. The weight loss associated with HIV disease is often severe and debilitating, producing a vicious cycle of anorexia, malnutrition, loss of tissue mass, muscle wasting, profound fatigue, and increased susceptibility to infections and drug interactions. Although typically seen in later stages HIV disease, malnutrition and wasting can occur in the early stages of HIV infection (Anastasi & Capili, 2001).

Neurological Complications

AIDS dementia. **HIV-associated cognitive motor complex** (previously known as AIDS dementia) is the term preferred by the WHO and the American Academy of Neurology (AAN) to describe a common CNS complication of HIV disease. The frequency is described as being anywhere between 20% and 33% of all adults and up to 50% of children with end-stage disease (i.e., AIDS) (Zwolski, 2001). This condition is a complex combination of signs and symptoms including dementia; impaired motor function; and, at times, characteristic behavioral changes that resemble an injury similar to a stroke or head trauma. The disease generally does not cause alterations in the level of consciousness or psychiatric disturbances. It is usually described as a triad of cognitive, motor, and behavioral dysfunction that slowly progresses over a period of weeks to months. The cognitive changes primarily involve a mental slowing and inattention. Patients typically lose their train of thought and complain of a slowness of thinking. They may miss appointments and find themselves making lists of tasks and chores that need completing. The symptoms of motor dysfunction ordinarily develop after those of cognitive impairment. They include poor balance and coordination (e.g., falling and tripping, dropping things); slower hand activities (e.g., writing, eating); and, ultimately, leg weakness that can limit ambulation. The diagnosis of this type of dementia can be made by conducting a simple physical examination, neurological testing, MRI/CT exams, and CSF analysis.

Nursing interventions for the treatment of neurocognitive dysfunction include the administration of anti-HIV medications and psychotropic medications (cautiously). Supervision of the patient, which includes a home safety assessment, is imperative. The nurse should ensure that orientation cues such as clocks and calendars are present, hallways and living areas are brightly lit, walkways are clear of electrical cords or throw rugs, and potentially dangerous objects (e.g., knives, poisons) are safely stored away.

Caring for patients with dementia is a collaborative effort between the health care provider and family. It is advisable to seek advice from a social worker, the home health care department, and a psychologist in developing a plan to care for an impaired individual.

AIDS-dementia complex (ADC), caused by HIV infection in the brain, is a common neurological disorder associated with HIV. Dementia symptoms are sometimes reversible if a treatable cause can be diagnosed. Treatable causes include dehydration, depression, and medication toxicity or side effects. Clinical manifestations of ADC include cognitive, behavioral, and motor abnormalities. Symptoms of ADC include decreased ability to concentrate, apathy, depression, social withdrawal, personality changes, confusion, hallucinations, altered levels of consciousness, and slowed response rates. ADC can lead to coma. Nursing interventions are focused on patient safety and caregiver support.

Peripheral neuropathy. Neuropathies are diseases that affect the peripheral nervous system. They can affect sensory, motor, or autonomic nerves. The causes of neuropathies can be related to HIV disease itself, or more frequently, the side effects of many anti-HIV medications (e.g., stavudine [d4T, Zerit], zalcitabine [ddC, Hivid], and didanosine [ddI, Videx]). Symptoms include numbness, localized tingling, hypesthesia (diminished sensitivity to stimulation) or anesthesia, loss of vibration and position sense (proprioception), and decreased or increased sensitivity to pain. In most cases, patients complain of numbness in the fingers, hands and feet, and pain on walking. Patients may also experience autonomic neuropathy. Symptoms such as mild positional hypotension to cardiovascular collapse, as well as chronic diarrhea, are suggestive of autonomic neuropathy.

Management of Opportunistic Infections

With the advent of effective antiretroviral therapy and better understanding of opportunistic infection prophylaxis, the frequency of opportunistic infections (OIs) has decreased dramatically. OIs still occur in severely immunocompromised patients; the nurse must be familiar with the recognition, treatment, and prophylaxis of these diseases. OIs are typically seen in individuals who are nonadherent to their antiretroviral regimen, nonadherent to OI prophylactic regimens, or at the end stage of HIV disease, and in individuals who do not consistently access the health care system. (See Table 16-6 for common OIs, treatment, and prevention.)

Health Promotion

Because patients with HIV disease are living longer, more productive lives, attention to the promotion of health and healthy behaviors is important (Health Promotion Considerations box). Patients should be encouraged to eat well-balanced meals, stop or at least reduce the number of cigarettes smoked, get adequate sleep and rest periods if possible, use stress-reduction modalities (e.g., biofeedback, referral for counseling), obtain dental care regularly, and keep scheduled appointments with all health care providers. Attention to comorbid conditions, such as hypertension and diabetes, is important to minimize additional health problems. Patients should be encouraged to get all immunizations and keep them up to date; female patients should regularly receive gynecologic care. If hospitalizations are necessary, encourage the participation of the patient and significant other(s) in treatment decision making and arrange for home care follow-up if indicated. Although some pets can pose risks for transmission of opportunistic infections, they are, overall, very therapeutic for the patient and healing. Only minor modifications need to be made for pet-owning HIV-infected people (e.g., bird cage and cat litter box cleaning). If possible, arrange pet visits to the hospital

or care facility if a long separation is anticipated—do not dismiss the idea of benefit because this practice is not acceptable at your health care facility. Speak with managers and supervisors to obtain permission, or help develop policies and procedures that allow the visitation of pets.

PREVENTION OF HIV INFECTION

HIV disease is **preventable.** However, prevention takes the cooperation and efforts of public health care providers, medical providers, nurses in all specialties, families, communities, churches, and schools (Box 16-7). Education on prevention is the only truly effective "vaccine" available to curb the HIV pandemic. Many patients admitted to acute-care facilities have unrecognized HIV disease or are at risk for HIV infection. Nurses have a responsibility to assess each patient's risk for HIV infection and counsel those at risk about HIV testing and the behaviors that put them at risk, and about how to reduce or eliminate those risks. Today, every nurse is an HIV nurse, implying that all nurses are responsible for teaching patients methods to reduce the risk of transmission. The nurse must be able to discuss the details of behaviors relating to sexual activity and drug use in a forthright, relaxed, and nonjudgmental manner. The nurse must be able to establish rapport before asking sensitive, explicit questions. One must be comfortable with the discussion of risk-reduction techniques (e.g., condom application, using clean "works).

Harm-reduction education is a fundamental element of HIV prevention methods. Harm reduction does not completely eliminate the risk of HIV transmission. Instead, it focuses on minimizing the personal and social harms and costs associated with these activities. The WHO and the Canadian government both endorse harm reduction as a method to help patients reduce their risk of exposure to HIV (Kirton, 2001). For example, asking patients to quit smoking two packs of cigarettes per day all at once almost always results in the patient failing. In harm reduction, the nurse can suggest to the patient to reduce the number of cigarettes smoked in a day from 40 to 30; although the ultimate goal is to have the patient stop smoking altogether, the patient has reduced the risk of long-term effects by at least limiting the number of cigarettes smoked. The same is true for HIV prevention. Encouraging patients to use protective barriers 50% of the time (although not ideal), still results in a reduced risk of HIV transmission.

HIV TESTING AND COUNSELING

HIV testing and counseling are an integral part in the prevention of HIV transmission (see Table 16-5 for important functions of HIV testing and counseling). Pa-

Health Promotion Considerations

The Patient Infected with HIV

- Remind patients that a positive diagnosis is not an immediate "death sentence." Patients are living increasingly longer after diagnosis because of medications, more specialized care, and decreased morbidity and mortality related to opportunistic diseases.
- Stress the importance of health-promoting behaviors to reduce the risk of comorbidity.
- Encourage patients to maintain good nutritional status by eating regular, well-balanced meals that are high in protein and calories. Increased protein is necessary for cell and tissue repair—especially in patients who may be hypermetabolic.
- Encourage patients to limit their intake of alcoholic beverages and avoid the use of illicit or recreational drugs.
- Encourage patients to maintain an adequate sleep schedule.
- Encourage patients to use stress reduction practices, such as biofeedback, massage, or progressive relaxation. Engage in relaxing or pleasurable activities.
- Encourage patients to use safer sexual practices to avoid reinfection and exposure to other sexually transmitted diseases.
- Encourage patients to establish an exercise regimen that includes aerobic activity as well as low-resistance weightlifting if possible.
- Most important, support patients in setting short- and long-term goals and assist them in achieving those goals.

| Box 16-7 | *Prevention Options* |

SEXUAL
No Risk

Abstinence from sexual contact in which there is exchange of semen, vaginal secretions, or blood.

Partners who are in a mutually monogamous (the state of having one mate) relationship in which neither partner is at risk of infection through IDU, and in which neither partner was previously exposed to HIV through drug use or sexual contact.

Reduced Risk

Limiting the number of partners, even though there would be a potential risk if there were sexual contact with one infected partner.

Protective measures through consistent and correct use of latex condoms with a spermicide in every act of sexual intercourse in which there would be exchange of semen, vaginal secretions, or blood. The correct use of condoms is as follows:

- Put on the condom as soon as erection occurs and before any sexual contact (anal, vaginal, oral).
- Leave space at the tip of the condom.
- Use only water-based lubricants.
- Hold the condom firmly to keep it from slipping off; withdraw from partner immediately after ejaculation.

INJECTING DRUG USE
No Risk

Stop the use of injectable drugs. Drug treatment opportunities should be provided.

If drugs are going to be injected, use sterile needles and equipment.

Reduced Risk

If needles and equipment are going to be shared, instructions on cleaning should be given.

Fill the syringe with sodium hypochlorite 5.25% (Clorox) bleach two times; empty two times. Fill the syringe with clean water two times; empty two times.

PERINATAL
No Risk

Avoidance of pregnancy is the only certain way to prevent transmission of HIV to a fetus or infant.

A woman of childbearing age of unknown HIV status should be counseled about behaviors that would put her at risk for HIV infection and about behaviors that would put her partner or spouse at risk for HIV infection. If risk factors are determined in either case, both individuals should be counseled about testing for HIV.

Reduced Risk

Adherence to barrier birth control measures, including use of condoms, to avoid pregnancy.

Use of zidovudine or other anti-HIV therapy given during pregnancy, and to infant for first 6 weeks of life.

---

tients should not be pressured to get tested. **Test decision counseling** is the process of assisting patients in making decisions about when, if, and how to be tested. It is important that the nurse take every opportunity to provide pretest counseling. As well as providing HIV testing information, the nurse must explain and obtain informed consent before actually drawing blood. This generally involves explaining the purpose, possible uses, limitations (window period, false-negative results, false-positive results), and meaning of the test results.

Consent policies are established by state laws and vary between states. The most common and acceptable policy is to obtain informed written consent before HIV antibody testing. All states have some exceptions to informed consent, usually relating to critical or emergency situations. For example, if a high-risk occupational exposure occurs and the patient is incapacitated and unable to give consent, most states allow the testing of the source patient's blood without the patient's consent. However, these situations are generally quite rare, and every effort should be made to obtain consent. When obtaining an informed consent, explain the applicable limits of confidentiality in the office, clinic, or hospital setting where the patient is being tested. The patient should be told who will have access to the test results, such as the health department or insurance company, and what will be done with that information (contact tracing or partner notification).

HIV antibody testing may take place in a physician's office or at designated HIV counseling and testing sites. When a therapeutic relationship exists between a health care provider and a patient, many patients feel more comfortable being tested by someone who knows their medical and social history. Conversely, other people prefer to be tested in a location where they will not be known. Nurses must be aware of the various options for HIV antibody testing in their state or community in order to advise patients appropriately.

HIV antibody testing can be done one of two ways—confidentially or anonymously. In **confidential testing,** individuals are asked to provide identifying information, including a name, address, and often demographic information such as age, sex, race, and occupation. Using this information, it is possible to locate and provide information to an individual who does not return for the test results or counseling. All records are kept strictly confidential, and testing in physicians' offices, clinics, and hospitals is conducted in a confidential manner. It is imperative the nurse maintain the results of confidential testing. There have been instances of litigation against health care providers who share or use this information inappropriately. Health care providers can be sued for negligence and invasion of privacy, and they may be disciplined by licensing boards for unauthorized disclosure or breach of confidentiality. Patients should be informed that the results of their HIV antibody test will be linked to the patient's medical record.

In **anonymous testing,** individuals are not asked to provide identifying information. Records are kept through assigned numbers, and the patient must retain this number to receive test results. It is not possible to locate and provide information to an individual who does not return for test results and counseling. In either form of testing, pretest and posttest counseling can be performed by the nurse.

RISK ASSESSMENT AND RISK REDUCTION

The nurse should encourage early detection of HIV infection. Testing for HIV is an important part of the public health response to HIV disease. Risk assessment should be patient centered, a joint process between the nurse and patient. The patient should take "ownership" of the risk for HIV infection. Patients need to be assessed for manifestations that would be indicative of risky behaviors, such as STDs. Risk assessment should be a continual process in patient care. However, a patient will not get tested unless there is a perceived need for testing and a feeling of safety in doing so. The nurse can help the patient assess the risks by asking some basic questions:

- Have you ever had a transfusion or used clotting factors? Was it before 1985?
- Have you ever shared needles, syringes, or other injecting equipment with anyone?
- Have you ever had a sexual experience in which your penis, vagina, rectum, or mouth came into contact with another person's penis, vagina, rectum, or mouth?

A positive response to any of the above questions will require the nurse to explore further with the patient. The nurse should be prepared to refer the patient to centers that provide testing and counseling services. All testing should include pretest and posttest counseling (see Table 16-5; Box 16-6).

HIV infection in women has been frequently overlooked for several reasons. First, in the United States, the disease initially occurred mostly in men, and treatment models were developed from the progression of disease in men. Second, providers did not assess the risks for women and women did not seek testing and counseling, due to denial or ignorance; thus, interventions have not been implemented effectively. Heterosexual transmission of HIV in women surpassed injecting drug use (IDU) as a vector for HIV transmission in the second decade of this pandemic and globally continues to be the highest risk factor in women (Dole, 2001). The 1993 CDC case definition includes at least one female-specific disease—cervical carcinoma. Women now need to be assessed for different manifestations, such as the common initial presenting condition for HIV-positive women—vaginal candidiasis.

BARRIERS TO PREVENTION

There are numerous barriers to HIV prevention, not the least of which is a denial of risk, an attitude that "it won't happen to me." Because the virus initially infected the MSM population in the United States, many other subpopulations have ignored their risks. Fear, misunderstanding, and the potential for social isolation and social stigma are significant barriers. Some individuals are so fearful that they will no longer give blood, and they will not eat at a restaurant if they think a homosexual food handler is employed. Fear and misinformation reinforce the need for consistent, accurate information about the virus, the risks of transmission, and HIV disease itself. Even today, more than 20 years into the epidemic, significant fear and inaccurate information exist among health care providers as well as the general public.

Cultural and community attitudes, values, and norms can affect the success of prevention efforts. A community may be opposed to HIV and AIDS education in the local school district because of the fear that values will be compromised. Those values may include views on sexuality, abstinence, the use of condoms, the use of drugs, and the provision of instructions on cleaning needles and syringes. Community organizations, churches, educators, and leaders can determine what the expectations or norms of that community will be. Cooperative efforts are essential for successful prevention of HIV transmission. The issues related to the HIV epidemic—sex, drug use, death, and homosexuality—are not easy issues for most cultures or communities.

Prevention of HIV transmission requires a commitment to change behaviors that put one at risk. Education to alter behaviors is a long-term process. Nurses need to take every opportunity to educate their patients on how to avoid or reduce the risk for HIV infection. Collective efforts will have the greatest effect (see Box 16-6).

Fear of alienation and discrimination are significant additional barriers to prevention. In some cases, individuals are reluctant to even pick up a pamphlet about HIV because they fear someone will believe they are gay or using illicit drugs. There is evidence that people will not go to a physician or to a testing and counseling site for HIV testing for fear of being seen. This fear is very real, particularly in rural parts of the country. Fear of discrimination includes fear of losing family, friends, prestige, job, housing, and insurance. Fortunately, many states have statutes in place to protect individuals with HIV disease from discrimination. Protection is also afforded by the ADA.

REDUCING RISKS RELATED TO SEXUAL TRANSMISSION

Safer sexual activities reduce the risk of exposure to HIV through semen and cervicovaginal secretions. Abstaining from all sexual activity is the most effective way to accomplish this goal. Limiting sexual behavior to activities in which the mouth, penis, vagina, or rectum do not come into contact with the partner's mouth, penis, vagina, or rectum is also safe, because there is no contact with blood, semen, or cervicovaginal secretions. These activities may include massage, masturbation, mutual masturbation, telephone sex, and many other activities. Insertive sex is considered to be safe only in a mutually monogamous relationship with a partner who is not infected with, or at risk of becoming infected with, HIV. The problem with mutual monogamy is that both partners need to follow all of the rules all of the time. Unfortunately, there are

a number of cases of HIV infection that occurred in individuals who were not aware that their partner had not remained monogamous. Serial monogamy (maintaining a monogamous relationship, including unprotected intercourse, with one partner for a short period of time, followed by another relationship, and then another) still presents an increased risk of HIV exposure (Box 16-8).

Risk-reducing sexual activities decrease the risk of contact with HIV through the use of barriers. Barriers should be used when engaging in sexual activity with a partner whose HIV status is not definitely known or with a partner who is known to be infected with HIV. The most commonly used barrier is the male condom. Although not 100% effective, when used correctly and consistently, male condoms are very effective in the prevention of HIV transmission. Other barriers include female condoms and latex dental dams. Female condoms consist of a vinyl sheath with two spring-form rings. The smaller ring is inserted into the vagina and holds the condom in place internally. The larger ring surrounds the opening to the condom. It functions to keep the condom in place externally while also protecting the external genitalia. Use can be complicated; careful instructions on its use are necessary. Female condoms can also be used for anal sex. Dental dams or microwave-safe plastic wrap can be used to cover the external genitalia or anus during oral sexual

---

| **Box 16-8** | ***Risk of HIV Transmission Associated with Sexual Practices*** |

HIGH RISK (IN DESCENDING ORDER OF RISK)
- Receptive anal intercourse with ejaculation (no condom)
- Receptive vaginal intercourse with ejaculation (no condom)
- Insertive anal intercourse (no condom)
- Insertive vaginal intercourse (no condom)
- Receptive anal intercourse with withdrawal before ejaculation
- Insertive anal intercourse with withdrawal before ejaculation
- Receptive vaginal intercourse (with spermicidal foam, no condom)
- Insertive vaginal intercourse (with spermicidal foam, no condom)
- Receptive anal or vaginal intercourse (with a condom)*
- Insertive anal or vaginal intercourse (with a condom)*

SOME RISK (IN DESCENDING ORDER OF RISK)
- Oral sex with men with ejaculation
- Oral sex with women

- Oral sex with men with preejaculate fluid (precum)
- Oral sex with men, no ejaculation or precum
- Oral sex with men (with a condom)

NO RISK
- Masturbating with another person without touching one another
- Hugging/massage/dry kissing, frottage (rubbing against each other)
- Masturbating alone
- Abstinence

UNRESOLVED ISSUES
- The role of preejaculate in transmission
- The protection offered by covering female genitals with a dental dam during oral sex
- The risk of transmission with wet kissing (French kissing)

Modified from Schram, N.R. Redefining safer sex, *Focus* 5(7):3, 1990. In Grimes D.E., & Grimes R.M. (1994). *AIDS and HIV infection.* St Louis, Mosby.
*Risk lower if no ejaculation and/or spermicidal foam used.

activity. Although the risk of HIV transmission is significantly reduced with the use of latex barriers, other STDs, such as human papillomavirus (HPV), warts, and HSV, can still be transmitted.

REDUCING RISKS RELATED TO DRUG ABUSE

The use of illicit or recreational drugs can cause immune suppression, malnutrition, and emotional difficulties. Although using illicit drugs can increase one's risk for acquiring an HIV infection, drug use itself does not cause HIV infection. The major risks of HIV transmission are related to sharing injecting equipment and having unsafe sexual experiences while under the influence of mood-altering chemicals. Essentially, one can reduce the risk of HIV infection by not using drugs. If injecting of drugs occurs, equipment should not be shared with others; sexual activity should not be engaged in while under the influence of any drug, including alcohol, that impairs decision-making ability.

The safest mechanism is to abstain from drugs, but this is not always a viable option for a user who has no access to drug treatment services or chooses not to quit. The risk of HIV for these individuals can be eliminated if they can find alternatives to injecting. Other routes of drug administration—such as smoking, snorting, or ingesting—are less risky, because they remove the risk of exposure to blood. Risk can also be eliminated if the user does not share injecting equipment. Injecting equipment includes needles, syringes, cookers, cotton, and rinse water. None of this equipment should be shared. Of course, the safest tactic is for the user to have ready access to sterile equipment. Many states have laws that prohibit over-the-counter sale of needles and syringes, such as diabetic supplies. Some communities have needle exchange programs that supply sterile equipment to users to help reduce the risk of HIV transmission. Opposition to these programs is supported by the fear that ready access to injecting supplies will increase drug use. However, studies have shown that in communities where exchange programs have been established, drug use does not increase and rates of HIV infection are controlled (Bradley-Springer, 1999).

Cleaning the equipment before use is a risk-reducing activity. It decreases the risk for those who must share equipment, particularly in "shooting galleries." To clean the equipment, used needles and syringes must be rinsed twice with tap water (using fresh tap water each time). Syringes must then be filled with full-strength household bleach, shaken for 30 seconds, and squirted clean; the bleaching process should be repeated. Then rinse the equipment twice with tap water. This process takes time and may be difficult for a person experiencing drug withdrawal and in need of drugs.

REDUCING RISKS RELATED TO OCCUPATIONAL EXPOSURE

As previously discussed, the risk of acquiring HIV through occupational exposure is quite rare. The CDC and Occupational Safety and Health Administration (OSHA) have instituted policies to ensure that employees are protected from exposure to blood and other potentially infectious fluids (CDC, 2001). The use of standard precautions and body substance isolation have been shown not only to reduce the risk of blood-borne pathogens, but also to reduce the risk of transmission of other diseases between the patient and the health care worker; it also reduces the risk of transmission between patients. Handwashing still remains the single most effective means of preventing the spread of infection.

The U.S. Public Health Service has published recommendations for the management of an occupational exposure to HIV (CDC, 2001). The current recommendations are to begin antiretroviral therapy with at least two or three medications (depending on the type and severity of exposure). The exposed health care worker should begin therapy with the appropriate medications within 1 to 4 hours following a high-risk exposure.

Epidemiologic and laboratory studies suggest that several factors might affect the risk of HIV transmission after an occupational exposure. In a retrospective study of health care workers who had percutaneous exposure to HIV, the risk of HIV infection was found to be increased with exposure to a larger quantity of blood from the source patient as indicated by (a) a device visibly contaminated with the patient's blood, (b) a procedure that involved a needle being placed directly in a vein or artery, or (c) a deep injury (Cardo et al, 1997). The risk is also increased for exposure to blood from a source person with terminal illness, possibly reflecting the higher viral load of the patient late in the course of HIV disease. A laboratory study that demonstrated more blood is transferred by deeper injuries and hollow-bore needles lends further support for the observed variation in risk related to blood quantity (Mast et al, 1993). Information about primary HIV infection (seroconversion) indicates that a systemic infection does not occur immediately, leaving a brief window of opportunity during which postexposure prophylaxis (PEP) might modify or prevent viral replication. Theoretically, initiation of antiretroviral PEP soon after exposure might prevent or inhibit systemic infection by limiting the proliferation of the virus in the initial target cells or lymph nodes.

For best prophylactic effect, initiation of PEP must occur within 36 hours—but preferably **within 1 to 4 hours**—of the exposure. Because the standard of care for pharmacologic intervention in patients with HIV disease is three or more anti-HIV medications (HAART), this same standard generally applies to health care providers who have a high-risk exposure.

Depending on the type of exposure and many other variables, either a two-drug or three-drug regimen is chosen. There have been reported failures of PEP after an exposure to HIV (Perdue et al, 1999). In addition to possible exposure to an antiretroviral-resistant strain of HIV, other factors that might have contributed to these apparent failures might include a high titer and/or large volume inoculum exposure, delayed initiation and/or short duration of PEP, and factors related to the exposed health care personnel (e.g., immune status).

Completion of a 4-week course of therapy after an occupational exposure is essential. The medications used have many side effects, and many health care workers have stopped PEP because of these. It is important to consult with experts in occupational exposure and seek expert opinion if side effects—headache, nausea, vomiting, diarrhea—become unbearable. The use of PEP regimens has been associated with new-onset diabetes mellitus, hyperglycemia, hypertriglyceridemia, pancreatitis, elevated lipids (cholesterol, low-density lipoproteins [LDL]), and kidney stones. Despite these serious side effects, the exposed health care worker must complete the prescribed 4-week therapy, or until a time it is determined that the source patient is not HIV infected.

Hospitals or agencies should have policies in place that specifically address occupational HIV exposure because instituting chemoprophylaxis needs to occur immediately—even before testing the source patient's and health care worker's blood for HIV or other bloodborne pathogens. Serial testing of the health care worker for HIV occurs at baseline, 6 months, and 12 months following the exposure. Optional HIV antibody testing may be done at 6 weeks and 3 months after exposure.

The maintaining of confidentiality for both the exposed health care worker and the source patient is of the utmost importance. Most states have separate, distinct consent forms that are required before HIV antibody testing can be performed. Only in rare circumstances, such as the inability to give consent, can HIV antibody testing be completed without the patient's informed consent. There are many ethical and legal issues surrounding HIV antibody testing, and it will benefit the nurse to be aware of what laws apply in the state in which he or she practices. In many states, charges of assault and battery can be brought against health care workers who perform HIV testing against a patient's will. Appropriate counseling and necessary referrals should be made for the health care worker and patient when HIV testing is indicated.

OTHER METHODS TO REDUCE RISK

HIV-infected people should be instructed not to give blood, donate organs, or donate semen for artificial insemination. They should not share razors, toothbrushes, or other household items that may contain blood or other body fluids. They should also avoid infecting sexual and needle-sharing partners, consider using birth control measures, and eliminate breastfeeding to avoid spreading the virus to infants.

OUTLOOK FOR THE FUTURE

As we enter the third decade of the HIV pandemic, much has been learned about transmission of the virus and ways to prevent infection. With no cure in sight, prevention of infection through education, prevention of mother-to-child transmission, and in some cases PEP can limit the effect this disease has on the human population. The dynamics of the pandemic have changed dramatically as well. In the United States, HIV has the characteristics of any other chronic illness: (1) the condition has no cure, (2) the condition continues throughout the life of the patient, (3) the condition causes increasing physical disability and dysfunction if not treated, and (4) the condition ultimately results in significant morbidity and mortality. Chronic diseases are characterized by acute exacerbations of cyclic problems that compound each other. Although there has been a significant decrease in the number of opportunistic infections, new complications have emerged. Health care providers today must address body composition changes, cardiac disease, neuropathies, and the long-term effects of the very medications that have kept HIV at bay. Despite this dismal outlook, there is much promise in the way of more treatments (e.g., new classes of medications, immunomodulators). Patients who had previously become disabled, quit jobs, and tended to end-of-life decisions are now reevaluating goals, returning to work, and rediscovering relative health.

HIV has become a disease whose face is represented by women and people of color. Early testing and diagnosis, followed by early intervention, are important activities; there is increasing evidence that HIV can be managed for several years before severe immune destruction occurs. Underdeveloped countries in Africa and Southeast Asia have been hardest hit; in fact, many villages have been destroyed because of HIV. The global threat of HIV is enormous, with nurses playing a key role in the care and treatment of HIV-infected individuals. For the best possible clinical, patient satisfaction, and financial outcomes, care must be received from HIV specialists. Always seek expert guidance when treating an individual with HIV disease because the care is very complex, and multiple needs arise.

The field of HIV and AIDS nursing changes frequently, and nurses must constantly refresh their base of knowledge. Resources for the nurse include local AIDS service organizations, and state and regional

AIDS education and training centers. As new therapies emerge, the nurse will be in the unique position to educate patients and the public regarding what is undoubtedly the most challenging infectious disease discovered in the twentieth century.

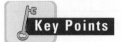

Key Points

- HIV, a retrovirus, is the agent that causes HIV disease and AIDS.
- Education and prevention are our only "vaccine" for preventing HIV disease and AIDS.
- Women and people of color constitute the fastest growing segment of the population with HIV disease.
- AIDS is the end stage of HIV infection.
- When HIV enters the body, its primary target is the immune system.
- HIV is transmitted by three major routes:
  1. Anal and vaginal intercourse
  2. Injecting drugs with contaminated needles/works
  3. From infected mother to child
- Blood, semen, vaginal secretions, and breast milk are the body fluids that most readily transmit HIV.
- Nurses have a responsibility to assess each patient's risks for HIV infection and counsel those at risk about testing, behaviors that put them at risk, and how to eliminate or reduce those risks.
- A positive HIV antibody test does not mean the patient has AIDS.
- A multidisciplinary care approach in which the patient is a primary member of the team is the most appropriate method to care for patients with HIV disease because of their complex needs.

- As HIV infection progresses, the immune system loses its ability to fight infectious agents and cancer cells.
- Patients at risk for HIV infection should be encouraged to know their HIV status.
- Whether or not signs and symptoms are present, a person infected with HIV virus can transmit the virus.
- Barriers to HIV prevention include denial, fear, misinformation, and cultural and community norms.
- CD_4^+ counts are important markers of disease progression and the status of the immune system.
- The stigma of HIV disease because of its association with drug use, homosexuality, and sexual transmission is a major concern.
- The 1993 expanded case definition of AIDS includes all HIV-infected people who have CD_4^+ T-lymphocyte counts of less than 200 cells/mm³; includes all people who have one or more of these three clinical conditions—pulmonary tuberculosis, recurrent pneumonia, or invasive cervical cancer; and retains the 23 clinical conditions listed in the 1987 AIDS case definition.
- Measuring viral load in the blood assesses effectiveness of therapy and possibly adherence.
- Adherence to medications is essential.

Go to your free CD-ROM for an Audio Glossary, animations, video clips, and Review Questions for the NCLEX-PN® Examination.

evolve Be sure to visit the companion Evolve site at http://evolve.elsevier.com/Christensen/adult/ for WebLinks and additional online resources.

CHAPTER CHALLENGE

1. The virus responsible for causing the majority of HIV disease/AIDS in human beings is:
   1. human immunodeficiency virus type 1.
   2. human immunodeficiency virus type 2.
   3. African immunodeficiency virus type 1.
   4. *Pneumocystis jiroveci* (formerly *carinii*) deficiency virus.

2. Vertical transmission of HIV occurs from:
   1. male to female.
   2. female to male.
   3. father to child.
   4. mother to child.

3. You are assessing a patient who has requested HIV testing. Which of the following would be considered to be the most risky behavior?
   1. Dry kissing a casual date
   2. Sharing a soda with an infected person
   3. Swimming with an infected person
   4. More than three sex partners in a year

4. Which of the following would be the most likely route of transmission of HIV?
   1. From infected female to noninfected male
   2. From infected male to noninfected female
   3. From infected father to child
   4. From infected mother to child

5. J., age 8, is diagnosed with hemophilia. His mother is very upset about the risk of her son acquiring HIV from blood products. Which of the following would be the nurse's best response?
   1. "All blood and blood products are screened for bloodborne diseases, so it is impossible for J. to be infected."
   2. "Many blood products are treated with heat or chemicals to inactivate the HIV virus."
   3. "We can talk about this if J. requires transfusions or blood products."
   4. "All blood donors are asked about HIV status and risk factors before giving blood."

6. The storage area in which HIV reproduces in the human body is:
   1. lymph glands.
   2. muscle tissues.
   3. bone marrow.
   4. B cells.

7. T., age 34, comes to the clinic requesting HIV testing. He is a gay man with two significant others in his lifetime. His lover was recently diagnosed with HIV. T. asks you how long it will take before the infection will show up in him. The best response of the nurse would be:
   1. "Antibodies usually are detected in the blood within 4 to 12 weeks of exposure."
   2. "It takes at least a year to know if you will be infected with HIV."
   3. "You'll have to ask your doctor the next time you go in for an appointment."
   4. "We don't know how long it will take to seroconvert to being HIV positive."

8. T. is concerned that he may be infected with HIV. Which of the following symptoms would alert the nurse to further assess T.?
   1. Night sweats
   2. Rash on the legs only
   3. Constipation
   4. Pruritus

9. The HIV factory of the human body is:
   1. infected CD_4 cells.
   2. infected macrophages.
   3. infected sweat glands.
   4. infected parotid glands.

10. T. is diagnosed with symptomatic HIV disease. The nurse would assess her regarding which of the following?
    1. T-cell count greater than 800
    2. WBC greater than 20,000
    3. Thrush
    4. Weight gain

11. HIV disease/AIDS is diagnosed according to:
    1. ELISA test.
    2. CD_4 counts.
    3. B-cell count.
    4. Western blot test.

12. B. is diagnosed with HIV disease. She visits the doctor today for her prescriptions. The nurse would expect the physician to order which of the following?
    1. Zidovudine (AZT)
    2. Lamivudine (Epivir)
    3. Nelfinavir (Viracept)
    4. Combination of these drugs

13. The nurse should instruct the patient with HIV on which of the following diets?
    1. High calorie, high fiber, low protein
    2. Low calorie, low fiber, high protein
    3. High calorie, high protein, low residue
    4. Low calorie, high fiber, high protein

14. The progression of HIV disease is very predictable in all patients. True or false?

15. HIV disease is diagnosed when the CD_4 cell count is 200 cells/mm^3 or fewer. True or false?

16. HIV disease in men who have sex with men is decreasing. True or false?

17. Ninety-nine percent seroconversion of exposed individuals occurs within 6 months of the exposure. True or false?

18. An HIV-infected person may appear to be very healthy. True or false?

19. It is not possible to become infected with HIV after one unprotected sexual encounter. True or false?

20. Most of the children infected with the HIV virus have some form of hemophilia. True or false?

21. The most common opportunistic infection and malignant neoplasm in the patient with advanced HIV disease (AIDS) are:
    1. streptococcal pneumonitis, myeloma
    2. *Pneumocsytis jiroveci* (formerly *carinii*) pneumonia, Kaposi's sarcoma
    3. *Streptococcus pneumoniae*, malignant melanoma
    4. *Mycoplasma* pneumonitis, Kaposi's sarcoma

22. For most people who are HIV positive, marker antibodies are usually present in 10 to 12 weeks after exposure. The development of these antibodies is called:
    1. immunocompetence.
    2. seroconversion.
    3. immunodeficient.
    4. viral load.

23. The expanded definition for AIDS is that the person will:
    1. have the HIV virus present.
    2. have a dysfunction of the immune system and be HIV positive.
    3. be HIV positive and have an opportunistic disease.
    4. be HIV positive with $CD_4{}^+$ lymphocyte count less than 200 mm^3.

Continued

CHAPTER CHALLENGE—cont'd

24. "Why should I use condoms? They don't work," retorts D., a young gay patient being treated for his third sexually transmitted disease. The nurse's most appropriate response should be:
    1. "Condoms may not provide 100% protection, but when used correctly and consistently with every act of sexual intercourse, they reduce your risk of getting infected with HIV or other sexually transmitted diseases."
    2. "You are correct: condoms don't always work. So your best protection is to limit your number of partners."
    3. "Condoms do not provide 100% protection, so you should always discuss with your sexual partners their HIV status or ask if they have any STDs."
    4. "Condoms do not provide 100% protection, but when used with a spermicide, you can be assured of complete protection against HIV and other STDs."

25. K. has been advised to be tested for HIV because of multiple sexual partners and intravenous illicit drug use. The nurse should make certain that K. understands the test by informing him that:
    1. the blood is tested with the highly sensitive test called the Western blot, then with ELISA.
    2. the blood is tested with ELISA; if positive, it is tested again with ELISA and then the Western blot.
    3. a series of HIV tests are performed to confirm if K. has AIDS.
    4. if the HIV tests are seronegative, K. can be assured that he isn't infected.

26. When the human immunodeficiency retrovirus enters the body, it attacks primarily which cells, resulting in an immunocompromised status?
    1. T-cell lymphocytes
    2. B-cell lymphocytes
    3. Neutrophils
    4. Monocytes

27. J., a 21 year-old patient, has been treated for *Chlamydia* and has a history of recurrent vaginal herpes. What would be the most appropriate action by the nurse?
    1. Counsel J. about her sexual and drug use history, risk reduction measures, and HIV testing.
    2. Refer J. to a family planning clinic.
    3. Counsel J. about testing for HIV and what the test results mean.
    4. Counsel J. about abstinence and a monogamous relationship.

28. If a person is infected with HIV and has not seroconverted to the HIV-specific antibody and will not test HIV antibody positive, this is referred to as:
    1. a "window-period."
    2. negative CD_4^+ count.
    3. positive CD_4^+ count.
    4. viral load.

29. In people who are HIV positive, the highest viral load is seen:
    1. at seroconversion time with CD_4^+ count less than 500.
    2. in symptomatic phase of HIV spectrum.
    3. at seroconversion time and in advanced HIV disease (AIDS).
    4. None of the above

30. The purpose of doing a viral load study once every 3 to 4 months in the HIV-positive person is to determine:
    1. the CD_4^+ count.
    2. the progression of the disease.
    3. what the CD_8 count is.
    4. the results of the Western blot test.

31. Dr. Q. asks you to talk with Mr. C. about how HIV is transmitted. Which of the following routes of transmission would you discuss with Mr. C.?
    1. Receiving blood, donating blood
    2. Food, water, air
    3. Sexual intercourse, sharing needles, mother-to-child transmission
    4. Dirty toilets, swimming pools, mosquitoes

32. C. asks the nurse, "How does HIV cause AIDS?" The nurse's response should be:
    1. "HIV attacks the immune system, a system that protects the body from foreign invaders, making it unable to protect the body from organisms that cause diseases."
    2. "HIV breaks down the circulatory system, making the body unable to assimilate oxygen and nutrients."
    3. "HIV attacks the respiratory system, making the lungs more susceptible to organisms, causing pneumonia."
    4. "HIV attacks the digestive system, decreasing the absorption of essential nutrients and resulting in weight loss and fatigue."

33. The pathophysiology of advanced HIV disease results from all of the following: (Choose all correct answers.)
    1. T-helper lymphocytes decreasing.
    2. T-suppressor lymphocytes dominating.
    3. profound immunosuppression noted.
    4. B lymphocyte unable to help with infection and antibody formation.
    5. T-helper lymphocytes increasing.

34. All of the following people are high risk for contracting HIV virus: (Choose all correct answers.)
    1. a monogamous partner.
    2. homosexuals.
    3. drug users.
    4. heterosexual partners of homosexuals or bisexuals.
    5. prostitutes.

17 Care of the Patient with Cancer

BARBARA LAURITSEN CHRISTENSEN

Objectives

After reading this chapter, the student should be able to do the following:

1. Define the key terms as listed.
2. List seven risk factors for the development of cancer.
3. State seven warning signs of cancer.
4. Indicate the incidence of cancer as one of the leading causes of death in the United States.
5. Discuss development, prevention, and detection of cancer.
6. Define the terminology used to describe cellular changes, characteristics of malignant cells, and types of malignancies.
7. Describe the pathophysiology of cancer, including the characteristics of malignant cells and the nature of metastasis.
8. Describe the major categories of chemotherapeutic agents.
9. Describe the process of metastasis.
10. Explain common reasons for delay in seeking medical care when a diagnosis of cancer is suspected.
11. List common diagnostic tests used to identify the presence of cancer.
12. Explain why biopsy is essential in confirming a diagnosis of cancer.
13. Discuss the American Cancer Society's recommendations for preventive behaviors and screening tests for men and women.
14. Define the systems of tumor classification: grading and staging.
15. Discuss six general guidelines for the use of pain relief measures for the patient with advanced cancer.
16. Describe nursing interventions for the individual undergoing surgery, radiation therapy, chemotherapy, bone marrow, or peripheral stem cell transplantation.
17. Explain the etiology/pathophysiology, clinical manifestations, diagnostic tests, medical management, and nursing interventions and prognosis for tumor lysis syndrome.

Key Terms

Be sure to check out the bonus material on the free CD-ROM, including selected audio pronunciations.

alopecia (ăl-ō-PĒ-shē-ă, p. 834)
autologous (aw-TŎL-ō-gŭs, p. 839)
benign (Bě-NĪN, p. 823)
biopsy (BĪ-ŏp-sē, p. 824)
carcinogen (kăr-SĬN-o-jen, p. 816)
carcinogenesis (kăr-sĭn-ō-JĔN-e-sis, p. 816)
carcinoma (kăr-sĭ-NŌ-mă, p. 823)
differentiated (dĭf-ĕr-ĔN-shă-ā-tĕd, p. 823)
immunosurveillance (ĭm-ū-nō-sĕr-VĀ-lĕns, p. 823)
leukopenia (loo-kō-PĒ-nē-ă, p. 831)
malignant (mă-LĬG-nănt, p. 823)
metastasis (mĕ-TĂS-tă-sĭs, p. 823)
neoplasm (NĒ-ō-plăzm, p. 823)
oncology (ŏn-KŎL-ō-jē, p. 815)
palliative (PĂL-ē-ă-tĭv, p. 827)
Papanicolaou's test (smear) (pă-pĕ-NĬ-kō-looz tĕst, smēr, p. 824)
sarcoma (săr-KŌ-mă, p. 823)
stomatitis (stō-mă-TĪ-tĭs, p. 835)
thrombocytopenia (thrŏm-bō-sīt-ō-PĒ-nē-ă, p. 834)
tumor lysis syndrome (TOO-mŏr LĪ-sĭs SĬN-drŏm, p. 838)

ONCOLOGY

Oncology is the sum of knowledge regarding tumors; it is the branch of medicine that deals with the study of tumors. Oncology nursing is the care of people with cancer.

Until the appearance of AIDS, probably no other medical diagnosis produced as much fear as a diagnosis of cancer. Cancer is feared far more than heart disease. The word *cancer* is viewed as synonymous with death, pain, and disfigurement. However, attitudes toward cancer do not fit today's status of the treatment and control of cancer. Education of health care professionals and the public is essential if current attitudes about cancer and cancer treatment are to become more positive and realistic (Lewis et al, 2004). The American Cancer Society indicates that in the United States men have a 1 in 2 lifetime risk of developing cancer; for women, the risk is 1 in 3. Of every five deaths in the United States, one is from cancer, making it the second leading cause of death (heart disease is the most common).

Cancer is not one disease, but a group of more than 200 diseases characterized by the uncontrolled and unregulated growth and spread of abnormal cells. Early detection and prompt treatment can cure some cancers and slow the progression of others. If not detected and controlled, cancer can result in death. Overall, it affects

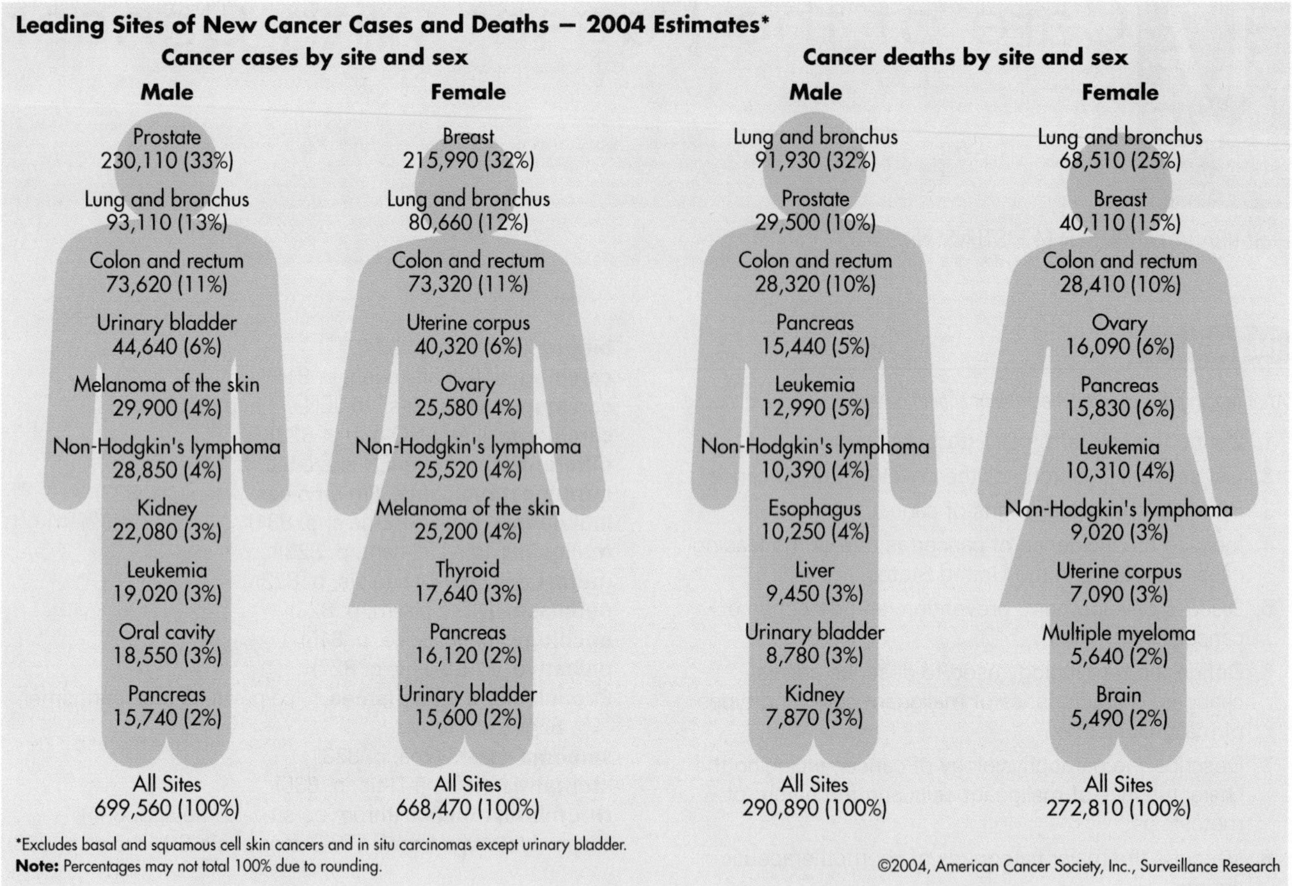

Leading Sites of New Cancer Cases and Deaths — 2004 Estimates*

Cancer cases by site and sex

Male	Female
Prostate 230,110 (33%)	Breast 215,990 (32%)
Lung and bronchus 93,110 (13%)	Lung and bronchus 80,660 (12%)
Colon and rectum 73,620 (11%)	Colon and rectum 73,320 (11%)
Urinary bladder 44,640 (6%)	Uterine corpus 40,320 (6%)
Melanoma of the skin 29,900 (4%)	Ovary 25,580 (4%)
Non-Hodgkin's lymphoma 28,850 (4%)	Non-Hodgkin's lymphoma 25,520 (4%)
Kidney 22,080 (3%)	Melanoma of the skin 25,200 (4%)
Leukemia 19,020 (3%)	Thyroid 17,640 (3%)
Oral cavity 18,550 (3%)	Pancreas 16,120 (2%)
Pancreas 15,740 (2%)	Urinary bladder 15,600 (2%)
All Sites 699,560 (100%)	All Sites 668,470 (100%)

Cancer deaths by site and sex

Male	Female
Lung and bronchus 91,930 (32%)	Lung and bronchus 68,510 (25%)
Prostate 29,500 (10%)	Breast 40,110 (15%)
Colon and rectum 28,320 (10%)	Colon and rectum 28,410 (10%)
Pancreas 15,440 (5%)	Ovary 16,090 (6%)
Leukemia 12,990 (5%)	Pancreas 15,830 (6%)
Non-Hodgkin's lymphoma 10,390 (4%)	Leukemia 10,310 (4%)
Esophagus 10,250 (4%)	Non-Hodgkin's lymphoma 9,020 (3%)
Liver 9,450 (3%)	Uterine corpus 7,090 (3%)
Urinary bladder 8,780 (3%)	Multiple myeloma 5,640 (2%)
Kidney 7,870 (3%)	Brain 5,490 (2%)
All Sites 290,890 (100%)	All Sites 272,810 (100%)

*Excludes basal and squamous cell skin cancers and in situ carcinomas except urinary bladder.
Note: Percentages may not total 100% due to rounding.

©2004, American Cancer Society, Inc., Surveillance Research

FIGURE **17-1** Leading sites of new cancer cases and deaths (2004 estimates).

people of all ages, but occurs more frequently in the aged and the very young. An estimated 30% of Americans now living will experience cancer at some point in their lives. The 5-year survival rate is now 62%.

Lung cancer is the leading cause of cancer-related death in both men and women. Other cancers, such as breast and prostate, occur more often than lung cancer, but they have better cure and survival rates due to early detection and treatment (Figure 17-1).

DEVELOPMENT, PREVENTION, AND DETECTION OF CANCER

CARCINOGENESIS AND THE PRIMARY PREVENTION OF CANCER

Carcinogenesis is the process by which normal cells are transformed into cancer cells. Although numerous theories have been proposed to explain it, no single unifying cause has been offered or accepted. The exact cause of most human cancers is still unknown. The cause and development of each type of cancer are likely to be multiple. It is not known how many tumors have a chemical, environmental, genetic, im-

munologic, or viral origin. Cancers may arise spontaneously from causes that are thus far unexplained.

Carcinogenesis is the term used for the various factors that are possible origins of cancer. Primary prevention of cancer consists of changes in lifestyle habits to eliminate or reduce exposure to carcinogens, substances known to increase the risk for developing cancer.

Risk factors include the following:
- Smoking: According to the American Cancer Society, smoking is the most preventable cause of death from lung cancer. It is estimated that 87% of people who develop lung cancer are smokers. Other cancers associated with smoking are bladder, kidney, mouth, pharynx, larynx, esophagus, pancreas, uterine, and cervix.
- Dietary habits: When it comes to preventing cancer, is diet really important? Experts believe diet is very important. It is estimated that one third of cancer deaths are attributable to nutritional factors such as high-fat, low-fiber diets (Cancer Facts and Figures, 2004). The National Cancer Institute estimates that dietary modifications could have saved 30,000 lives by the year 2000. Diet plays a role in the development of cancer of the colon, rectum, and breast. A diet high in fiber and

low in fat is recommended for prevention. To teach Americans how to improve their diets, the National Cancer Institute (NCI) has launched a program called "5 a Day for Better Health." It aims to show how easy it is to add at least five servings of fruits and vegetables to the daily diet as a way of reducing the risks of cancer (Health Promotion Considerations box). At present only 20% of the U.S. population consumes five daily servings of fruits and vegetables. Obesity is a risk factor for breast, prostate, gallbladder, ovarian, and uterine cancers.

- Exposure to radiation: Excessive exposure to the sun's ultraviolet rays is a factor in the development of basal and squamous cell skin cancers and melanoma. Sunlamps and tanning booth beds also emit ultraviolet rays and have the same risks as sunlight. In addition, the effects of radiation commonly used for medical diagnosis and treatment are known to be carcinogenic. Exposure should be limited and monitored.
- Exposure to environmental and chemical carcinogens: Some of these include fumes from rubber and chlorine and dust from cotton, coal, nickel, chromate, asbestos, and vinyl chloride. There is a greater incidence of bladder cancer among people who live in urban areas and among those who work with dyes, rubber, or leather.
- Smokeless tobacco: Use of smokeless tobacco increases the risk of cancer of the mouth, larynx, pharynx, and esophagus.
- Frequent heavy consumption of alcohol: Alcohol may result in oral cancer and cancer of the larynx, throat, esophagus, and liver.

HEREDITARY CANCERS

About 90% of cancers are not inherited. Hereditary cancers are those cancers that arise from germline mutations. Hereditary cancers are diagnosed at an earlier age—usually 15 to 20 years earlier than cancers that are not inherited. Often, several relatives have the same or related cancers; they are more likely to be bilateral, and multiple cancers are seen in single individuals. These multiple cancers are often seen in unusual organ combinations, such as breast and sarcoma, breast and thyroid, leukemia and brain tumors. Hereditary cancers are characterized by the presence of precursor lesions, such as polyps in colorectal cancer and dysplastic nevi in melanoma (Lewis et al, 2004).

GENETIC SUSCEPTIBILITY

For many years scientists have searched for genetic patterns in the most common cancer sites. The following patterns have emerged:

- The incidence of postmenopausal breast cancer is three times higher and the incidence of premenopausal breast cancer is five times higher in women with a family history of this disease. Breast cancer is rare in Asian women and common in white women.
- The incidence of lung cancer is greater in smokers with a family history of this disease than in smokers without a family history of the disease.
- The incidence of leukemia is greater in an identical twin of a person with the disease.
- Neuroblastoma occurs with increased frequency among siblings.
- Colon cancer is more likely to occur in women who have a history of breast cancer.

CANCER RISK ASSESSMENT AND CANCER GENETIC COUNSELING

When an individual or family is suspected of having a mutation in a cancer-causing gene, a cancer risk assessment is performed. This is the first step toward identifying hereditary cancer predisposition. The process of risk assessment begins with a comprehensive family history. Information is obtained from the individual regarding his or her first-, second-, and third-degree relatives. Once the detailed family history is completed, medical records are obtained. These records are necessary to confirm the cancer diagnoses identified in the

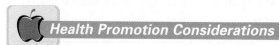

Health Promotion Considerations

Foods to Reduce Cancer Risk

- Vegetables from the cabbage family, such as:
  Broccoli
  Cauliflower
  Brussels sprouts
  All types of cabbage and kale
- Vegetables and fruits high in beta-carotene, such as:
  Carrots
  Peaches
  Apricots
  Squash
  Broccoli
- Rich sources of vitamin C, such as:
  Grapefruit
  Oranges
  Cantaloupe
  Strawberries
  Red and green peppers
  Broccoli
  Tomatoes
- The National Cancer Institute has recommended including at least five servings of fruits and vegetables in the daily diet.
- Lean meat, fish, skinned poultry
- Low-fat dairy products, including white cheese rather than yellow
- Avoid salt-cured, smoked, or nitrite-cured foods

family history. Confirmation is a critical step in the risk assessment process. The records usually requested include pathology reports, autopsy reports, death certificates, and discharge summaries from hospitalizations. Confirmation of cancer diagnoses through medical record analysis provides the patient with the most accurate risk analysis possible. Genetic counseling is an essential component of the genetic evaluation. It is comprehensive in its approach to provide education, health promotion, informed consent, and support to individuals and families facing the uncertainty of hereditary cancer and cancer syndromes.

CANCER PREVENTION AND EARLY DETECTION

Prevention and early detection of cancer includes recognition of cancer's warning signals (Box 17-1). The American Cancer Society advises specific preventive behaviors and screening tests for men and women, as shown in Tables 17-1 and 17-2. The nurse plays a prominent role in prevention and detection of cancer. Early detection and prompt treatment are directly responsible for increased survival rates in patients with

cancer (see Health Promotion Considerations box). It is reported that 62% who are diagnosed with cancer today will be alive 5 years after diagnosis.

Beginning at the high school years, all women should be taught to perform breast self-examination (BSE) each month, 2 or 3 days after the menstrual period ends. After menopause, a woman should choose a specific day to help remind her, such as the first day of each month. A woman needs to become familiar with the appearance and feel of her breasts. This will help her identify any change from one month to the next. Any abnormality—such as discharge from

| Box 17-1 | *Cancer's Seven Warning Signals* |

If you have a warning signal, see your doctor.
1. Changes in bowel or bladder habits
2. A sore that does not heal
3. Unusual bleeding or discharge
4. Thickening or lump in breast or elsewhere
5. Indigestion or difficulty in swallowing
6. Obvious change in warts or moles
7. Nagging cough or hoarseness

| Table 17-1 | *Cancer Prevention and Early Detection in the Female* |

The American Cancer Society recommends that all women get a cancer-related checkup every 3 years between the ages of 20 and 40, and every year thereafter. This checkup, depending on a person's age, might include examinations for cancer of the skin, thyroid, mouth, lymph nodes, and ovaries.

PREVENTIVE BEHAVIORS	SCREENING TESTS
COLORECTAL CANCER	
• Following screening guidelines to remove adenomatous polyps before they become cancer	Beginning at age 50, a woman should follow one of the five screening options below:
• Getting at least 30 minutes of physical activity on most days	• Yearly fecal occult blood test (FOBT)
• Achieving and maintaining a healthy weight	• Flexible sigmoidoscopy every 5 years
• Eating plenty of fruits, vegetables, and whole-grain foods, and limiting intake of high-fat foods	• Yearly fecal occult blood test plus flexible sigmoidoscopy every 5 years
• Quitting smoking	(Of the options above, the American Cancer Society prefers yearly FOBT combined with flexible sigmoidoscopy every 5 years)
	• Double–contrast barium enema every 5 years
	• Colonoscopy every 10 years
	Talk to physician about beginning screening earlier and/or more often if one has any of the following risk factors:
	• Strong family history of colorectal cancer or polyps (cancer of polyps in a first-degree relative younger than 60 or in two first-degree relatives of any age). NOTE: A first degree-relative is defined as a parent, sibling, or child.
	• A known family history of colorectal cancer syndromes
	• A personal history of colorectal cancer or adenomatous polyps
	• A personal history of chronic inflammatory bowel disease

Table 17-1 *Cancer Prevention and Early Detection in the Female—cont'd*

PREVENTIVE BEHAVIORS	SCREENING TESTS
CERVICAL CANCER • Abstaining from or practicing safer sex using barrier protection each time you have intercourse • Quitting smoking • Eating a diet rich in fruits and vegetables • Watching for and reporting signs and symptoms (although all of these can have other causes): Abnormal uterine bleeding or spotting Abnormal vaginal discharge Pain during intercourse	• Yearly pelvic examination with Pap test to begin at age 18 or when sexually active, whichever is earlier • After three or more consecutive satisfactory normal yearly examinations, the Pap test may be performed less frequently at the discretion of the physician
BREAST CANCER **Ages 20 to 39** • Breast self-examination each month • Clinical breast examination by health care professional every 3 years **Ages 40 and over** • Yearly mammogram • Yearly clinical breast examination by a health care professional, near the time of the mammogram • Breast self-examination every month	• Following recommended guidelines for early detection of breast cancer • Talking with your physician about the risks and benefits of hormone replacement therapy for your risk of cancer and other diseases (like heart disease and osteoporosis) • Getting at least 30 minutes of physical activity on most days • Achieving and maintaining a healthy weight • Eating plenty of fruits, vegetables, and whole-grain foods and limiting intake of high-fat foods • Decreasing your alcohol intake
ENDOMETRIAL CANCER • Watching for and reporting any abnormal uterine spotting or bleeding • Using oral contraceptives for many years • Talking with your doctor about the risks and benefits of hormone replacement therapy for your risk of cancer and other diseases (like heart disease and osteoporosis) • If taking hormone replacement therapy with your uterus still intact, take estrogen with progesterone	**Average Risk** • Talk with the physician especially at the time of menopause, about the risks and symptoms of endometrial cancer • Report any vaginal bleeding or spotting to your physician
OVARIAN CANCER • Using oral contraceptives for several years • Watching for and reporting signs and symptoms (although all of these can have other causes): Abdominal swelling Vaginal bleeding Back and/or leg pain Chronic stomach pain • Talking with your physician about the risks and benefits of hormone replacement therapy and your risks of cancer and other diseases, like heart disease and osteoporosis • Talking with your physician about having your ovaries removed, if you are at high risk (This surgery causes sudden menopause.)	There are no effective and proven tests for early detection of ovarian cancer. • As part of one's health maintenance, undergo a periodic and thorough pelvic examination as directed by the physician
SKIN CANCER • Staying out of the sun, especially between 10 AM and 4 PM • Wearing a broad-brimmed hat, a shirt, and sunglasses when out in the sun	• Skin examination **Older than age 20:** Every 3 years **Older than age 40:** Every year • Self-examination (monthly)

Continued

Table 17-1 *Cancer Prevention and Early Detection in the Female—cont'd*

PREVENTIVE BEHAVIORS	SCREENING TESTS
SKIN CANCER—cont'd • Using a sunscreen with an SPF of 15 or higher, and reapplying it often • Not using tanning beds or sunlamps • Protecting your young children from excessive sun exposure • Checking your skin regularly for abnormal or changing areas, especially moles, and having them examined by your physician	Become familiar with any moles, freckles, or other abnormalities on the skin; use a mirror or have a family member or close friend look at areas one can't see (ears, scalp, lower back) Check for changes once a month; show any suspicious or changing areas to the physician
LUNG CANCER • Quitting smoking • Encouraging those you live with or work with to quit • If you smoke, let your doctor know if you develop any of the following symptoms (some may have causes other than cancer): A cough that does not go away Chest pain, often aggravated by deep breathing Hoarseness Weight loss and loss of appetite Bloody or rust-colored sputum Shortness of breath Fever without a known reason Recurring infections such as bronchitis and pneumonia New onset of wheezing	None have been found to be effective; usually found on x-ray examination, but there are often no symptoms • Talk to the physician about possible screening if one has any of the risk factors listed below: Smoke tobacco Work around asbestos Exposed to radon Exposed to uranium Exposed to arsenic Exposed to vinyl chloride Smoke marijuana Regularly exposed to secondhand smoke

Table 17-2 *Cancer Prevention and Early Detection in the Male*

The American Cancer Society recommends a cancer-related checkup every 3 years between the ages of 20 and 40, and every year thereafter. Depending on the male's age, examinations might include examination for cancers of the skin, thyroid, mouth, lymph nodes, and testes.

PREVENTIVE BEHAVIORS	SCREENING TESTS
COLORECTAL CANCER • Following screening guidelines to remove adenomatous polyps before they become cancer • Getting at least 30 minutes of physical activity on most days • Achieving and maintaining a healthy weight • Eating plenty of fruits, vegetables, and whole grain foods, and limiting intake of high-fat foods • Quitting smoking	Beginning at age 50, the male should follow one of the five screening options below: • Yearly fecal occult blood test (FOBT) • Flexible sigmoidoscopy every 5 years • Yearly FOBT plus flexible sigmoidoscopy every 5 years (Of the options above, the American Cancer Society prefers yearly FOBT combined with flexible sigmoidoscopy every 5 years) • Double contrast barium enema every 5 years • Colonoscopy every 10 years Talk to physician about beginning screening earlier and/or more often if one has any of the following risk factors: • Strong family history of colorectal cancer or polyps (cancer of polyps in a first-degree relative younger than 60 or in two first-degree relatives of any age). NOTE: A first degree-relative is defined as a parent, sibling, or child.

Table 17-2 *Cancer Prevention and Early Detection in the Male—cont'd*

PREVENTIVE BEHAVIORS	SCREENING TESTS
COLORECTAL CANCER—cont'd	• A known family history of colorectal cancer syndromes • A personal history of colorectal cancer or adenomatous polyps • A personal history of chronic inflammatory bowel disease
PROSTATE CANCER • Eating a diet low in fat and high in vegetables, fruits, and grains • Getting at least 30 minutes of physical activity on most days • Achieving and maintaining a healthy weight	• The male should consider a yearly PSA blood test and digital rectal examination starting at age 50 or at age 45 if at high risk (African-American, or have a father or brother diagnosed with prostate cancer at a young age)
SKIN CANCER • Staying out of the sun, especially between 10 AM and 4 PM • Wearing a broad-brimmed hat, a shirt, and sunglasses when out in the sun • Using a sunscreen with an SPF of 15 or higher, and reapplying it often • Not using tanning beds or sunlamps • Protecting your young children from excessive sun exposure • Checking your skin regularly for abnormal or changing areas, especially moles, and having them examined by your physician	• Skin examination **Older than 20:** every 3 years **Older than 40:** every year • Self-examination (monthly) Become familiar with any moles, freckles or other abnormalities on the skin; use a mirror or have a family member or close friend look at areas one can't see (ears, scalp, lower back) Check for changes once a month; show any suspicious or changing areas to the physician
LUNG CANCER • Quitting smoking • Encouraging those you live with or work with to quit • If you smoke, let your physician know if you develop any of the following symptoms (some may have causes other than cancer): A cough that does not go away Chest pain, often aggravated by deep breathing Hoarseness Weight loss and loss of appetite Bloody or rust-colored sputum Shortness of breath Fever without a known reason Recurring infections such as bronchitis and pneumonia New onset of wheezing	None have been found to be effective. Usually found on x-ray examination, but there are often no symptoms. • Talk to the physician about possible screening if one has any of the risk factors listed below: Smoke tobacco Work around asbestos Exposed to radon Exposed to uranium Exposed to arsenic Exposed to vinyl chloride Smoke marijuana Regularly exposed to secondhand smoke

the nipples; puckering, dimpling, or scaling of the skin; and the palpation of a lump or thickness—is significant.

The following is a guide to examining the breasts:

1. Inspect the breasts before a mirror, arms raised behind the head; also place hands on hips with shoulders and elbows pulled forward. Gently squeeze the nipples to determine if any discharge is present.

2. While bathing, when the breasts and hands are wet, slide the fingers of each hand over the skin of the opposite breast. Use the flat surface of two or three fingers. This is a good practice for men as well as women.

3. In a prone position, place a towel or small pillow under the shoulder of the breast being examined to flatten the breast and make it easier to feel. Use the flat surface of two or three fingers of the hand opposite the side being examined. Gently palpate each breast, moving in at least three circles of different distances from the nipple, starting at different points—such as the 1 o'clock, 2 o'clock,

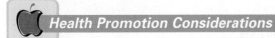

Prevention and Detection of Cancer

- Reduce or avoid exposure to known or suspected carcinogens and cancer-promoting agents, including cigarette smoke and sun exposure.
- Eat a balanced diet that includes vegetables (green, yellow, and orange), fresh fruits, whole grains, and adequate amounts of fiber, and reduce the amount of fat and preservatives, including smoked and salt-cured meats.
- Exercise regularly.
- Obtain adequate, consistent periods of rest (at least 6 to 8 hours per night).
- Have a health examination on a regular basis that includes a health history, a physical examination, and specific diagnostic tests for common cancers in accordance with the guidelines published by the American Cancer Society *(www.cancer.org)* (Tables 17-1 and 17-2).
- Eliminate, reduce, or change the perceptions of stressors and enhance the ability to effectively cope with stressors.
- Enjoy consistent periods of relaxation and leisure.
- Know the seven warning signs of cancer (Box 17-1). (These actually detect fairly advanced disease.)
- Learn and practice self-examination (e.g., breast self-examination, testicular self-examination).
- Seek immediate medical care if you notice a change in what is normal for you and if cancer is suspected. Early detection of cancer has a positive effect on prognosis.

---

or 3 o'clock position—and continuing to the 12 o'clock position.

The upper, outer tail of the breast that extends to the axilla, as well as the entire axillary area, must also be checked (see Chapter 12). Nurses should teach BSE to all patients (men and women), emphasizing that any identifiable problem should be brought to the attention of a physician. Any delay is a waste of valuable time if cancer is present.

Men should be taught to check the scrotum for enlargement, thickening, or the presence of a lump in the testicles. This should be done monthly, after a warm bath or shower. It should be emphasized that a physician must be contacted to determine the significance of any changes from the normal, smooth consistency of the testes (see Chapter 12). Men older than the age of 50 should be advised to have a prostate-specific antigen (PSA) test and rectal examination once a year. Symptoms of blood in the urine, difficulty starting to urinate, a weak flow of urine, or other urination problems should be reported to the physician.

A common reason for delay in diagnosing cancer is that early malignant changes do not produce pain. Cancer may be insidious at the onset, and it may often be far advanced before the individual experiences any symptoms.

PATHOPHYSIOLOGY OF CANCER

CELL MECHANISMS AND GROWTH

The basic unit of structure and function in all living things is the **cell.** Approximately 60,000 billion cells are in the adult human body and, although there are many different types of cells, all of them have certain common characteristics. For example, all cells need nourishment to maintain life, and all cells use almost identical nutri-ents. All cells use oxygen (O_2); the O_2 combines with fat, protein, or carbohydrates (CHOs) to release the energy needed for cells to function. The mechanisms for changing nutrients into energy are generally the same in all cells, and all cells deliver their end product of chemical reactions into the nearby fluids.

Most cells have the ability to reproduce. Whenever cells are destroyed, the remaining cells of the same type reproduce until the correct number have been replenished. This orderly replacement of cells is governed by a control mechanism that stops when the loss or damage has been corrected. Dynamic, active, and orderly, the healthy cell is a small powerhouse, laboratory, factory, and duplicating machine, perfectly copying itself over and over.

Cancer cells are not subject to the usual restrictions placed on cell proliferation by the host. When malignant cells change, they become unlike parent cells. They are not differentiated or recognizable as being the same in size or shape as normal cells. Cancer cells can divide and multiply, but not in a normal manner. Instead of limiting their growth to meet specific needs of the body, they continue to reproduce in a disorderly and unrestricted manner. The cellular features of cancer cells are a local increase in the number of cells, loss of normal cellular arrangement, variation in cell shape and size, increased nuclear size, increased miotic activity, and abnormal mitosis and chromosomes.

Proliferation is not always indicative of cancer, however. Abnormal cellular growth is classified as nonneoplastic growth and neoplastic growth. The four common nonneoplastic growth patterns are hypertrophy, hyperplasia, metaplasia, and dysplasia. Though not neoplastic conditions, these may precede the development of cancer. **Anaplasia** means "without form" and is an irreversible change in which the structures of adult cells regress to more primitive levels.

Neoplasm is the term for uncontrolled or abnormal growth of cells. Neoplasms may be **benign** (not recurrent or progressive; nonmalignant) or **malignant** (growing worse and resisting treatment, as in cancerous growths [Table 17-3]). The growths are also called **tumors,** which means swelling or enlargement. They may be localized or invasive. Benign tumors may become serious because of localized increase in growth with damage to surrounding tissues, as in a benign brain tumor. Malignant neoplasms may progress and destroy surrounding tissues. They may also metastasize from the primary site of origin to distant sites.

Metastasis (the process by which tumor cells are spread to distant parts of the body) is the term used to describe the movement of cancer cells from the primary site to a secondary site. Once cancer cells have moved to another area of the body, secondary tumors may grow in that area. Metastasis can occur by the following mechanisms:

- Direct spread of tumor cells by diffusion to other body cavities.
- Circulation by way of blood and lymphatic channels.
- Transplantation or direct transport of tumor cells from one site to another. Transplantation may occur accidentally during surgery or other procedures when cancer cells are "carried" on instruments or gloves.

In addition to the identified carcinogenic factors that may cause malignant cellular changes, certain viruses have been suspected. There is also evidence to suggest certain genetic factors that result in a predisposition to the development of cancer.

The body's immune system is responsible for recognizing and destroying malignant cells. The immune system may be weakened by cancer-producing substances, tumor cells, and the aging process.

Some T cells are responsible for **immunosurveillance** (the immune system's recognition and destruction of newly developed abnormal cells). When a cell becomes malignant, it carries a tumor-specific antigen on its membranes that is recognized by the body as nonself and destroyed. If T-cell function is suppressed by age, drugs (corticosteroids), poor nutrition, alcohol, serious infections, or certain disease processes (neoplastic invasion of bone and lymph tissue), the risk of cancer increases. To suppress T-cell rejection of a transplanted organ, steroids and other drugs are administered. The resultant loss of immunosurveillance increases the risk of certain cancers.

DESCRIPTION, GRADING, AND STAGING OF TUMORS

Tumors are described according to the parent tissue of the specific location in the body. **Carcinoma** is the term used for malignant tumors composed of epithelial cells, which have a tendency to metastasize. Carcinomas originate from embryonal ectoderm (skin and glands) and endoderm (mucous membrane linings of the respiratory tract, GI tract, and genitourinary [GU] tract). **Sarcoma** refers to malignant tumors of connective tissues; they originate from embryonal mesoderm, such as muscle, bone, or fat, usually presenting as a painless swelling. Sarcoma may affect the bone, bladder, kidneys, liver, lungs, parotids, and spleen. **Lymphomas** and **leukemias** originate from the hematopoietic system.

Tumors are classified grade 1 to grade 4 by the degree of malignancy. Grade 1 is the most **differentiated** (most like the parent tissue) tumor and the least malignant. Grade 4 is the least differentiated (unlike parent tissue) tumor and the most malignant. (Box 17-2).

The tumor, nodes, metastasis (TNM) staging system of staging cancer is used to indicate **tumor size,** spread to **lymph nodes,** and extent of **metastasis** (Box 17-2). This system is used to direct treatment, predict prognosis, and contribute to cancer research by ensuring reliable comparison of different patients.

Extent of Disease Classification

Classifying the extent and spread of disease is termed **staging.** This classification system is based on a description of the extent of the disease rather than on cell appearance. Although there are similarities in the staging of cancers, there are many differences, based on a thorough knowledge of the natural history of each specific type of cancer.

Clinical staging. The clinical staging classification system determines the extent of the disease process of cancer by stages.

Stage 0:	Cancer in situ
Stage I:	Tumor limited to the tissue of origin; localized tumor growth
Stage II:	Limited local spread
Stage III:	Extensive local and regional spread
Stage IV:	Metastasis

Table 17-3 *General Characteristics of Neoplasms*

BENIGN TUMORS	MALIGNANT TUMORS
Slow, steady growth	Rate of growth varies—usually rapid
Remains localized	Metastasizes
Usually contained within a capsule	Rarely contained within a capsule
Smooth, well defined; movable when palpated	Irregular; more immobile when palpated
Resembles parent tissue	Little resemblance to parent tissue
Crowds normal tissue	Invades normal tissue
Rarely recurs after removal	May recur after removal
Rarely fatal	Fatal without treatment

Box 17-2 *TNM Cancer Staging Classification System*

T* SUBCLASSES

T_x—tumor cannot be adequately assessed
T_0—no evidence of primary tumor
T_{is}—carcinoma in situ
T_1, T_2, T_3, T_4—progressive increase in tumor size and involvement

N† SUBCLASSES

N_x—regional lymph nodes cannot be assessed
N_0—no regional lymph node metastasis
N_1, N_2, N_3, N_4—increasing involvement regional lymph nodes

M‡ SUBCLASSES

M_x—not assessed
M_0—no (known) distant metastasis
M_1-M_4—distant metastasis present, specify site(s)

HISTOPATHOLOGY

G_1—well-differentiated grade—cells differ slightly from normal cells (mild dysplasia)
G_2—moderately well-differentiated grade—cells are more abnormal (moderate dysplasia)
G_3—poorly differentiated grade—cells are very abnormal (severe dysplasia)
G_4—undifferentiated—cells are immature and primative (anaplasia) a cell of this origin is difficult to determine

From American Joint Committee for Cancer. (1992). *AJCC manual for staging of cancer.* (4th ed.). Philadelphia: Lippincott.
*T—Primary tumor.
†N—Regional lymph nodes.
‡M—Distant metastasis.

TNM classification system. The *TNM classification system* represents the standardization of the clinical staging of cancer. This classification system is used to determine the extent of the disease process of cancer according to three parameters: tumor size (T), degree of regional spread to the lymph nodes (N), and metastasis (M). (An example of the TNM classification system can be found in Box 17-2).

A tumor may be named for its location, its cellular makeup, or the person by whom it was identified.

Exfoliative (pertaining to the shedding of something) cytology [e.g., Papanicolaou's test (smear) (Pap)] is a means of studying cells that the body has shed during the normal sequence of growth and replacement of body tissues. If cancer is present, cancer cells are also shed. It is most commonly used to detect cancers of the cervix, but it may be used for tissue specimens from any organ.

The results of the Pap test, as given by the **Bethesda system (the preferred system)**, are as follows:

Negative (normal), formerly class I
Probably negative, may indicate infection; atypical squamous cells; reactive changes, formerly class II
Suspicious, but not conclusive for malignancy; low-grade squamous intraepithelial lesion, formerly class III
More suspicious, strongly suggestive of malignancy; high-grade squamous intraepithelial lesion, formerly class IV
Conclusive for malignancy; invasive squamous cell carcinoma, formerly class V

DIAGNOSIS OF CANCER

BIOPSY

People who show signs of cancer should undergo diagnostic testing to confirm or rule out the diagnosis. The only definitive way to determine the presence of malignant cells is to perform a tissue biopsy (the removal of a small piece of living tissue from an organ or other part of the body for microscopic examination; used to confirm or establish a diagnosis, establish prognosis, or follow the course of a disease).

In general, the purpose of a biopsy is to obtain a sample of tissue for pathologic examination. The three types of biopsy are incisional, excisional, and needle aspiration (Figure 17-2). **Incisional** biopsy is the removal of a portion of tissue for examination, such as the bite biopsy performed during endoscopy. **Excisional** biopsy is the removal of the complete lesion, with little or no margin of surrounding normal tissue removed, as in polypectomy. Another example of excisional biopsy is the dissection of peripheral lymph nodes, such as those of the axilla for staging of breast cancer or those of the peritoneal region for staging of various abdominal cancers. **Needle aspiration** biopsy is the aspiration of fluid or tissue by means of a needle (breast biopsy is performed with an aspiration needle). Transcutaneous aspiration biopsy has eliminated most of the exploratory laparotomies for diagnosing metastatic cancer of the liver or for primary inoperable pancreatic cancer. Organs accessible to thin-needle biopsy under guidance of palpation include breasts, skin, thyroid gland, prostate, palpable lymph nodes, and salivary glands.

ENDOSCOPY

Cells or tissue can also be obtained using an **endoscope** to directly visualize an internal structure through a body cavity or through a small incision. Endoscopes are rigid or flexible tubes containing a magnifying lens and a light. Endoscopes vary in diameter and length according to the structure being examined—the bronchoscope is used to visualize the tracheobronchial tree; upper gastrointestinal (GI) endoscopy allows direct visualization of the upper GI

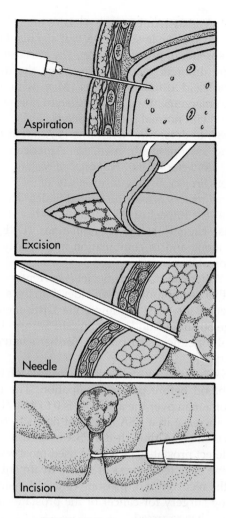

FIGURE **17-2** Types of biopsy.

tract (esophagus, stomach, duodenum); the colonoscopy is used to visualize the entire colon; and the sigmoidoscope is used to examine the sigmoid colon, rectum, and anus.

Other diagnostic studies determine the depth of the specific lesion and identify other structures that may have been invaded. These include radiographs and scanning procedures. Commonly ordered radiographic studies are the chest radiograph, mammography, bone scan, GI series, barium enema, and intravenous pyelogram.

DIAGNOSTIC IMAGING

Bone scanning involves several steps. First, a radioactive material is injected into a vein in the arm. The patient is encouraged to drink water over the next 1 to 3 hours to aid renal clearance of any radioisotope not picked up by the bone. Areas of concentrated uptake may represent a tumor or abnormality. These areas of concentration can be detected days or weeks before an ordinary radiograph could reveal a lesion. Bone scanning is indicated to detect metastatic tumors; all malignancies capable of metastasis may reach the bone,

especially those malignancies of the breasts, kidneys, lungs, prostate, thyroid gland, and urinary bladder.

Tomography is the special technique of making multiple radiographic films at different depths of a specific area, organ, or structure. The details of each thin section can be clearly visualized.

Computed tomography (CT) scan uses radiographs and a computed scanning system to produce and record images of specific structures at different angles. The entire body can be scanned to detect the presence of any abnormal lesion. CT scan is especially helpful to detect small lesions that may not be seen by radiographs or tomography.

Radioisotope studies require the injection or ingestion of a radioactive substance. A scanning device is used to identify the distribution of the substance in different areas of the body. Concentration of the radioisotope in a specific organ, such as the thyroid gland or brain, identifies a tumor in that location (may be primary or metastatic).

Ultrasound testing is a noninvasive procedure using high-frequency sound waves to examine internal structures of the body. As a transducer is moved over the area being studied, an ultrasound beam is directed through the tissues, which reflects back to the transducer. The sound waves are converted into electrical impulses, which produce an image on a display screen. Ultrasound can show the size, consistency, and shape of the structure being studied, and it is most helpful in distinguishing between cystic and solid tumors. Ultrasound is not used to examine bones or air-filled organs. The procedure is painless. People having ultrasonography will feel the transducer moving over their skin and may need to hold their breath for brief periods and remain still while the procedure is being done.

Magnetic resonance imaging (MRI) is a painless diagnostic procedure that does not involve any exposure to radiation. As the person reclines on a narrow surface that moves into a cylindrical tunnel containing magnetic coils, radiofrequency energy waves produce signals that are processed by a computer and displayed as images on a video monitor. The images can be recorded on film or magnetic tape for permanent storage. This test is currently used in the diagnosis of intracranial and spinal lesions and of cardiovascular and soft tissue abnormalities. The procedure also provides information about changes within the cells of soft tissues, arteries, veins, the brain, and spinal column.

The person having MRI must not have any metallic materials on the body during the test; no jewelry may be worn. MRI cannot be done if the person has any metallic implants in the body, such as a pacemaker, orthopedic nail, or aneurysm screw.

The person having the test can talk to those performing the test by means of a microphone placed inside the scanner tunnel. The person will hear the sound waves thumping on the magnetic field and must lie still while the test is being done; it may take more than an hour to obtain the images needed.

LABORATORY TESTS

Commonly used laboratory tests include the following.

Measurement of Alkaline Phosphatase Blood Levels

Alkaline phosphatase is elevated if there is metastasis to the bone or liver.

Serum Calcitonin Level

Calcitonin is a hormone secreted by the thyroid gland in response to a rising serum calcium level. The level is increased in the blood of people who have cancer of the thyroid. It may be elevated with breast cancer and oat cell cancer of the lung. Calcitonin stimulation testing may be used in addition to the baseline level testing to confirm a diagnosis. It is essential that the person having this test does not eat or drink during the night before the test.

Carcinoembryonic Antigen (CEA) Serum Level

Normally, production of CEA stops before birth, but may begin again if a neoplasm develops. This test cannot be used as a general indicator of cancer because there are other reasons why the level may be elevated; for example, the level is elevated in people who smoke. CEA is found in increased amounts in the blood of people with colorectal cancer. The test may assist in the evaluation of cancer treatment, in which a rising CEA may indicate tumor recurrence or metastatic disease. This test is used less frequently today, because research has found it less accurate than was previously thought.

PSA and CA-125

There are many different blood studies (markers) currently being evaluated to determine their usefulness in cancer screening and diagnosis. Two examples are the PSA for prostate cancer and the CA-125 for ovarian cancer. PSA is a biological marker, specific for cellular activity in the prostate gland.

PSA, the gold standard tumor marker for prostate cancer, is increasingly important in the diagnostic assessment and follow-up of patients with the disease. PSA also plays an important role in staging prostate cancer and in monitoring for recurrence. The American Cancer Society began recommending its use for screening asymptomatic men in November 1992.

Although PSA levels are usually elevated when cancer is present, PSA alone does not diagnose prostate cancer. Other common conditions, such as benign enlargement of the prostate, can also elevate PSA. The finding of elevated PSA requires further evaluation to assess the cause of the high levels. This may involve transrectal ultrasonography (TRUS) of the prostate gland.

The PSA assay requires a physician's interpretation. There is no specific level of PSA that signals the presence or absence of prostate cancer. The PSA test is produced by different manufacturers, and the different products yield different results. Men with benign prostate enlargement will have different normal levels than men with normal prostate glands.

In 1987, to determine what role PSA might play in screening asymptomatic men, the American Cancer Society undertook its National Prostate Cancer Detection Project, a long-term study of 2425 men at 10 clinical centers across the United States. This study looked at the impact of PSA and two other screening methods—digital rectal examination (DRE) and TRUS—alone and in combination in the early detection of prostate cancer.

The American Cancer Society currently recommends that asymptomatic men older than the age of 40 be screened for prostate cancer via DRE; men older than age 50 should undergo annual PSA and DRE. If the result of either is suspicious, further evaluation is necessary.

A PSA is done by collecting a sample of the patient's blood before prostate palpation. The normal range for a man over the age of 40 is 0 to 4 ng/L. Even a small increase in a PSA test level needs to be carefully evaluated. Although the PSA is used in screening to detect prostate cancer, it is used most widely to determine the effectiveness of cancer treatment and to assess the recurrence of prostate cancer. A rising PSA following surgery for cancer of the prostate suggests the cancer has recurred.

CA-125 is a cancer antigen detected in the blood and peritoneal ascites. The normal range is 35 units/mL. CA-125 may be elevated in gynecologic cancers (including ovarian cancer) and cancer of the pancreas.

A monoclonal antibody has been developed that reacts with this antigen, giving physicians a method to measure the amount of CA-125 present in blood samples. The amount of CA-125 in the blood is a useful test to monitor whether a cancer is growing or regressing.

CA-125 has been presented as a way to detect primary ovarian cancer. Although a detection test for ovarian cancer is desirable, CA-125 does not fit this category. CA-125 is useful mainly to signal a recurrence of ovarian cancer. Other conditions—such as endometriosis, hepatitis, pelvic inflammatory diseases, or pregnancy—may increase CA-125 levels in the blood.

Stool Examination for Blood

The cause of blood in the stool must be identified to rule out the possibility of cancer. The guaiac test is commonly used to detect occult (hidden) blood in the stools. Names of other commonly used tests for occult blood in the stool are Hematest, Occultest, and Hemoccult test. Early detection self-tests are available for home use. If blood is found, the person should seek immediate medical attention. For accurate test results for the presence of blood, it is essential that the person not have any of the following foods or medications for 4 days before the test: red meat; turnips; melons; aspirin; and vitamin C. The test must be performed on three consecutive bowel movements.

People must be urged to follow through with diagnostic tests recommended by their physician as a result of preliminary examinations and laboratory tests.

CANCER THERAPIES

SURGERY

By the time it is decided that surgery is needed to remove a cancerous lesion, cancer cells may already have spread to other areas. The goal of surgery is to remove all malignant cells; this may include the removal of the tumor, surrounding tissue, and regional lymph nodes. Surgery in conjunction with chemotherapy and/or radiation therapy may increase the destruction of cancer cells. The effects of cancer drugs and radiation treatments administered before, during, and after surgery are being investigated. A surgical cure may result from a well-isolated lesion removed in the very early stages, such as in cancer of the skin, testicle, breast, or cervix. Surgery may be performed for many reasons—preventive, diagnostic, curative, and palliative (therapy designed to relieve or reduce intensity of uncomfortable symptoms, but that does not produce a cure).

Surgery may be performed to remove polyps in the colon before they undergo any malignant changes. Occasionally, prophylactic mastectomy is done to prevent breast cancer in those identified to be at increased risk because of their family history or other factors.

A radical surgical approach to operable tumors is no longer routinely used because of more sensitive and accurate diagnosing methods, a greater variety of surgical procedures, more sophisticated staging techniques, and more available advanced treatment options. The more conservative surgical management of breast cancer is an excellent example of this trend.

If the cancerous lesion has already metastasized, surgery may provide palliation by relieving some of the associated problems, such as obstruction, ulceration, hemorrhage, and pain.

The pituitary, adrenal glands, ovaries, or testes may be surgically removed to help control the growth and spread of malignancies caused by hormonal stimulation.

Reconstructive surgery may be needed to improve body functions and appearance after some types of surgery, such as modified radical mastectomy. Breast reconstruction is an option for women whose disease and treatment enable the surgeon to implant a prosthesis or to transplant tissue from other areas of the body to create a more natural breast. When this is an-

ticipated, preoperative counseling by the surgeon and the nurse will help the patient consider the long-range outcome instead of the immediate surgical procedure.

Nursing Interventions

If the nurse is not present when the physician explains recommendations for care, the nurse must ask the physician what the patient and family have been told. This is essential to be able to reinforce the information given by the physician. Patients and families are usually frightened and may not remember all that the physician has explained to them (Older Adult Considerations box).

Patients should have confidence and trust in those responsible for their care. Positive feelings and attitudes promote relaxation and help reduce anxiety and fear (Therapeutic Dialogue box). The nurse should encourage the patient to ask the physician any questions concerning potential risks of a given treatment. A patient needs to feel comfortable with the decision to follow through with the physician's recommendations.

The following are nursing guidelines to ensure that patients get the information they need:

- Be present when patient and physician are discussing treatment decisions.

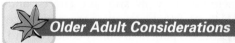

Older Adult Considerations

Cancer

- There are more cases of cancer among older adults than people of any other age group.
- The incidence of cancer increases with aging, possibly as a result of decreased effectiveness of the immune system and changes in deoxyribonucleic acid (DNA).
- The types of cancers seen in older adults are prostate, lung, breast, and colorectal cancer. Cancers of the skin, urinary bladder, vagina, and vulva are seen primarily in older adults. Chronic lymphocytic leukemia and multiple myeloma are seen more frequently in older adults than in younger people.
- Many of the early signs and symptoms of cancer may be misdiagnosed as normal changes of aging. The importance of routine medical screening and self-examination should be stressed to the aging adult.
- Because of fear or past experience, older adults may adopt a fatalistic frame of mind after hearing the diagnosis of cancer. Use of the terms "tumor" or "growth" may be more acceptable.
- The type of treatment for cancer should be based on the older person's wishes and overall state of health. Older individuals, their family members, and significant others should be presented with all options so that informed decisions regarding treatment can be made.

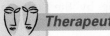

Therapeutic Dialogue

NURSE: *Good afternoon, Mrs. S. My name is J., and I will be your nurse this evening. How are you feeling? (introduction and general lead)*

PATIENT: *I'm feeling all right now. It's tomorrow I'm dreading.*

NURSE: *You're dreading tomorrow? (restatement)*

PATIENT: *Yes. My doctor told me he has to remove my entire breast and even cut under my arm to remove any malignant lymph nodes. I dread the thought that I'll look so different.*

NURSE: *You're anxious about the fact that you may look different. (reflection)*

PATIENT: *I'll be embarrassed to undress in front of my husband. He may think I'm no longer attractive.*

NURSE: *Have you had a chance to discuss your feelings with your husband? (clarification)*

PATIENT: *No, he's out of town but will be back tonight. I guess I could talk to him then. Maybe he will accept it better than I think.*

NURSE: *We'll talk more after you've had a chance to talk to him about your feelings. Is there anything else on your mind that you'd like to talk about now? (showing acceptance and general lead)*

- If it seems necessary, clarify explanations of treatments, including benefits and side effects, and help the patient formulate questions and voice concerns. Address patient or family concerns and questions concerning alternative treatments.
- Afterward, talk to the patient and his or her family about the information the doctor presented; assess their understanding of the treatment, as well as their goals and needs.
- Report any apparent misunderstandings, unrealistic expectations, or other problems to the physician.
- Talk to the patient to verify that his or her problem was resolved.
- Accept and support the patient's choice, regardless of personal opinion.

The use of laser beams as an alternative for some oncology surgical procedures is increasing. The laser beam vaporizes tissue with little bleeding and low risk of infection. Currently the major uses of laser surgery are in ophthalmology, gynecology, urology, neurosurgery, and otolaryngology. The chief discomfort while undergoing laser surgery is that the person must lie very still while the laser is in use.

Preparing the patient for a surgical procedure must include an explanation of what to expect postoperatively. Preoperative teaching is discussed in Chapter 2.

Whatever the surgical procedure, the patient's nutritional status, both before and after surgery, has been found to be a significant factor in the amount of surgery that can be tolerated, the rate of recovery from the surgery, the patient's role performance, and the adequacy of wound healing.

When surgery may result in a changed body image—as in mastectomy, laryngectomy, or the formation of an ostomy—the patient may benefit from talking with another person who has undergone the same type of surgery. The American Cancer Society sponsors support groups. They also specially prepare volunteers to visit individuals who need these types of surgical procedures. Reach to Recovery; the Lost Chord Club; I Can Cope; Look Good, Feel Good; and the Ostomy Club are some of the special groups available in some local communities.

RADIATION THERAPY

Radiation therapy can be used to cure or control cancer that has spread to local lymph nodes or to treat tumors that cannot be removed.

Radiation may be used preoperatively to reduce the size of a tumor. Postoperative radiation may be indicated to destroy malignant cells not removed by surgery. Radiation may also be used to slow the growth of malignant tumors.

Radiation may be delivered externally or internally. External therapy may be directed toward superficial lesions or may be targeted to deeper structures within the body. Normal cells are better able to recover from the damage caused by radiation than are cancer cells. Because malignant cells lack the capacity for repair, more cancer cells than normal cells are damaged by radiation. However, normal cells do have a maximum dose of radiation that they can tolerate before irreversible damage occurs. Treatment plans are designed to minimize the radiation dose to normal structures. Meticulous planning and recording of the dose are essential.

External Radiation Therapy

When external radiation is planned, the specific area on the body is marked to indicate the port at which external radiation will be directed. These markings must not be washed off. If the area becomes wet while bathing, the skin should be patted with an absorbent towel. The nurse should help the patient to understand the need to protect this area. The nurse should also instruct the patient to avoid the use of any ointments, lotions, or powder on this area. The physician may approve specific lotions or creams for drying skin. The patient should be told to protect the radiated area from direct sunlight and to avoid applications of heat or cold because these would increase erythema, drying, and pruritus of the skin, which is common over an irradiated area.

A diet high in protein and calories and a fluid intake of 2 or 3 quarts per day must be encouraged. The person undergoing radiation therapy should be assured that lethargy and fatigue are not uncommon during treatment, and that frequent rest periods are helpful.

Some 60% of all people with cancer are treated with radiation therapy at some point. For many of these, radiation therapy is the only therapy needed to destroy the cancer.

Internal Radiation Therapy

General principles to be followed when caring for the patient treated with internal radiation are the following:

1. Assemble materials and plan ahead to provide several nursing interventions at the same time upon entering the patient's room.
2. Stand at the greatest distance away from the site where an internal radiation device is in the patient's body.
3. Limit the time needed for close contact near the irradiated site. If direct, prolonged care is needed, nurses should wear a lead apron.

Unsealed internal radiation is administered intravenously or orally, so that it is distributed throughout the patient's body. Special precautions must be taken to prevent exposure to radiation from direct contact with the patient or any body tissue or fluid (Box 17-3).

Radioactive implant (brachytherapy) is the insertion of **sealed radioactive materials** temporarily or permanently into hollow cavities, within body tissues, or on the body's surface. The radioactive source delivers a specific radiation dose continuously over hours or days. A highly concentrated radiation dose is delivered in or near a tumor. This technique is generally combined with a course of external radiation therapy to increase the dosage to a specific site. Certain organs, such as the uterus and vagina, are natural receptacles for the placement of an applicator that can be loaded with radioactive material. Radioactive needles, wires, seeds, beads, or catheters may be inserted directly into tumor tissue.

Children younger than 18 years of age and pregnant women should not be allowed to visit implant patients. Approved visitors should be advised regarding the recommended limits on length of stay and on safe distance from the patient. Visitors shall be instructed to limit visits to 10 minutes when with the patient, always standing as far away from the pelvic area as possible.

When cancer of the cervix is treated with the use of an applicator containing a radioactive material, the applicator is placed in the vagina. The following special nursing measures are indicated:

1. Place "Radiation in Use" sign on the patient's door.
2. Prevent dislodgment. Keep the patient on strict bed rest. Instruct the patient not to turn from side to side or onto the abdomen. Do not raise the head of the bed more than 45 degrees.
3. Do not give a complete bed bath while the applicator is in place, and do not bathe the patient below the waist. Do not change bed linen unless necessary.

4. Encourage the patient to do active range-of-motion (ROM) exercises with both arms and mild foot and leg exercises to minimize the hazards of immobility. Patient will wear antiembolism stockings (thromboembolic disease [TED] hose) or pneumatic compression boots.
5. Monitor vital signs every 4 hours, observing for elevations in temperature, pulse, and respirations. A temperature greater than 100°F (37.7° C) should be reported to the physician.
6. Observe for and report the development of any rash or skin eruption, excessive vaginal bleeding, or vaginal discharge.
7. Keep accurate I&O record. Encourage a fluid intake of at least 3 L daily. An indwelling catheter will be in place to reduce the size of the bladder and decrease the effects of radiation on the bladder. Check to be sure it is draining well.
8. Serve diet as ordered—usually a low-residue diet to minimize peristalsis and bowel movement, which might lead to dislodgment of the applicator.
9. Check position of applicator every 4 hours.
10. Keep long-handled forceps and a special lead container in the patient's room for use by the radiologist, should the implant become dislodged. Never touch a dislodged applicator or any other materials that have fallen out of the patient. These may contain the radioactive sources. Any bed linens, dressings, or pads that have been changed for the patient must be checked with a radiation survey meter before they are removed from the patient's room.
11. After the applicator is removed, the indwelling catheter is usually removed, and a douche and enema are generally prescribed.
12. Precautions are no longer needed after removal of the applicator. Encourage ambulation and gradual resumption of activities.
13. Sexual intercourse is usually delayed for 7 to 10 days.
14. Instruct the patient to notify the physician of nausea, vomiting, diarrhea, frequent or painful urination, or a temperature more than 100° F (37.7° C).

The nurse should follow the principles of time limits and safe distance when caring for the patient with a radiation implant. Directions supplied by the hospital related to the radioactive substance being used should be followed. Generally, it is recommended that the nurse spend no more than 10 minutes at a time in the room of a patient with an implant. The nurse should stand at least 6 feet away from the patient when not giving direct care, and he or she should stand as far away from the pelvic area as possible when the cervical implant is in use.

Box 17-3 *Instructions for Nursing Interventions for Patients Treated with (Unsealed Internal Radiation) I¹³¹ for Thyroid Cancer*

Nurses should spend as little time as possible for ordinary nursing care. The patient must be as self-sufficient as possible. The patient is radioactive and exposes the nurse to radiation while caring for the patient. The radioactive I¹³¹ leaves the patient through urine and perspiration. Therefore the patient contaminates everything he or she touches and can spread contamination to the nurse in this way.

PRECAUTIONS THAT WILL REDUCE EXPOSURE TO THE NURSE

a. Limit the time spent in the room. Work quickly and only enter as necessary.
b. When in the room, maintain as much distance from the patient as possible. A few feet of distance makes a lot of difference in the amount of exposure to the nurse.
c. Wear shoe covers and disposable, fluidproof gloves, and avoid contact with all surfaces in the room.
d. When leaving the room:
   1. Wash hands with gloves on.
   2. Remove one shoe cover at the door, step that foot out, and drop that shoe cover into the trash.
   3. Remove the other shoe cover and step that foot out and drop that shoe cover into the trash.
   4. Remove gloves and drop them into the trash.
   5. Do not remove shoe covers or gloves from the room. All trash must stay in the room.
e. Always wear the dosimeter while in the room and log the exposure you receive at each visit. The dosimeter, log, and instructions are kept outside the door.
   1. No visitors are allowed.
   2. The patient is confined to the room.
   3. Nothing is to leave the room unless checked for contamination and released by the radiation safety officer (RSO)/designee. All trash and laundry are to remain in the special containers.
   4. Pregnant nursing or nuclear medicine personnel will not enter the area.
   5. Shoe covers and fluidproof disposable gloves (nonsterile type) are to be worn when entering the room. Gowns will be available.
   6. The dosimeter is to be worn in the room, and exposure is to be logged when leaving the room.
   7. All clothes and bed linens used by the patient should be placed in the laundry bag provided and should be left in the patient's room to be checked by the RSO/designee.
   8. No housekeeping is allowed until the room is officially released.
   9. Food is delivered only by nursing. It is delivered to the door and picked up by the patient. Mail, flowers, and other items are delivered in the same way.
   10. Whenever possible, only disposable items may be used in the care of these patients. These

items should be placed in the designated waste container. Contact the RSO/designee for proper disposal of the contents of the designated waste container.
11. Except in emergencies, urine collection or blood draws are not allowed after the patient has been dosed with I¹³¹. The urine and blood are radioactive.
12. The patient is to flush the toilet three times after each use, and males should sit down to void.
13. If the nurse helps to collect the excreta, disposable gloves should be worn. Afterward, hands should be washed with the gloves on and again after the gloves are removed. The gloves should be placed in the designated waste container for disposal by the RSO/designee.
14. Utmost precautions must be taken to see that no urine or vomitus is spilled on the floor or the bed. If any part of the patient's room is suspected to be contaminated, notify the RSO/designee in the Nuclear Medicine Department.
15. If a nurse, attendant, or anyone else knows or suspects that his or her skin or clothing, including shoes, is contaminated, notify the RSO/designee immediately. This person should remain in an area adjacent to the patient's room and should not walk about the hospital. If the hands become contaminated, wash them immediately with soap and water.
16. If a therapy patient should need emergency surgery or should die, notify the RSO or the Nuclear Medicine Department immediately.
17. Vomiting within 24 hours after oral administration, urinary incontinence, or excessive sweating within the first 48 hours may result in contamination of linen and floor. In any such situation, or if radioactive urine or feces is spilled during collection, call the RSO/designee. Meanwhile, handle all contaminated material with disposable gloves and avoid spreading contamination.
18. All vomitus must be kept in the patient's room for disposal by the RSO/designee only if the patient has vomited over the bed or the surrounding area. Otherwise, it will be flushed down the toilet with at least three volumes of water or more after it. Feces need not be routinely saved unless ordered on the chart. The same toilet should be used by the patient at all times, and it should be well flushed (at least three times).
19. The patient may not be discharged without prior approval of the RSO/designee. The room may not be remade, used, or entered by unauthorized people until released by the RSO. Nothing may leave the room unless it is checked for contamination and released by the RSO.

Courtesy Great Plains Regional Medical Center Nuclear Medicine Department, North Platte, Neb.

CHEMOTHERAPY

Chemotherapy drugs are used to reduce or slow the growth of metastatic cancer. Most chemotherapeutic agents work by interfering with the cells' ability to multiply or reproduce. Drugs that interfere with a cell's **replication** (duplicating or reproducing) process damage the cell and cause cellular death. Both malignant and normal cells are affected by chemotherapy. Cells that multiply rapidly are affected the most, such as cells of the **hematopoietic system,** the **hair follicles,** and the **GI system.** Most of the side effects from chemotherapeutic agents result from the destruction of normal cells in the above systems. Common side effects are listed below (Medications: Chemotherapy table).

Hematopoietic System

Leukopenia. Leukopenia (reduction in the number of circulating white blood cells due to depression of the bone marrow), a common problem for patients receiving chemotherapy, can lead to life-threatening infections. Normal value for white blood cells (WBCs) is

 MEDICATIONS | *Chemotherapy*

DRUG CLASS	MODE OF ACTION	DISEASE FOR WHICH COMMONLY USED	COMMON SIDE EFFECTS
ALKYLATING AGENTS			
Cyclophosphamide (Cytoxan)	Interfere with DNA replication, cell-cycle nonspecific	Leukemia, breast, lymphoma, lung, ovarian, myeloma	Myelosuppression, alopecia, hemorrhagic cystitis, nausea, vomiting, cardiotoxicity
Cisplatin (Platinol)	Interfere with DNA replication, cell-cycle nonspecific	Testicular, ovarian, lung, cervical, head, and neck	Nephrotoxicity, neurotoxicity, nausea, vomiting, ototoxicity
Carboplatin (Paraplatin)	Interfere with DNA replication, cell-cycle nonspecific	Ovarian, leukemia, lung	Myelosuppression, nausea, vomiting, nephrotoxicity, neurotoxicity
Chlorambucil (Leukeran)	Interfere with DNA replication, cell-cycle nonspecific	Lymphoma, chronic lymphocytic leukemia (CLL)	Myelosuppression, sterility, stomatitis, pulmonary infiltrates
ANTITUMOR ANTIBIOTICS			
Bleomycin (Blenoxane)	Inhibit DNA and RNA synthesis, cell-cycle nonspecific	Testicular, cervical, Hodgkin's, lymphoma	Anaphylaxis, nausea, vomiting, rash, pulmonary fibrosis, alopecia, stomatitis
Doxorubicin (Adriamycin)	Inhibit DNA and RNA synthesis, cell-cycle nonspecific	Breast, endometrial, leukemia, Hodgkin's melanoma, lymphoma	Myelosuppression, cardiotoxicity, extravasation, nausea, vomiting, alopecia, stomatitis, red urine (24 to 48 hours)
Mitoxantrone (Novantrone)	Inhibit DNA and RNA synthesis, cell-cycle nonspecific	Hodgkin's, lymphoma, leukemia, breast cancer	Myelosuppression, cardiotoxicity, nausea, vomiting, blue urine (immediate to 24 hours)
ANTIMETABOLITES			
Cytarabine (Ara-C, Cytosar)	Damage cell in 's' phase, cell-cycle specific	Leukemia, lymphoma	Myelosuppression, neurotoxicity, rash, nausea, vomiting, stomatitis, alopecia, anaphylaxis
Fludarabine (Fludara)	Damage cell in 's' phase, cell-cycle specific	Leukemia (CLL, hairy cell), low-grade lymphoma	Myelosuppression, CNS toxicity, visual disturbance, nausea and vomiting, renal damage (tumor lysis syndrome)
Fluorouracil (5-FU)	Damage cell in 's' phase, cell-cycle specific	Breast, colorectal, liver, endometrial, esophageal, pancreatic, bladder	Myelosuppression, nausea, vomiting, stomatitis, alopecia, diarrhea
Gemcitabine (Gemzar)	Damage cell in 's' phase, cell-cycle specific	Pancreatic, lung	Myelosuppression, fatigue
Methotrexate (MXT, amethopterin)	Damage cell in 's' phase, cell-cycle specific	Breast, lymphoma, leukemia, bladder, head and neck, esophageal	Myelosuppression, diarrhea, oral and GI ulcerations, pulmonary infiltrates, nausea and vomiting

Continued

MEDICATIONS | *Chemotherapy—cont'd*

DRUG CLASS	MODE OF ACTION	DISEASE FOR WHICH COMMONLY USED	COMMON SIDE EFFECTS
HORMONAL AGENTS			
Corticosteroids (Decadron, Solucortef, Solumedrol, Medrol, prednisone)	Alter hormonal environment that promotes cancer growth	Used in many chemotherapy disease protocols	Fluid and electrolyte disturbances, neuromuscular imbalances, changes in appetite and energy, requires glucose and insulin adjustment
Megestrol (Megace)	Alter hormonal environment that promotes cancer growth	Breast, prostate	Menstrual changes, hot flashes, nausea, vomiting, headache, weight gain, edema
Leuprolide (Lupron)	Alter hormonal environment that promotes cancer growth	Prostate	Impotence, testicular atrophy, hot flashes, gynecomastia, peripheral edema
Tamoxifen (Nolvadex)	Competes with estrogen for binding sites in breast and other tissues	Breast	Vaginal bleeding, hot flashes, rash, hypercalcemia, peripheral edema
VINCA ALKALOIDS			
Etoposide (VP-16)	Inhibit cell division, cell-cycle specific	Lung, testicular, leukemia, lymphoma, small cell carcinoma of the lung	Myelosuppression, nausea, vomiting, diarrhea, fever, hypotension, phlebitis, alopecia
Vinblastine (Velban)	Inhibit cell division, cell-cycle specific	Testicular, Hodgkin's, lung, lymphoma, bladder, renal	Myelosuppression, extravasation, nausea, vomiting, alopecia, loss of deep tendon reflex
Vincristine (Oncovin)	Inhibit cell division, cell-cycle specific	Leukemia (acute lymphocytic leukemia, chronic myelogenous leukemia)	Extravasation, alopecia, stomatitis, constipation, peripheral neuropathy, optic atrophy
Vinorelbine (Navelbine)	Inhibit cell division, cell-cycle specific	Breast, lung, Hodgkin's, head and neck	Myelosuppression, alopecia, injection site reaction (phlebitis), nausea, anorexia, constipation, peripheral neuropathy
MISCELLANEOUS ANTINEOPLASTIC AGENTS			
Asparaginase (Elspar)	Cell-cycle specific ('g' phase)	Leukemia (ALL)	Nausea, vomiting, chills, headache, CNS depression, abdominal pain, anaphylaxis
Paclitaxel (Taxol)	Mitotic inhibitor	Breast, lung, ovarian	Myelosuppression, dyspnea, hypotension, alopecia, cardiotoxicity, peripheral neuropathy anaphylaxis
Taxotere (Docetaxel)	Miotic inhibitor	Breast, lung, ovarian	Myelosuppression, fluid retention, mucositis, phlebitis, vomiting, diarrhea, anaphylaxis
Topotecan (HC) (Hycantin)	Interrupts DNA synthesis	Lung, breast, esophagus, tumor, lymphoma	Myelosuppression, nausea, vomiting, diarrhea, fever, fatigue, alopecia, elevated liver enzymes
Irinotecan—CPT-11 (Camptosar)	Interrupts DNA synthesis	Colorectal, pancreatic	Severe diarrhea, myelosuppression, nausea and vomiting

5000 to 10,000/mm³. A total WBC less than 4000/mm³ is leukopenia. Lack of neutrophils, the type of WBC most often suppressed in the differential WBC, is called **neutropenia.** Normal value for neutrophils is 60% to 70% or 3000 to 7000/mm³. Neutropenia is a neutrophil count less than 1000/mm³. Severe neutropenia is associated with a neutrophil count less than 500/mm³. Without enough neutrophils, the body's first line of defense collapses, opening the way for pneumonia, septicemia, or other potentially overwhelming infections.

The nurse needs to protect the patient against pathogens, monitor the patient for signs of infection, and respond aggressively if an infection occurs (Safety Considerations box). The patient's vital signs should be monitored every 4 hours and the physician notified if temperature starts to rise. A temperature of 100° F (38° C) or more is considered a sign of impending infection.

Fresh flowers or live plants should be discouraged in the room of the patient with neutropenia. Mites, gnats, and other microscopic organisms could be a potential source of infection for the patient. The patient's diet should also be monitored. Fresh fruits and vegetables should be avoided because of the presence of microscopic pathogens in uncooked produce—this is sometimes referred to as a neutropenic diet.

The nurse should take the following systematic approach to assessing the patient for infection.

Assessing the mouth. Stomatitis, an inflammation of the oral mucosa, is one of the most common complications of chemotherapy and can easily lead to severe swallowing problems and systemic infections. Use a penlight and tongue blade to look for lesions, ulcers, or white plaque.

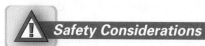

Safety Considerations

The Patient with Neutropenia

- Monitor for fever and neutrophil count to identify signs of and potential for infection.
- Evaluate for presence of chills. Take vital signs every 4 hours because fever may be only indication of infection and septic shock.
- Report temperature elevations >100.4° F (38° C) to health care provider immediately in order to promptly initiate antibiotic therapy due to the rapidly lethal effects of infection.
- Institute good handwashing technique with antiseptic solution for all people in contact with patient; place patient in private room; limit and/or screen visitors and hospital staff members with colds or potentially communicable illness to prevent transmission of harmful pathogens to patient.
- Teach patient necessary personal hygiene techniques, (e.g., handwashing, oral care, skin hygiene, pulmonary hygiene, and potential infection risks.)
- Avoid invasive procedures to the greatest extent possible (e.g., venipuncture, urinary catheter).
- Administer hematopoietic growth factors (e.g., G-CSF Neupogen]) to increase patient's WBC count and reduce infection risk during periods of neutropenia.
- Maintain neutropenic diet (avoid fresh fruits and vegetables because of presence of microscopic pathogens in uncooked produce.)

Teach the patient the importance of performing regular, but gentle, mouth care. Have the patient use a soft toothbrush and rinse the mouth with normal saline or sodium bicarbonate solution every 2 to 4 hours. A sponge-tipped applicator (Toothette) may help prevent bleeding gums, a common adverse effect of chemotherapy and radiation.

To reduce the risk of an oral *Candida* infection, the physician may order prophylactic antifungal medications such as an oral nystatin (Mycostatin) suspension, clotrimazole (Lotrimin) lozenges, or fluconazole (Diflucan). A soft or liquid diet may also be ordered

Assessing the skin. A rash or eruption may indicate that the patient has an infection or is predisposed to one.

Bacteria may flourish in skinfolds, such as in the groin and axillae, so clean these areas twice a day with soap and water. Water-soluble moisturizers may be used to keep the patient's skin from drying. To prevent cuts, advise the patient to shave with an electric razor.

Vascular access sites are common gateways to infection. Central and peripheral intravenous (IV) catheters should all be monitored carefully. Check for edema, drainage, erythema, or pain around catheter entry sites.

Organisms can also grow along catheter tracts and infect the blood, resulting in septicemia. Signs and symptoms of a catheter tract infection include tenderness around the catheter site and referred pain in the shoulder.

Administer oral drugs whenever possible. Try to avoid subcutaneous (subQ) or intramuscular (IM) injections, because they can cause abscesses in patients with neutropenia. Excessive bleeding is also a risk for these patients because of the potential for associated decreases in platelets and other formed elements in the blood.

Puncturing the skin is sometimes unavoidable, as when the patient needs a bone marrow biopsy. After a biopsy, carefully assess the site, swab it with an antibacterial solution (such as povidone-iodine [Betadine]), and apply an occlusive dressing until the skin heals.

Assessing for pulmonary function. Be aware that many neutropenic patients with lung infections do not have common signs and symptoms, such as sputum production or infiltrates demonstrable on chest radiographs. Therefore, be alert for other indications of an impending infection, including changes in lung sounds, respiratory rate and rhythm, and breathing effort. The patient may also complain of pain during inspiration or expiration.

To help prevent a lung infection, encourage the patient to be as active as able and to perform deep-breathing and coughing exercises. Use of an incentive spirometer can help by maximizing ventilatory capacity.

Assessing urinary and bowel function. Changes in urinary function can also warn of infection in a neutropenic patient. Assess for decreased urinary output, changes in the urine's odor or color, hematuria, or glycosuria—all possible signs of infection. The patient may also complain of urinary frequency, urgency, or pain.

To reduce the risk of urinary infection, avoid bladder catheterization. If catheterization is absolutely indicated, follow strict aseptic technique when inserting the catheter and perform catheter care according to the agency's guidelines.

Also routinely assess the patient's bowel function. Assess stool samples for color, consistency, and the presence of blood, and ask the patient to report any changes in bowel habits.

Does the patient need to strain when defecating? If so, the physician may prescribe a stool softener such as docusate (Colace). Straining can cause ulcerations or fissures in the rectum, creating ports of entry for bacteria. Avoid enemas, rectal medications, and rectal thermometers, which can break the mucosal lining. Be aware that neutropenia predisposes a patient to rectal abscesses. If the patient complains of perirectal pain, the physician should be notified immediately.

A breakthrough in treating patients with neutropenia is commercially made colony-stimulating factors (CSFs), the only therapy that can actually prevent or manage neutropenia. The two types of CSFs are granulocyte colony-stimulating factors (G-CSF) (filgrastim [Neupogen]) and granulocyte-macrophage colony-stimulating factors (GM-CSF) (sargramostim [Leukine or Prokine]). These CSFs are given subcutaneously or intravenously.

Although CSFs are extremely expensive, they are used prophylactically for patients at increased risk for neutropenia, such as those with a history of developing severe or prolonged neutropenia after chemotherapy.

Anemia. Anemia is a reduction in the number of circulating red blood cells, hemoglobin, and/or volume of packed red blood cells (RBCs) (hematocrit) due to depression of the bone marrow. Normal values are as follows:

	Male	Female
Erythrocytes (RBCs)	4.7 to 6.1 million/ mm³	4.2 to 5.4 million/ mm³
Hemoglobin (Hgb)	14-18 g/dL	12-16 g/dL
Hematocrit (Hct)	42%-52%	37%-47%

Hemoglobin levels of 10 to 14 g/dL indicate mild anemia, 6 to 10 g/dL indicate moderate anemia, and less than 6 g/dL severe anemia. Fatigue is a major problem for persons with anemia because of the decreased oxygenation to tissues from the decreased hemoglobin. For the hospitalized patient, care should be planned to balance activities and rest to prevent increased oxygen expenditure and hypoxemia. Persons at home need to plan activities of daily living (ADLs) to allow rest periods.

Recombinant human erythropoietin, or epoetin alfa (EPO; Epogen, Procrit), was initially approved by the U.S. Food and Drug Administration (FDA) in 1987 for management of chronic anemia associated with end-stage renal disease. In 1993, the FDA approval was expanded to include management of chemotherapy-related anemia. EPO is given subcutaneously or intravenously.

Transfusion of RBCs is indicated if there is evidence of cardiac decompensation or if low hemoglobin levels are combined with low platelet counts. Replacement of circulating red cell mass to improve oxygen-carrying capacity should be accomplished by transfusion of packed RBCs. This provides for more efficient use of blood components and less risk of volume overload.

Thrombocytopenia. Thrombocytopenia is a reduction in the number of circulating platelets, due to the depression of the bone marrow. Normal platelet values are 150,000 to 400,000/mm³. When the platelet count is less than 20,000/mm³, spontaneous bleeding can occur. Platelet transfusions may be necessary.

The following are patient teaching measures to prevent injury and hemorrhage due to decreased platelets:
- Use soft toothbrush or swab for mouth care.
- Keep mouth clean and free of debris.
- Avoid intrusions into rectum (such as rectal medications or enemas).
- Use electric shaver.
- Apply direct pressure for 5 to 10 minutes if any bleeding occurs.
- Avoid contact sports, elective surgery, and tooth extraction.
- Avoid picking or blowing nose forcefully.
- Avoid trauma, falls, bumps, and cuts.
- Avoid use of aspirin or aspirin preparations.
- Use adequate lubrication and gentleness during sexual intercourse.

Integumentary System

Alopecia. Alopecia is loss of hair due to the destruction of hair follicles. It may occur by two mechanisms. If the hair roots are atrophied, alopecia occurs readily. The hair falls out either spontaneously or during hair combing, often in large clumps. If the hair shaft is constricted because of atrophy or necrosis, the hair will break off very near the scalp. The root remains in the scalp and a patchy, thinning pattern of hair loss occurs. Hair loss may also occur on other parts of the body. Loss of leg, arm, pubic, axillary, and facial hair is seen less often, although loss of eyebrows and eyelashes may occur.

The pattern and extent of hair loss cannot be accurately predicted for a given patient. When treatment is given with a drug known to cause alopecia, the patient needs to be told that severe hair loss can begin within a few days or weeks of treatment and that partial or complete baldness can quickly ensue. Drug-induced alopecia is never permanent. The patient may experience a change in hair color or texture when regrowth occurs. Occasionally, hair growth may return while chemotherapy treatment continues. Given this perspective, coupled with the goal of disease control or cure, most patients tolerate the hair loss with minimal distress. However, many patients have difficulty adjusting to the change in body image due to hair loss. The hair is very much a part of the self-image.

To meet the patient's needs, an education program, written materials, and educational sessions with a hair stylist are valuable services for the patient. The patient should be informed about health care measures for scalp protection, such as the use of gentle shampoos; avoidance of hair dryers, curling irons, permanents, and hair coloring; protecting the scalp in winter and summer (cold or heat loss); and wearing protective covering when outdoors. The patient with long or thick hair may wish to trim or cut hair short to delay hair loss as long as possible. Sincere concern and emotional support should be provided for the patient.

Gastrointestinal System

Stomatitis. Stomatitis is a mouth inflammation due to destruction of normal cells of the oral cavity. It may range from an erythema of the oral mucosa to mild or severe ulceration. Methotrexate, 5-fluorouracil (5-FU), doxorubicin, dactinomycin, and bleomycin are the chemotherapeutic drugs that most frequently cause stomatitis. Patients may also develop a superimposed *Candida* infection of the mouth and esophagus, and oral nystatin is usually prescribed. Good mouth care is important.

Viscous lidocaine (Xylocaine) is used when stomatitis becomes intolerable to the patient. Light topical application can decrease pain so the patient may eat and drink. Usually a soft or liquid diet is encouraged to help maintain nutritional status.

Nausea, vomiting, and diarrhea. These are disorders of the GI tract due to the breakdown of normal GI cells. Nausea and vomiting are among the most uncomfortable and distressing side effects of chemotherapy. The onset and duration vary greatly among patients and with the drug given. For the ambulatory patient, nausea may interfere with the ability to continue daily work. Persistent vomiting may result in fluid and electrolyte imbalance, general weakness, and weight loss. Decline of nutritional status renders the patient more susceptible to infection and perhaps less able to tolerate therapy. Such physiologic symptoms can accompany or precipitate psychological responses that might include depression and withdrawal. Every effort must be made to minimize chemotherapy-induced nausea and vomiting.

Antiemetics vary in success. Tetrahydrocannabinol (THC) taken in pill form produces an antiemetic effect in some patients who have not benefited from the commonly prescribed prochlorperazine (Compazine). Metoclopramide (Reglan), ondansetron (Zofran), and granisetron (Kytril) are often helpful for people receiving chemotherapy, and lorazepam (Ativan) is often effective in producing a relaxed state during which an individual is less sensitive to nausea-inducing stimuli (Medications: Symptom Control of Cancer Treatment table).

It is imperative that patients receive antiemetic drugs to control the side effects of nausea and vomiting while undergoing chemotherapy. The patient may receive antiemetics orally, intramuscularly, rectally, or intravenously, as well as via pumps like those used in patient-controlled analgesia.

The development and use of the 5-HT$_3$ antagonists (ondansetron, granisetron) has resulted in effective antiemetic therapy. Prevention of nausea and vomiting will increase patient comfort as well as decrease or eliminate anxiety and fear. These antiemetics are given before chemotherapy to prevent nausea and vomiting as well as after chemotherapy as directed by the physician. The side effects are mild, and the drugs can be used safely in the outpatient setting. Metoclopramide (Reglan), a dopamine antagonist, has been proven effective in controlling mild to moderate nausea and vomiting. Metoclopramide blocks dopamine receptors in the chemoreceptor trigger zone of the central nervous system, stimulates motility of the upper GI tract, and accelerates gastric emptying (Medications table).

Changes in bowel habits commonly occur but usually do not require intervention. If diarrhea becomes marked or persistent, an antidiarrheal medication such as diphenoxylate with atropine (Lomotil) may be prescribed.

Combinations of chemotherapy agents, as well as chemotherapy combined with other treatments, have increased the number of cures, remissions, and palliative outcomes.

Many of the problems experienced by people undergoing chemotherapy are the same as those that may result from radiation therapy (depending on the target site and amount of radiation). The nurse must help the patient realize that some of the problems are the result of therapy and not a sign that the cancer is increasing.

MEDICATIONS | *Symptom Control of Cancer Treatment*

MEDICATION	TRADE NAME	ACTION	SIDE EFFECTS	NURSING IMPLICATIONS
Ondansetron	Zofran	Antiemetic	Headache, diarrhea, constipation, abdominal pain, transient increase in aspartate aminotransferase (AST) or alanine aminotransferase (ALT)	Dilute intravenous dose with D$_5$W or NaCl and give total dose (approximately 32 mg) 30 minutes before chemotherapy. Give 8 mg orally before chemotherapy and three times a day for 2 days.
Granisetron	Kytril	Antiemetic	Headache, constipation, somnolence, diarrhea, mild changes in blood pressure	Administer dose over 5-minute period, beginning 30 minutes before chemotherapy. Know that granisetron (Kytril) is given once a day in a 5-minute infusion, or give 2 mg by mouth 1 hour before chemotherapy and 1 mg bid × 2 days.
Metoclopramide	Reglan	Antiemetic	Drowsiness, extrapyramidal reactions, restlessness, dysrhythmias, anxiety	Administer IV dose 30 minutes before administration of chemotherapeutic agent. po: Administer doses 30 min before meals and at bedtime.
Prochlorperazine	Compazine	Antiemetic	Extrapyramidal symptoms, orthostatic hypotension, ocular changes (blurred vision), dry mouth, constipation, urine retention, photosensitivity	Use cautiously with other CNS depressants (alcohol) and medications that decrease blood pressure, as well as patients with liver disease. Decrease dose in older adults. Do not exceed recommended dose. Protect from light.
Diphenoxylate/ atropine	Lomotil	Antidiarrheal	Sedation, dizziness, dry mouth, urinary retention, rash	Watch for physical dependence. Know that it should work within 48 hours. Give naloxone as antidote for respiratory depression.
Morphine	Roxanol, MS Contin	Opioid analgesic	Decreased respiratory rate, euphoria, seizures, physical dependence, hypotension, bradycardia, miosis, drowsiness, dizziness, urinary retention, constipation, rash	Use cautiously with other CNS depressants (alcohol). Monitor respirations, heart rate, and mental status closely. Have naloxone available as antidote. Do not give sustained-release tablets for acute pain.

MEDICATIONS | *Symptom Control of Cancer Treatment—cont'd*

MEDICATION	TRADE NAME	ACTION	SIDE EFFECTS	NURSING IMPLICATIONS
Hydromorphone	Dilaudid	Opioid analgesic	Decreased respiratory rate, euphoria, seizures, physical dependence, hypotension, bradycardia, miosis, drowsiness, dizziness, urinary retention, constipation, rash	Use cautiously with other CNS depressants (alcohol). Monitor respirations, heart rate, and mental status closely. Have naloxone available as antidote. Do not give sustained-release tablets for acute pain. Have Dilaudid-HP (10 mg/mL) available for chronic pain.
Naproxen	Naprosyn, Anaprox	Nonsteroidal antiinflammatory agent (NSAID)	Agranulocytosis, headache, dizziness, drowsiness, peripheral edema, visual disturbances, GI upset (occult blood loss and peptic ulcers), prolonged bleeding time, tinnitus	Know that concurrent use of alcohol, acetylsalicylic acid, and steroids will increase chance of GI bleeding. Know that it may interact with warfarin sodium (Coumadin). Avoid use in patient allergic to acetylsalicylic acid. Give with food. Advise patient that it may take 4 weeks to show benefit.
Diphenhydramine	Benadryl	Antihistamine May also be used for antiemetic and sedation purposes	Drowsiness, dry mouth	Anticholinergic effect; used as an antiemetic.
Metoclopramide	Reglan	Antiemetic	Restlessness, dry mouth	Delayed gastric emptying, gastroesophageal reflux, antiemetic.
Amitriptyline	Elavil	Tricyclic antidepressant	Tremors, orthostatic hypertension, urinary retention	Used in combination with narcotics in neuropathies and postherpetic neuralgia (especially with burning pain). Therapeutic effect takes 2 to 3 weeks.
Dexamethasone	Decadron	Antiinflammatory and immune modifier	Hyperglycemia, mood swings, depression	Effective as antiemetic in chemotherapy: immunosuppression, palliation of selected neoplasms.
Lorazepam	Ativan	Antianxiety agent Antiemetic	Drowsiness, headache, diarrhea, respiratory depression	Smoking decreases effectiveness. Decreases nausea, especially when given before and during chemotherapy.

Nursing diagnoses and interventions for the patient undergoing chemotherapy include but are not limited to the following:

Nursing Diagnoses	Nursing Interventions
Impaired tissue integrity: oral mucous membrane, related to stomatitis (inflammation of the mouth); xerostomia (decreased salivation)	Assist with frequent, careful oral hygiene and hydration; use very soft toothbrush. Provide meticulous mouth care. Give soothing oral lozenges; use ice chips and frequent sips of ice water; avoid hot beverages; use lip balm for dryness.
Imbalanced nutrition: less than body requirements, related to anorexia (from changes in taste and smell); nausea/vomiting; dysphagia (difficulty in swallowing); aspiration; diarrhea; malabsorption; cachexia (general ill health and malnutrition, marked by weakness and emaciation, usually associated with a serious disease such as cancer)	Provide adequate, easily digestible, soft, bland diet; avoid spicy foods. Keep room free of odors and clutter. Give small, frequent, highly nutritional meals to meet the extra demands created by energy used by malignant cells; allow extra time to eat.
Risk for infection, related to weakened immune system; leukopenia	Protect against infections, especially from other people. Avoid crowds. Observe and promptly report to physician any signs of inflammation at injection sites or insertion sites of any peripheral or central IV lines; report any temperature greater than 100° F. Use sterile technique whenever possible. Initiate reverse isolation as indicated. Monitor temperature, leukocyte count. Discourage fresh-cut flowers. Avoid indwelling catheters and performing rectal procedures, or examinations. Administer antibiotics as prescribed.

Tumor Lysis Syndrome

Tumor lysis syndrome (TLS) is an oncologic emergency with rapid lysis of malignant cells.

Etiology/pathophysiology. Tumor lysis syndrome may occur spontaneously in patients with inordinately high tumor burdens. However, it is most commonly caused as a result of chemotherapy or irradiation treatment–related malignant cell death. It is most frequently associated with chemotherapy. It may occur anywhere from 24 hours to 7 days after antineoplastic therapy is initiated. Patients most at risk are those who have large tumor cell burdens such as with high-grade lymphomas or markedly elevated WBC level (acute leukemias). TLS is also seen in chronic lymphocytic leukemia in blast crisis and metastatic breast cancer.

The syndrome develops when chemotherapy or irradiation causes the destruction (or lysis) of a large number of rapidly dividing malignant cells.

As malignant cells are lysed, intracellular contents are rapidly released into the bloodstream. This results in high levels of potassium (hyperkalemia), phosphate (hyperphosphatemia), and uric acid (hyperuricemia). Hyperkalemia, hyperphosphatemia with secondary hypocalcemia, and hyperuricemia all put the patient at risk for renal failure and alterations in cardiac function.

Clinical manifestations. Early signs may include nausea, vomiting, anorexia, and diarrhea; these may be accompanied by muscle weakness and cramping. Later signs may progress to tetany, paresthesias, seizures, anuria, and cardiac arrest.

Diagnostic tests. Tumor lysis syndrome is diagnosed by observation of the signs and symptoms and by confirmation of abnormal laboratory values. Early symptoms of tumor lysis syndrome may not be readily apparent, and clinical manifestations appear rapidly; the syndrome is most frequently detected by abnormalities in blood chemistry. Serum potassium, phosphate, calcium, and uric acid are diagnostic. Other important values include serum creatinine, blood urea nitrogen (BUN), and urine pH. Metabolic abnormalities associated with tumor lysis syndrome include hyperkalemia, hyperphosphatemia with secondary hypocalcemia, and hyperuricemia.

Medical management. The best way to treat TLS is to prevent it by recognizing the patient population who is at risk and initiating prophylactic measures before antineoplastic therapy begins. This includes pretreatment **hydration** to maintain a urinary output of 150 mL/hour. Hydration should begin 24 to 48 hours before treatment and continue for at least 72 hours after treatment. **Diuretics** may be used to promote the excretion of phosphate and uric acid. **Allopurinol** prevents uric acid formation. It is begun a few days before treatment and should be continued for 3 to 5 days after treatment is completed. **Sodium bicarbonate** is used to maintain an alkaline urine (pH >7) to prevent uric acid crystallization. Diuretics are used to prevent volume overload and promote the excretion of potassium in the urine. Cation-exchange resins, such a kayexalate, are used to bind with potassium so it can be excreted through the bowel. **Calcium gluconate** given intravenously is used to correct hypocalcemia. Cardiac monitoring is required. Phosphate-binding gels, such as aluminum hydroxide, are given to form an insoluble complex that is excreted by the bowel. When these measures are not successful, renal dialysis may be necessary.

Nursing interventions. Nursing interventions include the following:

- Identify patients at risk for TLS.
- Initiate hydration 24 to 48 hours before initiating chemotherapy in high-risk patients.
- Administer allopurinol before and during chemotherapy to maintain alkaline urine.
- Assess medications for those that contain phosphate or spare potassium and discuss discontinuation with physician.
- Monitor potassium, phosphorus, calcium, and uric acid levels.
- Assess patient for signs and symptoms of TLS:

  Hyperkalemia: electrocardiographic changes, muscle weakness, twitching, paresthesia, paralysis, muscle cramps, nausea, vomiting, lethargy, and syncope

  Hyperphosphatemia: azotemia, oliguria, hypertension, and renal failure

  Hypocalcemia: electrocardiographic changes (heart block, dysrhythmias, and cardiac arrest), tetany, confusion, and hallucinations

  Hyperuricemia: renal failure, nausea, vomiting, flank pain, gout, and pruritus

- Administer diuretics, sodium bicarbonate, cation-exchange resins, and phosphate-binding gels as appropriate.
- Monitor intake and output and notify physician if urinary output is less than 100 mL/hour.
- Monitor urine pH and maintain at greater than 7 with sodium bicarbonate.
- Prepare the patient and family for dialysis if other measures are not effective.

Prognosis. Successful treatment of TLS depends on preventing renal failure. TLS typically resolves within 7 days, once appropriate treatment is initiated.

Chemotherapy has proven effective in treatment of many cancer patients. Many cancer patients can be cured with chemotherapy, whereas others will experience cancer-free intervals and/or control of cancer pain. Nurses must learn about each drug being administered to anticipate the expected side effects and plan the nursing interventions needed.

There are safety guidelines to be followed by the caregiver in preparing and administering chemotherapeutic agents because they may be absorbed into the skin or inhaled. The major types of chemotherapeutic agents used to treat cancer are given in the Medications table.

BIOTHERAPY

The observation of interactions between the immune system and malignant cells led to the development of therapies that could manipulate this natural process.

Traditionally, this field has been known as immunotherapy. It has led to the modern era of biotherapy. Since the 1980s, biotherapy or biologic therapy, has emerged as an important fourth modality for treating cancer. **Biotherapy** may be defined as treatment with agents derived from biologic sources or affecting biologic responses.

There are three major mechanisms by which **biologic response modifiers** (BRMs) work. The first mechanism increases, restores, or modifies the host defenses against the tumor (CSFs, Neupogen, erythropoietin, GM-CSFs). The second mechanism uses agents that are directly, toxic to tumors (interleukins, IL-2, bacille Calmette-Guérin vaccine [BCG]). The third mechanism modifies the tumor biology (interferons alpha, beta, and gamma).

Most of these therapies are IM or subQ injections and need to be given over an extended time. Compliance and motivation are important considerations when monitoring these patients. Side effects common to BMRs include fatigue, flulike symptoms, leukopenia, nausea, and vomiting.

For health care professionals it is imperative that these therapies be understood to help give the cancer patient the best chance available. These therapies and research are leading to the development of gene therapy today; this will lead to improved cancer therapy in the future.

BONE MARROW TRANSPLANTATION

Bone marrow transplantation is the process of replacing diseased or damaged bone marrow with normally functioning bone marrow. Bone marrow transplants (BMTs) are used in the treatment of a variety of diseases and offer a chance for long-term survival.

Stem cell transplants are being used in the adjuvant setting in some solid tumor cancers, such as high-risk breast cancer. Bone marrow harvests are becoming less frequent because many centers have turned to peripheral stem cell transplants for hematopoietic support after high-dose chemotherapy (Lewis et al, 2004).

Most transplantation bone marrow is obtained by multiple needle aspirations from the posterior iliac crest while the patient is under general or spinal anesthesia. The anterior iliac crest and sternum may also be used. The amount of marrow extracted ranges from 600 to 2500 mL for the average adult. After processing, the marrow is given to the patient intravenously through a transfusion bag, or it can be frozen (cryopreservation). Marrow may be kept for 3 or more years. When the bone marrow is infused, it is via a central line without a filter over 1 to 4 hours.

Bone marrow may be removed from an individual for personal use (autologous, indicating something that has its origin within an individual, especially a factor present in tissues or fluids) at a later time.

An individual may be given allogenic bone marrow (**allogenic,** meaning the transplant came from someone else). Three types of allogenic bone marrow transplants are (1) **syngenic** (donation came from the patient's identical twin), (2) **related** (donation came from a relative, usually a sibling), and (3) **unrelated** (donation came from a nonrelative). The patient is at increased risk for developing infection during the process of transplant because the immune defenses are weakened. These patients are cared for in special bone marrow units so they can be monitored closely.

Effects to prevent infections include protective isolation or laminar airflow rooms; prophylactic systemic antibiotics and antiviral agents (primarily acyclovir); and routine cultures of blood, urine, throat, and stool. Despite these and other interventions, the patient can become septic in hours, with multisystem failure.

Survival after bone marrow transplantation depends on the patient's age, remission, status, and clinical status at the time of transplantation.

Nurses should communicate genuine concern for cancer patients. This includes reinforcing information explained to patients by their physicians regarding the expectations of their specific treatments. Patients may become discouraged by toxic side effects and other problems they experience while undergoing conventional cancer therapies. Nurses should allow extra time to listen to patients with cancer express their feelings and to encourage them to follow the guidelines of conventional medical practice that offer the most hope.

The number of cancers that are being cured is rising daily. About 544,000 Americans (or 4 of 10 patients) who get cancer this year will be alive 5 years after diagnosis, if current therapy is used. The gain from 1 in 3 in the 1960s to 4 in 10 now represents more than 91,000 people each year. "Cured" means that a patient has no evidence of disease and has the same life expectancy as a person who never had cancer.

PERIPHERAL STEM CELL TRANSPLANTATION

An emerging and promising alternative to bone marrow transplantation is peripheral stem cell transplant (PSCT). This procedure is based on the fact that peripheral or circulating stem cells are capable of repopulating the bone marrow. PSCT is a type of transplant that differs from BMT primarily in the method of collection of stem cells. Because there are fewer stem cells in the blood than in the bone marrow, mobilization of stem cells from the bone marrow into the peripheral blood can be done using chemotherapy or hematopoietic growth factors. Common growth factors that are used are GM-CSF and G-CSF.

The donor's blood is collected via pheresis, in which the person is attached to a cell separator machine that removes peripheral stem cells and then returns the blood to the person. This procedure, called **leukapheresis,** usually takes 2 to 4 hours to complete. In autologous transplants the stem cells are purged to kill any cancer cells and then frozen and stored until used for transplantation. Although many of the same steps (harvesting, intensive chemotherapy, reinfusion) of BMT are used in PSCT, the hematologic recovery period in PSCT is shorter, and fewer, less severe complications are seen (Lewis et al, 2004).

ADVANCED CANCER

PAIN MANAGEMENT

Patients with cancer may have pain at any point during the course of the disease and its treatment. In fact, of the 4 million people throughout the world who die from cancer each year, 70% experience pain as a primary symptom. Unfortunately, many people believe that pain is an early symptom of cancer and do not seek diagnosis until pain occurs. In fact, pain is almost without exception a late symptom of cancer and indicates tumor obstruction, pressure on the nerves, invasion of bone, phantom sensation, peripheral neuropathy, and neuralgia.

It is estimated that 85% of patients with cancer pain can be managed effectively with appropriate therapy. The American Cancer Society, the American Pain Society, the World Health Organization, and the Oncology Nursing Society, as well as many other organizations, consider pain control to be a major issue in the management of a person with cancer.

One of the many challenges facing the nurse who cares for the patient with pain is the assessment of the pain. The nurse must accept the definition of pain as whatever the person experiencing the pain says it is, existing whenever the patient says it does.

Cultural and religious practices in one's family play an important role in the perception of pain or suffering as a weakness. Some families tend to minimize pain. Other cultures expect the expression of pain; therefore they may have a greater overt expression of pain (Cultural and Ethnic Considerations box).

Many nurses and physicians may doubt the presence and nature of the patient's pain when there are no physiologic parameters by which to measure it. The nurse must gather data and properly assess the patient. It is of extreme importance not to be judgmental concerning the patient's complaints of pain.

Opioids used in the management of cancer pain include morphine (the prototype), hydromorphone, fentanyl, and methadone. Sustained-release morphine in an oral form, such as MS Contin, Oramorph SR, Avinza, Kadian, or Roxanol SR, has been found to be of particular value in the management of the terminally ill person with pain. Administering opioids via transdermal method, by IV drips, intrathecally, and epidurally enhances the analgesic effect of the opioids. Avoiding the peaks and valleys of pain relief with bo-

Cultural and Ethnic Considerations

Cancer

- African-Americans have a higher incidence of cancer than whites.
- The death rate from the four most common cancers (lung, colorectal, breast, prostate) is highest among minorities (except Asian-Americans) than in whites.
- Asian-Americans have the lowest death rate from cancer of any ethnic group.
- African-American men have almost twice the rate of prostate cancer than white men and are more than twice as likely to die from the disease.
- Hispanic women have the highest rate of invasive cervical cancer of any group other than Vietnamese, and twice the incidence rate of non-Hispanic white women.
- Although African-American women are less likely than white women to develop breast cancer, they are more likely to die from the disease if they develop it.
- American Indians have a lower incidence of cancer than any other group in the United States but have the poorest survival rate when they do get cancer.

Source: *Cancer facts and figures.* (2003). Atlanta: American Cancer Society.

lus injections provides a more constant analgesic effect for patients with cancer pain. The need for around-the-clock dosage is clear. Fixed dosage schedules with adequate doses for pain relief provide more constant blood levels and predictable pain relief. Some patients have breakthrough pain that requires additional doses, but the fixed dosage schedule should be maintained. Opioid side effects that require monitoring and intervention by the nurse include constipation, vomiting, and respiratory and central nervous system depression.

Patient self-control methods include distraction, massage, relaxation, biofeedback, hypnosis, and imagery. Many patients respond positively to the opportunity for self-care in the management of pain and indicate that such self-control measures enhance the effectiveness of other prescribed pain interventions.

The nurse's unique contributions to pain management are in acting as key link between the patient and the health care team, in the amount of time spent with the patient, in the ability to assess the patient's response to the pain and its management, and in the role of patient and family educator. In addition, the nurse should be able to articulate a concise pain assessment and anticipate and address patient, family, and health care provider misconceptions about pain management. For example, many patients and their families have opioid phobia, the irrational and undocumented fear that even the appropriate use of opioids causes addiction. This fear of addiction

among both health care providers and the public seems to be a major reason for the undertreatment of pain. Fear of addiction should not enter into pain relief for the terminally ill. The nurse must understand and be able to articulate the necessity of opioids in terminally ill patients. The nurse must use pain management strategies appropriately to enable patients and their families to accept the therapeutic value of drugs such as opioids. Patients should not be subjected to severe suffering from potentially controllable pain.

General guidelines for the use of pain relief measures are:

1. Use a variety of pain relief measures.
2. Use pain relief measures before the patient's pain becomes severe.
3. Include pain relief measures that the patient believes will be helpful.
4. Determine the patient's ability or willingness to participate actively in the use of pain relief measures.
5. Rely on patient behavior to indicate pain severity rather than relying on known physical stimuli.
6. Encourage the patient to try a pain relief measure at least two times before abandoning it as ineffective.
7. Have an open mind as to what may relieve the patient's pain, including nonpharmacologic measures.
8. Keep trying to relieve the pain; do not become discouraged and do not stop working with the patient.

Chemical means of pain management include the use of opioids and nonopioids. Valuable nonopioid analgesics in the treatment of certain levels of cancer pain are acetaminophen; aspirin; and nonsteroidal antiinflammatory drugs (NSAIDs), such as ibuprofen, indomethacin, and naproxen.

Adequate rest, sleep, diversion, and other meaningful activities will also help in the management of the patient's pain.

Fear and anxiety increase as a result of pain. Many cancer patients believe increased pain is a sign their condition is worsening and death is imminent. Pain increases their fear, and the cycle of pain continues.

The combination of (1) appropriate pain relief methods, (2) the opportunity to make personal and spiritual peace if there are unresolved conflicts in relationships with others, and (3) someone to listen and offer comfort is probably the most effective pain reliever known. The patient with advanced cancer often experiences *cachexia,* a profound state of ill health, malnutrition, and wasting. Positioning, giving meticulous skin care, offering nutritious fluids and foods, and using other comfort measures to promote relaxation and rest will help to reduce pain and severe fatigue.

NUTRITIONAL THERAPY

Nutritional problems that most frequently occur in the patient with cancer are malnutrition, anorexia, altered taste sensation, nausea, vomiting, diarrhea, stomatitis, and mucositis. These problems can be caused by a combination of many factors, including drug toxicity, effects of radiation therapy, tumor involvement, recent surgery, emotional distress, or difficulty with ingestion or digestion of food. If the patient is inadequately nourished, the normal cells will not be able to recover from the effects of therapy, and the immune system will be depressed because of depletion of protein stores.

Malnutrition

The patient with cancer usually experiences protein and calorie malnutrition characterized by fat and muscle depletion. Foods suggested for increasing protein intake and facilitate repair and regeneration of cells are encouraged as well as high-calorie foods that provide energy and minimize weight loss.

The nurse should suggest to the physician the need for a nutritional supplement as soon as a 5% weight loss is noted or if the patient has the potential for protein and caloric malnutrition. Albumin and prealbumin levels should be monitored. Once a 10 pounds (4.5 kg) weight loss occurs, it is difficult to maintain the nutritional status. The patient can be taught to use nutritional supplements in place of milk when cooking or baking. Foods to which nutritional supplements can be easily added include scrambled eggs, pudding, custard, mashed potatoes, cereal, and cream sauces. Packages of instant breakfast can be used as indicated or sprinkled on cereals, desserts, and casseroles. If the malnutrition cannot be treated with dietary intake, it may be necessary to use enteral or parenteral nutrition as an adjunct nutritional measure.

Anorexia

It is important to realize that the anorexia experienced by the patient with cancer is a challenging problem. An intervention may be effective one day and ineffective the next. Continual assessment and intervention are necessary to successfully manage this problem. The nurse must develop the philosophy that something can be done to prevent or minimize anorexia, evaluate each intervention, and continue to use those interventions that have been successful in the past.

Altered Taste Sensation

It is theorized that cancer cells release substances that resemble amino acids and stimulate the bitter taste buds. The patient may also experience an alteration in the sweet taste sensation, as well as in the sour and salty taste sensations. Meat may also taste bitter to the patient. At this time the physiologic basis of these var-ied taste alterations is unknown. The patient with an altered taste problem should be instructed to avoid foods that are disliked. Frequently the patient may feel compelled to eat certain foods because those foods are believed to be beneficial. The patient can be taught to experiment with spices and other seasoning agents in an attempt to mask the taste alterations that are occurring. Lemon juice, onion, mint, basil, and fruit juice marinades may improve the taste of certain meats and fish. Bacon bits, onion, and pieces of ham may enhance the taste of vegetables. An additional amount of spice or seasoning agent is usually not an effective way to enhance the taste.

COMMUNICATION AND PSYCHOLOGICAL SUPPORT

The patient and the family may become irritable and angry with caregivers when suffering and progressive problems are experienced. Nurses should understand that these feelings are not directed toward them personally but have emerged from the circumstances associated with the patient's disease. A display of anger toward the staff may be caused by deep-seated frustration or anxiety. Understanding and continued warm, responsive caring are the best approaches. The patient may not hear the explanations that have been given when feelings are at a high level. By listening and administering kind and gentle nursing care, the nurse may communicate more effectively than with words. Touch may also be appropriate, adding the dimension of another human being's awareness of the emotional distress being experienced.

Nurses are in the enviable position of being able to make cancer's effects less traumatic through sensitivity and creativity. Nurses need to understand how much each patient needs a sense of control; some need it more than others. The health care system encourages dependency by stripping away most traces of a patient's identity. An adult is told when to get out of bed, have a drink, wash up, and even urinate. The nurse should be aware of the dynamics of what is happening to the patient and provide as many avenues of patient control as possible. It is important that nurses learn the art of talking to patients, not at patients. Nurses must stay watchful, for the family's and the patient's sake.

Psychological support of the patient is an important aspect of cancer care. Because of the effectiveness of cancer treatment, many patients with cancer are cured or their disease is controlled for long periods. In light of this trend in cancer treatment, emphasis must be placed on maintaining an optimal quality of life after the diagnosis of cancer. A positive attitude of patient, family, and caregivers toward cancer and cancer treatment has a significant positive effect on the quality of life that the patient experiences. A positive attitude may also influence the prognosis of the patient with cancer.

The diagnosis of cancer is viewed by most people as a crisis. The most common fears experienced by the patient with cancer include disfigurement, dependency, pain, emaciation, financial depletion, abandonment, and death.

To cope with these fears, the patient with cancer will use and experience different behavioral patterns: shock, anger, denial, bargaining, depression, helplessness, hopelessness, rationalization, acceptance, and intellectualization. These behavioral patterns may occur at any time during the process of cancer. However, some patterns appear to occur more frequently or at a greater intensity at certain specific stages of the disease process. The following factors may determine how the patient will cope with the diagnosis of cancer:

- Ability to cope with stressful events in the past (i.e., loss of job, major disappointment). By simply asking how the patient has coped with stressful events, the nurse can gain an understanding of the patient's coping patterns, the effectiveness of the usual coping patterns, and the usual coping time framework.
- **Availability of significant others.** The patient who has effective support systems tends to cope more effectively than the patient who does not have a meaningful, available support system.
- **Ability to express feelings and concerns.** The patient who is able to express feelings and needs and who seeks and asks for help appears to cope more effectively than the patient who internalizes feelings and needs.
- **Age at the time of diagnosis.** Age determines the coping strategies to a great degree. For example, a young mother with cancer may have concerns that differ from those of a 70-year-old woman with cancer.
- **Extent of disease.** Cure or control of the disease process is usually easier to cope with than the reality of terminal illness.
- **Disruption of body image.** Disruption of the body image (e.g., radical neck dissection, alopecia, mastectomy) may intensify the psychological effect of cancer.
- **Presence of symptoms.** Symptoms such as fatigue, nausea, diarrhea, and pain may intensify the psychological effect of cancer.
- **Past experience with cancer.** If past experiences with cancer have been negative, the patient will probably view the present status as negative.
- **Attitude associated with cancer.** A patient who feels in control and has a positive attitude about cancer and cancer treatment is better able to cope with the diagnosis and treatment of cancer than the patient who feels hopeless, helpless, and out of control.

To facilitate the development of a hopeful attitude about cancer and to support the patient and the family during the various stages of the process of cancer, the nurse should do the following:

- Be available and continue to be available, especially during difficult times.
- Exhibit a caring attitude.
- Listen actively to fears and concerns.
- Provide relief from distressing symptoms.
- Provide essential information regarding cancer and cancer care.
- Maintain a relationship based on trust and confidence, be open, honest, and caring in the approach.
- Use touch to exhibit caring. A squeeze of the hand may at times be more effective than words.
- Assist the patient in setting realistic, reachable short- and long-term goals.
- Assist the patient in maintaining usual lifestyle patterns.
- Maintain hope, which is the key to effective cancer care. Hope varies, depending on the status of the patient—hope that the symptoms are not serious, hope that the treatment is curative, hope for independence, hope for relief of pain, hope for a longer life, or hope for a peaceful death. Hope provides control over what is occurring and is the basis of a positive attitude toward cancer and cancer care (Lewis et al, 2004).

TERMINAL PROGNOSIS

Coping with the multiple problems experienced when one has advanced cancer can lead to a sense of helplessness and hopelessness in spite of all efforts. The patient and the family may look forward to death as a relief from unrelenting suffering.

Most patients with advanced cancer know that they are dying. Attempts at circumventing the truth are usually recognized by the patient and cause feelings of distrust and hostility toward the person who makes such attempts. Honesty and openness are the best approaches. Most patients will surprise caregivers by expressing relief at a willingness to discuss what is foremost in their minds—their imminent death.

Spiritual activities may provide mental and emotional strength in spite of physical deterioration. The patient may ask the nurse to read the Bible or to pray with him or her, or the patient may request that a minister, priest, or rabbi visit. Spiritual strength may help the patient and the family to cope with the continuing problems encountered in the cancer experience.

The hospital social worker assists the patient and family in planning to meet the immediate needs for home care. Arrangements for any special supplies and equipment are made before discharge. The nurse plays a major role in teaching the patient and at least one family member or significant other how to continue any special care needed at home, such as dressing changes, irrigations, the management of a feeding tube, or the care of a central venous line for administration of parenteral nutrition or medications.

Throughout the hospital stay, nurses must take advantage of time available to promote self-care to the greatest extent possible. Assessment of the readiness to learn and the ability to assume active participation in caring for self is a major responsibility of nurses. Advanced clinical nursing specialists may need to be consulted to provide individualized guidelines for teaching patients. Plans for patient education must be written on the nursing care plan. Evidence of the patient's comprehension of and ability to handle self-care must be documented, and assistance needed from others must be planned and provided for accordingly. Continuity of care is the goal in discharge planning. Hospice services can be arranged in most communities for those who have advanced cancer. There are free-standing hospices, hospices within a hospital or skilled nursing facility, or at-home arrangements. The primary focus of a hospice is enhancing the quality of life for the individual, not prolonging life. Efforts are directed toward relief from pain and other problems. Skilled professional care and voluntary support services are provided to assist the patient and family to live life to the fullest each day.

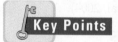

Key Points

- It is currently estimated that one of every five people in the United States will get cancer. The 5-year survival rate is 62%.
- There is strong evidence that what people eat or drink or their lifestyle habits may predispose them to the development of cancer.
- The American Cancer Society recommends specific preventive behaviors and screening tests for cancer prevention and early detection for males and females.
- It is imperative for the person to perform self-examination to detect any changes and report them to the physician immediately.
- It is important to have periodic physical examinations and to seek medical attention promptly if one of the warning signs of cancer develops.

- A common reason for a delay in diagnosing cancer is because early malignant changes are not accompanied by pain.
- Seeking medical attention when any warning signs occur is also frequently delayed because people fear the possible diagnosis of cancer and hope the signs and symptoms will just go away.
- The diagnosis of cancer has a profound effect on family members, as well as on the patient. Shock, disbelief, denial, anger, and fear are experienced. These feelings are accompanied by a high degree of anxiety and a sense of helplessness.
- Most of the side effects from chemotherapeutic agents result from the destruction of normal cells from the hematopoietic system, hair follicles, and the gastrointestinal system.
- Tumor lysis syndrome (TLS) is an oncologic emergency that occurs in cancer patients with heavy tumor burdens after they receive chemotherapy or irradiation, which causes rapid lysis of malignant cells.
- The American Cancer Society sponsors organized support groups for individuals with the same types of cancer; some of these are Reach to Recovery; the Lost Chord Club; I Can Cope; Look Good, Feel Good; and the Ostomy Club. Prepared volunteer visitors are available in most communities to visit a newly diagnosed patient on the approval of the responsible physician.
- Spiritual strength assists the patient and the family to cope with the problems experienced as a result of cancer. Based on the patient's preference, religious counsel may be helpful.
- The American Cancer Society, the American Pain Society, the World Health Organization, and the Oncology Nursing Society consider pain control to be a major issue in the management of a person with cancer.
- The concept of rehabilitation should be applied in planning care for the patient with cancer to promote the highest level of functioning possible.

Go to your free CD-ROM for an Audio Glossary, animations, video clips, and Review Questions for the NCLEX-PN® Examination.

evolve   Be sure to visit the companion Evolve site at http://evolve.elsevier.com/Christensen/adult/ for WebLinks and additional online resources.

CHAPTER CHALLENGE

1. Mr. P. presents with a complaint of mouth pain 10 days after receiving chemotherapy. On inspection, the nurse finds the inside of the mouth is erythematous, edematous, and dry. The most likely problem is:
   1. candidiasis.
   2. hypercalcemia.
   3. stomatitis.
   4. esophagitis.

2. Ms. J. has metastatic breast cancer with involvement in her L5 vertebral body. She is paralyzed from the waist down with incontinence of stool and urine. She is undergoing radiation therapy for spinal cord compression. Which of the following is an appropriate nursing diagnosis for Ms. J.?
   1. Risk for disturbed body image, related to alopecia
   2. Risk for deficient fluid volume, related to stool incontinence
   3. Risk for impaired skin integrity, related to prolonged immobility and incontinence
   4. All of the above

3. Mr. N., a 58-year-old patient with colon cancer, is receiving combined radiation and chemotherapy. He is suffering from diarrhea; this is related to the:
   1. diagnosis of the patient.
   2. patient's inability to eat and drink during treatment.
   3. treatment's irritating effect on the mucosa of the GI tract.
   4. fluid and electrolyte imbalance of the patient.

4. The current recommendation for *first-time baseline* mammogram in asymptomatic women is:
   1. at the onset of menopause.
   2. that it is not necessary if the patient has had a previous biopsy.
   3. at ages 35 to 39.
   4. at age 50.

5. Which of the following are considered cancer-screening activities?
   1. Performing a risk factor assessment and physical examination
   2. Giving a patient instruction for performing the test for fecal occult blood
   3. Instructing a patient in self-examination of the skin or oral cavity
   4. All of the above

6. Mr. S. has terminal lung cancer. To maintain optimal pain control, scheduling of oral analgesics generally should be:
   1. at scheduled intervals.
   2. every 2 hours.
   3. as required.
   4. related to a patient's activity level.

7. Cancer preventions and health promotion behaviors for patients with a diagnosis of cancer:
   1. will not decrease the risk of developing a second malignancy.
   2. will not be affected by personal choices related to diet and smoking.
   3. are increasingly important with the growing population of cancer survivors.
   4. would include only routine physical examinations.

8. Ms. B. has been diagnosed with stage I breast cancer. She is receiving adjuvant chemotherapy and radiation therapy following a lumpectomy. All the following points about alopecia would be made *except:*
   1. chemotherapy-related hair loss is reversible and temporary.
   2. all chemotherapeutic agents result in alopecia.
   3. hair that grows back may have a different texture and color.
   4. gentle shampooing is recommended.

9. Ms. N., a 61-year-old patient, is receiving chemotherapy. Ms. N. becomes anemic and has petechiae and ecchymoses scattered over her upper trunk, especially her arms. Which of the following side effects is Ms. N. experiencing?
   1. Bone marrow suppression
   2. Cardiac suppression
   3. Liver toxicity
   4. Pulmonary toxicity

10. Before the insertion of a cervical implant, the nurse tells Ms. P. what to expect while it is in place. Which statement is accurate?
    1. "Nurses will always be available, but they will spend only short periods of time at your bedside."
    2. "Personal cleanliness is essential, so you will be given a complete bed bath each day."
    3. "Pain or discomfort is a common side effect of this type of radiation."
    4. "Your bed linens will be completely changed each day to minimize radioactive contamination."

11. T.J., a 24-year-old patient, has been receiving chemotherapy for acute lymphoblastic leukemia. Which of the following statements would indicate that he understands discharge teaching concerning leukopenia?
    1. "I am cured and have no limitations."
    2. "My family can catch leukopenia, so I need to be careful to not get too close to any of them."
    3. "I should avoid close contact with people who might give me an infection."
    4. "I need to be careful not to cut myself when shaving, because I may not be able to stop the bleeding."

12. Ms. R., a 42-year-old patient, has palpated a small lump on her left breast during her monthly BSE. She has scheduled an appointment with her physician. Which of the following tests will be used to make a definite diagnosis of a benign or malignant tumor of her breast?
    1. Biopsy
    2. Mammography
    3. Tomography
    4. Ultrasound

13. The nurse educator is discussing the importance of the reduction of carcinogens in primary prevention of cancer. Which risk factor is considered significant in the cause of several types of cancer?
    1. Diet low in fat
    2. Occasional moderate use of alcohol
    3. High pollen count in the environment
    4. Smoking

Continued

14. A therapeutic approach by the nurse to assist Mr. B., a terminally ill cancer patient, in the management of his pain is that:

    1. antiinflammatory agents are effective analgesics for severe pain.
    2. opioids should be withheld because they are addictive.
    3. pain is what the patient says it is.
    4. one can increase one's tolerance for pain.

15. Which of the following statements by Ms. J., a chemotherapy patient with a low WBC count, a low platelet count, and a hemoglobin measurement of 5.6 g would indicate the need for further teaching?

    1. "I check my mouth and teeth after each meal."
    2. "I've been very constipated and need an enema."
    3. "My husband and I have been using a vaginal lubrication before intercourse."
    4. "My lips are dry and cracking. I need some lubricant."

16. Which of the following is a biologic modifier that is a breakthrough in treating patients with neutropenia and is used prophylactically for patients at risk for neutropenia?

    1. Lymphopenic stimulating factor (LSF)
    2. Erythropoietic stimulating factor (ESF)
    3. Neutropenic stimulating factor (NSF)
    4. Colony-stimulating factor (CSF)

17. According to the American Cancer Society, what is the most preventable cause of death from lung cancer?

    1. Five fruits and vegetables a day
    2. Yearly chest radiograph for those 50 years and older
    3. Cessation of smoking
    4. Reduction of environmental/chemical carcinogens

18. Aggressive chemotherapy to decrease the growth of rapidly progressive malignant tumors causes destruction of a large number of rapidly dividing malignant cells and increases the risk of which complication? (The drug allopurinol and hydration help control the metabolic complication that may occur.) _____

19. The nursing diagnosis of imbalanced nutrition: less than body requirements is often seen in chemotherapy patients as a result of:

    1. impaired tissue integrity, related to damage to integumentary tissue.
    2. alopecia and leukopenia.
    3. stomatitis, anorexia, vomiting, and diarrhea.
    4. myelosuppression.

20. Select all of the following important points for the nurse to educate the patient and family in prevention of constipation.

    1. Opioids may cause constipation, so laxatives must be given with opioids.
    2. Patients who are not eating continue to produce waste in the bowel and get impacted with feces.
    3. High fluid intake should be maintained.
    4. The patient should have a bowel movement at least every day.
    5. If possible, eating foods high in fiber is helpful.

21. Ms. B. has a vaginal radiation implant in place. The nurse would:

    1. instruct her to turn from side to side for comfort.
    2. restrict fluid intake to prevent bladder distention.
    3. promote intake of a high-residue diet to prevent constipation.
    4. monitor vital signs every 4 hours and report temperature greater than 100° F.

22. In the nursing interventions of a patient receiving external radiation therapy for a malignancy, the nurse must remember to:

    1. vigorously scrub the areas of entry of "ports" marked by the radiologist.
    2. apply some form of ointment with a metallic base to the area of entry each time the patient goes for radiation treatments.
    3. instruct the patient to avoid irritating the "ports" by not lying on that part of the body and not wearing constricting clothing.
    4. isolate the patient so he or she will not expose others to radiation.

23. Mr. O. is admitted with a history of oat cell carcinoma of the lung and is being treated with chemotherapy. His WBC count is 1.5 mm³. The nurse's primary concern would be:

    1. prevention of hemorrhage.
    2. prevention of infection.
    3. prevention of dehydration.
    4. prevention of electrolyte imbalance.

24. Mr. K, age 63, has a diagnosis of cancer of the prostate gland with metastasis and is experiencing cachexia. This state is best described by which of the following characteristics:

    1. Poor health, malnutrition, and wasting
    2. Increased appetite and nervousness
    3. Irritability and anger
    4. Depression, fear, and anxiety

Matching

25. _____ Carcinogen

26. _____ Mammography

27. _____ Pathogenesis

28. _____ Thrombocytopenia

29. _____ Leukopenia

A. Reduction of WBCs

B. Radiographic examination of the breast

C. The development of morbid conditions or of disease

D. Decrease in platelets

E. Any agent or substance that causes cancer

30. Metoclopramide (Reglan) is an antiemetic that is helpful in preventing chemotherapy-induced emesis. Choose all the correct answers that describe its action.

   1. Blocks dopamine receptors in chemoreceptor trigger zone of CNS
   2. Accelerates gastric emptying
   3. Blocks the effects of serotonin at 5-HT$_3$ receptor sites
   4. Stimulates motility of the upper GI tract

Common Abbreviations

°C	degrees Centigrade	ECG, EKG	electrocardiogram
°F	degrees Fahrenheit	EEG	electroencephalogram
℥*	dram	elix	elixir
@	at	ER	emergency room
♀	female	ESR	erythrocyte sedimentation rate
♂	male		
>	greater than	ETOH	ethyl alcohol
<	less than	f℥	fluid ounce
↑	increase	FUO	fever of unknown origin
↓	decrease	Fx, fx	fracture; fractional urine test
1°	primary	g, gm, Gm	gram
2°	secondary	GI	gastrointestinal
Δ	change	gr	grain
aa	indicating equal amounts of each	gt; gtt	drop; drops
		GTT	glucose tolerance test
ABGs	arterial blood gases	h, hr	hour
ac	before meals	H&P	history and physical examination
ad lib	freely as desired		
ADL	activities of daily living	HCT, Hct	hematocrit
ama, AMA	against medical advice	Hgb	hemoglobin
AND	allow natural death	HIV	human immunodeficiency virus (AIDS)
BE	barium enema		
bid	two times a day	hs*	at bedtime
BP	blood pressure	I&O	intake and output
BRP	bathroom privileges	IDDM	insulin-dependent diabetes mellitus
BUN	blood urea nitrogen		
c̄	with	IM	intramuscular
cap	capsule	IV	intravenous
CBC	complete blood count	IVP	intravenous push; intravenous pyelogram
cc*	cubic centimeter		
CDC	Centers for Disease Control and Prevention	IVU	intravenous urogram
		K	potassium
cm	centimeter	kg	kilogram
c/o	complains of	KUB	kidney, ureters, and bladder (radiograph)
CO	carbon monoxide		
CO₂	carbon dioxide	KVO	keep vein open
CPR	cardiopulmonary resuscitation	L	liter
		LOC	laxative of choice; level of consciousness
CT	computed tomography		
D₅W	5% dextrose in water	m	meter
dL	deciliter	mcg, μg*	microgram
DNR	do not resuscitate	mg	milligram
Dx, dx	diagnosis	mL	milliliter
		mm	millimeter
		mm Hg	millimeters of mercury
		MRI	magnetic resonance imaging

*On JCAHO's Lists of Dangerous Abbreviations, Acronyms, and Symbols, see pp. 851 to 852.

Ndx	nursing diagnoses	qd*	every day
NPO	nothing per os, nothing by mouth	qh	every hour
		qid*	four times a day
O_2	oxygen	qod*	every other day
OD	optical density; overdose	ROM	range of motion
O.D.*	right eye	Rx	take; treatment
O.S.*	left eye	s̄	without
O.U.*	both eyes	SC,* SQ,* Sub-Q, subQ	subcutaneous
oz, ℥	ounce	ss*	half
pc	after meals	SSE	soapsuds enema
PERRLA	pupils equal, round, and re-active to light and accom-modation	stat	immediately
		tid	three times a day
		TKO	to keep open
pH	hydrogen ion concentration (acidity and alkalinity)	TLC	tender loving care
		TPN	total parenteral nutrition
PO, po	orally, per os	TPR	temperature, pulse, and res-pirations
prn	as often as necessary, when required		
		WBC	white blood cell, white blood count
q	every		

B JCAHO Lists of Dangerous Abbreviations, Acronyms, and Symbols

A "minimum list" of dangerous abbreviations, acronyms, and symbols has been approved by the Joint Commission on Accreditation of Healthcare Organizations (JCAHO). Beginning January 1, 2004 the following items in Table 1 must be included on each accredited organization's Do Not Use list:

Table 1 *Minimum Do-Not-Use List of Abbreviations*

ABBREVIATION	POTENTIAL PROBLEM	PREFERRED TERM
U (for unit)	Mistaken as *zero*, *four*, or cc	Write *unit*
IU (for international unit)	Mistaken as IV (intravenous) or 10 (ten)	Write *international unit*
Q.D., Q.O.D., Q.I.D. (Latin abbreviations for once daily, every other day, and 4 times daily)	Mistaken for each other The period after the "Q" can be mistaken for an "I," and the "O" can be mistaken for "I"	Write *daily*, *every other day*, and *4 times daily*
Trailing zero (X.0 mg) *(Note: prohibited only for medication-related notations)* Lack of leading zero (.X mg)	Decimal point is missed	Never write a zero by itself after a decimal point (X mg), and always use a zero before a decimal point (0.X mg)
MS MSO$_4$ MgSO$_4$	Confused for one another Can mean morphine sulfate or magnesium sulfate	Write *morphine sulfate* or *magnesium sulfate*

From the Joint Commission on Accreditation of Healthcare Organizations, 2003.

Additional abbreviations, acronyms, and symbols for *possible* future inclusion in the official "Do Not Use" list are provided in Table 2.

Table 2	*Additional Abbreviations to Avoid*	
ABBREVIATION	**POTENTIAL PROBLEM**	**PREFERRED TERM**
μg (for microgram)	Mistaken for *mg* (milligrams) resulting in 1000-fold overdose	Write *mcg*
IN (intranasal)	Mistaken for *IM*	Write out *intranasal*
H.S. (for half-strength or Latin abbreviation for bedtime)	Mistaken for either half-strength or hour of sleep (at bedtime); *q.H.S.* mistaken for every hour All can result in a dosing error	Write out *half-strength* or *at bedtime*
T.I.W. (for 3 times a week)	Mistaken for 3 times a day or twice weekly resulting in an overdose	Write *3 times weekly* or *three times weekly*
S.C. or S.Q. for subcutaneous)	Mistaken for *SL* for sublingual, or *5 every*	Write *Sub-Q, subQ,* or *subcutaneously*
D/C (for discharge)	Interpreted as discontinue whatever medications follow (typically discharge meds)	Write *discharge*
c.c. (for cubic centimeter)	Mistaken for *U* (units) when poorly written	Write *ml* for milliliters
A.S., A.D., A.U. (Latin abbreviation for left, right, or both ears)	Mistaken for *OS, OD, OU,* etc.	Write *left ear, right ear,* or *both ears*
SS (half)	Read as *55*	Use metric system
℥ (dram)	Read as *3*	Use metric system
M (minim)	Misread as *ml*	Use metric system
Zero after decimal	*1.0,* for example, misread as *10*	Do not use trailing zero after whole numbers

From the Joint Commission on Accreditation of Healthcare Organizations, 2003.
Recommended precautions: Two nurses must double-check the following before administration: heparin, insulin, parenteral chemotherapeutic agents, patient-controlled analgesia, and epidural pumps.
HIPAA privacy requirements: Patient information concerning name, age, diagnosis, and so forth should not be posted. Charts and medication records must be kept in confidential area.
Also, the Institute for Safe Medication Practices (ISMP) has published a list of dangerous abbreviations relating to medication use that it recommends should be explicitly prohibited. This list is available on its website, http://www.ismp.org/ (revised November 3, 2003).

C Laboratory Reference Values*

Reference Intervals for Hematology

TEST	CONVENTIONAL UNITS	SI UNITS
Acid hemolysis (Ham test)	No hemolysis	No hemolysis
Alkaline phosphatase, leukocyte	Total score, 14-100	Total score, 14-100
Cell counts		
Erythrocytes		
Males	4.6-6.2 million/mm^3	4.6-6.2 × 10^{12}/L
Females	4.2-5.4 million/mm^3	4.2-5.4 × 10^{12}/L
Children (varies with age)	4.5-5.1 million/mm^3	4.5-5.1 × 10^{12}/L
Leukocytes, total	4500-11,000/mm^3	4.5-11.0 × 10^9/L
Leukocytes, differential counts*		
Myelocytes	0%	0/L
Band neutrophils	3%-5%	150-400 × 10^6/L
Segmented neutrophils	54%-62%	3000-5800 × 10^6/L
Lymphocytes	25%-33%	1500-3000 × 10^6/L
Monocytes	3%-7%	300-500 × 10^6/L
Eosinophils	1%-3%	50-250 × 10^6/L
Basophils	0%-1%	15-50 × 10^6/L
Platelets	150,000-400,000/mm^3	150-400 × 10^9/L
Reticulocytes	25,000-75,000/mm^3 (0.5%-1.5% of erythrocytes)	25-75 × 10^9/L
Coagulation tests		
Bleeding time (template)	2.75-8.0 min	2.75-8.0 min
Coagulation time (glass tube)	5-15 min	5-15 min
D-Dimer	<0.5 mcg/mL	<0.5 mg/L
Factor VIII and other coagulation factors	50%-150% of normal	0.5-1.5 of normal
Fibrin split products (Thrombo-Welco test)	<10 mcg/mL	<10 mg/L
Fibrinogen	200-400 mg/dL	2.0-4.0 g/L
Partial thromboplastin time, activated (aPTT)	20-25 sec	20-35 sec
Prothrombin time (PT)	12.0-14.0 sec	12.0-14.0 sec
Coombs' test		
Direct	Negative	Negative
Indirect	Negative	Negative
Corpuscular values of erythrocytes		
Mean corpuscular hemoglobin (MCH)	26-34 pg/cell	26-34 pg/cell
Mean corpuscular volume (MCV)	80-96 μm^3	80-96 fL
Mean corpuscular hemoglobin concentration (MCHC)	32-36 g/dL	320-360 g/L
Haptoglobin	20-165 mg/dL	0.20-1.65 g/L
Hematocrit		
Males	40-54 mL/dL	0.40-0.54
Females	37-47 mL/dL	0.37-0.47
Newborns	49-54 mL/dL	0.49-0.54
Children (varies with age)	35-49 mL/dL	0.35-0.49
Hemoglobin		
Males	13.0-18.0 g/dL	8.1-11.2 mmol/L
Females	12.0-16.0 g/dL	7.4-9.9 mmol/L
Newborns	16.5-19.5 g/dL	10.2-12.1 mmol/L
Children (varies with age)	11.2-16.5 g/dL	7.0-10.2 mmol/L

*Conventional units are percentages; SI units are absolute cell counts.

Continued

*From Rakel, R.E.; Bope, E.T. (2005). *Conn's current therapy* 2005. Philadelphia: Elsevier.

Reference Intervals for Hematology—cont'd

TEST	CONVENTIONAL UNITS	SI UNITS
Hemoglobin, fetal	<1.0% of total	<0.01 of total
Hemoglobin A$_{1C}$	3%-5% of total	0.03-0.05 of total
Hemoglobin A$_2$	1.5%-3.0% of total	0.015-0.03 of total
Hemoglobin, plasma	0.0-5.0 mg/dL	0.0-3.2 μmol/L
Methemoglobin	30-130 mg/dL	19-80 μmol/L
Erythrocyte sedimentation rate (ESR)		
Wintrobe		
Males	0-5 mm/hr	0-5 mm/hr
Females	0-15 mm/hr	0-15 mm/hr
Westergren		
Males	0-15 mm/hr	0-15 mm/hr
Females	0-20 mm/hr	0-20 mm/hr

Reference Intervals* for Clinical Chemistry (Blood, Serum, and Plasma)

ANALYTE	CONVENTIONAL UNITS	SI UNITS
Acetoacetate plus acetone		
Qualitative	Negative	Negative
Quantitative	0.3-2.0 mg/dL	30-200 μmol/L
Acid phosphatase, serum (thymolphthalein monophosphate substrate)	0.1-0.6 units/L	0.1-0.6 units/L
ACTH (see Corticotropin)		
Alanine aminotransferase (ALT, serum (SGPT)	1-45 units/L	1-45 units/L
Albumin, serum	3.3-5.2 g/dL	33-52 g/L
Aldolase, serum	0.0-7.0 units/L	0.0-7.0 units/L
Aldosterone, plasma		
Standing	5-30 ng/dL	140-830 pmol/L
Recumbent	3-10 ng/dL	80-275 pmol/L
Alkaline, phosphatase (ALP), serum		
Adult	35-150 units/L	35-150 units/L
Adolescent	100-500 units/L	100-500 units/L
Child	100-350 units/L	100-350 units/L
Ammonia nitrogen, plasma	10-50 μmol/L	10-50 μmol/L
Amylase, serum	25-125 units/L	25-125 units/L
Anion gap, serum calculated	8-16 mEq/L	8-16 mmol/L
Ascorbic acid, blood	0.4-1.5 mg/dL	23-85 μmol/L
Aspartate aminotransferase (AST), serum (SGOT)	1-36 units/L	1-36 units/L
Base excess, arterial blood, calculated	0 ±2 mEq/L	0 ±2 mmol/L
Bicarbonate		
Venous plasma	23-29 mEq/L	23-29 mmol/L
Arterial blood	21-27 mEq/L	21-27 mmol/L
Bile acids, serum	0.3-3.0 mg/dL	0.8-7.6 μmol/L
Bilirubin, serum		
Conjugated	0.1-0.4 mg/dL	1.7-6.8 μmol/L
Total	0.3-1.1 mg/dL	5.1-19.0 μmol/L
Calcium, serum	8.4-10.6 mg/dL	2.10-2.65 mmol/L
Calcium, ionized, serum	4.25-5.25 mg/dL	1.05-1.30 mmol/L
Carbon dioxide, total, serum or plasma	24-31 mEq/L	24-31 mmol/L
Carbon dioxide tension (P$_{CO_2}$), blood	35-45 mm Hg	35-45 mm Hg
β-Carotene, serum	60-260 mcg/dL	1.1-8.6 μmol/L
Ceruloplasmin, serum	23-44 mg/dL	230-440 mg/L
Chloride, serum or plasma	96-106 mEq/L	96-106 mmol/L

*Reference values may vary, depending on the method and sample source used.

Reference Intervals for Clinical Chemistry (Blood, Serum, and Plasma)—cont'd

ANALYTE	CONVENTIONAL UNITS	SL UNITS
Cholesterol, serum or EDTA plasma		
Desirable range	<200 mg/dL	<5.20 mmol/L
Low-density lipoprotein (LDL) cholesterol	60-180 mg/dL	1.55-4.65 mmol/L
High-density lipoprotein (HDL) cholesterol	30-80 mg/dL	0.80-2.05 mmol/L
Copper	70-140 mcg/dL	11-22 µmol/L
Corticotropin (ACTH), plasma, 8 AM	10-80 pg/mL	2-18 pmol/L
Cortisol, plasma		
8:00 AM	6-23 mcg/dL	170-630 nmol/L
4:00 PM	3-15 mcg/dL	80-410 nmol/L
10:00 PM	<50% of 8:00 AM value	<50% of 8:00 AM value
Creatine, serum		
Males	0.2-0.5 mg/dL	15-40 µmol/L
Females	0.3-0.9 mg/dL	25-70 µmol/L
Creatine kinase (CK), serum		
Males	55-170 units/L	55-170 units/L
Females	30-135 units/L	30-135 units/L
Creatinine kinase MB isoenzyme, serum	<5% of total CK activity	<5% of total CK activity
	<5% of ng/mL by immunoassay	<5% of ng/mL by immunoassay
Creatinine, serum	0.6-1.2 mg/dL	50-110 µmol/L
Estradiol-17β, adult		
Males	10-65 pg/mL	35-240 pmol/L
Females		
Follicular	30-100 pg/mL	110-370 pmol/L
Ovulatory	200-400 pg/mL	730-1470 pmol/L
Luteal	50-140 pg/mL	180-510 pmol/L
Ferritin, serum	20-200 ng/mL	20-200 mcg/L
Fibrinogen, plasma	200-400 mg/dL	2.0-4.0 g/L
Folate, serum	3-18 ng/mL	6.8-41 nmol/L
Erythrocytes	145-540 ng/mL	330-120 nmol/L
Follicle-stimulating hormone (FSH), plasma		
Males	4-25 mU/mL	4-25 units/L
Females, premenopausal	4-30 mU/mL	4-30 units/L
Females, postmenopausal	40-250 mU/mL	40-250 units/L
Gastrin, fasting, serum	0-100 pg/mL	0-100 mg/L
Glucose, fasting, plasma or serum	70-115 mg/dL	3.9-6.4 nmol/L
γ-Glutamyltransferase (GGT), serum	5-40 units/L	5-40 units/L
Growth hormone (hGH), plasma, adult, fasting	0-6 ng/mL	0-6 mcg/L
Haptoglobin, serum	20-165 mg/dL	0.20-1.65 g/L
Immunoglobulins, serum (see table of Reference Intervals for Tests of Immunologic Function)		
Iron, serum	75-175 mcg/dL	13-31 µmol/L
Iron-binding capacity, serum		
Total	250-410 mcg/dL	45-73 µmol/L
Saturation	20%-55%	0.20-0.55
Lactate		
Venous whole blood	5.0-20.0 mg/dL	0.6-2.2 mmol/L
Arterial whole blood	5.0-15.0 mg/dL	0.6-1.7 mmol/L
Lactate dehydrogenase (LD), serum	110-220 units/L	110-220 units/L
Lipase, serum	10-140 units/L	10-140 units/L
Lutropin (LH), serum		
Males	1-9 units/L	1-9 units/L
Females		
Follicular phase	2-10 units/L	2-10 units/L
Midcycle peak	15-65 units/L	15-65 units/L
Luteal phase	1-12 units/L	1-12 units/L
Postmenopausal	12-65 units/L	12-65 units/L

Continued

Reference Intervals* for Clinical Chemistry (Blood, Serum, and Plasma)—cont'd

ANALYTE	CONVENTIONAL UNITS	SL UNITS
Magnesium, serum	1.3-2.1 mg/dL	0.65-1.05 mmol/L
Osmolality	275-295 mOsm/kg water	275-295 mOsm/kg water
Oxygen, blood, arterial, room air		
Partial pressure (PaO_2)	80-100 mm Hg	80-100 mm Hg
Saturation (SaO_2)	95%-98%	95%-98%
pH, arterial blood	7.35-7.45	7.35-7.45
Phosphate, inorganic, serum		
Adult	3.0-4.5 mg/dL	1.0-1.5 mmol/L
Child	4.0-7.0 mg/dL	1.3-2.3 mmol/L
Potassium		
Serum	3.5-5.0 mEq/L	3.5-5.0 mmol/L
Plasma	3.5-4.5 mEq/L	3.5-4.5 mmol/L
Progesterone, serum, adult		
Males	0.0-0.4 ng/mL	0.0-1.3 mmol/L
Females		
Follicular phase	0.1-1.5 ng/mL	0.3-4.8 mmol/L
Luteal phase	2.5-28.0 ng/mL	8.0-89.0 mmol/L
Prolactin, serum		
Males	1.0-15.0 ng/mL	1.0-15.0 mcg/L
Females	1.0-20.0 ng/mL	1.0-20.0 mcg/L
Protein, serum, electrophoresis		
Total	6.0-8.0 g/dL	60-80 g/L
Albumin	3.5-5.5 g/dL	35-55 g/L
Globulins		
α_1	0.2-0.4 g/dL	2.0-4.0 g/L
α_2	0.5-0.9 g/dL	5.0-9.0 g/L
β	0.6-1.1 g/dL	6.0-11.0 g/L
γ	0.7-1.7 g/dL	7.0-17.0 g/L
Pyruvate, blood	0.3-0.9 mg/dL	0.03-0.10 mmol/L
Rheumatoid factor	0.0-30.0 IU/mL	0.0-30.0 kIU/L
Sodium, serum or plasma	135-145 mEq/L	135-145 mmol/L
Testosterone, plasma		
Males, adult	300-1200 ng/dL	10.4-41.6 nmol/L
Females, adult	20-75 ng/dL	0.7-2.6 nmol/L
Pregnant females	40-200 ng/dL	1.4-6.9 nmol/L
Thyroglobulin	3-42 ng/mL	3-42 mcg/L
Thyrotropin (hTSH), serum	0.4-4.8 µIU/mL	0.4-4.8 mIU/L
Thyrotropin-releasing hormone (TRH)	5-60 pg/mL	5-60 ng/L
Thyroxine (FT_4), free, serum	0.9-2.1 ng/dL	12-27 pmol/L
Thyroxine (T_4), serum	4.5-12.0 mcg/mL	58-154 nmol/L
Thyroxine-binding globulin (TBG)	15.0-34.0 mcg/mL	15.0-34.0 mg/L
Transferrin	250-430 mg/dL	2.5-4.3 g/L
Triglycerides, serum, after 12-hr fast	40-150 mg/dL	0.4-1.5 g/L
Triiodothyronine (T_3), serum	70-190 ng/dL	1.1-2.9 nmol/L
Triiodothyronine uptake, resin (T_3RU)	25%-38%	0.25-0.38
Urate		
Males	2.5-8.0 mg/dL	150-480 µmol/L
Females	2.2-7.0 mg/dL	130-420 µmol/L
Urea, serum or plasma	24-49 mg/dL	4.0-8.2 nmol/L
Urea, nitrogen, serum or plasma	11-23 mg/dL	8.0-16.4 nmol/L
Viscosity, serum	1.4-1.8 × water	1.4-1.8 × water
Vitamin A, serum	20-80 mcg/dL	0.70-2.80 µmol/L
Vitamin B_{12}, serum	180-900 pg/mL	133-664 pmol/L

*JCAHO requires IU to be spelled out as International Units when written by hand.

Reference Intervals for Therapeutic Drug Monitoring (Serum or Plasma)*

ANALYTE	THERAPEUTIC RANGE	TOXIC CONCENTRATIONS	PROPRIETARY NAME(S)
ANALGESICS			
Acetaminophen	10-40 mcg/mL	>150 mcg/mL	Tylenol
			Datril
Salicylate	100-250 mcg/mL	>300 mcg/mL	Aspirin
			Bufferin
ANTIBIOTICS			
Amikacin	20-30 mcg/mL	Peak >35 mcg/mL	Amkin
		Trough >10 mcg/mL	
Gentamicin	5-10 mcg/mL	Peak >10 mcg/mL	Garamycin
		Trough >2 mcg/mL	
Tobramycin	5-10 mcg/mL	Peak >10 mcg/mL	Nebcin
		Trough >2 mcg/mL	
Vancomycin	5-35 mcg/mL	Peak >40 mcg/mL	Vancocin
		Trough >10 mcg/mL	
ANTICONVULSANTS			
Carbamazepine	5-12 mcg/mL	>15 mcg/mL	Tegretol
Ethosuximide	40-100 mcg/mL	>250 mcg/mL	Zarontin
Phenobarbital	15-40 mcg/mL	40-100 ng/mL (varies widely)	Luminal
Phenytoin	10-20 mcg/mL	>20 mcg/mL	Dilantin
Primidone	5-12 mcg/mL	>15 mcg/mL	Mysoline
Valproic acid	50-100 mcg/mL	>100 mcg/mL	Depakene
ANTINEOPLASTICS AND IMMUNOSUPPRESSIVES			
Cyclosporine	100-300 ng/mL	>400 ng/mL	Sandimmune
Methotrexate, high-dose, 48 hr	Variable	>1 μmol/L, 48 hr after dose	
Tacrolimus (FK-506), whole blood	3-20 mcg/L	>15 mcg/L	Prograf
BRONCHODILATORS AND RESPIRATORY STIMULANTS			
Caffeine	3-15 ng/mL	>30 mcg/mL	Elixophyllin
Theophylline (aminophylline)	10-20 mcg/mL	>30 mcg/mL	Quibron
CARDIOVASCULAR DRUGS			
Amiodarone (obtain specimen more than 8 hr after last dose)	1.0-2.0 mcg/mL	>2.0 mcg/mL	Cordarone
Digoxin (obtain specimen more than 6 hr after last dose)	0.8-2.0 mcg/mL	>2.4 ng/mL	Lanoxin
Disopyramide	2-5 mcg/mL	>7 mcg/mL	Norpace
Flecainide	0.2-1.0 mcg/mL	>1 mcg/mL	Tambocor
Lidocaine	1.5-5.0 mcg/mL	>6 mcg/mL	Xylocaine
Mexiletine	0.7-2.0 mcg/mL	>2 mcg/mL	Mexitil
Procainamide	4-10 mcg/mL	>12 mcg/mL	Pronestyl
Procainamide plus NAPA (*N*-acetyl procainamide)	8-30 mcg/mL	>30 mcg/mL	
Propranolol	50-100 ng/mL	Variable	Inderal
Quinidine	2-5 mcg/mL	>6 mcg/mL	Cardioquin
			Quinaglute
Tocainide	4-10 ng/mL	>10 ng/mL	Tonocard
PSYCHOPHARMACOLOGICAL DRUGS			
Amitriptyline	120-150 ng/mL	>500 ng/mL	Elavil
			Triavil
Bupropion	25-100 ng/mL	Not applicable	Wellbutrin
Desipramine	150-300 ng/mL	>500 ng/mL	Norpramin
Imipramine	125-250 ng/mL	>400 ng/mL	Tofranil
Lithium (obtain specimen 12 hr after last dose)	0.6-1.5 mEq/L	>1.5 mEq/L	Lithobid
Nortriptyline	50-150 ng/mL	>500 ng/mL	Aventyl
			Pamelor

*Values may vary depending on the method and sample collection device used. Always consult the reference values provided by the laboratory performing the analysis.

Reference Intervals* for Clinical Chemistry (Urine)

ANALYTE	CONVENTIONAL UNITS	SI UNITS
Acetone and acetoacetate, qualitative	Negative	Negative
Albumin		
Qualitative	Negative	Negative
Quantitative	10-100 mg/24 hr	0.15-1.5 μmol/day
Aldosterone	3-20 mcg/24 hr	8.3-55 nmol/day
δ-Aminolevulinic acid (δ-ALA)	1.3-7.0 mg/24 hr	10-53 μmol/day
Amylase	<17 units/h	<17 units/h
Amylase/creatinine clearance ratio	0.01-0.04	0.01-0.04
Bilirubin, qualitative	Negative	Negative
Calcium (regular diet)	<250 mg/24 hr	<6.3 nmol/day
Catecholamines		
Epinephine	<10 mcg/24 hr	<55 nmol/day
Norepinephine	<100 mcg/24 hr	<590 nmol/day
Total free catecholamines	4-126 mcg/24 hr	24-745 nmol/day
Total metanephrines	0.1-1.6 mg/24 hr	0.5-8.1 μmol/day
Chloride (varies with intake)	110-250 mEq/24 hr	110-250 mmol/day
Copper	0-50 mcg/24 hr	0.0-0.80 μmol/day
Cortisol, free	10-100 mcg/24 hr	27.6-276 nmol/day
Creatine		
Males	0-40 mg/24 hr	0.0-0.30 mmol/day
Females	0-80 mg/24 hr	0.0-0.60 mmol/day
Creatinine	15-25 mg/kg/24 hr	0.13-0.22 mmol/kg/day
Creatinine clearance (endogenous)		
Males	110-150 mL/min/1.73 m²	110-150 mL/min/1.73 m²
Females	105-132 mL/min/1.73 m²	105-132 mL/min/1.73 m²
Cystine or cysteine	Negative	Negative
Dehydroepiandrosterone		
Males	0.2-2.0 mg/24h	0.7-6.9 μmol/day
Females	0.2-1.8 mg/24h	0.7-6.2 μmol/day
Estrogens, total		
Males	4-25 mcg/24 hr	14-90 nmol/day
Females	5-100 mcg/24 hr	18-360 nmol/day
Glucose (as reducing substance)	<250 mg/24 hr	<250 mg/day
Hemoglobin and myoglobin, qualitative	Negative	Negative
Hemogentisic acid, qualitative	Negative	Negative
17-Hydroxycorticosteroids		
Males	3-9 mg/24 hr	8.3-25 μmol/day
Females	2-8 mg/24 hr	5.5-22 μmol/day
5-Hydroxyindoleacetic acid		
Qualitative	Negative	Negative
Quantitative	2-6 mg/24 hr	10-31 μmol/day
17-Ketogenic steroids		
Males	5-23 mg/24 hr	17-80 μmol/day
Females	3-15 mg/24 hr	10-52 μmol/day
17-Ketosteroids		
Males	8-22 mg/24 hr	28-76 μmol/day
Females	6-15 mg/24 hr	21-52 μmol/day
Magnesium	6-10 mEq/24 hr	3-5 mmol/day
Metanephrines	0.05-1.2 ng/mg creatinine	0.03-0.70 mmol/mmol creatinine
Osmolality	38-1400 mOsm/kg water	38-1400 mOsm/kg water
pH	4.6-8.0	4.6-8.0
Phenylpyruvic acid, qualitative	Negative	Negative
Phosphate	0.4-1.3 g/24 hr	13-42 mmol/day

*Values may vary, depending on the method used.

Reference Intervals for Clinical Chemistry (Urine)—cont'd*

ANALYTE	CONVENTIONAL UNITS	SI UNITS
Porphobilinogen		
Qualitative	Negative	Negative
Quantitative	<2 mg/24 hr	<9 μmol/day
Porphyrins		
Coproporphyrin	50-250 mcg/24 hr	77-380 nmol/day
Uroporphyrin	10-30 mcg/24 hr	12-36 nmol/day
Potassium	25-125 mEq/24 hr	25-125 mmol/day
Pregnanediol		
Males	0.0-1.9 mg/24 hr	0.0-6.0 μmol/day
Females		
Proliferative phase	0.0-2.6 mg/24 hr	0.0-8.0 μmol/day
Luteal phase	2.6-10.6 mg/24 hr	8-33 μmol/day
Postmenopausal	0.2-1.0 mg/24 hr	0.6-3.1 μmol/day
Pregnanetriol	0.0-2.5 mg/24 hr	0.0-7.4 μmol/day
Protein, total		
Qualitative	Negative	Negative
Quantitative	10-150 mg/24 hr	10-150 mg/day
Protein/creatinine ratio	<0.2	<0.2
Sodium (regular diet)	60-260 mEq/24 hr	60-260 mmol/day
Specific gravity		
Random specimen	1.003-1.030	1.003-1.030
24-hr collection	1.015-1.025	1.015-1.025
Urate (regular diet)	250-750 mg/24 hr	1.5-4.4 mmol/day
Urobilinogen	0.5-4.0 mg/24 hr	0.6-6.8 μmol/day
Vanillylmandelic acid (VMA)	1.0-8.0 mg/24 hr	5-40 μmol/day

*Values may vary, depending on the method used.

Reference Intervals for Toxic Substances

ANALYTE	CONVENTIONAL UNITS	SI UNITS
Arsenic, urine	<130 mcg/24 hr	<1.7 μmol/day
Bromides, serum, inorganic	<100 mg/dL	<10 mmol/L
Toxic symptoms	140-1000 mg/dL	14-100 mmol/L
Carboxyhemoglobin, blood	Saturation, percent	
Urban environment	<5%	<0.05
Smokers	<12%	<0.12
Symptoms		
Headache	>15%	>0.15
Nausea and vomiting	>25%	>0.25
Potentially lethal	>50%	>0.50
Ethanol, blood	<0.05 mg/dL	<1.0 mmol/L
	<0.005%	
Intoxication	>100 mg/dL	>22 mmol/L
	>0.1%	
Marked intoxication	300-400 mg/dL	65-87 mmol/L
	0.3%-0.4%	
Alcoholic stupor	400-500 mg/dL	87-109 mmol/L
	0.4%-0.5%	
	>500 mg/dL	
Coma	>0.5%	>109 mmol/L
Lead, blood		
Adults	<20 mcg/dL	<1.0 μmol/L
Children	<10 mcg/dL	<0.5 μmol/L
Lead, urine	<80 mcg/24 hr	<0.4 μmol/day
Mercury, urine	<10 mcg/24 hr	<150 nmol/day

Reference Intervals for Tests Performed on Cerebrospinal Fluid

TEST	CONVENTIONAL UNITS	SI UNITS
Cells	<5 mm³; all mononuclear	<5 × 10⁶/L, all mononuclear
Protein electrophoresis	Albumin predominant	Albumin predominant
Glucose	50-75 mg/dL (20 mg/dL less than in serum)	2.8-4.2 mmol/L (1.1 mmol/L less than in serum)
IgG		
Children <14 yr	<8% of total protein	<0.08 of total protein
Adults	<14% of total protein	<0.14 of total protein
IgG index $\left(\dfrac{\text{CSF/serum IgG ratio}}{\text{CSF/serum albumin ratio}}\right)$	0.3-0.6	0.3-0.6
Oligoclonal banding on electrophoresis	Absent	Absent
Pressure, opening	70-180 mm H₂O	70-180 mm H₂O
Protein, total	15-45 mg/dL	150-450 mg/L

Reference Intervals for Tests of Gastrointestinal Function

TEST	CONVENTIONAL UNITS
Bentiromide	6-hr urinary arylamine excretion >57% excludes pancreatic insufficiency
β-Carotene, serum	60-250 ng/dL
Fecal fat estimation	
Qualitative	No fat globules seen by high-power microscope
Quantitative	<6 g/24 hr (>95% coefficient of fat absorption)
Gastric acid output	
Basal	
Males	0.0-10.5 mmol/hr
Females	0.0-5.6 mmol/hr
Maximum (after histamine or pentagastrin)	
Males	9.0-48.0 mmol/hr
Females	6.0-31.0 mmol/hr
Ratio: basal/maximum	
Males	0.0-0.31
Females	0.0-0.29
Secretion test, pancreatic fluid	
Volume	>1.8 mL/kg/hr
Bicarbonate	>80 mEq/L
D-Xylose absorption test, urine	>20% of ingested dose excreted in 5 hr

Reference Intervals for Tests of Immunologic Function

TEST	CONVENTIONAL UNITS	SI UNITS
Complement, serum		
C3	85-175 mg/dL	0.85-1.75 g/L
C4	15-45 mg/dL	150-450 mg/L
Total hemolytic (CH_{50})	150-250 units/mL	150-250 units/mL
Immunoglobulins, serum, adult		
IgG	640-1350 mg/dL	6.4-13.5 g/L
IgA	70-310 mg/dL	0.70-3.1 g/L
IgM	90-350 mg/dL	0.90-3.5 g/L
IgD	0.0-6.0 mg/dL	0.0-60 mg/L
IgE	0.0-430 ng/dL	0.0-430 mcg/L

Lymphocytes Subsets, Whole Blood, Heparinized

ANTIGEN(S) EXPRESSED	CELL TYPE	PERCENTAGE (%)	ABSOLUTE CELL COUNT
CD3	Total T cells	56-77	860-1880
CD19	Total B cells	7-17	140-370
CD3 and CD4	Helper-inducer cells	32-54	550-1190
CD3 and CD8	Suppressor-cytotoxic cells	24-37	430-1060
CD3 and DR	Activated T cells	5-14	70-310
CD2	E rosette T cells	73-87	1040-2160
CD16 and CD56	Natural killer (NK) cells	8-22	130-500
Helper/suppressor ratio: 0.8-1.8			

Reference Values for Semen Analysis

TEST	CONVENTIONAL UNITS	SI UNITS
Volume	2-5 mL	2-5 mL
Liquefaction	Complete in 15 min	Complete in 15 min
pH	7.2-8.0	7.2-8.0
Leukocytes	Occasional or absent	Occasional or absent
Spermatozoa		
Count	$60\text{-}150 \times 10^6$ mL	$60\text{-}150 \times 10^6$ mL
Motility	>80% motile	>0.80 motile
Morphology	80%-90% normal forms	>0.80-0.90 normal forms
Fructose	>150 mg/dL	>8.33 mmol/L

CHAPTER CHALLENGE ANSWERS

Chapter 1
1. 2
2. 3
3. 1
4. 4
5. 2
6. 4
7. 1
8. 3
9. 2
10. 2
11. 3
12. 4
13. 3
14. 2
15. e
16. d
17. a
18. c
19. b
20. f
21. k
22. a
23. i
24. b
25. g
26. c
27. j
28. d
29. e
30. h

Chapter 2
1. 4
2. 2
3. 3
4. 1
5. 1
6. 4
7. 3
8. 2
9. 1
10. 2
11. 3
12. 2
13. 4
14. 3
15. 3
16. 3
17. 3
18. 2
19. 2
20. 1

Chapter 3
1. 1
2. 2
3. 3
4. 3
5. 2
6. 1

7. 1
8. 1
9. 4
10. 2
11. 1
12. 2
13. 3
14. 1
15. 2
16. 1
17. 2
18. 2
19. 2
20. 1
21. 2
22. 2
23. 1, 2
24. 1
25. 3
26. papule
27. 2

Chapter 4
1. 2
2. 4
3. 4
4. 2
5. 3
6. 4
7. 2
8. 4
9. 3
10. 3
11. 2
12. 2
13. 1
14. 2
15. 2
16. 3
17. 3
18. 4
19. 1
20. 4
21. 3
22. 3
23. 4

Chapter 5
1. 2
2. 3
3. 2
4. 2
5. 2
6. 1
7. 4
8. 2
9. 2
10. 1
11. 1
12. 3
13. 3

14. 4
15. 4
16. 3
17. 3
18. 1
19. 3
20. 2
21. 4

Chapter 6
1. 1
2. 1
3. 2, 3, 4
4. 4
5. 2
6. 3
7. 2
8. 3
9. 3
10. 4
11. 4
12. 2
13. 3
14. 3
15. 2
16. 2
17. 4
18. 1
19. Reinfection, cirrhosis

Chapter 7
1. 3
2. 1
3. 2
4. 3
5. 4
6. 2
7. 3
8. 2
9. 4
10. 3
11. 1
12. 4
13. 3
14. 2
15. 3
16. 2
17. 2
18. 1
19. 2
20. 4
21. 3
22. 1
23. 2
24. 1
25. 1, 2, 3
26. 1, 2, 3, 5
27. 1, 2, 3, 5
28. 1, 2, 4, 5
29. 2

Chapter 8
1. 1
2. 2
3. 1
4. 3
5. 4
6. 3
7. 4
8. 1
9. 4
10. 4
11. 2
12. 2
13. 4
14. 2
15. 1
16. 3
17. 1
18. 2
19. 2
20. 2
21. 4
22. 3
23. 1
24. Troponin I

Chapter 9
1. 2
2. 3
3. 3
4. 4
5. 4
6. 1
7. 2
8. 3
9. 3
10. 3
11. 2
12. 1
13. 2
14. 4
15. 1
16. 3
17. 4
18. 3
19. 1
20. 3
21. 4
22. 1
23. 3
24. 3
25. 1
26. 1, 3, 4
27. 1, 2, 4
28. 2, 3, 4, 5
29. 1, 2, 4
30. 2
31. 1, 2, 3, 5
32. 1, 3, 4
33. 2, 3, 4, 5

34. 1, 2, 3, 4
35. 1, 2, 4, 5
36. 1, 2, 3, 5

Chapter 10
1. 4
2. 3
3. 1
4. 4
5. 1
6. 3
7. 4
8. 1
9. 3
10. 2
11. 2
12. 3
13. 1
14. 1
15. 1
16. 4
17. 2
18. 3
19. 2
20. 4
21. 4
22. 1
23. 1
24. 2
25. 2
26. 4
27. 1, 2, 3
28. 1, 2, 3
29. 1, 2, 4
30. 1, 3, 4

Chapter 11
1. 3
2. 1
3. 4
4. 3
5. 3
6. 4
7. 1
8. 4
9. 4
10. 1
11. 1
12. 4
13. 4
14. 2
15. 2
16. 4
17. 3
18. 4
19. 4
20. 3
21. 3
22. Regular or rapid acting
23. 1, 2, 3

Chapter 12
1. 1
2. 2
3. 3
4. 4
5. 3
6. 4
7. 2
8. 1
9. 1, 3, 4
10. 3
11. 2
12. 1
13. 3
14. 4
15. 1
16. 3
17. 4
18. 2, 3

Chapter 13
1. 3
2. 2
3. 1
4. 4
5. 3
6. 4
7. 1
8. 1
9. 2
10. 4
11. 2
12. 2
13. 1
14. 2
15. 3
16. 1
17. 3
18. 2
19. 3
20. 3
21. 2, 3, 4
22. 1
23. 1
24. 3
25. 3
26. 1
27. 1
28. 2
29. 4
30. Cochlear implant
31. 4

Chapter 14
1. 4
2. 3
3. 2
4. 2
5. 1
6. 4

7. 3
8. 1
9. 3
10. 3
11. 1
12. 1
13. 1, 2, 3
14. 1
15. 2
16. 2
17. 1
18. 4
19. 1
20. 3
21. 2, 3, 4
22. C
23. E
24. D
25. B
26. A

27. 1, 2, 3, 4
28. 2, 3, 4
29. 1, 2, 3, 5
30. 3
31. 4
32. 2

Chapter 15
1. 4
2. 2
3. 1
4. 2
5. 2
6. 1
7. 3
8. 3
9. 4
10. 2
11. 1
12. 1

13. 2, 3, 4
14. 3
15. 4
16. 3
17. **Natural rubber latex proteins**

Chapter 16
1. 1
2. 4
3. 4
4. 2
5. 2
6. 1
7. 1
8. 1
9. 1
10. 3

11. 2
12. 4
13. 3
14. False
15. True
16. True
17. True
18. True
19. False
20. False
21. 2
22. 2
23. 4
24. 1
25. 2
26. 1
27. 1
28. 1
29. 3

30. 2
31. 3
32. 1
33. 1, 2, 3, 4
34. 2, 3, 4, 5

Chapter 17
1. 3
2. 3
3. 3
4. 3
5. 4
6. 1
7. 3
8. 2
9. 1
10. 1
11. 3
12. 1

13. 4
14. 3
15. 2
16. 4
17. 3
18. **Tumor lysis syndrome**
19. 3
20. 1, 2, 3, 5
21. 4
22. 3
23. 2
24. 1
25. E
26. B
27. C
28. D
29. A
30. 1, 2, 4

NANDA Nursing Diagnoses 2005-2006*

Activity intolerance
Activity intolerance, Risk for
Adjustment, Impaired
Airway clearance, Ineffective
Allergy response, Latex
Allergy response, Risk for latex
Anxiety
Anxiety, Death
Aspiration, Risk for
Attachment, Risk for impaired
    parent/infant/child
Autonomic dysreflexia
Autonomic dysreflexia, Risk for
Body image, Disturbed
Body temperature, Risk for imbalanced
Bowel incontinence
Breastfeeding, Effective
Breastfeeding, Ineffective
Breastfeeding, Interrupted
Breathing pattern, Ineffective
Cardiac output, Decreased
Caregiver role strain
Caregiver role strain, Risk for
Communication, Impaired verbal
Communication, Readiness for
    enhanced
Conflict, Decisional
Conflict, Parental role
Confusion, Acute
Confusion, Chronic
Constipation
Constipation, Perceived
Constipation, Risk for
Coping, Compromised family
Coping, Defensive
Coping, Disabled family
Coping, Ineffective
Coping, Ineffective community
Coping, Readiness for enhanced
Coping, Readiness for enhanced
    community
Coping, Readiness for enhanced
    family
Denial, Ineffective
Dentition, Impaired
Development, Risk for delayed
Diarrhea
Disuse syndrome, Risk for
Diversional activity, Deficient
Energy field, Disturbed
Environmental interpretation
    syndrome, Impaired
Failure to thrive, Adult
Falls, Risk for
Family processes: Alcoholism,
    Dysfunctional
Family processes, Interrupted
Family processes, Readiness for
    enhanced
Fatigue
Fear
Fluid balance, Readiness for enhanced
Fluid volume, Deficient
Fluid volume, Excess
Fluid volume, Risk for deficient

Fluid volume, Risk for imbalanced
Gas exchange, Impaired
Grieving, Anticipatory
Grieving, Dysfunctional
Grieving, Risk for dysfunctional
Growth, Risk for disproportionate
Growth and development, Delayed
Health maintenance, Ineffective
Health-seeking behaviors
Home maintenance, Impaired
Hopelessness
Hyperthermia
Hypothermia
Identity, Disturbed personal
Incontinence, Functional urinary
Incontinence, Reflex urinary
Incontinence, Stress urinary
Incontinence, Total urinary
Incontinence, Urge urinary
Incontinence, Risk for urge urinary
Infant behavior, Disorganized
Infant behavior, Readiness for en-
    hanced organized
Infant behavior, Risk for disorganized
Infant feeding pattern, Ineffective
Infection, Risk for
Injury, Risk for
Injury, Risk for perioperative-positioning
Intracranial adaptive capacity,
    Decreased
Knowledge, Deficient
Knowledge, Readiness for enhanced
Lifestyle, Sedentary
Loneliness, Risk for
Memory, Impaired
Mobility, Impaired bed
Mobility, Impaired physical
Mobility, Impaired wheelchair
Nausea
Neglect, Unilateral
Noncompliance
Nutrition, Readiness for enhanced
Nutrition: less than body requirements,
    Imbalanced
Nutrition: more than body require-
    ments, Imbalanced
Nutrition: more than body require-
    ments, Risk for imbalanced
Oral mucous membrane, Impaired
Pain, Acute
Pain, Chronic
Parenting, Impaired
Parenting, Readiness for enhanced
Parenting, Risk for impaired
Peripheral neurovascular dysfunction,
    Risk for
Poisoning, Risk for
Post-trauma syndrome
Post-trauma syndrome, Risk for
Powerlessness
Powerlessness, Risk for
Protection, Ineffective
Rape-trauma syndrome
Rape-trauma syndrome, compound
    reaction

Rape-trauma syndrome, silent reaction
Religiosity, Impaired
Religiosity, Readiness for enhanced
Religiosity, Risk for Impaired
Relocation stress syndrome
Relocation stress syndrome, Risk for
Role performance, Ineffective
Self-care deficit, Bathing/hygiene
Self-care deficit, Dressing/grooming
Self-care deficit, Feeding
Self-care deficit, Toileting
Self-concept, Readiness for enhanced
Self-esteem, Chronic low
Self-esteem, Situational low
Self-esteem, Risk for situational low
Self-mutilation
Self-mutilation, Risk for
Sensory perception, Disturbed
Sexual dysfunction
Sexuality pattern, Ineffective
Skin integrity, Impaired
Skin integrity, Risk for impaired
Sleep, Readiness for enhanced
Sleep deprivation
Sleep pattern, Disturbed
Social interaction, Impaired
Social isolation
Sorrow, Chronic
Spiritual distress
Spiritual distress, Risk for
Spiritual well-being, Readiness for
    enhanced
Sudden Infant Death Syndrome,
    Risk for
Suffocation, Risk for
Suicide, Risk for
Surgical recovery, Delayed
Swallowing, Impaired
Therapeutic regimen management,
    Effective
Therapeutic regimen management,
    Ineffective
Therapeutic regimen management,
    Ineffective community
Therapeutic regimen management,
    Ineffective family
Therapeutic regimen management,
    Readiness for enhanced
Thermoregulation, Ineffective
Thought processes, Disturbed
Tissue integrity, Impaired
Tissue perfusion, Ineffective
Transfer ability, Impaired
Trauma, Risk for
Urinary elimination, Impaired
Urinary elimination, Readiness for
    enhanced
Urinary retention
Ventilation, Impaired spontaneous
Ventilatory weaning response,
    Dysfunctional
Violence, Risk for other-directed
Violence, Risk for self-directed
Walking, Impaired
Wandering

References & Suggested Readings

Chapter 1 Introduction to Anatomy and Physiology

Anderson, D.M., et al. (2002). *Mosby's medical, nursing, and allied health dictionary.* (6th ed.). St. Louis: Mosby.

Herlihy, B. & Maebius, N.K. (2004). *The human body in health and illness.* Philadelphia: Saunders.

Langford, R.W. & Thompson, J.M. (2004). *Mosby's handbook of diseases.* (3rd ed.). St. Louis: Mosby.

Lewis, S.L., et al. (2004). *Medical-surgical nursing: assessment and management of clinical problems.* (6th ed.). St. Louis: Mosby.

Memmler, R.L., et al. (2004). *Structure and function of the human body.* (8th ed.). Philadelphia: Lippincott.

Patton, K.T. & Thibodeau, G.A. (2000). *Mosby's handbook of anatomy and physiology.* St. Louis: Mosby.

Petti, K. (2003). *Anatomy and physiology.* (5th ed.). St. Louis: Mosby.

Phipps, W.J., et al. (2003). *Medical-surgical nursing: health and illness perspectives.* (7th ed.). St. Louis: Mosby.

Swisher, L. (2004). *Structure and function of the body.* (12th ed.). St. Louis: Mosby.

Thibodeau, G.A. & Patton, K.T. (2003). *Anatomy and physiology.* (5th ed.). St. Louis: Mosby.

Thibodeau, G.A. & Patton, K.T. (2004). *Structure and function of the body.* (12th ed.). St. Louis: Mosby.

Thibodeau, G.A. & Patton, K.T. (2005). *The human body in health and disease.* (4th ed.). St. Louis: Mosby.

Thompson, J.M., et al. (2001). *Mosby's clinical nursing.* (5th ed.). St. Louis: Mosby.

Chapter 2 Care of the Surgical Patient

Ackley, B.J. & Ladwig, G.B. (2005). *Nursing diagnosis handbook.* (6th ed.). St. Louis: Mosby.

Anderson, D.M., et al. (2002). *Mosby's medical, nursing, and allied health dictionary.* (6th ed.). St. Louis: Mosby.

Applying antioembolism stockings isn't just pulling on socks. *Nursing,* 34(8):48, 2004.

Banks, N. Preoperative stoma site assessment and marking. *American Journal of Nursing,* 103(3):82, 2003.

Chart smart: keeping tabs on arrhythmias. *Nursing,* 32(3):82, 2002.

Cofer, M. (2005). Unwelcome companion to older patients: postoperative delirium. *Nursing,* 35(1):32, 2005.

Dunn, D. Preventing perioperative complications in an older adult. *Nursing,* 34(11):36, 2004.

Elkin, M.K., et al. (2004). *Nursing interventions and clinical skills.* (3rd ed.). St. Louis: Mosby.

Ennis, D. Reducing the risk of surgical site infection: use these techniques to prevent postoperative infections. *Nursing,* 29(6):33, 1999.

Giger, J.M. & Davidhizar, R.E. (2004). *Transcultural nursing: assessment and intervention.* (4th ed.). St. Louis: Mosby.

Harkreader, H. & Hogan, M.A. (2004). *Fundamentals of nursing.* (2nd ed.). St. Louis: Saunders.

Kozier, B., et al. (2004). *Fundamentals of nursing concepts, process and practice.* (7th ed.). Upper Saddle River, NJ: Pearson/Prentice Hall.

Joint Commission on Accreditation of Healthcare Organizations: *Universal protocol for preventing wrong site, wrong procedure and wrong person surgery.* Available online at http://www.jcaho.org/accredited+organizations/patient+safety/universal+protocol/wss_universal+protocol.htm. Accessed August, 2004.

McConnell, E.A. Applying antiembolism stockings. *Nursing,* 32(4):17, 2002.

Moz, T. A stitch in time unravels. *Nursing Made Incredibly Easy,* November/December:52, 2004.

Moz, T. Wound dehiscence and evisceration. *Nursing,* 34(5):88, 2004.

Pagana, K.D. & Pagana, T.J. (2005). *Mosby's diagnostic and laboratory test reference.* (7th ed.). St. Louis: Mosby.

Phipps, W.J., et al. (2003). *Medical-surgical nursing: health and illness perspectives.* (7th ed.). St. Louis: Mosby.

Potter, P.A. & Perry A.G. (2003). *Basic nursing: essentials for practice.* (5th ed.). St. Louis: Mosby.

Potter, P.A. & Perry, A.G. (2005). *Fundamentals of nursing: concepts, process, and practice.* (6th ed.). St. Louis: Mosby.

Pullen, J. & Richard, L. Teaching bedside incentive spirometry. *Nursing,* 33(8):24, 2003.

Smith, S.F., et al. (2002). *Photo guide to nursing skills.* Upper Saddle River, NJ: Prentice Hall.

Smith, S.F., et al. (2004). *Clinical nursing skill:, basic to advanced skills.* (6th ed.). Upper Saddle River, NJ: Pearson/Prentice Hall.

Swearingen, P.L. (2004). *All-in-one care planning resource.* St. Louis: Mosby.

Williams, L.S. & Hopper, P.D. (2003). *Understanding medical surgical nursing.* (2nd ed.). Philadelphia: Davis.

Chapter 3 Care of the Patient with an Integumentary Disorder

Black, J.M. & Hawks, H.J. (2005). *Medical-surgical nursing: clinical management for positive outcomes.* (7th ed.). Philadelphia: Saunders.

Burn care. (2000). Available online at http://wfubmc.edu/burnunit/. Accessed July, 2005.

Callahan, E. Cutaneous (non-HIV) infections. *Dermatologic Clinics,* 18(3):497, 2000.

Danks, R.R. Burn management: a comprehensive review of the epidemiology and treatment of burn victims. *JEMS Journal of Emergency Medical Services,* 28(5):118, 122, 124, 2003.

DeBoer, S., et al. Burn care in EMS. *Emergency Medical Services,* 33(2):69, 72, 87, 2004.

D'Espiro, N.W. Deciphering autoimmune disease in women. *Patient Care,* 34(7):49, 2000.

Gatty, B. Initiatives outline future of skin disorders. *Dermatology Times,* 22(5), 2001.

Hess, C.T. Treating a fungal rash. *Nursing 2003,* 33(9):9, 2003.

Hockenberry, M. (2005). *Wong's essentials of pediatric nursing.* (7th ed.). St. Louis: Mosby.

Inglesby, T., et al. Anthrax as a biological weapon: medical and public health management. *Journal of the American Medical Association,* 281(18):1735, 1999.

Johnson, B. Clinical snapshot: systemic lupus erythematosus. *American Journal of Nursing,* 99(1):40, 1999.

Kagan, R.J. Evaluation and treatment of thermal injuries. *Dermatology Nursing,* 12(5):334, 2000.

Kent, H. PDT effective for inflammatory, viral skin lesions. *Dermatology Times,* 22(8):19, 2000.

Kleinpell, R. The role of the critical care nurse in the assessment and management of the patient with severe sepsis. *Critical Care Nursing Clinics of North America,* 15(1):27, 2003.

Lapka, D.V. Oncology today: skin cancer. *RN,* 63(7):32, 2000.

Lewis, S.M., et al. (2004). *Medical-surgical nursing: assessment and management of clinical problems.* (6th ed.). St. Louis: Mosby.

McCance, K.L. & Huether, S.E. (1998). *Pathophysiology: the biologic basis for disease in adults and children.* (4th ed.). St. Louis: Mosby.

Melnyk, B.M. & Ebling, A.M. Effectiveness of oral antibiotics and topical retinal therapy in the treatment of acne in adolescents. *Pediatric Nursing,* 27(4):41, 2001.

Morgan, E.D. Ambulatory management of burns. *American Family Physician,* 62(9):2015, 2000.

Mower-Wade, D. & Kang, T.M. Sepsis: when defense turns deadly. *Nursing 2004,* 34(7):30, 2004.

Myth and facts . . . about systemic lupus erythematosus. *Nursing,* 29(9):26, 1999.

Phipps, W.J., et al. (2003). *Medical-surgical nursing: health and illness perspectives.* (7th ed.). St. Louis: Mosby.

Quillen, T.F. Easing the heartbreak of psoriasis. *Nursing 2004,* 34(11):18, 2004.

Rhody, C. Bacterial infections of the skin. *Primary Care,* 27(2):459, 2000.

Rossiter, R. Improving lupus knowledge. *Australian Journal of Nursing,* 9(3):17, 2001.

Roy, D.E. & Stotts, N.A. Targeting cellulitis. *Nursing 2002,* 32(12):32, 2002.

Schmitt, B.D. (2001). *Your child's health.* San Francisco: Clinical Reference Systems.

Sheridan, R.L. Evaluating and managing burn wounds. *Dermatology Nursing,* 12(1), 2000.

Stalbow, J. Preventing cellulitis in older people with persistent lower limb edema. *British Journal of Nursing,* 13(12):725, 2004.

Swartz, M. Recognition and management of anthrax: an update. *New England Journal of Medicine,* 345(22):1621, 2001.

Thompson, J. A practical guide to wound care. *RN,* 63(1):48, 2000.

Ventura, M.J. A new option for burn victims. *RN,* 61(11):37, 1998.

Wiebelhaus, P. & Hansen, S.L. Burns. Handle with care. *RN,* 62(11):52, 1999.

Wiebelhaus, P. & Hansen, S.L. Another choice for burn victims. *RN,* 64(9):34, 2001.

Wiebelhaus, P. & Hansen, S.L. What you should know about managing burn emergencies. *Nursing,* 31(1):36, 2001.

Windham, S.T. (2001). Pathophysiology of thermal injuries. Presented at University of Alabama at Birmingham seminar, September 25. *Cutting edge information for critically injured burn survivors.*

Wright, J. Promoting healthy skin in older people. *Nursing Older People,* 15(8):22, 2002.

Chapter 4 Care of the Patient with a Musculoskeletal Disorder

Achenbrenner, D. New drug for osteoporosis. *American Journal of Nursing,* 103(3):27, 2003.

Anderson, D.M., et al. (2002). *Mosby's medical, nursing, and allied health dictionary.* (6th ed.). St. Louis: Mosby.

Arthritis Foundation Online Disease Center. Available online at www.arthritis.org/conditions/diseasecenter/. Accessed July, 2005.

Black J.M. & Hawks, H.J. (2005). *Medical-surgical nursing: clinical management for positive outcomes.* (7th ed.). Philadelphia: Saunders.

Blakeley, J. & Ribeiro, V. Glucosamine and osteoarthritis. *American Journal of Nursing,* 104(2):54, 2004.

Bryant, G. Stump care. *American Journal of Nursing,* 101(2):67, 2001.

Canobbio, J. (2000). *Mosby's handbook of patient teaching.* (2nd ed.). St. Louis: Mosby.

Danter, J. Geriatric assessment. *Nursing 2003,* 33(11):52, 2003.

Davis, M.P. & Srivastrava, M. Demographics, assessment and management of pain in the elderly. *Drugs Aging,* 20(1):23-57, 2003.

Deal, C. & Giddeon, J. Recombinant human PTH 1-34 (Forteo): an anabolic drug for osteoporosis. *Cleveland Clinic Journal of Medicine,* 70(7):585, 2003.

Dunkin, M.A. Drug guide: get smart about the drugs you take. *Arthritis Today,* 15(1):39, 2001.

Einhorn, T. Use of COX-2 inhibitors in patients with fractures. *American Academy of Orthopedic Surgeons Bulletin,* 50(5):1, 2002.

Fort, C. Getting a fix on long-bone fracture. *Nursing 2002,* 32(6):32hn1, 2002.

Gambaro, G. & Perazella, M.A. Adverse renal effects of inflammatory agents: evaluation of selective and nonselective cyclooxygenase inhibitors. *Journal of Internal Medicine,* 253(6):643, 2003.

Genesis Health Care System. (2002). *Clinical pathways.* Zanesville, Ohio: Genesis.

Gianakos, D. Acute knee pain. *Patient Care,* January:13, 2004.

Hatcher, T. The proverbial herb. *American Journal of Nursing,* 101(2):36, 2001.

Hodgson, B. & Kizior, R. (2005). *Saunders' nursing drug handbook 2005.* Philadelphia: Saunders.

Hoeman, S. (2001). *Rehabilitation nursing: process and application.* (3rd ed.). St. Louis: Mosby.

Hong, E. An approach to knee pain. *Patient Care,* January:42, 2003.

Hutchinson, R. COX-2 selective NSAIDs: a review and comparison with nonselective NSAIDs. *American Journal of Nursing,* 104(3):52, 2004.

Johnson S. Hormone replacement therapy: applying the results of the Women's Health Initiative. *Cleveland Clinic Journal of Medicine,* 69(9):682, 2002.

Klippel, J. On call: what is the difference between fibromyalgia and chronic fatigue syndrome? *Arthritis Today,* 15(1):86, 2001.

Leopold, S. (2003). *Unicompartmental knee arthroplasty: a patient's guide to partial knee replacement using minimally invasive surgery (MIS) techniques.* University of Washington Orthopaedics and Sports Medicine. Available online at www.orthop.washington. edu/faculty/Leopold/miniknee/01. Accessed August, 2004.

Licata, A. Osteoporosis in men: suspect secondary disease first. *Cleveland Clinic Journal of Medicine,* 70(3):247, 2003.

Ling, S. & Bathon, J. (2003). *Osteoarthritis pathophysiology.* Available online at arthritis.som.jhmi.edu/osteo/osteo_patho.html. Accessed August, 2004.

Maher, A. et al (eds.). (2002). *Orthopaedic nursing.* (3rd ed.). Philadelphia: Saunders.

McConnell, E. Assessing neurovascular status in a casted limb. *Nursing 2002,* 32(9):20, 2002.

McCormick, W., et al. Cervical spondylotic myelopathy: make the difficult diagnosis, then refer for surgery. *Cleveland Clinic Journal of Medicine,* 70(10):899, 2003.

Metules, T. Osteoporosis. *RN,* 66(11):56, 2003.

Moseley, J.B., et al. A controlled trial of arthroscopic surgery for osteoarthritis of the knee. *New England Journal of Medicine,* 347:81, 2002.

National Osteoporosis Foundation. *America's bone health: the state of osteoporosis and low bone mass.* Available online at www.nof.org/ advocacy/prevalence/index.htm. Accessed March, 2003.

Nelson, A., et al. Myths and facts about back injuries in nursing. *American Journal of Nursing,* 103(2):32, 2003.

Phipps, W.J., et al. (2003). *Medical-surgical nursing: health and illness perspectives.* (7th ed.). St. Louis: Mosby.

Reuben, D., et al. (2003). *Geriatrics at your fingertips.* (5th ed.). Malden, Mass: Blackwell.

Roll-a-bout. (2004). www. roll-a-bout.com. Accessed August, 2004.

Rooney, J. Don't get out of joint. *Nursing Made Incredibly Easy,* March/April:26, 2004.

Seidel H., et al. (2003). *Mosby's guide to physical examination.* (5th ed.). St Louis: Mosby.

Thibodeau, G.A. & Patton, K.T. (2004). *Structure and function of the body.* (12th ed.). St. Louis: Mosby.

Upshur, C. & Wooten, J. Chronic pain and depression: dual challenges in managing the older patient. *Clinical Geriatrics,* 11(11):30, 2003.

Williams, S.R. (2000). *Basic nutrition and diet therapy.* (11th ed.). St. Louis: Mosby.

Chapter 5 Care of the Patient with a Gastrointestinal Disorder

Ackley, B.J. & Ladwig, G.B. (2005). *Nursing diagnosis handbook.* (6th ed.). St. Louis: Mosby.

Anderson, D.M., et al. (2002). *Mosby's medical, nursing, and allied health dictionary.* (6th ed.). St. Louis: Mosby.

Ahlquist, D.A. & Shaber, A.P. Stool screening for colorectal cancer: evolution from occult blood to molecular markers. *Clinica Chimica Acta* 315:157, 2002.

American Cancer Society. (2004). *Cancer facts and figures 2004.* Atlanta: American Cancer Society.

Atassi, K. Appendicitis. *Nursing,* 32(8):96, 2002.

Barkausas, V.H., et al. (2002). *Health and physical assessment.* (3rd ed.). St Louis: Mosby.

Black, J.M. & Hawks, H.J. (2005). *Medical-surgical nursing: clinical management for positive outcomes.* (7th ed.). Philadelphia: Saunders.

Boyer, M.J. (2004). *Study guide to Brunner and Suddarth's textbook of medical-surgical nursing.* (10th ed.). Philadelphia: Lippincott.

Brunner, L.S. & Suddarth, D.S. (2004). *Textbook of medical-surgical nursing.* (10th ed.). Philadelphia: Lippincott.

Chan, H.L., et al. Is non-*Helicobacter pylori,* non-NSAID peptic ulcer a common cause of upper GI bleeding? *Gastrointestinal Endoscopy,* 53:438, 2001.

Deglin, J. & Vallerand, A. (2005). *Davis' drug guide for nurses.* (13th ed.). Philadelphia: Davis.

Dest, V. Colorectal cancer. *RN,* 63(3):54-59, 2000.

Gallagher, S. Taking the weight off with bariatric surgery. *Nursing,* 34(3):59, 2004.

Galvan, T. Dysphagia: going down and staying down. *American Journal of Nursing,* 101(1):37, 2001.

Heitkemper, M. & Jarrett, M. It's not all in your head: irritable bowel syndrome. *American Journal of Nursing,* 101(1):26, 2001.

Living with irritable bowel syndrome. *Nursing,* 29(9):20, 1999.

Ishigami, S., et al. Clinical importance of preoperative acarcinoembryonic antigen and carbohydrate antigen 19-9 levels in gastric cancer, *Journal of Clinical Gastroenterology,* 32:41, 2001.

Karlowicz, D. An endoscopic approach to GERD. *RN,* 66(12):56, 2004.

Klonowski, E. & Masoodi, J. The patient with Crohn's disease. *RN,* 62(3):32, 1999.

Lewis, S.M., et al. (2004). *Medical-surgical nursing: assessment and management of clinical problems.* (6th ed.). St. Louis: Mosby.

Livingston, C.D., et al. (2001). Laparoscopic hiatal hernia repair in patients with poor esophageal motility or paraesophageal herniation, *The American Surgeon,* 67:987, 2001.

Long, B., et al. (2001). *Medical-surgical nursing: a nursing process approach.* (5th ed.). St. Louis: Mosby.

MacKenzie, D. When *E. coli* turns deadly. *RN,* 62(7):28, 1999.

Memmler, R.I., et al. (2004). *Structure and function of the human body.* (8th ed.). Philadelphia: Lippincott.

Miller M.A., et al. Morbidity, mortality, and healthcare burden of nosocomial *Clostridium difficile*–associated diarrhea. *Infection Control: Hospital Epidemiology,* 23:137, 2002.

Muller-Lissner, S. General geriatrics and gastroenterology: constipation and fecal incontinence. *Best Practice & Research: Clinical Gastroenterology,* 16:115, 2002.

Pagana, K.D. & Pagana, T.J. (2005). *Mosby's diagnostic and laboratory test reference.* (7th ed.). St. Louis: Mosby.

Perry, A.G. & Potter, P.A. (2005). *Clinical nursing skills and techniques.* (6th ed.). St. Louis: Mosby.

Phipps, W.J., et al. (2003). *Medical-surgical nursing: health and illness perspectives.* (7th ed.). St. Louis: Mosby.

Potter, P.A. & Perry, A.G. (2003). *Basic nursing: essentials for practice.* (5th ed.). St. Louis: Mosby.

Potter, P.A., et al. (2004). *Nursing interventions and clinical skills.* (3rd ed.). St. Louis: Mosby.

Rayhorn, N. Understanding inflammatory bowel disease. *Nursing,* 29(12):57, 1999.

Rayhorn, N., et al. Understanding gastroesophageal reflux disease. *Nursing,* 33(10):36, 2003.

Rush, C. (1995). Gastrointestinal bleeding, preventing hypovolemic shock. *Nursing,* 25(8):33, 1995.

Seidel, H.M., et al. (2003). *Mosby's guide to physical examination.* (4th ed.). St. Louis: Mosby.

Sheff, B. Minimizing the threat of *C. difficile. Nursing,* 29 (2):34, 1999.

Thibodeau, G.A. & Patton, K.T. (2003). *Anatomy and physiology.* (5th ed.). St. Louis: Mosby.

Thibodeau, G.A. & Patton, K.T. (2004). *Structure and function of the body.* (12th ed.). St. Louis: Mosby.

Thibodeau, G.A. & Patton, K.T. (2005). *The human body in health and disease.* (4th ed.). St. Louis: Mosby.

Thompson, J., et al. (2005). *Mosby's clinical nursing.* (6th ed.). St. Louis: Mosby.

Tucker, S.M., et al. (2002). *Patient care standards: Collaborative practice planning.* (7th ed.). St. Louis: Mosby.

Vakil, N. Endoscopic treatments for gastro-esophageal reflux disease. *Alimentary Pharmacology & Therapeutics,* 17(12):1427, 2003.

Walker, B. (2004). Assessing gastrointestinal infections. *Nursing,* 34(5): 48, 2004.

Venes, D. (2005.) *Taber's cyclopedic medical dictionary.* (20th ed.). Philadelphia: Davis.

Additional Resources

Crohn's and Colitis Foundation of America
386 Park Ave. South, 17th Floor
New York, NY 10016-8804
800-932-2423 or 212-685-3440
Information hotline: 800-343-3637
www.ccfa.org

United Ostomy Association
19772 MacArthur Blvd., Suite 200
Irvine, CA 92612-2405
800-826-0826
www.uao.org

Chapter 6 Care of the Patient with a Gallbladder, Liver, Biliary Tract, or Exocrine Pancreatic Disorder

Ackley, B.J. & Ladwig, G.B. (2005). *Nursing diagnosis handbook.* (6th ed.). St. Louis: Mosby.

Anderson, D.M., et al. (2002). *Mosby's medical, nursing, and allied health dictionary.* (6th ed.). St. Louis: Mosby.

Black, J.M., & Hawks, H.J. (2005). *Medical-surgical nursing: clinical management for positive outcomes.* (7th ed.). Philadelphia: Saunders.

Boyer, M.J. (2004). *Study guide to Brunner and Suddarth's textbook of medical-surgical nursing.* (10th ed.). Philadelphia: Lippincott.

Centers for Disease Control and Prevention, National Center for Infectious Diseases: *Viral hepatitis.* Available online at www.cdc.gov/ncidod/diseases/hepatitis. Accessed April, 2004.

Durston, S. The ABC's and more of hepatitis. *Nursing Made Incredibly Easy,* July/August 22:31, 2004.

Farrar, J. Emergency: acute cholelithiasis. *American Journal of Nursing,* 101(1):35, 2001.

Gemcitabine (Gemzar) for pancreatic cancer: a new treatment option. *American Journal of Nursing,* 96(12):96, 1996.

Giger, J.M. & Davidhizar, R.E. (2004). *Transcultural nursing: assessment and intervention.* (4th ed.). St. Louis: Mosby.

Holcomb, S. Hepatitis: which types are trouble? *Nursing,* 32(6):32cc1, 2002.

Jones, S. (2003). When the liver fails: new help and hope. *RN,* 66(11):33, 2003.

Kjaergard, L.L., et al. (2003). Artificial and bioartificial support systems for acute and chronic liver failure. *Journal of the American Medical Association,* 289(2):217, 2003.

Lewis, S.M., et al. (2004). *Medical-surgical nursing: assessment and management of clinical problems.* (6th ed.). St. Louis: Mosby.

Organ procurement and transplantation network. Data, 2003. Available online at www.optn.org//atestdata/rptdata/asp. Access August, 2003.

Pagana, K.D. & Pagana, T.J. (2005). *Mosby's diagnostic and laboratory test reference.* (7th ed.). St. Louis: Mosby.

Parini, S. Hepatitis, speaking out about the silent epidemic. *Nursing,* 31(3):36, 2001.

Perry, A.G. & Potter, P.A. (2005). *Clinical nursing skills and techniques.* (6th ed.). St. Louis: Mosby.

Phipps, W.J., et al. (2003). *Medical-surgical nursing: health and illness perspectives.* (7th ed.). St. Louis: Mosby.

Potter, P.A. & Perry, A.G. (2003). *Basic nursing: essentials for practice.* (5th ed.). St. Louis: Mosby.

Potter, P.A. & Perry, A.G. (2005). *Fundamentals of nursing: concepts, process, and practice.* (6th ed.). St. Louis: Mosby.

Rosen, H.R. (2001). Hepatitis B and C in the liver transplant recipient: current understanding and treatment. *Liver Transplant,* 11 (suppl 11):S87, 2001.

Seidel, H.M., et al. (2003). *Mosby's guide to physical examination.* (5th ed.). St. Louis: Mosby.

Shapiro, C.N., et al. (1999). Hepatitis B. In *Centers for Disease Control and Prevention manual for the surveillance of vaccine-preventable diseases*. Atlanta: Centers for Disease Control and Prevention.

Thibodeau, G.A. & Patton, K.T. (2003). *Anatomy and physiology.* (5th ed.). St. Louis: Mosby.

Thibodeau, G.A. & Patton, K.T. (2004). *Structure and function of the body.* (12th ed.). St. Louis: Mosby.

Thibodeau, G.A. & Patton, K.T. (2005). *The human body in health and diseases.* (4th ed.). St. Louis: Mosby.

Thompson, J., et al. (2005). *Mosby's clinical nursing.* (6th ed.). St. Louis: Mosby.

Tucker, S.M., et al. (2004). *Patient care standards: collaborative practice planning.* (8th ed.). St. Louis: Mosby.

Venes, D. (2005.) *Taber's cyclopedic medical dictionary.* (20th ed.). Philadelphia: Davis.

Warren, M. Taking a hard look at cirrhosis. *Nursing,* 29(12):32, 1999.

Chapter 7 Care of the Patient with a Blood or Lymphatic Disorder

Ackley, B.J. & Ladwig, G.B. (2005). *Nursing diagnosis handbook.* (6th ed.). St. Louis: Mosby.

Anderson, D.M., et al. (2002). *Mosby's medical, nursing, and allied health dictionary.* (6th ed.). St. Louis: Mosby.

Armas-Loughran, B., et al. Evaluation and management of anemia and bleeding disorders in surgical patients. *Medical Clinics of North America,* 87(1):229, 2003.

Barkauskas, V., et al. (2002). *Health and physical assessment.* (3rd ed.). St. Louis: Mosby.

Black, J. M., & Hawks, H.J. (2004). *Medical surgical nursing: clinical management for positive outcomes.* (5th ed.). Philadelphia: Saunders.

Borton, D. WBC count and differential. *Nursing,* 26:11, 1996.

Clines, D.B. Immune thrombocytopenic purpura. *New England Journal of Medicine,* 356:995, 2002.

Cohen, H. Anemia in the elderly: clinical impact and practical diagnosis. *Journal of American Geriatrics Society,* 51(3)(suppl):51, 2003.

Day, M. Sickle-cell crisis. *Nursing,* 5:31, 2001.

Day, S.E. Sickle cell pain and hydroxyurea. *American Journal of Nursing,* 100(34), 2000.

Deglin, J. & Vallerand, A. (2005). *Davis's drug guide for nurses.* (13th ed.). Philadelphia: Davis.

Deziel, S. Anemia management in patients with chronic conditions that affect erythropoiesis. Case study of the anemic patient. *Nephrology Nursing Journal,* 29(6):582: 2002.

Diagnosis and management of multiple myeloma. *British Journal of Haematology,* 115:522, 2001.

Exposure safety—risky phlebotomy with a syringe. *Nursing,* 2: 31, 2001.

Fitzpatrick, L. When to administer modified blood products. *Nursing,* 32:36, 2002.

Geiter, H. Disseminated intravascular coagulopathy. *Dimensions of Critical Care Nursing,* 22(3):108, 2003.

Giger, J.M. & Davidhizar, R.E. (2004). *Transcultural nursing: assessment and intervention.* (4th ed.). St. Louis: Mosby.

Gorman, K. Sickle cell disease. *American Journal of Nursing,* 3:99, 1999.

Gutaj, D. Oncology today: Lymphoma. *RN,* 8:63, 2000.

Johnson, M., et al. (2000). *Nursing outcomes classification (NOC).* (2nd ed.). St. Louis: Mosby.

Kim, M.J., et al. (2005). *Pocket guide to nursing diagnoses.* (8th ed.). St. Louis: Mosby.

Levi, M., et al. The diagnosis of disseminated intravascular coagulation. *Blood Reviews,* 16(4):217, 2002.

Lewis, S.M., et al. (2004). *Medical-surgical nursing: assessment and management of clinical problems.* (6th ed.). St. Louis: Mosby.

Lipschitz, D. Medical and functional consequences of anemia in the elderly. *Journal of the American Geriatrics Society,* 51(3)(suppl):510, 2003.

Montoya, V., et al. Anemia, what lies beneath, *Nursing Made Incredibly Easy,* January/February:38, 2004.

Pagana, K.D. & Pagana, T.J. (2003). *Diagnostic testing and nursing implications: a case study approach.* (5th ed.). St. Louis: Mosby.

Pagana, K.D. & Pagana, T.J. (2005). *Mosby's diagnostic and laboratory test reference.* (7th ed.). St. Louis: Mosby.

Pear R. Understanding and managing anemia in cricially ill patients. *Critical Care Nurse,* (suppl):12, 2002

Perry, A.G. & Potter, P.A. (2005). *Clinical nursing skills and techniques.* (6th ed.). St. Louis: Mosby.

Phipps, W.J., et al. (2003). *Medical-surgical nursing: health and illness perspectives.* (7th ed.). St. Louis: Mosby.

Portielje, J.E., et al. Morbidity and mortality in adults with immune thrombocytopenic purpura. *Blood,* 97:2549, 2001.

Potter, P.A. & Perry, A.G. (2003). *Basic nursing: essentials for practice.* (5th ed.). St. Louis: Mosby.

Reviewing the basics: Blood group compatibility. (2000). *Nursing,* 12, 30.

Seidel, H.M., et al. (2003). *Mosby's guide to physical examination.* (5th ed.). St. Louis: Mosby.

Seiter, K.: Treatment of acute myelogenous leukemia in the elderly patients. *Clinical Geriatrics,* 10:41, 2002.

Skidmore-Roth, L. (2006). *Mosby's 2006 nursing drug reference.* St. Louis: Mosby.

Thibodeau, G.A. & Patton, K.T. (2003). *Anatomy and physiology.* (5th ed.). St. Louis: Mosby.

Thibodeau, G.A. & Patton, K.T. (2004). *Structure and function of the body.* (12th ed.). St. Louis: Mosby.

Thompson, J.M., et al. (2005). *Mosby's clinical nursing.* (6th ed.). St. Louis: Mosby.

Chapter 8 Care of the Patient with a Cardiovascular or a Peripheral Vascular Disorder

Anderson, D.M., et al. (2002). *Mosby's medical, nursing, and allied health dictionary.* (6th ed.). St. Louis: Mosby.

Artinian, N. (2003). The psychosocial aspects of heart failure. *American Journal of Nursing,* 103(12):32, 2003.

Beese-Bjurstrom, S. Aortic aneurysms and dissection. *Nursing,* 34(2):36, 2004.

Beltrami, A., et al. Evidence that human cardiac myocytes divide after myocardial infarction. *New England Journal of Medicine,* 344(6):1750, 2001.

Bengston, A. & Drevenhorn, E. The nurse's role and skills in hypertension care: a review. *Clinical Nurse Specialist,* 17(5):260, 2003.

Bittner, V. Women and coronary heart disease risk factors. *Journal of Cardiovascular Risk,* 9(6):315, 2002.

Black, J.H. & Hawks, H.J. (2005). *Medical-surgical nursing: clinical management for positive outcomes.* (7th ed.). Philadelphia: Saunders.

Braunwald, E., et al. (2003). *Harrison's principles of internal medicine.* (15th ed.). New York: McGraw-Hill.

Bosen, D. What you need to know about the new heart failure guidelines. *Nursing,* 32(6):32CC8, 2002.

Canobbio, M.M. (2004). *Mosby's handbook of patient teaching.* (3rd ed.). St. Louis: Mosby.

Chase, S. Hypertensive crisis, *RN,* 63(6):62, 2000.

Chiocca, E. & Russo, L. Superior vena cava syndrome. *Nursing,* 30(6):33, 2000.

Chojnowski, D. Putting together the pieces of cardiomyopathy. *Nursing Made Incredibly Easy,* May/June:18, 2004.

Church, V. DVT and PE. *Nursing,* 30(2):35, 2000.

Furry B., et al: Reviewing the drug line up against AMI. *Nursing,* 30:32, 2000.

Giger, J.M. & Davidhizar, R.E. (2004). *Transcultural nursing: assessment and intervention.* (4th ed.). St. Louis: Mosby.

Hayes, D. Stemming the tide of pleural effusions. *Nursing,* 31(5):49, 2001.

Hobbs, R.E. Using BNP to diagnose, manage, and treat heart failure. *Cleveland Clinics Journal of Medicine,* 70(4):333, 2003.

Holcomb, S. Recognizing and managing endocarditis. *Nursing,* 34(2):32, 2004.

Iyer, P.W. & Camp, N.H. (2003). *Nursing documentation: a nursing process approach.* (4th ed.). St. Louis: Mosby.

Langford, R. & Thompson, J. (2004). *Mosby's handbook of diseases.* (3rd ed.). St. Louis: Mosby.

Le, T. & Bayer, A. combination antibiotic therapy for infective endocarditis. *Clinical Infectious Diseases,* 36(5):615, 2003.

Lewis, S., et al. (2004). *Medical-surgical nursing: assessment and management of clinical problems* (6th ed.). St. Louis: Mosby.

Lloyd-Jones, D.M., et al. Lifetime risk for developing congestive heart failure: the Framingham heart study. *Circulation,* 106(24):3068, 2002.

McDonnell, E. Applying nitroglycerin ointment. *Nursing,* 31(6):3, 2001.

McFarland, G. & McFarland, E. (2001). *Nursing diagnosis and intervention: planning for patient care.* (4th ed.). St. Louis: Mosby.

Miracle, V. Put the brakes on pericarditis. *Nursing,* 31:4, 2001.

Moriarty, M. Heart disease. *RN,* 67(1):33, 2004.

Nagle, B. Acute myocardial infarction. *Nursing,* 32(10):50, 2002.

National Heart, Lung and Blood Institute. Available online at www.nhlbinih.gov.

Nienaber, C. & Eagle, K. Aortic dissection: new frontiers in diagnosis and management. Part I: from etiology to diagnostic strategies. *Circulation,* 108(5):628, 2003.

Nienaber, C. & Eagle, K. Aortic dissection: new frontiers in diagnosis and management. Part II: therapeutic management and follow-up. *Circulation,* 108(5):772, 2003.

Pagana, K.D. & Pagana, T.J. (2005). *Mosby's diagnostic and laboratory test reference.* (7th ed.). St. Louis: Mosby.

Palatnik, A. How cardiac drugs do what they do. *Nursing,* 31(5):54, 2001.

Phipps, W.J., et al. (2003). *Medical-surgical nursing: health and illness perspectives.* (7th ed.). St. Louis: Mosby.

Pope, B. What's at the heart of your patient's chest pain? *Nursing Made Incredibly Easy,* January/February 8:18, 2004.

Riggs, J. New therapies for heart failure. *RN,* 67(3):29, 2004.

The seventh report of the Joint National Committee on Prevention, Detection, Evaluation, and Treatment of High Blood Pressure, Bethesda, Md., U.S. Department of Health and Human Services, National Institutes of Health, National Heart, Lung and Blood Institute, May, 2003.

Shatzer, M. & Saul, L. What does BNP tell you? *Nursing Made Incredibly Easy,* May/June:7, 2004.

Simms, J. & Miracle, V. Fast facts about supraventricular tachycardia. *Nursing,* 31(6):44, 2001.

Skidmore-Roth, L. (2006). *Mosby's 2006 nursing drug reference.* St. Louis: Mosby.

Steinke, E. Sexual counseling after myocardial infarction. *American Journal of Nursing,* 100(12):38, 2000.

Thibodeau, G.A. & Patton, K.T. (2004). *Structure and function of the human body.* (12th ed.). St. Louis: Mosby.

Thibodeau, G.A. & Patton, K.T. (2005). *The human body in health and disease.* (4th ed.). St. Louis: Mosby.

Thomas, C.L. (2005). *Taber's cyclopedic medical dictionary.* (20th ed.). Philadelphia: Davis.

Thompson, J., et al. (2005). *Mosby's clinical nursing.* (8th ed.). St. Louis: Mosby.

Tucker, S.M., et al. (2004). *Patient care standards.* (8th ed.). St. Louis: Mosby.

Willis, K. Gaining perspective on peripheral vascular disease. *Nursing,* 31:2, 2001.

Chapter 9 Care of the Patient with a Respiratory Disorder

Anderson, D.M., et al. (2002). *Mosby's medical, nursing, and allied health dictionary.* (6th ed.). St. Louis: Mosby.

Assessing breath sounds. *Nursing* 96(6):26, 1996.

Barkauskas, V., et al. (2003). *Health and physician assessment.* (3rd ed.). St. Louis: Mosby.

Black, J.M. & Hawks, H.J. (2004). *Medical surgical nursing: clinical management for positive outcomes.* (7th ed.). Philadelphia: Saunders.

Bock-Avolos, S. The hard truth about the PPD skin test. *Nursing,* 31(6):56, 2001.

Carlson, B. (2003). Changes in sleep patterns in COPD. *American Journal of Nursing,* 103(12):71, 2003.

Covey, M. & Larson, J. Exercise and COPD. *American Journal of Nursing,* 104(5):40, 2003.

Davis, P. Guarding your patient against ARDS. *Nursing,* 32(3):36, 2002.

Deglin, J. & Vallerand, A. (2005). *Davis's drug guide for nurses.* (13th ed.). Philadelphia: Davis.

Dest, V. Oncology today: lung cancer. *RN,* 63(5):32, 2000.

Giger, J.M. & Davidhizar, R.E. (2004). *Transcultural nursing: assessment and intervention.* (4th ed.). St. Louis: Mosby.

Global initiative for chronic obstructive lung disease. Available online at http://goldcopd.com. Accessed August, 2005.

Goldrick, B. Adult respiratory infections. *American Journal of Nursing,* 103(10):65, 2003.

Goldrick, B. 21st-century emerging and reemerging infections. *American Journal of Nursing,* 104(1):67, 2004.

Ignatavicius, D., et al. (2003). *Medical-surgical nursing across the healthcare continuum.* (4th ed.). St. Louis: Mosby.

Inglesby, T., et al. Anthrax as a biological weapon: medical and public health management. *JAMA* 281(18), 1735-1745, 1999.

Katz, J. & Hirsch, A. When global health is local health (SARS). *American Journal of Nursing,* 103(12):75, 2003.

Koschel, M. Pulmonary embolism. *American Journal of Nursing,* 104(6):46, 2004.

Kreamer, K. Lung cancer. *Nursing,* 33(11):36, 2003.

Langford, R. & Thompson, J. (2004). *Mosby's handbook of diseases.* (3rd ed.). St. Louis: Mosby.

Lattavo, K. Pinpointing postoperative hypoxemia. *Nursing,* 31(1):32, 2001.

Lazzara, D. Respiratory distress, pulmonary embolism, pneumothorax and pulmonary edema. *Nursing,* 31(6):58, 2001.

Lazzara, D. Chest tubes. *Nursing,* 32(6):36, 2002.

Lewis, S.M., et al. (2004). *Medical-surgical nursing: assessment and management of clinical problems.* (6th ed.). St. Louis: Mosby.

Lezon, K. Teaching incentive spirometry. *Nursing,* 29(1):60, 1999.

Marion, B. A turn for the better: "prone positioning" of patient with ARDS. *American Journal of Nursing,* 101(5):26, 2001.

McConnell, E. Do's and don'ts, performing pulse oximetry. *Nursing,* 29(1):17, 1999.

McFarland, G. & McFarland, E. (2003). *Nursing diagnosis and intervention: planning for patient care.* (4th ed.). St. Louis: Mosby.

Miracle, V. & Winston, M. Take the wind out of asthma. *Nursing,* 30(8):34, 2000.

Otto, S. (2001). *Oncology nursing.* (4th ed.). St. Louis: Mosby.

Pagana, K.D. & Pagana, T.J. (2005). *Mosby's diagnostic and laboratory test reference.* (7th ed.). St. Louis: Mosby.

Parini, S. Severe acute respiratory syndrome. *Nursing,* 33(9):96, 2003.

Phipps, W.J., et al. (2003). *Medical-surgical nursing: health and illness perspectives.* (7th ed.). St. Louis: Mosby.

Pope, B. Asthma. *Nursing,* 32(5):44, 2002.

Potter, P.A. & Perry A.G. (2005). *Fundamentals of nursing: concepts, process, and practice.* (6th ed.). St. Louis: Mosby.

Potter, P.A. & Perry, A.G. (2003). *Basic nursing: essentials for practice.* (5th ed.). St. Louis: Mosby.

Price, S. & Wilson, L. (2003). *Pathophysiology: clinical concepts of disease processes.* (6th ed.). St. Louis: Mosby.

Ruppel, G. (2003). *Manual of pulmonary function testing.* (8th ed.). St. Louis: Mosby.

Schleder, B. Keeping hospital bugs at bay. *Nursing Made Incredibly Easy,* March/April:36, 2004.

Seidel, H.M., et al. (2003). *Mosby's guide to physical examination.* (5th ed.). St. Louis: Mosby.

Sin D., et al. Contemporary management of chronic obstructive pulmonary disease: scientific review. *Journal of the American Medical Association,* 290(17):2301, 2003.

Skidmore-Roth, L. (2006). *Mosby's 2006 nursing drug reference.* St. Louis: Mosby.

Swartz, M. (2001). Recognition and management of anthrax—an update. *New England Journal of Medicine,* 345(22):1621, 2001.

Swearingen, P.L. (2003). *Manual of medical-surgical nursing.* (5th ed.). St. Louis: Mosby.

Tate, J. & Tasota, F. Eye and diagnostics, using pulse oximetry. *Nursing,* 30(9):30, 2000.

Tate, J. & Tasota, F. More than a snore: recognizing the danger of sleep apnea. *Nursing,* 32(8):46, 2002.

Thibodeau, G.A. & Patton, K.T. (2004). *Structure and function of the human body.* (12th ed.). St. Louis: Mosby.

Thibodeau, G.A. & Patton, K.T. (2005). *The human body in health and disease.* (4th ed.). St. Louis: Mosby.

Thompson, J.M., et al. (2005). *Mosby's clinical nursing.* (6th ed.). St. Louis: Mosby.

Wisniewski, A. (2004). When air is rare—helping patients with chronic bronchitis or emphysema breathe easier. *Nursing Made Incredibly Easy,* January/February:20, 2004.

Chapter 10 Care of the Patient with a Urinary Disorder

Abrams, A.C. (2003). *Clinical drug therapy.* (5th ed.). Philadelphia: Lippincott.

Ackley, B.J. & Ladwig, G.B. (2005). *Nursing diagnosis handbook.* (6th ed.). St. Louis: Mosby.

Anderson, D.M., et al. (2002). *Mosby's medical, nursing, and allied health dictionary.* (6th ed.). St. Louis: Mosby.

Astle, S M. A new direction for dialysis. *RN,* 64(7):56, 2001.

Black, J.M. & Hawks, J.H. (2005). *Medical-surgical nursing: clinical management for positive outcomes.* (7th ed.). Philadelphia: Saunders.

Boggs, W. (2004). *Doxycycline improves cystitis symptoms in women.* www.nlm.nih.gov/medlineplus/news/fullstory_18649.html.

Bosch, R. (2000). *Use of neuromodulation in voiding dysfunction.* www.indianacontinencefoundation.org/clinupdate_files/8.html.

Bullock, B.L. & Henze, R. (2000). *Focus on pathology.* (5th ed.). Philadelphia: Lippincott.

Carpenito, L.J. (2003). *Handbook of nursing diagnoses.* (10th ed.). Philadelphia: Lippincott.

Chang, M. & Harden, J. Meeting the challenge of the new millennium: caring for culturally diverse patients. *Urologic Nursing,* 22(6):372, 2002.

Cheung, A. & Wong, L. Infections in diabetes and end-stage renal failure. *Infectious Diseases Clinics of North America,* 15(3): 2001.

Colella, KI. & DeLuca, G. Shared decision making in patients with newly diagnosed prostate cancer: a model for treatment education and support. *Urologic Nursing,* 24(3):187, 2004.

Crowe, H. & Costello, A. Prostate cancer: perspectives on quality of life and impact of treatment of patients and their partners. *Urologic Nursing,* 23(4):279, 2003.

Dinwiddie, L.C. Caring through the end of life. *Nephrology Nursing Journal,* 31(3):263, 2004.

Dirkes, S. & Kozlowski, C. Renal assist device therapy for acute renal failure. *Nephrology Nursing Journal,* 30(6):611, 2003.

Dixon, L., et al. Urinary diversions: a review of nursing care. *Urologic Nursing,* 21(5):37, 2001.

Early radiation therapy after prostatectomy may dramatically reduce cancer recurrence. *Urologic Nursing,* 22(3):197, 2002.

Eckler, J.A.L. Combating UTI. *Nursing* 30(6):1, 2000.

Feingold, M. & Crawford, J. Urologic management of a quadriplegic patient during pregnancy. *Infections in Urology,* 13(3):77, 2000.

Fischback, F. & Dunning, M. (2003). *A manual of laboratory and diagnostic tests.* (7th ed.). Philadelphia: Lippincott.

Gaines, K. Dutasteride (Avodart): new 5-alpha-reductase inhibitor for treating BPH. *Urologic Nursing,* 23(3):218, 2003.

Geerlings, S.E., et al. Asymptomatic bacteriuria may be considered a complication in women with diabetes. *Diabetes Care,* 23(6):744, 2000.

Gray, M. Urinary retention, part 1. *American Journal of Nursing,* 100(7):40, 2000.

Gray, M. Urinary retention, part 2. *American Journal of Nursing,* 100(8):36, 2000.

Gray, M. Gender, race, and culture in research on UI. In Newman D.K. & Palmer, M.H. (eds.). The state of the science on urinary incontinence. *American Journal of Nursing,* (suppl 3):20, 2003.

Grill, W., et al. Emerging clinical applications of electrical stimulation electrical stimulation: opportunities for restoration of function. *Journal of Rehabilitation Research and Development,* 38(6):2004.

Hall, G., et al. New directions in peritoneal training. *Nephrology Nursing Journal,* 31(2):149, 2004.

Hanson, K. Diagnostic tests and tools in the evaluation of urologic disease: part 11. *Urologic Nursing,* 23(6):405, 2003.

Hanson, K. Laboratory studies in the evaluation of urologic disease: part 1. *Urologic Nursing,* 23(6):400, 2003.

Hayes, D.D. Caring for your patient with a permanent hemodialysis access. *Nursing,* 30(3):41, 2000.

Held-Warmkessel, J. How to care for men with prostate cancer. *Nursing,* 29(11):51, 1999.

Held-Warmkessel, J. What your patient needs to know about prostate. *Nursing 2002,* 32(12):36, 2003.

Hinds, A. Obstructive uropathy: considerations for the nephrology nurse. *Nephrology Nursing Journal,* 31(2):166, 2004. http://gokind.org.

Hoffman, M.A. & Diamond, D. Do fluoroquinolones have a role in pediatric urinary tract infections? *Infections in Medicine,* 17(5):334, 2000.

Huether, S.E. & McCance, K.L. (2003). *Understanding pathophysiology.* (3rd ed.). St. Louis: Mosby.

Jackson, R. My prostate cancer's back. Now what? *Nursing 2002,* 32(4):32hn2, 2002.

Kay, B., et al. The role of ketorolac tromethamine in a clinical care pathway for men undergoing radical retropubic prostatectomy. *Urologic Nursing,* 22(6):392, 2002.

King, B. Meds and the dialysis patient. *RN,* 63(7):54, 2000.

Kuebler, K. Palliative nursing care for the patient experiencing end-stage renal failure. *Urologic Nursing,* 21(3):167, 2001.

Lehne, R.A. (2003). *Pharmacology for nursing care.* (5th ed.). Philadelphia: Elsevier.

Lehne, R.A. (2003). *Study guide for pharmacology in nursing care.* (5th ed.). Philadelphia: Elsevier.

Lekan-Rutledge, D. & Colling, J. Urinary incontinence in the frail elderly. In Newman, D.K. & Palmer, M.H. (eds). The state of the science on urinary incontinence. *American Journal of Nursing,* (suppl 3):36, 2003.

Lewis, S.M., et al. (2004). *Medical-surgical nursing: assessment and management of clinical problems.* (6th ed.). St. Louis: Elsevier.

Linton, A., et al. (2000). *Introductory nursing care of adults.* (2nd ed.). Philadelphia: Saunders.

Little, C. Renovascular hypertension. *American Journal of Nursing,* 100(2):46, 2001.

Maloney, C. Estrogen and recurrent UTI. *American Journal of Nursing,* 102(8):44, 2002.

Managing IC symptoms with neuromodulation devices. (1999). ICA update, 14(4). www.ichel.com/TreatmentAndSelfHelp/ManagingICSymptomsWithNeuromoulati…

Meloskey, J.C. & Blechek, G.M. (eds.). (2000). *Nursing interventions classification.* (3rd ed.). St. Louis: Mosby.

Metheny, N.M. (2000). *Fluid and electrolyte balance.* (4th ed.). Philadelphia: Lippincott.

Miller, D., et al. Challenges for nephrology nurses in the management of children with chronic kidney disease. *Nephrology Nursing Journal,* 31(3):287, 2004.

Moon, M. Neurostimulator advocated for incontinence—when other treatments fail. *OB/GYN News,* June 15, 2002.

Moore, M.C. (1997). *Mosby's nutritional care.* (3rd ed.). St. Louis: Mosby.

Moyad, M. Calcium oxalate kidney stones: another reason to encourage moderate calcium intakes and other dietary changes. *Urologic Nursing,* 23(4):310, 2003.

Munnings, L. & Cawood, C. Clinical study of a new urine collection bag. *Urologic Nursing,* 23(40):287, 2003.

National Kidney and Urologic Diseases Information clearinghouse. Available online at http://ikidney.com.

Newman, D. Stress urinary incontinence in women. *American Journal of Nursing,* 103(8):46, 2003.

Neyhart, C. current issues in transplant nursing. *Nephrology Nursing Journal,* 31(3):337. 2004.

Ostomies. Alternaive methods for waste elimination. *Mayo Clinic Health Letter,* May, 22(5):7, 2004.

Pentosan polysulfate sodium effective in treating interstitial cystitis. *Urologic Nursing,* 22(3):198, 2002.

Perry, A.G. & Potter, P.A. (2005). *Clinical nursing skills and techniques.* (6th ed.). St. Louis: Mosby.

Pile, C. Hemodialysis vascular access: how do practice patterns affect outcomes? *Nephrology Nursing Journal,* 31(3):305, 2004.

Polycystic kidney disease (NK012): The Medifocus Guide on Polycystic Kidney Disease. Available online at www.medivillage.com/guides/index.efm?Guide=K012. Accessed

Potter, P.A. & Perry A.G. (2005). *Fundamentals of nursing: concepts, process, and practice.* (6th ed.). St. Louis: Mosby.

Price, C.A. Resources for planning palliative and end-of-life care for patients with kidney disease. *Nephrology Nursing Journal,* 30(6):649, 2003.

Quallich, S. & Ohl, D. Artificial urinary sphincter, part II: patient teaching and perioperative care. *Urologic Nursing,* 23(4):269, 2003.

Rabetoy, C. & Colaneri, J. Living anonymous kidney donation: a solution to the organ donor shortage? No the research is incomplete. *Nephrology Nursing Journal,* 31(3):330, 2004.

Rabetoy, C. & Neyhart, C. Living anonymous kidney donation: a solution to the organ donor shortage? Yes, another availale resource. *Nephrology Nursing Journal,* 31(3):330, 2004.

Randall, S. Valrubicin: an alternative to radical cystectomy for carcinoma in situ of the bladder. *Urologic Nursing,* 21(1):30, 2001.

Razi, H., et al. Intracorporeal lithotripsy with the holmium:YAG laser. *Journal of Urology,* 156(3):912, 1996.

Robb-Nicholson, C. & Schatz, C. The mystery of cystitis. *Newsweek,* 143(19):77, 2004.

Sairanen, J., et al. Long-term outcome of patients with interstitial cystitis treated with low dose cyclosporine A. *Journal of Urology,* 171(6 Pt 1):2138, 2004.

Sampselle, C. Behavioral interventions in young and middle-age women. In Newman D.K. & Palmer, M.H. (eds.). The state of the science on urinary incontinence. *American Journal of Nursing,* (suppl 3):9, 2003.

Schiffl, H., et al. Daily hemodialysis and the outcome of acute renal failure, *The New England Journal of Medicine,* 346(5):305, 2002.

Selo-Ojeme, D.O. & Onwude, J.L. Interstitial cystitis. *Journal of Obstetrics & Gynaecology,* 24(3):216, 2004.

Skidmore-Roth, L. (2006). *Mosby's 2006 nursing drug reference.* St. Louis: Mosby.

Smeltzer, S.C., et al. (2003). *Brunner and Suddarth's textbook of medical-surgical nursing.* (9th ed.). Philadelphia: Lippincott Williams & Wilkins.

Transdermal oxybutnin reduces overactive bladder symptoms with low side effects. *Urologic Nursing,* 22(3):199, 2002.

Tucker, S.M., et al. (2000). *Patient care standards: collaborative practice planning.* (7th ed.). St. Louis: Mosby.

Urinary incontinence. Johns Hopkins–Brady Urological Institute. Available online at http://urology.jhu.edu/incontinence/index.php?var=faculty.php.

UTI-Zone, TSN Database-USA© 2000, Focus/MRL, Inc. (2001, April 4). Available online at www.mrlinfo.com. Accessed August, 2005.

Ward-Smith, P. Brachytherapy for prostate cancer: the patient's perspective. *Urologic Nursing,* 23(5):213. 2003.

Wells, C. Optimizing nutrition in patients with chronic kidney disease. *Nephrology Nursing Journal,* 30(6):637, 2003.

Woodward, S. Current management of neurogenic bladder in patients in MS. *British Journal of Nursing,* 13(7):362, 2004.

Wong, D.L., et al. (2001). *Maternal child nursing care.* (2nd ed.). St. Louis: Elsevier.

Wyman, J. Treatment of urinary incontinence in men and older women. In Newman, D.K. & Palmer, M.H. (eds.). The state of the science on urinary incontinence. *American Journal of Nursing,* (suppl 3):26, 2003.

Young, J. Kidney stone. *Nursing,* 30(7):33, 2000.

Zabat, E. When your patient needs peritoneal dialysis. *Nursing 2003,* 33(8):52, 2003.

Zaccagnini, M. Prostate cancer. *American Journal of Nursing,* 99(4):34, 1999.

Chapter 11 Care of the Patient with an Endocrine Disorder

American Diabetes Association. *All about diabetes.* Available online at www.diabetes.org/about-diabetes.jsp. Accessed August, 2005.

American Diabetes Association. Standards of medical care for patients with diabetes mellitus. *Diabetes Care,* 26(suppl 1):533, 2003.

Anderson, D.M., et al. (2002). *Mosby's medical, nursing, and allied health dictionary.* (6th ed.). St. Louis: Mosby.

Barkauskas, V., et al. (2002). *Health and physical assessment.* (3rd ed.). St. Louis: Mosby.

Bartol, T. Putting a patient with diabetes in the driver's seat. *Nursing,* 32(2):53, 2002.

Bjerkness, S. & Hagen, G. Switching from animal to human insulin. *Diabetes Self-Management,* 18(2):70, 2001.

Black, J.M. & Hawks, H.J. (2005). *Medical surgical nursing: clinical management for positive outcomes.* (7th ed.). Philadelphia: Saunders.

Bode, B., et al. Comparison of insulin aspart with buffered regular insulin and insulin lispro in continuous subcutaneous infusion: a randomized study in type 1 diabetes. *Diabetes Care,* 25(3):439, 2002.

Crump, V. Hyperglycemic crisis—regaining control. *RN,* 67(41):23, 2004.

Daub, K. Pheochromocytoma, up close and personal. *Nursing,* 32(3):32hn1, 2002.

Egede, L. & Zheng, D. Independent factors associated with major depressive disorder in a national sample of individuals with diabetes. *Diabetic Care,* 26(1):104, 2003.

Fain, J. Delivering insulin around the clock. *Nursing,* 32(8):54, 2002.

Fain, J. Unlock the mysteries of insulin therapy. *Nursing,* 34(3):41, 2004.

Funnel, M. & Barlage, D. Managing diabetes with "agent oral." *Nursing,* 34(3):36, 2002.

Holcomb, S. Stopping the cascade of diabetes insipidus. *Nursing,* 32(3):32cc1, 2002.

Holcomb, S. Detecting thyroid disease, part 2. *Nursing,* 33(9):32cc1, 2003.

Harberg, R. Making sense of dietary recommendations. *Diabetes Self-Management,* July/August, 52, 2003

Hieronymus, L. & O'Connell, B. Diabetes basics, understanding hypoglycemia. *Diabetes Self-Management,* November/December, 38, 2003.

Hieronymus, L. & O'Connell, B. Diabetes basics, managing hyperglycemia. *Diabetes Self-Management,* March/April, 2004.

Jacques, S. Diabetes under control: diabetes and depression. *American Journal of Nursing,* 104(9):56, 2004.

Lewis, S.M., et al. (2004). *Medical-surgical nursing: assessment and management of clinical problems.* (6th ed.). St. Louis: Mosby.

McCance, K.L. & Huether, S.E. (2002). *Pathophysiology: the biologic basis for disease in children and adults.* (4th ed.) St Louis: Mosby.

Moshang, J. What's your insulin IQ? The puzzle of type 1 diabetes. *Nursing Made Incredibly Easy,* May/June:4, 2004.

O'Connell, B. Herbal therapies and diabetes complications. *Diabetes Self-Management,* 18(1):87, 2001.

Olohan, K. The insulin pump. *American Journal of Nursing,* 103(4):48, 2003.

Pagana, K.D. & Pagana, T.J. (2005). *Mosby's diagnostic and laboratory test reference.* (7th ed.). St. Louis: Mosby.

Phipps, W.J., et al. (2003). *Medical-surgical nursing: health and illness perspectives.* (7th ed.).St. Louis: Mosby.

Potter, P.A. & Perry, A.G. (2003). *Basic nursing: essentials for practice.* (5th ed.). St. Louis: Mosby.

Potter, P.A. & Perry A.G. (2005). *Fundamentals of nursing: concepts, process, and practice.* (6th ed.). St. Louis: Mosby.

Report of the expert committee on the diagnosis and classification of diabetes mellitus. *Diabetic Care,* 25(suppl 1):5, 2002.

Retsinos, J. Type 2 diabetes. *Diabetes Self-Management,* May/June:27, 2003.

Seley, J. Commentary on the U.S. Preventive Services Task Force recommendations for screening for type 2 diabetes mellitus in adults. *American Journal of Nursing,* 104(31):93, 2004.

Simmons, S. Detecting thyroid disease, part 1. *Nursing,* 33(8):32cc1, 2003.

Skidmore-Roth, L. (2006). *Mosby's 2006 nursing drug reference.* St. Louis: Mosby.

Thibodeau, G.A. & Patton, K.T. (2004). *Structure and function of the human body.* (12th ed.). St. Louis: Mosby.

Thibodeau, G.A. & Patton, K.T. (2005). *The human body in health and disease.* (4th ed.). St. Louis: Mosby.

Thompson, J., et al. (2005). *Mosby's clinical nursing.* (6th ed.). St. Louis: Mosby.

White, J., et al. (2003). Pharmacologic therapies in a core curriculum for diabetes education. (5th ed.). In Franz, M. (ed.)., Chicago: The American Association of Diabetes Educators.

Wilson, S.F. & Gidden, J.F. (2005). *Health assessment for nursing practice,* 3rd ed.). St Louis: Mosby.

Chapter 12 Care of the Patient with a Reproductive Disorder

Ackley, B.J. & Ladwig, G.B. (2005). *Nursing diagnosis handbook.* (6th ed.). St. Louis: Mosby.

Akert, J. Hormone replacement therapy, *RN,* 66(12):40, 2003.

American Cancer Society. (2004). *Cancer facts and figures, 2004.* Atlanta: Author.

Anderson, D.M., et al. (2002). *Mosby's medical, nursing, and allied health dictionary.* (6th ed.). St. Louis: Mosby.

Aschenbrenner, D. Hormone replacement therapy (HRT): what should you tell patients about it now? *American Journal of Nursing,* 104(6):51, 2004.

Balzer-Riley, J. (2004). *Communication in nursing.* (5th ed.). St. Louis: Mosby.

Barkauskas, V., et al. (2002). *Health and physical assessment.* (3rd ed.). St. Louis: Mosby.

Baron, R. Sentinel lymph node biopsy in breast cancer and the role of the oncology nurse. *Clinical Journal of Oncology Nursing,* 3(1):17, 1999.

Black, J.M. & Hawks, H.J. (2004). *Medical surgical nursing: clinical management for positive outcomes.* (7th ed.). Philadelphia: Saunders.

Centers for Disease Control and Prevention. 1998 guidelines for treatment of sexually transmitted diseases. *Morbidity and Mortality Weekly Report,* 47, 1998.

Costantino, J.P., et al. Validation studies for models projecting the risk of invasive and total breast cancer incidence. *Journal of the National Cancer Institute,* 91(18):1541, 1999.

Deglin, J. & Vallerand, A. (2005). *Davis's drug guide for nurses.* (13th ed.). Philadelphia: Davis.

DuVal, S. Inflammatory breast cancer, *RN,* 67(2):43, 2004.

Editorial. Valacyclovir now approved for genital herpes, *American Journal of Nursing,* 103(12):65, 2003.

Elkin, M.K., et al. (2004). *Nursing interventions and clinical skills.* (3rd ed.). St. Louis: Mosby.

Giger, J.M. & Davidhizar, R.E. (2005). *Transcultural nursing: assessment and intervention.* (5th ed.). St. Louis: Mosby.

Greifzu, S. Breast cancer, *RN,* 67(2):35, 2004.

Langford, R. & Thompson, J. (2000). *Mosby's handbook of diseases.* (2nd ed.). St. Louis: Mosby.

Lewis, S., et al. (2004). *Medical-surgical nursing: assessment and management of clinical problems.* (6th ed.). St. Louis: Mosby.

Machia, J. Breast cancer: risk, prevention, and tamoxifen. *American Journal of Nursing,* 4:101, 2001.

McCaffery, M. & Pasero, C. (1999). *Pain: clinical manual.* (2nd ed.). St. Louis: Mosby.

Memmler, R.L., et al. (2004). *Structure and function of the human body.* (8th ed.). Philadelphia: Lippincott.

Noonon, D. Breast cancer's "new era." *Newsweek,* October 20:67, 2003.

Otto, S. (2001). *Oncology nursing.* (4th ed.). St. Louis: Mosby.

Pagana, K.D. & Pagana, T.J. (2005). *Mosby's diagnostic and laboratory test reference.* (7th ed.). St. Louis: Mosby.

Phipps, W.J., et al. (2003). *Medical-surgical nursing: health and illness perspectives.* (7th ed.).St. Louis: Mosby.

Potter, P.A. & Perry A.G. (2005). *Fundamentals of nursing: concepts, process, and practice.* (6th ed.). St. Louis: Mosby.

Rossouw, J. (2002). End of the age of estrogen. *Newsweek,* July 22 (editorial).

Seidel, H.M., et al. (2003). *Mosby's guide to physical examination.* (5th ed.). St. Louis: Mosby.

Shinn, S. Taking a stand against cervical cancer. *Nursing,* 34(5):36, 2004.

Skidmore-Roth, L. (2006). *Mosby's 2006 nursing drug reference.* St. Louis: Mosby.

Swayze, S. Preventing problems from tampon use. *Nursing,* 31(7):28. 2001.

Thibodeau, G.A. & Patton, K.T. (2003). *Anatomy and physiology.* (5th ed.). St. Louis: Mosby.

Thibodeau, G.A. & Patton, K.T. (2004). *Structure and function of the body.* (12th ed.). St. Louis: Mosby.

Thomas, S. Oncology today: breast cancer. *RN,* 63(4):40, 2000.

Thompson, J., et al. (2005). *Mosby's clinical nursing.* (6th ed.). St. Louis: Mosby.

Timby, B.K. & Lewis, L.W. (2004). *Fundamental skills and concepts in patient care.* (8th ed.). Philadelphia: Lippincott.

Uniformed Services University of the Health Sciences (USUHS) and the National Institutes of Health. (2004). Fibroid tumors lack crucial structural protein. National Institutes of Health. Available online at www.nichd.nih.gov.

Workman, L. Breast cancer—new strategies to beat an old enemy. *Nursing,* 32(10):58, 2002.

Writing Group for the Women's Health Initiative Investigators. Risk and benefits of estrogen plus progestin in healthy postmenopausal women. *Journal of the American Medical Association,* 288(3):321, 2002.

Additional Resources

Cancer Hope Network, 677-HOPENET, www.cancerhopenetwork.org. Accessed July, 2005.

Living Beyond Breast Cancer, 888-753-LBBC, www.lbbc.org. Accessed July, 2005.

The Linda Creed Breast Cancer Foundation, 888-CREED-4-U, www.lindacreed.org. Accessed July, 2005.

The Susan G. Komen Breast Cancer Foundation, 972-855-1600, www. komen.org. Accessed July, 2005.

Y-Me National Breast Cancer Organization, 800-221-2141, www. y-me.org. Accessed July, 2005.

Chapter 13 Care of the Patient with a Visual or Auditory Disorder

Albert, D. & Gragoudas, E. (2004). *Principles and practice of ophthalmology.* (3rd ed.). Philadelphia: Saunders.

Ball, K. (2003). *The perioperative challenge.* (4th ed.). St. Louis: Mosby.

Balzer-Riley, J. (2004). *Communication in nursing.* St. Louis: Mosby.

Black, J.M. & Hawks, H.J. (2005). *Medical surgical nursing: clinical management for positive outcomes.* (7th ed.). Philadelphia: Saunders.

Burke, M. & Walsh, M. (2005). *Gerontologic nursing.* (4th ed.). St. Louis: Mosby.

Ebersole, H. (2002). *Toward healthy aging.* (6th ed.). St. Louis: Mosby.

Edmunds, M. (2004). *Introduction to clinical pharmacology.* (4th ed.). St. Louis: Mosby.

Giger, J.M. & Davidhizar, R.E. (2004). *Transcultural nursing: assessment and intervention.* (4th ed.). St. Louis: Mosby.

Hard of Hearing Advocates. Available online at www. hohadvocates.org. Accessed August, 2005.

Jaffe, M. & Skidmore-Roth, L. (2005). *Home health nursing.* (5th ed.). St. Louis: Mosby.

Lewis, S.M., et al. (2004). *Medical-surgical nursing: assessment and management of clinical problems.* (6th ed.). St. Louis: Mosby.

Lucus, L. & Flint, L. Heed the word about hearing impairment. *Nursing,* 33(10):32hnl, 2003.

McConnell, E. How to converse with a hearing impaired patient. *Nursing,* 32(8):20, 2002.

Meeker, M. & Rothrock, J. (2003). *Alexander's care of the patient in surgery.* (12th ed.). St. Louis: Mosby.

Novak, J.C. & Broom, B.L. (2004). Ingalls and Salerno's maternal and child health nursing. (10th ed.). St Louis: Mosby.

Phipps, W.J., et al. (2003). *Medical-surgical nursing: health and illness perspectives.* (7th ed.). St. Louis: Mosby.

Potter, P.A. & Perry A.G. (2005). *Fundamentals of nursing: concepts, process, and practice.* (6th ed.). St. Louis: Mosby.

Schoofs, N. Sjögren's syndrome. *RN,* 62(4):45, 1999.

Seidel, H., et al. (2003). *Mosby's guide to physical examination.* (5th ed.). St. Louis: Mosby.

Skidmore-Roth, L. (2006). *Mosby's 2006 nursing drug reference.* St. Louis: Mosby.

Thibodeau, G.A. & Patton, K.T. (2003). *Anatomy and physiology.* (5th ed.). St. Louis: Mosby.

Thibodeau, G.A. & Patton, K.T. (2004). *Structure and function of the body.* (12th ed.). St. Louis: Mosby.

Thompson, J.M., et al. (2002). *Mosby's clinical nursing.* (5th ed.). St Louis: Mosby.

Watson, G. Low vision in the geriatric population: rehabilitation and management. *Journal of the American Geriatric Society, 49:*317, 2001.

Additional Resources

A special report, "The Aging Eye," is available from:
Harvard Health Publications
P.O. Box 421073
Palm Coast, FL 32142-1073
E-mail: harvardpro@palmcoastd.com

American Academy of Ophthalmology
P.O. Box 7424
San Francisco, CA 94120-7424
www.eyeorbit.org

American Foundation for the Blind
15 West 16th St.
New York, NY 10011
A list of free brochures.

American Optometric Association Communications Division
243 North Lindbergh Blvd.
St. Louis, MO 63141
Free brochures on eye care for the elderly.

Captioned Films for the Deaf: 800-237-6213.

National Eye Institute
2020 Vision Place
Bethesda, MD 20892
301-496-5248
www.nei.nih.gov (Accessed July, 2005)

National Institute to Prevent Blindness
79 Madison Ave.
New York, NY 10016
Free pamphlets on specific diseases affecting the eye.

Office of Scientific Reporting, National Eye Institute
Bldg. 31, Rm. 6A32
Bethesda, MD 20205
A list of free brochures on eye disorders.

Vision Foundation
2 Mt. Auburn St.
Watertown, MA 02172
No charge for a Vision Inventory List

Chapter 14 Care of the Patient with a Neurological Disorder

AANN (2000). *AANN's neuroscience nursing: human response to neurologic dysfunction.* (2nd ed.). Philadelphia: Saunders.

Anderson, D.M., et al. (2002). *Mosby's medical, nursing, and allied health dictionary.* (6th ed.). St. Louis: Mosby.

Bender, K. West Nile virus: a growing challenge. *American Journal of Nursing,* 103(6):32, 2003.

Black, J.M. & Hawks, H.J. (2005). *Medical-surgical nursing: clinical management for positive outcomes.* (7th ed.). Philadelphia: Saunders.

Blackwell, T., et al. (2001). *Spinal cord injury desk reference: guidelines for life care planning and case management.* New York: Demas.

Blumenfeld, H. (2002). *Neuroanatomy through clinical cases.* Sunderland, Mass: Sinauer.

Centers for Disease Control and Prevention. (2004). *Division of vector-borne infectious diseases: West Nile virus.* Available online at www.cdc.gov/ncidod/dvbid/westnile/qu/testing-treating.htm. Accessed January, 2004.

Craig Hospital, Englewood, Colo: *Bladder cancer (in SCI patients).* Available online at www.craighospital.org/sci/mets/bladder-cancer.asp. Accessed August, 2005.

Cunning, S. When the DX is myasthenia gravis. *RN,* 63(4):26, 2000.

Drug for migraine: eletriptan hydobromide (Replax). *Nursing,* 34(2):58, 2004.

Deuschl, G., et al. The pathophysiology of tremor. *Muscle Nerve,* 24(6):716, 2001.

Evans, R.W. (2003). *Saunders manual of neurologic practice.* Philadelphia: Saunders.

Fisher, D. Help your patient manage myasthenia gravis. *Nursing Made Incredibly Easy,* January/February:28, 2004.

Freeman, T.B., et al. Transplanted fetal striatum in Huntington's disease: phenotypic development and lack of pathology. *Proceedings of the National Academy of Sciences of the United States of America,* 97:13877, 2000.

Gibson, K. Caring for a patient with a spinal cord injury. *Nursing,* 33(7):36, 2003.

Giger, J.M. & Davidhizar, R.E. (2004). *Transcultural nursing: assessment and intervention.* (4th ed.). St. Louis: Mosby.

Goetz, C. (2003). *Textbook of clinical neurology.* (2nd ed.). Philadelphia: Saunders.

Goldrick, B. Keeping West Nile virus at bay. *Nursing,* 33(8):44, 2003.

Jarvis, C. (2004). *Physical examination and health assessment.* (4th ed.). Philadelphia: Saunders.

Kemp, B. & Thompson, L. Aging and spinal cord injury: medical, functional, and psychosocial changes. *SCI Nursing,* 19(2):51, 2002.

Lejeune, G. & Howard-Fain, T. Nursing assessment and management of patients with head injuries. *Dimensions of Critical Care Nursing,* 27(6):226, 2002.

Lewis, S.M., et al. (2004). *Medical-surgical nursing: assessment and management of clinical problems.* (6th ed.). St. Louis: Mosby.

Lower, J. Facing neuro assessment fearlessly. *Nursing,* 32(2):58, 2002.

Mower-Wade, D., et al. Protecting a patient with ruptured cerebral aneurysm. *Nursing,* 31(2):54, 2001.

National Institute of Neurological Disorders and Stroke. Available online at www.ninds.nih.gov. Accessed August, 2005.

Overstreet, M. When mosquitoes attack—an update on West Nile virus. *Nursing Made Incredibly Easy,* May/June:42, 2004.

Pagana, K.D. & Pagana, T.J. (2006). *Mosby's manual of diagnostic and laboratory tests.* (3rd ed.). St. Louis: Mosby.

Pullen, R. Assessing for signs of meningitis. *Nursing,* 34(3):18, 2004.

Pullen, R. Neurologic assessment for pronator drift. *Nursing,* 34(3):22, 2004.

Rice, R. (2000). *Home health nursing practice.* (3rd ed.). St. Louis: Mosby.

Roquer, J., et al. Stroke. *Nursing,* 34(7):84, 2003.

Seshadri, S., et al. Plasma homocysteine as a risk factor for dementia and Alzheimer's disease. *New England Journal of Medicine,* 346:476, 2002.

Smith, L. Steady the course of Parkinson's disease. *Nursing,* 32(3):43, 2002.

Spinal Cord Information Network: *Spinal cord injury: facts and figures at a glance.* University of Alabama at Birmingham. Available online at www.spinalcord.uab.edu. Accessed August, 2005.

Tanne, D., et al. Markers of increased risk of intracerebral hemorrhage after intravenous recombinant tissue plasminogen activator therapy for acute ischemic stroke in clinical practice. The multicenter rt-PA acute stroke survey. *Circulation,* 105:1679, 2002.

Tornqvist, A. Neurosurgery for movement disorders. *Journal of Neuroscience Nursing,* 33(2):79, 2001.

U.S. Food and Drug Administration. *FDA News: FDA approved memantine (Namenda) for Alzheimer's disease.* Available online at www.fda.gov/bbs/topics/NEWS/2003?NEW00961.html. Accessed August, 2005.

Weir, C.S., et al. Serum urate as an independent predictor of poor outcome and future vascular events after acute stroke. *Stroke,* 34(8):1951, 2003.

Williams, M. How to assess swallowing after a stroke. *Nursing,* 32hn5, 2002.

Worsham, T. Easing the course of Guillain-Barré syndrome. *RN,* 63(3):46, 2000.

Writing Group for the Women's Health Initiative Investigators. Risks and benefits of estrogen plus progestin in healthy post-menopausal women: principal results from the Women's Health Initiative randomized control trial. *Journal of the American Medical Association,* 288:321, 2002.

www.nih.gov/news/pr/Jul2004/nia-18.htm.

www.alz.org.

Chapter 15 Care of the Patient with an Immune Disorder

Anderson, D.M., et al. (2002). *Mosby's medical, nursing, and allied health dictionary.* (6th ed.). St. Louis: Mosby.

Barkauskas, V., et al. (2002). *Health and physical assessment.* (3rd ed.). St. Louis: Mosby.

Black, J.M. & Hawks, H.J. (2005). *Medical-surgical nursing: clinical management for positive outcomes.* (7th ed.). Philadelphia: Saunders.

Colletti, M., et al. (2001). Immunologic system. In Thompson, J., et al. (eds.), *Mosby's clinical nursing.* (5th ed.). St. Louis: Mosby.

Gulanick, M., et al. (2002). *Nursing care plans: nursing diagnoses and interventions.* (5th ed.). St. Louis: Mosby.

Handbook of allergic disorders. (2002). Philadelphia: Lippincott, Williams & Wilkins.

Hayden, M. In defense of the body: how the immune system protects us from harm. *Nursing Made Incredibly Easy,* May/June, 2004.

Kay, A.B. Allergy and allergic diseases. Part 1. *New England Journal of Medicine,* 344(1):30, 2001.

Kay, A.B. Allergy and allergic diseases. Part 2. *New England Journal of Medicine,* 344(2):109, 2001.

Lea, D.H. Ahead to the past: how genetics is changing your practice. *Nursing,* 32:48, 2002.

Lenehan, G. Latex allergy: separating fact from fiction. *Nursing,* 32:50, 2002.

Lewis, S.M., et al. (2004). *Medical-surgical nursing: assessment and management of clinical problems.* (6th ed.). St. Louis: Mosby.

Lieberman, P. and Anderson, J. (eds.). (2000). *Allergic diseases, diagnosis, and treatment.* Totowa, NJ: Humana.

Naguwa, S. & Gershwin, M. (2001). *Allergy and immunology secrets.* Philadelphia: Hanley & Belfus.

Pagana, K.D. & Pagana, T.J. (2005). *Mosby's diagnostic and laboratory test reference.* (7th ed.). St. Louis: Mosby.

Phipps, W.J., et al. (2003). *Medical-surgical nursing: health and illness perspectives.* (7th ed.). St. Louis: Mosby.

Potter, P.A. & Perry, A.G. (2003). *Basic nursing: essentials for practice.* (5th ed.). St. Louis: Mosby.

Rote, N.S. (2002). Alternations in immunity and inflammation. In McCance, K.L. & Huether, S.E. (eds.), *Pathophysiology: the biologic basis for disease in adults and children.* (4th ed.). St. Louis: Mosby.

Reviewing the immune system. *Nursing,* 31(3):70-71, 2001.

Roitt, I., et al. (2002). *Immunology.* (6th ed.). St. Louis: Mosby.

Seidel, H.B. (2003). *Mosby's guide to physical examination.* (5th ed.). St. Louis: Mosby.

Shearer, W. & Fleisher, T. (2003). The immune system. In Adkinson, N., et al. (eds.), *Middleton's allergy: principles and practice.* (6th ed.). Philadelphia: Mosby.

Venes, D. (2005.) *Taber's cyclopedic medical dictionary.* (20th ed.). Philadelphia: Davis.

Thompson, J.M., et al. (2001). *Mosby's clinical nursing.* (5th ed.). St. Louis: Mosby.

Zimmaro, D. & Lehmann, S. Immune-boosting formulas. *RN,* 62(8):26, 2001.

Chapter 16 Care of the Patient with HIV/AIDS

AmfAR. (n.d.). *Facts about HIV/AIDS.* Available online at www.amfar.org/cgi-bin/iowa/abouthiv/record.html?record=3 Accessed July, 2005.

Anastasi, J.K. & Capili, B. HIV-related diarrhea and outcome measures. *Journal of the Association of Nurses in AIDS Care,* 12(Suppl):44, 2001.

Bartlett, J.G. & Gallant, J.E. (2001). *Medical management of HIV injection (2001-2002).* Baltimore, MD: Johns Hopkins University, Division of Infectious Diseases.

Black J.M. & Hawks, H.J. (2005). *Medical-surgical nursing: clinical management for positive outcomes.* (7th ed.). Philadelphia: Saunders.

Bozzette, S.A., et al. Expenditures for the care of HIV-infected patients in the era of highly active antiretroviral therapy. *New England Journal of Medicine,* 344:817, 2001.

Bradley-Springer, L.A. Prevention: What works? *American Journal of Nursing,* 101(6):45, 2001.

Bradley-Springer, L.A. The complex realities of primary prevention for HIV infection in a "just do it" world. *Nursing Clinics of North America,* 34(1):49, 1999.

Cardo, D.M., et al. A case-control study of HIV seroconversion in health care workers after percutaneous exposure. *New England Journal of Medicine,* 337:1485, 1997.

Carr, A., et al. Pathogenesis of HIV-1 protease inhibitor–associated peripheral lipodystrophy, hyperlipidemia and insulin resistance. *Lancet,* 131:1881, 1998.

Centers for Disease Control and Prevention. *HIV/AIDS Surveillance Report,* 12(1):2, 2000.

Centers for Disease Control and Prevention. Updated U. S. Public Health Service guidelines for the management of occupational exposures to HBV, HCV, and HIV and recommendations for postexposure prophylaxis. *MMWR: Morbidity and Mortality Weekly Report,* 50 (No. RR-11):1, 2001.

Centers for Disease Control and Prevention. *HIV postexposure prophylaxis in the 21st century.* Available online at: www.cdc.gov. Accessed January, 2004.

Coffin J. The scoop on HIV mutations. *Journal of the International Association of Physicians in AIDS Care,* 2(7):45, 1996.

Crespo-Fierro, M. Compliance/adherence and care management in HIV disease. *Journal of the Association of Nurses in AIDS Care,* 8(4):43, 1997.

Dole, P.J. Primary care of HPV management in HIV-infected women. *Nurse Practitioner Forum,* 12(4):214, 2001.

Essex, M. & Kanki, P. J. The origins of the AIDS virus. *Scientific American,* 259(4):44, 1998.

Feng, Y., et al. HIV-1 entry cofactor: functional bDNA cloning of a seven-transmembrane G protein–coupled receptor. *Science,* 272:872, 1996.

Galvani, A.P. Emerging infections: what have we learned from SARS? *Emerging Infectious Diseases,* 10(7):1351, 2004.

Hellinger, F.J. & Fleishman, J.A. Estimating the national cost of treating people with HIV disease: patient, payer, and provider data. *Journal of Acquired Immune Deficiency Syndromes,* 24:182, 2000.

Henderson, D.K. Postexposure prophylaxis in the 21st century. *Emerging Infectious Diseases,* 7(2): 254, 2004.

Ho, D.D., et al. Rapid turnover of plasma virions and CD4 lymphocytes in HIV-1 infection. *Nature* 373:123, 1995.

Joint United Nations Programme on HIV/AIDS (UNAIDS) World Health Organization (WHO). (n. d.). *AIDS epidemic update: December 2000.* Available online at www.unaids.org/EN/other/functionalities/Search.asp Accessed July, 2005.

Kirton, C.A. Promoting healthy behaviors in HIV primary care. *Nurse Practitioner Forum,* 12(4):223, 2001.

Laurence, J. AIDS: 20th anniversary, June 2001. *The AIDS Reader,* 11(6):296, 2001.

Marlink, R., et al. Reduced rate of disease development after HIV-2 infections as compared to HIV-1. *Science,* 8:1587, 1994.

Marmor, M., et al. Homozygous and heterozygous CCR5-Δ32 genotypes are associated with resistance to HIV infection. *Journal of Acquired Immune Deficiency Syndromes,* 27(5):472, 2001.

Mast, S.T., et al. Efficacy of gloves in reducing blood volumes transferred during simulated needlestick injury. *Journal of Infectious Diseases*, 168:1589, 1993.

Miller, K.D., et al. Visceral fat accumulation associated with the use of indinavir therapy. *Lancet*, 315:871, 1998.

Mofenson, L.M. Interaction between timing of perinatal human immunodeficiency virus infection and the design of preventive and therapeutic interventions. *Acta Paediatrica Supplement*, 491:1, 1997.

Morbidity and Mortality Weekly Report. (1999). Increases in unsafe sex and rectal gonorrhea among men who have sex with men—San Francisco, California, 1994-1997. *MMWR Morbidity and Mortality Weekly Report*, 48(3):45, 1999.

Nelson, P.W., et al. Effect of drug efficacy and the eclipse phase of the viral life cycle on estimates of HIV viral dynamic parameters. *Journal of Acquired Immune Deficiency Syndromes*, 26(5):405, 2001.

Nielsen, C.E. HIV/AIDS update. *Nurse Practitioner Forum*, 12(4):179, 2001.

O'Neill, J. & Alexander, C. Palliative medicine and HIV/AIDS. *HIV/AIDS Management in Office Practice*, 24(3):607, 1997.

Perdue, B., et al. (1999). HIV-1 transmission by a needlestick injury despite rapid initiation of four drug postexposure prophylaxis [Abstract 210]. In Program and abstracts of the 6th Conference on Retroviruses and Opportunistic Infections. Chicago: Foundation for Retrovirology and Human Health in scientific collaboration with the National Institute of Allergy and Infectious Diseases and CDC.

Perinatal HIV Guidelines Working Group. (2001, May 4). *Public Health Service Task Force recommendations for use of antiretroviral drugs in pregnant HIV-1–infected women for maternal health and interventions to reduce perinatal HIV-1 transmission in the United States.* Available online at www.hivatis.org/guidelines/perinatal/May03_01/PerinatalMay04_01.pdf. Accessed December 10, 2001.

Santangelo, J. (2001). Acute seroconversion of HIV infection in the ambulatory care setting. *Nurse Practitioner*, 26(4):48, 2001.

Schacker, T., et al. Rapid accumulating of human immunodeficiency virus (HIV) in lymphatic tissue reservoirs during acute and early HIV infection: implications for timing of antiretroviral therapy. *Journal of Infectious Diseases*, 181:354, 2000.

Sherman, D. (2001). Palliative care. In C.A. Kirton, et al. (eds.), *Handbook of HIV/AIDS nursing*. St. Louis: Mosby.

Ungvarski, P.J. The past 20 years of AIDS. *American Journal of Nursing*, 101(6):26, 2001.

U.S. Department of Health and Human Services. Centers for Disease Control and Prevention (CDC). *HIV/AIDS Surveillance Report*, 10(2):24, 1998.

Winson, G. (2001). HIV/AIDS nutritional management. In C.A. Kirton, et al. (eds.), *Handbook of HIV/AIDS nursing*. St. Louis: Mosby.

Winson, G. Management of HIV-associated diarrhea and wasting. *Journal of the Association of Nurses in AIDS Care*, 12(Suppl):55, 2001.

Zwolski, K. (2001). HIV immunopathogenesis. In C.A. Kirton, et al. (eds.), *Handbook of HIV/AIDS nursing*. St. Louis: Mosby.

Zwolski, K. (2001). Neurological disorders in HIV/AIDS. In C.A. Kirton, et al. (eds.), *Handbook of HIV/AIDS nursing*. St. Louis: Mosby.

Chapter 17 Care of the Patient with Cancer

Acello, B. (2000). Controlling pain, facing fears about opioid addiction. *Nursing*, 30:5, 2000.

Acello, B. (2000). Controlling pain, switching to the patch. *Nursing*, 30:8, 2000.

Ackley, B.J. & Ladwig, G.B. (2005). *Nursing diagnosis handbook.* (6th ed.). St. Louis: Mosby.

Alfaro-Lefevre, R. (2003). *Critical thinking in nursing: a practical approach.* (3rd ed.). St. Louis: Mosby.

American Breast Cancer Society. (2003). *Tamoxifen and raloifene to reduce breast cancer risk: questions and answers.* Available online at www.cancer.org/docroot/CRI/content/CRI_2_6Xtamoxifen_and_Raloxifene_Question_and_Answers_5.asp. Accessed November 14, 2003.

American Cancer Society. (2000). Available online at www.cancer.org [see Statistics]. Accessed July, 2005.

American Cancer Society. (2004). *Cancer facts and figures.* Atlanta: American Cancer Society.

Anderson, D.M., et al. (2002). *Mosby's medical, nursing, and allied health dictionary.* (6th ed.). St. Louis: Mosby.

Anderson, D. Using hyperbaric oxygen therapy to heal radiation wounds. *Nursing*, 33(3):50, 2003.

Balzer-Riley, J. (2004). *Communication in nursing.* (5th ed.). St. Louis: Mosby.

Barkauskas, V., et al. (2002). *Health and physical assessment.* (3rd ed.). St. Louis: Mosby.

Black, J.M. & Hawks, H.J. (2004). *Medical-surgical nursing: clinical management for positive outcomes* (7th ed.). Philadelphia: Saunders.

Bradley, C.J., et al. Race, socioeconomic status, and breast cancer treatment and survival. *Journal of the National Cancer Institute*, 94(7):490, 2002.

Brown, C. Safeguarding chemotherapy. *Nursing*, 31(5):32, 2001.

Brunner, L., et al. (2004). *Textbook of medical-surgical nursing.* (10th ed.). Philadelphia: Lippincott.

Calle, E.E., et al. Overweight, obesity, and mortality from cancer in a prospectively studied cohort of US adults. *New England Journal of Medicine*, 348(17):1625, 2003.

Cantril, C. Emergency tumor lysis syndrome. *American Journal of Nursing*, 104(4):49, 2004.

Correa, P. *Helicobacter pylori* infection and gastric cancer. *Cancer Epidemiology, Biomarkers, and Prevention*, 12(3):238S, 2003.

Coyne, B. Chemo's toll on memory. *RN*, 67(4):40, 2004.

DuVal, S. Inflammatory breast cancer. *RN*, 67(2):43, 2004.

Freedman, G.M. & Anderson, P.R. Routine mammography is associated with earlier stage disease and greater eligiblity bor breast conservation in breast carcinoma patients age 40 years and older. *Cancer*, 98(5):918, 2003.

Giarelli, E., et al. Stable & able, a standardized nursing intervention protocol for patients with cancer. *American Journal of Nursing*, 1000(12):26, 2000.

Giger, J.M. & Davidhizar, R.E. (2004). *Transcultural nursing: assessment and intervention.* (4th ed.). St. Louis: Mosby.

Gordon, M. (2005). *Manual of nursing diagnosis.* (10th ed.). St. Louis: Mosby.

Gutaj, D. Oncology today: lymphoma, *EN*, 63(8):32, 2001.

Hughes, L.C., et al. Information needs of elderly postsurgical cancer patients during the transition from hospital to home. *Image—The Journal of Nursing Scholarship*, 32(1):25, 2000.

Lewis, S.M., et al. (2004). *Medical-surgical nursing: assessment and management of clinical problems.* (6th ed.). St. Louis: Mosby.

Lilley, L.L. & Aucker, R.S. (2001). *Pharmacology and the nursing process.* (2nd ed.). St. Louis: Mosby.

McCaffery, M. & Pasero, C. (2003). *Pain: clinical manual.* (3rd ed.). St. Louis: Mosby.

National Cancer Institute. (2003). *Cancer health disparities.* Available online at: www.cancer.gov/newcenter/healthdisparities. Accessed April, 2003.

National Center for Health Statistics. (2001). *Data file documentation, National Health Interview Survey 2000 (machine readable data file and documentation).* Hyattsville: National Center for Health Statistics.

Ngo-Metzger, Q., et al. Older Asian American and Pacific Islanders dying of cancer use hospice less frequently than older white patients. *American Journal of Medicine*, 115(1):47, 2003.

Noonon, D. Breast cancer's "new era." *Newsweek*, October 20:67, 2003.

Otto, S. (2001). *Oncology nursing.* (4th ed.). St. Louis: Mosby.

Pagana, K.D. & Pagana, T.J. (2005). *Mosby's diagnostic and laboratory test reference.* (7th ed.). St. Louis: Mosby.

Phipps, W.J., et al. (2003). *Medical-surgical nursing: health and illness perspectives.* (7th ed.). St. Louis: Mosby.

Rivera, P., et al. Hospital nursing, a team approach to managing pain. *Nursing*, 30:2, 2000.

Shinn, S. Cervical cancer. *Nursing,* 34(5):36, 2004.

Skidmore-Roth, L. (2006). *Mosby's 2006 nursing drug reference.* St. Louis: Mosby.

Smith, L. Shedding light of phodynamic therapy (cancer-fighting treatment). *Nursing,* 34(5):32hn2, 2004.

Thomas, S. Oncology today: breast cancer. *RN,* 63(4):40, 2000.

Thompson, J.M., et al. (2005). *Mosby's clinical nursing.* (6th ed.). St. Louis: Mosby.

Tucker, S.M., et al. (2004). *Patient care standards: nursing process, diagnosis and outcomes.* (7th ed.). St. Louis: Mosby.

U.S. Department of Health and Human Services. *Tracking Healthy People 2010.* Washington, DC: U.S. Government Printing Office.

Weaver, C. Life after breast cancer surgery. *Nursing,* (10):30, 2000.

Workman, L. Breast cancer—new strategies to beat an old enemy. *Nursing,* 32(10):58, 2002.

Illustration Credits

Chapter 1

1-1, 1-2, 1-3, 1-4, 1-5, 1-6, 1-9, 1-13, from Thibodeau, G.A. & Patton, K.T. (2004). *Structure and function of the body.* (12th ed.). St. Louis: Mosby. **1-7,** from Herlihy, B. & Maebius, N.K. (2003). *The human body in health and illness.* (2nd ed.). Philadelphia: Saunders. **1-8, 1-10, 1-11,** from Thibodeau, G.A. & Patton, K.T. (2003). *Anatomy and physiology.* (5th ed.). St. Louis: Mosby.

Chapter 2

2-1, 2-6, 2-9, 2-12, 2-17, 2-18, from Harkreader, H. & Hogan, M.A. (2004). *Fundamentals of nursing: caring and clinical judgment.* (2nd ed.). Philadelphia: Saunders. **2-2,** from Cole, G. (1996). *Fundamental nursing: concepts and skills.* (2nd ed.). St. Louis: Mosby. **2-3, 2-4, 2-7, 2-16,** from Elkin, M. K., et al. (2004). *Nursing interventions and clinical skills.* (3rd ed.). St. Louis: Mosby. **2-5,** from Potter, P.A. & Perry, A.G. (2003). *Basic nursing: essentials for practice.* (5th ed.). St. Louis: Mosby. **2-8,** from Meeker, M. H. & Rothrock, J. C. (1999). *Alexander's care of the patient in surgery.* (11th ed.). St. Louis: Mosby. **2-10, 2-14,** courtesy of Great Plains Regional Medical Center, North Platte, Nebraska. **2-11,** from Lewis, S.M., et al. (2004). *Medical-surgical nursing: assessment and management of clinical problems.* (6th ed.). St. Louis: Mosby. **2-13,** from Potter, P.A. & Perry, A.G. (2005). *Fundamentals of nursing.* (6th ed.). St. Louis: Mosby. **Skill 2-1 step 14,** from Sorrentino, S.A. (2004). *Mosby's textbook for nursing assistants.* (6th ed.). St. Louis: Mosby. **Skill 2-2 step 9a, step 10c; Skill 2-3 step 10; Skill 2-4 step 17, step 20,** from Potter, P.A. & Perry, A.G. (2005). *Fundamentals of nursing.* (6th ed.). St. Louis. Mosby. **Skill 2-3 step 8,** from Elkin, M.K., et al. (2004). *Nursing interventions and clinical skills.* (3rd ed.). St. Louis: Mosby.

Chapter 3

3-1, from Thibodeau, G.A. & Patton, K.T. (2005), *The human body in health and disease.* (4th ed.). St. Louis: Mosby. **3-2, 3-7, 3-8, 3-13, 3-18,** from Habif, T.P. (2004). *Clinical dermatology.* (4th ed.). St. Louis: Mosby. **3-3, 3-4, 3-5, 3-6, 3-10, 3-17,** courtesy of the Department of Dermatology, School of Medicine, University of Utah. **3-9** from Weston, W.L., et al. (1996). *Color textbook of pediatric dermatology.* St. Louis: Mosby. **3-11,** from Habif, T.P., et al. (2005). *Skin disease: diagnosis and treatment.* (2nd ed.). St. Louis: Mosby. **3-12,** from Baran R., et al. (1991). *Color atlas of the hair, scalp, and nails.* St. Louis: Mosby. **3-14,** courtesy of Department of Dermatology, University of North Carolina at Chapel Hill. **3-15,** from Zitelli, B.J. & Davis, H.W. (2002). *Atlas of pediatric physical diagnosis.* (4th ed.). St. Louis: Mosby. **3-16,** from Belcher, A.E. (1992). *Cancer nursing.* St. Louis: Mosby. **3-19,** from Wong, D. (1995). *Whaley & Wong's nursing care of infants and children.* (5th ed.). St. Louis: Mosby. **3-20, 3-21,** courtesy of Intermountain Burn Center, University of Utah. **3-22,** from Thibodeau, G.A. & Patton, K.T. (2003). *Anatomy and physiology.* (5th ed.). St. Louis: Mosby. **3-23, 3-24, 3-25,** courtesy of Burn Center, Cleveland Metropolitan General Hospital, Cleveland, Ohio.

Chapter 4

4-1, from Thibodeau, G.A. & Patton, K.T. (2004). *Structure and function of the body.* (12th ed.). St. Louis: Mosby. **4-2, 4-3, 4-41,** from Thibodeau, G.A. & Patton, K.T. (1997). *The human body in health and disease.* (2nd ed.). St. Louis: Mosby. **4-4,** from Thibodeau, G.A. & Patton, K.T. (1997). *Structure and function of the body.* (10th ed.). St. Louis, Mosby. **4-5, 4-6, 4-22, 4-24, 4-43,** from Thibodeau, G.A. & Patton, K.T. (2005). *The human body in health and disease.* (4th ed.). St. Louis: Mosby. **4-7, 4-8,** from Kamal, A. & Brocklehurst, J.C. (1991). *Color atlas of geriatric medicine.* (2nd ed.). St. Louis: Mosby. **4-9, 4-17, 4-25,** from Lewis, S. M., et al. (2004). *Medical-surgical nursing: assessment and management of clinical problems.* (6th ed.). St. Louis: Mosby.

4-10, 4-23, 4-35, from Ignatavicius, D.D. & Workman, M.L. (2002). *Medical-surgical nursing across the healthcare continuum.* (4th ed.). Philadelphia: Saunders. **4-11; 4-16; 4-20; 4-32, B,** from Phipps, W., et al. (2003). *Medical-surgical nursing: health and illness perspectives.* (7th ed.). St. Louis: Mosby. **4-12, 4-15, 4-33,** courtesy of Zimmer, Inc., Warsaw, Indiana. **4-13** courtesy of Orthologic Corporation, Phoenix, Arizona. **4-18; 4-28 B, C; 4-32, A** modified from Mourad, L. (1991). *Orthopedic disorders.* St. Louis: Mosby. **4-26, 4-30,** courtesy of Dr. Henry Bohlman, Cleveland, Ohio. **4-27, 4-42,** from Beare, P.G. & Myers, J.L. (1998). *Adult health nursing.* (3rd ed.). St. Louis: Mosby. **4-28, A,** from Stryker Howmedica Osteonics, Inc. **4-29, 4-40,** from Thompson, J.M., et al. (2002). *Mosby's clinical nursing.* (5th ed.). St. Louis: Mosby. **4-31,** from Elkin, M.K., et al. (1996). *Nursing interventions and clinical skills.* St. Louis: Mosby. **4-34,** from Harkness, G.A. & Dincher, J.R.: *Medical-surgical nursing: total patient care.* (10th ed.). St. Louis: Mosby. **4-36, 4-38,** from Potter, P.A. & Perry, A.G. (2003). *Basic nursing: essentials for practice.* (5th ed.). St. Louis: Mosby. **4-37,** from Elkin, M.K., et al. (2004). *Nursing interventions and clinical skills.* (3rd ed.). St. Louis: Mosby. **4-39,** courtesy of Roll-a-Bout Corporation, Frederica, Delaware. **Skill 4-1 step 8a,** from Phipps, W.J., et al. (1995). *Medical-surgical nursing: concepts and clinical practice.* (5th ed.). St. Louis: Mosby.

Chapter 5

5-1, 5-2, from Thibodeau, G.A. & Patton, K.T. (1987). *Anatomy and physiology.* St. Louis: Mosby. **5-3,** from Thibodeau, G.A. & Patton, K.T. (2004). *Structure and function of the body.* (12th ed.). St. Louis: Mosby. **5-4,** from Thibodeau, G.A. & Patton, K.T. (2003). *Anatomy and physiology.* (5th ed.). St. Louis: Mosby. **5-5, 5-8, 5-20,** from Phipps, W.J., et al. (2003). *Medical-surgical nursing: concepts and clinical practice.* (7th ed.). St. Louis: Mosby. **5-7, 5-12, 5-13, 5-14, 5-16,** from Beare, P.G. & Myers, J.L. (1998). *Adult health nursing.* (3rd ed.). St. Louis: Mosby.

Chapter 6

6-1, courtesy of Olympus America, Inc., Melville, New York. **6-2, 6-4, 6-7, 6-9,** from Lewis, S.M., et al. (2004). *Medical-surgical nursing: assessment and management of clinical problems.* (6th ed.). St. Louis: Mosby. **6-3, 6-8,** from Beare, P.G. & Myers, J.L. (1998). *Adult health nursing.* (3rd ed.). St. Louis: Mosby. **6-5,** from Kamal, A. & Brockelhurst, J.C. (1991). *Color atlas of geriatric medicine.* (3rd ed.). St. Louis: Mosby–Year Book, Europe. **6-6,** from Phipps, W.J., et al. (2003). *Medical-surgical nursing: health and illness perspectives.* (7th ed.). St. Louis: Mosby.

Chapter 7

7-1, 7-4, from Thibodeau, G.A. & Patton, K.T. (2003). *Anatomy and physiology.* (5th ed.). St. Louis: Mosby. **7-2, 7-3,** from Thibodeau, G.A. & Patton, K.T. (2005). *The human body in health and disease.* (4th ed.). St. Louis: Mosby. **7-5,** from Belcher, A.E. (1992). *Mosby's clinical nursing series: blood disorders.* St. Louis: Mosby.

Chapter 8

8-1, 8-2, 8-3, from Thibodeau, G.A. & Patton, K.T. (2003). *Anatomy and physiology.* (5th ed.). St. Louis: Mosby. **8-4, 8-5, 8-6, 8-17,** from Canobbio, M. (1990). *Mosby's clinical nursing series: cardiovascular disorders.* St. Louis: Mosby. **8-9, A,** courtesy of Medtronic, Inc., Minneapolis, Minnesota. **8-9, B; 8-10; 8-11; 8-12, B; 8-16; 8-18; 8-19; 8-20; 8-21, 8-23,** from Lewis, S.M., et al. (2004). *Medical-surgical nursing: assessment and management of clinical problems.* (6th ed.). St. Louis: Mosby. **8-12, A,** from Thelan, L., et al. (1998). *Critical care nursing.* (3rd ed.). St. Louis: Mosby. **8-13, 8-23,** from Phipps, W.J., et al. (1995). *Medical-surgical nursing: concepts and clinical practice.* (5th ed.). St. Louis: Mosby. **8-14,** from Beare, P.G. & Myers, J.L. (1998). *Adult health nursing.* (3rd ed.). St. Louis: Mosby. **8-15,** from *Heart disease and stroke,* 2:99, 1993. Copyright American Heart Association. **8-22, 8-24,** from Kamal, A. & Brockelhurst, J.C.: *Color atlas of geriatric medicine.* (3rd ed.). St. Louis: Mosby–Year Book, Europe.

Chapter 9

9-1, 9-2, 9-3, 9-4, 9-6, from Thibodeau, G.A. & Patton, K.T. (2004). *Structure and function of the body.* (12th ed.). St. Louis: Mosby. **9-5,** from Thibodeau, G.A. & Patton, K.T. (2005). *The human body in health and disease.* (4th ed.). St. Louis: Mosby. **9-7, A,** courtesy of Olympus America, Melville, New York. **9-7, B,** from Meduri, G.U., et al. Protected bronchoalveolar lavage. *American Review of Respiratory Disease,* 143:855, 1991, official journal of the American Thoracic Society, copyright American Lung Association. **9-8,** from Lewis, S.M., et al. (2004). *Medical-surgical nursing: assessment and management of clinical problems.* (6th ed.). St. Louis: Mosby. **9-9, 9-12, 9-13,** from Potter, P.A. & Perry, A.G. (2005). *Fundamentals of nursing.* (6th ed.). St. Louis: Mosby. **9-14,** from Wilson, S. & Thompson, J. (1991). *Mosby's clinical nursing series: respiratory disorders.* St. Louis: Mosby. **9-15,** from Lewis, S.M., et al. (1996). *Medical-surgical nursing: assessment and management of clinical problems.* (4th ed.). St. Louis: Mosby. **9-16,** from McCance, K.L. & Huether, S.E. (2002). *Pathophysiology: the biologic basis for disease in adults and children.* (4th ed.). St. Louis: Mosby.

Chapter 10

10-1, 10-2, 10-3, 10-5, from Thibodeau, G.A. & Patton, K.T. (2003). *Anatomy and physiology.* (5th ed.). St. Louis: Mosby. **10-6,** from Lewis, S.M., et al. (2004). *Medical-surgical nursing: assessment and management of clinical problems.* (6th ed.). St. Louis: Mosby. **10-7, 10-9,** from Beare, P.G. & Myers, J.L. (1998). *Adult health nursing.* (3rd ed.). St. Louis: Mosby. **10-10, 10-11,** from Tucker, S., et al. (1996). *Patient care standards: collaborative practice planning guides.* (6th ed.). St. Louis: Mosby. **10-12,** from Belcher, A.E. (1992). *Cancer nursing.* St. Louis: Mosby. **10-14,** from Thibodeau, G.A. & Patton, K.T. (2004). *Structure and function of the body.* (12th ed.). St. Louis: Mosby.

Chapter 11

11-1, 11-2, from Thibodeau, G.A. & Patton, K.T. (2004). *Structure and function of the body.* (12th ed.). St. Louis: Mosby. **11-4,** from Thibodeau, G.A. & Patton, K.T. (1997). *Structure and function of the body.* (10th ed.). St. Louis: Mosby. **11-5,** from Thibodeau, G.A. & Patton, K.T. (1996). *Anatomy and physiology.* (3rd ed.). St. Louis: Mosby. **11-6,** courtesy of the Group for Research in Pathology Education. **11-7, 11-8,** from Seidel, H.M., et al. (2003). *Mosby's guide to physical examination.* (5th ed.). St. Louis: Mosby. **11-9,** from Schneeburg, N.G. (1979). *Essentials of clinical endocrinology.* St. Louis: Mosby. **11-10,** courtesy of L.V. Bergman & Associates, Inc., Cold Springs, New York. **11-12,** from Lewis, S.M., et al. (2004). *Medical-surgical nursing: assessment and management of clinical problems.* (6th ed.). St. Louis: Mosby. **11-14,** from Potter, P.A. & Perry, A.G. (2003). *Basic nursing: essentials for practice.* (5th ed.). St. Louis: Mosby. **11-15,** from Phipps, W.J., et al. (2003). *Medical-surgical nursing: health and illness perspectives.* (7th ed.). St. Louis: Mosby.

Chapter 12

12-1, 12-2, 12-3, 12-5, 12-6, from Thibodeau, G.A. & Patton, K.T. (1987). *Anatomy and physiology.* St. Louis: Mosby. **12-4,** from Thibodeau, G.A. & Patton, K.T. (2004). *Structure and function of the body.* (12th ed.). St. Louis: Mosby. **12-7,** from Thibodeau, G.A. & Patton, K.T. (2003). *Anatomy and physiology.* (5th ed.). St. Louis: Mosby. **12-9, 12-11, 12-19, 12-20,** from Beare, P.G. & Myers, J.L. (1998). *Adult health nursing.* (3rd ed.). St. Louis: Mosby. **12-10,** from Herbst, A.L., et al. (1992). *Comprehensive gynecology.* (2nd ed.). St. Louis: Mosby. **12-12, 12-15, 12-16,** from Seidel, H.M, et al. (2003). *Mosby's guide to physical examination.* (5th ed.). St. Louis: Mosby. **12-13, 12-17,** from Lewis, S.M., et al. (2004). *Medical-surgical nursing: assessment and management of clinical problems.* (6th ed.). St. Louis: Mosby. **12-14,** redrawn from Novak, E.R. & Woodruff, J.D. (eds.). (1967). *Novak's gynecologic and obstetric pathology.* (6th ed.). Philadelphia: Saunders. (In K.L. McCance, & S. E. Huether [eds.]. [1998]. *Pathophysiology: the biologic basis for disease in adults and children.* [3rd ed.]. St. Louis: Mosby.) **12-18,** from Belcher, A.E. (1992). *Cancer nursing.* St. Louis: Mosby. **12-21, 12-22,** from Lowdermilk, D.L., et al. (2004). *Maternity and women's health care.* (8th ed.). St. Louis: Mosby.

Chapter 13

13-1, from Thibodeau, G.A. & Patton, K.T. (2004). *Anatomy and physiology.* (5th ed.). St. Louis: Mosby. **13-2, 13-3,** from Thibodeau, G.A. & Patton, K.T. (2004). *Structure and function of the body.* (12th ed.). St. Louis: Mosby. **13-4,** from Thibodeau, G.A. & Patton, K.T. (2005). *The human body in health and disease.* (4th ed.). St. Louis: Mosby. **13-5, 13-7, 13-8, 13-10, 13-12,** from Lewis, S.M., et al. (2004). *Medical-surgical nursing: assessment and management of clinical problems.* (6th ed.). St. Louis: Mosby. **13-6,** from Lowdermilk, D.L., et al. (1997). *Maternity & women's health care.* (6th ed.). St. Louis: Mosby. **13-9** from Havener, W.H. (1997). *Synopsis of ophthalmology.* St. Louis: Mosby. **13-11,** from Phipps, W.J., et al. (2003). *Medical-surgical nursing: concepts and clinical practice.* (7th ed.). St. Louis: Mosby (Photo by Stephen M. Beazley). **13-13, 13-14,** from Seidel, H.M, et al. (2003). *Mosby's guide to physical examination.* (5th ed.). St. Louis: Mosby. **13-15,** from Long, B., et al. (1995). *Medical-surgical nursing: a nursing process approach.* (3rd ed.). St. Louis: Mosby. **13-16,** from Lemmi, F.O. & Lemmi, C.A.E. (2000). *Physical assessment findings CD-ROM.* Philadelphia: Saunders.

Chapter 14

14-1, A, C, from Thibodeau, G.A. & Patton, K.T. (2003). *Anatomy and physiology.* (5th ed.). St. Louis: Mosby. **14-1, B,** courtesy of Brenda Russell, PhD, University of Illinois at Chicago. **14-2,** from Thibodeau, G.A. & Patton, K.T. (1987). *Anatomy and physiology.* St. Louis: Mosby. **14-3,** from Thibodeau, G.A. & Patton, K.T. (1990). *Anthony's textbook of anatomy and physiology.* (13th ed.). St. Louis: Mosby. **14-5,** from Elkin, M.K., et al. (2004). *Nursing interventions and clinical skills.* (3rd ed.). St. Louis: Mosby. **14-6,** from Long, B., et al. (1993). *Medical-surgical nursing: a nursing process approach.* (3rd ed.). St. Louis: Mosby. **14-7, 14-20, 14-23,** from Phipps, W.J., et al. (1995). *Medical-surgical nursing: concepts and clinical practice.* (5th ed.). St. Louis: Mosby. **14-8, 14-9,** from Rudy, E.B. (1984). *Advanced neurological and neurosurgical nursing.* St. Louis: Mosby. **14-10,** from Hoemann, S.P. (1996). *Rehabilitation nursing: process and application.* (2nd ed.). St. Louis: Mosby. **14-11, 14-12,** from Dittmar, S.S. (1989). *Rehabilitation nursing: process and application.* St. Louis: Mosby. **14-13, 14-14, 14-16, 14-17, 14-18, 14-19, 14-22,** from Lewis, S.M., et al. (2004). *Medical-surgical nursing: assessment and management of clinical problems.* (6th ed.). St. Louis: Mosby. **14-15,** redrawn from Rudy, E.B. (1984). *Advanced neurological and neurosurgical nursing.* St. Louis: Mosby. (In Lewis, S.M., et al. [2000]. *Medical-surgical nursing: assessment and management of clinical problems.* [5th ed.]. St. Louis: Mosby.) **14-21,** redrawn from Barker, E. (1994). *Neuroscience nursing.* St. Louis: Mosby. (In Lewis, S.M., et al. [2000]. *Medical-surgical nursing: assessment and management of clinical problems.* [5th ed.]. St. Louis: Mosby.) **14-24,** courtesy of Michael S. Clement, MD, Mesa, Arizona.

Chapter 15

15-2, from Grimes, D. (1991). *Infectious diseases.* St. Louis: Mosby. **15-3,** from Thibodeau, G.A. & Patton, K.T. (1996). *Anatomy and physiology.* (3rd ed.). St. Louis: Mosby.

Chapter 16

16-2, 16-4, redrawn from Gottfried, S.S. (1993). *Human biology.* Sudbury, Mass: Jones & Bartlett. **16-5,** from Friedman-Kien, A.E. & Cockerell, C.J. (1996). *Color atlas of AIDS.* (2nd ed.). Philadelphia: Saunders. **16-6,** redrawn from Martin, S., et al. (1998). *HIV/AIDS prevention: early intervention and health promotion.* Denver, Colo: Mountain-Plains Regional AIDS Education and Training Center, University of Colorado Health Sciences Center.

Chapter 17

17-1, from *Cancer facts & figures 2004.* © 2004, American Cancer Society, Inc., Surveillance Research. **17-2,** from Belcher, A.E. (1992). *Cancer nursing.* St. Louis: Mosby

Glossary

Pronunciation of Terms*

The markings ¯ and ˘ above the vowels (a, e, i, o, and u) indicate the proper sounds of the vowels.

When ¯ is above a vowel, its sound is long, that is, exactly like its name. For example:

ā as in āpe
ē as in ēven
ī as in īce
ō as in ōpen
ū as in ūnit

The ˘ marking indicates a short vowel sound, as in the following examples:

ă as in ăpple
ĕ as in ĕvery
ĭ as in ĭnterest
ŏ as in pŏt
ŭ as in ŭnder

A

ablation Amputation or excision of any part of the body; removal of a growth or harmful substance.

achalasia Abnormal condition characterized by the inability of a muscle, particularly the cardiac sphincter of the stomach, to relax.

achlorhydria Abnormal condition characterized by the absence of hydrochloric acid in the gastric secretions.

acquired immunodeficiency syndrome (AIDS) An acquired condition that impairs the body's ability to fight disease; it is the end stage of a continuum of HIV infection, in which the infected person has a CD_4^+ count of 200 cells/mm³ or less.

active transport The movement of materials across the membrane of a cell by means of chemical activity, which allows the cell to admit larger molecules than would otherwise be able to enter.

acute coryza Acute rhinitis, also known as the common cold; an inflammatory condition of the mucous membranes of the nose and accessory sinuses.

adaptive immunity Protection that provides a specific reaction to each invading antigen and has the unique ability to remember the antigen that caused the attack.

adherence Following a prescribed regimen of therapy or treatment for disease.

adventitious Abnormal sounds superimposed on breath sounds.

agnosia Total or partial loss of the ability to recognize familiar objects or people through sensory stimuli; results from organic brain damage.

allergen A substance that can produce a hypersensitive reaction in the body but is not necessarily inherently harmful.

From Chabner, D. (2004). *The language of medicine* (7th ed.). Philadelphia: Saunders.

alopecia Loss of hair resulting from destruction of the hair follicles.

amenorrhea Absence of menstrual flow.

anasarca Severe generalized edema.

anastomosis Surgical joining of two ducts or blood vessels to allow flow from one to the other.

anatomy The study, classification, and description of structures and organs of the body.

anemia Blood disorder characterized by red blood cell, hemoglobin, and hematocrit levels below normal range.

anesthesia Absence of sensation (*an-* meaning "without," and -*esthesia* meaning "awareness or feeling").

aneurysm A localized dilation of the wall of a blood vessel, usually caused by atherosclerosis, hypertension, and less commonly by a congenital weakness in a vessel wall.

angina pectoris Paroxysmal thoracic pain and choking feeling caused by decreased oxygen (anoxia) of the myocardium.

ankylosis Fixation of a joint, often in an abnormal position, usually resulting from destruction of articular cartilage and subchondral bone.

antigen A substance recognized by the body as foreign that can trigger an immune response.

anuria Urinary output of less than 100 to 250 mL in 24 hours.

aphasia Abnormal neurologic condition in which language function is defective or absent because of an injury to certain areas of the cerebral cortex.

aplasia In hematology, a failure of the normal process of cell generation and development.

apraxia Impairment of the ability to perform purposeful acts; inability to use objects properly.

arteriosclerosis Common arterial disorder characterized by thickening, loss of elasticity, and calcification of arterial walls, resulting in a decreased blood supply.

arthrocentesis Puncture of a joint with a needle to withdraw fluid; performed to obtain synovial fluid for diagnostic purposes.

arthrodesis Surgical fusion of a joint.

arthroplasty Surgical repair or refashioning of one of both sides, parts, or specific tissues within a joint.

ascites An accumulation of fluid and albumin in the peritoneal cavity.

asterixis Hand-flapping tremor usually induced by extending the arm and dorsiflexing the wrist; frequently seen in hepatic coma.

asthenia General feeling of tiredness and listlessness.

astigmatism Defect in the curvature of the eyeball surface.

ataxia Abnormal condition characterized by impaired ability to coordinate movement.

atelectasis Collapse of lung tissues, preventing the respiratory exchange of carbon dioxide and oxygen.

atherosclerosis A common arterial disorder characterized by yellowish plaques of cholesterol, lipids, and cellular debris in the inner layer of the walls of large and medium-sized arteries.

attenuation The process of weakening the degree of virulence of a disease organism.

audiometry Testing of hearing acuity.

aura Sensation, as of light or warmth, that may precede the onset of a migraine or an epileptic seizure. An epileptic aura may be psychic, or it may be sensory with olfactory, visual, auditory, or taste hallucinations.

autograft Surgical transplantation of any tissue from one part of the body to another location in the same individual.

autoimmune/autoimmunity Immune response (autoantibodies or cellular immune response) to one's own tissues.

autologous Something that has its origin within an individual, especially a factor present in tissues or fluids.

azotemia Retention of excessive amounts of nitrogenous compounds in the blood.

B

bacteriuria Presence of bacteria in the urine.

benign Not recurrent or progressive; opposite of malignant.

biopsy The removal of a small piece of living tissue from an organ or other part of the body for microscopic examination; used to confirm or establish a diagnosis, establish a prognosis, or follow the course of a disease.

bipolar hip replacement (hemiarthroplasty) Prosthetic implant used to replace the femoral head and neck in hip fractures when the vascular supply to the femoral head is or may become compromised.

blanching test A test of the rate of capillary refill; blanching means to cause to become pale by applying digital pressure.

bradycardia Slow rhythm characterized by a pulse of fewer than 60 beats per minute.

bradykinesia An abnormal condition characterized by slowness of voluntary movements and speech.

bronchoscopy Visual examination of the larynx, trachea, and bronchi using a standard rigid, tubular metal bronchoscope or a narrower, flexible fiberoptic bronchoscope.

B-type natriuretic peptide (BNP) A neurohormone secreted by the heart in response to ventricular expansion.

C

cachexia General ill health and malnutrition marked by weakness and emaciation; usually associated with a serious disease, such as cancer.

callus Bony deposits formed between and around the broken ends of a fractured bone during healing.

candidiasis Mild fungal infection that appears in men and women; usually caused by *Candida albicans* and *C. tropicalis.*

carcinoembryonic antigen (CEA) Oncofetal glycoprotein antigen found in colonic adenocarcinoma and other cancers; also found in nonmalignant conditions.

carcinogen Substance known to increase the risk for the development of cancer.

carcinogenesis Various factors that are possible origins of cancer.

carcinoma The term used for a malignant tumor composed of epithelial cells; it displays a tendency to metastasize.

carcinoma in situ Preinvasive, asymptomatic carcinoma that can be diagnosed only by microscopic examination of cervical cells.

cardiac arrest Sudden cessation of functional circulation.

cardioversion Restoration of the heart's normal sinus rhythm by delivery of a synchronized electric shock through two metal paddles placed on the patient's chest.

catabolism Breakdown or destructive phase of metabolism. Catabolism occurs when complex body substances are broken down to simpler ones; opposite of anabolism.

cataract Opacity or clouding of the lens.

$CD_4{}^+$ lymphocyte A type of white blood cell; a protein on the surface of cells that normally helps the body's immune system combat disease.

cell The fundamental unit of all living tissue.

cellular immunity Acquired immunity characterized by the dominant role of small T lymphocytes; also called cell-mediated immunity.

Centers for Disease Control and Prevention (CDC) Federal agency that provides facilities and services for investigation, identification, prevention, and control of disease; headquartered in Atlanta, Georgia.

chancre Painless erosion of a papule that ulcerates superficially with a scooped-out appearance.

Chlamydia trachomatis A gram-negative intracellular bacterium that causes several common sexually transmitted diseases.

Chvostek's sign Abnormal spasm of the facial muscles elicited by light taps on the facial nerve in patients who are hypocalcemic; seen in tetany.

circumcision Surgical procedure in which a part of the foreskin is removed, leaving the glans penis uncovered.

climacteric Phase of the aging process marking the transition from the reproductive phase to a nonreproductive stage of life.

Colles' fracture A fracture of the distal portion of the radius within 1 inch of the joint of the wrist.

colporrhaphy Surgical correction of cystocele and rectocele by shortening the muscles that support the bladder and repair the rectocele.

colposcopy Examination of the cervix and vagina using a colposcope.

compartment syndrome Pathologic condition caused by progressive development of arterial compression and reduced blood supply to an extremity. Increased pressure from external devices (casts, bulky dressings) causes decreased blood flow, resulting in ischemic tissue necrosis; most often occurs in the extremities.

conjunctivitis Inflammation of the conjunctiva.

conscious sedation Administration of central nervous system depressant drugs and/or analgesia to relieve anxiety and/or provide amnesia during surgical, diagnostic, or interventional procedures.

contracture Abnormal, usually permanent condition of a joint characterized by flexion and fixation and caused by atrophy and shortening of muscle fibers.

cor pulmonale Abnormal cardiac condition characterized by hypertrophy of the right ventricle of the heart as a result of hypertension of the pulmonary circulation.

coronary artery disease (CAD) Variety of conditions that obstruct blood flow in the coronary arteries.

coryza Acute inflammation of the mucous membranes of the nose and accessory sinuses, usually accompanied by edema of the mucosa and nasal discharge.

costovertebral angle Pertaining to a rib and a vertebra; one of two angles that outline a space over the kidneys.

crackle(s) Short, discrete, interrupted crackling or bubbling adventitious breath sounds heard on auscultation of the chest, most commonly upon inspiration. They are produced by passage of air through the bronchi that contain secretions of exudate or are constricted by spasms or thickening; usually heard during inspiration; formerly called rales.

crepitus Sound that resembles the crackling noise heard when rubbing hair between the fingers or throwing salt on an open fire. It is associated with gas gangrene, the rubbing of bone fragments, or the crackles of a consolidated area of the lungs in pneumonia.

cryosurgery Procedure to "freeze" the border of a retinal hole with a frozen-tipped probe.

cryotherapy A procedure in which a topical anesthetic is used so that a cryoprobe can be placed directly on the surface of the eye.

cryptorchidism Failure of testes to descend into the scrotum.

culdoscopy Diagnostic procedure that provides visualization of the uterus and adnexa (uterine appendages that include the ovaries and fallopian tubes).

curettage Scraping of material from the wall of a cavity or other surface; performed to remove tumors or other abnormal tissue for microscopic study.

Curling's ulcer Duodenal ulcer that develops 8 to 14 days after severe burns on the surface of the body; the first sign is usually vomiting of bright red blood.

cyanosis Slightly bluish, gray, slatelike, or dark purple discoloration of the skin resulting from the presence of abnormally reduced amounts of oxygenated hemoglobin in the blood.

cytology/cytologic evaluation Study of cells and their formation, origin, structure, biochemical activities, and pathology.

cytoplasm "Living matter"; a substance that exists only in cells, composed largely of a gel-like substance that contains water, minerals, enzymes, and other specialized materials.

D

debridement Removal of damaged cellular tissue from a wound or burn to prevent infection and promote healing.

defibrillation The termination of ventricular fibrillation by delivering a direct electrical countershock to the precordium.

dehiscence Partial or complete separation of a surgical incision or rupture of a wound closure.

dendrite Branching process that extends from the cell body of a neuron and receives impulses.

diabetic retinopathy Disorder of retinal blood vessels characterized by capillary microaneurysms, hemorrhage, exudates, and formation of new vessels and connective tissue.

dialysis Medical procedure for the removal of certain elements from the blood or lymph by virtue of the difference in their rates of diffusion through an external semipermeable membrane or, in the case of peritoneal dialysis, through the peritoneum.

differentiated Describes a tumor that is most like the parent tissue.

diffusion A process in which solid particles in a fluid move from an area of higher concentration to an area of lower concentration.

diplopia Double vision.

disseminated intravascular coagulation (DIC) Acquired hemorrhage syndrome of clotting, cascade overstimulation, and anticlotting processes.

diuresis Secretion and passage of large amounts of urine.

dorsal Toward the back.

drainage Free flow or withdrawal of fluids from a wound or cavity by some sort of system (such as a catheter or T-tube).

dysarthria Difficult, poorly articulated speech resulting from interference in the control over the muscles of speech.

dysmenorrhea Painful menstruation.

dysphagia Difficulty swallowing.

dyspnea Shortness of breath or difficulty in breathing; may be caused by disturbances in the lungs, certain heart conditions, and hemoglobin deficiency.

dysrhythmia Any disturbance or abnormality in a normal rhythmic pattern, specifically irregularity in the normal rhythm of the heart; also called *arrhythmia*.

dysuria Painful or difficult urination.

E

embolism An abnormal circulatory condition in which an embolus (e.g., a foreign substance, blood clot, fat, air, or amniotic fluid) travels through the bloodstream and becomes lodged in a blood vessel.

embolus A foreign object, quantity of air or gas, bit of tissue or tumor, or a piece of thrombus that circulates in the bloodstream until it becomes lodged in a vessel.

empyema Accumulation of pus in a body cavity, especially the pleural space, as a result of infection.

endarterectomy Surgical removal of the intimal lining of an artery.

endocrinologist Physician who specializes in endocrinology.

endometriosis Condition in which endometrial tissue appears outside the uterus.

enucleation Surgical removal of the eyeball.

enzyme-linked immunosorbent assay (ELISA) Antibody test that uses a rapid enzyme immunochemical assay method to detect HIV antibodies.

epididymitis Infection of the cordlike excretory duct of the testicles.

epistaxis Hemorrhage from the nose; nosebleed.

erythrocytosis Abnormal increase in the number of circulating red blood cells.

erythropoiesis The process of red blood cell production.

eschar Black, leathery crust; a slough that the body forms over burned tissue.

esophageal varices A complex of longitudinal, tortuous veins at the lower end of the esophagus.

evisceration Protrusion of an internal organ through a disrupted wound or surgical incision.

exacerbation An increase in the seriousness of a disease or disorder; marked by greater intensity in the signs or symptoms of the patient being treated.

excoriation Injury to the surface layer of skin caused by scratching or abrasion.

exophthalmos An abnormal condition characterized by a marked protrusion of the eyeballs.

extravasation The escape of fluids into surrounding tissue.

extrinsic Caused by external factors.

extubate To remove an endotracheal tube from an airway.

exudate Fluid, cells, or other substances that have been slowly exuded or discharged from body cells or blood vessels through small pores or breaks in cell membrane.

F

fibromyalgia A musculoskeletal chronic pain syndrome of unknown etiology that causes pain in muscles, bones, or joints.

filtration The transfer of water and dissolved substances from an area of higher pressure to an area of lower pressure.

fistula Abnormal opening between two organs.

flaccid Weak, soft, and flabby; lacking normal muscle tone.

flatulence Excessive formation of gases in the stomach or intestine.

G

Glasgow coma scale A quick, practical, standardized system for assessing the degree of conscious impairment in the critically ill; also used for predicting the duration and ultimate outcome of coma, primarily in patients with head injuries.

glaucoma An abnormal condition of elevated pressure within an eye because of obstruction of the outflow of aqueous humor.

global cognitive dysfunction Generalized impairment of intellect, awareness, and judgment.

glycosuria Abnormal presence of sugar, especially glucose in the urine.

H

heart failure (HF) Syndrome characterized by circulatory congestion due to the heart's inability to act as an effective pump; it should be viewed as a neurohormonal problem in which pathology progresses as a result of chronic release in the body of substances such as catecholamines (epinephrine and norepinephrine).

hemarthrosis Bleeding into a joint space, a hallmark of severe disease usually occurring in the knees, ankles, and elbow.

hematemesis Vomiting blood.

hematuria Blood in the urine.

hemianopia Defective vision or blindness in half of the visual field.

hemiplegia Paralysis of one side of the body.

hemophilia A Hereditary coagulation disorder; caused by a lack of antihemophilic factor VIII, which is needed to convert prothrombin to thrombin through thromboplastin component.

hemoptysis Expectorating blood from the respiratory tract.

hepatic encephalopathy A type of brain damage caused by a liver disease and consequent ammonia intoxication.

hepatitis Inflammation of the liver resulting from several causes, including several types of viral agents or exposure to toxic substances.

heterograft (xenograft) Tissue from another species, used as a temporary graft.

heterozygous Having two different genes.

hirsutism Excessive body hair in a masculine distribution.

HIV disease Symptomatic human immunodeficiency virus (HIV) infection that is not severe enough for a diagnosis of acquired immunodeficiency syndrome (AIDS); symptoms of HIV disease are persistent unexplained fever, night sweats, diarrhea, weight loss, and fatigue.

HIV infection The state in which HIV enters the body under favorable conditions and multiplies, producing injurious effects.

homeostasis A relative constancy in the internal environment of the body, naturally maintained by adaptive responses that promote healthy survival.

homograft (allograft) The transfer of tissue between two genetically dissimilar individuals of the same species, such as a skin transplant between two humans who are not identical twins.

homozygous Having two identical genes, inherited from each parent, for a given hereditary characteristic.

human immunodeficiency virus (HIV) An obligate virus; a retrovirus that causes AIDS.

humoral immunity One of the two forms of immunity that respond to antigens such as bacteria and foreign tissue. It is mediated by B cells.

hydronephrosis The dilation of the renal pelvis and calyces.

hypercapnia Greater than normal amounts of carbon dioxide in the blood.

hyperglycemia A greater than normal amount of glucose in the blood.

hyperopia Farsightedness; inability to see objects at close range.

hyperreflexia Neurologic condition characterized by increased reflex reactions.

hypersensitivity An abnormal condition characterized by an excessive reaction to a particular stimulus.

hypocalcemia A deficiency of calcium in serum.

hypoglycemia A lower than normal amount of glucose in the blood; usually caused by administration of too much insulin, excessive secretion of insulin by the islet cells of the pancreas, or dietary deficiency.

hypokalemia A condition in which an inadequate amount of potassium, the major intracellular cation, is found in the circulatory bloodstream.

hypoventilation An abnormal condition of the respiratory system that occurs when the volume of air is not adequate for the metabolic needs of the body.

hypoxemia An abnormal deficiency of oxygen in the arterial blood.

hypoxia An inadequate, reduced tension of cellular oxygen.

I

idiopathic Cause unknown.

idiopathic hyperplasia Increase, without any known cause, in the number of cells.

ileal conduit Ureters are implanted into a loop of the ileum that is isolated and brought to the surface of the abdominal wall.

immunity The quality of being insusceptible to or unaffected by a particular disease or condition.

immunization A process by which resistance to an infectious disease is induced or increased.

immunocompetence/immunocompetent The ability of an immune system to mobilize and deploy its antibodies and other responses to stimulation by an antigen.

immunodeficiency An abnormal condition of the immune system in which cellular or humoral immunity is inadequate and resistance to infection is decreased.

immunogen Any agent or substance capable of provoking an immune response or producing immunity.

immunology Study of the immune system; the reaction of tissues of the immune system of the body of antigenic stimulation.

immunosuppression/immunosuppressive The administration of agents that significantly interfere with the ability of the immune system to respond to antigenic stimulation by inhibiting cellular and humoral immunity.

immunosurveillance The immune system's recognition and destruction of newly developed abnormal cells.

immunotherapy A special treatment of allergic responses; involves the administration of increasingly larger doses of the offending allergens to gradually develop immunity.

incentive spirometry A procedure in which a device (spirometer) is used at the bedside at regular intervals to encourage a patient to breathe deeply.

incision Surgical cut produced by a sharp instrument to create an opening into an organ or space in the body.

infarct Localized area of necrosis in tissue, a vessel, or an organ resulting from tissue anoxia; caused by an interruption in the blood supply to an area.

informed consent Permission obtained from the patient to perform a specific test or procedure.

innate immunity The body's first line of defense; provides physical and chemical barriers to invading pathogens and protects the body against the external environment.

intermittent claudication A weakness of the legs accompanied by cramplike pains in the calves; caused by poor arterial circulation of the blood to the leg muscles.

intraoperative Pertaining to a period of time during a surgical procedure.

intrinsic Caused by internal factors.

introitus An entrance to a cavity (e.g., the vaginal introitus).

intussusception Infolding of one segment of the intestine into the lumen of another segment; occurs in children.

ischemia Decreased blood supply to a body organ or part; often marked by pain and organ dysfunction.

J

jaundice Yellow discoloration of the skin, mucous membranes, and sclera of the eyes, caused by greater than normal amounts of bilirubin in the blood.

K

Kaposi's sarcoma (KS) Rare cancer of the skin or mucous membranes; characterized by blue, red, or purple raised lesions and seen mainly in middle-aged Mediterranean men and those with HIV disease.

keloids Overgrowths of collagenous scar tissue at the site of a skin wound.

keratitis An inflammation of the cornea.

keratoplasty Excision of the corneal tissue, followed by surgical implantation of a cornea from another human donor.

ketoacidosis Acidosis accompanied by an accumulation of ketone in the blood resulting from faulty carbohydrate metabolism.

ketone bodies Normal metabolic products, β-hydroxybutyric and aminoacetic acid, from which acetone may spontaneously arise.

kyphosis An abnormal condition of the vertebral column; characterized by increased convexity in the curvature of the thoracic spine.

L

labyrinthitis Inflammation of the labyrinthine canals of the inner ear.

laparoscopy The examination of the abdominal cavity with a laparoscope through a small incision beneath the umbilicus.

leukemia Malignant disorder of the hematopoietic system in which an excess of leukocytes accumulates in the bone marrow and lymph nodes.

leukopenia An abnormal decrease in the number of white blood cells to fewer than 5000 cells/mm^3 due to depression of the bone marrow.

leukoplakia A white patch in the mouth or on the tongue.

lipodystrophy Abnormality in the metabolism or deposition of fats. Insulin lipodystrophy is the loss of local fat deposits in diabetic patients as a complication of repeated insulin injections.

lordosis An increase in the curve at the lumbar space region that throws the shoulder back, making the appearance "lordly or kingly."

lumen Space within an artery, vein, intestine, or tube such as a needle or catheter.

lymphangitis Inflammation of one or more lymphatic vessels or channels; usually results from an acute streptococcal or staphylococcal infection in an extremity.

lymphedema Primary or secondary disorder characterized by the accumulation of lymph in soft tissue and edema.

lymphokine One of the chemical factors produced and released by T lymphocytes that attract macrophages to the site of infection or inflammation and prepare them for attack.

M

macules Small, flat, discolored blemishes; flush with the skin surface.

malignant Growing worse, resisting treatment; said of cancerous growths. Also tending or threatening to produce death; harmful.

mammography Radiography of the soft tissue of the breast to allow identification of various benign and neoplastic processes.

mastoiditis Infection of one of the mastoid bones.

melena Abnormal, black, tarry stool containing digested blood.

membrane Thin sheet of tissue that serves many functions in the body; it covers surfaces, lines and lubricates hollow organs, and protects and anchors organs and bones.

menorrhagia Excessive menstrual flow.

metastasis The process by which tumor cells are spread to distant parts of the body.

metrorrhagia Excessive spotting between cycles.

micturition Urination.

miotic Causing constriction of the pupil of the eye.

mitosis Type of cell division of somatic (i.e., nonreproductive) cells in which each daughter cell contains the same number of chromosomes as the parent cell.

multiple myeloma A malignant neoplastic immunodeficiency disease of the bone marrow; the tumor is composed of plasma cells.

mydriatic Causing pupillary dilation.

myeloproliferative Excessive bone marrow production.

myocardial infarction An occlaion of a major coronary artery or one of its branches; it is caused by atherosclerosis or an embolus resulting in necrosis of a portion of cardiac muscle.

myopia Condition of nearsightedness; inability to see objects at a distance.

myringotomy A surgical incision of the tympanic membrane to relieve pressure and release purulent exudate from the middle ear.

N

neoplasm Uncontrolled or abnormal growth of cells.

nephrotoxin Substances with specific destructive properties for the kidneys, such as certain antibiotics, heavy metals, solvents, and chemicals.

neuropathy Any abnormal condition characterized by inflammation and degeneration of the peripheral nerves.

nevi Pigmented, congenital skin blemishes that are usually benign but may become cancerous.

nocturia Excessive urination at night.

nucleus Largest organelle within the cell; it is responsible for cell reproduction and control of the other organelles.

nystagmus Involuntary, rhythmic movement of the eyes. Oscillations may be horizontal, vertical, rotary, or mixed.

O

occlusion An obstruction or closing off in a canal, vessel, or passage of the body.

occult blood Blood that is hidden or obscured from view.

oliguria A diminished capacity to form and pass urine (less than 500 mL in 24 hours); result is that the end products of metabolism cannot be excreted efficiently.

oncology The sum of knowledge regarding tumors; the branch of medicine that deals with the study of tumors.

open reduction with internal fixation (ORIF) A surgical procedure allowing fracture alignment under direct visualization while using various internal fixation devices applied to the bone.

opportunistic Disease characteristic caused by a normally nonpathogenic organism in a host whose resistance has been decreased by a disorder such as AIDS.

organ A group of several different kinds of tissue arranged so that they can work together to perform a special function.

orthopnea An abnormal condition in which a person must sit or stand in order to breathe deeply or comfortably.

osmosis Passage of water across a selectively permeable membrane; the water moves from a less concentrated solution to a more concentrated solution.

P

palliative Designed to relieve pain and distress and to control the signs and symptoms of disease; not designed to produce a cure.

pancytopenia Deficient condition of all three major blood elements (red cells, white cells, and platelets); results from the bone marrow being reduced or absent.

panhysterosalpingo-oophorectomy The removal of the uterus, fallopian tubes, and the ovaries; also called total abdominal hysterectomy with bilateral salpingo-oophorectomy.

Papanicolaou test (Pap smear) A simple smear method of examining stained exfoliative cells; used most commonly to detect cancers of the cervix.

papules Palpable, circumscribed, red solid elevations in the skin; smaller than 0.5 cm.

paracentesis A procedure in which fluid is withdrawn from the abdominal cavity.

paralytic ileus Most common type of intestinal obstruction; a decrease in or absence of intestinal peristalsis that may occur after abdominal surgery.

parenchyma Tissue of an organ as distinguished from supporting or connective tissue.

paresis A lesser degree of movement deficit from partial or incomplete paralysis.

paresthesia Any subjective sensation, such as a prickling "pins and needles" feeling or numbness.

passive transport The movement of small molecules across the membrane of a cell by diffusion; no cellular energy is required.

pathognomonic Sign or symptom specific to a disease condition.

pediculosis Lice infestation.

perioperative Entire surgical inpatient period occurring immediately before, during, and immediately after surgery.

peripheral Pertaining to the outside, surface, or surrounding area of an organ, other structure or fluid of vision.

pernicious Capable of causing great injury or destruction; deadly, fatal.

phagocytic Refers to the ingestion and digestion of bacteria.

phagocytosis The process that permits a cell to surround or engulf any foreign material and digest it.

phimosis A condition in which the prepuce is too small to allow retraction of the foreskin over the glans penis.

physiology Explanation of the processes and functions of the various structures of the body and how they interrelate.

pinocytosis The process by which extracellular fluid is ingested by the cells.

plasmapheresis Removal of plasma that contains components causing or thought to cause disease. Also called *plasma exchange* because when the plasma is removed, it is replaced by substitution fluids such as saline or albumin.

pleural effusion An abnormal accumulation of fluid in the thoracic cavity between the visceral and parietal pleurae.

pleural friction rub Low-pitched, grating, or creaking lung sounds that occur when inflamed pleural surfaces rub together during respiration.

***Pneumocystis jiroveci* (formerly *carinii*) pneumonia (PCP)** An unusual pulmonary disease caused by a parasite that is primarily associated with people who have suppressed immune systems, especially in people with AIDS.

pneumothorax A collection of air or gas in the pleural space, causing the lung to collapse.

polycythemia Abnormal increase in the number of red blood cells in the blood.

polydipsia Excessive thirst.

polyphagia Eating to the point of gluttony.

polyuria Excretion of an abnormally large quantity of urine.

postictal period A rest period of variable length after a tonic-clonic seizure.

postoperative Pertaining to a period of time after surgery.

preoperative Pertaining to a period of time before surgery.

procidentia Protrusion of the entire uterus through the introitus.

proliferation Reproduction or multiplication of similar forms.

proprioception Sensation pertaining to stimuli originating from within the body regarding spatial position and muscular activity stimuli or to the sensory receptors that those stimuli activate. This sensation gives one the ability to know the position of the body without looking at it and the ability to "know objectively the sense of touch."

prostatodynia Pain in the prostate gland.

prosthesis Artificial replacement for a missing body part.

pruritus The symptoms of itching; an uncomfortable sensation leading to the urge to scratch; scratching often leads to secondary infection. Some causes of pruritus are allergy, infection, elevated serum urea, jaundice, and skin irritation.

pulmonary edema Accumulation of extravascular fluid in lung tissues and alveoli; caused most commonly by left-sided heart failure.

pustulant vesicles Small, circumscribed pus-containing elevations of the skin.

pyuria Pus in the urine.

R

radial keratotomy Microscopic incisions on the surface of the cornea outside the optical area. These eight spokelike incisions flatten the cornea to a more normal curvature, thus reducing or eliminating myopia.

Reed-Sternberg cells Atypical histiocytes; large, abnormal, multinucleated cells in the lymphatic system, found in Hodgkin's disease.

remission A decrease in the severity of a disease or any of its symptoms.

residual urine Urine remaining in the urinary tract after voiding.

retention The inability to void even in the presence of an urge to void.

retinal detachment Separation of the retina from the choroid in the posterior of the eye.

retrovirus Lentivirus that contains reverse transcriptase, which is essential for reverse transcription (the production of a deoxyribonucleic acid (DNA) molecule from a ribonucleic acid (RNA) model).

rule of nines Division of the body into multiples of nine; used to determine the total body surface area (BSA) involved in burn trauma.

S

sarcoma Malignant tumor of connective tissues such as muscle or bone; usually presents as a painless swelling.

scoliosis Curvature of the spine usually consisting of two curves: the original abnormal curve and a compensatory curve in the opposite direction.

sentinel lymph node mapping Diagnostic tool used before therapeutic surgery, which identifies the first lymph node most likely to drain cancerous cells; used in axillary lymph node biopsy, specifically in breast cancer staging.

sequestrum A fragment of necrotic bone that is partially or entirely detached from the surrounding or adjacent healthy bone.

seroconversion The development of detectable levels of antibodies; a change in serologic tests (e.g., ELISA and Western blot) from negative to positive as antibodies develop in reaction to an infection.

seronegative Negative result on serologic examination. The state of lacking HIV antibodies; confirmed by blood tests.

sibilant wheeze Musical, high-pitched, squeaking, or whistlelike sound caused by the rapid movement of air through narrowed bronchioles.

singultus Hiccup.

Sjögren syndrome Dry-eye syndrome; an immunologic disorder characterized by low fluid production by lacrimal (tear), salivary, and other glands, resulting in abnormal dryness of mouth, eyes, and other mucous membranes.

Snellen's test Eye chart test for visual acuity; letters, numbers, or symbols are arranged on the chart in decreasing size from top to bottom.

sonorous wheeze Low-pitched, loud, coarse, snoring sound.

spastic Involuntary, sudden movements or muscular contractions with increased reflexes.

spider telangiectases Dilated superficial arterioles.

stapedectomy The removal of the stapes of the middle ear and insertion of a graft and prosthesis.

steatorrhea Excessive fat in the feces.

stertorous Pertaining to a respiratory effort that is strenuous and struggling, which provokes a snoring sound.

stoma Combining form meaning a mouth or opening.

stomatitis Inflammation of the mouth due to destruction of normal cells of the oral cavity that may result from infection by bacteria, viruses, or fungi from exposure to certain chemicals or drugs, vitamin deficiency, or systemic inflammatory disease.

strabismus Condition in which the eyes are unable to focus in the same direction; commonly called *cross-eyed*.

stroke An abnormal condition of the blood vessels of the brain characterized by hemorrhage into the brain; formation of an embolus or thrombus resulting in ischemia of the brain tissues normally perfused by the damaged vessels. The sequelae depend on the location and extent of ischemia.

subluxation Partial dislocation.

suppuration To produce purulent material.

surgery Branch of medicine concerned with diseases and trauma requiring operative procedures.

surgical asepsis A group of techniques that destroy all microorganisms and their spores (sterile technique).

system An organization of varying numbers and kinds of organs arranged so that they can work together to perform complex functions for the body.

T

tachycardia An abnormal condition in which the myocardium contracts regularly but at a rate greater than 100 beats per minute.

tachypnea An abnormally rapid rate of breathing.

tenesmus Persistent, ineffectual spasms of the rectum or bladder, accompanied by the desire to empty the bowel or bladder.

thoracentesis The surgical perforation of the chest wall and pleural space with a needle for the aspiration of fluid for diagnostic or therapeutic purposes.

thrombocytopenia An abnormal hematologic condition in which the number of platelets is reduced to fewer than 100,000/mm^3.

thrombus Of or pertaining to a clot.

tinnitus A subjective noise sensation in one or both ears; ringing or tinkling sound in the ear.

tissue An organization of many similar cells that act together to perform a common function.

tophi Calculi containing sodium urate deposits that develop in periarticular fibrous tissue; typically found in patients with gout.

trichomoniasis A sexually transmitted disease caused by the protozoan *Trichomonas vaginalis*.

Trousseau's sign A test for latent tetany in which carpal spasms are induced by inflating a sphygmomanometer cuff on the upper arm to a pressure exceeding systolic blood pressure for 3 minutes; used in hypocalcemia and hypomagnesemia.

tumor lysis syndrome Oncologic emergency that occurs with rapid lysis of malignant cells; most frequently associated with chemotherapy treatment. It is most commonly a result of treatment-related malignant cell death in patients with large tumor cell burdens.

turgor The normal resiliency of the skin caused by the outward pressure of the cells and interstitial fluid; may be assessed as increased or decreased skin turgor.

tympanoplasty One of several operative procedures on the eardrum or ossicles of the middle ear designed to restore or improve hearing in patients with conductive hearing loss.

type 1 diabetes mellitus Condition in which impaired glucose tolerance results because of destruction of beta cells in the pancreatic islets; results in deficient insulin production, but the patient retains normal sensitivity to insulin action; also called insulin-dependent diabetes mellitus.

type 2 diabetes mellitus Condition in which impaired glucose tolerance results from an abnormal resistance to insulin action; also called non–insulin-dependent diabetes mellitus.

U

unilateral neglect Condition in which an individual is perceptually unaware of and inattentive to one side of the body.

urolithiasis Formation of urinary calculi.

urticaria Itching skin eruption characterized by welts of varying sizes with well-defined inflamed margins and pale centers (also called *hives*).

V

ventral Facing forward; the front of the body.

verruca Benign, viral, warty skin lesion with a rough, papillomatous (nipplelike) growth.

vertical transmission Transmission of HIV from a mother to a fetus; can occur during pregnancy, during delivery, or through postpartum breastfeeding.

vertigo The sensation that the outer world is revolving about oneself or that one is moving in space.

vesicle Circumscribed elevation of skin filled with serous fluid.

viral load Amount of measurable HIV virions.

virulent Having the power to produce disease; of or pertaining to a very pathogenic or rapidly progressive condition.

Volkmann's contracture A permanent contracture with clawhand, flexion of wrist and finger, and atrophy of the forearm; can occur as a result of compartment syndrome.

volvulus Twisting of the bowel on itself, causing intestinal obstruction.

W

Western blot A laboratory blood test to detect the presence of antibodies to a specific antigen; used in diagnosing HIV.

wheals Irregularly shaped, elevated areas, white in the center with a pale red periphery, with superficial localized edema; vary in size (hives, mosquito bite).

Index

Page numbers followed by b indicate boxes; f, figures; t, tables.